Recommended Dietary Allowances (RDA) and Adequate Intakes (AI) for Vitamins

Age (yr)	Thiamin RDA (mg/day)	Riboflavin RDA (mg/day)	Niacin RDA (mg/day)[a]	Biotin AI (µg/day)	Pantothenic acid AI (mg/day)	Vitamin B_6 RDA (mg/day)	Folate RDA (µg/day)[b]	Vitamin B_{12} RDA (µg/day)	Choline AI (mg/day)	Vitamin C RDA (mg/day)	Vitamin A RDA (µg/day)[c]	Vi RD	Vi RD da	Vit AI
Infants														
0–0.5	0.2	0.3	2	5	1.7	0.1	65	0.4	125	40	400	10	4	2.0
0.5–1	0.3	0.4	4	6	1.8	0.3	80	0.5	150	50	500	10	5	2.5
Children														
1–3	0.5	0.5	6	8	2	0.5	150	0.9	200	15	300	15	6	30
4–8	0.6	0.6	8	12	3	0.6	200	1.2	250	25	400	15	7	55
Males														
9–13	0.9	0.9	12	20	4	1.0	300	1.8	375	45	600	15	11	60
14–18	1.2	1.3	16	25	5	1.3	400	2.4	550	75	900	15	15	75
19–30	1.2	1.3	16	30	5	1.3	400	2.4	550	90	900	15	15	120
31–50	1.2	1.3	16	30	5	1.3	400	2.4	550	90	900	15	15	120
51–70	1.2	1.3	16	30	5	1.7	400	2.4	550	90	900	15	15	120
>70	1.2	1.3	16	30	5	1.7	400	2.4	550	90	900	20	15	120
Females														
9–13	0.9	0.9	12	20	4	1.0	300	1.8	375	45	600	15	11	60
14–18	1.0	1.0	14	25	5	1.2	400	2.4	400	65	700	15	15	75
19–30	1.1	1.1	14	30	5	1.3	400	2.4	425	75	700	15	15	90
31–50	1.1	1.1	14	30	5	1.3	400	2.4	425	75	700	15	15	90
51–70	1.1	1.1	14	30	5	1.5	400	2.4	425	75	700	15	15	90
>70	1.1	1.1	14	30	5	1.5	400	2.4	425	75	700	20	15	90
Pregnancy														
≤18	1.4	1.4	18	30	6	1.9	600	2.6	450	80	750	15	15	75
19–30	1.4	1.4	18	30	6	1.9	600	2.6	450	85	770	15	15	90
31–50	1.4	1.4	18	30	6	1.9	600	2.6	450	85	770	15	15	90
Lactation														
≤18	1.4	1.6	17	35	7	2.0	500	2.8	550	115	1200	15	19	75
19–30	1.4	1.6	17	35	7	2.0	500	2.8	550	120	1300	15	19	90
31–50	1.4	1.6	17	35	7	2.0	500	2.8	550	120	1300	15	19	90

NOTE: For all nutrients, values for infants are AI. The glossary on the inside back cover defines units of nutrient measure.

[a]Niacin recommendations are expressed as niacin equivalents (NE), except for recommendations for infants younger than 6 months, which are expressed as preformed niacin.

[b]Folate recommendations are expressed as dietary folate equivalents (DFE).

[c]Vitamin A recommendations are expressed as retinol activity equivalents (RAE).

[d]Vitamin D recommendations are expressed as cholecalciferol and assume minimal sunlight.

[e]Vitamin E recommendations are expressed as α-tocopherol.

Recommended Dietary Allowances (RDA) and Adequate Intakes (AI) for Minerals

Age (yr)	Sodium AI (mg/day)	Chloride AI (mg/day)	Potassium AI (mg/day)	Calcium RDA (mg/day)	Phosphorus RDA (mg/day)	Magnesium RDA (mg/day)	Iron RDA (mg/day)	Zinc RDA (mg/day)	Iodine RDA (µg/day)	Selenium RDA (µg/day)	Copper RDA (µg/day)	Manganese AI (mg/day)	Fluoride AI (mg/day)	Chromium AI (µg/day)	Molybdenum RDA (µg/day)
Infants															
0–0.5	120	180	400	200	100	30	0.27	2	110	15	200	0.003	0.01	0.2	2
0.5–1	370	570	700	260	275	75	11	3	130	20	220	0.6	0.5	5.5	3
Children															
1–3	1000	1500	3000	700	460	80	7	3	90	20	340	1.2	0.7	11	17
4–8	1200	1900	3800	1000	500	130	10	5	90	30	440	1.5	1.0	15	22
Males															
9–13	1500	2300	4500	1300	1250	240	8	8	120	40	700	1.9	2	25	34
14–18	1500	2300	4700	1300	1250	410	11	11	150	55	890	2.2	3	35	43
19–30	1500	2300	4700	1000	700	400	8	11	150	55	900	2.3	4	35	45
31–50	1500	2300	4700	1000	700	420	8	11	150	55	900	2.3	4	35	45
51–70	1300	2000	4700	1000	700	420	8	11	150	55	900	2.3	4	30	45
>70	1200	1800	4700	1200	700	420	8	11	150	55	900	2.3	4	30	45
Females															
9–13	1500	2300	4500	1300	1250	240	8	8	120	40	700	1.6	2	21	34
14–18	1500	2300	4700	1300	1250	360	15	9	150	55	890	1.6	3	24	43
19–30	1500	2300	4700	1000	700	310	18	8	150	55	900	1.8	3	25	45
31–50	1500	2300	4700	1000	700	320	18	8	150	55	900	1.8	3	25	45
51–70	1300	2000	4700	1200	700	320	8	8	150	55	900	1.8	3	20	45
>70	1200	1800	4700	1200	700	320	8	8	150	55	900	1.8	3	20	45
Pregnancy															
≤18	1500	2300	4700	1300	1250	400	27	12	220	60	1000	2.0	3	29	50
19–30	1500	2300	4700	1000	700	350	27	11	220	60	1000	2.0	3	30	50
31–50	1500	2300	4700	1000	700	360	27	11	220	60	1000	2.0	3	30	50
Lactation															
≤18	1500	2300	5100	1300	1250	360	10	13	290	70	1300	2.6	3	44	50
19–30	1500	2300	5100	1000	700	310	9	12	290	70	1300	2.6	3	45	50
31–50	1500	2300	5100	1000	700	320	9	12	290	70	1300	2.6	3	45	50

NOTE: For all nutrients, values for infants are AI. The glossary on the inside back cover defines units of nutrient measure.

Tolerable Upper Intake Levels (UL) for Vitamins

Age (yr)	Niacin (mg/day)[a]	Vitamin B_6 (mg/day)	Folate (µg/day)[a]	Choline (mg/day)	Vitamin C (mg/day)	Vitamin A (µg/day)[b]	Vitamin D (µg/day)	Vitamin E (mg/day)[c]
Infants								
0–0.5	—	—	—	—	—	600	25	—
0.5–1	—	—	—	—	—	600	38	—
Children								
1–3	10	30	300	1000	400	600	63	200
4–8	15	40	400	1000	650	900	75	300
9–13	20	60	600	2000	1200	1700	100	600
Adolescents								
14–18	30	80	800	3000	1800	2800	100	800
Adults								
19–70	35	100	1000	3500	2000	3000	100	1000
>70	35	100	1000	3500	2000	3000	100	1000
Pregnancy								
≤18	30	80	800	3000	1800	2800	100	800
19–50	35	100	1000	3500	2000	3000	100	1000
Lactation								
≤18	30	80	800	3000	1800	2800	100	800
19–50	35	100	1000	3500	2000	3000	100	1000

[a]The UL for niacin and folate apply to synthetic forms obtained from supplements, fortified foods, or a combination of the two.
[b]The UL for vitamin A applies to the preformed vitamin only.
[c]The UL for vitamin E applies to any form of supplemental α-tocopherol, fortified foods, or a combination of the two.

Tolerable Upper Intake Levels (UL) for Minerals

Age (yr)	Sodium (mg/day)	Chloride (mg/day)	Calcium (mg/day)	Phosphorus (mg/day)	Magnesium (mg/day)[d]	Iron (mg/day)	Zinc (mg/day)	Iodine (µg/day)	Selenium (µg/day)	Copper (µg/day)	Manganese (mg/day)	Fluoride (mg/day)	Molybdenum (µg/day)	Boron (mg/day)	Nickel (mg/day)	Vanadium (mg/day)
Infants																
0–0.5	—	—	1000	—	—	40	4	—	45	—	—	0.7	—	—	—	—
0.5–1	—	—	1500	—	—	40	5	—	60	—	—	0.9	—	—	—	—
Children																
1–3	1500	2300	2500	3000	65	40	7	200	90	1000	2	1.3	300	3	0.2	—
4–8	1900	2900	2500	3000	110	40	12	300	150	3000	3	2.2	600	6	0.3	—
9–13	2200	3400	3000	4000	350	40	23	600	280	5000	6	10	1100	11	0.6	—
Adolescents																
14–18	2300	3600	3000	4000	350	45	34	900	400	8000	9	10	1700	17	1.0	—
Adults																
19–50	2300	3600	2500	4000	350	45	40	1100	400	10,000	11	10	2000	20	1.0	1.8
51–70	2300	3600	2000	4000	350	45	40	1100	400	10,000	11	10	2000	20	1.0	1.8
>70	2300	3600	2000	3000	350	45	40	1100	400	10,000	11	10	2000	20	1.0	1.8
Pregnancy																
≤18	2300	3600	3000	3500	350	45	34	900	400	8000	9	10	1700	17	1.0	—
19–50	2300	3600	2500	3500	350	45	40	1100	400	10,000	11	10	2000	20	1.0	—
Lactation																
≤18	2300	3600	3000	4000	350	45	34	900	400	8000	9	10	1700	17	1.0	—
19–50	2300	3600	2500	4000	350	45	40	1100	400	10,000	11	10	2000	20	1.0	—

[d]The UL for magnesium applies to synthetic forms obtained from supplements or drugs only.
NOTE: An Upper Limit was not established for vitamins and minerals not listed and for those age groups listed with a dash (—) because of a lack of data, not because these nutrients are safe to consume at any level of intake. All nutrients can have adverse effects when intakes are excessive.

SOURCE: Adapted from the *Dietary Reference Intakes series*, National Academies Press. National Academies of Sciences.

Understanding Nutrition

Fifteenth Edition

Ellie Whitney
Sharon Rady Rolfes

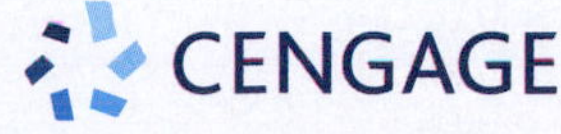

Australia • Brazil • Mexico • Singapore • United Kingdom • United States

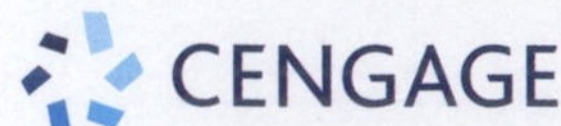

***Understanding Nutrition,* Fifteenth Edition**
Ellie Whitney, Sharon Rady Rolfes

Product Manager: Krista Mastroianni

Content Developer: Miriam Myers

Product Assistant: Marina Starkey

Content Project Manager: Carol Samet

Art Director: Michael Cook

Manufacturing Planner: Karen Hunt

Production Service: MPS Limited

Photo Researcher: Lumina Datamatics Ltd.

Text Researcher: Lumina Datamatics Ltd.

Text Designer: Diane Beasley

Cover Designer: Michael Cook

Cover Image: Patrizia Savarese/Digital Vision/ Getty Images

Compositor: MPS Limited

Library of Congress Control Number: 2017935637

Student Edition:
ISBN: 978-1-337-39269-3

Loose-leaf Edition:
ISBN: 978-1-337-55631-6

Cengage
20 Channel Center Street
Boston, MA 02210
USA

Printed in the United States of America
Print Number: 01 Print Year: 2017

To the memory of Eva May Nunnelly Hamilton, who first undertook to write this book with me in 1975. Her scholarship, enthusiasm, and warmth pervade its pages still.

Ellie Whitney

Nourishment means more than providing food; it also means giving love. Anyone joining my family at one of our gatherings would see an abundance of both. I dedicate this book to all the members of my family—including those who have departed and those who have yet to arrive.

Sharon Rady Rolfes

About the Authors

Ellie Whitney grew up in New York City and received her BA and PhD degrees in English and Biology at Harvard and Washington Universities. She taught at both Florida State University and Florida A&M University, wrote newspaper columns on environmental matters for the *Tallahassee Democrat*, and coauthored almost a dozen college textbooks on nutrition, health, and related topics, many of which repeatedly reappear as new editions. She spent three decades exploring outdoor Florida and studying its ecology, and then cowrote *Priceless Florida: Natural Ecosystems and Native Species* (Pineapple Press, 2004). Now retired, and more concerned about climate change than any other issue, she volunteers full-time for the nonpartisan national nonprofit Citizens Climate Lobby.

Sharon Rady Rolfes received her MS in nutrition and food science from Florida State University. She is a founding member of Nutrition and Health Associates, an information resource center that maintains a research database on more than 1000 nutrition-related topics. She has taught at Florida State University and coauthored several other college textbooks, including *Understanding Normal and Clinical Nutrition*. In addition to writing, she serves as a consultant for various educational projects. Her volunteer work includes serving on the board of Working Well, a community initiative dedicated to creating a healthy workforce. She maintains her registration as a dietitian nutritionist and membership in the Academy of Nutrition and Dietetics.

Brief Contents

Table of Contents

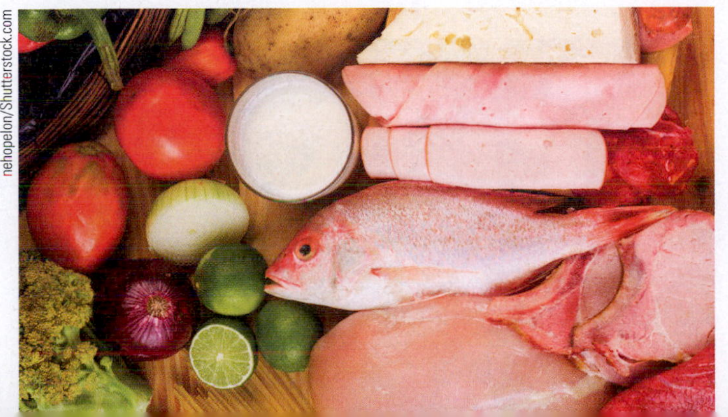

nehopelon/Shutterstock.com

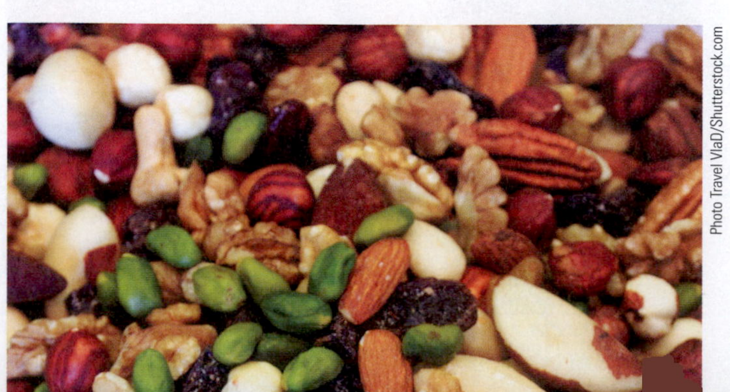
Photo Travel VlaD/Shutterstock.com

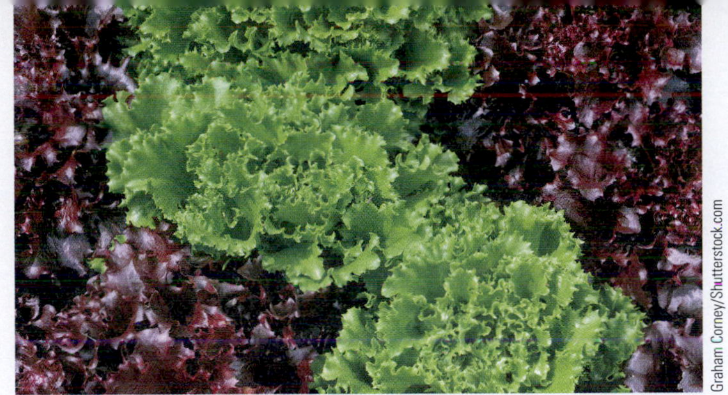
Graham Corney/Shutterstock.com

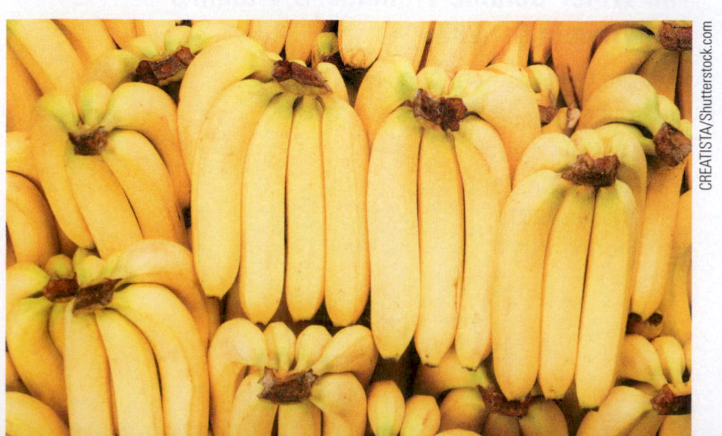
CREATISTA/Shutterstock.com

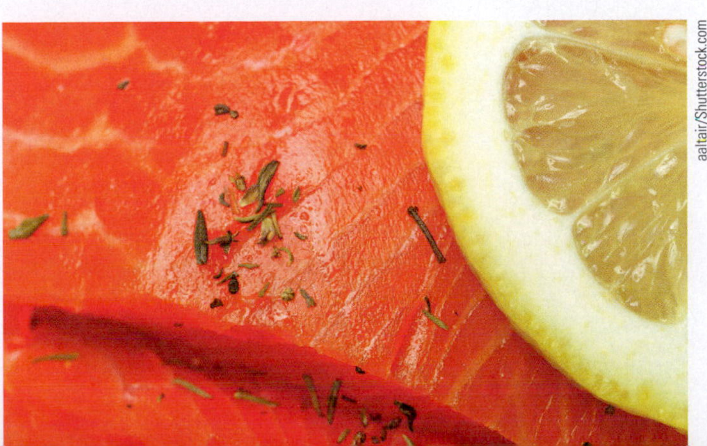
aaltair/Shutterstock.com

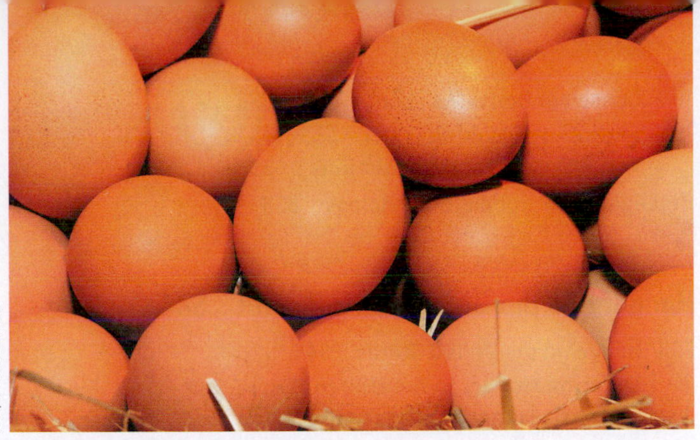
Nito/Shutterstock.com

Preface

Nutrition is a science. The details of a nutrient's chemistry or a cell's biology can be overwhelming and confusing to some, but it needn't be. When the science is explained step by step and the facts are connected one by one, the details become clear and understandable. By telling stories about fat mice, using analogies of lamps, and applying guidelines to groceries, we make the science of nutrition meaningful and memorable. That has been our mission since the first edition—to reveal the fascination of science and share the excitement of nutrition with readers. We have learned from the thousands of professors and more than a million students who have used this book through the years that readers want an *understanding* of nutrition so they can make healthy choices in their daily lives. We hope that this book serves you well.

A Book Tour of This Edition

Understanding Nutrition presents the core information of an introductory nutrition course. The early chapters introduce the nutrients and their work in the body, and the later chapters apply that information to people's lives—describing the role of foods and nutrients in energy balance and weight control, in physical activity, in the life cycle, in disease prevention, in food safety, and in hunger.

The Chapters Chapter 1 begins by exploring why we eat the foods we do and continues with a brief overview of the nutrients, the science of nutrition, recommended nutrient intakes, assessment, and important relationships between diet and health. Chapter 2 describes the diet-planning principles and food guides used to create eating patterns that support good health and includes instructions on how to read a food label. In Chapter 3 readers follow the journey of digestion and absorption as the body breaks down foods into nutrients. Chapters 4, 5, and 6 describe carbohydrates, fats, and proteins—their chemistry, roles in the body, and places in the diet. Then Chapter 7 shows how the body derives energy from these three nutrients. Chapters 8 and 9 continue the story with a look at energy balance, the factors associated with overweight and underweight, and the benefits and dangers of weight loss and weight gain. Chapters 10, 11, 12, and 13 complete the introductory lessons by describing the vitamins, the minerals, and water—their roles in the body, deficiency and toxicity symptoms, and sources.

The next seven chapters weave that basic information into practical applications, showing how nutrition influences people's lives. Chapter 14 describes how physical activity and nutrition work together to support fitness. Chapters 15, 16, and 17 present the special nutrient needs of people through the life cycle—pregnancy and lactation; infancy, childhood, and adolescence; and adulthood and the later years. Chapter 18 focuses on the dietary risk factors and recommendations associated with chronic diseases, and Chapter 19 addresses consumer concerns about the safety of the food and water supply. Chapter 20 closes the book by examining hunger, agriculture, and the environment.

The Highlights Every chapter is followed by a highlight that provides readers with an in-depth look at a current, and often controversial, topic that relates to its companion chapter. Each highlight closes with Critical Thinking Questions designed to encourage readers to develop clear, rational, open-minded, and informed thoughts based on the evidence presented in the text.

Special Features The art and layout in this edition have been carefully designed to be inviting while enhancing student learning. In addition, special features help readers identify key concepts and apply nutrition knowledge. When a new term is introduced, it is printed in bold type, and a **definition** is provided in the margin nearby. These definitions often include pronunciations and derivations to facilitate understanding. The glossary at the end of the book includes all defined terms.

definition (DEF-eh-NISH-en): the meaning of a word.
- **de** = from
- **finis** = boundary

LEARNING GUIDE

The opening page of each chapter provides a Learning Guide that serves as an outline and directs readers to the main heads within the chapter. Each main head is followed by a Learn It—a learning objective for the content covered in that section. The Learn It also appears within the text at the start of each main section as well as at the start of each Review It. After reading the chapter, students will be able to demonstrate competency in the Learn It objectives.

Nutrition in Your Life

The opening paragraph of each chapter—called Nutrition in Your Life—introduces the chapter's content in a friendly and familiar way. This short paragraph closes with a preview of how readers might apply that content to their daily lives.

> How To

Many of the chapters include "How To" features that guide readers through problem-solving tasks. For example, a "How To" in Chapter 1 presents the steps in calculating energy intake from the grams of carbohydrate, fat, and protein in a food.

> TRY IT Each "How To" feature ends with a "Try It" activity that gives readers an opportunity to practice these new lessons.

REVIEW IT Each major section within a chapter concludes with a Review It paragraph that summarizes key concepts. Similarly, Review It tables cue readers to important summaries.

Each chapter ends with an invitation to explore activities in the *Understanding Nutrition* MindTap.

What's Online

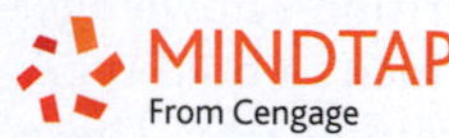
MINDTAP
From Cengage

Visit **www.cengagebrain.com** to access MindTap, a complete digital course that includes Diet & Wellness Plus, interactive quizzes, videos, and more.

The Appendixes

The appendixes are valuable references for a number of purposes. Appendix A summarizes background information on the hormonal and nervous systems, complementing Appendixes B and C on basic chemistry, the chemical structures of nutrients, and major metabolic pathways. Appendix D describes measures of protein quality. Appendix E provides detailed coverage of nutrition assessment, and Appendix F presents the estimated energy requirements for men and women at various levels of physical activity. Appendix G presents the 2014 publication *Choose Your Foods: Food Lists for Diabetes and Weight Management.* Appendix H features aids to calculations, a short tutorial on converting metric measures and handling basic math problems commonly found in the world of nutrition. Appendix I lists nutrition recommendations from the World Health Organization (WHO), and Appendix J presents the 2020 Healthy People nutrition-related objectives.

The Inserts

The inserts put commonly used information at your fingertips. Insert pages A-C present the current nutrient recommendations. The Daily Values used on food labels plus a glossary of nutrient measures are shown on page Y, and suggested weight ranges for various heights are shown on page Z.

Notable Changes in This Edition

Because nutrition is an active science, staying current is paramount. Just as nutrition research continuously adds to and revises the accepted body of knowledge, this edition builds on the science of previous editions with the latest in nutrition research. Much has changed in the world of nutrition and in our daily lives since the first edition. The number of foods has increased dramatically—even as we spend less time than ever in the kitchen preparing meals. The connections between diet and disease have become more apparent—and consumer interest in making smart health choices has followed. More people are living longer and healthier lives. The science of nutrition has grown rapidly, with new understandings emerging daily. In this edition, as with all previous editions, every chapter has been revised to enhance learning by presenting current information accurately and attractively. For all chapters and highlights we have:

- Reviewed and updated content
- Created several new figures and tables and revised others to enhance learning

Chapter 1

- Added new section on marketing to the food choices section
- Expanded discussion on processed foods, clarifying the distinction between minimally processed and ultra-processed foods
- Simplified figure comparing inaccurate and accurate view of nutrient intakes
- Created new figure illustrating how energy nutrients contribute to the total
- Expanded discussion on misinformation from TV talk shows and ads in fitness magazines
- Added short section on critical thinking

Chapter 2

- Revised entire section on Dietary Guidelines for Americans, including texts, tables, and figures to reflect 2015–2020 edition
- Updated and simplified figure comparing recommended and actual intakes from food groups
- Created new figure illustrating how the US population exceeds recommended limits for added sugars, saturated fats, and sodium

- Added more details on food allergens and front-of-label ingredients

Chapter 3

- Expanded discussion on microbiota
- Expanded discussion on celiac disease and introduced nonceliac gluten sensitivity

Chapter 4

- Introduced FODMAP—fermentable oligosaccharides, disaccharides, monosaccharides, and polyols
- Simplified figure on glucose homeostasis
- Created new figure illustrating high- vs. low-glycemic response

Chapter 5

- Revised recommendations and discussion for cholesterol based on the 2015–2020 *Dietary Guidelines for Americans*
- Added a new table for the USDA Healthy Mediterranean Eating Pattern

Chapter 6

- Reorganized the preview of protein metabolism
- Shortened sections on heart disease and osteoporosis
- Rewrote much of the supplement section
- Created new figure illustrating how genetics and lifestyle factors influence health and longevity

Chapter 7

- Added a new paragraph on intermittent fasting
- Revised the table of blood alcohol effects

Chapter 8

- Introduced the term *ectopic fat* and expanded discussion on obesity's role in inflammation and the metabolic syndrome
- Revised and expanded discussion on "healthy obese" and "metabolically normal obese"
- Introduced the term *orthorexia nervosa*

Chapter 9

- Updated figure of maps showing prevalence of obesity among US adults
- Revised figure of surgical procedures for severe obesity to include sleeve gastrectomy
- Created new table to summarize ghrelin and leptin
- Added new drugs to table of FDA-approved weight-loss drugs
- Added new discussion of other medical procedures to treat obesity, including endoscopic procedures, intragastric balloons, and gastric aspiration
- Created new table to introduce SMART goals

Chapter 10

- Added a brief review of DRI terms to the introduction
- Deleted How To Estimate Niacin Equivalents
- Added a figure showing folate in its polyglutamate and monoglutamate forms; deleted the figure showing decline in neural tube defects since folate fortification
- Deleted How To Estimate Dietary Folate Equivalents

Chapter 11

- Simplified the figure showing the blood-clotting process

Chapter 12

- Reorganized water section
- Added new figure illustrating the color of urine in relation to hydration
- Deleted How To Estimate Your Calcium Intake

Chapter 13

- Deleted How To Estimate the Recommended Daily Intake for Iron

Chapter 14

- Defined and discussed myokines
- Reorganized the section on glucose use during physical activity
- Created a table of carbohydrate recommendations for physical activities
- Updated protein recommendations for athletes and created a table of food sources
- Added discussion of dietary nitrate as an ergogenic aid; removed carnitine and chromium picolinate

Chapter 15

- Created new table of advice for pregnant (and lactating) women eating fish
- Added discussions on dietary factors related to postpartum depression, benefits of lactation in delaying onset of type 2 diabetes in women with gestational diabetes, and use of breast pumps

Chapter 16

- Updated table of supplements for infants
- Included current recommendations about peanut allergy during infancy
- Added discussion about zinc when introducing complementary foods during infancy
- Updated the table of energy needs for children
- Revised section on children's dietary patterns
- Created a "How To" feature for the figure of body mass index for age percentiles

Chapter 17

- Added discussion about influence of obesity on the aging brain

Chapter 18

- Removed short discussion of HIV from the infectious disease section
- Added brief discussion emphasizing the importance of lifestyle choices to disease prevention, even in those who are at a high genetic risk of disease
- Included new information about the importance of assessing cardiorespiratory fitness as an indicator of heart disease risk
- Added How To Count Carbohydrates feature in the section on diabetes
- Added discussions about sugar alcohols and artificial sweeteners in the diabetes section and about nitrites and nitrates in processed meats in the cancer section

Chapter 19

- Expanded discussion on product date labeling
- Removed discussion on dioxin

Chapter 20

- Expanded discussion on sustainable diets
- Refocused section on agriculture and the environment

Student and Instructor Resources

MindTap: A new approach to highly personalized online learning. Beyond an eBook, homework solution, digital supplement, or premium website, MindTap is a digital learning platform that works alongside your campus LMS to deliver course curriculum across the range of electronic devices in your life. MindTap is built on an "app" model allowing enhanced digital collaboration and delivery of engaging content accross a spectrum of Cengage and non-Cengage resources.

Instructor Companion Site: Everything you need for your course in one place! This collection of book-specific lecture and class tools is available online via www.cengage.com/login. Access and download PowerPoint presentations, images, instructor's manual, videos, and more.

Test Bank with Cognero: Cengage Learning Testing Powered by Cognero is a flexible, online system that allows you to:

- write, edit, and manage test bank content from multiple Cengage Learning solutions
- create multiple test versions in an instant
- deliver tests from your LMS, your classroom, or wherever you want

Diet & Wellness Plus: Diet & Wellness Plus helps you understand how nutrition relates to your personal health goals. Track your diet and activity, generate reports, and analyze the nutritional value of the food you eat. Diet & Wellness Plus includes over 75,000 foods as well as custom food and recipe features. The Behavior Change Planner helps you identify risks in your life and guides you through the key steps to make positive changes. Diet & Wellness Plus is also available as an app that can be accessed from the app dock in MindTap.

Global Nutrition Watch: Bring currency to the classroom with Global Nutrition Watch from Cengage Learning. This user-friendly website provides convenient access to thousands of trusted sources, including academic journals, newspapers, videos, and podcasts, for you to use for research projects or classroom discussion. Global Nutrition Watch is updated daily to offer the most current news about topics related to nutrition.

Closing Comments

We have taken great care to provide accurate information and have included many references at the end of each chapter and highlight. To keep the number of references manageable over the decades, however, many statements that appeared in previous editions with references now appear without them. All statements reflect current nutrition knowledge, and the authors will supply references upon request. In addition to supporting text statements, the end-of-chapter references provide readers with resources for finding a good overview or more details on the subject. Nutrition is a fascinating subject, and we hope our enthusiasm for it comes through on every page.

Ellie Whitney
Sharon Rady Rolfes
January 2018

Acknowledgments

To produce a book requires the coordinated effort of a team of people—and, no doubt, each team member has another team of support people as well. We salute, with a big round of applause, everyone who has worked so diligently to ensure the quality of this book.

We thank our partners and friends, Linda DeBruyne and Fran Webb, for their valuable consultations and contributions; working together over the past 30+ years has been a most wonderful experience. We especially appreciate Linda's research assistance on several chapters. Special thanks to our colleagues Kathy Pinna for her insightful comments and Sylvia Crews for her careful review of the math explanations in Appendix H. Thank you to Lauren Smith for clarifying content and providing a student's perspective, and Christopher Rolfes for assisting in numerous office tasks.

Our heartfelt thanks to our publishing team for their efforts in creating an outstanding nutrition textbook—Krista Mastroianni, Miriam Myers, and Carol Samet. Thank you to Tom Ziolkowski for his energetic efforts in marketing; Reba Frederics and Christine Myaskovsky for their assistance in obtaining permissions; and Thalia E. Prum and Lumina Datamatics Ltd. for their help in preparing content for the instructor and student resources.

We also thank Michael Cook, our art director, for creatively designing these pages; Lori Hazzard for her diligent attention to the innumerable details involved in production; Nisha Bhanu Beegum for selecting photographs that deliver nutrition messages attractively; Debbie Stone for copyediting close to 1000 manuscript pages; A. Nayyer Shamsi for proofreading close to 1000 final text pages; and Edwin Durbin for composing a thorough and useful index. To the hundreds of others involved in production and sales, we tip our hats in appreciation.

We are especially grateful to our friends and families for their continued encouragement and support. As always, we are grateful for the instructors who took the time to comment and contribute to this revision. Such suggestions are invaluable in strengthening the book and are always welcomed.

Reviewers of Recent Editions

Dr. Chris Adamson
Seminole State College of Florida

Becky Alejandre
American River College

Janet B. Anderson
Utah State University

Sandra D. Baker
University of Delaware

Angelina Boyce
Hillsborough Community College

Lynn S. Brann
Syracuse University

Shalon Bull
Palm Beach Community College

Dorothy A. Byrne
University of Texas, San Antonio

John R. Capeheart
University of Houston, Downtown

Leah Carter
Bakersfield College

Dr. Carrie A. Cate
Diné College

James F. Collins
University of Florida

Diane Curis
Los Rios Community College District

Ruth Davies
Florida Southwestern State College

Lisa K. Diewald
Montgomery County Community College

Kristine Duncan, MS, RDN, CDE
Skagit Valley College

Kelly K. Eichmann
Fresno City College

Shannon Fenster
Bellevue College

Katie Ferraro, MPH, RDN, CDE
San Diego State University

Shawn W. Flanagan, Ph.D
The University of Iowa

Shawn Flanagan
University of Iowa

Mary Flynn
Brown University

Betty J. Forbes
West Virginia University

Sue Fredstrom
Minnesota State University, Mankato

Trish Froehlich
Palm Beach Community College

Stephen P. Gagnon
Hillsborough Community College

Leonard Gerber
University of Rhode Island

Jill Golden
Orange Coast College

Barbara J. Goldman
Palm Beach State College

Kathleen Gould
Towson University

Margaret Gunther
Palomar College

Charlene Hamilton
University of Delaware

D. J. Hennager
Kirkwood Community College

Catherine Hagen Howard
Texarkana College

James W. Haynes
Glendale Community College

Ernest B. Izevbigie
Jackson State University

Craig Kasper
Hillsborough Community College

Shawnee Kelly
Pennsylvania State University

Carrie King, PhD, RD, CDE, LD
University of Alaska Anchorage

Younghee Kim
Bowling Green State University

Rebecca A. Kleinschmidt
University of Alaska Southeast

Vicki Kloosterhouse
Oakland Community College

Donna M. Kopas
Pennsylvania State University

Susan M. Krueger
University of Wisconsin, Eau Claire

Barbara Lange
College of Central Florida

Melissa Langone
Pasco-Hernando Community College

Grace Lasker
Lake Washington Institute of Technology

Darlene M. Levinson
Oakland Community College, Orchard Ridge

Kimberly Lower
Collin County Community College

Elizabeth F. Lowe, MS, RD, LDN
East Tennessee State University

Melissa B. McGuire
Maple Woods Community College

Diane L. McKay
Tufts University

Anne Miller
De Anza College

Anahita M. Mistry
Eastern Michigan University

Lisa Morse
Arizona State University

Mithia Mukutmoni
Sierra College

Lisa M. Murray, MS
Pierce College

Steven Nizielski
Grand Valley State University

Yvonne Ortega
Santa Monica College

Jane M. Osowski
University of Southern Mississippi

Sarah Panarello
Yakima Valley Community College

Ryan Paruch
Tulsa Community College

Jill Patterson
Pennsylvania State University

Gina Pazzaglia
West Chester University

Julie Priday
Centralia College

Thalia E. Prum
San Diego Mesa College

Kelsey Rami
South Dakota State University

Jennifer Rogers
University of Iowa

Kathy L. Sedlet
Collin County Community College

Vidya Sharma
San Antonio College

Melissa Shock
University of Central Arkansas

Krista M. Simonetti
Maricopa County College

LuAnn Soliah
Baylor University

Amanda B. Stewart, PhD
Bethany College

Kenneth Strothkamp
Lewis & Clark College

Andrea Villarreal
Phoenix College

Terry Weideman
Oakland Community College, Highland Lake

H. Garrison Wilkes
University of Massachusetts, Boston

Lynne C. Zeman
Kirkwood Community College

Maureen Zimmerman
Mesa Community College

1 An Overview of Nutrition

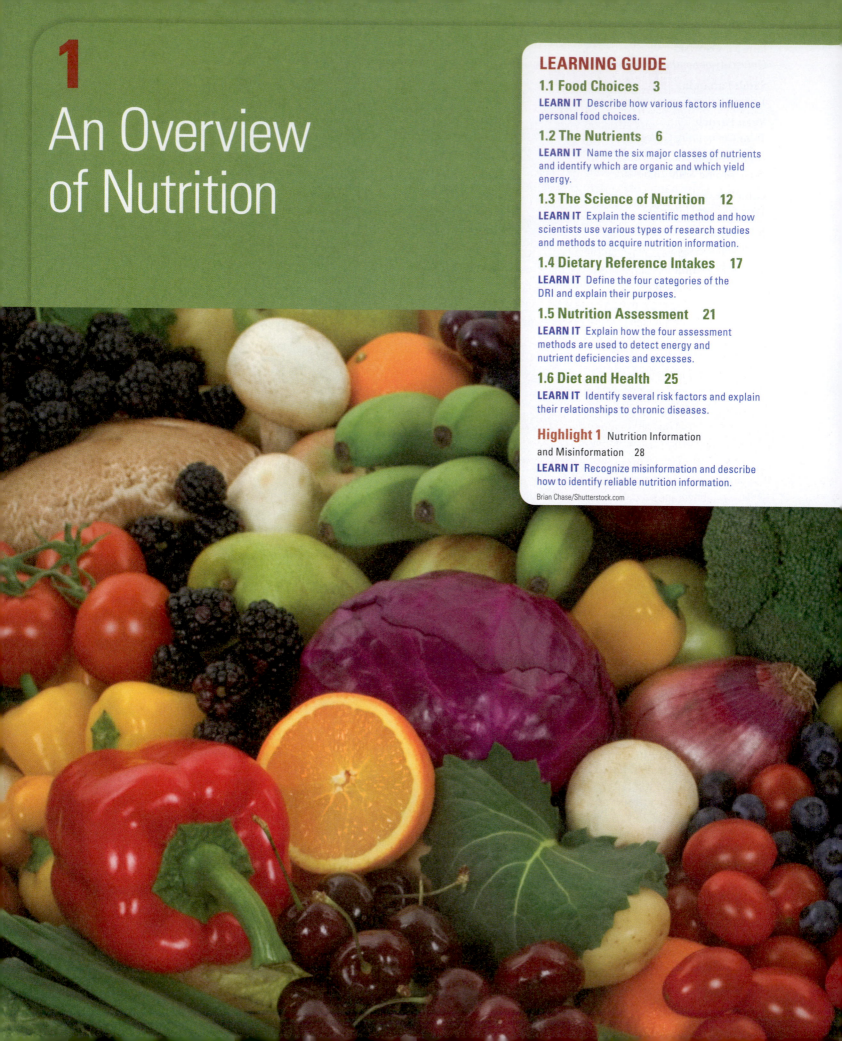

LEARNING GUIDE

Brian Chase/Shutterstock.com

Nutrition in Your Life

Believe it or not, you have probably eaten at least 20,000 meals in your life. Without any conscious effort on your part, your body uses the nutrients from those foods to make all its components, fuel all its activities, and defend itself against diseases. How successfully your body handles these tasks depends, in part, on your food choices. Nutritious food choices support healthy bodies. As you read this chapter, consider how your current food choices are influencing your health and risk of chronic diseases.

Nutrition has always played a significant role in your life. Every day, several times a day, you select **foods** that influence your body's health. Each day's food choices may benefit or harm health only a little, but over time, the consequences of these choices become major. That being the case, paying close attention to good eating habits now supports health benefits later. Conversely, carelessness about food choices can contribute to **chronic diseases**. Of course, some people will become ill or die young no matter what choices they make, and others will live long lives despite making poor choices. For most of us, however, the food choices we make will benefit or impair our health in proportion to how well those choices meet the body's needs.

Although most people realize food habits affect health, they often choose foods for other reasons. After all, foods bring pleasures, traditions, and associations as well as nourishment. The challenge, then, is to combine favorite foods and fun times with a nutritionally balanced **diet**. Take a moment to review the definition and note that *diet* does *not* mean a restrictive food plan designed for weight loss. It simply refers to the foods and beverages a person consumes. Whether it's a vegetarian diet, a weight-loss diet, or any other kind of diet depends on the types of foods and beverages a person chooses. Importantly, diets can change over time.

1.1 Food Choices

LEARN IT Describe how various factors influence personal food choices.

People decide what to eat, when to eat, how much to eat, and even whether to eat in highly personal ways. A variety of food choices can support good health, and an understanding of human nutrition can help a person make healthy selections more often.

Preferences As you might expect, the number one reason most people choose certain foods is taste—they like the flavor. Two widely shared preferences are for the sweetness of sugar and the savoriness of salt.[1] High-fat foods also appear to be a universally common preference.[2] Other preferences might be for the hot peppers common in Mexican cooking or the curry spices of Indian cuisine. Research suggests that genetics may influence taste perceptions and therefore food likes and dislikes.[3] Similarly, the hormones of pregnancy seem to influence food cravings and aversions (see Chapter 15).

Habit People sometimes select foods out of habit. They eat cereal every morning, for example, simply because they have always eaten cereal for breakfast. Eating a familiar food and not having to make any decisions can be comforting. Similarly, people may find certain foods and beverages most appropriate at certain times of day—orange juice in the morning, for example.

Ethnic Heritage and Regional Cuisines Among the strongest influences on food choices are ethnic heritage and regional cuisines. People tend to prefer the foods

nutrition: the science of the nutrients in foods and their actions within the body. A broader definition includes the study of human behaviors related to food and eating.

foods: products derived from plants or animals that can be taken into the body to yield energy and nutrients for the maintenance of life and the growth and repair of tissues.

chronic diseases: diseases characterized by slow progression and long duration. Examples include heart disease, diabetes, and some cancers.

- **chronos** = time

diet: the foods and beverages a person eats and drinks.

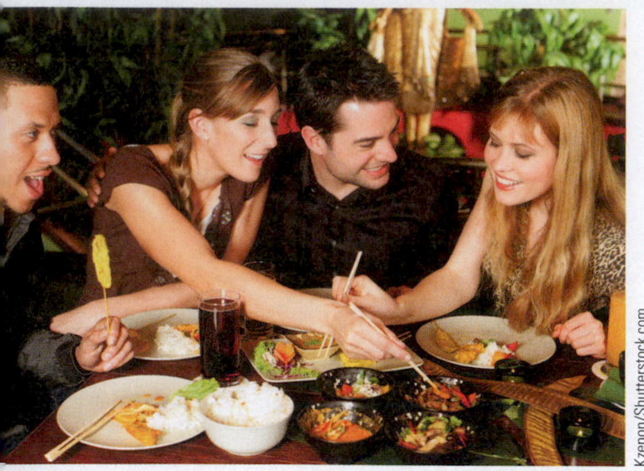
Kzenon/Shutterstock.com

> **PHOTO 1-1** An enjoyable way to learn about a culture is to taste the ethnic foods.

they grew up eating, but they may also be willing to try new foods, especially when traveling. Every country, and in fact every region of a country, has its own typical foods and ways of combining them into meals. These cuisines reflect a unique combination of local ingredients and cooking styles. Chowder in New England is made with clams, but in the Florida Keys conch is the featured ingredient. The Pacific Northwest is as famous for its marionberry pie as Georgia is for its peach cobbler. Philly has its cheesesteaks and New Orleans has its oyster po'boys. The "American diet" includes many ethnic foods and regional styles, all adding variety to the diet.

Enjoying traditional **ethnic foods** provides an opportunity to celebrate a person's cultural heritage (Photo 1-1). People offering ethnic foods share a part of their culture with others, and those accepting the foods learn about another's way of life. Developing **cultural competence** honors individual preferences and is particularly important for professionals who help others plan healthy diets.[4]

Social Interactions Meals are often social events, and sharing food is part of hospitality. Social customs invite people to accept food or drink offered by a host or shared by a group—regardless of hunger signals. Such social interactions can be a challenge for people trying to limit their food intake; Chapter 9 describes how people tend to eat more food when socializing with others. People also tend to eat the kinds of foods eaten by those in their social circles, thus helping to explain why obesity seems to spread in social networks and weight loss is easier with a partner.[5]

Marketing Another major influence on food choices is marketing. The food industry competes for our food dollars, persuading consumers to eat more—more food, more often. These marketing efforts pay off well, generating more than $900 billion in sales each year. In addition to building brand loyalty, food companies attract busy consumers with their promises of convenience.

Availability, Convenience, and Economy People often eat foods that are accessible, quick and easy to prepare, and within their financial means. Consumers who value convenience frequently eat out, bring home ready-to-eat meals, or have food delivered. Even when they venture into the kitchen, they want to prepare a meal in 15 to 20 minutes, using less than a half dozen ingredients—and those ingredients are often semiprepared foods, such as canned soups and frozen foods. Whether decisions based on convenience meet a person's nutrition needs depends on the choices made. Eating a banana or a candy bar may be equally convenient, but the fruit provides more vitamins and minerals and less sugar and fat.

Given the abundance of convenient food options, fewer adults are learning the cooking skills needed to prepare meals at home, which has its downside. People who are competent in their cooking skills and frequently eat their meals at home tend to make healthier food choices.[6] Not surprisingly, when eating out, consumers often choose low-cost fast-food outlets over more expensive fine-dining restaurants. Foods eaten away from home, especially fast-food meals, tend to be high in nutrients that Americans overconsume (saturated fat and sodium) and low in nutrients that Americans underconsume (calcium, fiber, and iron)—all of which can contribute to a variety of health problems.[7]

Unfortunately, healthful diets that include plenty of fruits, vegetables, fish, and nuts tend to cost a little more (about $1.50 per person per day more) than less healthful diets that feature meats, refined grains, and processed foods; also, milk is more expensive than soda.[8] Strategies to help consumers improve diet quality include reducing the price of fruits and vegetables, taxing processed foods, placing healthy options in strategic locations, and limiting discounts on less-healthy foods.[9]

Positive and Negative Associations People tend to like particular foods associated with happy occasions—such as hot dogs at ball games or cake and ice cream

ethnic foods: foods associated with particular cultural groups.

cultural competence: having an awareness and acceptance of cultures and the ability to interact effectively with people of diverse cultures.

at birthday parties. By the same token, people can develop aversions to and dislike foods that they ate when they felt sick or that they were forced to eat in negative situations.[10] Similarly, children learn to like and dislike certain foods when their parents use foods as rewards or punishments. Negative experiences can have long-lasting influences on food preferences. More than 50 years after World War II, veterans who had experienced intense combat in the Pacific dislike Asian food significantly more than their peers who were not engaged in battle or those who fought elsewhere.

Emotions Emotions guide food choices and eating behaviors.[11] Some people cannot eat when they are emotionally upset. Others may eat in response to a variety of emotional stimuli—for example, to relieve boredom or depression or to calm anxiety. A lonely person may choose to eat rather than to call a friend. A person who has returned home from an exciting evening out may unwind with a late-night snack. These people may find emotional comfort, in part, because foods can influence the brain's chemistry and the mind's response. Carbohydrates and alcohol, for example, tend to calm, whereas proteins and caffeine are more likely to stimulate. Eating in response to emotions and stress can easily lead to overeating and obesity, but it may be helpful at times. For example, sharing food at times of bereavement serves both the giver's need to provide comfort and the receiver's need to be cared for and to interact with others as well as to take nourishment.

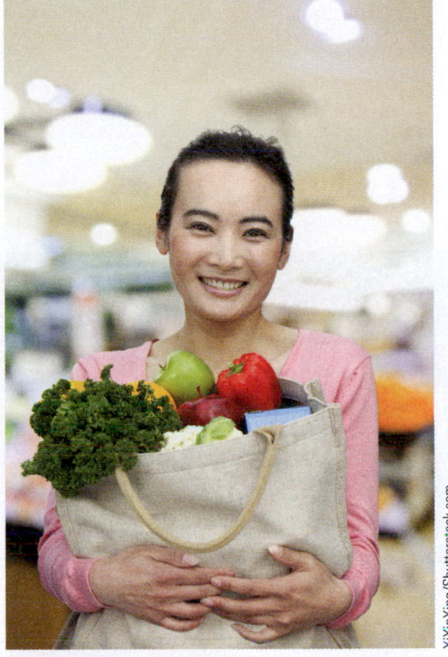
XiXinXing/Shutterstock.com

> **PHOTO 1-2** To protect the environment, shop at local markets and reuse cloth shopping bags. To enhance your health, keep nutrition in mind when selecting foods.

Values Food choices may reflect people's religious beliefs, political views, or environmental concerns. For example, some Christians forgo meat on Fridays during Lent (the period prior to Easter), Jewish law includes an extensive set of dietary rules that govern the use of foods derived from animals, and Muslims fast between sunrise and sunset during Ramadan (the ninth month of the Islamic calendar). Some vegetarians select foods based on their support for animal rights. A concerned consumer may boycott fruit picked by migrant workers who have been exploited. People may buy vegetables from local farmers to save the fuel and environmental costs of foods shipped long distances (see Photo 1-2). They may also select foods packaged in containers that can be reused or recycled. Some consumers accept or reject foods that have been irradiated, grown organically, or genetically modified, depending on their approval of these processes (see Chapter and Highlight 19 for a complete discussion).

Body Weight and Health Sometimes people select certain foods and supplements that they believe will improve their body weight, health, or allergies and avoid those they believe might be detrimental. Such decisions can be beneficial when based on nutrition science, but decisions based on fads or carried to extremes undermine good health, as pointed out in later discussions of eating disorders (Highlight 8) and dietary supplements commonly used by athletes (Highlight 14).

Nutrition Finally, of course, many consumers make food choices they believe are nutritious and healthy. Making healthy food choices 100 years ago was rather easy; the list of options was relatively short and markets sold mostly fresh, **whole foods**. Examples of whole foods include vegetables and legumes; fruits; seafood, meats, poultry, eggs, nuts, and seeds; milk; and whole grains. Today, tens of thousands of food items fill the shelves of super-grocery stores and most of those items are **processed foods**. Whether a processed food is a healthy choice depends, in part, on how extensively the food was processed. When changes are minimal, processing can provide an abundant, safe, convenient, affordable, and nutritious product.[12] Examples of minimally processed foods include frozen vegetables, fruit juices, smoked salmon, cheeses, and breads. The nutritional value diminishes, however, when changes are extensive, creating **ultra-processed foods**. Ultra-processed foods no longer resemble whole foods; they are made from substances

whole foods: fresh foods such as vegetables, grains, legumes, meats, and milk that are unprocessed or minimally processed.

processed foods: foods that have been intentionally changed by the addition of substances, or a method of cooking, preserving, milling, or such.

ultra-processed foods: foods that have been made from substances that are typically used in food preparation, but not consumed as foods by themselves (such as oils, fats, flours, refined starches, and sugars) that undergo further processing by adding a little, if any, minimally processed foods, salt and other preservatives, and additives such as flavors and colors.

that are typically used in food preparation, but not consumed as foods themselves (such as oils, fats, flours, refined starches, and sugars). These substances undergo further processing by adding a little, if any, processed foods, salt and other preservatives, and additives such as flavors and colors. Examples of ultra-processed foods include soft drinks, corn chips, fruit gummies, chicken nuggets, canned cheese spreads, and toaster pastries. Notably, these foods cannot be made in a home kitchen using common grocery ingredients. Dominating the global market, ultra-processed foods tend to be attractive, tasty, and cheap—as well as high in fat and sugar.[13] Consumers who want to make healthy food choices will select fewer ultra-processed foods and more whole foods and minimally processed foods.[14]

REVIEW IT Describe how various factors influence personal food choices.

A person selects foods for a variety of reasons. Whatever those reasons may be, food choices influence health. Individual food selections neither make nor break a diet's healthfulness, but the balance of foods selected over time can make an important difference to health.[15] For this reason, people are wise to think "nutrition" when making their food choices.

1.2 The Nutrients

LEARN IT Name the six major classes of nutrients and identify which are organic and which yield energy.

Biologically speaking, people eat to receive nourishment. Do you ever think of yourself as a biological being made of carefully arranged atoms, molecules, cells, tissues, and organs? Are you aware of the activity going on within your body even as you sit still? The atoms, molecules, and cells of your body continuously move and change, even though the structures of your tissues and organs and your external appearance remain relatively constant. The ongoing growth, maintenance, and repair of the body's tissues depend on the **energy** and the **nutrients** received from foods (see Photo 1-3).

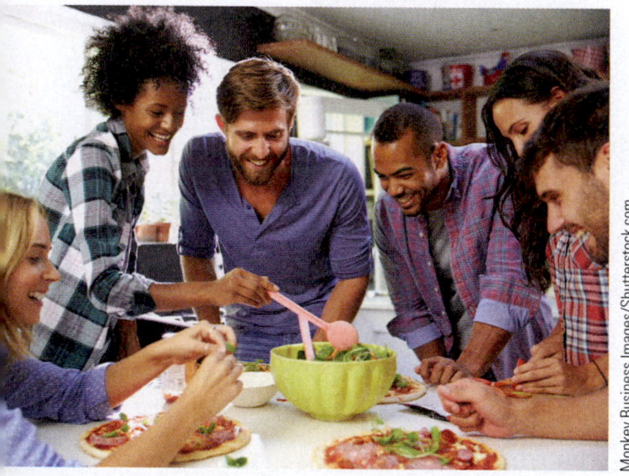

Monkey Business Images/Shutterstock.com

> **PHOTO 1-3** Find pleasure in eating well. Enjoy foods that meet both your nutrient needs and dietary preferences.

Nutrients in Foods and in the Body

Amazingly, our bodies can derive all the energy, structural materials, and regulating agents we need from the foods we eat. This section introduces the nutrients that foods deliver and shows how they participate in the dynamic processes that keep people alive and well.

Nutrient Composition of Foods Chemical analysis of a food such as a tomato shows that it is composed primarily of water (95 percent). Most of the solid materials are carbohydrates, lipids (fats), and proteins. If you could remove these materials, you would find a tiny residue of vitamins, minerals, and other compounds. Water, carbohydrates (including fibers), lipids, proteins, vitamins, and some of the minerals found in foods represent the six classes of nutrients—substances the body uses for the growth, maintenance, and repair of its tissues.

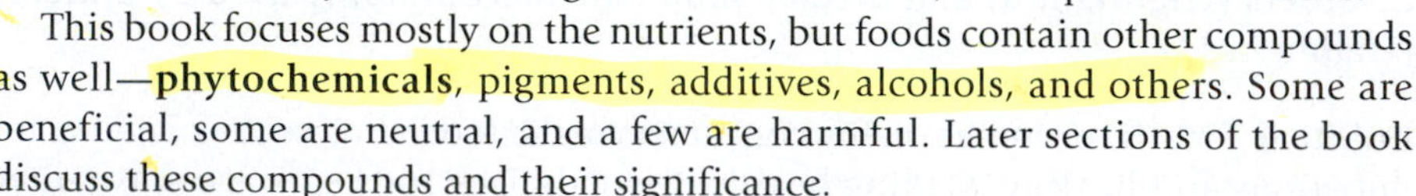

This book focuses mostly on the nutrients, but foods contain other compounds as well—**phytochemicals**, pigments, additives, alcohols, and others. Some are beneficial, some are neutral, and a few are harmful. Later sections of the book discuss these compounds and their significance.

Nutrient Composition of the Body A chemical analysis of your body would show that it is made of materials similar to those found in foods (see Figure 1-1). A healthy 150-pound body contains about 90 pounds of water and about 20 to 45 pounds of fat. The remaining pounds are mostly protein, carbohydrate, and the major minerals of the bones. Vitamins and other minerals constitute a fraction of a pound.

Chemical Composition of Nutrients The simplest of the nutrients are the minerals. Each mineral is a chemical element; its atoms are all alike. As a result, its identity never changes. For example, iron may have different electrical charges, but the individual iron atoms remain the same when they are in a food, when a person eats the food, when the iron becomes part of a red blood cell, when the cell is broken

energy: the capacity to do work. The energy in food is chemical energy. The body can convert this chemical energy to mechanical, electrical, or heat energy.

nutrients: chemical substances obtained from food and used in the body to provide energy, structural materials, and regulating agents to support growth, maintenance, and repair of the body's tissues. Nutrients may also reduce the risks of some diseases.

phytochemicals (FIE-toe-KEM-ih-cals): nonnutrient compounds found in plants. Some phytochemicals have biological activity in the body.

- **phyto** = plant

> **FIGURE 1-1 Body Composition of Healthy-Weight Men and Women**

The human body is made of compounds similar to those found in foods—mostly water (60 percent) and some fat (18 to 21 percent for young men, 23 to 26 percent for young women), with carbohydrate, protein, vitamins, minerals, and other minor constituents making up the remainder. (Chapter 8 describes the health hazards of too little or too much body fat.)

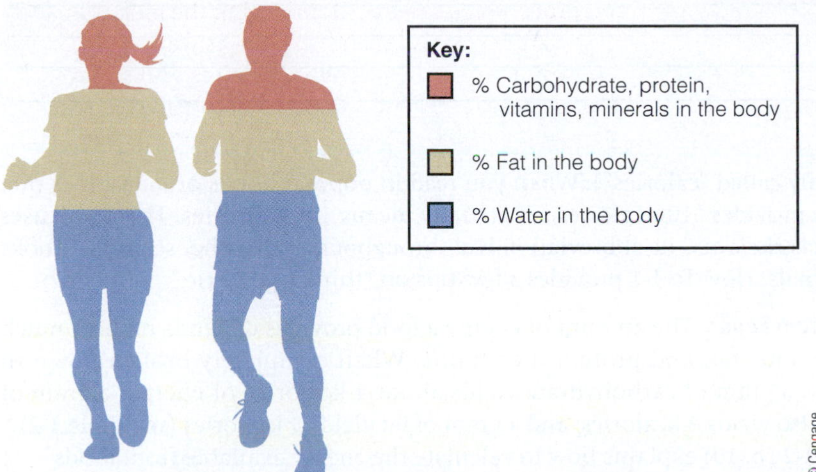
Key:
% Carbohydrate, protein, vitamins, minerals in the body
% Fat in the body
% Water in the body
© Cengage

down, and when the iron is lost from the body by excretion. The next simplest nutrient is water, a compound made of two elements—hydrogen and oxygen. Minerals and water are **inorganic** nutrients—which means they do not contain carbon.

The other four classes of nutrients (carbohydrates, lipids, proteins, and vitamins) are more complex. In addition to hydrogen and oxygen, they all contain carbon, an element found in all living things; they are therefore called **organic compounds** (meaning, literally, "alive").* This chemical definition of *organic* differs from the agricultural definition. As Chapter 19 explains, organic farming refers to growing crops and raising livestock according to standards set by the US Department of Agriculture (USDA). Protein and some vitamins also contain nitrogen and may contain other elements such as sulfur as well.

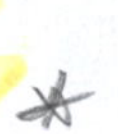

Essential Nutrients The body can make some nutrients, but it cannot make all of them. Also, it makes some in insufficient quantities to meet its needs and, therefore, must obtain these nutrients from foods. The nutrients that foods must supply are **essential nutrients**. When used to refer to nutrients, the word *essential* means more than just "necessary"; it means "needed from outside the body"—normally, from foods.

The Energy-Yielding Nutrients: Carbohydrate, Fat, and Protein

In the body, three of the organic nutrients can be used to provide energy: carbohydrate, fat, and protein. In contrast to these **energy-yielding nutrients**, vitamins, minerals, and water do not yield energy in the human body.

Carbohydrate, fat, and protein are sometimes called *macronutrients* because the body requires them in relatively large amounts (many grams daily). In contrast, vitamins and minerals are *micronutrients*, required only in small amounts (milligrams or micrograms daily). Table 1-1 (p. 8) summarizes some of the ways the six classes of nutrients can be described.

Energy Measured in kCalories The energy released from carbohydrate, fat, and protein can be measured in **calories**—tiny units of energy so small that a single apple provides tens of thousands of them. To ease calculations, energy is expressed in 1000-calorie metric units known as kilocalories (shortened to **kcalories**, but

* Note that this definition of *organic* excludes coal, diamonds, and a few carbon-containing compounds that contain only a single carbon and no hydrogen, such as carbon dioxide (CO_2), calcium carbonate ($CaCO_3$), magnesium carbonate ($MgCO_3$), and sodium cyanide (NaCN).

inorganic: not containing carbon or pertaining to living organisms. The two classes of nutrients that are inorganic are minerals and water.

- **in** = not

organic: in chemistry, substances or molecules containing carbon-carbon bonds or carbon-hydrogen bonds that are characteristic of living organisms. The four classes of nutrients that are organic are carbohydrates, lipids (fats), proteins, and vitamins.

essential nutrients: nutrients a person must obtain from food because the body cannot make them for itself in sufficient quantity to meet physiological needs; also called *indispensable nutrients*. About 40 nutrients are currently known to be essential for human beings.

energy-yielding nutrients: the nutrients that break down to yield energy the body can use:

- carbohydrate
- fat
- protein

calories or **kcalories:** a measure of *heat* energy. Energy provided by foods and beverages is measured in *kilocalories* (1000 calories equal 1 kilocalorie), abbreviated *kcalories* or *kcal*. One kcalorie is the amount of heat necessary to raise the temperature of 1 kilogram (kg) of water 1°C. The scientific use of the term *kcalorie* is the same as the popular use of the term *calorie*.

TABLE 1-1 The Six Classes of Nutrients

Nutrient	Organic	Inorganic	Energy-yielding	Macronutrient	Micronutrient
Carbohydrates	✓		✓	✓	
Lipids (fats)	✓		✓	✓	
Proteins	✓		✓	✓	
Vitamins	✓				✓
Minerals		✓			✓
Water		✓			

commonly called "calories"). When you read in popular books or magazines that an apple provides "100 calories," it actually means 100 kcalories. This book uses the term *kcalorie* and its abbreviation *kcal* throughout, as do other scientific books and journals. How To 1-1 provides a few tips on "thinking metric."

Energy from Foods The amount of energy a food provides depends on how much carbohydrate, fat, and protein it contains. When completely broken down in the body, a gram of carbohydrate yields about 4 kcalories of energy; a gram of protein also yields 4 kcalories; and a gram of fat yields 9 kcalories (see Table 1-2).* How To 1-2 (p. 10) explains how to calculate the energy available from foods.

TABLE 1-2 kCalorie Values of Energy Nutrients

Nutrients	Energy
Carbohydrate	4 kcal/g
Fat	9 kcal/g
Protein	4 kcal/g

NOTE: Alcohol contributes 7 kcal/g that can be used for energy, but it is not considered a nutrient because it interferes with the body's growth, maintenance, and repair.

Because fat provides more energy per gram, it has a greater **energy density** than either carbohydrate or protein. Figure 1-2 compares the energy density of two breakfast options, and later chapters describe how foods with a high energy density contribute to weight *gain*, whereas those with a low energy density help with weight *loss*.

One other substance contributes energy—alcohol. Alcohol, however, is not considered a nutrient. Unlike the nutrients, alcohol does not sustain life. In fact, it interferes with the growth, maintenance, and repair of the body. Its only common

> FIGURE 1-2 Energy Density of Two Breakfast Options Compared

Gram for gram, ounce for ounce, and bite for bite, foods with a high energy density deliver more kcalories than foods with a low energy density. Both of these breakfast options provide 500 kcalories, but the cereal with milk, fruit salad, scrambled egg, turkey sausage, and toast with jam offers three times as much food as the doughnuts (based on weight); it has a lower energy density than the doughnuts. Selecting a variety of foods also helps ensure nutrient adequacy.

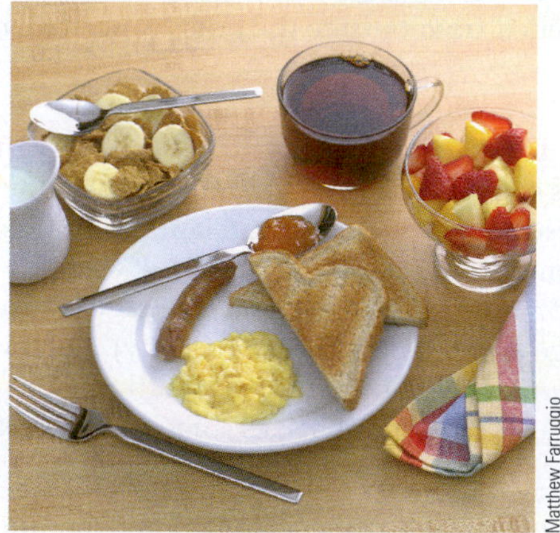

LOWER ENERGY DENSITY
This 450-gram breakfast delivers 500 kcalories, for an energy density of 1.1 (500 kcal ÷ 450 g = 1.1 kcal/g).

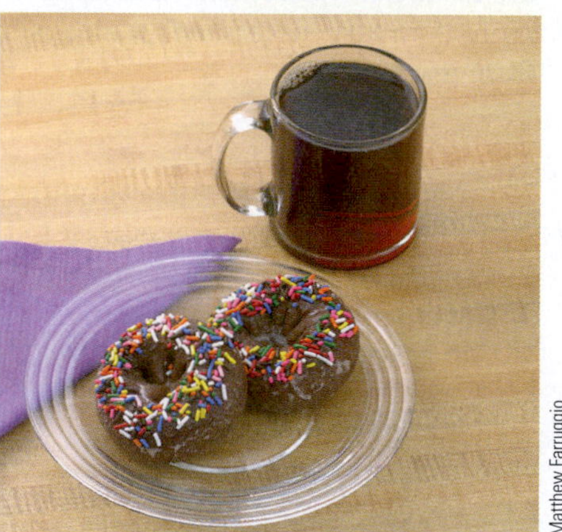

HIGHER ENERGY DENSITY
This 144-gram breakfast delivers 500 kcalories, for an energy density of 3.5 (500 kcal ÷ 144 g = 3.5 kcal/g).

energy density: a measure of the energy a food provides relative to the weight of the food (kcalories per gram).

*For those using kilojoules: 1 g carbohydrate = 17 kJ; 1 g protein = 17 kJ; 1 g fat = 37 kJ; and 1 g alcohol = 29 kJ.

>How To 1-1 Think Metric

Like other scientists, nutrition scientists use metric units of measure. They measure food energy in kilocalories, people's height in centimeters, people's weight in kilograms, and the weights of foods and nutrients in grams, milligrams, or micrograms. For ease in using these measures, it helps to remember that the prefixes imply 1000. For example, a *kilo*gram is 1000 grams, a *milli*gram is 1/1000 of a gram, and a *micro*gram is 1/1000 of a milligram (or 1/1,000,000 of a gram).

Most food labels and many recipes provide dual measures, listing both household measures, such as cups, quarts, and teaspoons, and metric measures, such as milliliters, liters, and grams. This practice gives people an opportunity to gradually learn to "think metric."

A person might begin to "think metric" by simply observing the measure—by noticing the amount of soda in a 2-liter bottle, for example. Through such experiences, a person can become familiar with a measure without having to do any conversions.

The international unit for measuring food energy is the joule—the amount of energy expended when 1 kilogram is moved 1 meter by a force of 1 newton. The joule is thus a measure of *work* energy, whereas the kcalorie is a measure of *heat* energy. While many scientists and journals report their findings in kilojoules (kJ), many others, particularly those in the United States, use kcalories (kcal). To convert energy measures from kcalories to kilojoules, multiply by 4.2; to convert kilojoules to kcalories, multiply by 0.24. For example, a 50-kcalorie cookie provides 210 kilojoules:

$$50 \text{ kcal} \times 4.2 = 210 \text{ kJ}$$

Appendix H provides math assistance and conversion factors for these and other units of measure.

Volume: Liters (L)

1 L = 1000 milliliters (mL)
0.95 L = 1 quart
1 mL = 0.03 fluid ounces
240 mL = 1 cup

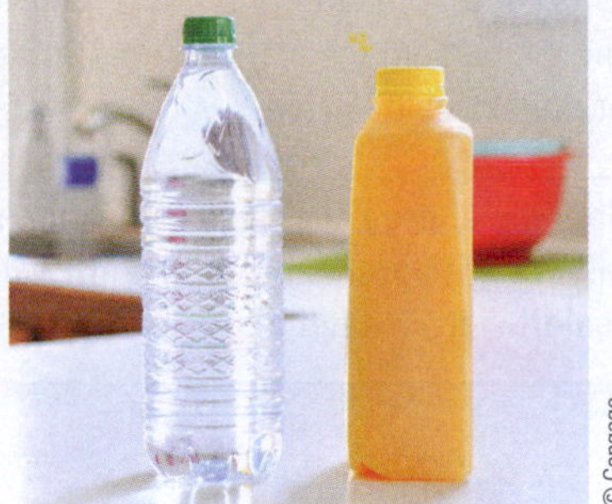

© Cengage

A liter of liquid is approximately one US quart. (Four liters are only about 5 percent more than a gallon.)

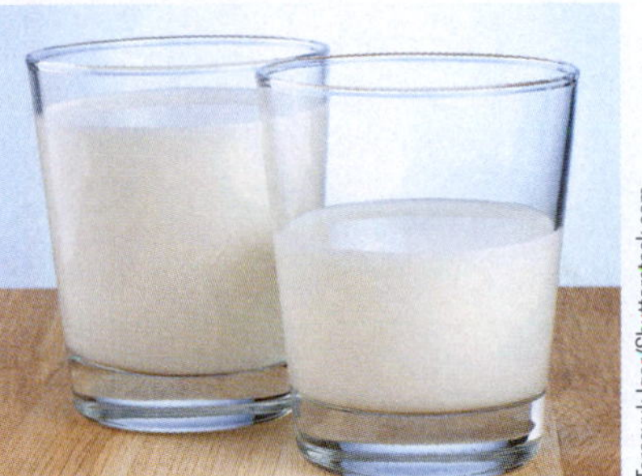

Tarasyuk Igor/Shutterstock.com

One cup of liquid is about 240 milliliters; a half-cup of liquid is about 120 milliliters.

Weight: Grams (g)

1 g = 1000 milligrams (mg)
1 g = 0.04 ounce (oz)
1 oz = 28.35 g (or 30 g)
100 g = 3½ oz
1 kilogram (kg) = 1000 g
1 kg = 2.2 pounds (lb)
454 g = 1 lb

Length: Centimeters (cm)

1 cm = 0.39 inches (in.)
1 in. = 2.54 cm

A kilogram is slightly more than 2 lb; conversely, a pound is about ½ kg.

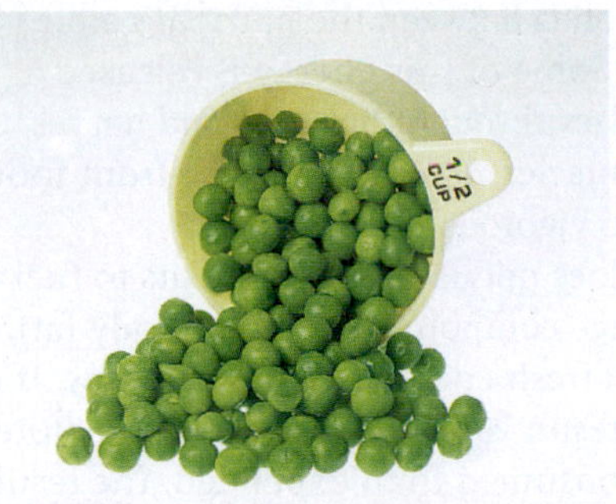
1/2 CUP

© Thomas Harm & Tom Peterson/Quest Photographic, Inc.

A half-cup of vegetables weighs about 100 grams; one pea weighs about ½ gram.

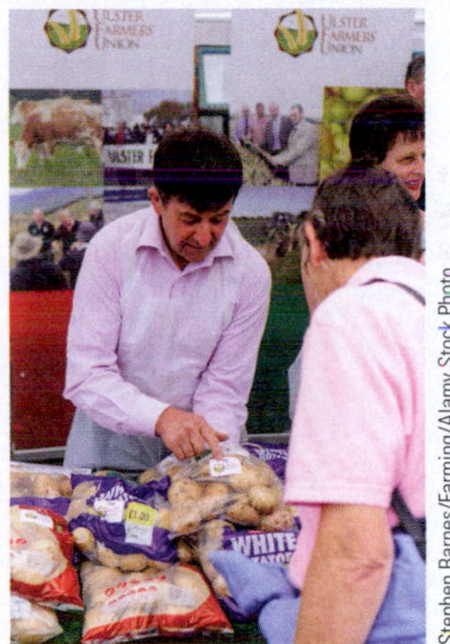
ULSTER FARMERS UNION
ULSTER FARMERS UNION
WHITE

Stephen Barnes/Farming/Alamy Stock Photo

A 5-pound bag of potatoes weighs about 2 kilograms, and a 176-pound person weighs 80 kilograms. The height of a person 5 feet 10 inches tall (70 inches) is 178 centimeters.

> TRY IT Convert your body weight from pounds to kilograms and your height from inches to centimeters.

characteristic with nutrients is that it yields energy (7 kcalories per gram) when metabolized in the body.

Most foods contain a mixture of the energy-yielding nutrients, vitamins, minerals, water, and other substances. For example, meat contains water, fat, vitamins,

>How To 1-2 Calculate the Energy Available from Foods

To calculate the energy available from a food, multiply the number of grams of carbohydrate, protein, and fat by 4, 4, and 9, respectively. Then add the results together. For example, 1 slice of bread with 1 tablespoon of peanut butter on it contains 16 grams carbohydrate, 7 grams protein, and 9 grams fat:

$$\begin{aligned} 16 \text{ g carbohydrate} \times 4 \text{ kcal/g} &= 64 \text{ kcal} \\ 7 \text{ g protein} \times 4 \text{ kcal/g} &= 28 \text{ kcal} \\ 9 \text{ g fat} \times 9 \text{ kcal/g} &= 81 \text{ kcal} \\ \text{Total} &= 173 \text{ kcal} \end{aligned}$$

From this information, you can calculate the percentage of kcalories each of the energy nutrients contributes to the total. To determine the percentage of kcalories from fat, for example, divide the 81 fat kcalories by the total 173 kcalories:

$$81 \text{ fat kcal} \div 173 \text{ total kcal} = 0.468 \text{ (rounded to 0.47)}$$

Then multiply by 100 to get the percentage:

$$0.47 \times 100 = 47\%$$

Dietary recommendations that urge people to limit fat intake to 20 to 35 percent of kcalories refer to the day's total energy intake, not to individual foods. Still, if the proportion of fat in each food choice throughout a day exceeds 35 percent of kcalories, then the day's total surely will, too. Knowing that this snack provides 47 percent of its kcalories from fat alerts a person to the need to make lower-fat selections at other times that day.

> TRY IT Calculate the energy available from a bean burrito with cheese (55 grams carbohydrate, 15 grams protein, and 12 grams fat). Determine the percentage of kcalories from each of the energy nutrients.

and minerals as well as protein. Bread contains water, a trace of fat, a little protein, and some vitamins and minerals in addition to its carbohydrate. Only a few foods are exceptions to this rule, the common ones being sugar (pure carbohydrate) and oil (essentially pure fat).

Energy in the Body When the body uses carbohydrate, fat, or protein to fuel its activities, the bonds between the nutrient's atoms break. As the bonds break, they release energy. Some of this energy is released as heat, but some is used to send electrical impulses through the brain and nerves, to synthesize body compounds, and to move muscles. Thus the energy from food supports every activity from quiet thought to vigorous sports.

If the body does not use these nutrients to fuel its current activities, it converts them into storage compounds (such as body fat), to be used between meals and overnight when fresh energy supplies run low. If more energy is consumed than expended, the result is an increase in energy stores and weight gain. Similarly, if less energy is consumed than expended, the result is a decrease in energy stores and weight loss.

When consumed in excess of energy needs, alcohol, too, can be converted to body fat and stored. When alcohol contributes a substantial portion of the energy in a person's diet, the harm it does far exceeds the problems of excess body fat. Highlight 7 describes the effects of alcohol on health and nutrition.

Other Roles of Energy-Yielding Nutrients In addition to providing energy, carbohydrates, fats, and proteins provide the raw materials for building the body's tissues and regulating its many activities. In fact, protein's role as an energy source is relatively minor compared with both the other two energy-yielding nutrients and its other roles. Proteins are found in structures such as the muscles and skin and help to regulate activities such as digestion and energy metabolism. Chapters 4, 5, and 6 present a full discussion on carbohydrates, fats, and proteins.

The Vitamins The **vitamins** are also organic, but they do not provide energy. Instead, they facilitate the release of energy from carbohydrate, fat, and protein and participate in numerous other activities throughout the body.

Each of the 13 vitamins has its own special roles to play.* One vitamin enables the eyes to see in dim light, another helps protect the lungs from air pollution, and still another helps make the sex hormones—among other things. When you cut yourself, one vitamin helps stop the bleeding and another helps repair the skin. Vitamins busily help replace old red blood cells and the lining of the digestive tract. Almost every action in the body requires the assistance of vitamins.

Vitamins can function only if they are intact, but because they are complex organic molecules, they are vulnerable to destruction by heat, light, and chemical agents. This is why the body handles them carefully, and why nutrition-wise cooks do, too. The strategies of cooking vegetables at moderate temperatures for short times and using small amounts of water help preserve the vitamins.

The Minerals In the body, some **minerals** are put together in orderly arrays in such structures as bones and teeth. Minerals are also found in the fluids of the body, which influences fluid balance and distribution. Whatever their roles, minerals do not yield energy.

Only 16 minerals are known to be essential in human nutrition.** Others are being studied to determine whether they play significant roles in the human body. Still other minerals, such as lead, are environmental contaminants that displace the nutrient minerals from their workplaces in the body, disrupting body functions. The problems caused by contaminant minerals are described in Chapter 13.

Because minerals are inorganic, they are indestructible and need not be handled with the special care that vitamins require. Minerals can, however, be bound by substances that interfere with the body's ability to absorb them. They can also be lost during food processing or during cooking when they leach into water that is discarded.

Water Water provides the environment in which nearly all the body's activities take place. It participates in many metabolic reactions and supplies the medium for transporting vital materials to cells and carrying waste products away from them. Water is discussed fully in Chapter 12, but it is mentioned in every chapter (see Photo 1-4). If you watch for it, you cannot help but be impressed by water's participation in all life processes.

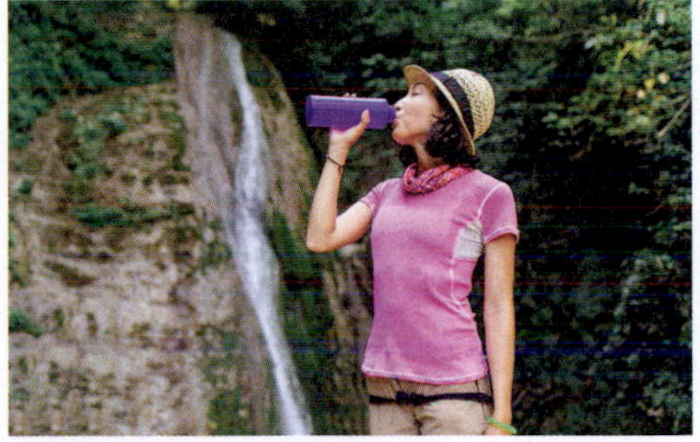
frantic00/Shutterstock.com

> **PHOTO 1-4** Water is an essential nutrient and naturally carries varying amounts of several minerals.

REVIEW IT Name the six major classes of nutrients and identify which are organic and which yield energy.

Foods provide nutrients—substances that support the growth, maintenance, and repair of the body's tissues. The six classes of nutrients include:

- Carbohydrates
- Lipids (fats)
- Proteins
- Vitamins
- Minerals
- Water

Foods rich in the energy-yielding nutrients (carbohydrate, fat, and protein) provide the major materials for building the body's tissues and yield energy for the body's use or storage. Energy is measured in kcalories—a measure of heat energy. Vitamins, minerals, and water do not yield energy; instead they facilitate a variety of activities in the body.

*The water-soluble vitamins are vitamin C and the eight B vitamins: thiamin, riboflavin, niacin, vitamins B_6 and B_{12}, folate, biotin, and pantothenic acid (see Chapter 10). The fat-soluble vitamins are vitamins A, D, E, and K (see Chapter 11).

**The major minerals are calcium, phosphorus, potassium, sodium, chloride, magnesium, and sulfate (see Chapter 12). The trace minerals are iron, iodine, zinc, chromium, selenium, fluoride, molybdenum, copper, and manganese (see Chapter 13).

vitamins: organic, essential nutrients required in small amounts by the body for health. Vitamins regulate body processes that support growth and maintain life.

minerals: inorganic elements. Some minerals are essential nutrients required in small amounts by the body for health.

Without exaggeration, nutrients provide the physical and metabolic basis for nearly all that we are and all that we do. The next section introduces the science of nutrition with emphasis on the research methods scientists have used in uncovering the wonders of nutrition.

1.3 The Science of Nutrition

LEARN IT Explain the scientific method and how scientists use various types of research studies and methods to acquire nutrition information.

The science of nutrition is the study of the nutrients and other substances in foods and the body's handling of them. Its foundation depends on several other sciences, including biology, biochemistry, and physiology. Nutrition is a relatively young science, but much has happened in its short life. And it is currently experiencing a tremendous growth spurt as scientists apply knowledge gained from sequencing the human **genome**. The integration of nutrition, genomics, and molecular biology has opened a whole new world of study called **nutritional genomics**—the science of how nutrients affect the activities of genes and how genes affect the interactions between diet and disease. Highlight 6 describes how nutritional genomics is shaping the science of nutrition, and examples of nutrient–gene interactions appear throughout later chapters.

Conducting Research Consumers sometimes depend on personal experience or social media to gather information on nutrition. Such a personal account of an experience or event is known as an **anecdote** and is not accepted as reliable scientific information (see Glossary 1-1 for definitions of research terms). In contrast, researchers use the scientific method to guide their work (see Figure 1-3). As the figure shows, research always begins with a problem or a question. For example, "What foods or nutrients might protect against the common cold?" In search of an answer, scientists make an educated guess **(hypothesis)**, such as "foods rich in vitamin C reduce the number of common colds." Then they systematically conduct research studies to collect data that will test the hypothesis. Some examples of various types of research designs are presented in Figure 1-4 (p. 14). Because each type of study has strengths and weaknesses, some provide stronger evidence than others, as Figure 1-4 explains.

In attempting to discover whether a nutrient relieves symptoms or cures a disease, researchers deliberately manipulate one variable (for example, the amount of vitamin C in the diet) and measure any observed changes (perhaps the number of colds). As much as possible, all other conditions are held constant.

Controls In studies examining the effectiveness of vitamin C, researchers typically divide the **subjects** into two groups. One group (the **experimental group**) receives a vitamin C supplement, and the other (the **control group**) does not. Researchers observe both groups to determine whether one group has fewer, milder, or shorter colds than the other.

In sorting subjects into two groups, researchers must ensure that each person has an equal chance of being assigned to either the experimental group or the control group. This is accomplished by **randomization**; that is, the subjects are chosen randomly from the same population by flipping a coin or some other method involving chance. Randomization helps to eliminate bias and ensure that the two groups are "equal" and that observed differences reflect the treatment and not other factors.[16]

Importantly, the two groups of subjects must be similar and must have the same track record with respect to colds to rule out the possibility that observed differences in the rate, severity, or duration of colds might have occurred anyway. If, for example, the control group would normally catch twice as many colds as the experimental group, then the findings prove nothing.

In experiments involving a nutrient, the diets of both groups must also be similar, especially with respect to the nutrient being studied. If those in the

genome (GEE-nome): the complete set of genetic material (DNA) in an organism or a cell. The study of genomes is called *genomics*.

nutritional genomics: the science of how nutrients affect the activities of genes (*nutrigenomics*) and how genes affect the activities of nutrients (*nutrigenetics*).

> FIGURE 1-3 The Scientific Method

Research scientists follow the scientific method. Note that most research generates new questions, not final answers. Thus, the sequence begins anew, and research continues in a somewhat cyclical way.

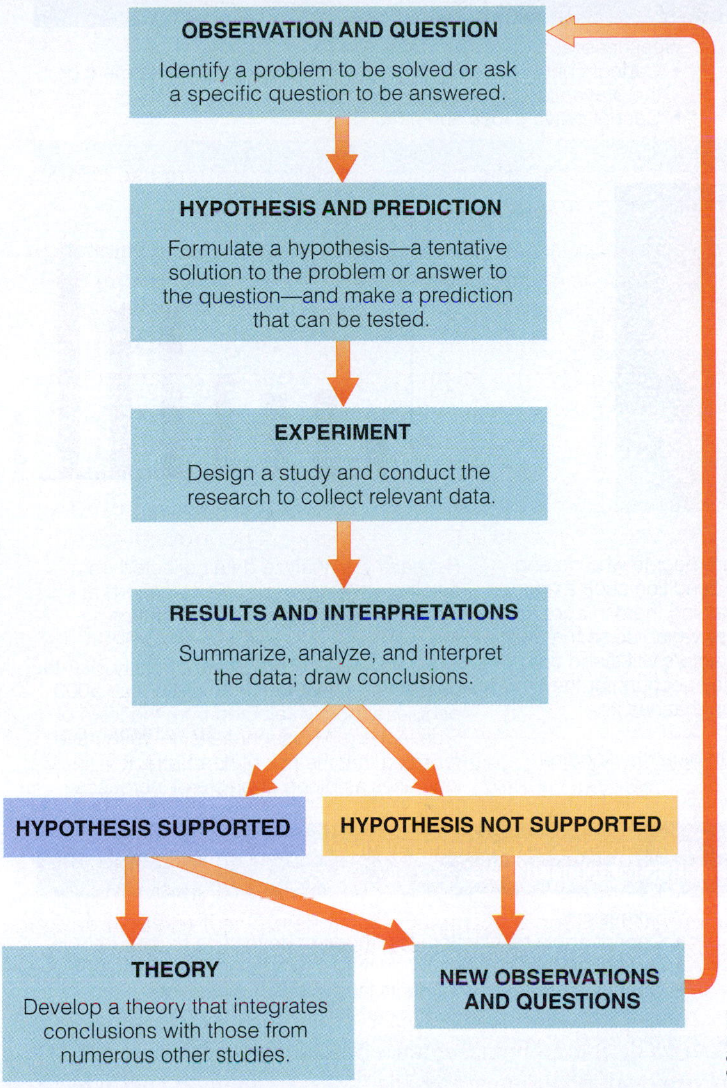

OBSERVATION AND QUESTION
Identify a problem to be solved or ask a specific question to be answered.
HYPOTHESIS AND PREDICTION
Formulate a hypothesis—a tentative solution to the problem or answer to the question—and make a prediction that can be tested.
EXPERIMENT
Design a study and conduct the research to collect relevant data.
RESULTS AND INTERPRETATIONS
Summarize, analyze, and interpret the data; draw conclusions.
HYPOTHESIS SUPPORTED
HYPOTHESIS NOT SUPPORTED
THEORY
Develop a theory that integrates conclusions with those from numerous other studies.
NEW OBSERVATIONS AND QUESTIONS
© Cengage

GLOSSARY 1-1
RESEARCH TERMS

anecdote: a personal account of an experience or event; not reliable scientific information.

blind experiment: an experiment in which the subjects do not know whether they are members of the experimental group or the control group.

control group: a group of individuals similar in all possible respects to the experimental group except for the treatment. Ideally, the control group receives a placebo while the experimental group receives a real treatment.

correlation (CORE-ee-LAY-shun): the simultaneous increase, decrease, or change in two variables. If A increases as B increases, or if A decreases as B decreases, the correlation is *positive.* (This does not mean that A causes B or vice versa.) If A increases as B decreases, or if A decreases as B increases, the correlation is *negative.* (This does not mean that A prevents B or vice versa.) Some third factor may account for both A and B.

double-blind experiment: an experiment in which neither the subjects nor the researchers know which subjects are members of the experimental group and which are serving as control subjects, until after the experiment is over.

experimental group: a group of individuals similar in all possible respects to the control group except for the treatment. The experimental group receives the real treatment.

hypothesis (hi-POTH-eh-sis): an unproven statement that tentatively explains the relationships between two or more variables.

peer review: a process in which a panel of scientists rigorously evaluates a research study to ensure that the scientific method was followed.

placebo (pla-SEE-bo): an inert, harmless medication given to provide comfort and hope; a sham treatment used in controlled research studies.

placebo effect: a change that occurs in response to expectations about the effectiveness of a treatment that actually has no pharmaceutical effects.

randomization (RAN-dom-ih-ZAY-shun): a process of choosing the members of the experimental and control groups without bias.

replication (REP-lih-KAY-shun): repeating an experiment and getting the same results.

subjects: the people or animals participating in a research project.

theory: a tentative explanation that integrates many diverse findings to further the understanding of a defined topic.

validity (va-LID-ih-tee): having the quality of being founded on fact or evidence.

variables: factors that change. A variable may depend on another variable (for example, a child's height depends on his age), or it may be independent (for example, a child's height does not depend on the color of her eyes). Sometimes both variables correlate with a third variable (a child's height and eye color both depend on genetics).

> FIGURE 1-4 Examples of Research Designs

EPIDEMIOLOGICAL STUDIES research the incidence, distribution, and control of diseases in a population. Epidemiological studies include cross-sectional, case-control, and cohort studies.

Strengths:
- Can narrow down the list of possible causes
- Can raise questions to pursue through other research

Weaknesses:
- Cannot control variables that may influence the development or the prevention of a disease
- Cannot prove cause and effect

CROSS-SECTIONAL STUDIES

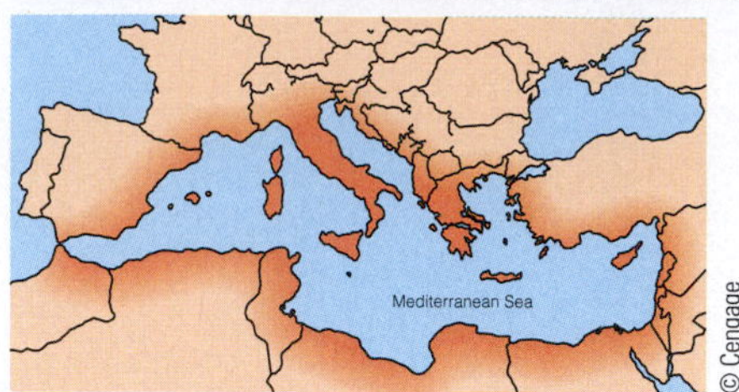
Mediterranean Sea

© Cengage

Researchers observe how much and what kinds of foods a group of people eat and how healthy those people are. Their findings identify factors that might influence the incidence of a disease in various populations.

Example. Many people in the Mediterranean region drink more wine, eat more fat from olive oil, and yet have a lower incidence of heart disease than northern Europeans and North Americans.

CASE-CONTROL STUDIES

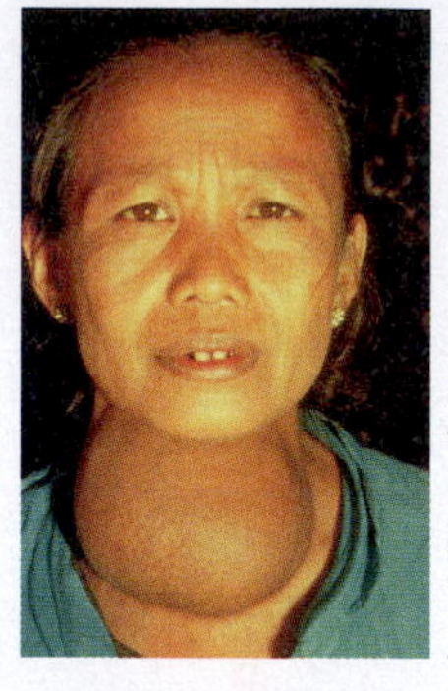

Lester V. Bergman/Getty Images

Researchers compare people who do and do not have a given condition such as a disease, closely matching them in age, gender, and other key variables so that differences in other factors will stand out. These differences may account for the condition in the group that has it.

Example. People with goiter lack iodine in their diets.

COHORT STUDIES

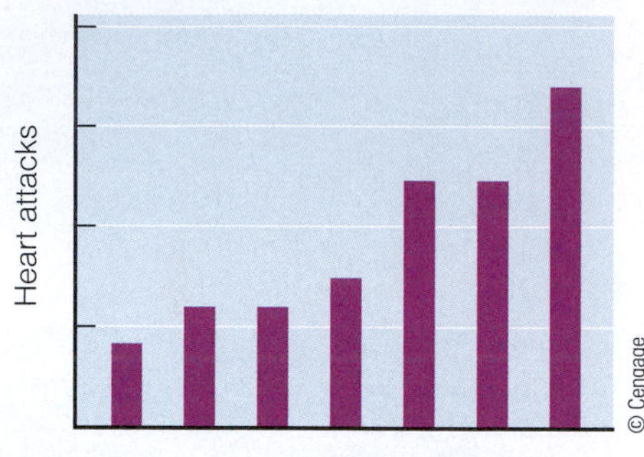
Heart attacks
Blood cholesterol

© Cengage

Researchers analyze data collected from a selected group of people (a cohort) at intervals over a certain period of time.

Example. Data collected periodically over the past several decades from more than 5000 people randomly selected from the town of Framingham, Massachusetts, in 1948 have revealed that the risk of heart attack increases as blood cholesterol increases.

EXPERIMENTAL STUDIES test cause-and-effect relationships between variables. Experimental studies include laboratory-based studies—on animals or in test tubes (in vitro)—and human intervention (or clinical) trials.

Strengths:
- Can control conditions (for the most part)
- Can determine effects of a variable
- Can apply some findings on human beings to some groups of human beings

Weaknesses:
- Cannot apply results from test tubes or animals to human beings
- Cannot generalize findings on human beings to all human beings
- Cannot use certain treatments for clinical or ethical reasons

LABORATORY-BASED ANIMAL STUDIES

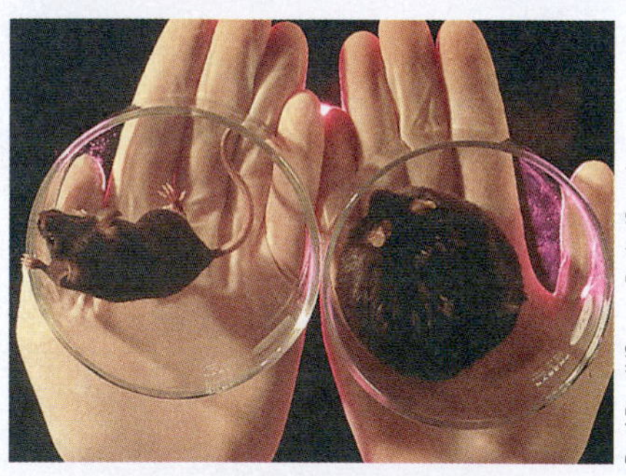

Remi Benali/Gamma-Rapho/Getty Images

Researchers feed animals special diets that provide or omit specific nutrients and then observe any changes in health. Such studies test possible disease causes and treatments in a laboratory where conditions can be controlled.

Example. Mice fed a high-fat diet eat less food than mice given a lower-fat diet, so they receive the same number of kcalories—but the mice eating the high-fat diet become obese.

LABORATORY-BASED IN VITRO STUDIES

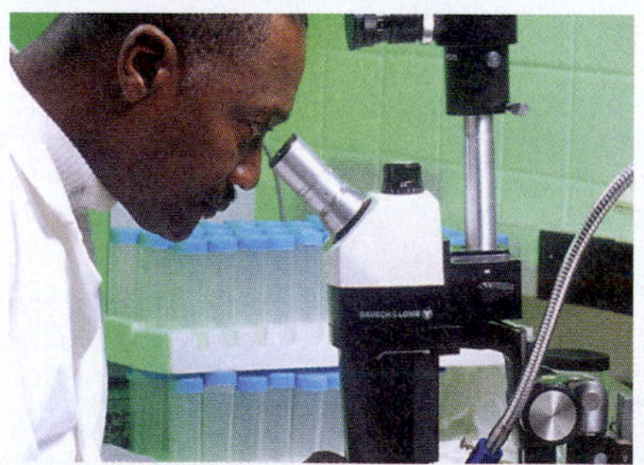

USDA Agricultural Research Service

Researchers examine the effects of a specific variable on a tissue, cell, or molecule isolated from a living organism.

Example. Laboratory studies find that fish oils inhibit the growth and activity of the bacteria implicated in ulcer formation.

HUMAN INTERVENTION (OR CLINICAL) TRIALS

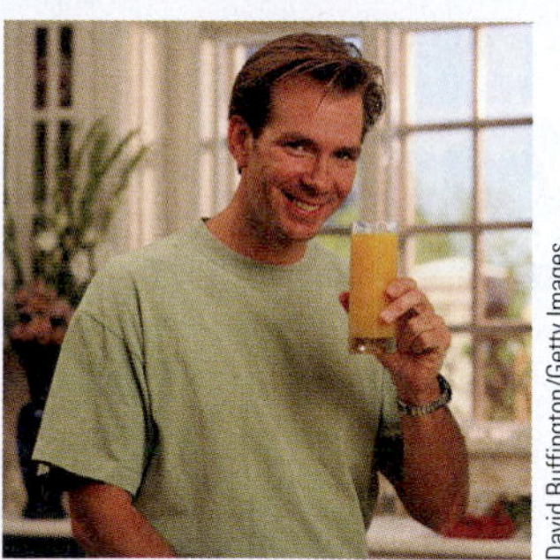

David Buffington/Getty Images

Researchers ask people to adopt a new behavior (for example, eat a citrus fruit, take a vitamin C supplement, or exercise daily). These trials help determine the effectiveness of such interventions on the development or prevention of disease.

Example. Heart disease risk factors improve when men drink fresh-squeezed orange juice daily for 2 months compared with those on a diet low in vitamin C—even when both groups follow a diet high in saturated fat.

experimental group are receiving less vitamin C from their usual diet, then any effects of the supplement may not be apparent.

Sample Size To ensure that chance variation between the two groups does not influence the results, the groups must be large. For example, if one member of a group of five catches a bad cold, he will pull the whole group's average toward bad colds; but if one member of a group of 500 catches a bad cold, she will not unduly affect the group average. Statistical methods are used to determine whether differences between groups of various sizes support a hypothesis.

Placebos If people who take vitamin C for colds *believe* it will cure them, their chances of recovery may improve. Taking pills believed to be beneficial may shorten the duration and lessen the severity of illness regardless of whether the pills contain active ingredients. This phenomenon, the result of expectations, is known as the **placebo effect.** In experiments designed to determine vitamin C's effect on colds, this mind-body effect must be rigorously controlled. Severity of symptoms is often a subjective measure, and people who believe they are receiving treatment may report less severe symptoms.

One way experimenters control for the placebo effect is to give pills to all participants. Those in the experimental group, for example, receive pills containing vitamin C, and those in the control group receive a **placebo**—pills of similar appearance and taste containing an inactive ingredient. This way, the expectations of the two groups will be equal. It is not necessary to convince all subjects that they are receiving vitamin C, but the extent of belief or nonbelief must be the same in both groups. A study conducted under these conditions is called a **blind experiment**—that is, the subjects do not know (are blind to) whether they are members of the experimental group (receiving treatment) or the control group (receiving the placebo).

Double Blind When both the subjects and the researchers do not know which subjects are in which group, the study is called a **double-blind experiment.** Being fallible human beings and having an emotional and sometimes financial investment in a successful outcome, researchers might record and interpret results with a bias in the expected direction. To prevent such bias, the pills are coded by a third party, who does not reveal to the experimenters which subjects are in which group until all results have been recorded.

Analyzing Research Findings

Research findings must be analyzed and interpreted with an awareness of each study's limitations. Scientists must be cautious about drawing any conclusions until they have accumulated a body of evidence from multiple studies that have used various types of research designs. As evidence accumulates, scientists begin to develop a **theory** that integrates the various findings and explains the complex relationships.

Correlations and Causes Researchers often examine the relationships between two or more **variables**—for example, daily vitamin C intake and the number of colds or the duration and severity of cold symptoms. Importantly, researchers must be able to observe, measure, or verify the variables selected. Findings sometimes suggest no **correlation** between variables (regardless of the amount of vitamin C consumed, the number of colds remains the same). Other times, studies find either a **positive correlation** (the more vitamin C, the more colds) or a **negative correlation** (the more vitamin C, the fewer colds). Notice that in a positive correlation, both variables change in the same direction, regardless of whether the direction is "more" or "less"—"the more vitamin C, the more colds" is a positive correlation, just as is "the less vitamin C, the fewer colds." In a negative correlation, the two variables change in opposite directions: "the less vitamin C, the more colds" or "the more vitamin C, the fewer colds." Also notice that a positive correlation does not necessarily reflect a desired outcome, nor does a negative correlation always reflect an undesirable outcome.

Correlational evidence proves only that variables are associated, not that one is the cause of the other. To actually prove that A causes B, scientists have to find evidence of the *mechanism*—that is, an explanation of how A might cause B.

Cautious Conclusions When researchers record and analyze the results of their experiments, they must exercise caution in their interpretation of the findings. For example, in an epidemiological study, scientists may use a specific segment of the population—say, men 18 to 30 years old. When the scientists draw conclusions, they are careful not to generalize the findings to older men or women of any age. Similarly, animals may provide a suitable model for some human studies but scientists must be cautious in applying animal findings to human beings.[17] Conclusions from any one research study are always tentative and take into account findings from studies conducted by other scientists as well. As evidence accumulates, scientists gain confidence about drawing conclusions and making recommendations. Even then, their statements are worded cautiously, such as "A diet high in fruits and vegetables *may* protect against *some* cancers."

Publishing Research The findings from a research study are submitted to a board of reviewers composed of other scientists who rigorously evaluate the study to ensure that the scientific method was followed—a process known as **peer review.** The reviewers critique the study's hypothesis, methodology, statistical significance, and conclusions. They also note the funding source, recognizing that financial support and other conflicts of interest may bias scientific conclusions.[18] If the reviewers consider the conclusions to be well supported by the evidence—that is, if the research has **validity**—they endorse the work for publication in a scientific journal where others can read it. This raises an important point regarding information found on the Internet: much gets published without the rigorous scrutiny of peer review. Consequently, readers must assume greater responsibility for examining the data and conclusions presented. Highlight 1 offers guidance in determining whether Internet information is reliable. Table 1-3 describes the parts of a typical research article.

Even when a new finding is published or released to the media, it is still only preliminary and not very meaningful by itself. Other scientists will need to confirm or disprove the findings through **replication** and reanalysis.[19] To be accepted into the body of nutrition knowledge, findings must stand up to rigorous, repeated testing in experiments conducted by other researchers. What we "know" in nutrition results from years of research findings. Communicating the latest finding in its proper context without distorting or oversimplifying the message is a challenge for scientists and journalists alike.[20] For a helpful scientific overview of topics in nutrition, look for review articles in scholarly journals such as *Nutrition Reviews.* Reviews may be either a **systematic review**, which provides a qualitative summary of the evidence or a **meta-analysis**, which provides a quantitative summary.[21]

With each report from scientists, the field of nutrition changes a little—each finding contributes another piece to the whole body of knowledge (see Photo 1-5). People who know how science works understand that single findings, like single

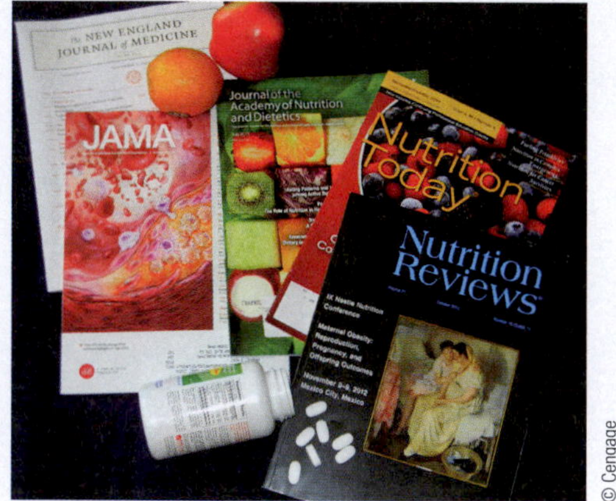
THE NEW ENGLAND JOURNAL of MEDICINE
JAMA
Journal of the Academy of Nutrition and Dietetics
Nutrition Today
Nutrition Reviews
© Cengage

> PHOTO 1-5 Knowledge about the nutrients and their effects on health comes from scientific studies.

TABLE 1-3 Parts of a Typical Research Article

- *Abstract:* The abstract provides a brief overview of the article.
- *Introduction:* The introduction clearly states the purpose of the current study and provides a comprehensive review of the relevant literature.
- *Methodology:* The methodology section defines key terms and describes the study design, subjects, and procedures used in conducting the study.
- *Results:* The results report the findings and may include tables and figures that summarize the information.
- *Discussion*: The discussion draws tentative conclusions that are supported by the data and reflect the original purpose as stated in the introduction. Usually, it answers a few questions and raises several more.
- *References*: The references reflect the investigator's knowledge of the subject and should include an extensive list of relevant studies.

© Cengage

systematic review: a critical and integrative summary of evidence gathered from multiple selected studies to answer a specific question and develop a *qualitative* review.

meta-analysis: an objective and statistical summary of evidence gathered from multiple selected studies to develop a *quantitative* review; often derived from a systematic review.

frames in a movie, are just small parts of a larger story. Over years, nutrition knowledge gradually changes, and dietary recommendations change to reflect the current understanding of scientific research. Highlight 5 provides a detailed look at how dietary fat recommendations have evolved over the past several decades as researchers have uncovered the relationships between the various kinds of fat and their roles in supporting or harming health.

REVIEW IT Explain the scientific method and how scientists use various types of research studies and methods to acquire nutrition information.

Scientists learn about nutrition by conducting experiments that follow the protocol of scientific research. In designing their studies, researchers randomly assign control and experimental groups, seek large sample sizes, provide placebos, and remain blind to treatments. Their findings must be reviewed and replicated by other scientists before being accepted as valid.

The characteristics of well-designed research have enabled scientists to study the actions of nutrients in the body. Such research has laid the foundation for quantifying how much of each nutrient the body needs.

1.4 Dietary Reference Intakes

LEARN IT Define the four categories of the DRI and explain their purposes.

Using the results of thousands of research studies, nutrition experts have produced a set of standards that define the amounts of energy, nutrients, and other dietary components that best support health. These recommendations are called **Dietary Reference Intakes (DRI)**, and they reflect the collaborative efforts of researchers in both the United States and Canada.* The insert of this book provides a handy reference for DRI values.

Establishing Nutrient Recommendations

The DRI Committee consists of highly qualified scientists who base their estimates of nutrient needs on careful examination and interpretation of scientific evidence. These recommendations apply to healthy people and may not be appropriate for people with diseases that increase or decrease nutrient needs. The next several paragraphs introduce the four categories of the DRI, explain their purposes, and discuss specific aspects of how the committee goes about establishing these values:

- Estimated Average Requirements (EAR)
- Recommended Dietary Allowances (RDA)
- Adequate Intakes (AI)
- Tolerable Upper Intake Levels (UL)

Estimated Average Requirements (EAR) The committee reviews hundreds of research studies to determine the **requirement** for a nutrient—how much is needed in the diet. The committee selects a specific criterion for each nutrient based on its roles in supporting various activities in the body and in reducing disease risks.

An examination of all the available data reveals that each person's body is unique and has its own set of requirements. Men differ from women, and needs change as people grow from infancy through old age. For this reason, the committee clusters its recommendations for people into groups based on gender and age. Even so, the exact requirements for people of the same gender and age are likely to be different. Person A might need 40 units of a particular nutrient each day; person B might need 35; and person C might need 57. Looking at enough people might reveal that their individual requirements fall into a symmetrical distribution, with most near the midpoint and only a few at the extremes (see the left side of Figure 1-5, p. 18). Using this information, the committee determines an **Estimated Average Requirement (EAR)**

*The DRI reports are produced by the Food and Nutrition Board, Institute of Medicine of the National Academies, with active involvement of scientists from the United States and Canada.

Dietary Reference Intakes (DRI): a set of nutrient intake values for healthy people in the United States and Canada. These values are used for planning and assessing diets and include:

- Estimated Average Requirements (EAR)
- Recommended Dietary Allowances (RDA)
- Adequate Intakes (AI)
- Tolerable Upper Intake Levels (UL)

requirement: the lowest continuing intake of a nutrient that will maintain a specified criterion of adequacy.

Estimated Average Requirement (EAR): the average daily amount of a nutrient that will maintain a specific biochemical or physiological function in half the healthy people of a given age and gender group.

> **FIGURE 1-5 Estimated Average Requirements (EAR) and Recommended Dietary Allowances (RDA) Compared**

Each square in the graphs below represents a person with unique nutritional requirements. (The text discusses three of these people—A, B, and C.) Some people require only a small amount of nutrient X and some require a lot. Most people, however, fall somewhere in the middle.

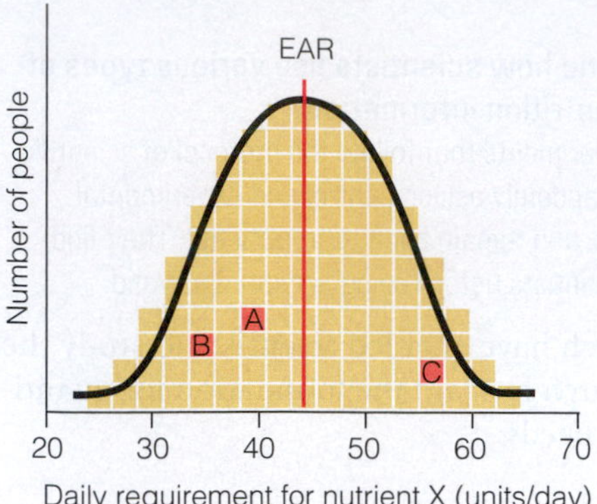

EAR
Number of people
A
B
C
20
30
40
50
60
70
Daily requirement for nutrient X (units/day)

The Estimated Average Requirement (EAR) for a nutrient is the amount that meets the needs of about half of the population (shown here by the red line).

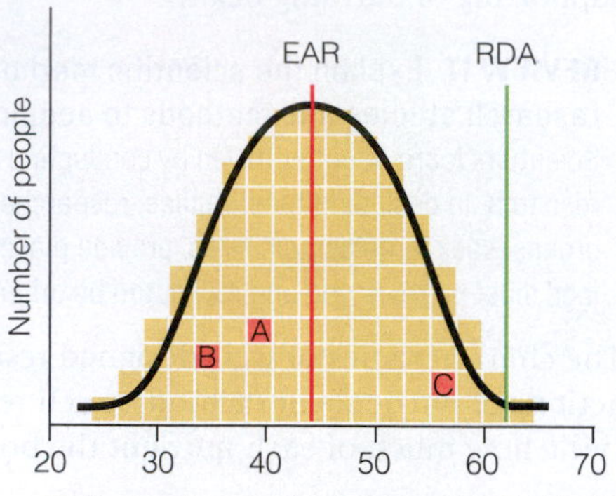

EAR
RDA
Number of people
A
B
C
20
30
40
50
60
70
Daily requirement for nutrient X (units/day)

The Recommended Dietary Allowance (RDA) for a nutrient (shown here in green) is set well above the EAR, meeting the needs of about 98% of the population.

for each nutrient—the average amount that appears sufficient for half of the population. In Figure 1-5, the EAR is shown as 45 units.

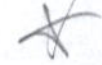

Recommended Dietary Allowances (RDA) Once a nutrient *requirement* is established, the committee must decide what intake to *recommend* for everybody—the **Recommended Dietary Allowance (RDA).** As you can see by the distribution in Figure 1-5, the EAR (shown in the figure as 45 units) is probably closest to everyone's need. If people consumed exactly the average requirement of a given nutrient each day, however, approximately half of the population would develop deficiencies of that nutrient—in Figure 1-5, for example, person C would be among them. Recommendations are therefore set greater than the EAR to meet the needs of most healthy people.

Small amounts greater than the daily requirement do no harm, whereas amounts less than the requirement may lead to health problems. When people's nutrient intakes are consistently **deficient** (less than the requirement), their nutrient stores decline, and over time this decline leads to poor health and deficiency symptoms. Therefore, to ensure that the nutrient RDA meet the needs of as many people as possible, the RDA are set near the top end of the range of the population's estimated requirements.

In this example, a reasonable RDA might be 63 units a day (see the right side of Figure 1-5). Such a point can be calculated mathematically so that the needs of about 98 percent of a population are included. Almost everybody—including person C, whose needs were more substantial than the average—would consume enough of the nutrient if they met this dietary goal. Relatively few people's requirements would exceed this recommendation, and even then, they wouldn't exceed it by much. Notice that Figure 1-5 illustrates how the EAR meets the needs of about half of the population, whereas the RDA meets the needs of about 98 percent of the population.

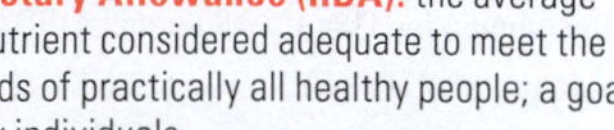

Adequate Intakes (AI) For some nutrients, such as vitamin K, there is insufficient scientific evidence to determine an EAR (which is needed to set an RDA). In these cases, the committee establishes an **Adequate Intake (AI)** instead of an RDA. An AI reflects the average amount of a nutrient that a group of healthy people consumes. Like the RDA, the AI may be used as a nutrient intake goal for individuals.

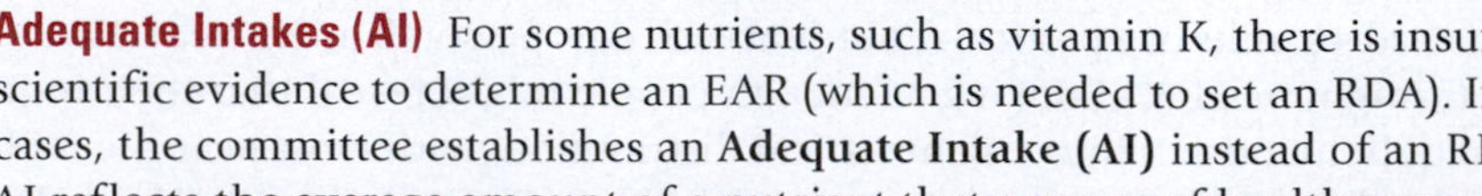

Although both the RDA and the AI serve as nutrient intake goals for individuals, their differences are noteworthy. An RDA for a given nutrient is based on enough scientific evidence to expect that the needs of almost all healthy people

Recommended Dietary Allowance (RDA): the average daily amount of a nutrient considered adequate to meet the known nutrient needs of practically all healthy people; a goal for dietary intake by individuals.

deficient: inadequate; a nutrient amount that fails to meet the body's needs and eventually results in deficiency symptoms.

Adequate Intake (AI): the average daily amount of a nutrient that appears sufficient to maintain a specified criterion; a value used as a guide for nutrient intake when an RDA cannot be determined.

> FIGURE 1-6 Inaccurate versus Accurate View of Nutrient Intakes

The RDA (or AI) for a given nutrient represents a point that lies within a range of appropriate and reasonable intakes between toxicity and deficiency. Both of these recommendations are high enough to provide reserves in times of short-term dietary inadequacies, but not so high as to approach toxicity. Nutrient intakes above or below this range may be equally harmful.

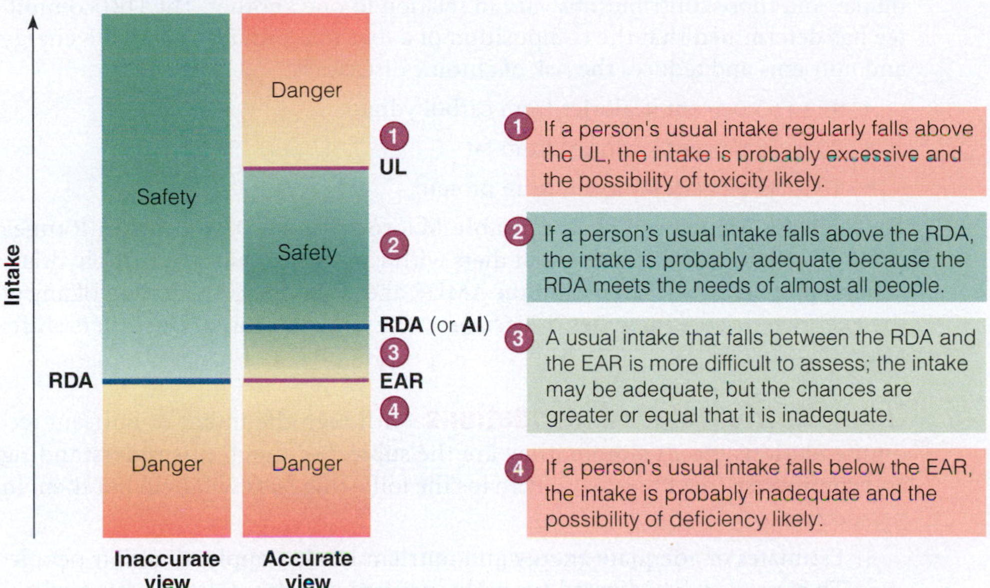

Intake
Safety
RDA
Danger
Danger
Safety
Danger
1
UL
2
RDA (or AI)
3
EAR
4
Inaccurate view
Accurate view
1 If a person's usual intake regularly falls above the UL, the intake is probably excessive and the possibility of toxicity likely.
2 If a person's usual intake falls above the RDA, the intake is probably adequate because the RDA meets the needs of almost all people.
3 A usual intake that falls between the RDA and the EAR is more difficult to assess; the intake may be adequate, but the chances are greater or equal that it is inadequate.
4 If a person's usual intake falls below the EAR, the intake is probably inadequate and the possibility of deficiency likely.

will be met. An AI, on the other hand, must rely more heavily on scientific judgments because sufficient evidence is lacking. For this reason, AI values are more tentative than RDA values. The insert (p. A) identifies which nutrients have an RDA and which have an AI. Later chapters present the RDA and AI values for vitamins and minerals.

Tolerable Upper Intake Levels (UL) As mentioned earlier, the recommended intakes for nutrients are generous, yet they may not be sufficient for every individual for every nutrient. Nevertheless, it is probably best not to exceed these recommendations by very much or very often. Individual tolerances for high doses of nutrients vary, and somewhere greater than the recommended intake is a point beyond which a nutrient is likely to become toxic. This point is known as the **Tolerable Upper Intake Level (UL).** It is naïve—and inaccurate—to think of recommendations as minimum amounts. A more accurate view is to see a person's nutrient needs as falling within a range, with marginal and danger zones at each end for intakes that are either inadequate or excessive (see Figure 1-6).

Paying attention to the UL is particularly useful in guarding against the overconsumption of nutrients, which may occur when people use large-dose dietary supplements and fortified foods regularly. Later chapters discuss the dangers associated with excessively high intakes of vitamins and minerals, and the insert (p. C) presents tables of the UL for selected nutrients.

Establishing Energy Recommendations

In contrast to the RDA and AI values for nutrients, the recommendation for energy is not generous. Excess energy cannot be readily excreted and is eventually stored as body fat. These reserves may be beneficial when food is scarce, but they can also lead to obesity and its associated health consequences.

Estimated Energy Requirement (EER) The energy recommendation—called the **Estimated Energy Requirement (EER)**—represents the average dietary energy intake (kcalories per day) that will maintain energy balance in a person who has a healthy body weight and level of physical activity. Balance is key to the energy recommendation. Enough food energy is needed to sustain a healthy and active life.

Tolerable Upper Intake Level (UL): the maximum daily amount of a nutrient that appears safe for most healthy people and beyond which there is an increased risk of adverse health effects.

Estimated Energy Requirement (EER): the average dietary energy intake that maintains energy balance and good health in a person of a given age, gender, weight, height, and level of physical activity.

Because *any* amount in excess of energy needs will result in weight gain, no UL for energy has been determined.

Acceptable Macronutrient Distribution Ranges (AMDR) People don't eat energy directly; they derive energy from foods containing carbohydrates, fats, and proteins. Each of these three energy-yielding nutrients contributes to the total energy intake, and those contributions vary in relation to one another. The DRI committee has determined that the composition of a diet that provides adequate energy and nutrients and reduces the risk of chronic diseases is:

- 45 to 65 percent kcalories from carbohydrate
- 20 to 35 percent kcalories from fat
- 10 to 35 percent kcalories from protein

These values are known as **Acceptable Macronutrient Distribution Ranges (AMDR).** Figure 1-7 illustrates that diets with varying amounts of carbohydrate, fat, and protein can all fall within the AMDR and when the contribution of any of the energy nutrients increases or decreases, the contribution of the others shifts as well.

Using Nutrient Recommendations

Although the intent of nutrient recommendations seems simple, they are the subject of much misunderstanding and controversy (see Photo 1-6). Perhaps the following facts will help put them in perspective:

1. Estimates of adequate energy and nutrient intakes apply to *healthy* people. They need to be adjusted for malnourished people or those with medical problems who may require supplemented or restricted dietary intakes.
2. *Recommendations* are not minimum requirements, nor are they necessarily optimal intakes for all individuals. Recommendations target most of the people and cannot account for individual variations in nutrient needs.
3. Most nutrient goals are intended to be met through diets composed of a variety of *foods* whenever possible. Excess intakes of vitamins and minerals are unlikely when they come from foods. Using dietary supplements to meet nutrient goals raises the risks of toxicity.

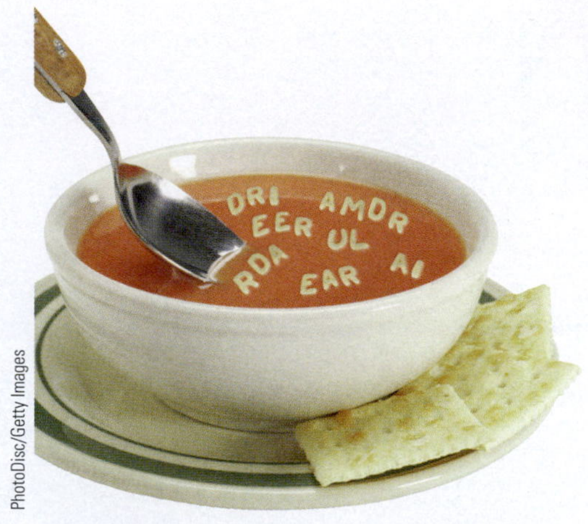
DRI
AMDR
EER
UL
RDA
AI
EAR
PhotoDisc/Getty Images

> **PHOTO 1-6** The DRI "alphabet soup" of nutrient intake standards makes sense when you learn their purposes.

> **FIGURE 1-7 Energy Nutrient Contributions to the Total**

The three energy nutrients—carbohydrate, fat, and protein—all contribute to the total energy (kcalorie) intake. Each of these three bars illustrates percentages that fall within the Acceptable Macronutrient Distribution Ranges (AMDR). Notice that whenever the percentage of any one of them increases or decreases, the percentages from the others change as well.

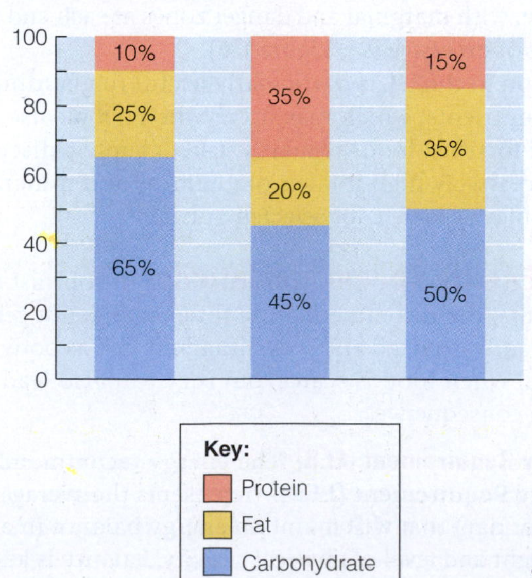
100
80
60
40
20
0
10%
25%
65%
35%
20%
45%
15%
35%
50%
Key:
Protein
Fat
Carbohydrate
© Cengage

Acceptable Macronutrient Distribution Ranges (AMDR): ranges of intakes for the energy nutrients that provide adequate energy and nutrients and reduce the risk of chronic diseases.

4. Recommendations apply to *average* daily intakes. Trying to meet the recommendations for every nutrient every day is difficult and unnecessary. The length of time over which a person's intake can deviate from the average without risk of deficiency or toxicity varies for each nutrient, depending on how the body uses and stores the nutrient. For most nutrients (such as thiamin and vitamin C), deprivation would lead to rapid development of deficiency symptoms (within days or weeks); for others (such as vitamin A and vitamin B_{12}), deficiencies would develop more slowly (over months or years).
5. Each of the DRI categories serves a unique purpose. For example, the EAR are most appropriately used to develop and evaluate nutrition programs for *groups* such as schoolchildren or military personnel. The RDA (or AI if an RDA is not available) can be used to set goals for *individuals*. The UL serve as a reminder to keep nutrient intakes less than amounts that increase the risk of toxicity—not a common problem when nutrients derive from foods, but a real possibility for some nutrients if supplements are used regularly.

With these understandings, professionals can use the DRI for a variety of purposes.[22]

Comparing Nutrient Recommendations More than 80 nations have published nutrient standards similar to those used in the United States. Slight differences may be apparent, reflecting differences both in the interpretation of the data from which the standards were derived and in the food habits and physical activities of the populations they serve.

Many countries use the recommendations developed by two international groups: FAO (Food and Agriculture Organization) and WHO (World Health Organization). The FAO/WHO nutrient recommendations are considered sufficient to maintain health in nearly all healthy people worldwide and are provided in Appendix I.

REVIEW IT Define the four categories of the DRI and explain their purposes.

The Dietary Reference Intakes (DRI) are a set of nutrient intake values that can be used to plan and evaluate diets for healthy people. The Estimated Average Requirement (EAR) defines the amount of a nutrient that supports a specific function in the body for half of the population. The Recommended Dietary Allowance (RDA) is based on the Estimated Average Requirement and establishes a goal for dietary intake that will meet the needs of about 98 percent of the population. An Adequate Intake (AI) serves a similar purpose when an RDA cannot be determined. The Estimated Energy Requirement (EER) defines the average amount of energy intake needed to maintain energy balance, and the Acceptable Macronutrient Distribution Ranges (AMDR) define the proportions contributed by carbohydrate, fat, and protein to a healthy diet. The Tolerable Upper Intake Level (UL) establishes the highest amount that appears safe for regular consumption.

1.5 Nutrition Assessment

LEARN IT Explain how the four assessment methods are used to detect energy and nutrient deficiencies and excesses.

What happens when a person doesn't consume enough or consumes too much of a specific nutrient or energy? If the deficiency or excess is significant over time, the person experiences symptoms of **malnutrition**. With a deficiency of energy, the person may display the symptoms of **undernutrition** by becoming extremely thin, losing muscle tissue, and becoming prone to infection and disease. With a deficiency of a nutrient, the person may experience skin rashes, depression, hair loss, bleeding gums, muscle spasms, night blindness, or other symptoms. Similarly, over time, regular intakes in excess of needs may also have adverse effects. With an excess of energy, the person may become obese and vulnerable to diseases associated with **overnutrition**, such as heart disease and diabetes. With a sudden nutrient overdose, the person may experience hot flashes, yellowing skin, a rapid heart rate, low blood pressure, or other symptoms.

Malnutrition symptoms—such as diarrhea, skin rashes, and fatigue—are easy to miss because they resemble the symptoms of other diseases. But a person who

malnutrition: any condition caused by excess or deficient food energy or nutrient intake or by an imbalance of nutrients.
- **mal** = bad

undernutrition: deficient energy or nutrients.

overnutrition: excess energy or nutrients.

has learned how to use assessment techniques to detect malnutrition can identify when these conditions are caused by poor nutrition and can recommend steps to correct it. This discussion presents the basics of nutrition assessment; many more details are offered in later chapters and in Appendix E.

Nutrition Assessment of Individuals

To prepare a **nutrition assessment,** a trained health-care professional uses:

- Historical information
- Anthropometric measurements
- Physical examinations
- Laboratory tests

Each of these methods involves collecting data in various ways and interpreting each finding in relation to the others to create a total picture.[23]

Historical Information

One step in evaluating nutrition status is to obtain information about a person's history with respect to health status, socioeconomic status, drug use, and diet. The **health history** reflects a person's medical record and may reveal a disease that interferes with the person's ability to eat or the body's use of nutrients. The person's family history of major diseases is also noteworthy, especially for conditions such as heart disease that have a genetic tendency to run in families. Economic circumstances may show a financial inability to buy foods or inadequate kitchen facilities in which to prepare them. Social factors such as marital status, ethnic background, and educational level also influence food choices and nutrition status. A **drug history**, including all prescribed and over-the-counter medications, may highlight possible interactions that lead to nutrient deficiencies (as described in Highlight 17). A **diet history** that examines a person's intake of foods, beverages, and dietary supplements may reveal either excess or inadequate intakes of nutrients or energy.

To take a diet history, the assessor collects data about the foods a person eats. The data may be collected by recording the foods the person has eaten over a period of 24 hours, 3 days, or a week or more or by asking what foods the person typically eats and how much of each. The days in the record must be fairly typical of the person's diet, and portion sizes must be recorded accurately. To determine the amounts of nutrients consumed, the assessor usually enters the foods and their portion sizes into a computer using a diet analysis program. The assessor then compares the calculated nutrient intakes with the DRI to determine the probability of adequacy. Alternatively, the diet history might be compared against standards such as the USDA Food Patterns or *Dietary Guidelines for Americans* (described in Chapter 2).

An estimate of energy and nutrient intakes from a diet history, when combined with information from other assessment results, can help confirm or rule out the *possibility* of suspected nutrition problems. A sufficient intake of a nutrient does not guarantee adequacy, and an insufficient intake does not always indicate a deficiency. Such findings, however, warn of possible problems.

Anthropometric Measurements

A second technique that may help reveal nutrition problems is taking **anthropometric** measures such as height and weight. The assessor compares a person's measurements with standards specific for gender and age or with previous measures on the same individual. (Chapter 8 presents information on body weight and its standards; Chapter 16 and Appendix E include growth charts for children.)

Measurements taken periodically and compared with previous measurements reveal patterns and indicate trends in a person's overall nutrition status, but they provide little information about specific nutrients. Instead, measurements out of line with expectations may reveal such problems as growth failure in children, wasting or swelling of body tissues in adults, and obesity—conditions that may reflect energy or nutrient deficiencies or excesses.

nutrition assessment: a comprehensive analysis of a person's nutrition status that uses health, socioeconomic, drug, and diet histories; anthropometric measurements; physical examinations; and laboratory tests.

health history: an account of a client's current and past health status and disease risks.

drug history: a record of all the drugs, over-the-counter and prescribed, that a person takes routinely.

diet history: a record of eating behaviors and the foods a person eats.

anthropometric (AN-throw-poe-MET-rick): relating to measurement of the physical characteristics of the body, such as height and weight.

- **anthropos** = human
- **metric** = measuring

Physical Examinations A third nutrition assessment technique is a physical examination looking for clues to poor nutrition status. Visual inspection of the hair, eyes, skin, posture, tongue, and fingernails can provide such clues (see Photo 1-7). In addition, information gathered from an interview can help identify physical symptoms. The examination requires skill because many physical signs and symptoms reflect more than one nutrient deficiency or toxicity—or even nonnutrition conditions. Like the other assessment techniques, a physical examination alone does not yield firm conclusions. Instead, physical examinations reveal possible imbalances that must be confirmed by other assessment techniques, or they confirm results from other assessment measures.

Laboratory Tests A fourth way to detect a developing deficiency, imbalance, or toxicity is to take samples of blood or urine, analyze them in the laboratory, and compare the results with normal values for a similar population. Laboratory tests are most useful in uncovering early signs of malnutrition before symptoms appear. In addition, they can confirm suspicions raised by other assessment methods.

Iron, for Example The mineral iron can be used to illustrate the stages in the development of a nutrient deficiency and the assessment techniques useful in detecting them. The **overt**, or outward, signs of an iron deficiency appear at the end of a long sequence of events. Figure 1-8 describes what happens in the body as a nutrient deficiency progresses and shows which assessment methods can reveal those changes.

First, the body has too little iron—either because iron is lacking in the person's diet (a **primary deficiency**) or because the person's body doesn't absorb enough, excretes too much, or uses iron inefficiently (a **secondary deficiency**). A diet history provides clues to primary deficiencies; a health history provides clues to secondary deficiencies.

Next, the body begins to use up its stores of iron. At this stage, the deficiency might be described as a **subclinical deficiency.** It exists as a **covert** condition, and although it might be detected by laboratory tests, outward signs are not yet apparent.

Finally, the body's iron stores are exhausted. Now, it cannot make enough iron-containing red blood cells to replace those that are aging and dying. Iron is needed in red blood cells to carry oxygen to all the body's tissues. When iron is lacking, fewer red blood cells are made, the new ones are pale and small, and every part of the body feels the effects of oxygen shortage. At this point in time, the overt symptoms of deficiency appear—weakness, fatigue, pallor, and headaches, reflecting the iron-deficient state of the blood. A physical examination and interview will reveal these symptoms.

Nutrition Assessment of Populations

To assess a population's nutrition status, researchers conduct surveys using techniques similar to those used on

> **FIGURE 1-8 Stages in the Development of a Nutrient Deficiency**

Internal changes precede outward signs of deficiencies. Outward signs of sickness, however, need not appear before a person takes corrective measures. Laboratory tests can help determine nutrient status in the early stages.

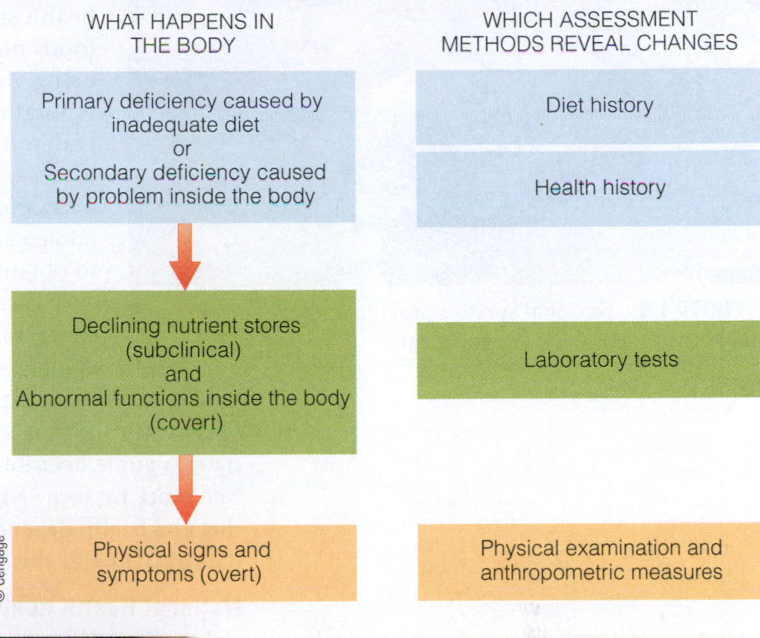
WHAT HAPPENS IN THE BODY
WHICH ASSESSMENT METHODS REVEAL CHANGES
Primary deficiency caused by inadequate diet
or
Secondary deficiency caused by problem inside the body
Diet history
Health history
Declining nutrient stores (subclinical)
and
Abnormal functions inside the body (covert)
Laboratory tests
Physical signs and symptoms (overt)
Physical examination and anthropometric measures
© Cengage

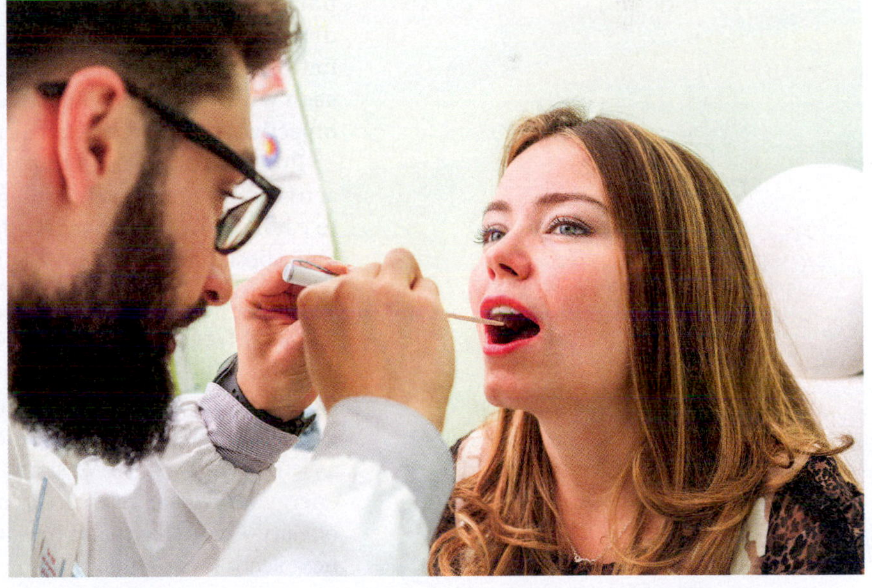
massimofusaro/Shutterstock.com

> **PHOTO 1-7** A peek inside the mouth provides clues to a person's nutrition status. An inflamed tongue may indicate a deficiency of one of the B vitamins, and mottled teeth may reveal fluoride toxicity, for example.

overt (oh-VERT): out in the open and easy to observe.
- **ouvrir** = to open

primary deficiency: a nutrient deficiency caused by inadequate dietary intake of a nutrient.

secondary deficiency: a nutrient deficiency caused by something other than an inadequate intake, such as a disease condition or drug interaction that reduces absorption, accelerates use, hastens excretion, or destroys the nutrient.

subclinical deficiency: a deficiency in the early stages, before the outward signs have appeared.

covert (KOH-vert): hidden, as if under covers.
- **couvrir** = to cover

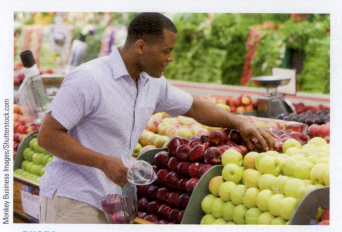
Monkey Business Images/Shutterstock.com

> **PHOTO 1-8** National surveys provide valuable information about the kinds of foods people eat.

individuals. The data collected are then used by various agencies for numerous purposes, including the development of national health goals.

National Nutrition Surveys National nutrition surveys gather information about the population's dietary, nutritional, and related health status. One survey collects data on the kinds and amounts of foods people eat.* Another survey examines the people themselves, using anthropometric measurements, physical examinations, and laboratory tests.** The data provide valuable information on several nutrition-related conditions, such as growth impairments, heart disease, and nutrient deficiencies. National nutrition surveys often oversample high-risk groups (low-income families, pregnant women, adolescents, the elderly, African Americans, and Mexican Americans) to obtain an accurate estimate of their health and nutrition status.

The resulting wealth of information from the national nutrition surveys is used for a variety of purposes (see Photo 1-8). For example, Congress uses this information to establish public policy on nutrition education, food assistance programs, and the regulation of the food supply. Scientists use the information to establish research priorities. The food industry uses these data to guide decisions in public relations and product development. The Dietary Reference Intakes and other major reports that examine the relationships between diet and health depend on information collected from these nutrition surveys. These data also provide the basis for developing and monitoring national health goals.

National Health Goals The **Healthy People** program sets priorities and guides policies that "increase the quality and years of healthy life" and "eliminate health disparities." At the start of each decade, the program sets goals for improving the nation's health during the next ten years. Nutrition is one of many topic areas, each with numerous objectives. Appendix J lists the nutrition and weight status objectives for 2020, as well as nutrition-related objectives from other topic areas.

Progress in meeting the 2020 goals is mixed. The objective to meet physical activity and muscle-strengthening guidelines has been achieved, but the objective to eat more fruits and vegetables showed no improvement.[24] Trends in overweight and obesity actually worsened. Clearly, "what we eat in America" must change if we hope to meet the Healthy People goals.

National Trends What do we eat in America and how has it changed over the past 45 years? The short answer to both questions is "a lot." We eat more meals away from home, particularly at fast-food restaurants. We eat larger portions. We drink more sweetened beverages and eat more energy-dense, nutrient-poor foods such as candy and chips. We snack frequently. As a result of these dietary habits, our energy intake has risen and, consequently, so has the incidence of overweight and obesity. Overweight and obesity, in turn, profoundly influence our health—as the next section explains.

REVIEW IT **Explain how the four assessment methods are used to detect energy and nutrient deficiencies and excesses.**

People become malnourished when they get too little or too much energy or nutrients. Deficiencies, excesses, and imbalances of nutrients lead to malnutrition diseases. To detect malnutrition in individuals, health-care professionals use a combination of four nutrition assessment methods. Reviewing historical information on diet and health may suggest a possible nutrition problem. Laboratory tests may detect a possible nutrition problem in its earliest stages, whereas anthropometric measurements and physical examinations pick up on the problem only after it causes symptoms. National surveys use similar assessment methods to measure people's food consumption and to evaluate the nutrition status of populations.

Healthy People: a national public health initiative under the jurisdiction of the US Department of Health and Human Services (DHHS) that identifies the most significant preventable threats to health and focuses efforts to eliminate them.

*This survey is called *What We Eat in America*.

**This survey is known as the National Health and Nutrition Examination Survey (NHANES).

1.6 Diet and Health

LEARN IT Identify several risk factors and explain their relationships to chronic diseases.

Foods play a vital role in supporting health. Early nutrition research focused on identifying the nutrients in foods that would prevent such common diseases as rickets (the vitamin D–deficiency disease) and scurvy (the vitamin C–deficiency disease). With this knowledge, developed countries have successfully defended against nutrient deficiency diseases. World hunger and nutrient deficiency diseases still pose a major health threat in developing countries, however, but not because of a lack of nutrition knowledge (as Chapter 20 explains). More recently, nutrition research has focused on obesity and chronic diseases associated with energy and nutrient excesses.[25] Chronic diseases are responsible for 7 out of 10 deaths among US adults and account for more than 85 percent of US health care costs.[26] Once thought to be "rich countries' problems," overconsumption of unhealthy foods and chronic diseases have escalated worldwide in recent decades.[27]

Chronic Diseases Table 1-4 lists the ten leading causes of death in the United States. These "causes" are stated as if a single condition such as heart disease caused death, but most chronic diseases arise from multiple factors over many years. A person who died of heart disease may have been overweight, had high blood pressure, been a cigarette smoker, and spent years eating a diet high in saturated fat and getting too little exercise.

Of course, not all people who die of heart disease fit this description, nor do all people with these characteristics die of heart disease. People who are overweight might die from the complications of diabetes instead, or those who smoke might die of cancer. They might even die from something totally unrelated to any of these factors, such as an automobile accident. Still, statistical studies have shown that certain conditions and behaviors are linked to certain diseases.

Table 1-4 highlights four of the top seven causes of death as having a link with diet. Notice that these four diseases—heart disease, cancers, strokes, and diabetes—account for more than half of the deaths each year.

TABLE 1-4 Leading Causes of Death in the United States

	Percentage of Total Deaths
1. **Heart disease**	23.5
2. **Cancers**	22.5
3. Chronic lung diseases	5.7
4. Accidents	5.0
5. **Strokes**	5.0
6. Alzheimer's disease	3.3
7. **Diabetes mellitus**	2.9
8. Pneumonia and influenza	2.2
9. Kidney disease	1.8
10. Suicide	1.6

NOTE: The diseases highlighted in bold have relationships with diet.

SOURCE: J. Q. Xu and coauthors, Deaths: Final data for 2013, *National Vital Statistics Reports* 64 (Hyattsville, MD: National Center for Health Statistics, 2016).

Risk Factors for Chronic Diseases Factors that increase or reduce the *risk* of developing chronic diseases can be identified by analyzing statistical data. A strong association between a **risk factor** and a disease means that when the factor is present, the *likelihood* of developing the disease increases. It does not mean that all people with the risk factor will develop the disease. Similarly, a lack of risk factors does not guarantee freedom from a given disease. On the average, though, the more risk factors in a person's life, the greater that person's chances of developing the disease. Conversely, the fewer risk factors in a person's life, the better the chances for good health.

Risk Factors Persist Risk factors tend to persist over time. Without intervention, a young adult with high blood pressure will most likely continue to have high blood pressure as an older adult, for example. Thus, to minimize the damage, early intervention is most effective.

Risk Factors Cluster Risk factors tend to cluster. For example, a person who is obese may be physically inactive, have high blood pressure, and have high blood cholesterol—all risk factors associated with heart disease. Multiple risk factors act synergistically to increase the risk of disease dramatically. Intervention that focuses on one risk factor often benefits the others as well. For example, physical activity can help reduce weight. Physical activity and weight loss will, in turn, help lower blood pressure and blood cholesterol (see Photo 1-9).

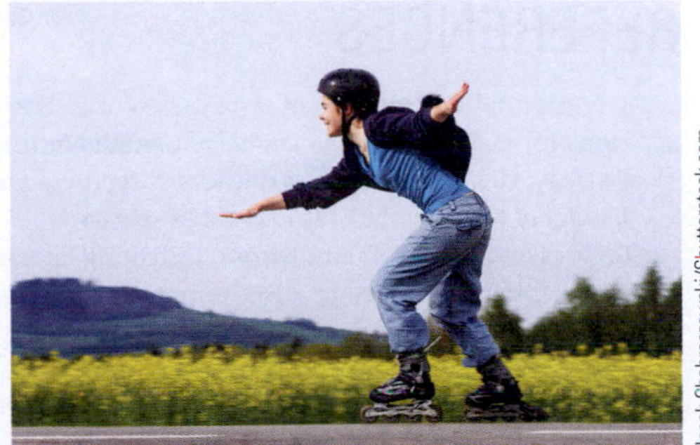

Jacek Chabraszewski/Shutterstock.com

> **PHOTO 1-9** Physical activity can be both fun and beneficial.

risk factor: a condition or behavior associated with an elevated frequency of a disease but not proved to be causal. Leading risk factors for chronic diseases include obesity, cigarette smoking, high blood pressure, high blood cholesterol, physical inactivity, and a diet high in added fats and low in vegetables, fruits, and whole grains.

Risk Factors in Perspective The most prominent risk factor—contributing to one of every five deaths each year in the United States—is tobacco use, followed

TABLE 1-5 Factors Contributing to Deaths in the United States

Factors	Percentage of Deaths
Tobacco	18
Poor diet/inactivity	15
Alcohol	4
Microbial agents	3
Toxic agents	2
Motor vehicles	2
Firearms	1
Sexual behavior	<1
Illicit drugs	<1

SOURCE: A. H. Mokdad and coauthors, Actual causes of death in the United States, 2000, *Journal of the American Medical Association* 291 (2004): 1238–1245, with corrections from *Journal of the American Medical Association* 293 (2005): 298.

closely by diet and activity patterns, and then alcohol use (see Table 1-5). Risk factors such as smoking, poor dietary habits, physical inactivity, and alcohol consumption are personal behaviors that can be changed. Decisions to not smoke, to eat a well-balanced diet, to engage in regular physical activity, and to drink alcohol in moderation (if at all) improve the likelihood that a person will enjoy good health. Other risk factors, such as genetics, gender, and age, also play important roles in the development of chronic diseases, but they cannot be changed. Health recommendations acknowledge the influence of such factors on the development of disease, but they must focus on the factors that are changeable.

Health Behaviors in the United States Despite evidence linking certain behaviors with chronic diseases, many Americans continue to engage in unhealthy behaviors. An estimated 35 percent of US adults consume more than moderate amounts of alcohol; 20 percent smoke cigarettes; 50 percent are physically inactive; 60 percent are either overweight or obese; and 30 percent obtain 7 hours or less of sleep per day.[28] For those who do not smoke or drink alcohol excessively, the one choice that can influence chronic disease risks more than any other is diet.[29]

REVIEW IT Identify several risk factors and explain their relationships to chronic diseases.

Diet has no influence on some diseases but is linked closely to others. Other life choices, such as engaging in physical activity and using tobacco or alcohol, also affect health for the better or worse.

The next several chapters provide many more details about nutrients and how they support health. Whenever appropriate, the discussion shows how diet influences each of today's major diseases. Dietary recommendations appear again and again, as each nutrient's relationships with health are explored. Most people who follow the recommendations will benefit and can enjoy good health into their later years.

What's Online

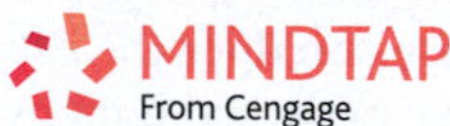
MINDTAP
From Cengage

Visit **www.cengagebrain.com** to access MindTap, a complete digital course that includes Diet & Wellness Plus, interactive quizzes, videos, and more.

REFERENCES

1. J. A. Mennella, Ontogeny of taste preferences: Basic biology and implications for health, *American Journal of Clinical Nutrition* 99 (2014): 704S–711S; A. Drewnowski and coauthors, Sweetness and food preference, *Journal of Nutrition* 142 (2012): 1142S–1148S.
2. S. Boesveldt and J. N. Lundström, Detecting fat content of food from a distance: Olfactory-based fat discrimination in humans, *PloS One* 9 (2014): e85977.
3. H. B. Loper and coauthors, Taste perception, associated hormonal modulation, and nutrient intake, *Nutrition Reviews* 73 (2015): 83–91; R. Negri and coauthors, Taste perception and food choices, *Journal of Pediatric Gastroenterology and Nutrition* 54 (2012): 624–629.
4. Think globally, practice locally: Culturally competent dietetics, *Journal of the Academy of Nutrition and Dietetics* 115 (2015): entire supplement; M. Truong, Y. Paradies, and N. Priest, Interventions to improve cultural competency in healthcare: A systematic review of reviews, *BMC Health Services Research* 14 (2014): 99. doi 10.1186/1472-6963-14-99.
5. E. Robinson and coauthors, What everyone else is eating: A systematic review and meta-analysis of the effect of informational eating norms on eating behavior, *Journal of the Academy of Nutrition and Dietetics* 114 (2014): 414–429.
6. J. A. Wolfson and S. N. Bleich, Is cooking at home associated with better diet quality or weight-loss intention? *Public Health Nutrition* 18 (2015): 1397–1406; C. Hartmann, S. Dohle, and M. Siegrist, Importance of cooking skills for balanced food choices, *Appetite* 65 (2013): 125–131.
7. L. E. Urban and coauthors, Temporal trends in fast-food restaurant energy, sodium, saturated fat, and *trans* fat content, United States, 1996–2013, *Preventing Chronic Disease* 11 (2014): E229; B. T. Nguyen and L. M. Powell, The impact of restaurant consumption among US adults: Effects on energy and nutrient intakes, *Public Health Nutrition* 17 (2014): 2445–2452; C. D. Fryar and R. B. Ervin, Caloric intake from fast food among adults: United States, 2007–2010, *NCHS Data Brief* 114 (February 2013); A. Jaworowska and coauthors, Nutritional challenges and health implications of takeaway and fast food, *Nutrition Reviews* 71 (2013): 310–318.
8. D. M. Kern and coauthors, Neighborhood variation in the price of soda relative to milk and its association neighbourhood socio-economic status and race, *Public Health Nutrition* 30 (2016): 1–11; M. Rao and coauthors, Do healthier foods and diet patterns cost more than less healthy options? A systematic review and meta-analysis, *BMJ Open* 3 (2013): e004277.
9. R. Nakamura and coauthors, Price promotions on healthier compared with less healthy foods: A hierarchical regression analysis of the impact

on sales and social patterning of responses to promotions in Great Britain, *American Journal of Clinical Nutrition* 101 (2015): 808–816; K. Ball and coauthors, Influence of price discounts and skill-building strategies on purchase and consumption of healthy food and beverages: Outcomes of the Supermarket Healthy Eating for Life randomized controlled trial, *American Journal of Clinical Nutrition* 101 (2015): 1055–1064; D. Mozaffarian, K. S. Rogoff, and D. S. Ludwig, The real cost of food: Can taxes and subsidies improve public health? *Journal of the American Medical Association* 312 (2014): 889–890; G. D. Foster and coauthors, Placement and promotion strategies to increase sales of healthier products in supermarkets in low-income, ethnically diverse neighborhoods: A randomized controlled trial, *American Journal of Clinical Nutrition* 99 (2014): 1359–1368.

10. A. K. Ventura and J. Worobey, Early influences on the development of food preferences, *Current Biology* 23 (2013): R401–R408.
11. C. Jacquier and coauthors, Improving the effectiveness of nutritional information policies: Assessment of unconscious pleasure mechanisms involved in food-choice decisions, *Nutrition Reviews* 70 (2012): 118–131.
12. C. M. Weaver and coauthors, Processed foods: Contributions to nutrition, *American Journal of Clinical Nutrition* 99 (2014): 1525–1542.
13. C. A. Monteiro and coauthors, Ultra-processed products are becoming dominant in the global food system, *Obesity Reviews* 14 (2013): 21–28.
14. E. M. Steele and coauthors, Ultra-processed foods and added sugars in the US diet: Evidence from a nationally representative cross-sectional study, *BMJ Open* 6 (2016): e009892.
15. Position of the Academy of Nutrition and Dietetics: Total diet approach to healthy eating, *Journal of the Academy of Nutrition and Dietetics* 113 (2013): 307–317.
16. L. Mauri, Why we still need randomized trials to compare effectiveness, *New England Journal of Medicine* 366 (2012): 1538–1540.
17. M. Lai, P. C. Chandrasekera, and N. D. Barnard, You are what you eat, or are you? The challenges of translating high-fat-fed rodents to human obesity and diabetes, *Nutrition and Diabetes* 4 (2014): e135; K. L. Nielsen and coauthors, Similar metabolic responses in pigs and humans to breads with different contents and compositions of dietary fibers: A metabolomics study, *American Journal of Clinical Nutrition* 99 (2014): 941–949.
18. S. B. Soumerai and coauthors, How do you know which health care effectiveness research you can trust? A guide to study design for the perplexed, *Preventing Chronic Disease* 12 (2015): 150187; L. Rosenbaum, Understanding bias: The case for careful study, *New England Journal of Medicine* 372 (2015): 1959–1963; D. M. Shaw, Beyond conflicts of interest: Disclosing medical biases, *Journal of the American Medical Association* 312 (2014) 697–698.
19. S. Ebrahim and coauthors, Reanalyses of randomized clinical trial data, *Journal of the American Medical Association* 312 (2014): 1024–1032.
20. R. H. Nagler, Adverse outcomes associated with media exposure to contradictory nutrition messages, *Journal of Health Communication* 19 (2014): 24–40.
21. A. Satija and F. B. Hu, Big data and systematic reviews in nutritional epidemiology, *Nutrition Reviews* 72 (2014): 737–740.
22. P. R. Trumbo and coauthors, Dietary Reference Intakes: Cases of appropriate and inappropriate uses, *Nutrition Reviews* 71 (2013): 657–664; Practice paper of the American Dietetic Association: Using the Dietary Reference Intakes, *Journal of the American Dietetic Association* 111 (2011): 762–770.
23. Practice paper of the Academy of Nutrition and Dietetics abstract: Critical thinking skills in nutrition assessment and diagnosis, *Journal of the Academy of Nutrition and Dietetics* 113 (2013): 1545.
24. US Department of Health and Human Services, *Healthy People 2020 Midcourse Review*, November 2016. https://www.cdc.gov/nchs/healthy_people/hp2020/hp2020_midcourse_review.htm
25. D. Raubenheimer and S. J. Simpson, Nutritional ecology and human health, *Annual Review of Nutrition* 36 (2016): 603–626.
26. Chronic disease prevention and health promotion, www.cdc.gov/chronicdisease, updated regularly.
27. F. Imamura and coauthors, Dietary quality among men and women in 187 countries in 1990 and 2010: A systematic assessment, *The Lancet Global Health* 3 (2015): e132–e142; L. J. Cobiac, L. Veerman, and T. Vos, The role of cost-effectiveness analysis in developing nutrition policy, *Annual Review of Nutrition* 33 (2013): 373–393.
28. Y. Liu and coauthors, Clustering of five health-related behaviors for chronic disease prevention among adults, United States, 2013, *Preventing Chronic Disease* 13 (2016): 160054.
29. V. Kontis and coauthors, Contribution of six risk factors to achieving the 25 × 25 non-communicable disease mortality reduction target: A modeling study, *Lancet* 384 (2014): 427–437.

HIGHLIGHT > 1

LEARN IT Recognize misinformation and describe how to identify reliable nutrition information.

Nutrition Information and Misinformation

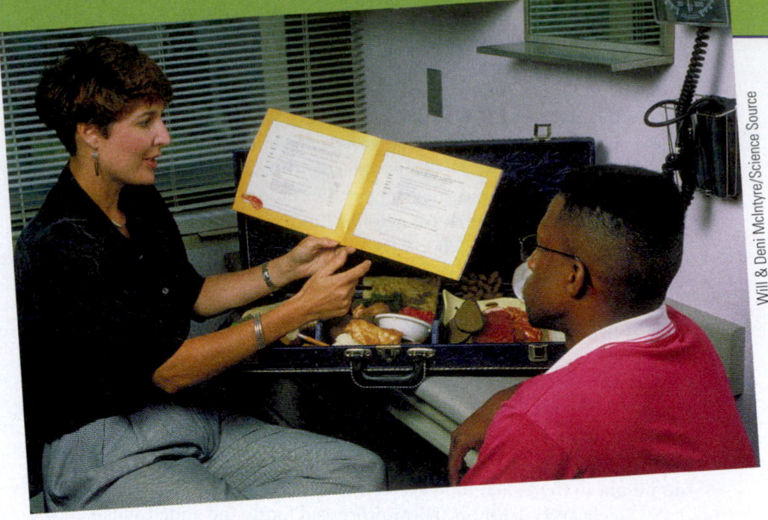
Will & Deni McIntyre/Science Source

How can people distinguish valid nutrition information from misinformation? One excellent approach is to notice *who* is providing the information. The "who" behind the information is not always evident, though, especially in the world of electronic media. Keep in mind that *people* create websites on the Internet, just as people write books and report the news. In all cases, consumers need to determine whether the person is qualified to provide nutrition information.

This highlight begins by examining the unique potential as well as the problems of relying on the Internet and the media for nutrition information. It continues with a discussion of how to identify reliable nutrition information that applies to all resources, including the Internet and the news. (Glossary H1-1 defines related terms.)

This discussion recognizes that identifying nutrition misinformation requires more than simply gathering accurate information, although that is a good start; it requires **critical thinking.** Critical thinking allows a person who has gathered information to:

- Understand the connections between concepts
- Identify and evaluate the pros and cons of an argument
- Detect inconsistencies and errors
- Solve problems
- Identify the relevance of information

To that end, the questions at the end of the highlights that follow all chapters are intended to help develop critical thinking skills.

Nutrition on the Internet

Got a question? The Internet has an answer. Almost 75 percent of Internet users look online for health information.[1] The Internet offers endless opportunities to obtain high-quality information, but it also delivers an abundance of incomplete, misleading, and inaccurate information.[2] Simply put: anyone can publish anything.

With hundreds of millions of websites, searching for nutrition information can be an overwhelming experience, with no guarantees of finding accurate information. When using the Internet, keep in mind that the quality of health-related information available covers a broad range. You must evaluate websites for their accuracy, just as you would any other source. How To H1-1 provides tips for determining whether a website is reliable.

One of the most trustworthy sites used by scientists and others is the US National Library of Medicine's PubMed, which provides free access to more than 25 million abstracts of research papers published in scientific journals around the world. Many abstracts provide links to the full articles. Figure H1-1 (p. 30) introduces this valuable resource.

Did you receive an e-mail warning of the health dangers associated with reusing or freezing plastic water bottles? If so, you've been

GLOSSARY H1-1

Academy of Nutrition and Dietetics: the professional organization of dietitians in the United States; formerly the American Dietetic Association.

accredited: approved; in the case of medical centers or universities, certified by an agency recognized by the US Department of Education.

certified nutritionist or **certified nutritional consultant** or **certified nutrition therapist:** a person who has been granted a document declaring his or her authority as a nutrition professional.

critical thinking: the mental activity of rationally and skillfully analyzing, synthesizing, and evaluating information to reach an informed conclusion based on evidence.

dietetic technician: a person who has completed a minimum of an associate's degree from an accredited university or college and an approved dietetic technician program that includes a supervised practice experience. See also *dietetic technician, registered.*

dietetic technician, registered (DTR): a dietetic technician who has passed a national examination and maintains registration through continuing professional education.

dietitian: a person trained in nutrition, food science, and diet planning. See also *registered dietitian nutritionist.*

diploma mills: entities without valid accreditation that provide worthless degrees.

DTR: see *dietetic technician, registered.*

fraudulent: the promotion, for financial gain, of devices, treatments, services, plans, or products (including diets and supplements) that alter or claim to alter a human condition without proof of safety or effectiveness.

license to practice: permission under state or federal law, granted on meeting specified criteria, to use a certain title (such as dietitian) and offer certain services. *Licensed dietitians* may use the initials *LD* after their names.

misinformation: false or misleading information.

public health dietitians: dietitians who specialize in providing nutrition services through organized community efforts.

RDN: see *registered dietitian nutritionist.*

registered dietitian nutritionist (RDN): a person who has completed a minimum of a bachelor's degree from an accredited university or college, has completed approved course work and a supervised practice program, has passed a national examination, and maintains registration through continuing professional education; also called *registered dietitian (RD).*

registration: listing; with respect to health professionals, listing with a professional organization that requires specific course work, experience, and passing of an examination.

a victim of urban scarelore. When nutrition information arrives in unsolicited e-mails, be suspicious if:

- The person sending it to you didn't write it and you cannot determine who did or if that person is a nutrition expert
- The phrase "Forward this to everyone you know" appears
- The phrase "This is not a hoax" appears, because chances are good that it is
- The news is sensational and you've never heard about it from legitimate sources
- The language is emphatic and the text is sprinkled with capitalized words and exclamation marks
- No references are given or, if present, are of questionable validity when examined
- The message has been debunked on websites such as www.quackwatch .org, www.snopes.com, or www.urbanlegends.about.com

>How To H1-1 Determine Whether a Website Is Reliable

To determine whether a website offers reliable nutrition information, ask the following questions:

- **Who?** Who is responsible for the site? Is it staffed by qualified professionals? Look for the authors' names and credentials. Have experts reviewed the content for accuracy?
- **When?** When was the site last updated? Because nutrition is an ever-changing science, sites need to be dated and updated frequently.
- **Where?** Where is the information coming from? The three letters following the dot in a Web address identify the site's affiliation. Addresses ending in "gov" (government), "edu" (educational institute), and "org" (organization) generally provide reliable information; "com" (commercial) sites represent businesses and, depending on their qualifications and integrity, may or may not offer dependable information.
- **Why?** Why is the site giving you this information? Is the site providing a public service or selling a product? Many commercial sites provide accurate information, but some do not. When money is the prime motivation, be aware that the information may be biased.

If you are satisfied with the answers to all of the previous questions, then ask this final question:

- **What?** What is the message, and is it in line with other reliable sources? Information that contradicts common knowledge should be questioned. Many reliable sites provide links to other sites to facilitate your quest for knowledge, but this provision alone does not guarantee a reputable intention. Be aware that any site can link to any other site without permission.

› TRY IT Visit a nutrition website and answer the five "W" questions to determine whether it is a reliable resource.

Nutrition in the News

Consumers get much of their nutrition information from Internet websites, television programs, and magazine articles, which have heightened awareness of how diet influences the development of diseases. Consumers benefit from news coverage of nutrition when they learn to make lifestyle changes that will improve their health. Sometimes, however, popular reports mislead consumers and create confusion. They often tell a lopsided story quickly instead of presenting the integrated results of research studies or a balance of expert opinions.

Tight deadlines and limited understanding sometimes make it difficult to provide a thorough report. Hungry for the latest news, the media often report scientific findings quickly and prematurely—without benefit of careful interpretation, replication, or peer review. Biases influence choices and perspectives.[3] Usually, the reports present findings from a single, recently released study, making the news current and controversial. Consequently, the public receives diet and health news fast, but not always in perspective. Reporters may twist inconclusive findings into "meaningful discoveries" when pressured to write catchy headlines and sensational stories.

As a result "surprising new findings" sometimes seem to contradict one another, and consumers may feel frustrated and betrayed. Occasionally, the reports are downright false, but more often the apparent contradictions are simply the normal result of science at work. A single study contributes to the big picture, but when viewed alone, it can easily distort the image. To be meaningful the conclusions of any study must be presented cautiously within the context of other research findings.

Televised talk shows frequently offer health advice—most commonly, dietary advice. Such advice may sound valid, especially when delivered by a doctor, but viewers need to remember that the primary purpose of these programs is entertainment. One study examining 160 episodes of two popular medical talk shows found that fewer than half of the recommendations were based on evidence.[4]

Fitness magazines and Internet websites are particularly troublesome because many of them present both valid and invalid nutrition information along with slick advertisements for nutrition products. Advertisements often feature colorful anatomical figures, graphs, and tables that appear scientific. Some ads even include references, citing or linking to such credible sources as the *American Journal of Clinical Nutrition* and the *Journal of the American Medical Association.* These ads create the illusion of endorsement and credibility. Keep in mind, however, that ads are created to sell products, not to teach. A careful reading of the cited research might reveal that the ads have exaggerated the significance of the findings or presented them out of context. For example, an ad might claim that its dietary supplement increases lean body mass, when in fact, the researchers concluded that "supplement use is not justified."

> **FIGURE H1-1 PubMed: Internet Resource for Scientific Nutrition References**

The US National Library of Medicine's PubMed website (www.ncbi.nlm.nih.gov/pubmed) offers tutorials to help beginners use the search system effectively. Often, simply visiting the site, typing a query in the "Search for" box, and clicking "Go" will yield satisfactory results.

For example, to find research concerning calcium and bone health, typing "calcium bone" yields more than 55,000 results. Try setting limits on publication dates, types of articles, languages, and other criteria to obtain a more manageable number of abstracts and articles to peruse.

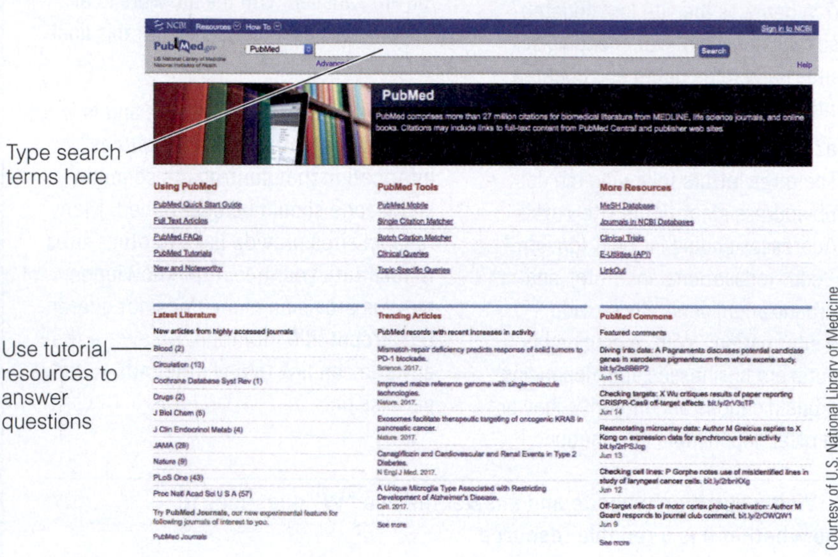
Type search terms here
Use tutorial resources to answer questions
PubMed
Using PubMed
PubMed Tools
More Resources
Latest Literature
Trending Articles
PubMed Commons

Courtesy of U.S. National Library of Medicine

Identifying Nutrition Experts

Regardless of whether the source is electronic, print, or video, consumers need to ask whether the person behind the information is qualified to speak on nutrition. If the creator of an Internet website recommends eating three pineapples a day to lose weight, a trainer at the gym praises a high-protein diet, or a health-food store clerk suggests an herbal supplement, should you believe these people? Can you distinguish between accurate news reports and infomercials on television? Have you noticed that many televised nutrition messages are presented by celebrities, athletes, psychologists, food editors, and chefs—that is, almost anyone except a **dietitian**? When you are confused or need sound dietary advice, whom should you ask?

Physicians and Other Health-Care Professionals

Many people turn to physicians or other health-care professionals for dietary advice, expecting them to know about all health-related matters. But are they the best sources of accurate and current information on nutrition?

Most physicians and other health-care professionals appreciate the connections between health and nutrition. Those who have specialized in clinical nutrition are especially well qualified to speak on the subject. Few, however, have the education, time, or experience to provide adequate nutrition care.[5] Often they wisely refer clients to a qualified nutrition expert—a **registered dietitian nutritionist (RDN).**

Registered Dietitian Nutritionist (RDN)

A registered dietitian nutritionist (RDN) has the educational background and clinical experience necessary to deliver reliable nutrition advice and care.[6] To become an RDN, a person must earn a degree from an accredited school based on course work that typically includes food and nutrition sciences, foodservice systems management, business, economics, computer science, sociology, biochemistry, physiology, microbiology, and chemistry; complete an accredited and supervised practice program; pass a national examination administered by the **Academy of Nutrition and Dietetics**; and maintain **registration** by participating in required continuing education activities.

Many states provide a further guarantee: a state registration, certification, or **license to practice.** In this way, states identify people who have met minimal standards of education and experience. Still, these state standards may fall short of those defining an RDN. Similarly, some alternative educational programs qualify a graduate as a **certified nutritionist, certified nutritional consultant,** or **certified nutrition therapist**—terms that sound authoritative but lack the credentials of an RDN.

Dietitians perform a multitude of duties in many settings in most communities.[7] They work in the food industry, pharmaceutical companies, home health agencies, long-term care institutions, private practice, public health departments, research centers, education settings, fitness centers, and hospitals. Depending on their work settings, dietitians can assume a number of different job responsibilities and positions. In the food industry, dietitians conduct research, develop products, and market services. In hospitals, administrative dietitians manage the foodservice system; clinical dietitians provide client care; and nutrition support team dietitians coordinate nutrition care with other health-care professionals. Recent rulings now allow qualified dietitians to order therapeutic diets and nutrition-related lab tests without the supervision or approval of a physician, thus improving the nutritional diagnosis and treatment plans of hospitalized patients.[8]

Public health dietitians who work in government-funded agencies such as health departments or clinics play a key role in delivering nutrition services to people in the community. Among their many roles, public health dietitians help plan, coordinate, and evaluate food assistance programs; act as consultants to other agencies; manage finances; and much more.

Dietetic Technician, Registered (DTR)

In some facilities, a **dietetic technician** assists an RDN in both administrative and clinical responsibilities. A dietetic technician has been educated and trained to work under the guidance of an RDN; upon passing a national examination, the title changes to **dietetic technician, registered (DTR).**

Other Dietary Employees

In addition to the dietetic technician, other dietary employees may include clerks, aides, cooks, porters, and assistants. These dietary employees do not have extensive formal training in nutrition, and their ability to provide accurate information may be limited.

Identifying Fake Credentials

In contrast to an RDN, thousands of people obtain fake nutrition degrees and claim to be nutrition consultants or doctors of "nutrimedicine." These and other such titles may sound meaningful, but most of these people lack the established credentials and training of an RDN. If you look closely, you can see signs of their fake expertise.

Consider educational background, for example. The minimum standards of education for an RDN specify a degree in food science and human nutrition or related fields from an **accredited** college or university.* Unfortunately, fake nutrition degrees are available from schools "accredited" by phony accrediting agencies. Acquiring false degrees and credentials is especially easy today, with **diploma mills** and **fraudulent** businesses operating via the Internet.

Knowing the qualifications of someone who provides nutrition information can help you determine whether that person's advice might be harmful or helpful. Don't be afraid to ask for credentials. Table H1-1 lists credible sources of nutrition information.

Red Flags of Nutrition Quackery

Figure H1-2 (p. 32) features eight red flags consumers can use to identify nutrition **misinformation.** Sales of unproven and dangerous products have always been a concern, but the Internet now provides merchants with an easy and inexpensive way to reach millions of customers around the world. Because of the difficulty in regulating the Internet, fraudulent and illegal sales of medical products have hit a bonanza. As is the case with the air, no one owns the Internet, and similarly, no one has control over the pollution. Countries have different laws regarding sales of drugs, dietary supplements, and other health products, but applying these laws to the Internet marketplace is almost impossible. Even if illegal activities could be defined and identified, finding the person responsible for a particular website is not always possible. Websites can appear and disappear in a blink of a cursor. Now, more than ever, consumers must heed the caution "Buyer beware."

In summary, when you hear nutrition news, consider its source. Ask yourself these two questions: Is the person providing the information qualified to speak on nutrition? Is the information based on valid scientific research? If not, find a better source. After all, your health depends on it.

TABLE H1-1 Credible Sources of Nutrition Information

Government agencies, volunteer associations, consumer groups, and professional organizations provide consumers with reliable health and nutrition information. Credible sources of nutrition information include:

- Nutrition and food science departments at a university or community college
- Local agencies such as the health department or County Cooperative Extension Service
- Government resources such as:

Centers for Disease Control and Prevention (CDC)	**www.cdc.gov**
Department of Agriculture (USDA)	**www.usda.gov**
Department of Health and Human Services (DHHS)	**www.hhs.gov**
Dietary Guidelines for Americans	**fnic.nal.usda.gov /dietary-guidance**
Food and Drug Administration (FDA)	**www.fda.gov**
Health Canada	**www.hc-sc.gc.ca/index-eng.php**
Healthy People	**www.healthypeople.gov**
Let's Move!	**www.letsmove.gov**
MyPlate	**www.choosemyplate.gov**
National Institutes of Health	**www.nih.gov**
Physical Activity Guidelines for Americans	**www.health.gov/paguidelines**

- Volunteer health agencies such as:

American Cancer Society	**www.cancer.org**
American Diabetes Association	**www.diabetes.org**
American Heart Association	**www.heart.org/HEARTORG**

- Reputable consumer groups such as:

American Council on Science and Health	**www.acsh.org**
International Food Information Council	**www.foodinsight.org**

- Professional health organizations such as:

Academy of Nutrition and Dietetics	**www.eatright.org**
American Medical Association	**www.ama-assn.org**
Dietitians of Canada	**www.dietitians.ca**

- Journals such as:

American Journal of Clinical Nutrition	**ajcn.nutrition.org**
Journal of the Academy of Nutrition and Dietetics	**www.andjrnl.org**
New England Journal of Medicine	**www.nejm.org**
Nutrition Reviews	**www.ilsi.org**

*To ensure the quality and continued improvement of nutrition and dietetics education programs, an agency of the Academy of Nutrition and Dietetics known as the Accreditation Council for Education in Nutrition and Dietetics (ACEND) establishes and enforces eligibility requirements and accreditation standards for programs preparing students for careers as registered dietitian nutritionists or dietetics technicians. Programs meeting those standards are accredited by ACEND.

> **FIGURE H1-2** **Red Flags of Nutrition Quackery**

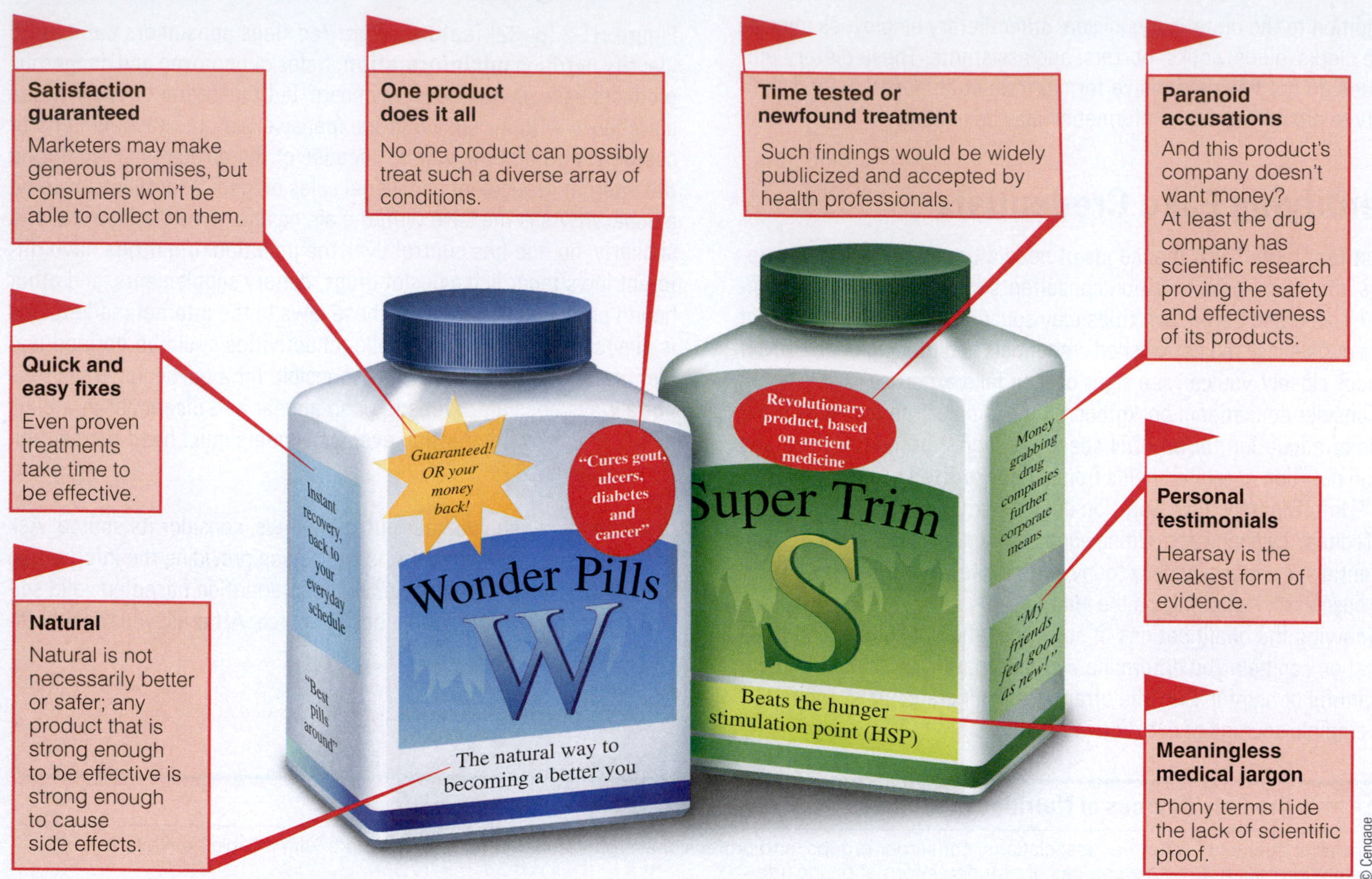
Satisfaction guaranteed
Marketers may make generous promises, but consumers won't be able to collect on them.
One product does it all
No one product can possibly treat such a diverse array of conditions.
Time tested or newfound treatment
Such findings would be widely publicized and accepted by health professionals.
Paranoid accusations
And this product's company doesn't want money? At least the drug company has scientific research proving the safety and effectiveness of its products.
Quick and easy fixes
Even proven treatments take time to be effective.
Natural
Natural is not necessarily better or safer; any product that is strong enough to be effective is strong enough to cause side effects.
Personal testimonials
Hearsay is the weakest form of evidence.
Meaningless medical jargon
Phony terms hide the lack of scientific proof.
Guaranteed! OR your money back!
"Cures gout, ulcers, diabetes and cancer"
Revolutionary product, based on ancient medicine
Instant recovery, back to your everyday schedule
"Best pills around"
Wonder Pills
W
The natural way to becoming a better you
Super Trim
S
Money grabbing drug companies further corporate means
"My friends feel good as new!"
Beats the hunger stimulation point (HSP)
© Cengage

CRITICAL THINKING QUESTIONS

A. How would you judge the accuracy or validity of nutrition information?

B. You have just received a forwarded e-mail from a friend warning that the artificial sweetener aspartame is a TOXIN that causes muscle spasms, leg numbness, stomach cramps, vertigo, dizziness, headaches, tinnitus, joint pain, depression, anxiety, slurred speech, blurred vision, and memory loss. It goes on to say that this DEADLY POISON causes blindness, multiple sclerosis, brain tumors, and cancer! The message alleges that aspartame remains on the market because of a conspiracy between the FDA and the manufacturer to keep these dangers hidden from the public. How can you determine whether these claims are legitimate warnings or an irresponsible hoax?

REFERENCES

1. Pew Research Center, The social life of health information, www.pewresearch.org/fact-tank/2014/01/15/the-social-life-of-health-information, January 15, 2014.
2. Practice paper of the Academy of Nutrition and Dietetics abstract: Communicating accurate food and nutrition information, *Journal of the Academy of Nutrition and Dietetics* 112 (2012): 759.
3. S. Rowe and N. Alexander, Conflicted science: Can nutrition communicators be biased too? *Nutrition Today* 50 (2015): 8–11.
4. C. Korownyk and coauthors, Televised medical talk shows—What they recommend and the evidence to support their recommendations: A prospective observational study, *British Medical Journal* 349 (2014): doi 10.1136/bmj.g7346.
5. P. M. Kris-Etherton and coauthors, Introduction to nutrition education in training medical and other health care professionals, *American Journal of Clinical Nutrition* 99 (2014): 1151S–1152S.
6. Position of the Academy of Nutrition and Dietetics: The role of nutrition in health promotion and chronic disease prevention, *Journal of the Academy of Nutrition and Dietetics* 113 (2013): 972–979.
7. Comprehensive scope of practice resources for the registered dietitian or registered dietitian nutritionist, *Journal of the Academy of Nutrition and Dietetics*, June 2013, Supplement 2.
8. B. Boyce, CMS final rule on therapeutic diet orders means new opportunities for RDNs, *Journal of the Academy of Nutrition and Dietetics* 114 (2014): 1326–1328.

2

Planning a Healthy Diet

LEARNING GUIDE

nehopelon/Shutterstock.com

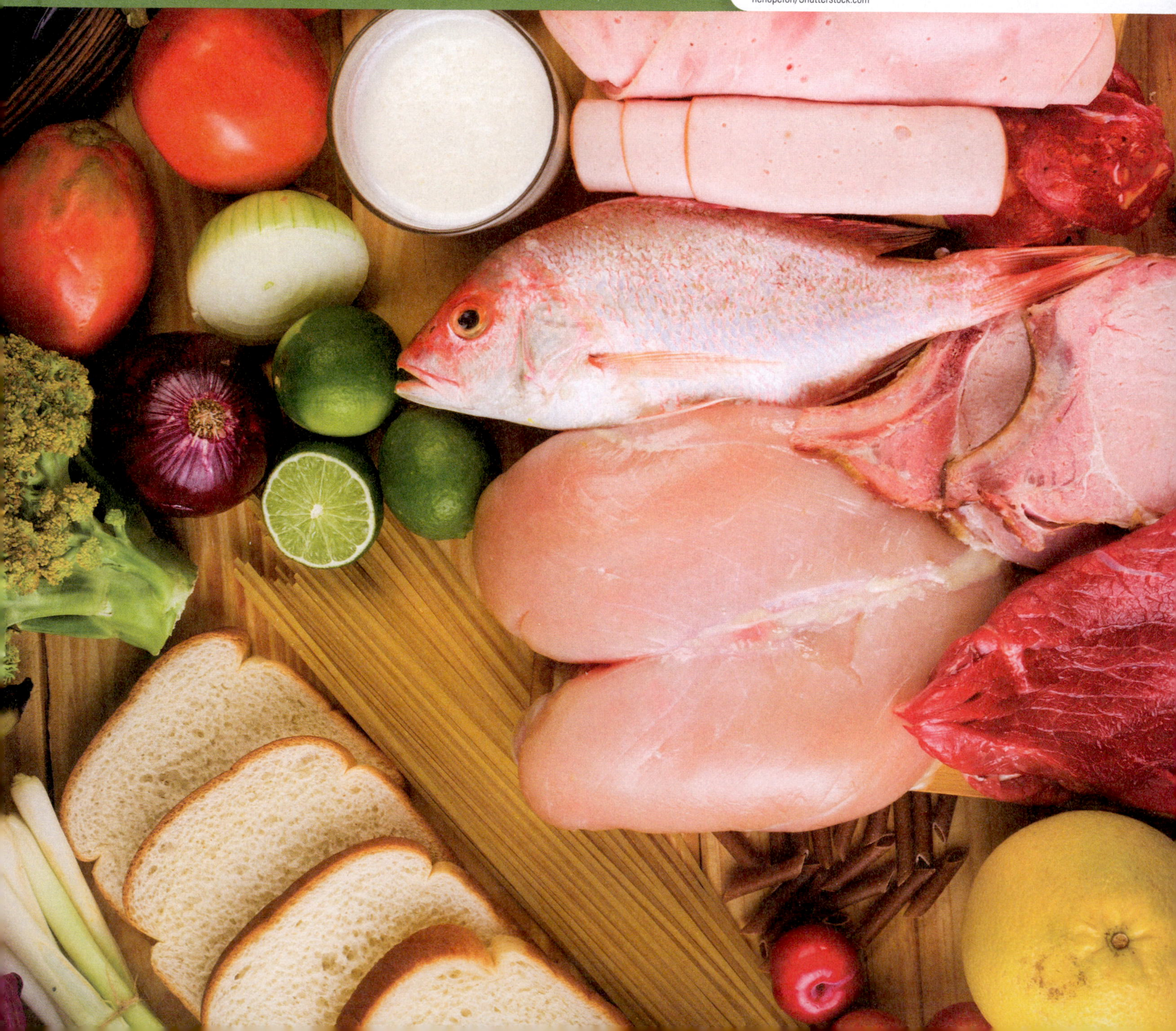

Nutrition in Your Life

You make food choices—deciding what to eat and how much to eat—more than 1000 times every year. We eat so frequently that it's easy to choose a meal without giving any thought to its nutrient contributions or health consequences. Even when we want to make healthy choices, we may not know which foods to select or how much to consume. With a few tools and tips, you can learn to plan a healthy diet. As you read this chapter, consider how your current diet compares with a healthy eating plan.

Chapter 1 explained that the nutrients delivered by the foods people eat support the body's many activities. Food choices made over years and decades influence the body's health, and consistently poor choices increase the risks of developing chronic diseases. Stated positively, optimal nourishment supports a robust life of vigorous activity and good health. This chapter shows how a person can select from the tens of thousands of available foods to create a nutritionally balanced diet that meets the body's nutrient and energy needs. Fortunately, most foods provide several nutrients, so one trick for wise diet planning is to select a combination of foods that deliver a full array of nutrients.

This chapter begins by introducing the diet-planning principles and dietary guidelines that promote good health and reduce disease risks. It continues by showing how people can use diet-planning guides to create eating patterns that will deliver sufficient nutrients without excess energy (kcalories). Learning how to read food labels eases the task of making healthy selections at the market.

2.1 Principles and Guidelines

LEARN IT Explain how each of the diet-planning principles can be used to plan a healthy diet.

How well you nourish yourself does not depend on the selection of any one food (see Photo 2-1). Instead, it depends on the overall **eating pattern**—the combination of many different foods and beverages at numerous meals over days, months, and years.[1] Diet-planning principles and dietary guidelines are key concepts to keep in mind whenever you are selecting foods—whether shopping at the grocery store, choosing from a restaurant menu, or preparing a home-cooked meal.

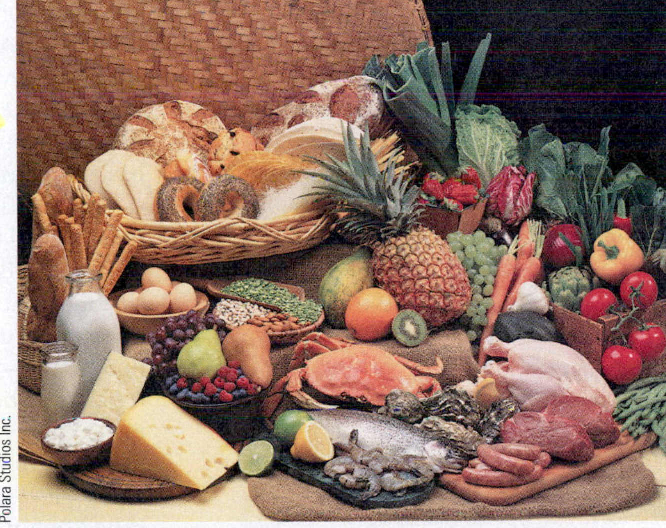

Polara Studios Inc.

> **PHOTO 2-1** To ensure an adequate and balanced diet, eat a variety of foods daily, choosing different foods from each group.

Diet-Planning Principles Diet planners have developed several ways to select foods. Whatever plan or combination of plans they use, though, they keep in mind these basic diet-planning principles:

- Adequacy
- Balance
- kCalorie (energy) control
- Nutrient density
- Moderation
- Variety

Adequacy Adequacy reflects a diet that provides sufficient energy and enough of all the nutrients to meet the needs of healthy people. Take the essential nutrient iron, for example. Because the body loses some iron each day, people have to replace it by eating foods that contain iron. A person whose diet fails to provide

eating pattern: customary quantities, proportions, and frequencies of consuming various foods and beverages over time.

adequacy (dietary): providing all the essential nutrients, fiber, and energy in amounts sufficient to maintain health.

enough iron-rich foods may develop the symptoms of iron-deficiency anemia: the person may feel weak, tired, and listless; have frequent headaches; and find that even the smallest amount of muscular work brings disabling fatigue. To prevent these deficiency symptoms, a person must include foods that supply adequate iron. The same is true for all the other essential nutrients introduced in Chapter 1.

Balance **Balance** in the diet helps to ensure adequacy. The art of balancing the diet involves consuming enough—but not too much—of different types of foods in proportion to one another. In a balanced diet, foods rich in some nutrients do not crowd out foods that are rich in other nutrients. The essential minerals calcium and iron, taken together, illustrate the importance of dietary balance. Meat is rich in iron but poor in calcium. Conversely, milk is rich in calcium but poor in iron. Eat some meat for iron; drink some milk for calcium; and be sure to include other foods, too, because a diet consisting of milk and meat alone would not be adequate. For the other nutrients, people need to eat other protein foods, whole grains, vegetables, and fruits.

kCalorie (Energy) Control Designing an adequate diet within a reasonable kcalorie allowance requires careful planning. Once again, balance plays a key role. The amount of energy coming into the body from foods should balance with the amount of energy being used by the body to sustain its metabolic and physical activities. Upsetting this balance leads to gains or losses in body weight. The discussion of energy balance and weight control in Chapters 8 and 9 examines this issue in more detail, but one key to **kcalorie control** is to select foods of high nutrient density.

Nutrient Density **Nutrient density** promotes adequacy and kcalorie control. To eat well without overeating, select nutrient-dense foods—that is, foods that deliver the most nutrients for the least food energy.[2] Consider foods containing calcium, for example. You can get about 300 milligrams of calcium from either 1½ ounces of cheddar cheese or 1 cup of fat-free milk, but the cheese delivers about twice as much food energy (kcalories) as the milk. The fat-free milk, then, is twice as calcium-dense as the cheddar cheese; it offers the same amount of calcium for half the kcalories. Both foods are excellent choices for adequacy's sake alone, but to achieve adequacy while controlling kcalories, the fat-free milk is the better choice. (Alternatively, a person could select a low-fat cheddar cheese with kcalories comparable to fat-free milk.) How To 2-1 describes how to compare foods based on nutrient density.

Just as a financially responsible person pays for rent, food, clothes, and tuition on a limited budget, healthy people obtain iron, calcium, and all the other essential nutrients on a limited energy (kcalorie) allowance. Success depends on getting many nutrients for each kcalorie "dollar." As Figure 2-1 illustrates, a breakfast of cereal, fruit, egg, and sausage delivers many more nutrients than a couple of doughnuts—even though they both provide about the same number of kcalories. A person who makes nutrient-dense choices can meet daily nutrient needs on a lower energy budget. Such choices support good health.

Foods that are notably low in nutrient density—such as potato chips, candy, and colas—are called **empty-kcalorie foods.** The kcalories these foods provide are called "empty" because they deliver a lot of energy (from added sugars, solid fats, or both) but little, or no, protein, vitamins, or minerals.

The concept of nutrient density is relatively simple when examining the contributions of one nutrient to a food or diet. With respect to calcium, milk ranks high and meats rank low. With respect to iron, meats rank high and milk ranks low. But it is a more complex task to answer the question, which food is more nutritious? To answer that question, we need to consider several nutrients—including both nutrients to encourage as well as those to limit. Ranking foods based on their overall nutrient composition is known as **nutrient profiling.** Researchers have yet to determine the best system to rate foods based on nutrient

balance (dietary): providing foods in proportion to one another and in proportion to the body's needs.

kcalorie (energy) control: management of food energy intake.

nutrient density: a measure of the nutrients a food provides relative to the energy it provides. The more nutrients and the fewer kcalories, the higher the nutrient density.

empty-kcalorie foods: a popular term used to denote foods that contribute energy but lack protein, vitamins, and minerals.

nutrient profiling: ranking foods based on their nutrient composition.

How To 2-1 Compare Foods Based on Nutrient Density

One way to evaluate foods is simply to notice their nutrient contribution *per serving:* 1 cup of milk provides about 300 milligrams of calcium, and ½ cup of fresh, cooked turnip greens provides about 100 milligrams. Thus a serving of milk offers three times as much calcium as a serving of turnip greens. To get 300 milligrams of calcium, a person could choose either 1 cup of milk or 1½ cups of turnip greens.

Another valuable way to evaluate foods is to consider their nutrient density—their nutrient contribution *per kcalorie*. Fat-free milk delivers about 85 kcalories with its 300 milligrams of calcium. To calculate the nutrient density, divide milligrams by kcalories:

$$\frac{300 \text{ mg calcium}}{85 \text{ kcal}} = 3.5 \text{ mg per kcal}$$

Do the same for the fresh turnip greens, which provide 15 kcalories with the 100 milligrams of calcium:

$$\frac{100 \text{ mg calcium}}{15 \text{ kcal}} = 6.7 \text{ mg per kcal}$$

The more milligrams per kcalorie, the greater the nutrient density. Turnip greens are more calcium-dense than milk. They provide more calcium *per kcalorie* than milk, but milk offers more calcium *per serving*. Both approaches offer valuable information, especially when combined with a realistic appraisal. What matters most is which are you more likely to consume—1½ cups of turnip greens or 1 cup of milk? You can get 300 milligrams of calcium from either, but the greens will save you about 40 kcalories (the savings would be even greater if you usually use whole milk).

Keep in mind, too, that calcium is only one of the many nutrients that foods provide. Similar calculations for protein, for example, would show that fat-free milk provides more protein both *per kcalorie* and *per serving* than turnip greens—that is, milk is more protein-dense. Combining variety with nutrient density helps ensure the adequacy of all nutrients.

› TRY IT Compare the thiamin density of 3 ounces of lean T-bone steak (174 kcalories, 0.09 milligrams thiamin) with ½ cup of fresh cooked broccoli (27 kcalories, 0.05 milligrams thiamin).

profiling, but when they do, nutrient profiling will be most helpful in identifing nutritious foods and planning healthy diets.[3]

moderation (dietary): providing enough but not too much of a substance.

solid fats: fats that are not usually liquid at room temperature; commonly found in most foods derived from animals and vegetable oils that have been hydrogenated. Solid fats typically contain more saturated and *trans* fats than most oils (Chapter 5 provides more details).

added sugars: sugars and other kcaloric sweeteners that are added to foods during processing, preparation, or at the table. Added sugars do not include the naturally occurring sugars found in fruits and milk products.

Moderation Moderation contributes to adequacy, balance, and kcalorie control. Foods rich in **solid fats** and **added sugars** often provide some enjoyment and lots of energy (kcalories) but relatively few nutrients; in addition, they promote weight gain when eaten in excess. A person practicing moderation eats such foods only on occasion and regularly selects foods low in solid fats and added sugars, a practice that automatically improves nutrient density. Returning to the example of cheddar cheese versus fat-free milk, the fat-free milk not only offers the same amount of calcium for less energy, but it also contains much less saturated fat than the cheese.

› FIGURE 2-1 Nutrient Density of Two Breakfast Options Compared

Chapter 1 presented these two breakfasts to illustrate energy density—that for the same number of kcalories, the breakfast on the left delivered less energy per gram of food, which benefits weight management. These two breakfasts also illustrate nutrient density—that for the same number of kcalories, the breakfast on the left delivers more nutrients per kcalorie.

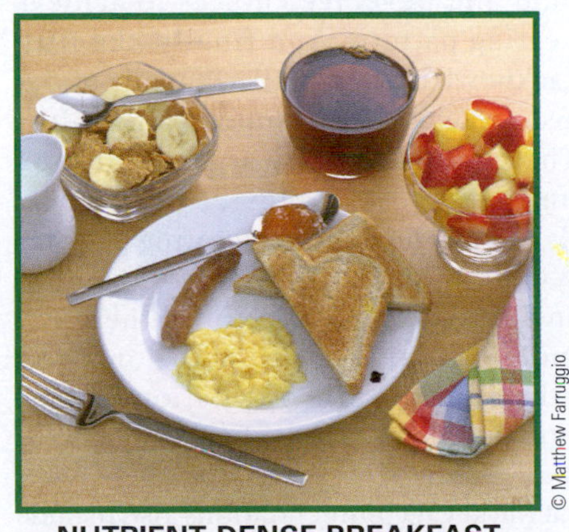

NUTRIENT-DENSE BREAKFAST

© Matthew Farruggio

Daily recommendations (%)

Key:
Nutrient-dense breakfast
Nutrient-poor breakfast

100, 80, 60, 40, 20, 0

Protein, Fiber, Vitamin D, Calcium, Iron, Potassium

© Cengage

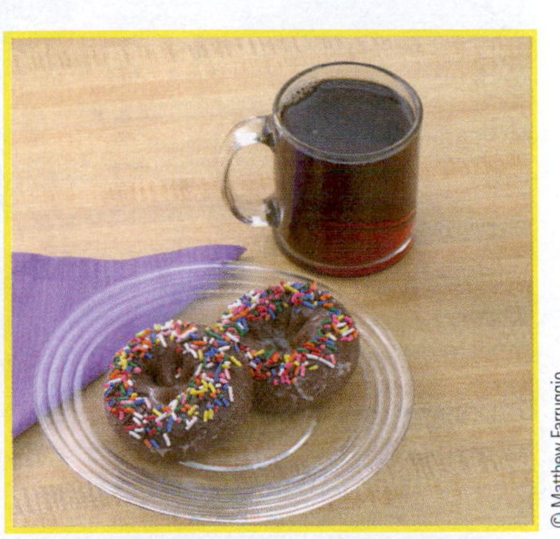

NUTRIENT-POOR BREAKFAST

© Matthew Farruggio

Variety Variety improves nutrient adequacy. A diet may have all of the virtues just described and still lack variety, if a person eats the same foods day after day. People should select foods from each of the food groups daily and vary their choices within each food group from day to day for several reasons. First, different foods within the same group contain different arrays of nutrients. Among the fruits, for example, strawberries are especially rich in vitamin C while apricots are rich in vitamin A. Second, no food is guaranteed to be entirely free of substances that, in excess, could be harmful. The strawberries might contain trace amounts of one contaminant, the apricots another. By alternating fruit choices, a person will ingest very little of either contaminant. (Contamination of foods is discussed in Chapter 19.) Third, as the adage goes, variety is the spice of life. A person who eats beans frequently can enjoy pinto beans in Mexican burritos today, garbanzo beans in a Greek salad tomorrow, and baked beans with barbecued chicken on the weekend. Eating nutritious meals need never be boring.

Dietary Guidelines for Americans

What should a person eat to stay healthy? The answers can be found in the *Dietary Guidelines for Americans*, an evidence-based document used to develop federal food, nutrition, and health policies and programs. These guidelines help translate the *nutrient* recommendations of the DRI (presented in Chapter 1) into *food* recommendations.

By law, the *Dietary Guidelines for Americans* are reviewed and revised as needed every 5 years. Each edition shares some similarities with previous editions but also sets precedent in new ways. Perhaps most noteworthy to the current edition is the focus on eating patterns—the foods and beverages a person consumes over time. The *2015–2020 Dietary Guidelines for Americans* recognize that "healthy eating patterns and regular physical activity can help people achieve and maintain good health and reduce the risk of chronic disease throughout all stages of the lifespan."[4]

Table 2-1 presents the current guidelines and key recommendations. The first guideline encourages a healthy eating pattern at an appropriate kcalorie level to support adequate nutrition, good health, and a healthy body weight throughout life. The second guideline notes that a focus on variety, nutrient density, and amounts help a person meet nutrient needs within kcalorie limits. The third guideline advises people to limit their intake of added sugars, saturated fats, sodium, and alcoholic beverages (for adults of legal age who partake). The fourth guideline recognizes that people will need to make shifts in their food and beverage choices to achieve a healthy eating pattern. And finally, the fifth guideline acknowledges that all segments of our society have a role to play in supporting healthy choices. These guidelines are accompanied by key recommendations that provide tips on how individuals can establish healthy eating patterns by specifying which foods and food components to include and which to limit; these key recommendations, along with additional recommendations for specific population groups, appear throughout the text as their subjects are discussed.

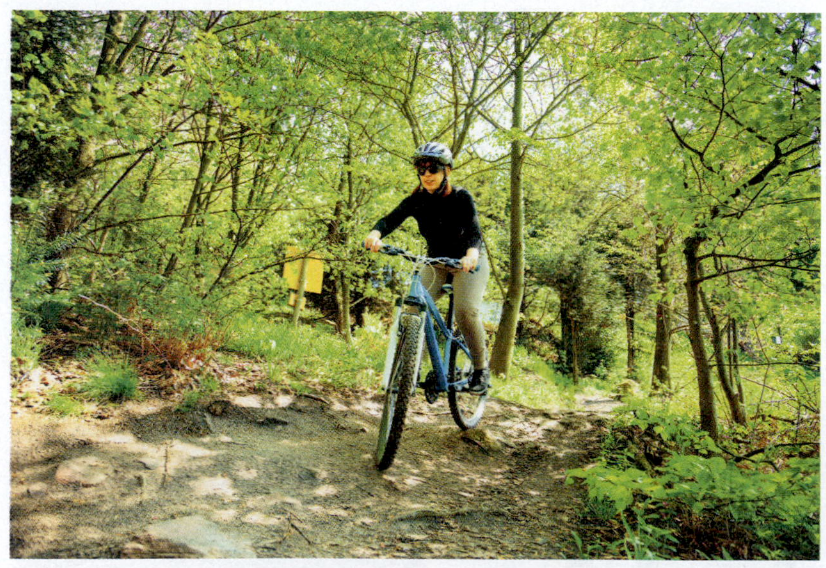

nullplus/Shutterstock.com

> **PHOTO 2-2** The *Dietary Guidelines* encourage Americans to increase the energy (kcalories) they expend through physical activity.

Note that the key recommendations also include encouragement to meet the *Physical Activity Guidelines for Americans*.[5] Some people might wonder why *dietary* recommendations refer to physical activity (see Photo 2-2). The simple answer is that most people who maintain a healthy body weight do

variety (dietary): eating a wide selection of foods within and among the major food groups.

TABLE 2-1 2015–2020 Dietary Guidelines for Americans: The Guidelines and Key Recommendations

The Guidelines

The following guidelines "encourage healthy eating patterns, recognize that individuals will need to make shifts in their food and beverage choices to achieve a healthy pattern, and acknowledge that all segments of our society have a role to play in supporting healthy choices."

1. **Follow a healthy eating pattern across the lifespan.** All food and beverage choices matter. Choose a healthy eating pattern at an appropriate kcalorie level to help achieve and maintain a healthy body weight, support nutrient adequacy, and reduce the risk of chronic disease.
2. **Focus on variety, nutrient density, and amount.** To meet nutrient needs within kcalorie limits, choose a variety of nutrient-dense foods across and within all food groups in recommended amounts.
3. **Limit kcalories from added sugars and saturated fats and reduce sodium intake.** Adopt an eating pattern low in added sugars, saturated fats, and sodium. Cut back on foods and beverages higher in these components to amounts that fit within healthy eating patterns.
4. **Shift to healthier food and beverage choices.** Choose nutrient-dense foods and beverages across and within all food groups in place of less healthy choices. Consider cultural and personal preferences to make these shifts easier to accomplish and maintain.
5. **Support healthy eating patterns for all.** Everyone has a role in helping to create and support healthy eating patterns in multiple settings nationwide, from home to school to work to communities.

Key Recommendations

The following key recommendations provide more detailed tips on how individuals can establish healthy eating patterns to meet the guidelines.

Adopt a healthy eating pattern that accounts for all foods and beverages within an appropriate kcalorie level.

A healthy eating pattern includes:

- A variety of vegetables from all of the subgroups—dark green, red and orange, legumes (beans and peas), starchy, and other.
- Fruits, especially whole fruits.
- Grains, at least half of which are whole grains.
- Fat-free or low-fat dairy, including milk, yogurt, cheese, and/or fortified soy beverages.
- A variety of protein foods, including seafood, lean meats and poultry, eggs, legumes (beans and peas), and nuts, seeds, and soy products.
- Oils.

A healthy eating pattern limits:

- Saturated fats and *trans* fats to less than 10 percent of kcalories per day.
- Added sugars to less than 10 percent of kcalories per day.
- Sodium to less than 2300 milligrams per day.
- If alcohol is consumed, it should be consumed in moderation—up to one drink per day for women and up to two drinks per day for men—and only by adults of legal drinking age.

Meet the *Physical Activity Guidelines for Americans* (https://health.gov/paguidelines).

NOTE: These guidelines and key recommendations are designed for individuals 2 years of age or older and should be applied in their entirety; they are interconnected, and each dietary component can affect the others.

SOURCE: U.S. Department of Health and Human Services and U.S. Department of Agriculture, *2015-2020 Dietary Guidelines for Americans*, 8th ed. (2015), https://health.gov/dietaryguidelines/2015/guidelines/.

more than just eat right. They also exercise—the equivalent of 30 to 60 minutes or more of moderately intense physical activity on most days. As you will see throughout this text, food and physical activity choices are integral partners in supporting good health, reducing the risk of chronic disease, and maintaining a healthy body weight.

Much controversy surrounded the release of the *2015–2020 Dietary Guidelines for Americans*. Most nutrition professionals applauded the work of the committee and its scientific report, but many objected to the final report, which had been substantially revised, claiming that those revisions reflected the special interests of food industries and politicians. Specific wording became vague and a new chapter on **sustainable diets** had been deleted. Food sustainability recognizes that foods and beverages have a large environmental impact—from farm to plate to waste—and that a sustainable food supply is essential to a healthy population and planet both for today and in the future. Many of those in the food industry opposed the inclusion of sustainability and convinced politicians that sustainability was outside the scope of providing dietary guidance. Such controversies remind us that food politics plays an ongoing role in defining nutrition policy and health recommendations.[6] The food labels illustrated in Figure 2-10 later in this chapter provide an example. Chapter 20 revisits the topic of food sustainability in its discussion of hunger and the environment.

sustainable diets: patterns of eating that promote health and provide food security for the present population while sustaining environmental resources for future generations.

REVIEW IT Explain how each of the diet-planning principles can be used to plan a healthy diet.

A well-planned diet delivers adequate nutrients, a balanced array of nutrients, and an appropriate amount of energy. It is based on nutrient-dense foods, moderate in substances that can be detrimental to health, and varied in its selections. The *Dietary Guidelines* apply these principles, offering practical tips on how individuals can establish healthy eating patterns by specifying which foods and food components to include and which to limit.

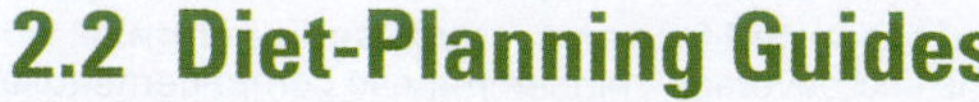

2.2 Diet-Planning Guides

LEARN IT Use the USDA Food Patterns to develop a meal plan within a specified energy allowance.

To plan a diet that achieves all of the dietary ideals just outlined, a person needs tools as well as knowledge. Among the most widely used tools for diet planning are **food group plans** that build a diet from clusters of foods that are similar in nutrient content. Thus each food group represents a set of nutrients that differs somewhat from the nutrients supplied by the other groups. Selecting foods from each of the groups eases the task of creating an adequate and balanced diet.

USDA Food Patterns The *Dietary Guidelines* encourage consumers to adopt a balanced eating pattern, using the USDA's Food Patterns. Eating patterns that follow USDA Food Patterns support good health—increasing life expectancy and reducing risks of chronic diseases. Notably, no one eating pattern is "the best."[7] Healthy eating patterns can be flexible enough to accommodate an individual's personal, cultural, and traditional preferences within a reasonable budget.

The USDA Food Patterns assign foods to five major groups—fruits, vegetables, grains, protein foods, and milk and milk products—and recommend daily amounts of foods from each group to meet nutrient needs. Figure 2-2 (pp. 42–43) presents the food groups, the most notable nutrients of each group, the serving equivalents, and the foods within each group. Chapter 16 provides a food guide for young children.

Recommended Amounts All food groups offer valuable nutrients, and people should make selections from each group daily. The amounts from each food group needed daily to create a healthful diet differ depending on a person's energy (kcalorie) needs. Energy needs, in turn, vary depending on a person's age, sex, height, weight, and level of physical activity. Table 2-2 presents estimated daily energy needs for sedentary adults; people who are more physically active need more kcalories per day (see Chapter 8 and Appendix F). Table 2-3 presents the recommended daily amounts from each food group for one of the USDA Food Patterns—the Healthy US-Style Eating Pattern. (Highlight 2 includes the Healthy Vegetarian Eating Pattern and Highlight 5 introduces the Healthy Mediterranean-Style Eating Pattern.) As Table 2-3 shows, an adult needing 2000 kcalories a day, for example, would select 2 cups of fruit; 2½ cups of vegetables; 6 ounces of grain foods; 5½ ounces of protein foods; and 3 cups of milk or milk products.* Additionally, a small amount of unsaturated oil, such as vegetable oil, or the oils of nuts, olives, or fatty fish, is required to supply needed nutrients.

All vegetables provide an array of nutrients, but some vegetables are especially good sources of specific nutrients. For this reason, the vegetable group is sorted into five subgroups. The dark-green vegetables deliver the B vitamin folate; the red and orange vegetables provide vitamin A; legumes supply iron and protein; the starchy vegetables contribute carbohydrate energy; and the other vegetables fill in the gaps and add more of these same nutrients.

*Milk and milk products also can be referred to as dairy products. Recommendations are based on age rather than on kcalorie level: 2 cups for children 2 to 3 years; 2½ cups for children 4 to 8 years; and 3 cups for older children, adolescents, and adults.

TABLE 2-2 Estimated Energy Needs for Sedentary Adults

	Energy (kcal/day)
Women	
19–25 yr	2000
26–50 yr	1800
51+ yr	1600
Men	
19–20 yr	2600
21–40 yr	2400
41–60 yr	2200
61+ yr	2000

NOTE: Sedentary describes a lifestyle that includes only the activities typical of independent living.

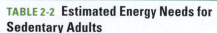

food group plans: diet-planning tools that sort foods into groups based on nutrient content and then specify that people should eat certain amounts of foods from each group.

TABLE 2-3 USDA Food Patterns: Healthy US-Style Eating Pattern

	1600 kcal	1800 kcal	2000 kcal	2200 kcal	2400 kcal	2600 kcal	2800 kcal	3000 kcal
Fruits	1½ c	1½ c	2 c	2 c	2 c	2 c	2½ c	2½ c
Vegetables	2 c	2½ c	2½ c	3 c	3 c	3½ c	3½ c	4 c
Grains	5 oz	6 oz	6 oz	7 oz	8 oz	9 oz	10 oz	10 oz
Protein foods	5 oz	5 oz	5½ oz	6 oz	6½ oz	6½ oz	7 oz	7 oz
Milk and milk products	3 c	3 c	3 c	3 c	3 c	3 c	3 c	3 c
Oils	5 tsp	5 tsp	6 tsp	6 tsp	7 tsp	8 tsp	8 tsp	10 tsp
Limit on kcalories available for other uses*	130 kcal	170 kcal	270 kcal	280 kcal	350 kcal	380 kcal	400 kcal	470 kcal

*The limit on kcalories for other uses describes how many kcalories are available for foods that are not in nutrient-dense forms; these kcalories may also be referred to as *discretionary kcalories* (discussed on p. 44).

In a 2000-kcalorie diet, then, the recommended 2½ cups of daily vegetables should be varied among the subgroups over a week's time. In other words, consuming 2½ cups of potatoes or even nutrient-rich spinach every day for seven days does *not* meet the recommended amounts for vegetables. Potatoes and spinach make excellent choices when consumed in balance with vegetables from the other subgroups. One way to help ensure selections for all of the subgroups is to eat vegetables of various colors—for example, green broccoli, orange sweet potatoes, black beans, yellow corn, and white cauliflower. Intakes of vegetables are appropriately averaged over a week's time—it is not necessary to include every subgroup every day.

For similar reasons, the protein foods group is sorted into three subgroups. Perhaps most notably, each of these subgroups contributes a different assortment of fats. Table 2-4 presents the recommended *weekly* amounts for each of the subgroups for vegetables and protein foods.

Notable Nutrients As Figure 2-2 notes, each food group contributes key nutrients. This feature provides flexibility in diet planning because a person can select any food from a food group (or its subgroup) and receive similar nutrients. For example, a person can choose milk, cheese, or yogurt and receive the same key nutrients. Importantly, foods provide not only these key nutrients, but small amounts of other nutrients as well.

Legumes contribute the same key nutrients—notably, protein, iron, and zinc—as meats, poultry, and seafood. They are also excellent sources of fiber, folate, and

legumes (lay-GYOOMS or LEG-yooms): plants of the bean and pea family, with seeds that are rich in protein compared with other plant-derived foods.

TABLE 2-4 Recommended Weekly Amounts from the Vegetables and Protein Foods Subgroups

Table 2-3 specifies the recommended amounts of total vegetables and protein foods per *day*. This table shows those amounts dispersed among five vegetable and three protein foods subgroups per *week*.

	1600 kcal	1800 kcal	2000 kcal	2200 kcal	2400 kcal	2600 kcal	2800 kcal	3000 kcal
Vegetable Subgroups								
Dark green	1½ c	1½ c	1½ c	2 c	2 c	2½ c	2½ c	2½ c
Red and orange	4 c	5½ c	5½ c	6 c	6 c	7 c	7 c	7½ c
Legumes	1 c	1½ c	1½ c	2 c	2 c	2½ c	2½ c	3 c
Starchy	4 c	5 c	5 c	6 c	6 c	7 c	7 c	8 c
Other	3½ c	4 c	4 c	5 c	5 c	5½ c	5½ c	7 c
Protein Foods Subgroups								
Seafood	8 oz	8 oz	8 oz	9 oz	10 oz	10 oz	10 oz	10 oz
Meats, poultry, eggs	23 oz	23 oz	26 oz	28 oz	31 oz	31 oz	33 oz	33 oz
Nuts, seeds, soy products	4 oz	4 oz	5 oz	5 oz	5 oz	5 oz	6 oz	6 oz

> FIGURE 2-2 USDA Food Patterns: Food Groups and Subgroups

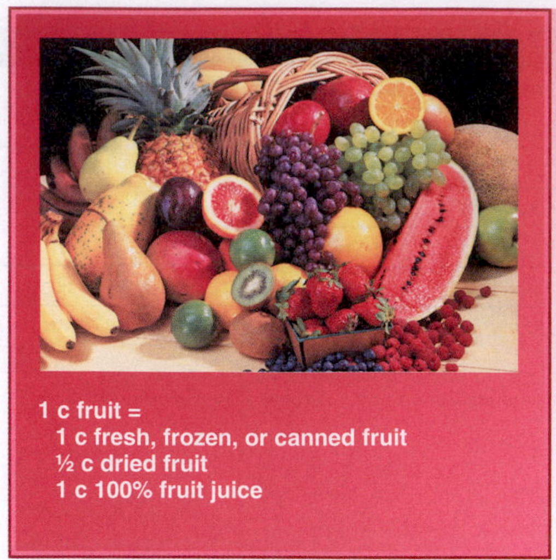

1 c fruit =
- 1 c fresh, frozen, or canned fruit
- ½ c dried fruit
- 1 c 100% fruit juice

Polara Studios Inc.

Fruits contribute folate, vitamin A, vitamin C, potassium, and fiber.

Consume a variety of fruits, and choose whole or cut-up fruits more often than fruit juice.

Apples, apricots, avocados, bananas, blueberries, cantaloupe, cherries, grapefruit, grapes, guava, honeydew, kiwi, mango, nectarines, oranges, papaya, peaches, pears, pineapples, plums, raspberries, strawberries, tangerines, watermelon; dried fruit (dates, figs, prunes, raisins); 100% fruit juices

Limit these fruits that contain solid fats and/or added sugars:
Canned or frozen fruit in syrup; juices, punches, ades, and fruit drinks with added sugars; fried plantains

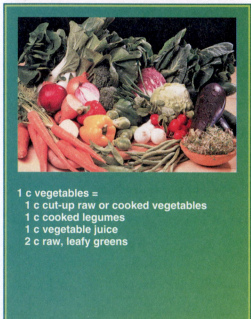

1 c vegetables =
- 1 c cut-up raw or cooked vegetables
- 1 c cooked legumes
- 1 c vegetable juice
- 2 c raw, leafy greens

Polara Studios Inc.

Vegetables contribute folate, vitamin A, vitamin C, vitamin K, vitamin E, magnesium, potassium, and fiber.

Consume a variety of vegetables each day, and choose from all five subgroups several times a week.

Dark-green vegetables: Broccoli and leafy greens such as arugula, beet greens, bok choy, collard greens, kale, mustard greens, romaine lettuce, spinach, turnip greens, watercress

Red and orange vegetables: Carrots, carrot juice, pumpkin, red bell peppers, sweet potatoes, tomatoes, tomato juice, vegetable juice, winter squash (acorn, butternut)

Legumes: Black beans, black-eyed peas, garbanzo beans (chickpeas), kidney beans, lentils, navy beans, pinto beans, soybeans and soy products such as tofu, split peas, white beans

Starchy vegetables: Cassava, corn, green peas, hominy, lima beans, potatoes

Other vegetables: Artichokes, asparagus, bamboo shoots, bean sprouts, beets, brussels sprouts, cabbages, cactus, cauliflower, celery, cucumbers, eggplant, green beans, green bell peppers, iceberg lettuce, mushrooms, okra, onions, seaweed, snow peas, zucchini

Limit these vegetables that contain solid fats and/or added sugars:
Baked beans, candied sweet potatoes, coleslaw, french fries, potato salad, refried beans, scalloped potatoes, tempura vegetables

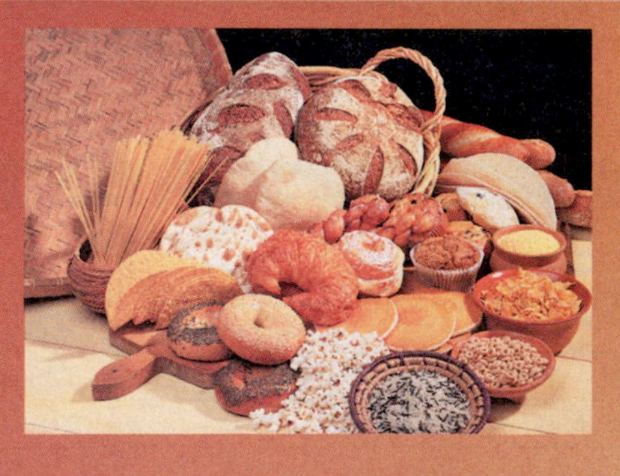

1 oz grains =
- 1 slice bread
- ½ c cooked rice, pasta, or cereal
- 1 oz dry pasta or rice
- 1 c ready-to-eat cereal
- 3 c popped popcorn

Polara Studios Inc.

Grains contribute folate, niacin, riboflavin, thiamin, iron, magnesium, selenium, and fiber.

Make most (at least half) of the grain selections whole grains.

Whole grains: amaranth, barley, brown rice, buckwheat, bulgur, cornmeal, millet, oats, quinoa, rye, wheat, wild rice and whole-grain products such as breads, cereals, crackers, and pastas; popcorn

Enriched refined products: bagels, breads, cereals, pastas (couscous, macaroni, spaghetti), pretzels, white rice, rolls, tortillas

Limit these grains that contain solid fats and/or added sugars:
Biscuits, cakes, cookies, cornbread, crackers, croissants, doughnuts, fried rice, granola, muffins, pastries, pies, presweetened cereals, taco shells

> FIGURE 2-2 USDA Food Patterns: Food Groups and Subgroups (*continued*)

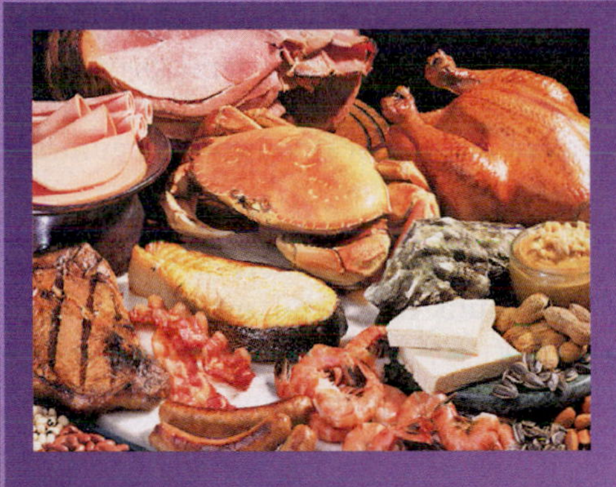

1 oz protein foods =
- 1 oz cooked lean meat, poultry, or seafood
- 1 egg
- ¼ c cooked legumes or tofu
- 1 tbs peanut butter
- ½ oz nuts or seeds

Polara Studios Inc.

Protein foods contribute protein, essential fatty acids, niacin, thiamin, vitamin B_6, vitamin B_{12}, iron, magnesium, potassium, and zinc.

Choose a variety of protein foods from the three subgroups, including seafood in place of meat or poultry twice a week.

Seafood: Fish (catfish, cod, flounder, haddock, halibut, herring, mackerel, pollock, salmon, sardines, sea bass, snapper, trout, tuna), shellfish (clams, crab, lobster, mussels, oysters, scallops, shrimp)

Meats, poultry, eggs: Lean or low-fat meats (fat-trimmed beef, game, ham, lamb, pork, veal), poultry (no skin), eggs

Nuts, seeds, soy products: Unsalted nuts (almonds, cashews, filberts, pecans, pistachios, walnuts), seeds (flaxseeds, pumpkin seeds, sesame seeds, sunflower seeds), legumes, soy products (textured vegetable protein, tofu, tempeh), peanut butter, peanuts

Limit these protein foods that contain solid fats and/or added sugars:
Bacon; baked beans; fried meat, seafood, poultry, eggs, or tofu; refried beans; ground beef; hot dogs; luncheon meats; marbled steaks; poultry with skin; sausages; spare ribs

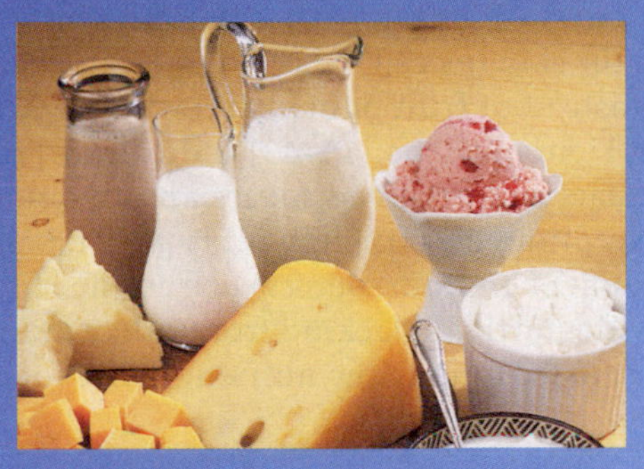

1 c milk or milk product =
- 1 c milk, yogurt, or fortified soy milk
- 1½ oz natural cheese
- 2 oz processed cheese

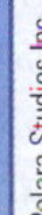
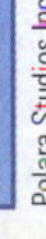

Polara Studios Inc.

Milk and milk products contribute protein, riboflavin, vitamin B_{12}, calcium, potassium, and, when fortified, vitamin A and vitamin D.

Make fat-free or low-fat choices. Choose other calcium-rich foods if you don't consume milk.

Fat-free or 1% low-fat milk and fat-free or 1% low-fat milk products such as buttermilk, cheeses, cottage cheese, yogurt; fat-free fortified soy milk

Limit these milk products that contain solid fats and/or added sugars:
2% reduced-fat milk and whole milk; 2% reduced-fat and whole-milk products such as cheeses, cottage cheese, and yogurt; flavored milk with added sugars such as chocolate milk, custard, frozen yogurt, ice cream, milk shakes, pudding, sherbet; fortified soy milk

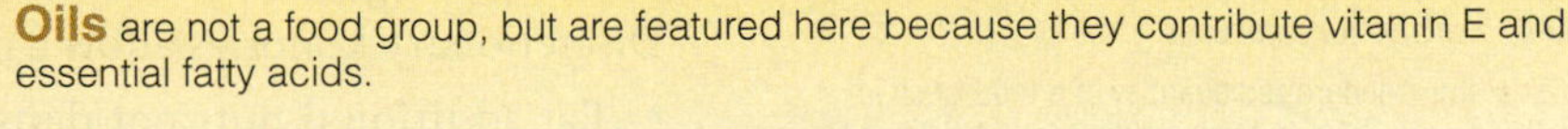

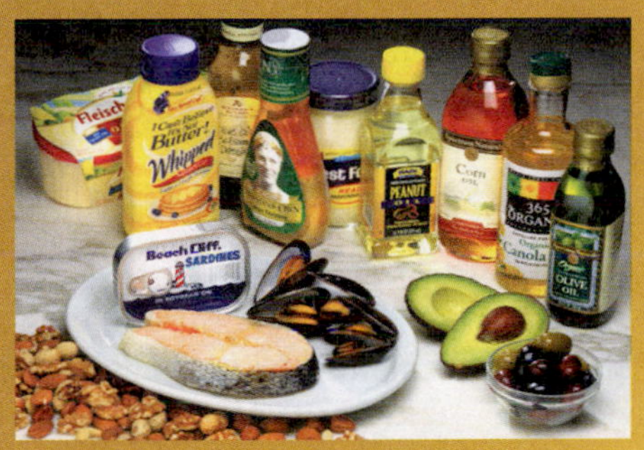

1 tsp oil =
- 1 tsp vegetable oil
- 1 tsp soft margarine
- 1 tbs low-fat mayonnaise
- 2 tbs light salad dressing

© Matthew Farruggio

Oils are not a food group, but are featured here because they contribute vitamin E and essential fatty acids.

Use oils instead of solid fats, when possible.

Liquid vegetable oils such as canola, corn, flaxseed, nut, olive, peanut, safflower, sesame, soybean, sunflower oils; mayonnaise, oil-based salad dressing, soft *trans*-fat-free margarine; unsaturated oils that occur naturally in foods such as avocados, fatty fish, nuts, olives, seeds (flaxseeds, sesame seeds), shellfish

Limit these solid fats:
Butter, animal fats, stick margarine, shortening

potassium, which are commonly found in vegetables. To encourage frequent consumption of these nutrient-rich foods, legumes are included as a subgroup of both the vegetable group and the protein foods group. Thus legumes can be counted in either the vegetable group or the protein foods group. In general, people who regularly eat meat, poultry, and seafood count legumes as a vegetable, and vegetarians and others who seldom eat meat, poultry, or seafood count legumes in the protein foods group.

The USDA Food Patterns encourage greater consumption from certain food groups to provide the nutrients most often lacking in the diets of Americans—dietary fiber, vitamin D, calcium, and potassium. In general, most people need to eat:

- *More* vegetables, fruits, whole grains, seafood, and milk and milk products.
- *Less* sodium, saturated fat, and *trans* fat and *fewer* refined grains and foods and beverages with solid fats and added sugars.

Nutrient-Dense Choices A healthy eating pattern emphasizes nutrient-dense options within each food group. By consistently selecting nutrient-dense foods, a person can obtain all the nutrients needed and still keep within kcalorie limits. In contrast, eating foods that are low in nutrient density makes it difficult to get enough nutrients without exceeding energy needs and gaining weight. For this reason, consumers should select nutrient-dense foods from each group and foods without solid fats or added sugars—for example, fat-free milk instead of whole milk, baked chicken without the skin instead of hot dogs, green beans instead of french fries, orange juice instead of fruit punch, and whole-wheat bread instead of biscuits. Notice that Figure 2-2 (pp. 42–43) indicates which foods *within each group* contain solid fats and/or added sugars and therefore should be limited. Oil is a notable exception: even though oil is pure fat and therefore rich in kcalories, a small amount of oil from sources such as nuts, fish, or vegetable oils is necessary to provide nutrients lacking from other foods. Consequently, these high-fat foods are listed among the nutrient-dense foods (see Highlight 5 to learn why).

Discretionary kCalories It takes a certain number of kcalories to keep our bodies functioning. Ideally, the foods providing those kcalories will also deliver all the nutrients needed to keep our bodies functioning optimally. People who consistently choose nutrient-dense foods may be able to meet their nutrient needs without consuming their full allowance of kcalories. Still, relatively few kcalories will be available for other uses; these kcalories may be referred to as **discretionary kcalories** (see Figure 2-3).

Discretionary kcalories allow a person to choose whether to:

- Eat additional nutrient-dense foods, such as an extra serving of skinless chicken or a second ear of corn.
    - Select a few foods with solid fats or added sugars, such as cheddar cheese or sweetened cereal.
    - Add a little fat or sugar to foods, such as butter or jelly on toast.
    - Consume some alcohol. (Highlight 7 explains why this may not be a good choice for some individuals.)

Alternatively, a person wanting to lose weight might choose to:

- *Not* use discretionary kcalories.

Table 2-3 (p. 41) includes these kcalories that are available for other uses, which reflect about 5 to 15 percent of total kcalories.

discretionary kcalories: the kcalories remaining in a person's energy allowance after consuming enough nutrient-dense foods to meet all nutrient needs for a day; also referred to as *kcalories available for other uses*.

serving sizes: the standardized quantity of a food; such information allows comparisons when reading food labels and consistency when following the *Dietary Guidelines*.

> FIGURE 2-3 Discretionary kCalories in a 2000-kCalorie Diet

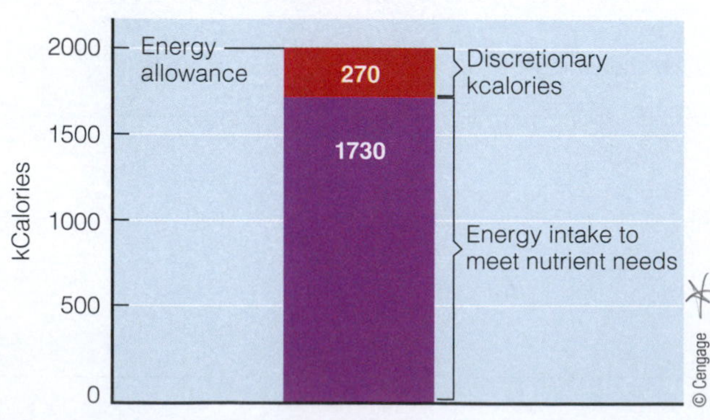

2000
1500
1000
500
0
kCalories
Energy allowance
270
1730
Discretionary kcalories
Energy intake to meet nutrient needs
© Cengage

Serving Equivalents Recommended serving amounts for fruits, vegetables, and milk are measured in cups, and those for grains and protein foods, in ounces. Figure 2-2 (pp. 42–43) provides the **serving sizes** and equivalent measures for foods in each group specifying, for example, that 1 ounce of grains is equivalent to 1 slice of bread or ½ cup of cooked rice.

Consumers using the USDA Food Patterns can learn how standard serving sizes compare with their personal **portion sizes** by determining the answers to questions such as these: What portion of a cup is a small handful of raisins? Is a "helping" of mashed potatoes more or less than a half cup? How many ounces of cereal do you typically pour into the bowl? How many ounces is the steak at your favorite restaurant? How many cups of milk does your glass hold? Photo 2-3 illustrates the difference between serving sizes and portion sizes.

Ethnic Food Choices People can use the USDA Food Patterns and still enjoy a diverse array of culinary styles by sorting ethnic foods into their appropriate food groups. For example, a person eating Mexican foods would find tortillas in the grains group, jicama in the vegetable group, and guava in the fruit group. Table 2-5 features some ethnic foods sorted into food groups.

Vegetarian Food Guide Vegetarian diets are plant-based eating patterns that rely mainly on grains, vegetables, legumes, fruits, seeds, and nuts. Some vegetarian diets include eggs, milk products, or both. People who do not eat meats or milk products can use the USDA Healthy Vegetarian Eating Pattern to create an adequate diet.[8] Highlight 2 defines vegetarian terms and provides details on planning healthy vegetarian diets.

Mixtures of Foods Some foods—such as casseroles, soups, and sandwiches—fall into two or more food groups. With a little practice, consumers can learn to see these mixtures of foods as items from various food groups. For example, from the

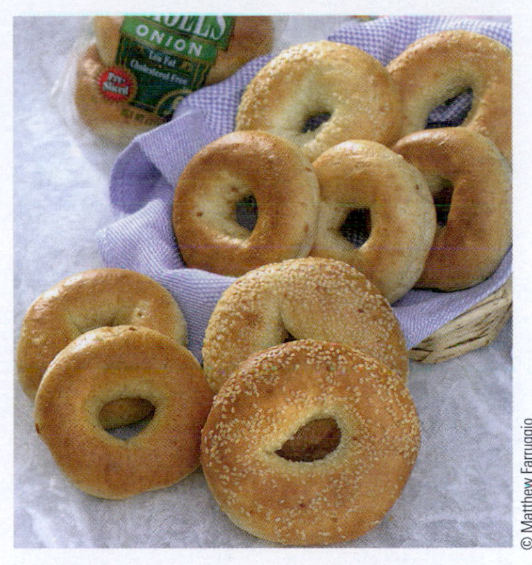

ONION

© Matthew Farruggio

> **PHOTO 2-3** Most bagels today weigh in at 4 ounces or more—meaning that a person eating one portion of these large bagels for breakfast is actually getting four or more grain servings, not one.

portion sizes: the quantity of a food served or eaten at one meal or snack; *not* a standard amount.

TABLE 2-5 Ethnic Food Choices

	Grains	Vegetables	Fruits	Protein Foods	Milk and Milk Products
Asian (Joshua Resnick/Shutterstock.com)	Rice, noodles, millet	Amaranth, baby corn, bamboo shoots, chayote, bok choy, mung bean sprouts, sugar peas, straw mushrooms, water chestnuts, kelp	Carambola, guava, kumquat, lychee, persimmon, melons, mandarin orange	Soybeans and soy products such as soy milk and tofu, squid, duck eggs, pork, poultry, fish and other seafood, peanuts, cashews	Usually excluded
Mediterranean (PhotoDisc/Getty Images)	Pita pocket bread, pastas, rice, couscous, polenta, bulgur, focaccia, Italian bread	Eggplant, tomatoes, peppers, cucumbers, grape leaves	Olives, grapes, figs	Fish and other seafood, gyros, lamb, chicken, beef, pork, sausage, lentils, fava beans	Ricotta, provolone, parmesan, feta, mozzarella, and goat cheeses; yogurt
Mexican (PhotoDisc/Getty Images)	Tortillas (corn or flour), taco shells, rice	Chayote, corn, jicama, tomato salsa, cactus, cassava, tomatoes, yams, chilies	Guava, mango, papaya, avocado, plantain, bananas, oranges	Refried beans, fish, chicken, chorizo, beef, eggs	Cheese, custard

> **FIGURE 2-4 MyPlate**

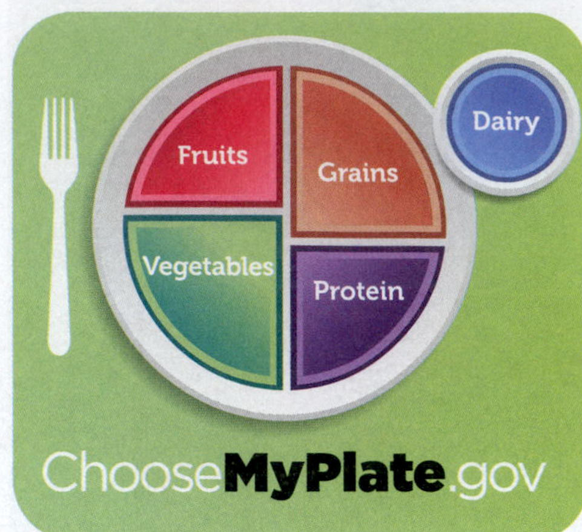
Dairy
Fruits
Grains
Vegetables
Protein
ChooseMyPlate.gov

SOURCE: USDA, www.choosemyplate.gov.

USDA Food Patterns point of view, a taco represents four different food groups: the taco shell from the grains group; the onions, lettuce, and tomatoes from the vegetables group; the ground beef from the protein foods group; and the cheese from the milk group.

MyPlate The USDA created an educational tool called MyPlate to illustrate the five food groups. Figure 2-4 shows the MyPlate icon, which was designed to remind consumers to make healthy food choices from all food groups.

The MyPlate icon divides a plate into four sections, each representing a food group—fruits, vegetables, grains, and protein foods. The sections vary in size, indicating the relative proportion each food group contributes to a healthy diet. A circle next to the plate represents the milk group (dairy).

The MyPlate icon does not stand alone as an educational tool. A wealth of information can be found at the website (www.choosemyplate.gov). Consumers can choose the kinds and amounts of foods they need to eat each day based on their height, weight, age, gender, and activity level. Information is also available for children, pregnant and breastfeeding women, and college students. In addition to creating a personal plan, consumers can find daily tips to help them improve their diet and increase physical activity. A key message of the website is to enjoy food, but eat less by avoiding oversized portions.

Recommendations versus Actual Intakes The USDA Food Patterns and MyPlate were developed to help people choose a balanced and healthful diet. Are consumers actually eating according to these recommendations? The short answer is "not really."[9] In general, consumers are not selecting the most nutrient-dense items from the food groups.[10] Instead, they are consuming too many foods high in solid fats and added sugars—soft drinks, desserts, whole milk products, and fatty meats. They are also not selecting the suggested quantities from each of the food groups, typically eating too few fruits, vegetables, whole grains, and milk products (see Figure 2-5).

> **FIGURE 2-5 Actual Intakes Compared with Recommended Intakes (100%)**

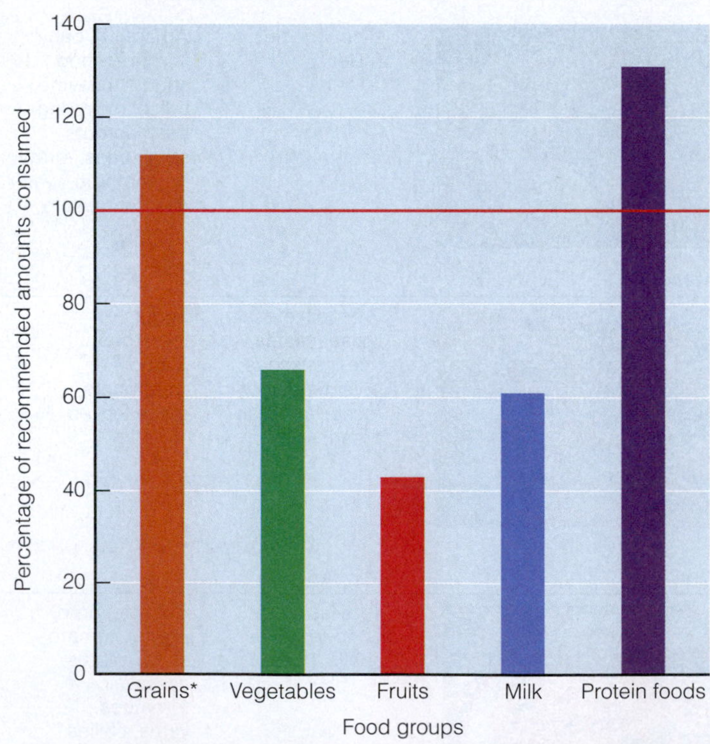
140
120
100
80
60
40
20
0
Percentage of recommended amounts consumed
Grains*
Vegetables
Fruits
Milk
Protein foods
Food groups

*Whole grains account for about 10 percent of grain servings.

SOURCE: U.S. Department of Health and Human Services and U.S. Department of Agriculture. 2015–2020 Dietary Guidelines for Americans. 8th ed. (December 2015), http://health.gov/dietaryguidelines/2015/guidelines/.

An assessment tool, called the **Healthy Eating Index,** can be used to measure how well a diet meets the recommendations of the *Dietary Guidelines*.[11] Various components of the diet are given scores that reflect the quantities consumed. For most components, higher intakes result in higher scores. For example, selecting at least 1.5 ounces of whole grains (per 1000 kcalories) gives a score of 5 points, whereas selecting no whole grains gives a score of 0 points. For a few components, lower intakes provide higher scores. For example, less than 0.7 grams of sodium (per 1000 kcalories) receives 10 points, but more than 2 grams gets 0 points. An assessment of recent nutrition surveys using the Healthy Eating Index reports that the American diet scores about 58 out of a possible 100 points.[12] To improve this score, the American diet needs to decrease kcalories from solid fats and added sugars; increase fruits, vegetables, and milk products; maintain the quantity of grains but shift the quality to more whole grains; and reduce salt. Eating patterns with high scores are associated with a lower risk of chronic diseases and mortality.[13]

MyPlate Shortcomings MyPlate is not perfect, and critics are quick to point out its flaws. The first main criticism is that MyPlate fails to convey enough information to help consumers choose a healthy diet. MyPlate contains few words and depends on its website to provide key information—which is helpful for those who have Internet access and are willing to take the time to become familiar with its teachings. The second main criticism is that MyPlate fails to recognize that some foods within a food group are healthier choices than others. For example, MyPlate does not distinguish between fish sticks and salmon or between broccoli and french fries. Many of the upcoming chapters examine the links between diet and health, and Chapter 18 presents a complete summary, including a look at an alternative Healthy Eating Plate created by the faculty members in the Harvard School of Public Health.

Food Lists

Food group plans are particularly well suited to help a person achieve dietary adequacy, balance, and variety. **Food lists**, formerly known as exchange lists, provide additional help in achieving kcalorie control and moderation. Originally developed as a meal planning guide for people with diabetes, food lists have proved useful for general diet planning and weight management as well.

Unlike the USDA Food Patterns, which sort foods primarily by their vitamin and mineral contents, the food lists group foods according to their energy-nutrient contents. Consequently, foods do not always appear on the food list where you might first expect to find them. For example, cheeses are grouped with meats on the protein list because, like meats, cheeses contribute energy from protein and fat but provide negligible carbohydrate. (In the USDA Food Patterns presented earlier, cheeses are grouped with milk because they are milk products with similar calcium contents.)

For similar reasons, starchy vegetables such as corn, green peas, and potatoes are listed with grains on the starch list in the food list system, rather than with the vegetables. Likewise, olives are not classed as a "fruit" as a botanist would claim; they are classified as a "fat" because their fat content makes them more similar to oil than to berries. Cream cheese, salt pork, and nuts are also on the fat list to remind users of their high fat content. These groupings highlight the characteristics of foods that are significant to energy intake. To learn more about this useful diet-planning tool, study Appendix G, which gives details of the 2014 publication *Choose Your Foods: Food Lists for Diabetes and Weight Management*.

Putting the Plan into Action

Familiarizing yourself with each of the food groups is the first step in diet planning. Table 2-6 (p. 48) shows how to use the 2000-kcalorie USDA Food Pattern to plan a diet. The amounts listed from each of the food groups (see the second column of the table) were taken from Table 2-3 (p. 41). The next step is to assign the food groups to meals (and snacks), as shown in the remaining columns of Table 2-6.

Healthy Eating Index: a measure that assesses how well a diet meets the recommendations of the *Dietary Guidelines for Americans*.

food lists: diet-planning tools that organize foods by their proportions of carbohydrate, fat, and protein; formerly known as *exchange lists*. Foods on any single list can be used interchangeably.

TABLE 2-6 Diet Planning Using the 2000-kCalorie USDA Food Pattern

This diet plan is one of many possibilities. It follows the amounts of foods suggested for a 2000-kcalorie diet as shown in Table 2-3 (p. 41), with a little less oil.

Food Group	Amounts	Breakfast	Lunch	Snack	Dinner	Snack
Fruits	2 c	½ c		½ c	1 c	
Vegetables	2½ c		1 c		1½ c	
Grains	6 oz	1 oz	2 oz	½ oz	2 oz	½ oz
Protein foods	5½ oz		2 oz		3½ oz	
Milk and milk products	3 c	1 c		1 c		1 c
Oils	6 tsp		1½ tsp		4 tsp	

© Cengage

At this point, a person can begin to fill in a plan with real foods to create a menu. For example, the breakfast calls for 1 ounce grain, ½ cup fruit, and 1 cup milk. A person might select a bowl of cereal with banana slices and milk:

1 cup cereal = 1 ounce grain

½ large banana = ½ cup fruit

1 cup fat-free milk = 1 cup milk

Or ½ English muffin and a bowl of strawberries topped with yogurt:

½ English muffin = 1 ounce grain

½ cup strawberries = ½ cup fruit

1 cup fat-free plain yogurt = 1 cup milk

Then the person can continue to create a diet plan by creating menus for lunch, dinner, and snacks. The final menu might look like the one presented in Table 2-7.

TABLE 2-7 A Sample Menu

This sample menu provides about 1850 kcalories and meets the recommendations to provide 45 to 65 percent of kcalories from carbohydrate, 20 to 35 percent from fat, and 10 to 35 percent from protein.

Amounts	Sample Menu	Energy (kcal)
	Breakfast	
1 oz whole grains	1 c whole-grain cereal	108
1 c milk	1 c fat-free milk	100
½ c fruit	1 medium banana (sliced)	105
	Lunch	
2 oz meats, 2 oz whole grains	1 turkey sandwich on whole-wheat roll	272
1½ tsp oils	1½ tbs low-fat mayonnaise	71
1 c vegetables	1 c vegetable juice	50
	Snack	
½ oz whole grains	4 whole-wheat reduced-fat crackers	86
1 c milk	1½ oz low-fat cheddar cheese	74
½ c fruit	1 medium apple	72
	Dinner	
½ c vegetables	1 c raw spinach leaves	8
¼ c vegetables	¼ c shredded carrots	11
1 oz meats	¼ c garbanzo beans	71
2 tsp oils	2 tbs oil-based salad dressing and olives	76
¾ c vegetables, 2½ oz meat, 2 oz enriched grains	Spaghetti with meat and tomato sauce	425
½ c vegetables	½ c green beans	22
2 tsp oils	2 tsp soft margarine	67
1 c fruit	1 c strawberries	49
	Snack	
½ oz whole grains	3 graham crackers	90
1 c milk	1 c fat-free milk	100

© Cengage

As you can see, we all make countless food-related decisions daily—whether we have a plan or not. Following an eating pattern that incorporates health recommendations and diet-planning principles helps a person make wise nutrition decisions.

From Guidelines to Groceries Dietary guidelines emphasize nutrient-dense foods such as whole grains, fruits, vegetables, lean meats, poultry, seafood, and low-fat milk products. You can design such a diet for yourself, but how do you begin? Start with the foods you regularly enjoy eating and then try to make a few improvements. For most people that will mean eating less red meat, cheeses, and salted snacks and more fruits, vegetables, whole grains, legumes, nuts, milk products, and seafood. Such changes can dramatically improve the diet. When shopping, think of the food groups, and choose nutrient-dense foods within each group.

Be aware that many of the tens of thousands of food options available today are processed foods that have lost valuable nutrients and gained sugar, fat, and salt as they were transformed from farm-fresh foods to those found in the bags, boxes, and cans that line grocery-store shelves. As Chapter 1 explains, their value in the diet depends on the original food and how extensively it was processed. Frozen corn, for example, is a minimally processed food that closely resembles farm-fresh corn on the cob in appearance, flavor, and nutrients. In contrast, caramel corn and corn chips are ultra-processed foods that have little in common with corn on the cob and deliver few nutrients and an abundance of sugar, fats, and salt. Such food choices have resulted in most of the US population exceeding the recommended limits for added sugars, saturated fats, and sodium (see Figure 2-6). By eating fewer ultra-processed foods and more fresh foods and minimally processed foods, consumers can reduce their intakes of added sugars, solid fats, and sodium for relatively little effort. Minimally processed foods that have been **fortified** to improve their nutrient contents can be helpful in increasing dietary intake of specific vitamins and minerals.

Grains When shopping for grain products, you will find them described as *refined*, *enriched*, or *whole grain*—terms that refer to the milling process and the making of grain products (see Figure 2-7, p. 50). **Refined** grains have lost many nutrients during processing; **enriched** grains have had some nutrients added back; and **whole-grain** products have all the nutrients and fiber found in the original grain.

> **FIGURE 2-6 Actual Intakes Compared with Recommended Intakes: Added Sugars, Saturated Fats, and Sodium**

Most of the US population exceeds the recommended limits for added sugars, saturated fats, and sodium. Each figure in the graph represents 10 percent of the population.

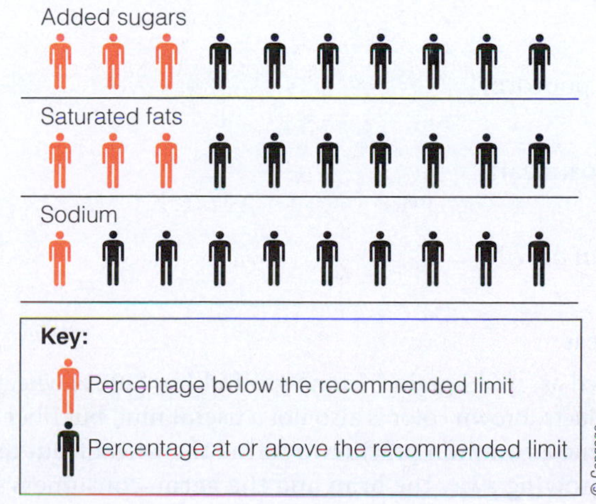
Added sugars
Saturated fats
Sodium
Key:
Percentage below the recommended limit
Percentage at or above the recommended limit
© Cengage

fortified: the addition to a food of nutrients that were either not originally present or present in insignificant amounts. Fortification can be used to correct or prevent a widespread nutrient deficiency or to balance the total nutrient profile of a food.

refined: the process by which the coarse parts of a food are removed. When wheat is refined into flour, the bran, germ, and husk are removed, leaving only the endosperm.

enriched: the addition to a food of specific nutrients to replace losses that occur during processing so that the food will meet a specified standard.

whole grain: a grain that maintains the same relative proportions of starchy endosperm, germ, and bran as the original (all but the husk); not refined.

> **FIGURE 2-7 A Wheat Plant**

The protective coating of **bran** around the kernel of grain is rich in nutrients and fiber.

The **endosperm** contains starch and proteins.

The **germ** is the seed that grows into a wheat plant, so it is especially rich in vitamins and minerals to support new life.

The outer **husk** (or **chaff**) is the inedible part of a grain.

Whole-grain products contain much of the germ and bran, as well as the endosperm; that is why they are so nutritious. Refined grain products contain only the endosperm. Even with nutrients added back, they are not as nutritious as whole-grain products, as shown in Figure 2-8 (p. 51).

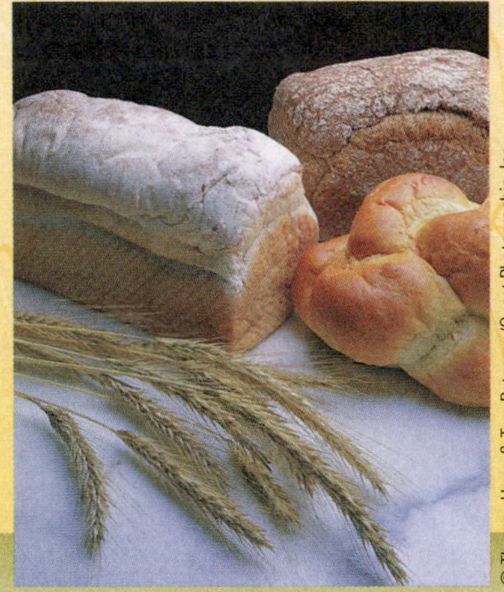

© Thomas Harm & Tom Peterson/Quest Photographic, Inc.

Common types of flour:

- **Refined flour:** finely ground endosperm that is usually enriched with nutrients and bleached for whiteness; sometimes called *white flour*.
- **Wheat flour:** any flour made from the endosperm of the wheat kernel.
- **Whole-wheat flour:** any flour made from the entire wheat kernel.

The difference between *white flour* and *white wheat* is noteworthy. Typically, *white flour* refers to refined flour (as defined above). Most flour—whether refined, white, or whole wheat—is made from red wheat. Whole-grain products made from red wheat are typically brown and full flavored.

To capture the health benefits of whole grains for consumers who prefer white bread, manufacturers use an albino variety of wheat called *white wheat*. Whole-grain products made from white wheat provide the nutrients and fiber of a whole grain with a light color and natural sweetness. Read labels carefully—white bread is a whole-grain product only if it is made from whole white wheat.

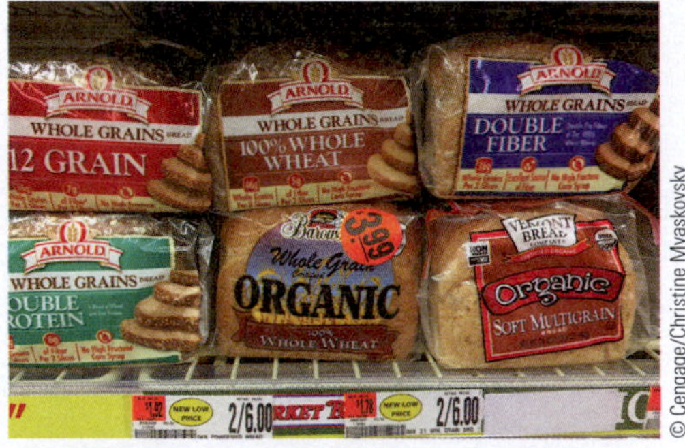
ARNOLD
WHOLE GRAINS
12 GRAIN
ARNOLD
WHOLE GRAINS
100% WHOLE WHEAT
ARNOLD
WHOLE GRAINS
DOUBLE FIBER
ARNOLD
WHOLE GRAINS
DOUBLE PROTEIN
ORGANIC
Organic
SOFT MULTIGRAIN
2/6.00
2/6.00

© Cengage/Christine Myaskovsky

> **PHOTO 2-4** When shopping for bread, look for the descriptive words *whole grain* or *whole wheat* and check the fiber content on the Nutrition Facts panel of the label—the more fiber, the more likely the bread is a whole-grain product.

As such, whole-grain products support good health and should account for at least half of the grains daily. Adding more whole grains to the diet can be as easy as eating oatmeal for breakfast and popcorn for a snack or substituting brown rice for white rice and whole-wheat bread for enriched white bread. To find whole-grain products, read food labels and select those that name a whole-grain first in the ingredient list (see Photo 2-4). Examples of whole grains include:

- Amaranth
- Barley
- Buckwheat
- Bulgur
- Corn (and popcorn)
- Millet
- Oats (and oatmeal)
- Quinoa
- Rice (brown or wild)
- Whole rye
- Whole wheat

Products described as "multi-grain," "stone-ground," or "100% wheat" are usually *not* whole-grain products. Brown color is also not a useful hint, but fiber content often is.

When it became a common practice to refine the wheat flour used for bread by milling it and throwing away the **bran** and the **germ**, consumers suffered a tragic

bran: the protective coating around the kernel of grain, rich in nutrients and fiber.

germ: the seed that grows into a mature plant, especially rich in vitamins and minerals.

loss of many nutrients. As a consequence, in the early 1940s Congress passed legislation requiring that all grain products that cross state lines be enriched with iron, thiamin, riboflavin, and niacin. In 1996, this legislation was amended to include folate, a vitamin considered essential in the prevention of some birth defects. Most grain products that have been refined, such as rice, pastas such as macaroni and spaghetti, and cereals (both cooked and ready-to-eat types), have subsequently been enriched. Food labels must specify that products have been enriched and include the enrichment nutrients in the ingredients list.

Even though the enrichment of flour helps prevent deficiencies of these added nutrients, it fails to compensate for the losses of many other nutrients and fiber. As Figure 2-8 shows, whole-grain items deliver many more nutrients than the enriched ones. Whole-grain products, such as brown rice and oatmeal, provide more nutrients and fiber and contain less salt, sugar, and fat than refined grain products, which helps explain why diet quality tends to be better for consumers who eat more whole grains.

Speaking of processed foods, ready-to-eat breakfast cereals are the most highly fortified foods on the market. Like an enriched food, a *fortified* food has had nutrients added during processing, but in a fortified food, the added nutrients may not have been present in the original product. (The terms *fortified* and *enriched* may be used interchangeably.) Some breakfast cereals made from refined flour and fortified with high doses of vitamins and minerals are actually more like dietary supplements disguised as cereals than they are like whole grains. They may be nutritious—with respect to the nutrients added—but they still may fail to convey the full spectrum of nutrients that a whole-grain food or a mixture of such foods might provide. Still, fortified foods help people meet their vitamin and mineral needs and improve the overall nutritional quality of diets.[14]

> **FIGURE 2-8 Nutrients in Bread**

Whole-grain bread is more nutritious than other breads, even enriched bread. For iron, thiamin, riboflavin, niacin, and folate, enriched bread provides about the same quantities as whole-grain bread and significantly more than unenriched bread. For fiber and the other nutrients (those shown here as well as those not shown), enriched bread provides less than whole-grain bread.

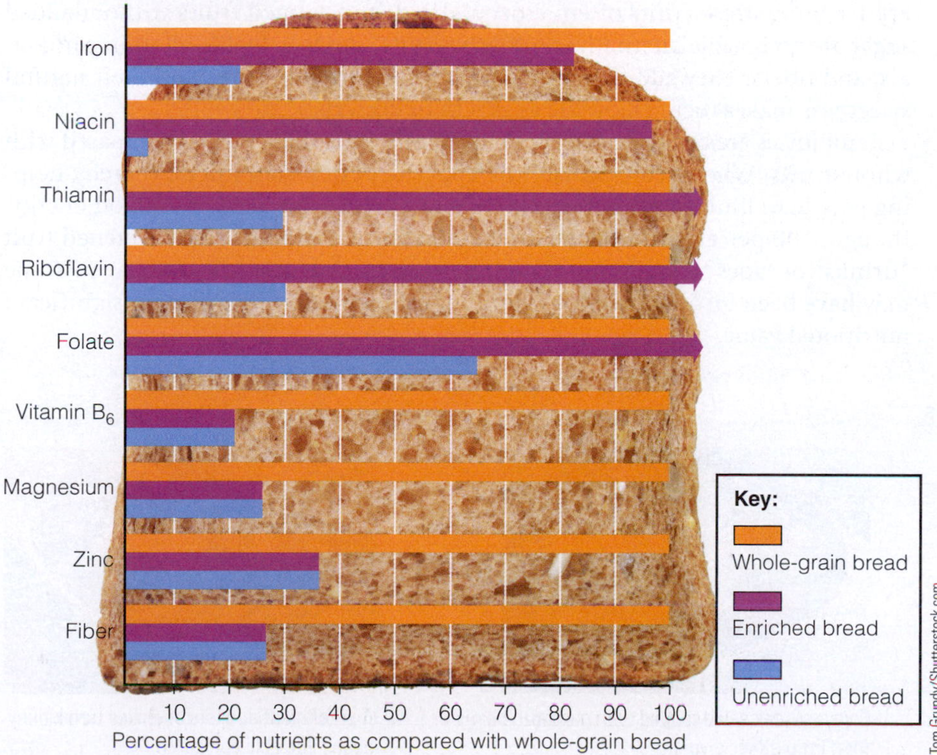

Iron
Niacin
Thiamin
Riboflavin
Folate
Vitamin B_6
Magnesium
Zinc
Fiber
10 20 30 40 50 60 70 80 90 100
Percentage of nutrients as compared with whole-grain bread
Key:
Whole-grain bread
Enriched bread
Unenriched bread

Tom Grundy/Shutterstock.com

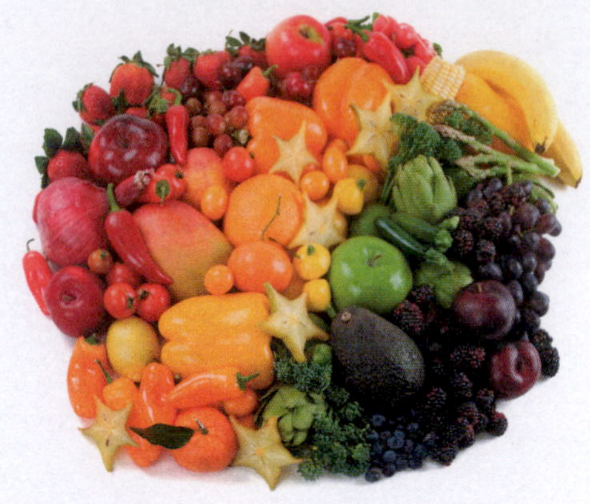

© iStock.com/kcline

> **PHOTO 2-5** Consumers can remember to eat a variety of fruits and vegetables every day by selecting from each of five colors.

Vegetables Posters in the produce section of grocery stores encourage consumers to "think variety, think color" (see Photo 2-5). Such efforts are part of a national educational campaign to increase fruit and vegetable consumption. Easy ways to effectively increase vegetable consumption include serving a variety of vegetables at meals, increasing the portion sizes, and adding pureed vegetables to recipes such as muffins or casseroles.

Choose fresh vegetables often, especially dark-green leafy and red and orange vegetables such as spinach, broccoli, tomatoes, and sweet potatoes. Cooked or raw, vegetables are good sources of vitamins, minerals, and fiber. Frozen and canned vegetables without added salt are acceptable alternatives to fresh. To control fat, energy, and sodium intakes, limit butter and salt on vegetables.

Choose often from the variety of legumes available:

- Adzuki beans
- Black beans
- Black-eyed peas
- Fava beans
- Garbanzo beans
- Great northern beans
- Kidney beans
- Lentils
- Lima beans
- Navy beans
- Peanuts
- Pinto beans
- Soybeans
- Split peas

Legumes are an economical, low-fat, nutrient- and fiber-rich food choice. Combining legumes with foods from other food groups creates delicious meals (see Figure 2-9).

Fruit Choose fresh fruits often. Frozen, dried, and canned fruits without added sugar are acceptable alternatives to fresh. Fruits supply valuable vitamins, minerals, and fibers. They add flavors, colors, and textures to meals, and their natural sweetness makes them enjoyable as snacks or desserts.

Fruit juices are healthy beverages but contain little dietary fiber compared with whole fruits. Whole fruits satisfy the appetite better than juices, thereby helping people to limit food energy intakes. For people who need extra food energy, though, 100 percent fruit juices are a good choice. Be aware that sweetened fruit "drinks" or "ades" contain mostly water, sugar, and a little juice for flavor. Some may have been fortified with vitamin C or calcium but lack any other significant nutritional value.

> **FIGURE 2-9 Meals Featuring Legumes**

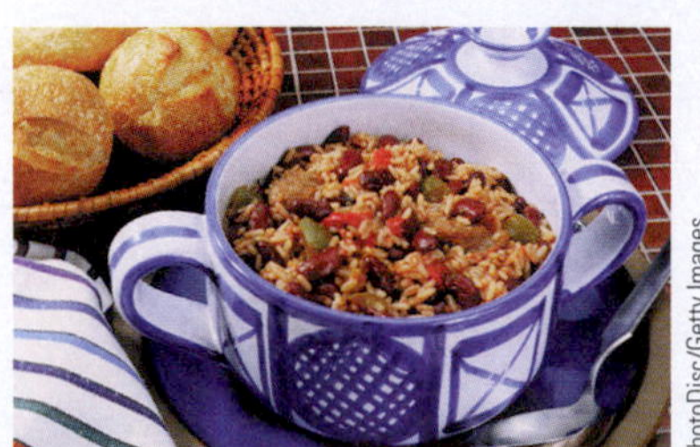

PhotoDisc/Getty Images

Add rice to red beans for a hearty meal.

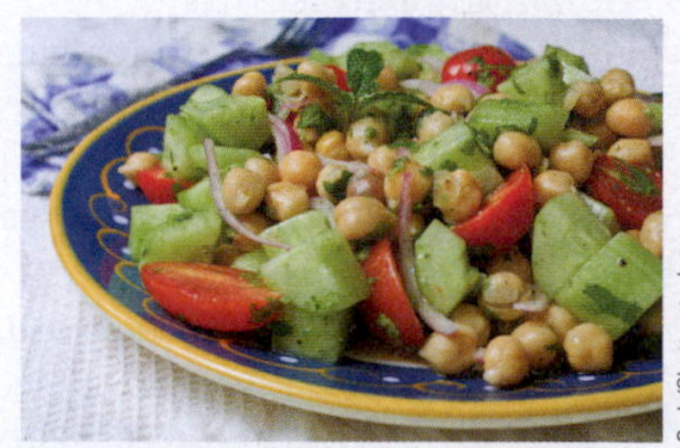

Cwb/Shutterstock.com

Enjoy a Greek salad topped with garbanzo beans for a little ethnic diversity.

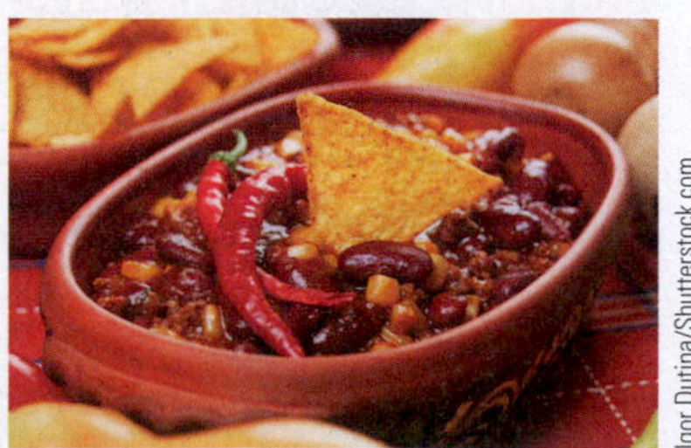

Igor Dutina/Shutterstock.com

A bit of meat and lots of spices turn kidney beans into chili con carne.

Protein Foods Protein foods include seafood, meats, poultry, eggs, legumes, soy products, nuts, and seeds. In addition to protein, these foods provide B vitamins, vitamin E, iron, zinc, and magnesium.

Serving sizes for meats, poultry, and seafood reflect weight after cooking and without bones. In general, 4 ounces of raw meat is equal to about 3 ounces of cooked meat. Some examples of 3-ounce portions include 1 medium pork chop, ½ chicken breast, or 1 steak or fish filet about the size of a deck of cards. When cooking meats, poultry, and seafood, bake, roast, broil, grill, or braise them (but do not fry them in fat); remove the skin from poultry after cooking; trim visible fat before cooking; and drain fat after cooking. Chapter 5 offers many additional strategies for making heart-healthy choices.

Milk and Milk Products Shoppers find a variety of fortified foods in the dairy case. Examples are milk, to which vitamins A and D have been added, and soy milk, to which calcium, vitamin D, and vitamin B_{12} have been added. Be aware that not all soy beverages have been fortified. Read labels carefully.

Milk is often described by its fat contents:

- Fat-free milk (also called nonfat, skim, zero-fat, or no-fat)
- Low-fat milk (also called 1% milk)
- Reduced-fat milk (also called 2% milk)
- Whole milk

When shopping, choose fat-free or low-fat milk, yogurt, and cheeses. Such selections help consumers meet their vitamin and mineral needs within their energy and saturated fat allowances.

REVIEW IT Use the USDA Food Patterns to develop a meal plan within a specified energy allowance.

Food group plans such as the USDA Food Patterns help consumers select the types and amounts of foods to provide adequacy, balance, and variety in the diet. They make it easier to plan a diet that includes a balance of grains, vegetables, fruits, protein foods, and milk and milk products. In making any food choice, remember to view the food in the context of the total diet. The combination of many different foods provides the array of nutrients that is so essential to a healthy diet.

2.3 Food Labels

LEARN IT Compare the information on food labels to make selections that meet specific dietary and health goals.

Many consumers, especially those interested in preventing chronic diseases, read food labels to help them make healthy choices. Food labels appear on virtually all packaged foods, and posters or brochures provide similar nutrition information for fresh fish, fruits, and vegetables. A few foods need not carry nutrition labels: those contributing few nutrients, such as plain coffee, tea, and spices; those produced by small businesses; and those prepared and sold in the same establishment. Markets selling nonpackaged items may voluntarily present nutrient information, either in brochures or on signs posted at the point of purchase.

Restaurants with 20 or more locations will provide menu listings of an item's kcalories, grams of saturated fat, and milligrams of sodium. In addition, kcalorie information will be provided for prepared foods and beverages at supermarkets, convenience stores, movie theaters, and vending machines. Other restaurants need not supply nutrition information for menu items unless claims such as "low-fat" or "heart healthy" have been made. When ordering from menus, keep in mind that restaurants tend to serve large portions—two to three times standard serving sizes. In general, most consumers support restaurant menu labeling and use the kcalorie information when making selections.[15] Menu labeling is especially helpful when comparing two unlike items—for example, a bacon cheeseburger with fettuccine Alfredo.[16]

The Ingredient List

All packaged foods must list *all* ingredients—including additives used to preserve or enhance foods, such as vitamins and minerals added to enrich or fortify products. The ingredients are listed on the label in descending order of predominance by weight. Knowing that the first ingredient predominates by weight, consumers can learn much about the product. Compare these products, for example:

- A beverage powder that contains "sugar, citric acid, natural flavors . . ." versus a juice that contains "water, tomato concentrate, concentrated juices of carrots, celery . . ."
- A cereal that contains "puffed milled corn, sugar, corn syrup, molasses, salt . . ." versus one that contains "100 percent rolled oats"
- A canned fruit that contains "sugar, apples, water" versus one that contains simply "apples, water"

In each of these comparisons, consumers can see that the second product is more nutrient dense.

The small type size and unfamiliar words on ingredients lists can overwhelm and confuse even the most conscientious consumer. One suggestion to ease decision making is to list the top three ingredients on the front of packages with a comment about how many total ingredients are in the product.[17] For example, a cereal might claim whole grain wheat, raisins, and wheat bran on the front of the box with the added comment "+5 more ingredients (see side panel for details)." Another cereal might claim sugar, corn flour blend, and wheat flour with the added comment "+18 more ingredients (see side panel for details)." Such an approach quickly shows consumers whether a cereal choice is mostly whole grain wheat or sugar and whether it is manufactured from fewer than 10, or more than 20, ingredients. In general, the longer the ingredient list, the more processed the product.

Food labels must also list the presence of common allergens in plain language, using the names of the eight most common allergy-causing foods. For example, a food containing "textured vegetable protein" must say "soy" on its label. Similarly, "casein" must be identified as "milk." Food producers must also prevent cross contamination during production and clearly label foods in which it is likely to occur. For example, equipment used for making peanut butter cookies must be scrupulously clean before being used to make oatmeal cookies; even then, the oatmeal cookie label warns consumers that this product "may contain peanuts" or "was made in a facility that uses peanuts."

Nutrition Facts Panel

The Nutrition Facts panel provides valuable nutrition information such as serving sizes, nutrient quantities, and Daily Values. Updated revisions to the nutrition facts panel reflect current nutrition science, actual serving sizes, and an improved design (see Figure 2-10).

Serving Sizes

Because labels present nutrient information based on one serving, they must identify the size of the serving. The Food and Drug Administration (FDA) has established serving sizes for various foods and requires that all labels for a given product use the same serving size. These serving sizes reflect typical eating habits, not recommended portion sizes. The proposed standard serving size for all ice creams, for example, is 2/3 cup. This facilitates comparison shopping. Consumers can see at a glance which brand has more or fewer kcalories or grams of saturated fat, for example.

When examining the nutrition facts on a food label, consumers need to compare the serving size on the label with how much they actually eat and

> FIGURE 2-10 Example of a Food Label

The original food label first appeared about 20 years ago; the updated label was approved and scheduled to be on the market by July 2018, but this deadline may be delayed.

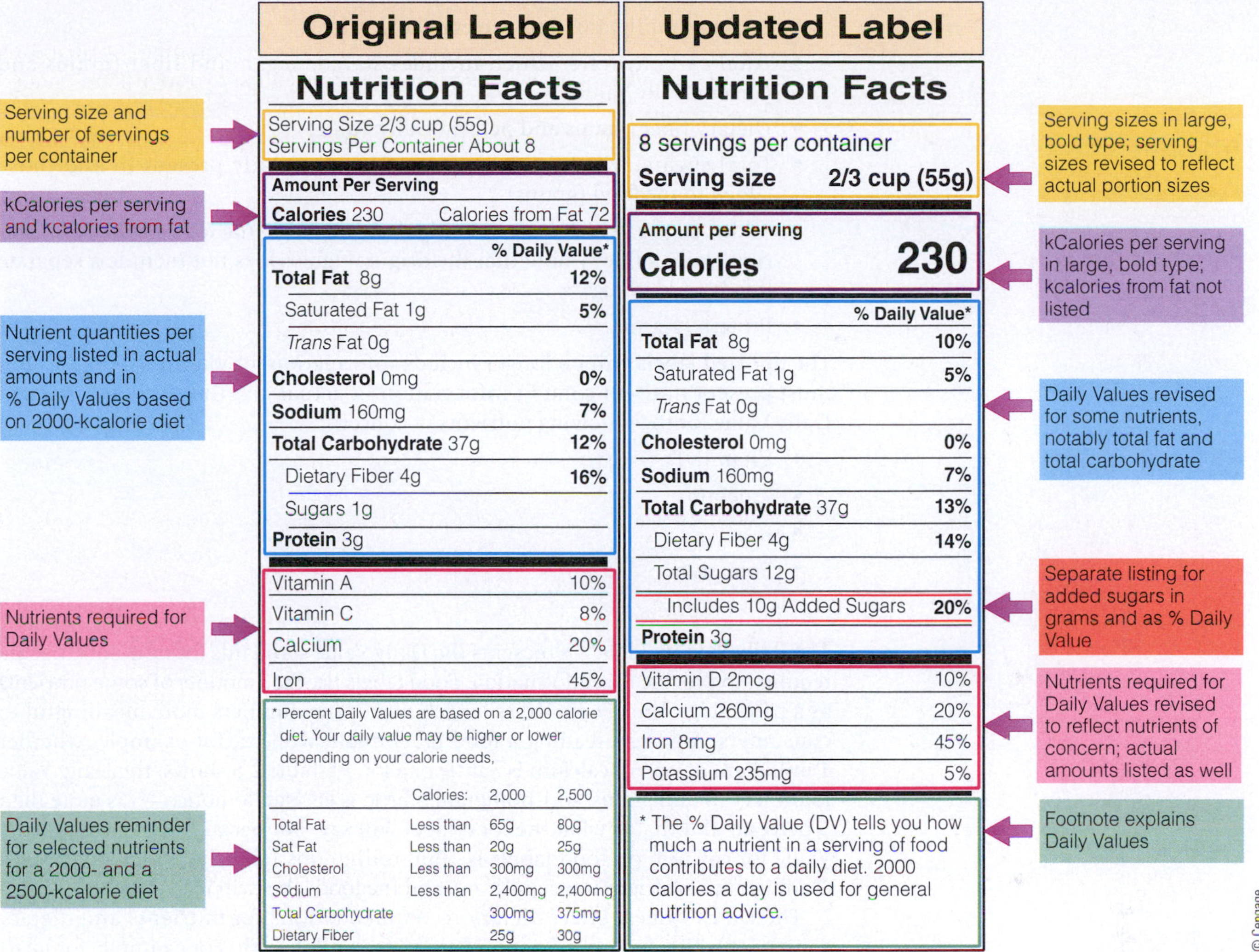

Original Label
Updated Label
Serving size and number of servings per container
kCalories per serving and kcalories from fat
Nutrient quantities per serving listed in actual amounts and in % Daily Values based on 2000-kcalorie diet
Nutrients required for Daily Values
Daily Values reminder for selected nutrients for a 2000- and a 2500-kcalorie diet
Nutrition Facts
Serving Size 2/3 cup (55g)
Servings Per Container About 8
Amount Per Serving
Calories 230 Calories from Fat 72
% Daily Value*
Total Fat 8g 12%
Saturated Fat 1g 5%
Trans Fat 0g
Cholesterol 0mg 0%
Sodium 160mg 7%
Total Carbohydrate 37g 12%
Dietary Fiber 4g 16%
Sugars 1g
Protein 3g
Vitamin A 10%
Vitamin C 8%
Calcium 20%
Iron 45%
* Percent Daily Values are based on a 2,000 calorie diet. Your daily value may be higher or lower depending on your calorie needs.
Calories: 2,000 2,500
Total Fat Less than 65g 80g
Sat Fat Less than 20g 25g
Cholesterol Less than 300mg 300mg
Sodium Less than 2,400mg 2,400mg
Total Carbohydrate 300mg 375mg
Dietary Fiber 25g 30g
Nutrition Facts
8 servings per container
Serving size 2/3 cup (55g)
Amount per serving
Calories 230
% Daily Value*
Total Fat 8g 10%
Saturated Fat 1g 5%
Trans Fat 0g
Cholesterol 0mg 0%
Sodium 160mg 7%
Total Carbohydrate 37g 13%
Dietary Fiber 4g 14%
Total Sugars 12g
Includes 10g Added Sugars 20%
Protein 3g
Vitamin D 2mcg 10%
Calcium 260mg 20%
Iron 8mg 45%
Potassium 235mg 5%
* The % Daily Value (DV) tells you how much a nutrient in a serving of food contributes to a daily diet. 2000 calories a day is used for general nutrition advice.
Serving sizes in large, bold type; serving sizes revised to reflect actual portion sizes
kCalories per serving in large, bold type; kcalories from fat not listed
Daily Values revised for some nutrients, notably total fat and total carbohydrate
Separate listing for added sugars in grams and as % Daily Value
Nutrients required for Daily Values revised to reflect nutrients of concern; actual amounts listed as well
Footnote explains Daily Values
© Cengage

adjust their calculations accordingly. For example, if the serving size is four cookies and you eat only two, then you need to cut the nutrient and kcalorie values in half; similarly, if you eat eight cookies, then you need to double the values. Packages, such as a 15-ounce can of soup, that contain more than one but less than two servings and are commonly eaten at one time will be labeled as one serving. For packages that contain two to four servings, food labels will present two columns, listing information both "per serving" and "per package." Such dual listings are particularly helpful for people who may consume the entire package in a single sitting. Examples include pints of ice cream and 20-ounce sodas.

Nutrient Quantities In addition to the serving size and the servings per container, the Nutrition Facts panel presents nutrient information in two ways—in quantities (such as grams) and as percentages of standards called the **Daily Values.** The proposed Nutrition Facts panel must provide the nutrient amount, **percent Daily Value,** or both for the following:

- Total food energy (kcalories)
- Total fat (grams and percent Daily Value)—note that the updated label does not include kcalories from fat

Daily Values (DV): reference values developed by the FDA specifically for use on food labels.

percent Daily Value (%DV): the percentage of a Daily Value recommendation found in a specified serving of food for key nutrients based on a 2000-kcalorie diet.

- Saturated fat (grams and percent Daily Value)
- *Trans* fat (grams)
- Cholesterol (milligrams and percent Daily Value)
- Sodium (milligrams and percent Daily Value)
- Total carbohydrate, which includes starch, sugar, and fiber (grams and percent Daily Value)
- Dietary fiber (grams and percent Daily Value)
- Total sugars, which includes both those naturally present in and those added to the food (grams)
- Added sugars, which includes only those added to the food (grams and percent Daily Value)—note that the original label does not include a separate line for added sugars
- Protein (grams)

The updated labels will no longer include information for vitamins A and C, but must present nutrient content information in actual amounts and as a percent Daily Value for the following nutrients of concern:

- Vitamin D
- Calcium
- Iron
- Potassium

The Daily Values Table 2-8 presents the Daily Value standards for nutrients that are required to provide this information. Food labels list the amounts of some nutrients as a percentage of its Daily Value, which makes the numbers more meaningful to consumers. A person reading a food label might wonder, for example, whether 1 milligram of iron or calcium is a little or a lot. As Table 2-8 shows, the Daily Value for iron is 18 milligrams, so 1 milligram of iron is enough to notice—it is more than 5 percent, and that is what the food label will say. But because the current Daily Value for calcium on food labels is 1000 milligrams (and the updated is 1300), 1 milligram of calcium is insignificant, and the food label will read "0%."

The Daily Values reflect dietary recommendations for nutrients and dietary components that have important relationships with health. For example, for heart health, consumers are advised to limit saturated fat to 10 percent of energy intake. For a 2000-kcalorie diet, 10 percent is 200 kcalories, or 22 grams of fat. (Remember that fats deliver 9 kcalories per gram.) As Table 2-8 shows, the Daily Value for saturated fat has been rounded down to 20 grams.

The "% Daily Value" column on a label provides a ballpark estimate of how individual foods contribute to the total diet. It compares key nutrients in a serving of food with the goals of a person consuming 2000 kcalories per day. A 2000-kcalorie diet is considered about right for sedentary younger women, active older women, and sedentary older men. Young children and sedentary older women may need fewer kcalories. By comparison, a 2500-kcalorie diet is considered about right for many men, teenage boys, and active younger women. People who are exceptionally active may have still higher energy needs.

People who consume 2000 kcalories a day can simply add up all of the "% Daily Values" for a particular nutrient to see if their diet for the day fits recommendations. People who require more or less than 2000 kcalories daily must do some calculations to see how foods compare with their personal nutrition goals. Those interested can use the Calculation Factors column on the insert (p. Y) or the suggestions presented in How To 2-2.

TABLE 2-8 Daily Values for Food Labels

Food labels must present the "% Daily Value" for these nutrients.

Nutrient	Original Daily Values	Updated Daily Values
Fat (total)	65 g	78 g
Saturated fat	20 g	20 g
Cholesterol	300 mg	300 mg
Sodium	2400 mg	2300 mg
Carbohydrate (total)	300 g	275 g
Fiber	25 g	28 g
Protein	50 g	50 g
Added sugars	—	50 g
Vitamin D	10 µg	20 µg
Calcium	1000 mg	1300 mg
Iron	18 mg	18 mg
Potassium	3500 mg	4700 mg

NOTE: Daily Values were established for adults and children aged 4 years and older and are based on an energy intake of 2000 kcalories a day. The %DV for protein is only required when a protein claim is made or the food is intended for young children.

> How To 2-2 Calculate Personal Daily Values

The Daily Values on food labels are designed for a 2000-kcalorie intake, but you can calculate a personal set of Daily Values based on your energy allowance. Consider a 1500-kcalorie intake, for example. To calculate a daily goal for fat, multiply energy intake by 30 percent:

$$1500 \text{ kcal} \times 0.30 \text{ kcal from fat} = 450 \text{ kcal from fat}$$

$$450 \text{ kcal from fat} \div 9 \text{ kcal/g} = 50 \text{ g fat}$$

Alternatively, a person can calculate that 1500 kcalories is 75 percent of the 2000-kcalorie intake used for Daily Values:

$$1500 \text{ kcal} \div 2000 \text{ kcal} = 0.75$$

$$0.75 \times 100 = 75\%$$

Then, instead of using 100 percent of the Daily Value, a person consuming 1500 kcalories will aim for 75 percent (or less, in this example). Similarly, a person consuming 2800 kcalories would use 140 percent:

$$2800 \text{ kcal} \div 2000 \text{ kcal} = 1.40 \text{ or } 140\%$$

> TRY IT Calculate the Daily Values for a 1800-kcalorie diet and revise the Daily Value percentages on one of the food labels found on p. 55.

Daily Values help consumers readily see whether a food contributes "a little" or "a lot" of a nutrient. For example, the "% Daily Value" column on a package of frozen macaroni and cheese may say 20 percent for saturated fat. This tells the consumer that each serving of this food contains about 20 percent of the day's allotted 20 grams of saturated fat. Be aware that for some nutrients (such as saturated fat and sodium) you will want to select foods with a low "% Daily Value" and for others (such as calcium and fiber) you will want a high "% Daily Value." To determine whether a particular food is a wise choice, a consumer needs to consider its place in the diet among all the other foods eaten during the day.

Daily Values also make it easy to compare foods. For example, a consumer might discover that frozen macaroni and cheese has a Daily Value for saturated fat of 20 percent, whereas macaroni and cheese prepared from a boxed mix has a Daily Value of 15 percent. By comparing labels, consumers can make informed decisions.

Front-of-Package Labels Some consumers find the many numbers on Nutrition Facts panels overwhelming. They want an easier and quicker way to interpret information and select products. Some food manufacturers responded by creating front-of-package labels that incorporate text, color, and icons to present key nutrient facts.[18] Without any regulations or oversight, however, different companies used a variety of different symbols to describe how healthful their products were. To calm the chaos and maintain the voluntary status of front-of-package labels, major food industry associations created a standardized presentation of nutrient information called Facts Up Front (see Figure 2-11). In general, consumers find front-of-package labeling to be a quick and easy way to select products.[19]

Claims on Labels

In addition to the Nutrition Facts panel, consumers may find various claims on food labels. These claims include nutrient claims, health claims, and structure-function claims.

> FIGURE 2-11 Facts Up Front

This example of front-of-package labeling (created by Grocery Manufacturers Association and the Food Marketing Institute) presents key nutrient facts.

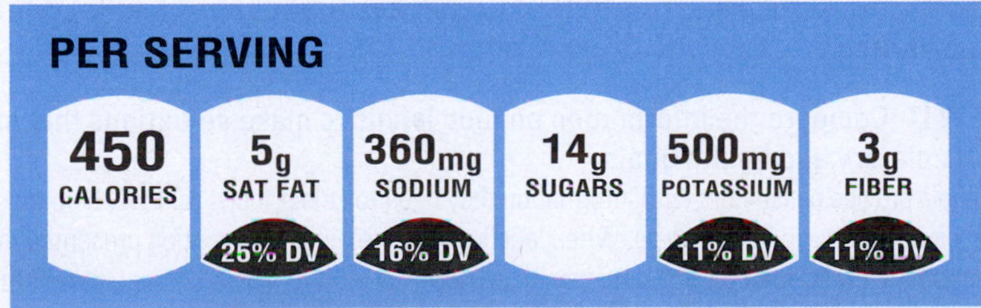
PER SERVING
450 CALORIES
5g SAT FAT 25% DV
360mg SODIUM 16% DV
14g SUGARS
500mg POTASSIUM 11% DV
3g FIBER 11% DV

Nutrient Claims Have you noticed phrases such as "good source of fiber" on a box of cereal or "rich in calcium" on a package of cheese? These and other **nutrient claims** may be used on labels so long as they meet FDA definitions, which include the conditions under which each term can be used. For example, in addition to having less than 2 milligrams of cholesterol, a "cholesterol-free" product may not contain more than 2 grams of saturated fat and *trans* fat combined per serving. Glossary 2-1 defines nutrient terms on food labels, including criteria for foods described as "low," "reduced," and "free." When nutrients have been added to enrich or fortify products, they must appear in the ingredients list.

Some descriptions *imply* that a food contains, or does not contain, a nutrient. Implied claims are prohibited unless they meet specified criteria. For example, a claim that a product "contains no oil" *implies* that the food contains no fat. If the product is truly fat-free, then it may make the no-oil claim, but if it contains another source of fat, such as butter, it may not.

Health Claims **Health claims** describe a relationship between a food (or nutrient) and a disease or health-related condition. In some cases, the FDA authorizes health claims based on an extensive review of the scientific literature. For example, the health claim that "Diets low in sodium may reduce the risk of high blood pressure" is based on enough scientific evidence to establish a clear link between diet and health. In cases where there is emerging—but not established—evidence for a relationship between a food or nutrient and disease, the FDA allows the use of *qualified* health claims that must use specific language indicating that the evidence supporting the claim is limited. A qualified health claim might read: "Very limited and preliminary research suggests that eating one-half to one cup of tomatoes and/or tomato sauce a week may reduce the risk of prostate cancer. The FDA concludes that there is little scientific evidence supporting the claim."

WavebreakMediaMicro/Fotolia LLC

> **PHOTO 2-6** Consumers can read food labels to learn about the nutrient contents of a food or to compare similar foods.

Structure-Function Claims Unlike health claims, which require food manufacturers to collect scientific evidence and petition the FDA, **structure-function claims** can be made without any FDA approval. Product labels can claim to "slow aging," "improve memory," and "build strong bones" without any proof. The only criterion for a structure-function claim is that it must not mention a disease or symptom. Unfortunately, structure-function claims can be deceptively similar to health claims, and most consumers do not distinguish between different types of claims.[20] Consider these statements:

- "May reduce the risk of heart disease"
- "Promotes a healthy heart"

The first is a health claim that requires FDA approval and the second is an unproven, but legal, structure-function claim. Figure 2-12 compares label claims.

Consumer Education

Food labels are a primary source of information for consumers trying to make healthy diet choices (see Photo 2-6), which is why FDA recently updated labels to place a bigger emphasis on total kcalories, added sugars, and nutrients of concern, such as vitamin D and potassium. In addition, the FDA has designed several programs to educate consumers. Consumers who understand how to read labels are best able to use the information to establish healthful eating patterns. Table 2-9 (p. 60) shows how the key recommendations from the *Dietary Guidelines*, the USDA Food Patterns, and food labels coordinate with one another.

nutrient claims: statements that characterize the quantity of a nutrient in a food.

health claims: statements that characterize the relationship between a nutrient or other substance in a food and a disease or health-related condition.

structure-function claims: statements that characterize the relationship between a nutrient or other substance in a food and its role in the body.

REVIEW IT Compare the information on food labels to make selections that meet specific dietary and health goals.

Food labels provide consumers with information they need to select foods that will help them meet their nutrition and health goals. When labels contain relevant information presented in a standardized, easy-to-read format, consumers are well prepared to plan and create healthful diets.

> **FIGURE 2-12 Label Claims**

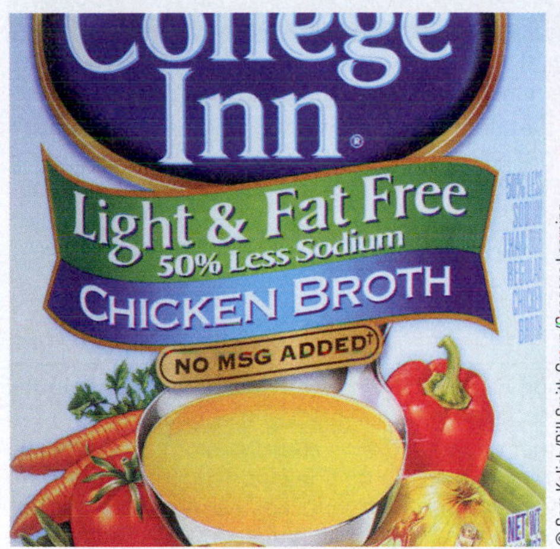
College Inn
Light & Fat Free
50% Less Sodium
CHICKEN BROTH
NO MSG ADDED

© Sam Kolich/Bill Smith Group/Cengage Learning

Nutrient claims characterize the level of a nutrient in the food—for example, "fat free" or "less sodium."

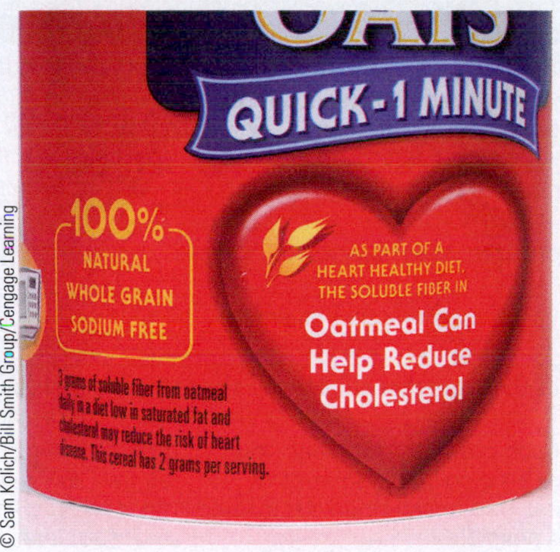
QUICK-1 MINUTE
100% NATURAL WHOLE GRAIN SODIUM FREE
AS PART OF A HEART HEALTHY DIET, THE SOLUBLE FIBER IN
Oatmeal Can Help Reduce Cholesterol

© Cengage

Health claims characterize the relationship of a food or nutrient to a disease or health-related condition—for example, "soluble fiber from oatmeal daily in a diet low in saturated fat and cholesterol may reduce the risk of heart disease" or "a diet low in total fat may reduce the risk of some cancers."

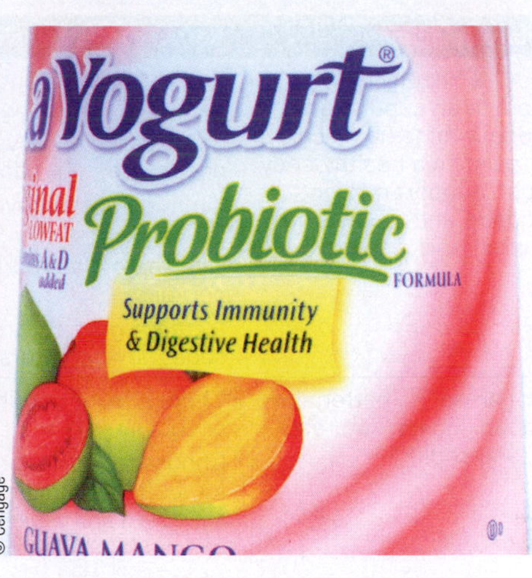
Yogurt
Probiotic
FORMULA
Supports Immunity & Digestive Health

© Sam Kolich/Bill Smith Group/Cengage Learning

Structure-function claims describe the effect that a substance has on the structure or function of the body and do not make reference to a disease—for example, "supports immunity and digestive health" or "calcium builds strong bones."

GLOSSARY 2-1
FOOD LABEL TERMS

GENERAL TERMS

free: "nutritionally trivial" and unlikely to have a physiological consequence; synonyms include *without, no,* and *zero.* A food that does not contain a nutrient naturally may make such a claim, but only as it applies to all similar foods (for example, "applesauce, a fat-free food").

gluten-free: a food that contains less than 20 parts per million of gluten from any source; synonyms include *no gluten, free of gluten,* or *without gluten.*

good source of: the product provides between 10 and 19 percent of the Daily Value for a given nutrient per serving.

healthy: a food that is low in fat, saturated fat, cholesterol, and sodium and that contains at least 10 percent of the Daily Values for vitamin D, potassium, iron, calcium, protein, or fiber.

high: 20 percent or more of the Daily Value for a given nutrient per serving; synonyms include *rich in* or *excellent source of.*

less: at least 25 percent less of a given nutrient or kcalories than the comparison food (see individual nutrients); synonyms include *fewer* and *reduced.*

light or lite: one-third fewer kcalories than the comparison food; 50 percent or less of the fat or sodium than the comparison food; any use of the term other than as defined must specify what it is referring to (for example, "light in color" or "light in texture").

low: an amount that would allow frequent consumption of a food without exceeding the Daily Value for the nutrient. A food that is naturally low in a nutrient may make such a claim, but only as it applies to all similar foods (for example, "fresh cauliflower, a low-sodium food"); synonyms include *little, few,* and *low source of.*

more: at least 10 percent more of the Daily Value for a given nutrient than the comparison food; synonyms include *added* and *extra.*

organic: on food labels, that at least 95 percent of the product's ingredients have been grown and processed according to USDA regulations defining the use of fertilizers, herbicides, insecticides, fungicides, preservatives, and other chemical ingredients.

ENERGY

kcalorie-free: fewer than 5 kcalories per serving.

low kcalorie: 40 kcalories or less per serving.

reduced kcalorie: at least 25 percent fewer kcalories per serving than the comparison food.

FAT AND CHOLESTEROL[a]

cholesterol-free: less than 2 milligrams of cholesterol per serving and 2 grams or less of saturated fat and *trans* fat combined per serving.

extra lean: less than 5 grams of fat, 2 grams of saturated fat and *trans* fat combined, and 95 milligrams of cholesterol per serving and per 100 grams of meat, poultry, and seafood.

lean: less than 10 grams of fat, 4.5 grams of saturated fat and *trans* fat combined, and 95 milligrams of cholesterol per serving and per 100 grams of meat, poultry, and seafood. For mixed dishes such as burritos and sandwiches, less than 8 grams of fat, 3.5 grams of saturated fat, and 80 milligrams of cholesterol per reference amount customarily consumed.

fat-free: less than 0.5 gram of fat per serving (and no added fat or oil); synonyms include *zero-fat, no-fat,* and *nonfat.*

less cholesterol: 25 percent or less cholesterol than the comparison food (reflecting a reduction of at least 20 milligrams per serving), and 2 grams or less of saturated fat and *trans* fat combined per serving.

less fat: 25 percent or less fat than the comparison food.

less saturated fat: 25 percent or less of saturated fat and *trans* fat combined than the comparison food.

low cholesterol: 20 milligrams or less of cholesterol per serving and 2 grams or less of saturated fat and *trans* fat combined per serving.

low fat: 3 grams or less of fat per serving.

low saturated fat: 1 gram or less of saturated fat and less than 0.5 gram of *trans* fat per serving.

percent fat-free: may be used only if the product meets the definition of *low fat* or *fat-free* and must reflect the amount of fat in 100 grams (for example, a food that contains 2.5 grams of fat per 50 grams can claim to be "95 percent fat-free").

saturated fat-free: less than 0.5 gram saturated fat and 0.5 gram of *trans* fat per serving.

***trans* fat-free:** less than 0.5 gram of *trans* fat and less than 0.5 gram of saturated fat per serving.

CARBOHYDRATES: FIBER AND SUGAR

high fiber: 5 grams or more of fiber per serving. A high-fiber claim made on a food that contains more than 3 grams of fat per serving and per 100 grams of food must also declare total fat.

sugar-free: less than 0.5 gram of sugar per serving.

SODIUM

low sodium: 140 milligrams or less per serving.

sodium-free and **salt-free:** less than 5 milligrams of sodium per serving.

very low sodium: 35 milligrams or less per serving.

[a]Foods containing more than 13 grams of total fat per serving or per 50 grams of food must indicate those contents immediately after a cholesterol claim. As you can see, all cholesterol claims are prohibited when the food contains more than 2 grams of saturated fat and *trans* fat combined per serving.

TABLE 2-9 From Guidelines to Groceries

Dietary Guidelines	USDA Food Patterns/MyPlate	Food Labels
Choose a healthy eating pattern at an appropriate kcalorie level to help achieve and maintain a healthy body weight, support nutrient adequacy, and reduce the risk of chronic disease.	Enjoy your food, but eat less. Select the recommended amounts from each food group at the energy level appropriate for your energy needs; meet, but do not exceed, energy needs. Limit foods and beverages with solid fats and added sugars. Use appropriate portion sizes; avoid oversized portions. Increase physical activity and reduce time spent in sedentary behaviors.	Read the Nutrition Facts to see how many kcalories are in a serving and the number of servings that are in a package. Look for foods that describe their kcalorie contents as *free, low, reduced, light*, or *less*.
Adopt an eating pattern low in added sugars, saturated fats, and sodium.	Choose foods within each group that are low in salt or sodium. Choose foods within each group that are lean, low fat, or fat free and have little solid fat (sources of saturated and *trans* fats); use unsaturated oils instead of solid fats whenever possible. Choose foods and beverages within each group that have little added sugars; drink water instead of sugary beverages. If alcohol is consumed by adults, use in moderation (no more than one drink a day for women and two drinks a day for men).	Read the Nutrition Facts to see how much sodium, saturated fat, *trans* fat, and cholesterol is in a serving of food. Look for foods that describe their salt and sodium contents as *free, low*, or *reduced*; foods that describe their saturated fat, *trans* fat, and cholesterol contents as *free, less, low, light, reduced, lean*, or *extra lean;* foods that describe their added sugar contents as *free* or *reduced*. Look for foods that provide no more than 5 percent of the Daily Value for sodium, saturated fat, and cholesterol. A food may be high in solid fats if its ingredients list begins with or contains several of the following: *beef fat (tallow, suet), butter, chicken fat, coconut oil, cream, hydrogenated oils, palm kernel oil, palm oil, partially hydrogenated oils, pork fat (lard), shortening*, or *stick margarine*. A food most likely contains trans fats if its ingredients list includes: *partially hydrogenated oils*. A food may be high in added sugars if its ingredients list begins with or contains several of the following: *brown sugar, confectioner's powdered sugar, corn syrup, dextrin, fructose, high-fructose corn syrup, honey, invert sugar, lactose, malt syrup, maltose, molasses, nectars, sucrose, sugar*, or *syrup*. Light beverages contain fewer kcalories and less alcohol than regular versions.
To meet nutrient needs within kcalorie limits, choose a variety of nutrient-dense foods across and within all food groups in recommended amounts.	Make half your plate fruits and vegetables. Choose a variety of vegetables from all five subgroups (dark green, red and orange, legumes, starchy vegetables, and other vegetables) several times a week. Choose a variety of fruits; consume whole or cut-up fruits more often than fruit juice. Choose potassium-rich foods such as fruits and vegetables often. Choose fiber-rich fruits, vegetables, and whole grains often. Choose whole grains; make at least half of the grain selections whole grains by replacing refined grains with whole grains whenever possible. Choose fat-free or low-fat milk and milk products. Choose a variety of protein foods; increase the amount and variety of seafood by choosing seafood in place of some meat and poultry.	Look for foods that describe their fiber, calcium, potassium, iron, and vitamin D contents as *good, high*, or *excellent*. Look for foods that provide at least 10 percent of the Daily Value for fiber, calcium, potassium, iron, and vitamin D from a variety of sources. A food may be a good source of whole grains if its ingredients list begins with or contains several of the following: *barley, brown rice, buckwheat, bulgur, corn, millet, oatmeal, popcorn, quinoa, rolled oats, rye, sorghum, triticale, whole wheat*, or *wild rice*.
Choose nutrient-dense foods and beverages across and within all food groups in place of less-healthy choices.	Select nutrient-dense foods and beverages within and among the food groups. Keep foods safe.	Look for foods that describe their vitamin, mineral, or fiber contents as a *good source* or *high*. Follow the *safe handling instructions* on packages of meat and other safety instructions, such as *keep refrigerated*, on packages of perishable foods.

This chapter provides practical information on implementing the dietary guidelines and offers helpful tips for selecting nutritious foods. For additional information on foods, including organic foods, irradiated foods, genetically modified foods, and more, turn to Chapter 19.

What's Online

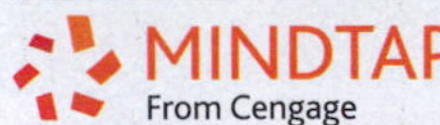

Visit **www.cengagebrain.com** to access MindTap, a complete digital course that includes Diet & Wellness Plus, interactive quizzes, videos, and more.

REFERENCES

1. Position of the Academy of Nutrition and Dietetics: Total diet approach to healthy eating, *Journal of the Academy of Nutrition and Dietetics* 113 (2013): 307–317.
2. Practice paper of the Academy of Nutrition and Dietetics: Selecting nutrient-dense foods for good health, *Journal of the Academy of Nutrition and Dietetics* 116 (2016): 1473–1479.
3. A. Drewnowski and V. L. Fulgoni III, Nutrient density: Principles and evaluation tools, *American Journal of Clinical Nutrition* 99 (2014): 1223S–1228S.
4. U.S. Department of Health and Human Services and U.S. Department of Agriculture, *2015–2020 Dietary Guidelines for Americans*, 8th ed. (2015): health.gov/dietaryguidelines/2015/guidelines/.
5. US Department of Health and Human Services, *Physical Activity Guidelines*, https://www.health.gov/paguidelines.
6. Marion Nestle, *Food Politics: How the Food Industry Influences Nutrition and Health* (University of California Press, 2007), www.foodpolitics.com.
7. K. L. Katz and S. Meller, Can we say what diet is best for health? *Annual Review of Public Health* 35 (2014): 83–103.
8. Position of the Academy of Nutrition and Dietetics, Vegetarian diets, *Journal of the Academy of Nutrition and Dietetics* 116 (2016): 1970–1980; U.S. Department of Health and Human Services and U.S. Department of Agriculture, *2015–2020 Dietary Guidelines for Americans*, 8th ed. (2015), http://health.gov/dietaryguidelines/2015/guidelines.
9. M. M. Wilson, J. Reedy, and S. M. Krebs-Smith, American diet quality: Where it is, where it is heading, and what it could be, *Journal of the Academy of Nutrition and Dietetics* 116 (2016): 302–310; S. A. Haack and C. J. Byker, Recent population adherence to and knowledge of United States federal nutrition guides, 1992–2013: A systematic review, *Nutrition Reviews* 72 (2014): 613–626.
10. P. Britten and coauthors, Impact of typical rather than nutrient-dense food choices in the US Department of Agriculture food patterns, *Journal of the Academy of Nutrition and Dietetics* 112 (2012): 1560–1569.
11. P. M. Guenther and coauthors, Update of the Healthy Eating Index: HEI-2010, *Journal of the Academy of Nutrition and Dietetics* 113 (2013): 569–580.
12. Analyses of *What We Eat in America, National Health and Nutrition Examination Survey (NHANES)* data from 1999-2000 through 2009-2010 as published in U.S. Department of Health and Human Services and U.S. Department of Agriculture, *2015–2020 Dietary Guidelines for Americans*, 8th ed. (2015), http://health.gov/dietaryguidelines/2015/guidelines.
13. B. E. Harmon and coauthors, Associations of key diet-quality indexes with mortality in the Multiethnic Cohort: The Dietary Patterns Methods Project, *American Journal of Clinical Nutrition* 101 (2015): 587–597; J. Mursu and coauthors, Diet quality indexes and mortality in postmenopausal women: The Iowa Women's Health Study, *American Journal of Clinical Nutrition* 98 (2013): 444–453.
14. J. T. Dwyer and coauthors, Fortification: New findings and implications, *Nutrition Reviews* 72 (2014): 127–141.
15. S. H. Lee-Kwan and coauthors, Restaurant menu labeling use among adults—17 states, 2012, *Morbidity and Mortality Weekly Report* 63 (2014): 581–584; J. P. Block and C. A. Roberto, Potential benefits of calorie labeling in restaurants, *Journal of the American Medical Association* 312 (2014): 887–888.
16. H. Stewart, J. Hyman, and D. Dong, *Menu Labeling Imparts New Information About the Calorie Content of Restaurant Foods*, ERR-179. Washington, DC: US Department of Agriculture, Economic Research Service, December 2014.
17. D. A. Kessler, Toward more comprehensive food labeling, *New England Journal of Medicine* 371 (2014): 193–195.
18. J. C. Hersey and coauthors, Effects of front-of-package and shelf nutrition labeling systems on consumers, *Nutrition Reviews* 71 (2013): 1–14.
19. M. S. Edge and coauthors, The impact of variations in a fact-based front-of-package nutrition labeling system on consumer comprehension, *Journal of the Academy of Nutrition and Dietetics* 114 (2014): 843–854.
20. C. L. Wong and coauthors, Consumer attitudes and understanding of low-sodium claims on food: An analysis of healthy and hypertensive individuals, *American Journal of Clinical Nutrition* 97 (2013): 1288–1298.

HIGHLIGHT > 2

LEARN IT Develop a well-balanced vegetarian meal plan.

Vegetarian Diets

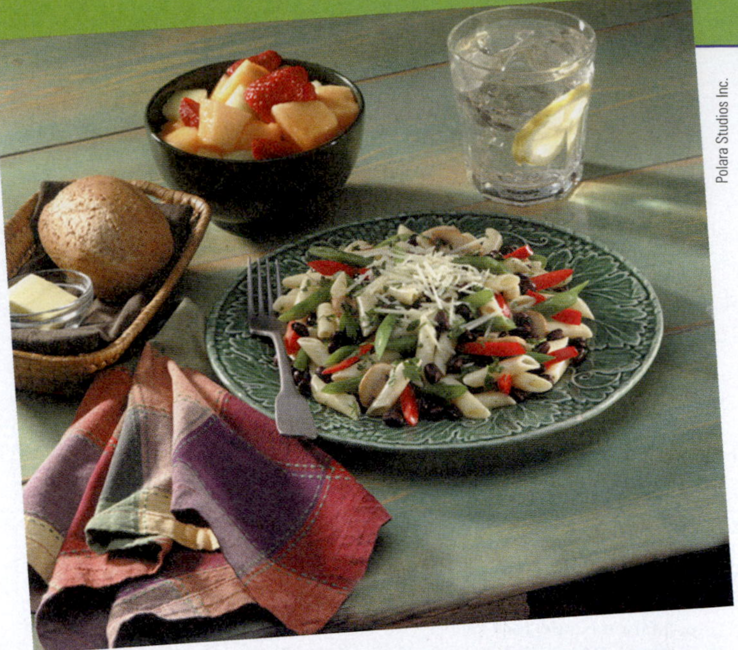
Polara Studios Inc.

The waiter presents this evening's specials: a fresh spinach salad topped with mandarin oranges, raisins, and sunflower seeds, served with a bowl of pasta smothered in a mushroom and tomato sauce and topped with grated parmesan cheese. Then this one: a salad made of chopped parsley, scallions, celery, and tomatoes mixed with bulgur wheat and dressed with olive oil and lemon juice, served with a spinach and feta cheese pie. Do these meals sound good to you? Or is something missing . . . a pork chop or chicken breast, perhaps?

Would vegetarian fare be acceptable to you some of the time? Most of the time? Ever? The health benefits of a primarily **vegetarian diet** seem to have encouraged many people to eat more plant-based meals. The popular press sometimes refers to individuals who eat small amounts of meat, seafood, or poultry from time to time as "flexitarians."

People who choose to exclude meat and other animal-derived foods from their diets today do so for many of the same reasons the Greek philosopher Pythagoras cited in the sixth century B.C.: physical health, ecological responsibility, and philosophical concerns. They might also cite world hunger issues, economic reasons, ethical concerns, or religious beliefs as motivating factors.[1] Whatever their reasons—and even if they don't have a particular reason—people who exclude meat will be better prepared to plan well-balanced meals if they understand the nutrition and health implications of their choices.

Vegetarian diets generally are categorized, not by a person's motivations but by the foods that are excluded (see Glossary H2-1). Some diets exclude red meat only; some also exclude poultry or seafood; others also exclude eggs; and still others exclude milk and milk products as well. In contrast, **omnivorous** diets do not exclude foods, but include many foods derived from both animals and plants.

As you will see, though, the foods a person *excludes* are not nearly as important as the foods a person *includes* in the diet. **Plant-based diets** that include a variety of whole grains, vegetables, legumes, fruits, and nuts and seeds offer abundant complex carbohydrates and fibers, an assortment of vitamins and minerals, a mixture of phytochemicals, and little saturated fat—characteristics that reflect current dietary recommendations aimed at maintaining good health and an appropriate body weight. This highlight examines the health benefits and potential problems of vegetarian diets and shows how to plan a well-balanced vegetarian diet. Highlight 20 includes a discussion of the environmental benefits of a sustainable plant-based diet.

Health Benefits of Vegetarian Diets

Research findings suggest that well-planned vegetarian (and vegan) diets offer sound nutrition and health benefits to adults.[2] Eating patterns that include very little, if any, meat are associated with a lower rate of death from all causes.[3] Some researchers estimate that eliminating even one serving of red meat per day would lower mortality risk by 7 to 19 percent.[4]

Obesity

Vegetarians tend to maintain a lower and healthier body weight than nonvegetarians. In general, red and processed meat intake is associated with an increased risk of obesity and the prevalence of obesity is lower among vegetarians.[5] Because obesity impairs health in a number of ways, vegetarian diets offer several health advantages.

GLOSSARY H2-1

lactovegetarian diet: an eating pattern that includes milk and milk products, but excludes meat, poultry, seafood, and eggs from the diet.

- **lacto** = milk

lacto-ovo-vegetarian diet: an eating pattern that includes milk, milk products, and eggs, but excludes meat, poultry, and seafood from the diet.

- **ovo** = egg

macrobiotic diet: a philosophical eating pattern based on mostly plant foods such as whole grains, legumes, and vegetables, with small amounts of fish, fruits, nuts, and seeds.

- **macro** = large, great
- **biotic** = life

meat replacements: products formulated to look and taste like meat, seafood, or poultry; usually made of textured vegetable protein.

omnivorous: an eating pattern that includes foods derived from both animals and plants.

- **omni** = all
- **vores** = to eat

plant-based diets: an eating pattern that derives most of its protein from plant products (although some animal products may be included).

tempeh (TEM-pay)**:** a fermented-soybean food, rich in protein and fiber.

tofu (TOE-foo)**:** a curd made from soybeans, rich in protein and often fortified with calcium; used in many Asian and vegetarian dishes in place of meat.

vegan (VEE-gan) **diet:** an eating pattern that excludes all animal-derived foods (including meat, poultry, fish, eggs, and dairy products); also called *pure vegetarian, strict vegetarian,* or *total vegetarian.*

vegetarian diet: a general term used to describe an eating pattern that excludes meat, poultry, fish, or other animal-derived foods from the diet.

Diabetes

Obesity and weight gains are strong risk factors for diabetes, which partially explains why nonvegetarian diets are more often associated with diabetes than vegetarian diets. Even when body weight and lifestyle factors are taken into account, vegetarian eating patterns seem to protect against diabetes.[6]

Hypertension

Vegetarians tend to have lower blood pressure and lower rates of hypertension than nonvegetarians.[7] Appropriate body weight helps maintain a healthy blood pressure, as does a diet high in fiber, fruits, vegetables, whole grains, low-fat milk products, and protein from plant sources. Lifestyle factors also influence blood pressure: smoking and alcohol intake raise blood pressure, and physical activity lowers it.

Heart Disease

Meat -based diets are associated with an increased risk of heart disease and related deaths.[8] The dietary factor most directly related to heart disease is saturated fat, and in general, meat-based diets are higher in saturated fat than typical plant-based diets. The fats common in plant-based diets—the monounsaturated fats of olives, seeds, and nuts and the polyunsaturated fats of vegetable oils—are associated with a decreased risk of heart disease. Furthermore, vegetarian diets are generally higher in dietary fiber, antioxidant vitamins, and phytochemicals—all factors that help control blood lipids and protect against heart disease. These plant-based diets may also reduce the risk of heart disease (and diabetes) by promoting a favorable population of microbes in the gastrointestinal tract (Chapter 3 provides more details).[9]

Cancer

Vegetarians (and fish eaters) have a lower risk of cancer than meat eaters.[10] Their low cancer rates may be due to their high intakes of fruits and vegetables (as Highlight 11 explains).[11] In fact, the ratio of vegetables to meat may be the most relevant dietary factor responsible for cancer prevention.

Some scientific findings indicate that vegetarian diets are associated not only with lower cancer rates in general, but also with lower incidence of cancer at specific sites as well, most notably, colon cancer.[12] Evidence for an association between red and processed meats and colon cancer is convincing.[13] The Healthy US-Style Eating Pattern introduced earlier in the chapter recommends 26 ounces per week of meats, poultry, and eggs (for a 2000-kcalorie diet). Some cancer experts recommend limiting consumption of red meat to no more than 11 ounces a week, with very little (if any) processed meat.

Other Diseases

In addition to obesity, diabetes, hypertension, heart disease, and some cancers, vegetarian diets may help prevent osteoporosis, diverticular disease, gallstones, cataracts, and rheumatoid arthritis. Health benefits of a vegetarian diet depend on wise diet planning.

Vegetarian Diet Planning

The vegetarian has the same meal-planning task as everyone else—using a variety of foods to deliver all the needed nutrients within an energy allowance that maintains a healthy body weight. Vegetarians who include milk, milk products, and eggs can meet recommendations for most nutrients about as easily as nonvegetarians. Such eating patterns may rely on some fortified foods, but generally provide enough energy, protein, and other nutrients to support the health of adults and the growth of children and adolescents. The USDA Healthy Vegetarian Eating Pattern is flexible enough that a variety of people can use it: people who have adopted various vegetarian diets, those who want to make the transition to a vegetarian diet, and those who simply want to reduce their meat intake and include more plant-based meals in their diets. The Healthy Vegetarian Eating Pattern is similar to the Healthy US-Style Eating Pattern presented earlier in the chapter, with a slight increase in grain servings and notable differences in the protein foods quantities and subgroups, as shown in Table H2-1 (p. 64).

Vegan diets exclude milk, milk products, and eggs and include protein foods such as legumes, nuts, and seeds as well as foods made from them, such as peanut butter, **tempeh,** and **tofu**. Vegans who do not use milk can use soy "milk"—a product made from soybeans that provides similar nutrients if fortified with calcium, vitamin D, and vitamin B_{12} (see Figure H2-1). Similarly, "milks"

> **FIGURE H2-1 Low-Fat Milk and Soy Milk Compared**

A comparison of low-fat milk and enriched soy milk shows that they provide similar amounts of key nutrients.

Low-Fat Milk

Nutrition Facts	
8 servings per container	
Serving size	1 cup (240 mL)
Amount per serving	
Calories	102
	% DV*
Total Fat 8g	10%
Saturated Fat 1g	5%
Trans Fat 0g	
Cholesterol 12mg	4%
Sodium 107mg	5%
Total Carbs 12g	4%
Dietary Fiber 0g	0%
Sugars 1g	
Includes 0g Added Sugars	0%
Protein 8g	
Vitamin D 3µg	15%
Calcium 305mg	23%
Iron 0mg	0%
Potassium 366mg	8%

Soy Milk

Nutrition Facts	
8 servings per container	
Serving size	1 cup (240 mL)
Amount per serving	
Calories	100
	% DV*
Total Fat 8g	10%
Saturated Fat 1g	5%
Trans Fat 0g	
Cholesterol 0mg	0%
Sodium 120mg	5%
Total Carbs 37g	13%
Dietary Fiber 1g	4%
Sugars 1g	
Includes 0g Added Sugars	0%
Protein 7g	
Vitamin D 2.9µg	15%
Calcium 299mg	23%
Iron 1mg	6%
Potassium 299mg	6%
Riboflavin 0.5mg	38%
Vitamin B12 3µg	125%

TABLE H2-1 USDA Food Patterns: Healthy Vegetarian Eating Pattern

The table first lists recommended amounts from each food group *per day* and then shows the amounts for vegetables and protein foods dispersed among subgroups *per week*. The highlighted rows indicate which food groups and serving sizes differ from the Healthy US-Style Eating Pattern (see Tables 2-3 and 2-4, p. 41).

Recommended Daily Amounts from Each Food Group

Food Group	1600 kcal	1800 kcal	2000 kcal	2200 kcal	2400 kcal	2600 kcal	2800 kcal	3000 kcal
Fruits	1½ c	1½ c	2 c	2 c	2 c	2 c	2½ c	2½ c
Vegetables	2 c	2½ c	2½ c	3 c	3 c	3½ c	3½ c	4 c
Grains	5½ oz	6½ oz	6½ oz	7½ oz	8½ oz	9½ oz	10½ oz	10½ oz
Protein foods	2½ oz	3 oz	3½ oz	3½ oz	4 oz	4½ oz	5 oz	5½ oz
Milk and milk products	3 c	3 c	3 c	3 c	3 c	3 c	3 c	3 c
Oils	5 tsp	5 tsp	6 tsp	6 tsp	7 tsp	8 tsp	8 tsp	10 tsp
Limit on kcalories available for other uses[a]	180 kcal	190 kcal	290 kcal	330 kcal	390 kcal	390 kcal	400 kcal	440 kcal

Recommended Weekly Amounts from Each Food Group

	1600 kcal	1800 kcal	2000 kcal	2200 kcal	2400 kcal	2600 kcal	2800 kcal	3000 kcal
Vegetables Subgroups								
Dark green	1½ c	1½ c	1½ c	2 c	2 c	2½ c	2½ c	2½ c
Red and orange	4 c	5½ c	5½ c	6 c	6 c	7 c	7 c	7½ c
Legumes	1 c	1½ c	1½ c	2 c	2 c	2½ c	2½ c	3 c
Starchy	4 c	5 c	5 c	6 c	6 c	7 c	7 c	8 c
Other	3½ c	4 c	4 c	5 c	5 c	5½ c	5½ c	7 c
Protein Foods Subgroups								
Eggs	3 oz	3 oz	3 oz	3 oz	3 oz	3 oz	4 oz	4 oz
Legumes[b]	4 oz	6 oz	6 oz	6 oz	8 oz	9 oz	10 oz	11 oz
Soy products	6 oz	6 oz	8 oz	8 oz	9 oz	10 oz	11 oz	12 oz
Nuts and seeds	5 oz	6 oz	7 oz	7 oz	8 oz	9 oz	10 oz	12 oz

[a]The limit on kcalories for other uses describes how many kcalories are available for foods that are not in nutrient-dense forms; these kcalories may also be referred to as discretionary kcalories (discussed on p. 44).

[b]About half of total legumes are listed as vegetables (measured in cup-equivalents) and half as protein foods (measured in ounce-equivalents); an ounce-equivalent of legumes in the protein foods subgroup is equal to ¼ cup. To convert legumes from the protein foods subgroup from ounce-equivalents to cups, divide by 4. Using the 1600-kcalorie recommendations for an example, the total legumes would be 2 cups—1 cup from the vegetable subgroup and the 1 cup from the protein foods subgroup (1 oz = ¼ cup; therefore, 4 oz = 1 cup).

NOTE: Milk and eggs are included in the Healthy Vegetarian Eating Pattern because they are commonly consumed as part of most vegetarian diets. To plan vegan diets, use fortified soy beverages (soymilk) or other plant-based dairy substitutes instead of milk and milk products and replace eggs with legumes, soy products, and nuts and seeds.

SOURCE: U.S. Department of Health and Human Services and U.S. Department of Agriculture. *2015–2020 Dietary Guidelines for Americans*. 8th ed. (December 2015), http://health.gov/dietaryguidelines/2015/guidelines/.

made from rice, almonds, and oats are reasonable alternatives, if adequately fortified. Vegan eating patterns must include fortified foods or supplements to provide adequate intakes of all essential nutrients.

MyPlate includes tips for planning vegetarian diets. When selecting from the vegetable and fruit groups, vegetarians may want to emphasize particularly good sources of calcium and iron. Green leafy vegetables provide almost five times as much calcium per serving as other vegetables. Similarly, dried fruits deserve special notice in the fruit group because they deliver six times as much iron as other fruits.

The nutrient profiles of vegetarian and nonvegetarian eating patterns differ markedly, which may explain some of the differences in the risks for obesity and chronic diseases mentioned earlier.[14] Nonvegetarians tend to have higher intakes of animal protein, saturated fat, and *trans* fat, whereas vegetarians tend to have higher intakes of plant proteins and fiber. In addition, vegetarians easily obtain large quantities of other nutrients that are abundant in plant foods, including folate, vitamin C, vitamin A, and vitamin E. Well-planned vegetarian eating patterns help ensure adequate intakes of the nutrients vegetarian diets might otherwise lack, including protein, iron, zinc, calcium, vitamin B_{12}, vitamin D, and omega-3 fatty acids. Table H2-2 presents good vegetarian sources of these key nutrients.

Protein

The protein RDA for vegetarians is the same as for those consuming other types of diets. **Lacto-ovo-vegetarian diets** that include animal-derived foods such as milk and eggs, deliver high-quality proteins and are likely to meet protein needs. Even vegans who adopt

TABLE H2-2 Good Vegetarian Sources of Key Nutrients

Nutrients	Grains	Vegetables	Fruits	Protein Foods	Milk	Oils
Protein[a]	Whole grains			Legumes, seeds, nuts, soy products (tempeh, tofu, veggie burgers) Eggs (for ovo-vegetarians)	Milk, cheese, yogurt (for lactovegetarians)	
Iron	Fortified cereals, enriched and whole grains	Dark green leafy vegetables (spinach, turnip greens)	Dried fruits (apricots, prunes, raisins)	Legumes (black-eyed peas, kidney beans, lentils)		
Zinc	Fortified cereals, whole grains			Legumes (garbanzo beans, kidney beans, navy beans), nuts, seeds (pumpkin seeds)	Milk, cheese, yogurt (for lactovegetarians)	
Calcium	Fortified cereals	Dark-green leafy vegetables (bok choy, broccoli, collard greens, kale, mustard greens, turnip greens, watercress)	Fortified juices, figs	Fortified soy products, nuts (almonds), seeds (sesame seeds)	Milk, cheese, yogurt (for lactovegetarians) Fortified soy milk	
Vitamin B_{12}	Fortified cereals			Eggs (for ovo-vegetarians) Fortified soy products	Milk, cheese, yogurt (for lactovegetarians) Fortified soy milk	
Vitamin D					Milk, cheese, yogurt (for lactovegetarians) Fortified soy milk	
Omega-3 fatty acids				Flaxseed, walnuts, soybeans		Flaxseed oil, walnut oil, soybean oil

[a]As Chapter 6 explains, many plant proteins do not contain all the essential amino acids in the amounts and proportions needed by human beings. To improve protein quality, vegetarians can eat grains and legumes together, for example, although it is not necessary if protein intake is varied and energy intake is sufficient.

only plant-based diets can readily meet protein needs provided that their energy intakes are adequate and the protein sources varied. The proteins of whole grains, vegetables, legumes, and nuts and seeds can provide adequate amounts of all the amino acids. An advantage of many vegetarian sources of protein is that they are generally lower in saturated fat than meats and are often higher in fiber and richer in some vitamins and minerals.

Vegetarians sometimes use **meat replacements** made of textured vegetable protein (soy protein). These foods are formulated to look and taste like meat, seafood, or poultry. Many of these products are fortified to provide the vitamins and minerals found in animal sources of protein. Some of these products may be high in salt, sugars, and saturated fats. A wise vegetarian learns to read labels and use a variety of whole, and minimally processed foods often and commercially fabricated foods less frequently. Vegetarians may also use soy products such as tofu to bolster protein intake.

Iron

Getting enough iron can be a problem even for meat eaters, and those who eat no meat must pay special attention to their iron intake. The iron in plant foods such as legumes, dark-green leafy vegetables, iron-fortified cereals, and whole-grain breads and cereals is poorly absorbed. Because iron absorption from a vegetarian diet is low, the iron RDA for vegetarians is higher than for others (see Chapter 13 for more details).

Fortunately, the body seems to adapt to a low-iron vegetarian diet by increasing iron absorption and decreasing iron losses. Furthermore, iron absorption is enhanced by vitamin C, and vegetarians typically eat many vitamin C–rich fruits and vegetables. Consequently, vegetarians tend to be no more iron deficient than other people.

Zinc

Zinc is similar to iron in that meat is its richest food source, and zinc from plant sources is not well absorbed. In addition, phytates and fiber, which are common in vegetarian diets, interfere with zinc absorption. Consequently, poor zinc intakes and mild deficiencies are prevalent.[15] Perhaps the best advice to vegetarians regarding zinc is to eat a variety of nutrient-dense foods; include whole grains, nuts, and legumes such as black-eyed peas, pinto beans, and kidney beans; and maintain an adequate energy intake. Those who include seafood in their diets should keep in mind that oysters, crabmeat, and shrimp are rich in zinc.

Calcium

The calcium intakes of those following a **lactovegetarian diet** are similar to those of the general population, but vegans who use no milk or milk products may not get enough calcium to defend against bone fractures.[16] To ensure adequate intakes, vegans can select calcium-rich foods, such as calcium-fortified juices, soy milk, and breakfast cereals, in ample quantities regularly. This advice is especially important for children and adolescents. Other good calcium sources include figs, some legumes, some green vegetables such as broccoli and turnip greens, some nuts such as almonds, certain seeds such as sesame seeds, and calcium-set tofu.* The choices should be varied because calcium absorption from some plant foods may be limited (as Chapter 12 explains).

Vitamin B_{12}

The requirement for vitamin B_{12} is small, but this vitamin is found only in animal-derived foods. Consequently, the risk of deficiency is relatively high among vegetarians, in general, and vegans who eat no foods of animal original, in particular.[17] Fermented soy products such as tempeh may contain some vitamin B_{12} from the bacteria, but unfortunately, much of the vitamin B_{12} found in these products may be an inactive form. Seaweeds such as nori and chlorella supply some vitamin B_{12}, but not much, and excessive intakes of these foods can lead to iodine toxicity. To defend against vitamin B_{12} deficiency, vegans must rely on vitamin B_{12}–fortified sources (such as soy milk or breakfast cereals) or supplements. Without vitamin B_{12}, the nerves suffer damage, leading to such health consequences as loss of vision.

Vitamin D

The vitamin D status of vegetarians is similar to that of nonvegetarians. People who do not use vitamin D–fortified foods and do not receive enough exposure to sunlight to synthesize adequate vitamin D may need supplements to defend against bone loss. This is particularly important for infants, children, and older adults. In northern climates during winter months, young children on vegan diets can readily develop rickets, the vitamin D–deficiency disease.

Omega-3 Fatty Acids

Both Chapter 5 and Highlight 5 describe the health benefits of unsaturated fats, most notably the omega-3 fatty acids commonly found in fatty fish. A diet that includes some fish provides more omega-3 fatty acids than a vegetarian diet.[18] Vegetarians can obtain the essential omega-3 fatty acids from plant sources such as flaxseed, walnuts, soy, and canola oil; supplements derived from marine algae that contain omega-3 fatty acids may also be beneficial.[19]

Healthy Food Choices

Later chapters provide details on how vegetarian diets can meet nutrient needs for various stages of the life cycle, including pregnancy, lactation, infancy, childhood, and adolescence. As mentioned earlier, well-planned vegetarian eating patterns may lower the risk of mortality and several chronic diseases, including obesity, diabetes, high blood pressure, heart disease, and some cancers. But there is nothing mysterious or magical about a vegetarian eating pattern. A dietary pattern that includes small amounts of meat can be equally healthy.[20] The quality of the diet depends not on whether it includes meat but on whether the other food choices are nutritionally sound. A plant-based eating pattern that includes ample fruits, vegetables, whole grains, legumes, nuts, and seeds is higher in fiber, antioxidant vitamins, and phytochemicals and lower in saturated fats than meat-based diets. Variety is key to nutritional adequacy in a vegetarian diet. Restrictive plans that limit selections to a few grains and vegetables cannot possibly deliver a full array of nutrients.

Some religions practice vegetarianism, but vegetarianism itself is not a religion; it is merely an eating pattern that selects plant foods to deliver needed nutrients. That said, some vegetarians choose to follow a **macrobiotic diet**; they select natural, organic foods and embrace a Zen-like spirituality. In other words, a macrobiotic diet represents a way of life, not just an eating pattern. Such a diet emphasizes whole grains, legumes, and vegetables, with small amounts of fish, fruits, nuts, and seeds. Practices include selecting locally grown foods, eating foods in their most natural state, and balancing cold, sweet, and passive foods with hot, salty, and aggressive ones. Some items, such as processed foods, alcohol, hot spices, and potatoes are excluded from the diet. Early versions of the macrobiotic diet followed a progression that ended with the "ultimate" diet of brown rice and water—a less than nutritionally balanced diet. Today's version reflects a modified vegetarian approach with an appreciation of how foods can enhance health. With careful planning, a macrobiotic diet can provide an array of nutrients that support good health.

If not properly balanced, any diet—vegetarian, macrobiotic, or otherwise—can lack nutrients. Poorly planned vegetarian diets typically lack iron, zinc, calcium, vitamin B_{12}, and vitamin D; without planning, meat-based diets may lack vitamin A, vitamin C, folate, and fiber, among others. Quite simply, the negative health aspects of any diet, including vegetarian diets, reflect poor diet planning. Careful attention to energy intake and specific nutrients of concern can ensure adequacy.

Keep in mind, too, that diet is only one factor influencing health. Whatever a diet consists of, its context is also important: no smoking, alcohol consumption in moderation (if at all), regular physical activity, adequate rest, and medical attention when needed all contribute to good health. Establishing these healthy habits early in life seems to be the most important step one can take to reduce the risks of chronic diseases later in life (as Highlight 16 explains).

*Calcium salts are often added during processing to coagulate the tofu.

CRITICAL THINKING QUESTIONS

A. What are the strengths and weaknesses of vegetarian diets?

B. Your interest in nutrition has been piqued by the concept of a vegetarian diet, and you wisely recognize that a well-planned diet involves more than simply replacing a turkey sandwich with peanut butter crackers. Design and follow a vegetarian meal plan for 3 days, including at least 1 vegan day. Outline the social, personal, and nutritional challenges you faced and describe how you might partially or fully integrate vegetarian meals into your current meal plan.

REFERENCES

1. C. Leitzmann, Vegetarian nutrition: Past, present, future, *American Journal of Clinical Nutrition* 100 (2014): 496S–502S.
2. Position of the Academy of Nutrition and Dietetics: Vegetarian diets, *Journal of the Academy of Nutrition and Dietetics* 116 (2016): 1970–1980; M. J. Orlich and G. E. Fraser, Vegetarian diets in the Adventist Health Study 2: A review of initial published findings, *American Journal of Clinical Nutrition* 100 (2014): 353S–358S; L. T. Le and J. Sabaté, Beyond meatless, the health effects of vegan diets: Findings from the Adventist cohorts, *Nutrients* 6 (2014): 2131–2147.
3. M. Song and coauthors, Association of animal and plant protein intake with all-cause and cause-specific mortality, *JAMA Internal Medicine* 176 (2016): 1453–1463; E. B. Richi and coauthors, Health risks associated with meat consumption: A review of epidemiological studies, *International Journal for Vitamin and Nutrition Research* 85 (2015): 70–78; M. J. Orlich and coauthors, Vegetarian dietary patterns and mortality in Adventist Health Study 2, *JAMA Internal Medicine* 173 (2013): 1230–1238.
4. A. Pan and coauthors, Red meat consumption and mortality, *Archives of Internal Medicine* 172 (2012): 555–563.
5. P. N. Appleby and T. J. Key, The long-term health of vegetarians and vegans, *Proceedings of the Nutrition Society* 28 (2015): 1–7.
6. A. Satija and coauthors, Plant-based dietary patterns and incidence of type 2 diabetes in US men and women: Results from three prospective cohort studies, *PLoS Medicine* 13 (2016): e1002039; S. Tonstad and coauthors, Vegetarian diets and incidence of diabetes in the Adventist Health Study-2, *Nutrition, Metabolism, and Cardiovascular Diseases* 23 (2013): 292–299.
7. Y. Yokoyama, Vegetarian diets and blood pressure: A meta-analysis, *JAMA Internal Medicine* 174 (2014): 577–587; B. J. Pettersen and coauthors, Vegetarian diets and blood pressure among white subjects: Results from the Adventist Health Study-2 (AHS-2), *Public Health Nutrition* 15 (2012): 1909–1916.
8. P. Tuso, S. R. Stoll, and W. W. Li, A plant-based diet, atherogenesis, and coronary artery disease prevention, *Permanente Journal* 19 (2015): 62–67.
9. J. M. W. Wong, Gut microbiota and cardiometabolic outcomes: Influences of dietary patterns and their associated components, *American Journal of Clinical Nutrition* 100 (2014): 369S–377S.
10. T. J. Key and coauthors, Cancer in British vegetarians: Updated analyses of 4998 incident cancers in a cohort of 32,491 meat eaters, 8612 fish eaters, 18,298 vegetarians, and 2246 vegans, *American Journal of Clinical Nutrition* 100 (2014): 378S–385S; T. Huang and coauthors, Cardiovascular disease mortality and cancer incidence in vegetarians: A meta-analysis and systematic review, *Annals of Nutrition and Metabolism* 60 (2012): 233–240.
11. K. E. Bradbury, P. N. Appleby, and T. J. Key, Fruit, vegetable, and fiber intake in relation to cancer risk: Findings from the European Prospective Investigation into Cancer and Nutrition (EPIC), *American Journal of Clinical Nutrition* 100 (2014): 394S–398S.
12. M. J. Orlich and coauthors, Vegetarian dietary patterns and the risk of colorectal cancers, *JAMA Internal Medicine* 175 (2015): 767–776; T. T. Fung and L. S. Brown, Dietary patterns and the risk of colorectal cancer, *Current Nutrition Reports* 2 (2013): 48–55.
13. Z. Abid, A. J. Cross, and R. Sinha, Meat, dairy, and cancer, *American Journal of Clinical Nutrition* 100 (2014): 386S–393S.
14. N. S. Rizzo and coauthors, Nutrient profiles of vegetarian and nonvegetarian dietary patterns, *Journal of the Academy of Nutrition and Dietetics* 113 (2013): 1610–1619.
15. M. Foster and coauthors, Effect of vegetarian diets on zinc status: A systematic review and meta-analysis of studies in humans, *Journal of the Science of Food and Agriculture* 93 (2013): 2362–2371.
16. K. L. Tucker, Vegetarian diets and bone status, *American Journal of Clinical Nutrition* 100 (2014): 329S–335S.
17. R. Pawlak, S. E. Lester, and T. Babatunde, The prevalence of cobalamin deficiency among vegetarians assessed by serum vitamin B12: A review of literature, *European Journal of Clinical Nutrition* 68 (2014): 541–548.
18. T. A. B. Sanders, Plant compared with marine n-3 fatty acid effects on cardiovascular risk factors and outcomes: What is the verdict? *American Journal of Clinical Nutrition* 100 (2014): 453S–458S.
19. W. S. Harris, Achieving optimal n-3 fatty acid status: The vegetarian's challenge . . . or not, *American Journal of Clinical Nutrition* 100 (2014): 449S–452S; K. Lane and coauthors, Bioavailability and potential uses of vegetarian sources of omega-3 fatty acids: A review of the literature, *Critical Reviews in Food Science and Nutrition* 54 (2014): 572–579; A. M. Bernstein and coauthors, A meta-analysis shows that docosahexaenoic acid from algal oil reduces serum triglycerides and increases HDL-cholesterol and LDL-cholesterol in persons without coronary heart disease, *Journal of Nutrition* 142 (2012): 99–104.
20. C. T. McEvoy, N. Temple, and J. V. Woodside, Vegetarian diets, low-meat diets and health: A review, *Public Health Nutrition* 15 (2012): 2287–2294.

3

Digestion, Absorption, and Transport

LEARNING GUIDE

meaofoto/Shutterstock.com

Nutrition in Your Life

Have you ever wondered what happens to the food you eat after you swallow it? Or how your body extracts nutrients from food? Have you ever marveled at how it all just seems to happen? Follow foods as they travel through the digestive system. Learn how a healthy digestive system takes whatever food you give it—whether sirloin steak and potatoes or tofu and brussels sprouts—and extracts the nutrients that will nourish the cells of your body. As you read this chapter, consider whether your current eating habits are supporting a healthy digestive system.

Each cell in the body needs a continuous supply of many specific nutrients to maintain itself and carry out its work. These nutrients derive from the foods a person eats, but before the body's cells can use the nutrients, foods must first be broken down mechanically and chemically. This chapter follows the journey that breaks down foods into the nutrients featured in the later chapters. Then it follows the nutrients as they travel through the intestinal cells and into the body to do their work.

As you read about the complexities and intricacies of these processes, take a moment to appreciate the beauty and wisdom of the body. Recognize that the activities of the **digestive system** are finely coordinated and fully integrated with those of the circulatory, nervous, and hormonal systems. Then be thankful that your body can efficiently take care of its business without any direction from you, but know that it performs its best when you have given it optimal nourishment. This introduction presents a general overview of the processes common to all nutrients; later chapters discuss the specifics of digesting and absorbing individual nutrients.

3.1 Digestion

LEARN IT Explain how foods move through the digestive system, describing the actions of the organs, muscles, and digestive secretions along the way.

Digestion is the body's ingenious way of breaking down foods into nutrients in preparation for **absorption** (see Photo 3-1). In the process, the body overcomes many challenges without any conscious effort. Consider these challenges:

1. Human beings breathe, eat, and drink through their mouths. Air taken in through the mouth must go to the lungs; food and beverages must go to the stomach. The throat must be arranged so that swallowing and breathing don't interfere with each other.
2. Positioned below the lungs is the diaphragm, a dome of muscle that separates the upper half of the torso from the lower half. The body needs a passageway that will allow food from the mouth to pass through the diaphragm to reach the stomach below.
3. The contents of the digestive tract should be kept moving forward, slowly but steadily, at a pace that permits all reactions to reach completion.
4. To move through the system, food must be lubricated with fluids. Too much would form a liquid that would flow too rapidly; too little would form a paste too dry and compact to move at all. The amount of fluids must be regulated to keep the intestinal contents at the right consistency to move along smoothly.
5. For digestive enzymes to work, foods must be broken down into small particles and suspended in enough liquid so that every particle is accessible. Once digestion is complete and nutrients have been absorbed from the GI tract into the body, the remaining waste must be excreted. Excreting all the water along with

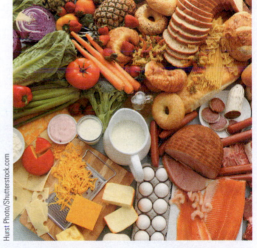

Hurst Photo/Shutterstock.com

> **PHOTO 3-1** The process of digestion breaks down all kinds of *foods* into *nutrients*.

digestive system: all the organs and glands associated with the ingestion and digestion of food.

digestion: the process by which food is broken down into absorbable units.

- **digest** = take apart

absorption: the uptake of nutrients by the cells of the small intestine for transport into either the blood or the lymph.

- **absorb** = suck in

the solid residue, however, would be both wasteful and messy. Some water must be withdrawn, leaving a solid waste product that is easy to pass.

6. The digestive enzymes are designed to digest carbohydrate, fat, and protein. The cells of the GI tract are also made of carbohydrate, fat, and protein. These cells must be protected against the powerful digestive juices that they secrete.
7. Once waste matter has reached the end of the GI tract, it must be excreted, but it would be inconvenient and embarrassing if this function occurred continuously. Evacuation needs to occur periodically.

The following sections show how the body elegantly and efficiently handles these challenges. Each section follows the GI tract from one end to the other—first describing its anatomy, then its muscular actions, and finally its secretions.

Anatomy of the Digestive Tract The **gastrointestinal (GI) tract** is a flexible muscular tube that extends from the mouth, through the esophagus, stomach, small intestine, large intestine, and rectum to the anus. Figure 3-1 traces the path followed by food from one end to the other. In a sense, the human body surrounds the GI tract. The inner space within the GI tract, called the **lumen,** is continuous from one end to the other. (GI anatomy terms appear in boldface type and are defined in Glossary 3-1.) A nutrient or other substance must pass through the GI tract's wall to enter the body proper; some materials pass through the GI tract without being digested or absorbed.

Mouth The process of digestion begins in the **mouth.** During chewing, teeth crush large pieces of food into smaller ones, and fluids from foods, beverages, and salivary glands blend with these pieces to ease swallowing.* Fluids also help dissolve the food so that the tongue can taste it; only particles in solution can react with taste buds. When stimulated, the taste buds detect one, or a combination, of the five basic taste sensations: sweet, sour, bitter, salty and umami (oo-MOM-ee), a savory flavor commonly associated with monosodium glutamate. In addition to these chemical triggers, aroma, appearance, texture, and temperature also influence a person's taste perceptions.

The tongue provides taste sensations and moves food around the mouth, facilitating chewing and swallowing. When a mouthful of food is swallowed, it passes through the **pharynx,** a short tube that is shared by both the digestive system and

gastrointestinal (GI) tract: the digestive tract. The principal organs are the stomach and intestines.
- **gastro** = stomach
- **intestinalis** = intestine

GLOSSARY 3-1
GI ANATOMY TERMS

anus (AY-nus)**:** the terminal outlet of the GI tract.

appendix: a narrow blind sac extending from the beginning of the colon that contains bacteria and lymph cells.

duodenum (doo-oh-DEEN-um or doo-ODD-num)**:** the top portion of the small intestine (about "12 fingers' breadth" long in ancient terminology).
- **duodecim** = twelve

epiglottis (epp-ih-GLOTT-iss)**:** cartilage in the throat that guards the entrance to the trachea and prevents fluid or food from entering it when a person swallows.
- **epi** = upon (over)
- **glottis** = back of tongue

esophageal (ee -SOFF-ah-GEE-al) **sphincter:** the circular muscle at the upper or lower end of the esophagus. The *lower esophageal sphincter* is also called the *cardiac sphincter* because of its proximity to the heart.

esophagus (ee-SOFF-ah-gus)**:** the food pipe; the conduit from the mouth to the stomach.

gallbladder: the organ that stores and concentrates bile. When it receives the signal that fat is present in the duodenum, the gallbladder contracts and squirts bile through the bile duct into the duodenum.

ileocecal (ill-ee-oh-SEEK-ul) **valve:** the sphincter separating the small and large intestines.

ileum (ILL-ee-um)**:** the last segment of the small intestine.

jejunum (je-JOON-um)**:** the first two-fifths of the small intestine beyond the duodenum.

large intestine or **colon** (COAL-un)**:** the lower portion of intestine that completes the digestive process. Its segments are the *ascending colon*, the *transverse colon*, the *descending colon*, and the *sigmoid colon*.
- **sigmoid** = shaped like the letter S (sigma in Greek)

lumen (LOO-men)**:** the space within a vessel such as the intestine.

mouth: the oral cavity containing the tongue and teeth.

pancreas: a gland that secretes digestive enzymes and juices into the duodenum. (The pancreas also secretes hormones into the blood that help maintain glucose homeostasis.)

pharynx (FAIR-inks)**:** the passageway leading from the nose and mouth to the larynx and esophagus, respectively.

pyloric (pie-LORE-ic) **sphincter:** the circular muscle that separates the stomach from the small intestine and regulates the flow of partially digested food into the small intestine; also called *pylorus* or *pyloric valve*.
- **pylorus** = gatekeeper

rectum: the muscular terminal part of the intestine, extending from the sigmoid colon to the anus.

small intestine: a 10-foot length of small-diameter intestine that is the major site of digestion of food and absorption of nutrients. Its segments are the *duodenum*, *jejunum*, and *ileum*.

sphincter (SFINK-ter)**:** a circular muscle surrounding, and able to close, a body opening. Sphincters are found at specific points along the GI tract and regulate the flow of food particles.
- **sphincter** = band (binder)

stomach: a muscular, elastic, saclike portion of the digestive tract that grinds and churns swallowed food, mixing it with acid and enzymes to form chyme.

*The process of chewing is called *mastication* (mass-tih-KAY-shun).

> **FIGURE 3-1 The Gastrointestinal Tract**

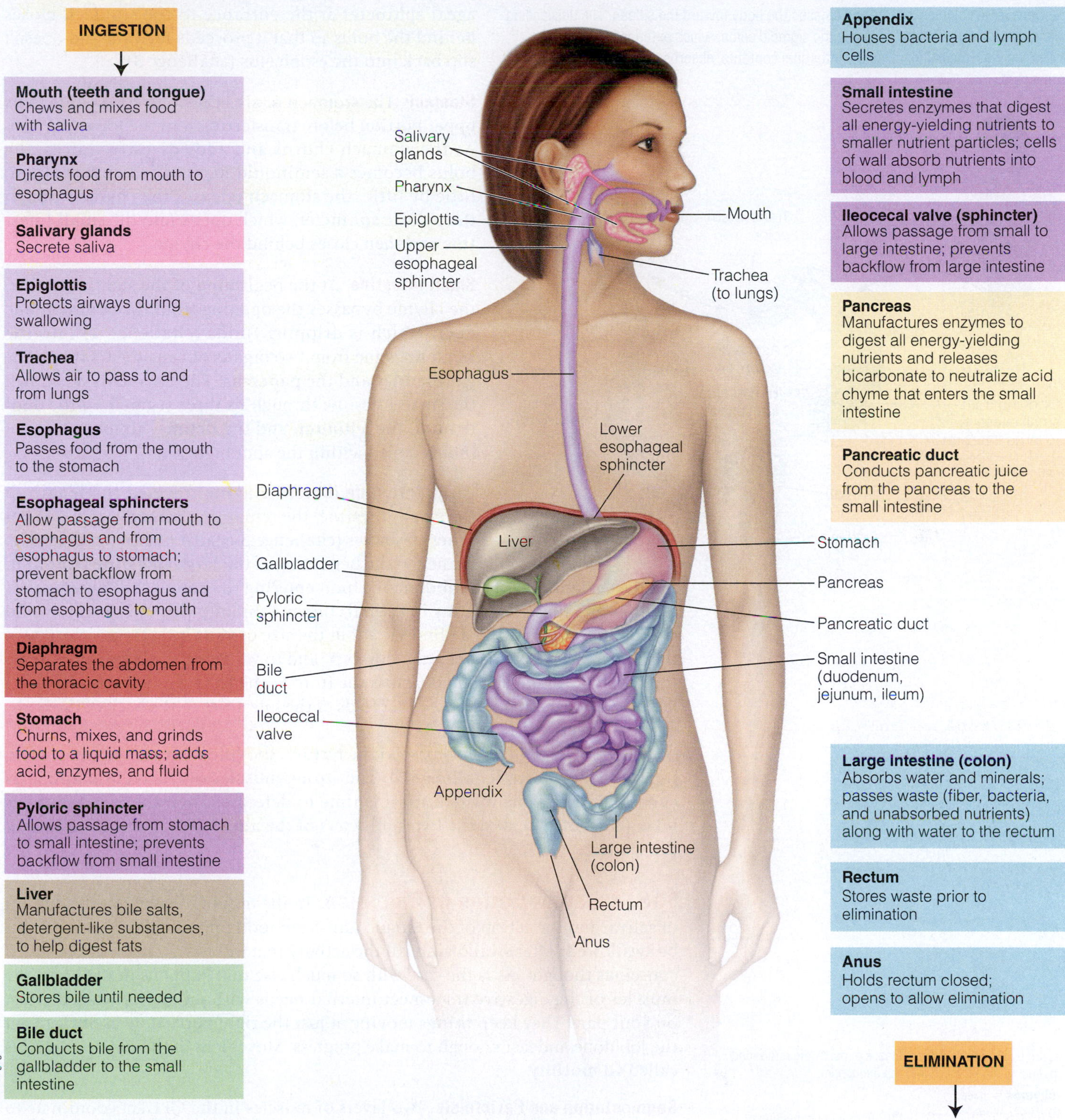

INGESTION
Mouth (teeth and tongue)
Chews and mixes food with saliva
Pharynx
Directs food from mouth to esophagus
Salivary glands
Secrete saliva
Epiglottis
Protects airways during swallowing
Trachea
Allows air to pass to and from lungs
Esophagus
Passes food from the mouth to the stomach
Esophageal sphincters
Allow passage from mouth to esophagus and from esophagus to stomach; prevent backflow from stomach to esophagus and from esophagus to mouth
Diaphragm
Separates the abdomen from the thoracic cavity
Stomach
Churns, mixes, and grinds food to a liquid mass; adds acid, enzymes, and fluid
Pyloric sphincter
Allows passage from stomach to small intestine; prevents backflow from small intestine
Liver
Manufactures bile salts, detergent-like substances, to help digest fats
Gallbladder
Stores bile until needed
Bile duct
Conducts bile from the gallbladder to the small intestine
Salivary glands
Pharynx
Epiglottis
Upper esophageal sphincter
Mouth
Trachea (to lungs)
Esophagus
Lower esophageal sphincter
Diaphragm
Liver
Gallbladder
Pyloric sphincter
Bile duct
Ileocecal valve
Appendix
Stomach
Pancreas
Pancreatic duct
Small intestine (duodenum, jejunum, ileum)
Large intestine (colon)
Rectum
Anus
Appendix
Houses bacteria and lymph cells
Small intestine
Secretes enzymes that digest all energy-yielding nutrients to smaller nutrient particles; cells of wall absorb nutrients into blood and lymph
Ileocecal valve (sphincter)
Allows passage from small to large intestine; prevents backflow from large intestine
Pancreas
Manufactures enzymes to digest all energy-yielding nutrients and releases bicarbonate to neutralize acid chyme that enters the small intestine
Pancreatic duct
Conducts pancreatic juice from the pancreas to the small intestine
Large Intestine (colon)
Absorbs water and minerals; passes waste (fiber, bacteria, and unabsorbed nutrients) along with water to the rectum
Rectum
Stores waste prior to elimination
Anus
Holds rectum closed; opens to allow elimination
ELIMINATION

the respiratory system. To bypass the entrance to the lungs, the **epiglottis** closes off the airway so that choking doesn't occur when swallowing, thus resolving the first challenge. (Choking is discussed on pp. 87–88.) After a mouthful of food has been chewed and swallowed, it is called a **bolus**.

Esophagus The **esophagus** has a **sphincter** muscle at each end. During a swallow, the upper **esophageal sphincter** opens. The bolus then slides down the

bolus (BOH-lus): a portion; with respect to food, the amount swallowed at one time.
- **bolos** = lump

> **FIGURE 3-2 The Colon**

The colon begins with the ascending colon rising upward toward the liver. It becomes the transverse colon as it turns and crosses the body toward the spleen. The descending colon turns downward and becomes the sigmoid colon, which extends to the rectum. Along the way, the colon mixes the intestinal contents, absorbs water and salts, and forms stool.

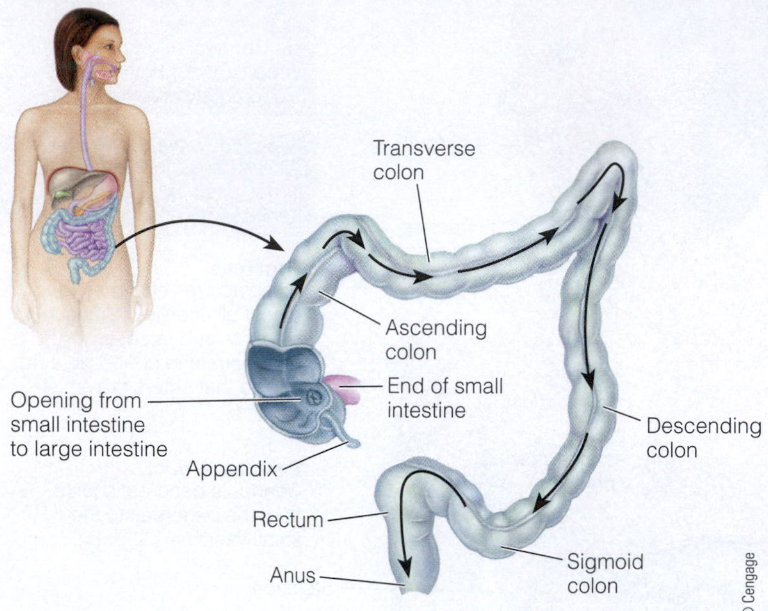

Transverse colon
Ascending colon
End of small intestine
Opening from small intestine to large intestine
Appendix
Descending colon
Rectum
Anus
Sigmoid colon
© Cengage

esophagus, which passes through a hole in the diaphragm (challenge 2) to the stomach. The lower esophageal sphincter at the entrance to the stomach closes behind the bolus so that it proceeds forward and doesn't slip back into the esophagus (challenge 3).

Stomach The **stomach** retains the bolus for a while in its upper portion before transferring it to the lower portion. As the stomach churns and adds digestive juices, the bolus becomes a semiliquid mass called **chyme.** Then, little by little, the stomach releases the chyme through the **pyloric sphincter,** which opens into the **small intestine** and then closes behind the chyme.

Small Intestine At the beginning of the small intestine, the chyme bypasses the opening from the common bile duct, which is dripping fluids (challenge 4) into the small intestine from two organs outside the GI tract—the **gallbladder** and the **pancreas.** The chyme travels down the small intestine through its three segments—the **duodenum,** the **jejunum,** and the **ileum**—almost 10 feet of tubing coiled within the abdomen.

Large Intestine (Colon) Having traveled the length of the small intestine, the remaining contents arrive at another sphincter (challenge 3 again): the **ileocecal valve,** located at the beginning of the **large intestine (colon)** in the lower right side of the abdomen. Upon entering the colon, the contents pass another opening. Should any intestinal contents slip into this opening, it would end up in the **appendix,** a blind sac about the size of your little finger. Normally, the contents bypass this opening, however, and travel along the large intestine up the right side of the abdomen, across the front to the left side, down to the lower left side, and finally below the other folds of the intestines to the back of the body, above the **rectum** (see Figure 3-2).

As the intestinal contents pass to the rectum, the colon withdraws water, leaving semisolid waste (challenge 5). The strong muscles of the rectum and anal canal hold back this waste until it is time to defecate. Then the rectal muscles relax (challenge 7), and the two sphincters of the **anus** open to allow passage of the waste.

The Muscular Action of Digestion

In the mouth, chewing, the addition of saliva, and the action of the tongue transform food into a coarse mash that can be swallowed. After swallowing, all the activity that follows occurs without much conscious thought. As is the case with so much else that happens in the body, the muscles of the digestive tract meet internal needs without any concerted effort on your part. They keep things moving at just the right pace, slow enough to get the job done and fast enough to make progress. Movement of the digestive tract is called **GI motility.**

Segmentation and Peristalsis Two layers of muscles in the GI tract coordinate to produce two kinds of action—**segmentation** and **peristalsis**. In segmentation, the inner circular muscles contract and relax in a way that churns the chyme. This churning action mixes the chyme with digestive juices and puts it in close contact with the absorbing cells of the intestinal wall. In peristalsis, the outer longitudinal muscles rhythmically contract in a way that moves chyme forward. These rhythmic contractions occur continuously at varying rates and intensities, depending on the section of the GI tract and on whether food is present. Factors such as stress, drugs, and illness may interfere with normal GI tract contractions.

chyme (KIME): the semiliquid mass of partly digested food expelled by the stomach into the duodenum.

- **chymos** = juice

GI motility (moh-TIL-ih-tee): the spontaneous movement of the GI tract that aids in the digestion and transit of the contents within it.

segmentation (SEG-men-TAY-shun): a periodic squeezing or partitioning of the intestine at intervals along its length by its circular muscles.

peristalsis (per-ih-STALL-sis): wavelike muscular contractions of the GI tract that push its contents along.

- **peri** = around
- **stellein** = wrap

Stomach Action The stomach has the thickest walls and strongest muscles of all the GI tract organs. In addition to the circular and longitudinal muscles, it has a third layer of diagonal muscles that also alternately contract and relax (see Figure 3-3). These three sets of muscles work to force the chyme downward, but the pyloric sphincter (at the bottom of the stomach) usually remains tightly closed, preventing the chyme from passing into the duodenum of the small intestine. As a result, the chyme is churned and forced down, hits the pyloric sphincter, and remains in the stomach. Meanwhile, the stomach wall releases gastric juices. When the chyme is completely liquefied with gastric juices, the pyloric sphincter opens briefly, about three times a minute, to allow small portions of chyme to pass through. At this point, the chyme no longer resembles food in the least.

> **FIGURE 3-3 Stomach Muscles**
The stomach has three layers of muscles.

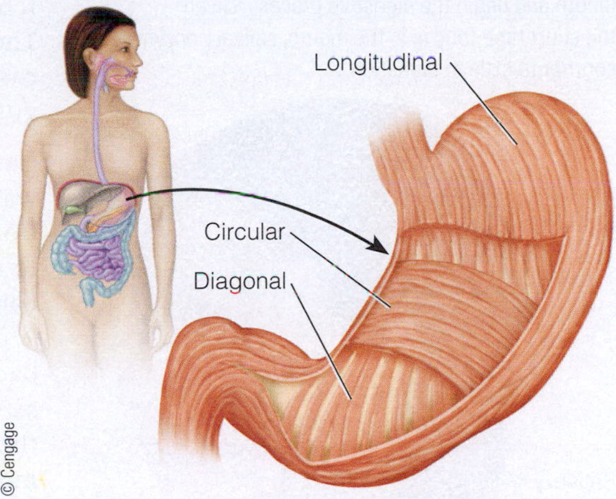
Longitudinal
Circular
Diagonal
© Cengage

Sphincter Contractions Sphincter muscles periodically open and close, allowing the contents of the GI tract to move along at a controlled pace (challenge 3 again). At the top of the esophagus, the upper esophageal sphincter opens in response to swallowing. At the bottom of the esophagus, the lower esophageal sphincter (sometimes called the cardiac sphincter because of its proximity to the heart) prevents **reflux** of the stomach contents. At the bottom of the stomach, the pyloric sphincter, which stays closed most of the time, holds the chyme in the stomach long enough for it to be thoroughly mixed with gastric juice and liquefied. The pyloric sphincter also prevents the intestinal contents from backing up into the stomach. At the end of the small intestine, the ileocecal valve performs a similar function, allowing the contents of the small intestine to empty into the large intestine. Finally, the tightness of the rectal muscle acts as a kind of safety device; together with the two sphincters of the anus, it prevents continuous elimination (challenge 7). Figure 3-4 illustrates how sphincter muscles contract and relax to close and open passageways.

The Secretions of Digestion

The breakdown of food into nutrients requires secretions from five different organs: the salivary glands, the stomach, the pancreas, the liver (via the gallbladder), and the small intestine. These secretions enter the GI tract at various points along the way, bringing an abundance of fluids (challenge 4) and a variety of enzymes.

Enzymes are formally introduced in Chapter 6, but for now a simple definition will suffice. An enzyme is a protein that facilitates a chemical reaction—making a molecule, breaking a molecule apart, changing the arrangement of a molecule, or exchanging parts of molecules. As a **catalyst**, the enzyme itself remains unchanged. The enzymes involved in digestion facilitate a chemical reaction known as **hydrolysis**—the addition of water *(hydro)* to break *(lysis)* a molecule into smaller pieces. Glossary 3-2 (p. 74) describes how to identify some of the common **digestive enzymes** and related terms; later chapters introduce specific enzymes. When learning about enzymes, it helps to know that the word ending *-ase* denotes an enzyme. Enzymes are often identified by the organ they come from and the compounds they work on. *Gastric lipase*, for example, is a stomach enzyme that acts on lipids, whereas *pancreatic lipase* comes from the pancreas (and also works on lipids).

> **FIGURE 3-4 An Example of a Sphincter Muscle**
When the circular muscles of a sphincter contract, the passage closes; when they relax, the passage opens.

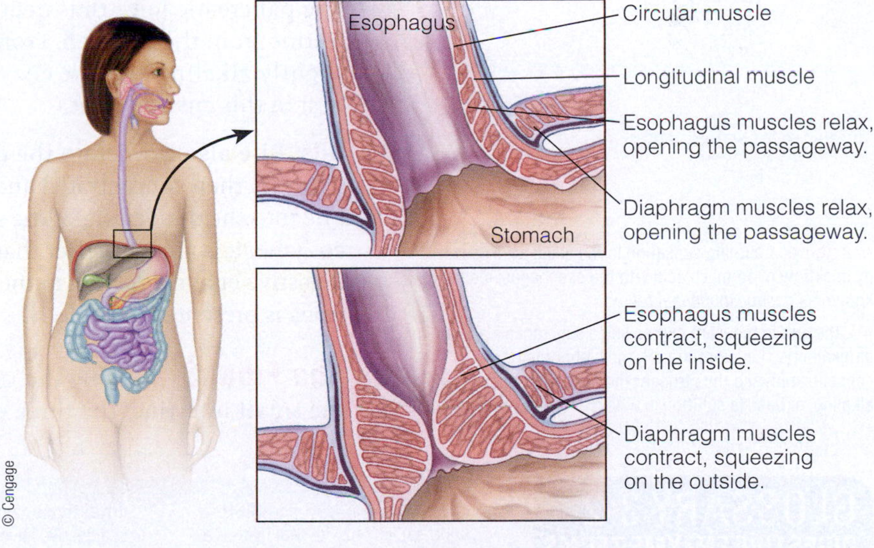
Esophagus
Stomach
Circular muscle
Longitudinal muscle
Esophagus muscles relax, opening the passageway.
Diaphragm muscles relax, opening the passageway.
Esophagus muscles contract, squeezing on the inside.
Diaphragm muscles contract, squeezing on the outside.
© Cengage

reflux: a backward flow.
- **re** = back
- **flux** = flow

catalyst (CAT-uh-list)**:** a compound that facilitates chemical reactions without itself being changed in the process.

> **FIGURE 3-5 The Salivary Glands**

The salivary glands secrete enzyme-rich saliva into the mouth and begin the digestive process. Given the short time food is in the mouth, salivary enzymes contribute little to digestion.

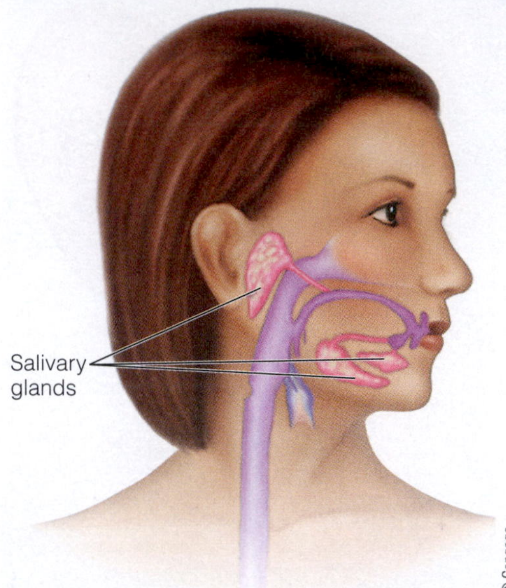
Salivary glands
© Cengage

Saliva The **salivary glands,** shown in Figure 3-5, squirt just enough **saliva** to moisten each mouthful of food so that it can pass easily down the esophagus (challenge 4). (Digestive **glands** and their secretions are defined in Glossary 3-3.) The saliva contains water, salts, mucus, and enzymes that initiate the digestion of carbohydrates. Saliva also protects the teeth and the linings of the mouth, esophagus, and stomach from substances that might cause damage.

Gastric Juice In the stomach, **gastric glands** secrete **gastric juice,** a mixture of water, enzymes, and **hydrochloric acid,** which acts primarily in protein digestion. The acid is so strong that it causes the sensation of **heartburn** if it happens to reflux into the esophagus. Highlight 3 discusses heartburn, ulcers, and other common digestive problems.

The strong acidity of the stomach prevents bacterial growth and kills most bacteria that enter the body with food. It would destroy the cells of the stomach as well, but for their natural defenses. To protect themselves from gastric juice, the cells of the stomach wall (in fact, of the entire gastrointestinal lining) secrete **mucus,** a thick, slippery, white substance that coats the cells, protecting them from stomach acid, enzymes, and disease-causing bacteria that might otherwise cause harm (challenge 6).

Figure 3-6 shows how the strength of acids is measured—in **pH** units. Note that the acidity of gastric juice registers below 2 on the pH scale—stronger than vinegar. The stomach enzymes work most efficiently in the stomach's strong acid, but the salivary enzymes, which are swallowed with food, do not work in acid this strong. Consequently, the salivary digestion of carbohydrates ceases as stomach acid penetrates each newly swallowed bolus of food. Once in the stomach, salivary enzymes simply become proteins to be digested.

Pancreatic Juice and Intestinal Enzymes By the time food leaves the stomach, digestion of all three energy nutrients (carbohydrates, fats, and proteins) has begun, and the action gains momentum in the small intestine. There the pancreas contributes digestive juices by way of ducts leading into the duodenum. The **pancreatic juice** contains enzymes that act on all three energy nutrients, and the cells of the intestinal wall also possess digestive enzymes on their surfaces.

In addition to enzymes, the pancreatic juice contains sodium **bicarbonate,** which is basic or alkaline—the opposite of the stomach's acid (review Figure 3-6). The pancreatic juice thus neutralizes the acidic chyme arriving in the small intestine from the stomach. From this point on, the chyme remains at a neutral or slightly alkaline pH. The enzymes of both the intestine and the pancreas work best in this environment.

Bile Bile also flows into the duodenum. The **liver** continuously produces bile, which is then concentrated and stored in the gallbladder. The gallbladder squirts bile into the duodenum of the small intestine when fat arrives there. Bile is not an enzyme; it is an **emulsifier** that disperses fats in watery solutions, which gives the digestive enzymes access to them. A summary of digestive secretions and their actions is presented in Table 3-1.

heartburn: a burning sensation in the chest area caused by backflow of stomach acid into the esophagus; medically known as *gastroesophageal reflux*.

pH: the unit of measure expressing a substance's acidity or alkalinity. The lower the pH, the higher the H^+ ion concentration and the stronger the acid. A pH above 7 is alkaline, or base (a solution in which OH^- ions predominate).

The Final Stage

By the time the contents of the GI tract reach the end of the small intestine, the three energy-yielding nutrients—carbohydrate, fat, and

GLOSSARY 3-2 DIGESTIVE ENZYME TERMS

-ase (ACE): suffix denoting an enzyme. The root of the word often identifies the compound the enzyme works on. Examples include:

- *carbohydrase* (KAR-boe-HIGH-drase), an enzyme that hydrolyzes carbohydrates.
- *lipase* (LYE-pase), an enzyme that hydrolyzes lipids (fats).
- *protease* (PRO-tee-ase), an enzyme that hydrolyzes proteins.

digestive enzymes: proteins found in digestive juices that act on food substances, causing them to break down into simpler compounds.

hydrolysis (high-DROL-ih-sis): a chemical reaction in which one molecule is split into two molecules, with hydrogen (H) added to one and a hydroxyl group (OH) added to the other (from water, H_2O). (The noun is *hydrolysis*; the verb is *hydrolyze*.)

- **hydro** = water
- **lysis** = breaking

TABLE 3-1 Summary of Digestive Secretions and Their Major Actions

Organ or Gland	Target Organ	Secretion	Action
Salivary glands	Mouth	Saliva	Fluid eases swallowing; salivary enzyme breaks down some *carbohydrate*.*
Gastric glands	Stomach	Gastric juice	Fluid mixes with bolus; hydrochloric acid uncoils *proteins;* enzymes break down proteins; mucus protects stomach cells.*
Pancreas	Small intestine	Pancreatic juice	Bicarbonate neutralizes acidic gastric juices; pancreatic enzymes break down *carbohydrates, fats,* and *proteins.*
Liver	Gallbladder	Bile	Bile is stored until needed.
Gallbladder	Small intestine	Bile	Bile emulsifies *fat* so that enzymes can have access to break it down.
Intestinal glands	Small intestine	Intestinal juice	Intestinal enzymes break down *carbohydrate, fat,* and *protein* fragments; mucus protects the intestinal wall.

*Saliva and gastric juice also contain lipases, but most fat breakdown occurs in the small intestine.

protein—have been digested. Some vitamins and minerals are altered slightly during digestion, but most are absorbed as they are. All that remains—fluids, a few dissolved salts, and undigested materials such as fiber—enters the large intestine (colon). Fiber carries with it some fat, cholesterol, and a few minerals and retains water as well, accounting for the consistency of **stool**. Intestinal bacteria ferment some fibers, producing water, gas, and small fragments of fat that provide energy for the cells of the colon. The colon itself retrieves the fluids and salts that the body can recycle. The waste that is finally excreted has little or nothing of value left in it. The body has extracted all that it can use from the food. Figure 3-7 (p. 76) summarizes digestion by following a sandwich through the GI tract and into the body.

REVIEW IT Explain how foods move through the digestive system, describing the actions of the organs, muscles, and digestive secretions along the way.

As Figure 3-1 (p. 71) shows, food enters the mouth and travels down the esophagus and through the upper and lower esophageal sphincters to the stomach, then through the pyloric sphincter to the small intestine, on through the ileocecal valve to the large intestine, past the appendix to the rectum, ending at the anus. The wavelike contractions of peristalsis and the periodic squeezing of segmentation keep things moving at a reasonable pace. Along the way, secretions from the salivary glands, stomach, pancreas, liver (via the gallbladder), and small intestine deliver fluids and digestive enzymes.

> FIGURE 3-6 The pH of Common Substances

A substance's acidity or alkalinity is measured in pH units. The pH is the negative logarithm of the hydrogen ion concentration. Each increment represents a tenfold increase in concentration of hydrogen ions, meaning, for example, that a pH of 2 is 1000 times stronger than a pH of 5.

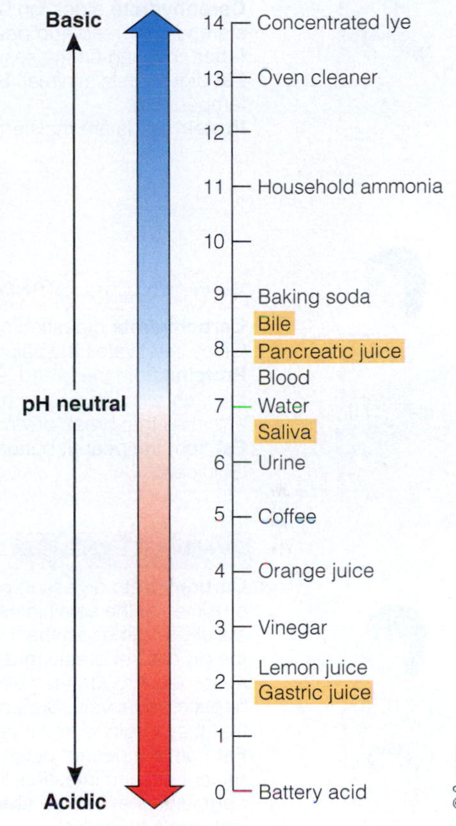

Basic
pH neutral
Acidic
14 Concentrated lye
13 Oven cleaner
12
11 Household ammonia
10
9 Baking soda
Bile
8 Pancreatic juice
Blood
7 Water
Saliva
6 Urine
5 Coffee
4 Orange juice
3 Vinegar
Lemon juice
2 Gastric juice
1
0 Battery acid
© Cengage

stool: waste matter discharged from the colon; also called *feces* (FEE-seez).

GLOSSARY 3-3
DIGESTIVE GLAND AND SECRETION TERMS

bicarbonate: an alkaline compound with the formula HCO_3 that is secreted from the pancreas as part of the pancreatic juice. (Bicarbonate is also produced in all cell fluids from the dissociation of carbonic acid to help maintain the body's acid-base balance.)

bile: an emulsifier that prepares fats and oils for digestion; an exocrine secretion made by the liver, stored in the gallbladder, and released into the small intestine when needed.

emulsifier (ee-MUL-sih-fire): a substance with both water-soluble and fat-soluble portions that promotes the mixing of oils and fats in a watery solution.

gastric glands: exocrine glands in the stomach wall that secrete gastric juice into the stomach.

- **gastro** = stomach

gastric juice: the digestive secretion of the gastric glands of the stomach.

glands: cells or groups of cells that secrete materials for special uses in the body. Glands may be *exocrine* (EKS-oh-crin) *glands*, secreting their materials "out" (into the digestive tract or onto the surface of the skin), or *endocrine* (EN-doe-crin) *glands*, secreting their materials "in" (into the blood).

- **exo** = outside
- **endo** = inside
- **krine** = to separate

hydrochloric acid: an acid composed of hydrogen and chloride atoms (HCl) that is normally produced by the gastric glands.

liver: the organ that manufactures bile, among many other functions (described in Chapter 7).

mucus (MYOO-kus): a slippery substance secreted by cells of the GI lining (and other body linings) that protects the cells from exposure to digestive juices (and other destructive agents). The lining of the GI tract with its coat of mucus is a *mucous membrane*. (The noun is *mucus;* the adjective is *mucous.*)

pancreatic (pank-ree-AT-ic) **juice:** the exocrine secretion of the pancreas that contains both enzymes for the digestion of carbohydrate, fat, and protein as well as bicarbonate, a neutralizing agent. The juice flows from the pancreas into the small intestine through the pancreatic duct. (The pancreas also has an endocrine function, the secretion of insulin and other hormones.)

saliva: the secretion of the salivary glands. Its principal enzyme begins carbohydrate digestion.

salivary glands: exocrine glands that secrete saliva into the mouth.

> **FIGURE 3-7 The Digestive Fate of a Sandwich**

To review the digestive processes, follow a peanut butter and banana sandwich on whole-wheat, sesame seed bread through the GI tract. As the graph on the right illustrates, digestion of the energy nutrients begins in different parts of the GI tract, but all are ready for absorption by the time they reach the end of the small intestine.

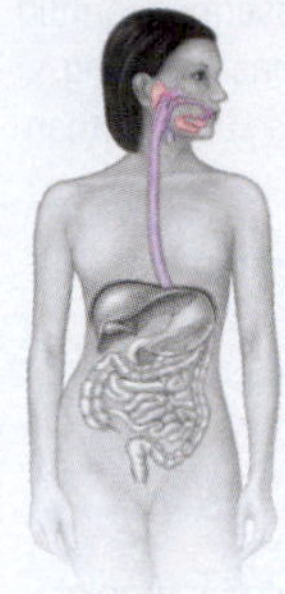

MOUTH: CHEWING AND SWALLOWING, WITH LITTLE DIGESTION

Carbohydrate digestion begins as salivary amylase breaks down starch from bread and peanut butter.
Fiber covering on the sesame seeds is crushed by the teeth.
Fat digestion is minimal. Some hard fats melt as they reach body temperature.
Protein foods are moistened by saliva.

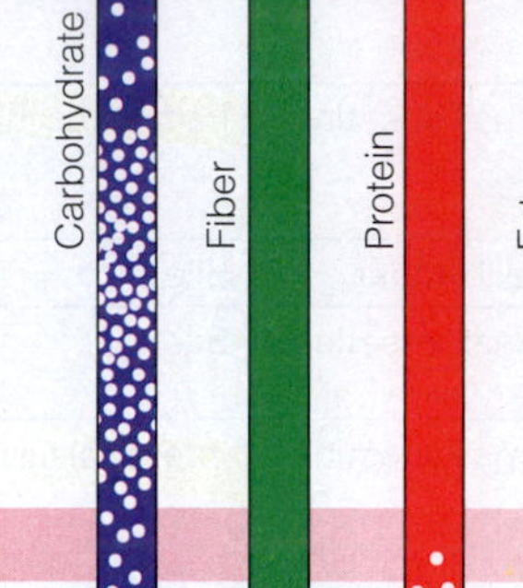

Carbohydrate
Fiber
Protein
Fat

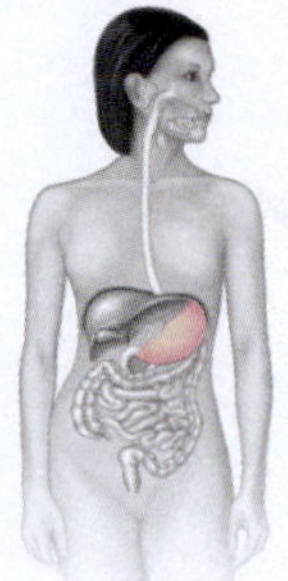

STOMACH: COLLECTING AND CHURNING, WITH SOME DIGESTION

Carbohydrate digestion ceases when the stomach acid of the gastric juices inactivates the salivary amylase.
Proteins from the bread, seeds, and peanut butter begin to uncoil when they mix with the gastric acid, exposing them to the gastric protease enzymes that break down proteins.
Fat from the peanut butter and seeds tends to separate from the watery GI juices.

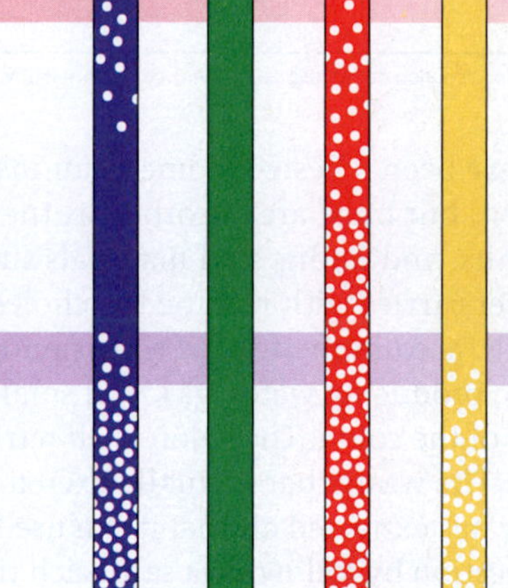

SMALL INTESTINE: DIGESTING AND ABSORBING

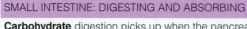

Carbohydrate digestion picks up when the pancreas sends pancreatic enzymes to the small intestine via the pancreatic duct to break down starch. Enzymes on the surfaces of the small intestinal cells complete the process of breaking down starch into small fragments that can be absorbed through the cells of the small intestine walls and into the hepatic portal vein. Sugars from the banana require so little digestion that they begin to traverse the intestinal cells immediately on contact.
Fat from the peanut butter and seeds is emulsified by bile. Now pancreatic and intestinal lipases can break down the fat to smaller fragments that can be absorbed through the cells of the small intestine wall and into the lymph.
Protein breakdown depends on the pancreatic and intestinal proteases. Small fragments of protein are absorbed through the cells of the small intestine wall and into the hepatic portal vein.
Vitamins and minerals are absorbed.

Note: Sugars and starches are members of the carbohydrate family.

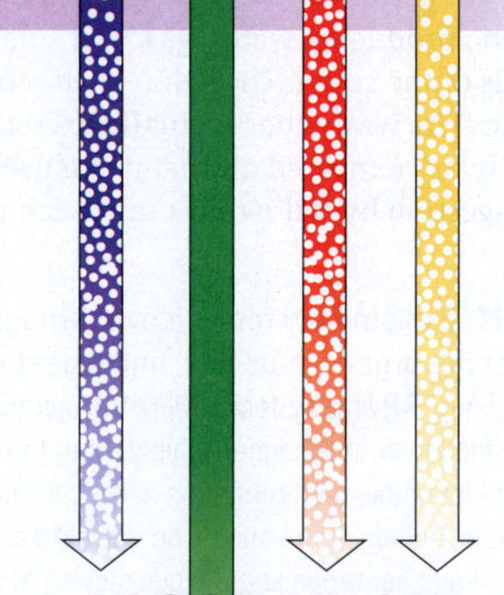

ABSORPTION

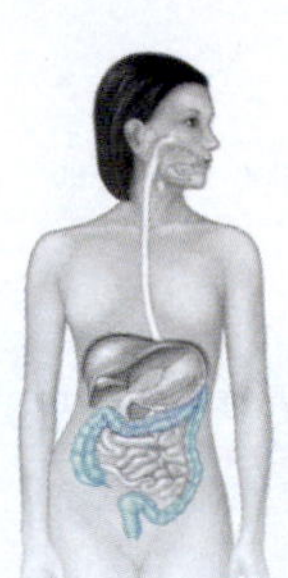

LARGE INTESTINE: ABSORBING AND ELIMINATING

Fluids and some minerals are absorbed.
Some fibers from the seeds, whole-wheat bread, peanut butter, and banana are partly digested by the bacteria living in the large intestine, and some of these products are absorbed.
Most fibers pass through the large intestine and are excreted as feces; some fat, cholesterol, and minerals bind to fiber and are also excreted.

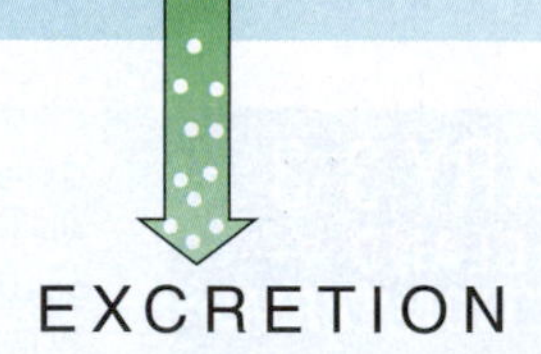

EXCRETION

3.2 Absorption

LEARN IT Describe the anatomical details of the intestinal cells that facilitate nutrient absorption.

Within three or four hours after a person has eaten a dinner of beans and rice (or spinach lasagna, or steak and potatoes) with vegetable, salad, beverage, and dessert, the body must find a way to absorb the molecules derived from carbohydrate, protein, and fat digestion—and the vitamin and mineral molecules as well. Most absorption takes place in the small intestine, one of the most elegantly designed organ systems in the body. Within its 10-foot length, which provides a surface area equivalent to 1.5 bowling lanes, the small intestine traps and absorbs the nutrient molecules.[1] To remove the absorbed molecules rapidly and provide room for more to be absorbed, a rush of circulating blood continuously washes the underside of this surface, carrying the absorbed nutrients away to the liver and other parts of the body. Figure 3-8 describes how most nutrients are absorbed by simple diffusion, facilitated diffusion, or active transport. Later chapters provide details on specific nutrients. Before following nutrients through the body, we must look more closely at the anatomy of the absorptive system.

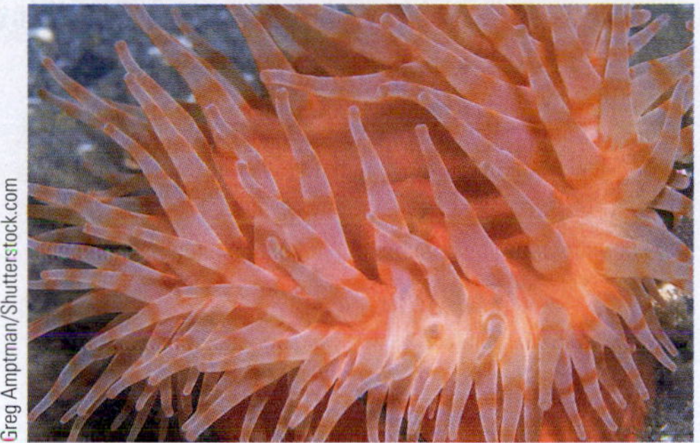
Greg Amptman/Shutterstock.com

> **PHOTO 3-2** If you have ever watched a sea anemone with its fingerlike projections in constant motion, you have a good picture of how the intestinal villi move.

Anatomy of the Absorptive System The inner surface of the small intestine looks smooth and slippery, but when viewed through a microscope, it turns out to be wrinkled into hundreds of folds. Each fold is contoured into thousands of fingerlike projections, as numerous as the hairs on velvet fabric. These small intestinal projections are called **villi.** A single villus, magnified still more, turns out to be composed of hundreds of cells, each covered with its own microscopic hairs, called **microvilli** (see Figure 3-9, p. 78). In the crevices between the villi lie the **crypts**—tubular glands that secrete the intestinal juices into the small intestine. Nearby **goblet cells** secrete mucus.

The villi are in constant motion. Each villus is lined by a thin sheet of muscle, so it can wave, squirm, and wriggle like the tentacles of a sea anemone (see Photo 3-2). Any nutrient molecule small enough to be absorbed is trapped among the microvilli and then drawn into the cells. Some partially digested nutrients are caught in the microvilli, digested further by enzymes there, and then absorbed into the cells.

A Closer Look at the Intestinal Cells The cells of the villi are among the most amazing in the body, for they recognize and select the nutrients the body needs and regulate their absorption. As already described, each cell of a villus is coated with thousands of microvilli, which project from the cell's membrane (review Figure 3-9 and see Photo 3-3, p. 78). In these microvilli, and in the membrane,

villi (VILL-ee or VILL-eye): fingerlike projections from the folds of the small intestine; singular *villus.*

microvilli (MY-cro-VILL-ee or MY-cro-VILL-eye): tiny, hairlike projections on each cell of every villus that can trap nutrient particles and transport them into the cells; singular *microvillus.*

crypts (KRIPTS): tubular glands that lie between the intestinal villi and secrete intestinal juices into the small intestine.

goblet cells: cells of the GI tract (and lungs) that secrete mucus.

> **FIGURE 3-8 Absorption of Nutrients**

Absorption of nutrients into intestinal cells typically occurs by simple diffusion, facilitated diffusion, or active transport. Occasionally, a large molecule is absorbed by *endocytosis*—a process in which the cell membrane engulfs the molecule, forming a sac that separates from the membrane and moves into the cell.

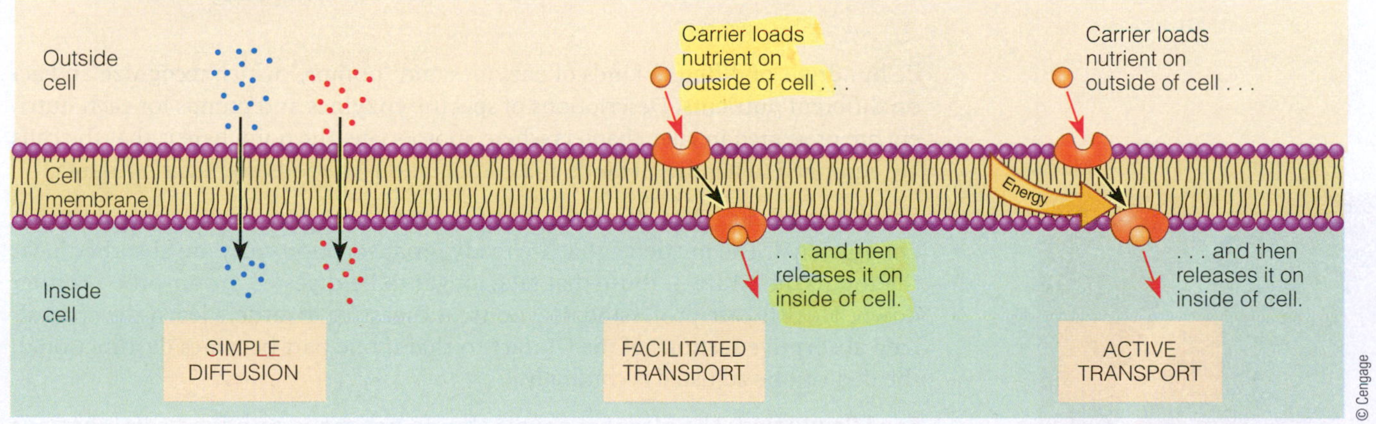
Outside cell
Cell membrane
Inside cell
Carrier loads nutrient on outside of cell . . .
. . . and then releases it on inside of cell.
Carrier loads nutrient on outside of cell . . .
Energy
. . . and then releases it on inside of cell.
SIMPLE DIFFUSION
FACILITATED TRANSPORT
ACTIVE TRANSPORT
© Cengage

Some nutrients (such as water and small lipids) are absorbed by simple diffusion. They cross into intestinal cells freely.

Some nutrients (such as the water-soluble vitamins) are absorbed by facilitated transport. They need a specific carrier to transport them from one side of the cell membrane to the other. (Alternatively, facilitated transport may occur when the carrier changes the cell membrane in such a way that the nutrients can pass through.)

Some nutrients (such as glucose and amino acids) are absorbed actively. These nutrients move against a concentration gradient, which requires energy.

> **FIGURE 3-9 The Small Intestine**

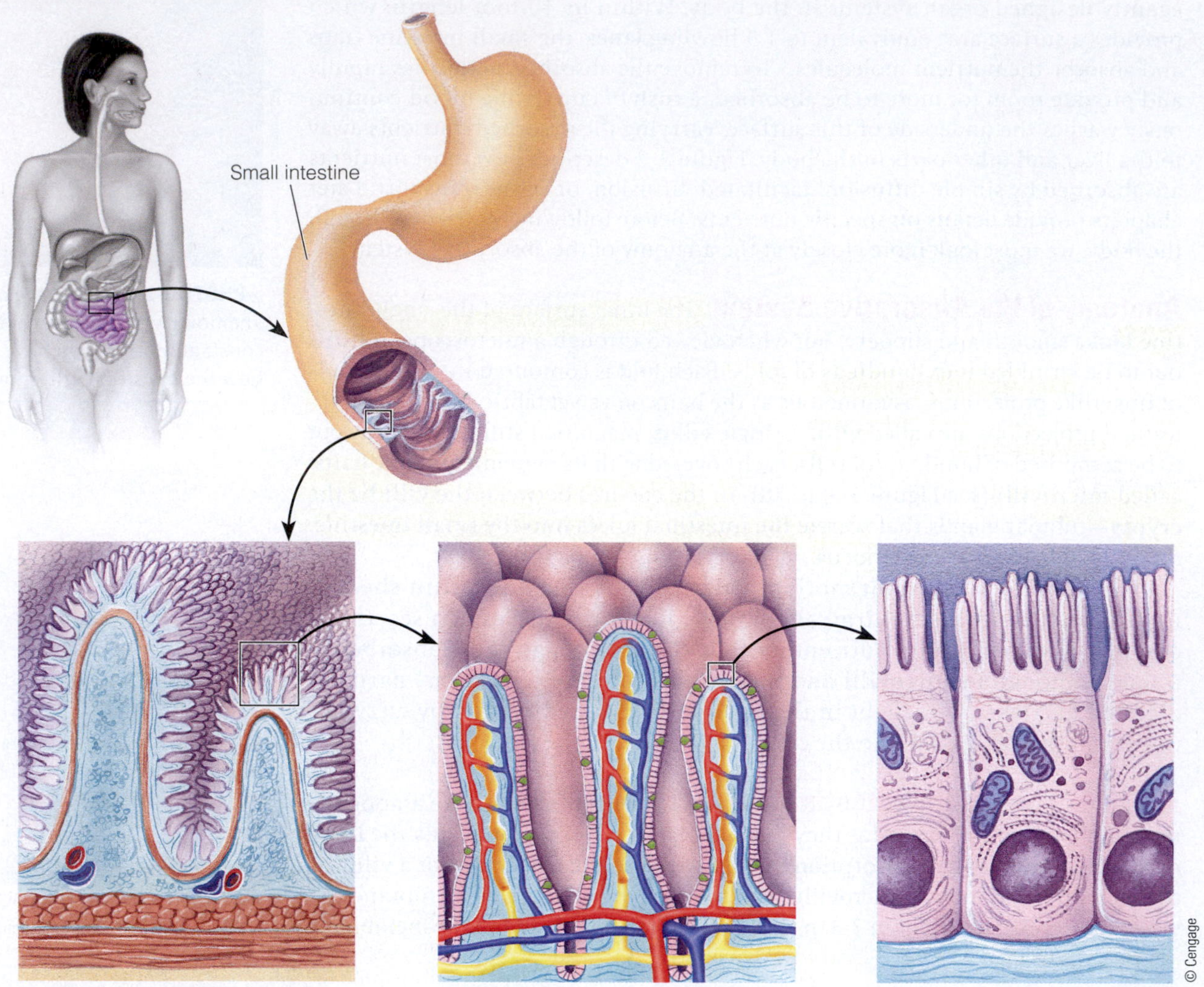

Small intestine

The walls of the small intestine are wrinkled into thousands of folds covered with villi.

Each villus contains a network of capillaries and lymphatic vessels for transporting nutrients out of the intestinal cells.

Each villus is made of absorptive cells that are covered with even smaller projections—the microvilli—that trap and absorb the nutrients.

lie hundreds of different kinds of enzymes and "pumps," which recognize and act on different nutrients. Descriptions of specific enzymes and pumps for each nutrient are presented in later chapters where appropriate; the point here is that the cells are equipped to handle all kinds and combinations of foods and their nutrients.

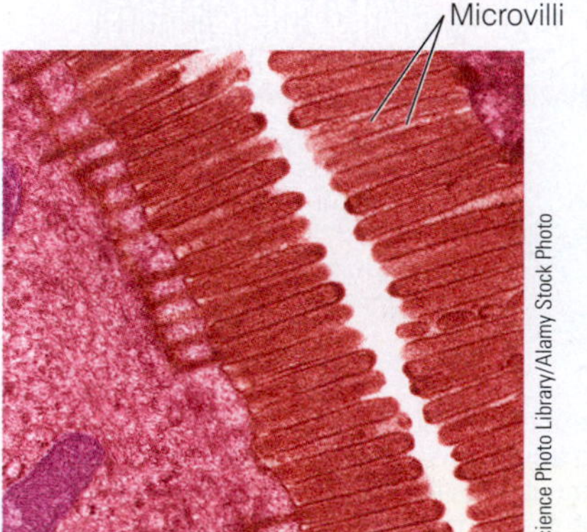
Microvilli

> **PHOTO 3-3** A human intestinal cell is lined with microvilli.

Specialized Cells The cells of the intestinal tract are specialized to absorb different nutrients. The nutrients that are ready for absorption early are absorbed near the top of the GI tract; those that take longer to be digested are absorbed farther down. Health-care professionals who treat digestive disorders learn the specialized absorptive sections of the GI tract so that if one part becomes dysfunctional, the diet can be adjusted accordingly.

Food Combining The idea that people should not eat certain food combinations (for example, fruit and meat) at the same meal, because the digestive system cannot handle more than one task at a time, is a myth. The art of "food combining"—which actually emphasizes "food separating"—is based on this myth, and it represents faulty logic and a gross underestimation of the body's capabilities. In fact, the contrary is often true; foods eaten together can enhance each other's use by the body. For example, vitamin C in bell peppers and tomatoes can enhance the absorption of iron from a meal of beans and rice or other iron-containing foods. Many other examples of mutually beneficial interactions are presented in later chapters.

Preparing Nutrients for Transport When a nutrient molecule has been absorbed and has crossed into the cell of a villus, it enters either the bloodstream or the lymphatic system (see Photo 3-4). Both transport systems supply vessels to each villus, as shown in Figure 3-9. The water-soluble nutrients and the smaller products of fat digestion are released directly into the bloodstream and guided directly to the liver, where their fate and destination will be determined.

The larger fats and the fat-soluble vitamins are insoluble in water, however, and blood is mostly water. The intestinal cells assemble many of the products of fat digestion into larger molecules. These larger molecules cluster together with special proteins, forming chylomicrons. Chylomicrons (kye-lo-MY-cronz) are defined and described in more detail in Chapter 5. For now, keep in mind that because chylomicrons carry fats, they are released into the lymphatic system. They move through the lymph until they can enter the bloodstream at a point near the heart. Consequently, chylomicrons bypass the liver at first. Details follow.

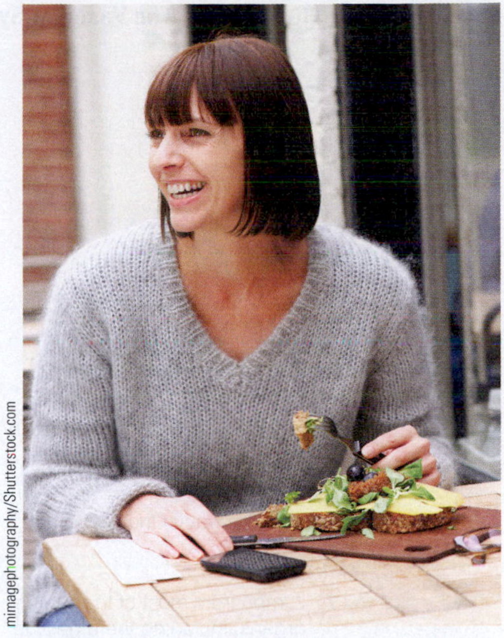

mimagephotography/Shutterstock.com

> **PHOTO 3-4** For the body to use nutrients from food, they must first be digested and absorbed.

REVIEW IT Describe the anatomical details of the intestinal cells that facilitate nutrient absorption.

The many folds and villi of the small intestine dramatically increase its surface area, facilitating nutrient absorption. Nutrients pass through the cells of the villi and enter either the blood (if they are water soluble or small fat fragments) or the lymph (if they are fat soluble).

3.3 The Circulatory Systems

LEARN IT Explain how nutrients are routed in the circulatory systems from the GI tract into the body and identify which nutrients enter the blood directly and which must first enter the lymph.

Once a nutrient has entered the bloodstream, it may be transported to any of the cells in the body, from the tips of the toes to the roots of the hair. The circulatory systems deliver nutrients wherever they are needed.

The Vascular System The vascular, or blood circulatory, system is a closed system of vessels through which blood flows continuously, with the heart serving as the pump (see Figure 3-10, p. 80). As the blood circulates through this system, it picks up and delivers materials as needed.

Nutrient Transport All the body tissues derive nutrients and oxygen from the blood and deposit carbon dioxide and other wastes back into the blood. The digestive system supplies the nutrients. The lungs exchange oxygen (which enters the blood to be delivered to all cells) and carbon dioxide (which leaves the blood to be exhaled). The kidneys filter wastes other than carbon dioxide out of the blood to be excreted in the urine.

Blood leaving the right side of the heart circulates through the lungs and then back to the left side of the heart. The left side of the heart then pumps the blood out of the **aorta** through **arteries** to all systems of the body. The blood circulates in the **capillaries**, where it exchanges material with the cells and then collects into **veins**, which return it again to the right side of the heart. In short, blood travels this simple route:

Heart to arteries to capillaries to veins to heart

The routing of the blood leaving the digestive system has a special feature. The blood is carried to the digestive system (as to all organs) by way of an artery, which (as in all organs) branches into capillaries to reach every cell. Blood leaving the digestive system, however, goes by way of a vein. The **hepatic portal vein** directs blood not back to the heart but to another organ, the liver. This vein

aorta (ay-OR-tuh): the large, primary artery that conducts blood from the heart to the body's smaller arteries.

arteries: vessels that carry blood from the heart to the tissues.

capillaries (CAP-ill-aries): small vessels that branch from an artery. Capillaries connect arteries to veins. Exchange of oxygen, nutrients, and waste materials takes place across capillary walls.

veins (VANES): vessels that carry blood to the heart.

hepatic portal vein: the vein that collects blood from the GI tract and conducts it to the liver.

- **portal** = gateway

> **FIGURE 3-10 The Vascular System**

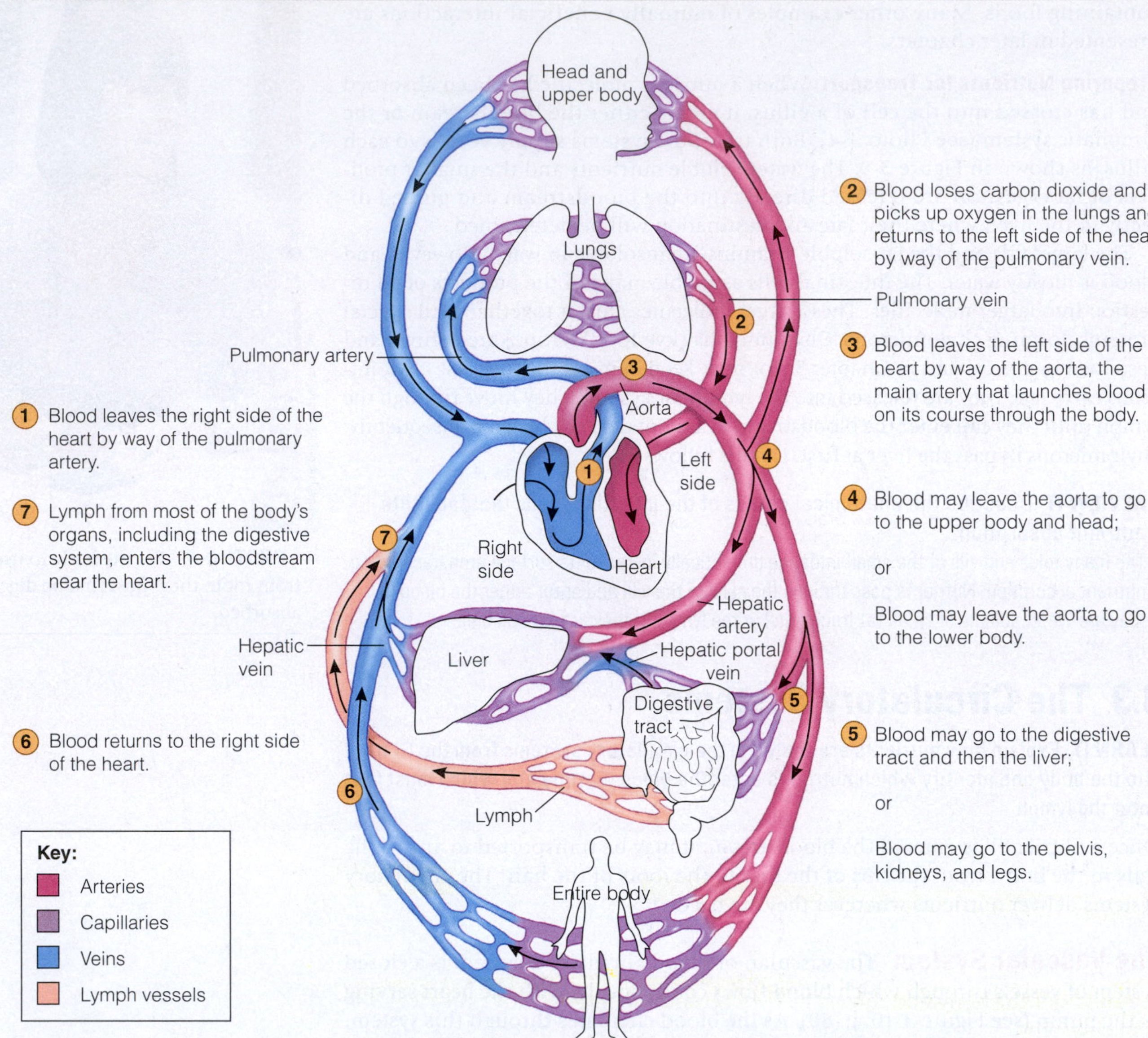

Head and upper body
Lungs
Pulmonary artery
Pulmonary vein
Aorta
Left side
Right side
Heart
Hepatic artery
Hepatic vein
Liver
Hepatic portal vein
Digestive tract
Lymph
Entire body
1 Blood leaves the right side of the heart by way of the pulmonary artery.
2 Blood loses carbon dioxide and picks up oxygen in the lungs and returns to the left side of the heart by way of the pulmonary vein.
3 Blood leaves the left side of the heart by way of the aorta, the main artery that launches blood on its course through the body.
4 Blood may leave the aorta to go to the upper body and head;
or
Blood may leave the aorta to go to the lower body.
5 Blood may go to the digestive tract and then the liver;
or
Blood may go to the pelvis, kidneys, and legs.
6 Blood returns to the right side of the heart.
7 Lymph from most of the body's organs, including the digestive system, enters the bloodstream near the heart.
Key:
Arteries
Capillaries
Veins
Lymph vessels

branches into a network of large capillaries so that every cell of the liver has access to the blood. Blood leaving the liver then collects into the **hepatic vein,** which returns blood to the heart. The route is:

Heart to arteries to capillaries (in intestines) to hepatic portal vein to capillaries (in liver) to hepatic vein to heart

The Liver Figure 3-11 shows the liver's key position in nutrient transport. An anatomist studying this system knows there must be a reason for this special arrangement. The liver's placement ensures that it will be first to receive the nutrients absorbed from the GI tract. In fact, the liver busily prepares carbohydrates, fats, proteins, and other absorbed nutrients for use by the rest of the body. Of all the body's organs, the liver is the most metabolically active, as Chapter 7 describes.

In addition, the liver defends the body by detoxifying substances that might cause harm and preparing waste products for excretion. This is why, when people ingest poisons that succeed in passing the first barrier (the intestinal cells), the liver quite often suffers the damage—from viruses such as hepatitis, from drugs such as barbiturates or alcohol, from toxins such as pesticide residues, and from contaminants such as mercury. Perhaps, in fact, you have been undervaluing your liver, not knowing what heroic tasks it quietly performs for you.

hepatic vein: the vein that collects blood from the liver and returns it to the heart.
- **hepatic** = liver

> **FIGURE 3-11 The Liver**

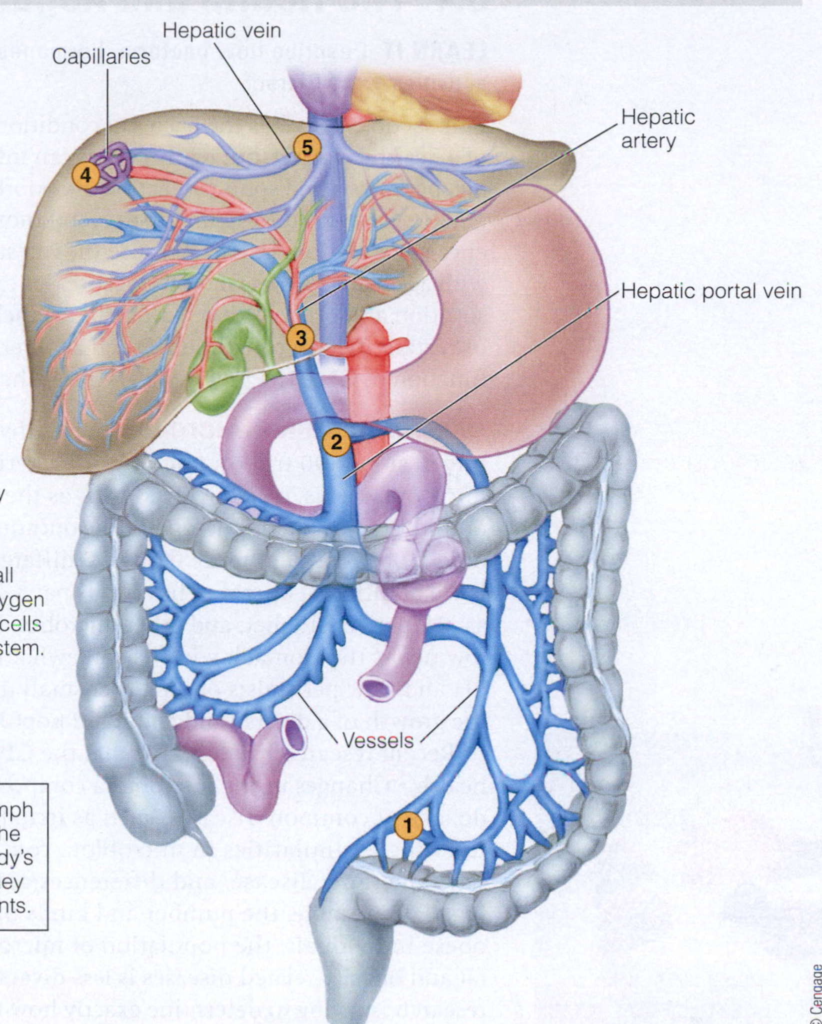

Hepatic vein
Capillaries
Hepatic artery
Hepatic portal vein
Vessels
© Cengage

1. Vessels gather up nutrients from the digestive tract.

Not shown here: Parallel to these vessels (veins) are other vessels (arteries) that carry oxygen-rich blood from the heart to the intestines.

2. The vessels merge into the hepatic portal vein, which conducts all absorbed materials to the liver.

3. The hepatic artery brings a supply of freshly oxygenated blood (not loaded with nutrients) from the lungs to supply oxygen to the liver's own cells.

4. A network of large capillaries branch all over the liver, making nutrients and oxygen available to all its cells and giving the cells access to blood from the digestive system.

5. The hepatic vein gathers up blood in the liver and returns it to the heart.

In contrast, nutrients absorbed into lymph do not go to the liver first. They go to the heart, which pumps them to all the body's cells. The cells remove the nutrients they need, and the liver handles the remnants.

The Lymphatic System The **lymphatic system** collects fluid from tissues throughout the body and directs its flow toward the heart. Unlike the cardiovascular system, the lymphatic system has no central pump; instead, **lymph** moves through the vessels in response to body movements—either voluntary actions of skeletal muscles (as when we walk) or involuntary actions of smooth muscles (as when we breathe). Ultimately, much of the lymph collects in the **thoracic duct** behind the heart. The thoracic duct opens into the **subclavian vein**, where the lymph enters the bloodstream. Thus, nutrients from the GI tract that enter lymphatic vessels (large fats and fat-soluble vitamins) ultimately enter the bloodstream, circulating through arteries, capillaries, and veins like the other nutrients, with a notable exception—they bypass the liver at first.*

Once inside the cardiovascular system, the nutrients can travel all over the body, where they can be taken into cells and used as needed. What becomes of them is described in later chapters.

REVIEW IT Explain how nutrients are routed in the circulatory systems from the GI tract into the body and identify which nutrients enter the blood directly and which must first enter the lymph.

Nutrients leaving the digestive system via the blood are routed directly to the liver before being transported to the body's cells. Those leaving via the lymphatic system (large fats and fat-soluble vitamins) eventually enter the vascular system but bypass the liver at first.

*The lymphatic vessels of the intestine that take up nutrients and pass them to the lymph circulation are called *lacteals* (LACK-tee-als).

lymphatic (lim-FAT-ic) **system:** a network of tissues and organs that transport fluids toward the heart. The GI part of the lymphatic system carries the products of fat digestion into the bloodstream.

lymph (Limf): a clear fluid that contains infection-fighting white blood cells. Lymph from the GI tract transports fat and fat-soluble vitamins to the bloodstream via lymphatic vessels.

thoracic (thor-ASS-ic) **duct:** the main lymphatic vessel that collects lymph and drains into the left subclavian vein.

subclavian (sub-KLAY-vee-an) **vein:** the vein that provides passageway from the lymphatic system to the vascular system.

3.4 The Health and Regulation of the GI Tract

LEARN IT Describe how bacteria, hormones, and nerves influence the health and activities of the GI tract.

This section describes the bacterial conditions and hormonal and nerve regulation of a healthy GI tract, but many factors can influence normal GI function. For example, peristalsis and sphincter action are poorly coordinated in newborns, so infants tend to "spit up" during the first several months of life. Older adults often experience constipation, in part because the intestinal wall loses strength and elasticity with age, which slows GI motility. Diseases can also interfere with digestion and absorption and often lead to malnutrition. Lack of nourishment, in general, and lack of certain dietary constituents such as fiber, in particular, alter the structure and function of GI cells. Quite simply, GI tract health depends on adequate nutrition.

Gastrointestinal Microbes A healthy GI tract is home to a vibrant community of some 100 trillion **microbes**—bacteria, viruses, fungi, protozoa, and other microorganisms, collectively known as the **GI microbiota**. Weighing less than a pound in total, these microbial cells outnumber the body's cells tenfold. The bacteria alone represent more than 400 different species and subspecies. The prevalence of different microbes in various parts of the GI tract depends on such factors as pH, peristalsis, diet, and other microbes. Relatively few microbes can live in the low pH of the stomach with its somewhat rapid peristalsis, whereas the neutral pH and slow peristalsis of the lower small intestine and the large intestine permit the growth of a diverse and abundant population.

Recent research has revealed that the GI microbiota may play a critical role in health.[2] Changes in the microbiota composition and activity are associated with dozens of common diseases, such as irritable bowel syndrome and obesity.[3] Interestingly, similarities in microbiota composition are apparent in people who have the same disease, and differences are noted when their health status differs. For example, the number and kinds of GI microbes differ in nonobese and obese individuals; the population of microbes in obese people with more body fat and obesity-related diseases is less diverse than in nonobese people.[4] Ongoing research is trying to determine exactly how the GI microbiota might contribute to the development of obesity and other metabolic diseases.[5]

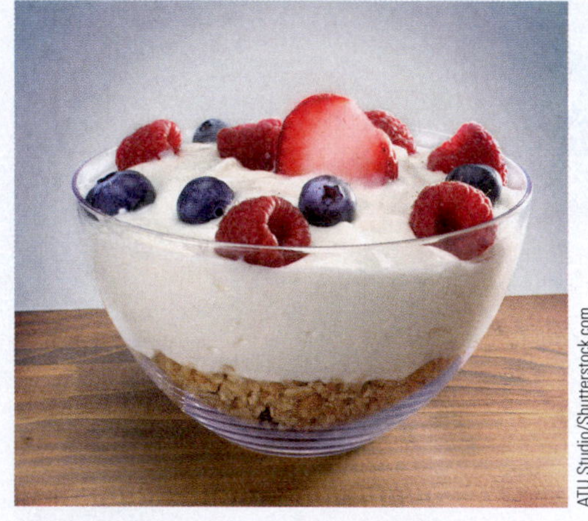
ATU Studio/Shutterstock.com

> PHOTO 3-5 Eaten regularly, yogurt may alleviate common digestive problems.

The GI microbiota changes in response to diet—both in the short term (daily meals) and in the long term (habitual diet patterns).[6] In fact, one of the ways diet may help manage diseases is by changing the microbiota.[7] Consider, for example, that the most recommended diet strategy to improve health—plant-based eating patterns—promotes the most favorable changes in the GI microbiota.[8] Such diets are high in fibers that cannot be digested by the human body but can provide a major source of energy for bacteria, fostering their growth. As GI bacteria digest and metabolize fibers, they produce short fragments of fat, which influence metabolism, inflammation, and disease.[9] These actions may help explain how dietary fiber protects against colon cancer.[10]

Fibers and some other food components are called **prebiotics** because they encourage the growth and activity of bacteria. Research suggests that prebiotics may reduce the risk of GI infections, inflammation, and disorders; increase the bioavailability of nutrients; and regulate appetite and satiety.[11]

Some foods contain **probiotics,** live microbes that change the conditions in the GI tract in ways that seem to benefit health. For example, **yogurt**, with its live bacterial strains, has been used for thousands of years for its health-promoting properties (see Photo 3-5).[12] The potential GI health benefits of probiotics (or products of their metabolism) include helping to alleviate diarrhea, constipation, inflammatory bowel syndrome, ulcers, allergies, lactose intolerance, and infant colic; enhance immune function; and protect against colon cancer.[13] Research studies continue to explore how diet influences GI bacteria and which foods—with their prebiotics and probiotics—affect GI health. In addition, research studies are

microbes (MY-krobes): microscopically small organisms including bacteria, viruses, fungi, and protozoa; also called *microorganisms.*
- **mikros** = small

GI microbiota: the collection of microbes found in the GI tract; sometimes called the *microflora* or *gut flora.* The collection of genes and genomes of the microbiota is called the *microbiome.*

prebiotics: food components (such as fibers) that are not digested by the human body but are used as food by the GI bacteria to promote their growth and activity.

probiotics: living microorganisms found in foods and dietary supplements that, when consumed in sufficient quantities, are beneficial to health.
- **pro** = for
- **bios** = life

yogurt: milk product that results from the fermentation of lactic acid in milk by *Lactobacillus bulgaricus* and *Streptococcus thermophilus.*

beginning to reveal several health benefits beyond the GI tract—such as lowering blood cholesterol, blood pressure, and inflammation.[14]

Bacteria in the GI tract also produce several vitamins, including biotin, folate, pantothenic acid, riboflavin, thiamin, vitamin B_6, vitamin B_{12}, and vitamin K. Because the amount produced is insufficient to meet the body's needs fully, these vitamins are considered essential nutrients and must be provided by the diet.

Gastrointestinal Hormones and Nerve Pathways The ability of the digestive tract to handle its ever-changing contents illustrates an important physiological principle that governs the way all living things function—the principle of **homeostasis.** Simply stated, survival depends on body conditions staying about the same; if they deviate too far from the norm, the body must "do something" to bring them back to normal. The body's regulation of digestion is one example of homeostatic regulation. The body also regulates its temperature, its blood pressure, and all other aspects of its blood chemistry in similar ways.

Two intricate and sensitive systems coordinate all the digestive and absorptive processes: the hormonal (or endocrine) system and the nervous system. Even before the first bite of food is taken, the mere thought, sight, or smell of food can trigger a response from these systems. Then, as food travels through the GI tract, it either stimulates or inhibits digestive secretions by way of messages that are carried from one organ to another by both **hormones** and nerve pathways. (Appendix A presents a brief summary of the body's hormonal system and nervous system.)

Notice that the kinds of regulation described in the following paragraphs are all examples of *feedback* mechanisms. A certain condition demands a response. The response changes that condition, and the change then cuts off the response. Thus, the system is self-correcting.

- *The stomach normally maintains a pH between 1.5 and 1.7. How does it stay that way?* Food entering the stomach stimulates cells in the stomach wall to release the hormone **gastrin.** Gastrin, in turn, stimulates the stomach glands to secrete the components of hydrochloric acid. When pH 1.5 is reached, the acid itself turns off the gastrin-producing cells; they stop releasing gastrin, and the glands stop producing hydrochloric acid. Thus, the system adjusts itself, as Figure 3-12 shows.

Nerve receptors in the stomach wall also respond to the presence of food and stimulate the gastric glands to secrete juices and the muscles to contract. As the stomach empties, the receptors are no longer stimulated, the flow of juices slows, and the stomach quiets down.

- *The pyloric sphincter opens to let out a little chyme, then closes again. How does it know when to open and close?* When the pyloric sphincter relaxes, acidic chyme slips through. The cells of the pyloric muscle on the intestinal side sense the acid, causing the pyloric sphincter to close tightly. Only after the chyme has been neutralized by pancreatic bicarbonate and the juices surrounding the pyloric sphincter have become alkaline can the muscle relax again. This process ensures that the chyme will be released slowly enough to be neutralized as it flows through the small intestine. This is important because the small intestine has less of a mucous coating than the stomach does and so is not as well protected from acid.

- *As the chyme enters the small intestine, the pancreas adds bicarbonate to it so that the intestinal contents always remain at a slightly alkaline pH. How does the pancreas know how much to add?* The presence of chyme stimulates the cells of the duodenual wall to release the hormone **secretin** into the blood. When secretin reaches the pancreas, it stimulates the pancreas to release its bicarbonate-rich juices. Thus, whenever the duodenum signals that acidic chyme is present, the pancreas responds by sending bicarbonate to neutralize it. When the need has been met, the cells of the duodenal wall are no longer stimulated to release secretin, the hormone no longer flows through the blood, and the pancreas no longer receives the message and stops sending pancreatic juice. Nerves also regulate pancreatic secretions.

> FIGURE 3-12 **An Example of a Negative Feedback Loop**

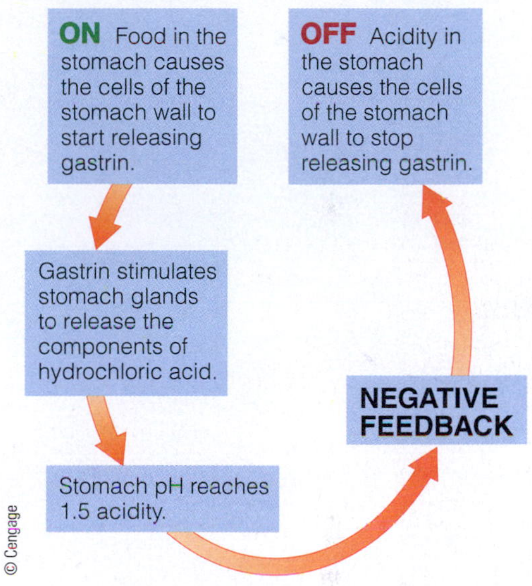

ON Food in the stomach causes the cells of the stomach wall to start releasing gastrin.
OFF Acidity in the stomach causes the cells of the stomach wall to stop releasing gastrin.
Gastrin stimulates stomach glands to release the components of hydrochloric acid.
NEGATIVE FEEDBACK
Stomach pH reaches 1.5 acidity.
© Cengage

homeostasis (HOME-ee-oh-STAY-sis): the maintenance of constant internal conditions (such as blood chemistry, temperature, and blood pressure) by the body's control systems. A homeostatic system is constantly reacting to external forces to maintain limits set by the body's needs.
- **homeo** = like, similar
- **stasis** = staying

hormones: chemical messengers. Hormones are secreted by a variety of glands in response to altered conditions in the body. Each hormone travels to one or more specific target tissues or organs, where it elicits a specific response to maintain homeostasis. The study of hormones and their actions is called *endocrinology*.

gastrin: a hormone secreted by cells in the stomach wall. Target organ: the glands of the stomach. Response: secretion of gastric acid.

secretin (see-CREET-in): a hormone produced by cells in the duodenum wall. Target organ: the pancreas. Response: secretion of bicarbonate-rich pancreatic juice.

• *Pancreatic secretions contain a mixture of enzymes to digest carbohydrate, fat, and protein. How does the pancreas know how much of each type of enzyme to provide?* This is one of the most interesting questions physiologists have asked. Clearly, the pancreas does know what its owner has been eating, and it secretes enzyme mixtures tailored to handle the food mixtures that have been arriving recently (over the past several days). Enzyme activity changes proportionately in response to the amounts of carbohydrate, fat, and protein in the diet. If a person has been eating mostly carbohydrates, the pancreas makes and secretes mostly carbohydrases; if the person's diet has been high in fat, the pancreas produces more lipases; and so forth. Hormones from the GI tract, secreted in response to meals, keep the pancreas informed as to its digestive tasks. The day or two lag between the time a person's diet changes dramatically and the time digestion of the new diet becomes efficient explains why dietary changes can "upset digestion" and should be made gradually.

• *Why don't the digestive enzymes damage the pancreas?* The pancreas protects itself from harm by producing an inactive form of the enzymes.* It releases these proteins into the small intestine, where they are activated to become enzymes. In pancreatitis, the digestive enzymes become active within the infected pancreas, causing inflammation and damaging the delicate pancreatic tissues.

• *When fat is present in the intestine, the gallbladder contracts to squirt bile into the intestine to emulsify the fat. How does the gallbladder get the message that fat is present?* Fat in the intestine stimulates cells of the intestinal wall to release the hormone **cholecystokinin (CCK).** This hormone travels by way of the blood to the gallbladder and stimulates it to contract, which releases bile into the small intestine. Cholecystokinin also travels to the pancreas and stimulates it to secrete its juices, which releases bicarbonate and enzymes into the small intestine. Once the fat in the intestine is emulsified and enzymes have begun to work on it, the fat no longer provokes release of the hormone, and the message to contract is canceled. (By the way, fat emulsification can continue even after a diseased gallbladder has been surgically removed because the liver can deliver bile directly to the small intestine.)

• *Fat and protein take longer to digest than carbohydrate does. When fat or protein is present, intestinal motility slows to allow time for its digestion. How does the intestine know when to slow down?* Cholecystokinin is released in response to fat or protein in the small intestine. In addition to its role in fat emulsification and digestion, cholecystokinin slows GI tract motility. Slowing the digestive process helps maintain a pace that allows all reactions to reach completion. Hormonal and nervous mechanisms like these account for much of the body's ability to adapt to changing conditions.

Table 3-2 summarizes the actions of these three GI hormones. Gastrin, secretin, and cholecystokinin are among the most studied GI hormones, but the GI tract releases more than 50 hormones. In addition to assisting with digestion and absorption, many of these hormones regulate food intake and influence satiation—the feeling of satisfaction and fullness that occurs during a meal and

cholecystokinin (COAL-ee-SIS-toe-KINE-in), or **CCK:** a hormone produced by cells of the intestinal wall. Target organ: the gallbladder. Response: release of bile and slowing of GI motility.

TABLE 3-2 The Primary Actions of Selected GI Hormones

Hormone	Responds to	Secreted from	Stimulates	Response
Gastrin	Food in the stomach	Stomach wall	Stomach glands	Hydrochloric acid secreted into the stomach to maintain an acidic pH
Secretin	Acidic chyme in the small intestine	Duodenal wall	Pancreas	Bicarbonate-rich juices secreted into the small intestine to maintain a slightly alkaline pH
Cholecystokinin	Fat or protein in the small intestine	Intestinal wall	Gallbladder	Bile secreted into the duodenum to emulsify fats
			Pancreas	Bicarbonate- and enzyme-rich juices secreted into the small intestine to maintain a slightly alkaline pH, digest fats and proteins, and slow GI tract motility

*The inactive precursor of an enzyme is called a *zymogen* (ZYE-mo-jen).

halts eating. Current research is focusing on the roles these hormones may play in the development of obesity and its treatments (Chapter 8 provides more details).

Discovering the answers to questions like these has led some people to devote their entire lives to the study of physiology. For now, however, these few examples illustrate how all the processes throughout the digestive system are precisely and automatically regulated without any conscious effort.

The System at Its Best This chapter describes the anatomy of the digestive tract on several levels: the sequence of digestive organs, the muscular actions, the digestive secretions, and the absorptive surfaces. The intricate architecture of the digestive system makes it sensitive and responsive to conditions in its environment. Several different kinds of GI tract cells confer specific immunity against intestinal diseases such as inflammatory bowel syndrome. In addition, secretions from the GI tract—saliva, mucus, gastric acid, and digestive enzymes—not only help with digestion, but also defend against foreign invaders. Together the GI's team of bacteria, cells, and secretions defend the body against many illnesses.

One indispensable condition is good health of the digestive system itself. Like all the other organs of the body, the GI tract depends on a healthy supply of blood. The cells of the GI tract become weak and inflamed when blood flow is diminished, as may occur in heart disease when arteries become clogged or blood clots form. Just as a diminished blood flow to the heart or brain can cause a heart attack or stroke, respectively, too little blood to the intestines can also be damaging—or even fatal. A diminished blood flow to the intestines—called **intestinal ischemia**—is characterized by abdominal pain, forceful bowel movements, and blood in the stool.

The health of the digestive system is also affected by such lifestyle factors as sleep, physical activity, and state of mind (see Photo 3-6). Adequate sleep allows for repair and maintenance of tissue and removal of wastes that might impair efficient functioning. Activity promotes healthy muscle tone. Stress alters GI motility, secretions, permeability, blood flow, and bacteria. For healthy digestion, mealtimes should be relaxed and tranquil. Pleasant conversations and peaceful environments during meals ease the digestive process.

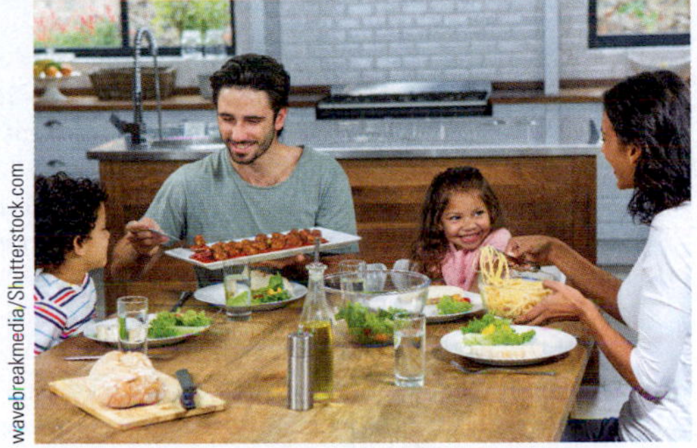

wavebreakmedia/Shutterstock.com

> **PHOTO 3-6** Nourishing foods and pleasant conversations support a healthy digestive system.

Another factor in GI health is the kind of foods eaten. Among the characteristics of meals that promote optimal absorption of nutrients are those mentioned in Chapter 2: balance, moderation, variety, and adequacy. Balance and moderation require having neither too much nor too little of anything. For example, too much fat can be harmful, but some fat is beneficial in slowing down intestinal motility and providing time for absorption of some of the nutrients that are slow to be absorbed.

Variety is important for many reasons, but one is that some food constituents interfere with nutrient absorption. For example, some compounds common in high-fiber foods such as whole-grain cereals, certain leafy green vegetables, and legumes bind with minerals. To some extent, then, the minerals in those foods may become unavailable for absorption. These high-fiber foods are still valuable, but they need to be balanced with a variety of other foods that can provide the minerals.

As for adequacy—in a sense, this entire book is about dietary adequacy. A diet must provide all the essential nutrients, fiber, and energy in amounts sufficient to maintain health. But here, at the end of this chapter, is a good place to emphasize the interdependence of the nutrients. It could almost be said that every nutrient depends on every other. All the nutrients work together, and all are present in the cells of a healthy digestive tract. To maintain health and promote the functions of the GI tract, make balance, moderation, variety, and adequacy features of every day's meals.

REVIEW IT **Describe how bacteria, hormones, and nerves influence the health and activities of the GI tract.**

A diverse and abundant microbiome supports GI health. The regulation of GI processes depends on the coordinated efforts of the hormonal system and the nervous system. Together, digestion and absorption break down foods into nutrients for the body's use. To function optimally, a healthy GI tract needs a balanced diet, adequate rest, and regular physical activity.

intestinal ischemia (is-KEY-me-ah): a diminished blood flow to the intestines that is characterized by abdominal pain, forceful bowel movements, and blood in the stool.

What's Online

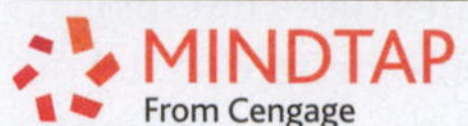

Visit **www.cengagebrain.com** to access MindTap, a complete digital course that includes Diet & Wellness Plus, interactive quizzes, videos, and more.

REFERENCES

1. H. F. Helander and L. Fändriks, Surface area of the digestive tract—revisited, *Scandinavian Journal of Gastroenterology* 49 (2014): 681–689.
2. S. V. Lynch and O. Pedersen, The human intestinal microbiome in health and disease, *New England Journal of Medicine* 375 (2016): 2369–2379; D. S. Spasova and C. D. Surh, Blowing on embers: Commensal microbiota and our immune system, *Frontiers in Immunology* 5 (2014): 1–20; D. A. Relman, The human microbiome: Ecosystem resilience and health, *Nutrition Reviews* 70 (2012): S2–S9.
3. D. A. Relman, The human microbiome and the future practice of medicine, *Journal of the American Medical Association* 314 (2015): 1127–1128; C. M. Ferreira and coauthors, The central role of the gut microbiota in chronic inflammatory diseases, *Journal of Immunology Research* 2014 (2014): 689492; F. Bäckhed, Host responses to the human microbiome, *Nutrition Reviews* 70 (2012): S14–S17; W. M. deVos and E. A. J. deVos, Role of the intestinal microbiome in health and disease: From correlation to causation, *Nutrition Reviews* 70 (2012): S45–S56.
4. E. LeChatelier and coauthors, Richness of human gut microbiome correlates with metabolic markers, *Nature* 500 (2013): 541–546.
5. I. Moreno-Indias and coauthors, Impact of the gut microbiota on the development of obesity and type 2 diabetes mellitus, *Frontiers in Microbiology* 5 (2014): 1–10.
6. L. A. David and coauthors, Diet rapidly and reproducibly alters the human gut microbiome, *Nature* 505 (2014): 559–563; N. Voreades, A. Kozil, and T. L. Weir, Diet and the development of the human intestinal microbiome, *Frontiers in Microbiology* 5 (2014): 1–9; Y. K. Lee, Effects of diet on gut microbiota profile and the implications for health and disease, *Bioscience of Microbiota, Food and Health* 32 (2013): 1–12; T. Peregrin, The inside tract: What RDs need to know about the gut microbiome, *Journal of the Academy of Nutrition and Dietetics* 113 (2013): 1019–1023.
7. O. O. Erejuwa, S. A. Sulaiman, and M. S. Ab Wahab, Modulation of gut microbiota in the management of metabolic disorders: The prospects and challenges, *International Journal of Molecular Sciences* 15 (2014): 4158–4188.
8. V. A. do Rosario, R. Fernandes, and E. B. S. de M. Trindade, Vegetarian diets and gut microbiota: Important shifts in markers of metabolism and cardiovascular disease, *Nutrition Reviews* 74 (2016): 444-454; J. M. W. Wong, Gut microbiota and cardiometabolic outcomes: Influence of dietary patterns and their associated components, *American Journal of Clinical Nutrition* 100 (2014): 369S–377S.
9. J. Tan and coauthors, The role of short-chain fatty acids in health and disease, *Advances in Immunology* 121 (2014): 91–119.
10. H. Zeng, D. L. lazarova, M. Bordonaro, Mechanisms linking dietary fiber, gut microbiota and colon cancer prevention, *World Journal of Gastrointestinal Oncology* 6 (2014): 41–51.
11. J. Breton and coauthors, Gut commensal E. coli proteins activate host satiety pathways following nutrient-induced bacterial growth, *Cell Metabolism* 23 (2016): 324–334; A. Perez-Cornago and coauthors, Prebiotic consumption and the incidence of overweight in a Mediterranean cohort: The Seguimiento Universidad de navarra Project, *American Journal of Clinical Nutrition* 102 (2015): 1554–1562; A. M. Brownawell and coauthors, Prebiotics and the health benefits of fiber: Current regulatory status, future research, and goals, *Journal of Nutrition* 142 (2012): 962–974.
12. M. Fisberg and R. Machado, History of yogurt and current patterns of consumption, *Nutrition Reviews* 73 (2015): 4–7.
13. S. Lohner and coauthors, Prebiotics in healthy infants and children for prevention of acute infectious diseases: A systematic review and meta-analysis, *Nutrition Reviews* 72 (2014): 523–531; E. Dimidi and coauthors, The effect of probiotics on functional constipation in adults: A systematic review and meta-analysis of randomized controlled trials, *American Journal of Clinical Nutrition* 100 (2014): 1075S–1084S; S. Hempel and coauthors, Probiotics for the prevention and treatment of antibiotic-associated diarrhea: A systematic review and meta-analysis, *Journal of the American Medical Association* 307 (2012): 1959–1969; B. C. Johnston and coauthors, Probiotics for the prevention of *Clostridium difficile*–associated diarrhea: A systematic review and meta-analysis, *Annals of Internal Medicine* 157 (2012): 878–888; M. Kumar and coauthors, Probiotic metabolites as epigenetic targets in the prevention of colon cancer, *Nutrition Reviews* 71 (2012): 23–34.
14. D. B. DiRienzo, Effect of probiotics on biomarkers of cardiovascular disease: Implications for heart-healthy diets, *Nutrition Reviews* 72 (2014): 18–29.

LEARN IT Outline strategies to prevent or alleviate common GI problems.

Common Digestive Problems

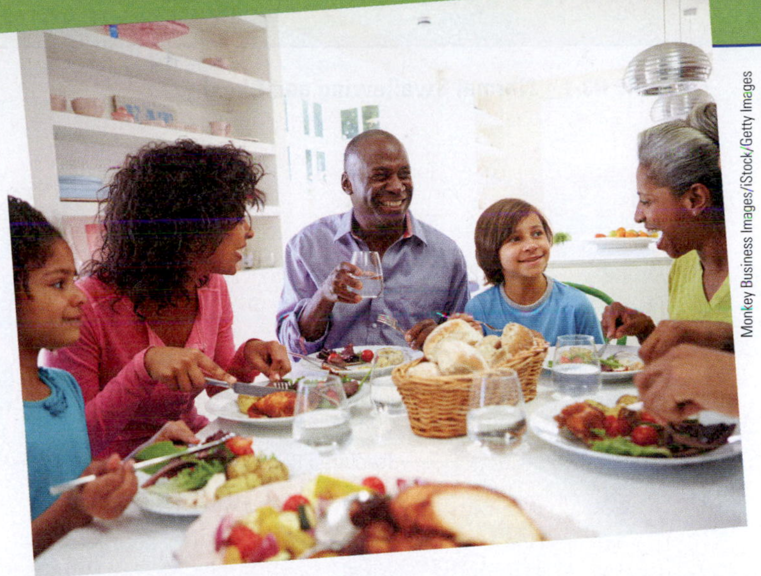
Monkey Business Images/iStock/Getty Images

The facts of anatomy and physiology presented in Chapter 3 permit easy understanding of some common problems that occasionally arise in the digestive tract. Food may slip into the airways instead of the esophagus, causing choking. Bowel movements may be loose and watery, as in diarrhea, or painful and hard, as in constipation. Some people complain about belching, while others are bothered by intestinal gas. Sometimes people develop medical problems such as ulcers. This highlight describes some of the symptoms of these common digestive problems and suggests strategies for preventing them (Glossary H3-1 defines related terms).

Choking

Sometimes a sip of a beverage or a tiny bit of food "slips down the wrong pipe." The body's first response is to cough, and quite often coughing clears the passage. When someone is truly choking, however, food has slipped into the **trachea** and completely blocked the air passageways (see Figure H3-1, p. 88). Thus, the person cannot cough—or even breathe. Without oxygen, the person may suffer permanent brain damage within 5 minutes or may even die. For this reason, it is imperative that everyone learn to recognize the universal distress signal for choking (shown in Figure H3-2, p. 88) and act promptly.

Because the **larynx** is in the trachea and makes sounds only when air is pushed across it, a person choking will be unable to speak. For this reason, to help a person who is choking, first ask "Can you speak?" If the person is coughing, breathing adequately, or able to speak, do not interfere. Whatever you do, do not hit him on the back as the particle may become lodged more firmly in his air passageway. If the person cannot speak or cough, shout for help and perform the **Heimlich maneuver** (described in Figure H3-2). Almost any food can cause choking, although some are cited more often than others: chunks of meat, hot dogs, nuts, whole grapes, raw carrots, marshmallows, hard or sticky candies, gum, popcorn, and peanut butter. These foods are particularly difficult for young children (especially those 4 years of age

GLOSSARY H3-1

acid controllers: medications used to prevent or relieve indigestion by suppressing production of acid in the stomach; also called *H2 blockers*.

antacids: medications used to relieve indigestion by neutralizing acid in the stomach.

belching: the release of air or gas from the stomach through the mouth.

bloating: uncomfortable abdominal fullness or distention.

celiac (SEE-lee-ak) **disease:** an intestinal disorder in which the inability to absorb gluten results in an immune response that damages intestinal cells; also called *celiac sprue, nontropical sprue,* or *gluten-sensitive enteropathy*.

colitis (ko-LYE-tis): inflammation of the colon.

colonic irrigation: the popular, but potentially harmful practice of "washing" the large intestine with a powerful enema machine; also called *colonic hydrotherapy*.

constipation: the condition of having infrequent or difficult bowel movements.

defecate (DEF-uh-cate): to move the bowels and eliminate waste.

- **defaecare** = to remove dregs

diarrhea: the frequent passage of watery bowel movements.

diverticula (dye-ver-TIC-you-la): sacs or pouches that develop in the weakened areas of the intestinal wall (like bulges in an inner tube where the tire wall is weak).

- **divertir** = to turn aside

diverticulitis (DYE-ver-tic-you-LYE-tis): infected or inflamed diverticula.

- **itis** = infection or inflammation

diverticulosis (DYE-ver-tic-you-LOH-sis): the condition of having diverticula.

- **osis** = condition

enema: solution inserted into the rectum and colon to stimulate a bowel movement and empty the lower large intestine.

flatulence: passage of excessive amounts of intestinal gas.

FODMAP: a collective term used to describe **f**ermentable **o**ligosaccharides, **d**isaccharides, **m**onosaccharides, **a**nd **p**loyols that are commonly found in such foods as wheat, onions, some fruits and vegetables, sorbitol, and some dairy.

gastroesophageal reflux: the backflow of stomach acid into the esophagus, causing damage to the cells of the esophagus and the sensation of heartburn; commonly known as *heartburn* or *acid indigestion*.

gluten (GLOO-tuhn): proteins in grains that give dough its elastic texture; in people with celiac disease, gluten damages the small intestine.

Heimlich (HIME-lick) **maneuver (abdominal thrusts):** a technique for dislodging an object from the trachea of a choking person (see Figure H3-2); named for the physician who developed it.

hemorrhoids (HEM-oh-royds): painful swelling of the veins surrounding the rectum.

indigestion: incomplete or uncomfortable digestion, usually accompanied by pain, nausea, vomiting, heartburn, intestinal gas, or belching.

- **in** = not

irritable bowel syndrome: an intestinal disorder of unknown cause. Symptoms include abdominal discomfort and cramping, diarrhea, constipation, or alternating diarrhea and constipation.

larynx (LAIR-inks): the entryway to the trachea that contains the vocal cords; also called the *voice box* (see Figure H3-1).

laxatives: substances that loosen the bowels and thereby prevent or treat constipation.

mineral oil: a purified liquid derived from petroleum and used to treat constipation.

nonceliac gluten sensitivity: a poorly defined cluster of digestive symptoms that seem to improve with the elimination of gluten from the diet.

peptic ulcer: a lesion in the mucous membrane of either the stomach (a *gastric ulcer*) or the duodenum (a *duodenal ulcer*).

- **peptic** = concerning digestion

stool softeners: substances that increase the amount of water the stool absorbs in the GI tract, making the stool softer and easier to pass.

trachea (TRAKE-ee-uh): the air passageway from the larynx to the lungs; also called the *windpipe*.

ulcer: a lesion of the skin or mucous membranes characterized by inflammation and damaged tissues. See also *peptic ulcer*.

vomiting: expulsion of the contents of the stomach up through the esophagus to the mouth.

> **FIGURE H3-1 Normal Swallowing and Choking**

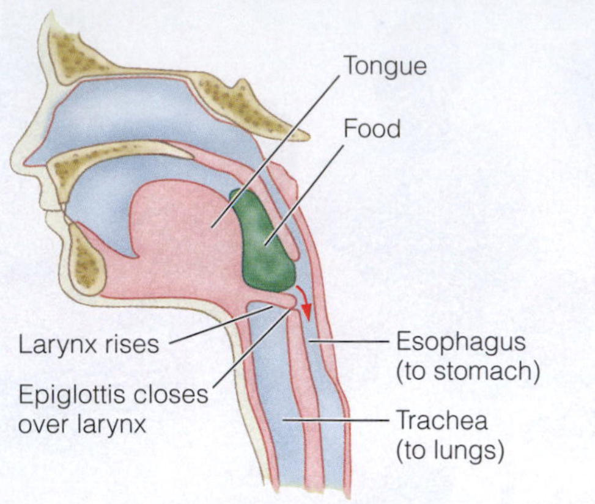

Tongue
Food
Larynx rises
Epiglottis closes over larynx
Esophagus (to stomach)
Trachea (to lungs)

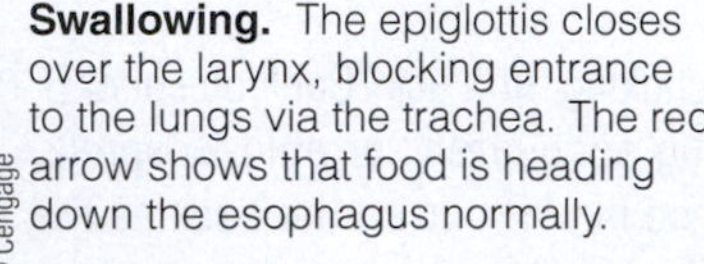

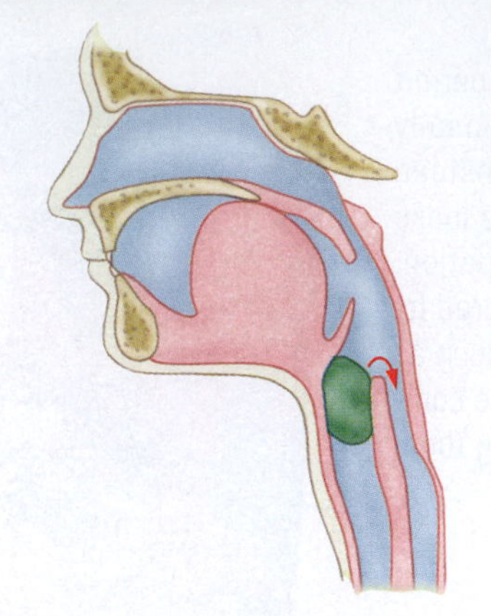

Swallowing. The epiglottis closes over the larynx, blocking entrance to the lungs via the trachea. The red arrow shows that food is heading down the esophagus normally.

Choking. A choking person cannot speak or gasp because food lodged in the trachea blocks the passage of air. The red arrow points to where the food should have gone to prevent choking.

and younger) to safely chew and swallow. Each year more than 10,000 children (14 years old or younger) in the United States choke; more than half choke on food. Every 5 days, a child in the United States chokes to death on food.[1] An adult should be present and alert to the dangers of choking whenever young children are eating. Older adults are also vulnerable to choking, especially those who have Alzheimer's disease, Parkinson's disease, or pneumonia.[2] To prevent choking, cut food into small pieces, chew thoroughly before swallowing, don't talk or laugh with food in your mouth, and don't eat when breathing hard.

Vomiting

Vomiting can be a symptom of many different diseases or may arise in situations that upset the body's equilibrium, such as car, air, or sea travel. For whatever reason, the contents of the stomach are propelled up through the esophagus to the mouth and expelled. Sometimes the muscular contractions will extend beyond the stomach

> **FIGURE H3-2 First Aid for Choking**

First aid for choking relies on abdominal thrusts, sometimes called the Heimlich maneuver. If abdominal thrusts are not successful and the person loses consciousness, lower him to the floor, call 911, remove the object blocking the airway if possible, and begin CPR. Because there is no time for hesitation when called upon to perform this death-defying act, you would do well to take a life-saving course to learn these techniques.

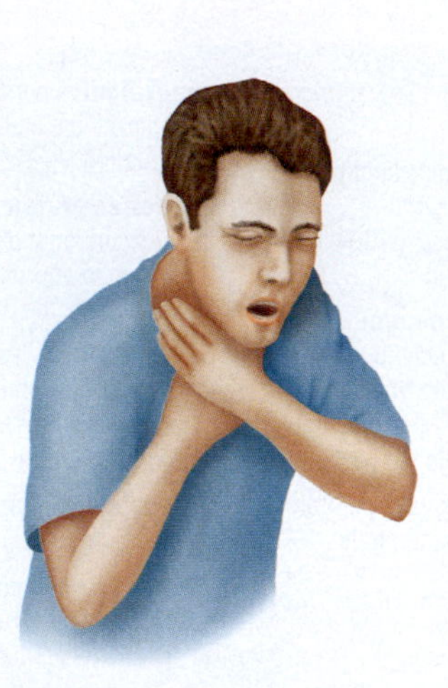

The universal signal for choking alerts others to the need for assistance.

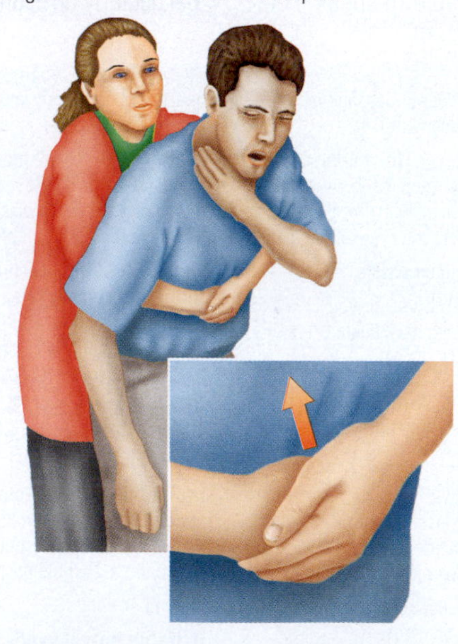

Stand behind the person with your arms wrapped around him. Make a fist with one hand and place the thumb side snugly against the body, slightly above the navel and below the breastbone.

Grasp the fist with your other hand and make a quick upward and inward thrust. Repeat thrusts until the object is dislodged.

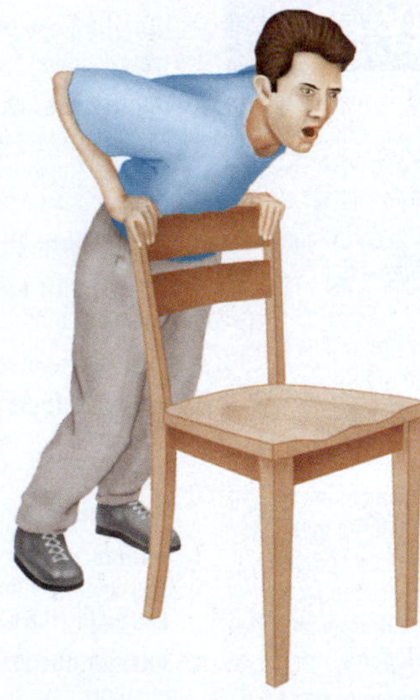

To perform abdominal thrusts on yourself, make a fist and place the thumb below your breastbone and above your navel. Grasp your fist with your other hand and press inward with a quick upward thrust. Alternatively, quickly thrust your upper body against a table edge, chair, or railing.

and carry the contents of the duodenum, with its green bile, into the stomach and then up the esophagus. Although certainly unpleasant and wearying for the nauseated person, vomiting is often not a cause for alarm. Vomiting is one of the body's adaptive mechanisms to rid itself of something irritating. The best advice is to rest and drink small amounts of liquids as tolerated until the nausea subsides.

If vomiting incurs such large losses of fluid as to cause dehydration, a physician's care may be needed. As fluid is lost from the GI tract, the body's other fluids redistribute themselves, taking fluid from every cell of the body. Fluid leaving the cells is accompanied by salts that are absolutely essential to the life of the cells. Replacing salts and fluid is difficult if the vomiting continues, and intravenous feedings of saline and glucose may be necessary. Vomiting and dehydration are especially serious in an infant, and a physician should be contacted without delay.

Self-induced vomiting, such as occurs in bulimia nervosa, also has serious consequences. In addition to fluid and salt imbalances, repeated vomiting can cause irritation and infection of the pharynx, esophagus, and salivary glands; erosion of the teeth and gums; and dental caries. The esophagus may rupture or tear, as may the stomach. Sometimes the eyes become red from pressure during vomiting. Bulimic behavior reflects underlying psychological problems that require intervention. (Bulimia nervosa is discussed fully in Highlight 8.)

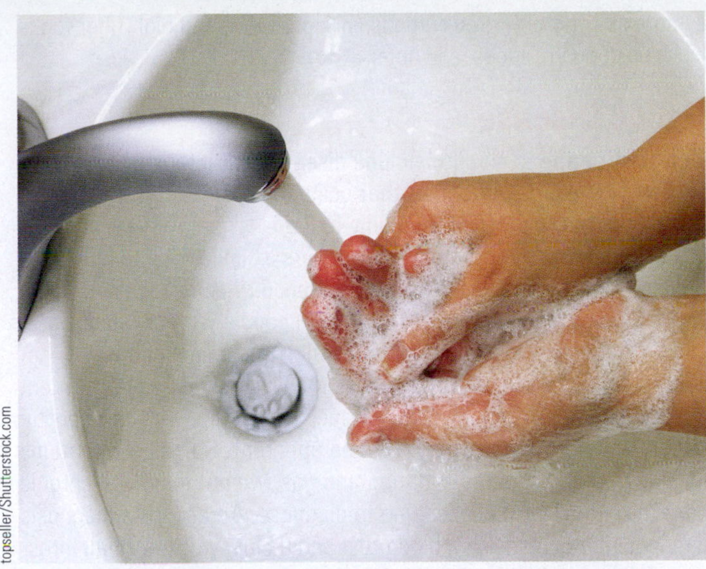

topseller/Shutterstock.com

> **PHOTO H3-1** Personal hygiene (such as regular hand washing with soap and water) and safe food preparation (as described in Chapter 19) are easy and effective steps to take in preventing diarrheal diseases.

Diarrhea

Diarrhea is characterized by frequent, loose, watery stools. Such stools indicate that the intestinal contents have moved too quickly through the intestines for fluid absorption to take place or that water has been drawn from the cells lining the intestinal tract and added to the food residue. Like vomiting, diarrhea can lead to life-threatening dehydration. An estimated half-million children under age 5 die each year from diarrhea-related causes. A strategy as simple as hand washing might reduce the incidence of diarrhea among children by 30 percent (see Photo H3-1).[3]

Diarrhea is a symptom of various medical conditions and treatments. It may occur abruptly in a healthy person as a result of infections (such as foodborne illness) or as a side effect of medications. When used in large quantities, food ingredients such as the sugar alternative sorbitol and the fat alternative olestra may also cause diarrhea in some people. If a food is responsible, then that food must be omitted from the diet, at least temporarily. If medication is responsible, a different medicine, when possible, or a different form (injectable versus oral, for example) may alleviate the problem. Diarrhea may also occur as a result of disorders of the GI tract, such as irritable bowel syndrome or colitis.

Treatment for diarrhea depends on its cause and severity, but it always begins with rehydration.[4] Mild diarrhea may subside with simple rest and extra liquids (such as clear juices and soups) to replace fluid losses. If diarrhea is bloody or if it worsens or persists—especially in an infant, young child, elderly person, or person with a compromised immune system—call a physician. Severe diarrhea can be life-threatening. Notice that the following disorders all include diarrhea as a symptom, but their treatments differ.

Irritable Bowel Syndrome

Irritable bowel syndrome is one of the most common GI disorders and is characterized by frequent or severe abdominal pain or cramping and a disturbance in the motility of the GI tract.[5] In most cases, GI contractions are stronger and last longer than normal, forcing intestinal contents through quickly and causing gas, **bloating,** and diarrhea. In some cases, however, GI contractions are weaker than normal, slowing the passage of intestinal contents and causing constipation. The exact cause of irritable bowel syndrome is not known, but researchers are actively investigating the role of the nervous system and stress.[6] The condition seems to worsen for some people when they eat certain foods or during stressful events. These triggers seem to aggravate symptoms but not cause them. Dietary treatment hinges on identifying and avoiding individual foods that aggravate symptoms, using probiotics, and eating small meals. Emerging evidence suggests some benefit from diets that are free of **gluten** and low in specific carbohydrates referred to as **FODMAP** (Chapter 4 describes these in more detail). Other treatments that may be effective include exercise; antispasmodic and antidiarrheal drugs for diarrhea and fiber supplements and laxatives for constipation; and psychological and behavioral therapies to reduce stress.[7]

Colitis

People with **colitis,** an inflammation of the large intestine, may also suffer from severe diarrhea, abdominal pain, and bloating. Depending on the cause, treatment generally focuses on hydration and medication to control diarrhea, abdominal pain, and inflammation. Some people find some relief by avoiding certain foods that tend to worsen symptoms—notably greasy foods, milk products, and high-fiber foods (such as popcorn, seeds, and nuts).

Celiac Disease

Celiac disease is an autoimmune disease characterized by inflammation of the small intestine that occurs in response to foods that contain gluten, a protein commonly found in wheat, barley, and rye. Oats contain a similar protein that triggers a similar reaction in some people with celiac disease.[8] The prevalence of celiac disease in the United States is estimated at 1 in 141.[9] In people with celiac disease, gluten triggers an immune system reaction in the small intestine that causes inflammation, which damages the villi and decreases nutrient absorption. Signs of malnutrition—such as anemia, weak and brittle bones, and dermatitis—may become apparent. Common symptoms include abdominal pains, bloating and gas, weight loss, and chronic diarrhea—making it challenging to diagnose. An accurate diagnosis depends on results from a blood test and a biopsy of the small intestine. Treatment focuses on a gluten-free diet, which allows the small intestine to heal. A gluten-free diet must eliminate not only wheat, barley, rye, and oats, but also many processed items made with these grains, such as bouillon cubes, hot dogs, gravies, salad dressings, soups, and dietary supplements. People with celiac disease learn to read food labels at grocery stores and ask questions at restaurants in their search for gluten-free foods.

Some people who do not test positive for celiac disease seem to have similar symptoms that tend to diminish when on a gluten-free diet and return when gluten is reintroduced into the diet. These people may be described as having **nonceliac gluten sensitivity**.[10] Quite often, they tend to self-diagnose and self-treat, which presents a problem because a gluten-free diet interferes with an accurate diagnosis of celiac disease.[11] Whether the symptoms in nonceliac gluten sensitivity are responding to gluten or FODMAP in similar foods is unclear.[12]

The popularity of gluten-free diets and products has grown dramatically in recent years, in part because of nonceliac gluten sensitivity.[13] In addition, some consumers seem a bit confused and mistakenly believe that if a product is free of something, then that missing something must be bad. Another common misconception is that a gluten-free diet is a weight-loss diet. Despite claims that eliminating gluten from the diet helps with a variety of ailments, there is no evidence to suggest that a gluten-free diet is beneficial for the general population, and it may even have unintended consequences.[14]

Constipation

Like diarrhea, **constipation** describes a symptom, not a disease. Each person's GI tract has its own cycle of waste elimination, which depends on its owner's health, the type of food eaten, when it was eaten, and when the person takes time to **defecate.** What's normal for some people may not be normal for others. Some people have bowel movements three times a day; others may have them three times a week. The symptoms of constipation include straining during bowel movements, hard stools, and infrequent bowel movements (fewer than three per week).[15] Abdominal discomfort, headaches, backaches, and the passing of gas sometimes accompany constipation.

Often a person's lifestyle may cause constipation. Being too busy to respond to the defecation signal is a common complaint. If a person receives the signal to defecate and ignores it, the signal may not return for several hours. In the meantime, fluids continue to be withdrawn from the fecal matter, so when the person does defecate, the stools are dry and hard. In such a case, a person's daily regimen may need to be revised to allow time to have a bowel movement when the body sends its signal.

Although constipation usually reflects lifestyle habits, in some cases it may be a side effect of medication or a medical problem such as bowel obstruction. If discomfort is associated with passing fecal matter, seek medical advice to rule out disease. Once this has been done, simple treatments, such as increased fiber, fluids, and exercise, are recommended before medications are introduced.

One dietary measure that may be appropriate is to increase dietary fiber to 25 to 28 grams per day gradually over the course of a week or two. Fibers found in fruits, vegetables, and whole grains help prevent constipation by increasing fecal mass. In the GI tract, fiber attracts water, creating soft, bulky stools that stimulate bowel contractions to push the contents along. These contractions strengthen the intestinal muscles. The improved muscle tone, together with the water content of the stools, eases elimination, reducing the pressure in the rectal veins and helping to prevent **hemorrhoids.** Chapter 4 provides more information on fiber's role in maintaining a healthy colon and reducing the risks of colon cancer and diverticulosis. **Diverticulosis** is a condition in which the intestinal walls develop bulges in weakened areas, most commonly in the colon (see Figure H3-3). These bulging pockets, known as **diverticula,** can worsen constipation, entrap feces, and become painfully infected and inflamed **(diverticulitis).** Treatment may require hospitalization, antibiotics, or surgery.

Drinking plenty of water in conjunction with eating high-fiber foods also helps prevent constipation. The increased bulk physically stimulates the upper GI tract, promoting peristalsis throughout. Similarly,

> **FIGURE H3-3 Diverticula in the Colon**

Diverticula may develop anywhere along the GI tract, but they are most common in the colon.

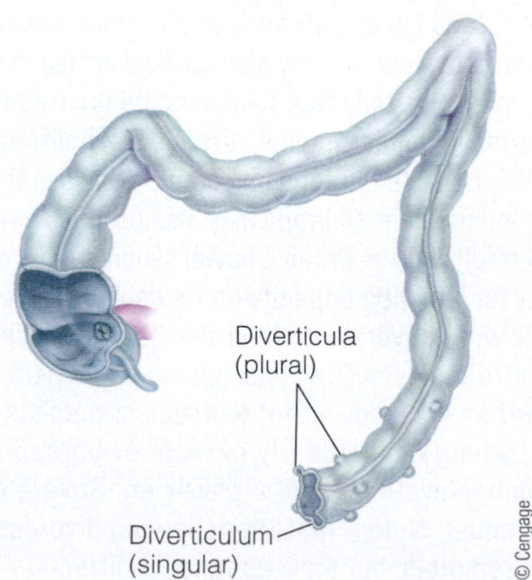
Diverticula
(plural)
Diverticulum
(singular)
© Cengage

physical activity improves the muscle tone and motility of the digestive tract. As little as 30 minutes of physical activity a day can help prevent or alleviate constipation.

Eating prunes—or "dried plums" as some have renamed them—can also be helpful. Prunes are high in fiber and also contain a laxative substance.* Similarly, probiotics may help alleviate constipation by improving GI motility and stool consistency.[16]

If these suggested changes in lifestyle and diet do not correct constipation, then a physician might recommend the use of **stool softeners, laxatives,** or **mineral oil.** These products are best used for brief periods. If needed for extended times, they should be used under physician supervision. Stool softeners may cause stomach pain, diarrhea, or cramping. Frequent use of laxatives can lead to dependency and upset the body's fluid, salt, and mineral balances. Mineral oil interferes with the absorption of fat-soluble vitamins.

One potentially harmful but currently popular practice is **colonic irrigation**—the internal washing of the large intestine with a powerful **enema** machine. Such an extreme cleansing is not only unnecessary, but it can be hazardous, especially for those with a history of digestive diseases. Side effects may be relatively minor (cramping, abdominal pain, bloating, nausea, and vomiting) or quite severe (infections, kidney failure, pancreatitis, and heart failure), sometimes leading to death. Common problems include equipment contamination, electrolyte abnormalities, and intestinal perforation. Less extreme practices can cause problems, too.

Belching and Gas

Many people complain of problems that they attribute to excessive gas. For some, belching is the complaint. Others blame intestinal gas for abdominal discomforts and embarrassment.

Belching

Belching results from swallowing air. Everyone swallows a little bit of air with each mouthful of food, but people who eat too fast may swallow too much air. Ill-fitting dentures, carbonated beverages, and chewing gum can also contribute to the swallowing of air with resultant belching. The best advice for belching seems to be to eat slowly, chew thoroughly, and relax while eating.

Intestinal Gas

Although **flatulence** can be an embarrassing experience, it is quite normal. (People who experience painful bloating from GI diseases, however, require medical treatment.) Healthy people expel several hundred milliliters of intestinal gas several times a day. Almost all (99 percent) of the gases expelled—nitrogen, oxygen, hydrogen, methane, and carbon dioxide—are odorless. The remaining "volatile" gases are the infamous ones.

Foods that produce gas usually must be determined individually (see Photo H3-2). The most common offenders are foods rich in the carbohydrates—sugars, starches, and fibers. When partially digested carbohydrates reach the large intestine, bacteria digest them, giving off gas as a by-product. People can test foods suspected of forming gas by omitting them individually for a trial period to see if there is any improvement.

*This laxative substance is *dihydroxyphenyl isatin.*

Gastroesophageal Reflux

Almost everyone has experienced heartburn at one time or another, usually soon after eating a meal. Medically known as **gastroesophageal reflux,** heartburn is the painful sensation a person feels behind the breastbone when the lower esophageal sphincter allows the stomach contents to reflux into the esophagus (see Figure H3-4, p. 92). This may happen if a person eats or drinks too much (or both). Tight clothing and even changes of position (lying down, bending over) can cause it, too, as can some medications and smoking. Weight gain and overweight increase the frequency, severity, and duration of heartburn symptoms. A defect of the sphincter muscle itself is a possible, but less common, cause.

If heartburn is not caused by an anatomical defect, treatment is fairly simple. To avoid such misery in the future, the person needs to learn to eat less at a sitting, chew food more thoroughly, and eat more slowly. Additional strategies are presented in Table H3-1 (p. 92).

People who overeat or eat too quickly are likely to suffer from **indigestion.** The muscular reaction of the stomach to unchewed lumps or to being overfilled may be so intense that it upsets normal peristalsis. When this happens, overeaters may taste the stomach acid and feel pain. Over-the-counter **antacids** and **acid controllers** may provide relief but should be used only infrequently for

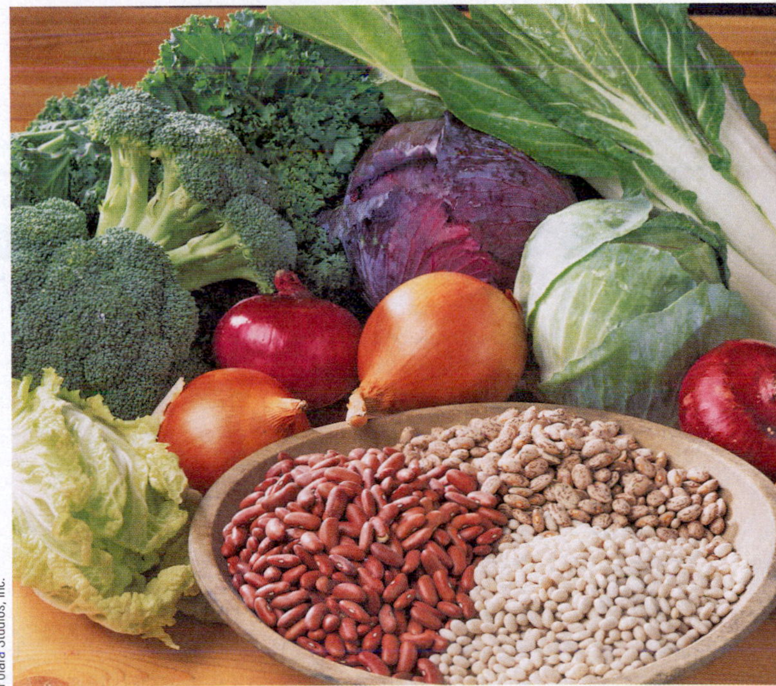
Polara Studios, Inc.

> **PHOTO H3-2** People troubled by intestinal gas need to determine which foods bother them and then eat those foods in moderation.

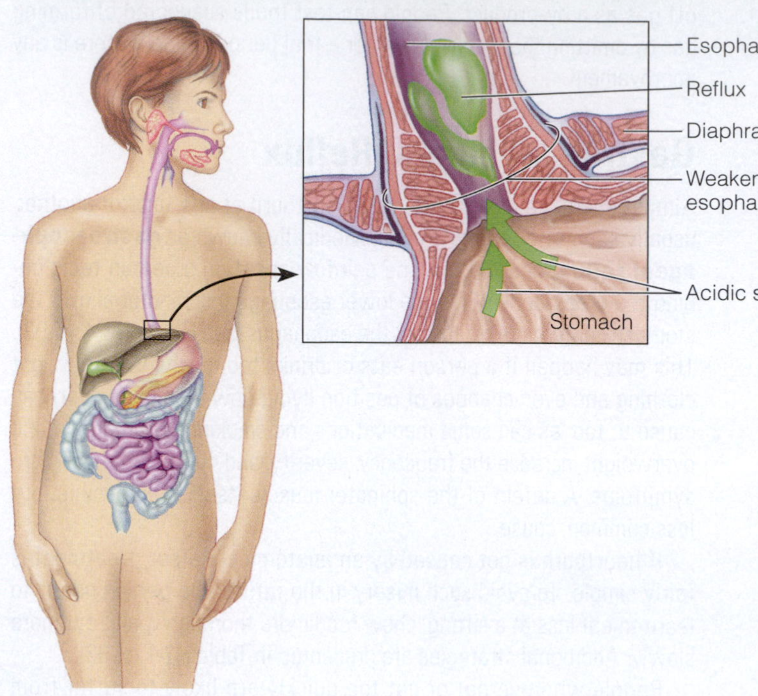
Esophagus
Reflux
Diaphragm
Weakened lower esophageal sphincter
Acidic stomach contents
Stomach
© Cengage

> **FIGURE H3-4 Gastroesophageal Reflux**

occasional heartburn; they may mask or cause problems if used regularly without medical supervision. If problems continue, people who suffer from frequent and regular bouts of heartburn and indigestion may need to see a physician, who can prescribe specific medication to control gastroesophageal reflux. Without treatment, the repeated splashes of acid can severely damage the cells of the esophagus, creating a condition known as Barrett's esophagus. At that stage, the risk of cancer in the esophagus increases dramatically.[17] To repeat, if symptoms persist, see a doctor—don't self-medicate.

Ulcers

Ulcers are another common digestive problem, affecting an estimated 10 percent of adults in the United States. An **ulcer** is a lesion (a sore), and a **peptic ulcer** is a lesion in the lining of the stomach (gastric ulcers) or the duodenum of the small intestine (duodenal ulcers). The compromised lining is left unprotected and exposed to gastric juices, which can be painful. In some cases, ulcers can cause internal bleeding. GI bleeding from ulcers is responsible for more than 250,000 hospitalizations in the United States each year.[18] Excessive blood loss may create an iron deficiency. Ulcers that perforate the GI lining can pose life-threatening complications.

Many people naively believe that an ulcer is caused by stress or spicy foods, but this is not the case. The stomach lining in a healthy person is well protected by its mucous coat. What, then, causes ulcers to form?

Three major causes of ulcers have been identified: bacterial infection with *Helicobacter pylori* (commonly abbreviated *H. pylori*); the use of certain anti-inflammatory drugs such as aspirin, ibuprofen, and naproxen; and disorders that cause excessive gastric acid secretion.

TABLE H3-1 Strategies to Prevent or Alleviate Common GI Problems

GI Problem	Strategies
Choking	• Take small bites of food. • Chew thoroughly before swallowing. • Don't talk or laugh with food in your mouth. • Don't eat when breathing hard.
Diarrhea	• Avoid strenuous activity. • Rest. • Drink fluids to replace losses. • Call for medical help if diarrhea persists.
Constipation	• Eat a high-fiber diet. • Drink plenty of fluids. • Exercise regularly. • Respond promptly to the urge to defecate.
Belching	• Eat slowly. • Chew thoroughly. • Relax while eating.
Intestinal gas	• Eat bothersome foods in moderation.
Heartburn	• Eat small meals. • Drink liquids between meals. • Sit up while eating; elevate your head when lying down. • Wait 3 hours after eating before lying down. • Wait 2 hours after eating before exercising. • Refrain from wearing tight-fitting clothing. • Avoid foods, beverages, and medications that aggravate your heartburn. Common irritants include foods that are fried or high in fat; chocolate and peppermint; coffee, alcoholic beverages, and carbonated beverages; mustard, ketchup, and tomato sauces; acidic substances such as vinegar, citrus juices, and citrus fruits. • Refrain from smoking cigarettes or using tobacco products. • Lose weight if overweight. • Take medicine as prescribed by your physician.
Ulcer	• Avoid coffee and caffeine- and alcohol-containing beverages. • Avoid foods that aggravate your ulcer. • Minimize aspirin, ibuprofen, and naproxen use. • Refrain from smoking cigarettes.

Most commonly, ulcers develop in response to *H. pylori* infection. The cause of the ulcer dictates the type of medication used in treatment. For example, people with ulcers caused by infection receive antibiotics, whereas those with ulcers caused by medicines discontinue their use. In addition, all treatment plans aim to relieve pain, heal the ulcer, and prevent recurrence.

The regimen for ulcer treatment is to treat for infection, eliminate any food that routinely causes indigestion or pain, and avoid coffee and caffeine- and alcohol-containing beverages. Both regular and decaffeinated coffee stimulate acid secretion and so aggravate *existing* ulcers.

Ulcers and their treatments highlight the importance of not self-medicating when symptoms persist. People with *H. pylori* infection often take over-the-counter acid controllers to relieve the pain of their ulcers when, instead, they need physician-prescribed antibiotics. Suppressing gastric acidity not only fails to heal the ulcer, but it also actually worsens inflammation during an *H. pylori* infection. Furthermore, *H. pylori* infection has been linked with stomach cancer, making prompt diagnosis and appropriate treatment essential.[19]

Table H3-1 summarizes strategies to prevent or alleviate common GI problems. Many of these problems reflect hurried lifestyles. For this reason, many of their remedies require that people slow down and take the time to eat at a leisurely pace; chew food thoroughly to prevent choking, heartburn, and acid indigestion; rest until vomiting and diarrhea subside; and heed the urge to defecate. In addition, people must learn how to handle life's day-to-day problems and challenges without overreacting and becoming upset; learn how to relax, get enough sleep, and enjoy life. Remember, "what's eating you" may cause more GI distress than what you eat.

CRITICAL THINKING QUESTIONS

A. What strategies would be most helpful in preventing common digestive problems?

B. You've noticed the abundance of gluten-free foods on the grocery store shelves. The demand for gluten-free products has increased dramatically over the past decade as gluten-free diets have gained in popularity. Although a gluten-free diet is the best treatment for people with celiac disease, it has been adopted by millions of other people for a variety of other reasons. Compare the kcalories, fiber, added sugars, and saturated fat on the labels of two similar products—one whole grain and the other gluten free—and determine what benefits and risks might accompany a gluten-free diet for those with celiac disease and for others. Which product would you now be more likely to buy? Why?

REFERENCES

1. American Academy of Pediatrics, Policy statement: Prevention of choking among children, *Pediatrics* 125 (2010): 601–607.
2. E. Kramarow, M. Warner, and L. H. Chen, Food-related choking deaths among the elderly, *Injury Prevention* 20 (2014): 200–203.
3. R. I. Ejemot-Nwadiaro and coauthors, Hand washing promotion for preventing diarrhoea, *Cochrane Database of Systematic Reviews* 9 (2015): CD004265.
4. K. G. Brandt, M. M. Castro Antunes, and G. A. Silva, Acute diarrhea: Evidence-based management, *Journal of Pediatrics* 91 (2015): S36–S43.
5. Y. J. Lee and K. S. Park, Irritable bowel syndrome: Emerging paradigm in pathophysiology, *World Journal of Gastroenterology* 20 (2014): 2456–2469; D. Keszthelyi, F. J. Troost, and A. A. Masclee, Irritable bowel syndrome: Methods, mechanisms, and pathophysiology. Methods to assess visceral hypersensitivity in irritable bowel syndrome, *American Journal of Physiology: Gastrointestinal and Liver Physiology* 303 (2012): G141–G154; M. Camilleri, Peripheral mechanisms in irritable bowel syndrome, *New England Journal of Medicine* 367 (2012): 1626–1635.
6. C. Stasi and coauthors, Serotonin receptors and their role in the pathophysiology and therapy of irritable bowel syndrome, *Techniques in Coloproctology* 18 (2014): 613–621.
7. W. D. Chey, J. Kurlander, and S. Eswaran, Irritable bowel syndrome: A clinical review, *Journal of the American Medical Association* 313 (2015): 949–958; T. Wilkins and coauthors, Diagnosis and management of IBS in adults, *American Family Physician* 86 (2012): 419–426.
8. M. Y. Hardy and coauthors, Ingestion of oats and barley in patients with celiac disease mobilizes cross-reactive T cells activated by avenin peptides and immuno-dominant hordein peptides, *Journal of Autoimmunity* 56 (2015): 56–65.
9. A. Rubio-Tapia and coauthors, The prevalence of celiac disease in the United States, *American Journal of Gastroenterology* 107 (2012): 1538–1544.
10. A. Fasano and coauthors, Nonceliac gluten sensitivity, *Gastroenterology* 148 (2015): 1195–1204; L. Elli, L. Roncoroni, and M. T. Bardella, Non-celiac gluten sensitivity: Time for sifting the grain, *World Journal of Gastroenterology* 21 (2015): 8221–8226.
11. M. El-Salhy and coauthors, The relation between celiac disease, nonceliac gluten sensitivity and irritable bowel syndrome, *Nutrition Journal* 14 (2015): 92–100.
12. M. Vazquez-Roque and A. S. Oxentenko, Nonceliac gluten sensitivity, *Mayo Clinic Proceedings* 90 (2015): 1272–1277.
13. B. Lebwohl, J. F. Ludvigsson, and P. H. Green, Celiac disease and non-celiac gluten sensitivity, *British Medical Journal* 351 (2015): h4347.
14. K. Stein, Severely restricted diets in the absence of medical necessity: The unintended consequences, *Journal of the Academy of Nutrition and Dietetics* 114 (2014): 986–994; G. A. Gaesser and S. S. Angadi, Gluten-free diet: Imprudent dietary advice for the general population? *Journal of the Academy of Nutrition and Dietetics* 112 (2012): 1330–1333.
15. G. Basilisco and M. Coletta, Chronic constipation: A critical review, *Digestive and Liver Disease* 45 (2013): 886–893.
16. E. Dimidi and coauthors, The effect of probiotics on functional constipation in adults: A systematic review and meta-analysis of randomized controlled trials, *American Journal of Clinical Nutrition* 100 (2014): 1075–1084.
17. S. J. Spechler and R. F. Souza, Barrett's esophagus, *New England Journal of Medicine* 371 (2014): 836–845.
18. L. Laine, Upper gastrointestinal bleeding due to a peptic ulcer, *New England Journal of Medicine* 374 (2016): 2367–2376.
19. R. Herrero, J. Parsonnet, and E. R. Greenberg, Prevention of gastric cancer, *Journal of the American Medical Association* 312 (2014): 1197–1198; A. Axon, Helicobacter pylori and public health, *Helicobacter* 19 (2014): 68–73.

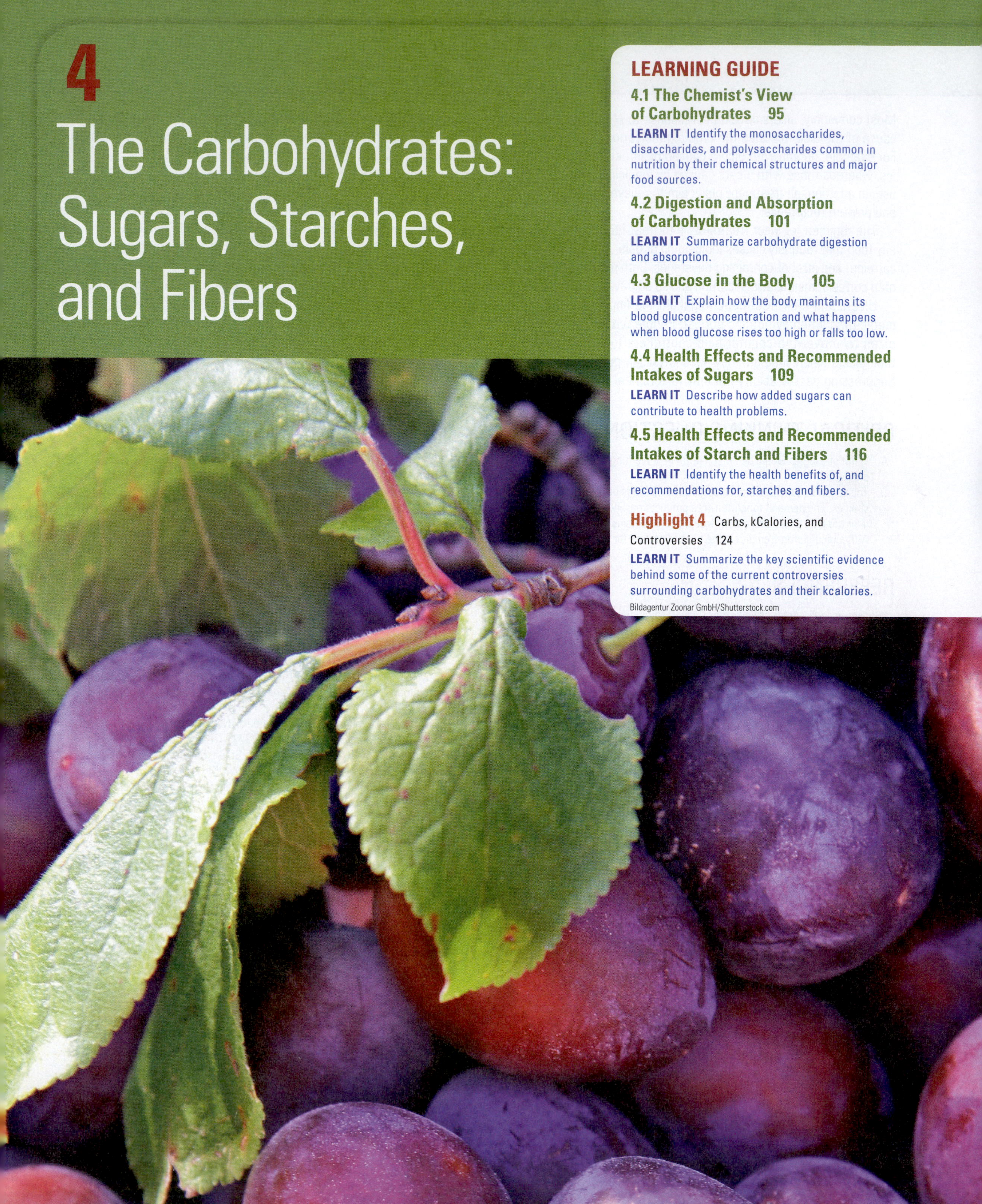

4

The Carbohydrates: Sugars, Starches, and Fibers

LEARNING GUIDE

Bildagentur Zoonar GmbH/Shutterstock.com

Nutrition in Your Life

Whether you are studying for an exam or daydreaming about your next vacation, your brain needs carbohydrate to power its activities. Your muscles need carbohydrate to fuel their work, too, whether you are racing up the stairs to class or moving on the dance floor to your favorite music. Where can you get carbohydrate? Are some foods healthier choices than others? As you will learn from this chapter, grains, vegetables, legumes, and fruits naturally deliver ample carbohydrate and fiber along with valuable vitamins and minerals. Milk products typically lack fiber, but they also provide carbohydrate along with an assortment of vitamins and minerals. As you read this chapter, consider whether your current carbohydrate choices are meeting dietary goals.

A student, quietly studying, is seldom aware of the billions of glucose molecules in his brain cells that provide the energy to learn. Yet glucose fuels nearly all of the brain's activities. Similarly, a marathon runner, triumphantly crossing the finish line, seldom gives credit to the glycogen her muscles have used to fuel the race. Yet, together, these two **carbohydrates**—glucose and its storage form glycogen—provide about half of all the energy muscles and other body tissues use. (The other half comes mostly from fat.) People don't eat glucose and glycogen. When they eat foods rich in carbohydrates, their bodies receive glucose for immediate energy and convert some glucose into glycogen for reserve energy.

The carbohydrate family includes sugars, starches, and fibers. Foods rich in carbohydrates include all plant foods—grains, vegetables, legumes, and fruits as well as milk. Notably, these foods deliver valuable vitamins and minerals along with their sugars, starches, and fibers; processed foods—such as soft drinks, candies, and cookies—deliver an abundance of added sugars with few, if any, nutrients of value.

As the next section explains, the members of the carbohydrate family differ in their chemical structures and food sources; later sections describe their health consequences. Clearly, not all carbohydrates are created equal.

4.1 The Chemist's View of Carbohydrates

LEARN IT Identify the monosaccharides, disaccharides, and polysaccharides common in nutrition by their chemical structures and major food sources.

The dietary carbohydrate family includes:

- Monosaccharides: single sugars
- Disaccharides: pairs of monosaccharides
- Polysaccharides: chains of monosaccharides

Monosaccharides and disaccharides (the sugars) are sometimes called *simple carbohydrates,* and polysaccharides (starches and fibers) are sometimes called *complex carbohydrates.*

To understand the structure of carbohydrates, look at the atoms within them. Each atom can form a certain number of chemical bonds with other atoms:

- Hydrogen atoms, one
- Oxygen atoms, two
- Nitrogen atoms, three
- Carbon atoms, four

Chemists represent the bonds as lines between the chemical symbols (such as H, O, N, and C) that stand for the atoms (see Figure 4-1).

> **FIGURE 4-1 Atoms and Their Bonds**

The four main types of atoms found in nutrients are hydrogen (H), oxygen (O), nitrogen (N), and carbon (C).

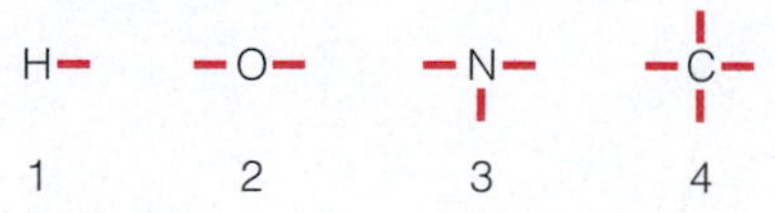

H— (1)   —O— (2)   —N— (3)   —C— (4)

Each atom has a characteristic number of bonds it can form with other atoms.

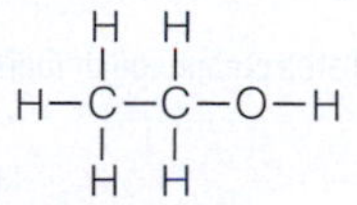

```
   H  H
   |  |
H—C—C—O—H
   |  |
   H  H
```

Notice that in this simple molecule of ethyl alcohol, each H has one bond, O has two, and each C has four.

carbohydrates: compounds composed of carbon, oxygen, and hydrogen arranged as monosaccharides or multiples of monosaccharides. Most, but not all, carbohydrates have a ratio of one carbon molecule to one water molecule: $(CH_2O)_n$.

- **carbo** = carbon (C)
- **hydrate** = with water (H_2O)

> **FIGURE 4-2 Chemical Structure of Glucose**

The diagram of a glucose molecule on the left shows all the bonds between the 6 carbon (C), 12 hydrogen (H), and 6 oxygen (O) atoms. It proves simple on examination, but chemists have adopted shortcuts to depict chemical structures. The middle and right diagrams also present the chemical structure of glucose, but as simplified versions with fewer symbols and bonds showing.

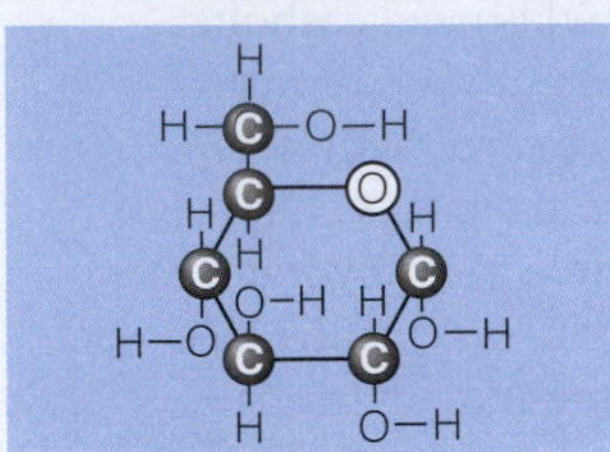

The structure of glucose has to be drawn flat, but in nature the five carbons and oxygen are roughly in a plane. The atoms attached to the ring carbons extend up and down from the plane.

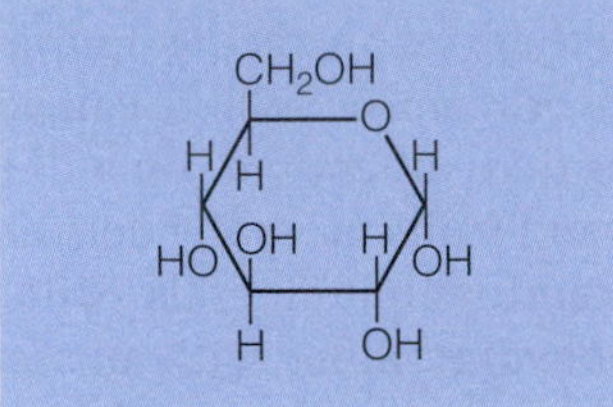

CH_2OH

The lines representing some of the bonds and the carbons at the corners are not shown.

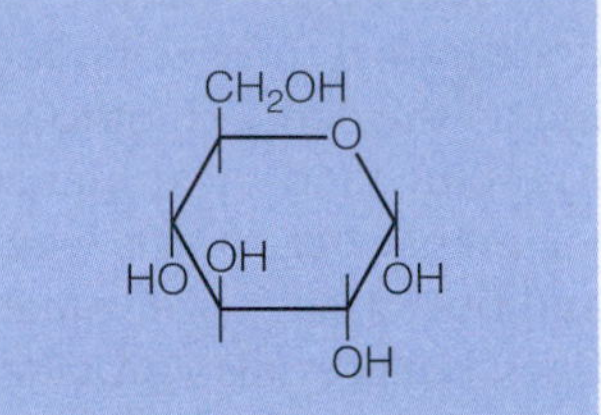

CH_2OH

Now the single hydrogens are not shown, but lines still extend upward or downward from the ring to show where they belong.

Atoms form molecules in ways that satisfy the bonding requirements of each atom. Figure 4-1 includes the structure of ethyl alcohol, the active ingredient of alcoholic beverages, as an example. The two carbons each have four bonds represented by lines; the oxygen has two; and each hydrogen has one bond connecting it to other atoms. Chemical structures always bond according to these rules.

The following list of the most important **sugars** in nutrition symbolizes them as hexagons and pentagons of different colors.* Three are monosaccharides:

- Glucose
- Fructose
- Galactose

Three are disaccharides:

- Maltose (glucose + glucose)
- Sucrose (glucose + fructose) 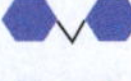
- Lactose (glucose + galactose) 

Monosaccharides

The three **monosaccharides** most important in nutrition all have the same numbers and kinds of atoms—each contains 6 carbon atoms, 12 hydrogens, and 6 oxygens (written in shorthand as $C_6H_{12}O_6$). The monosaccharides differ in their arrangements of the atoms. These chemical differences account for the differing sweetness of the monosaccharides. A pinch of purified glucose on the tongue gives only a mild sweet flavor, and galactose hardly tastes sweet at all. Fructose, however, is as intensely sweet as honey and, in fact, is the sugar primarily responsible for honey's sweetness.

Glucose

Chemically, **glucose** is a larger and more complicated molecule than the ethyl alcohol shown in Figure 4-1, but it obeys the same rules of chemistry: each carbon atom has four bonds; each oxygen, two bonds; and each hydrogen, one bond. Figure 4-2 illustrates the chemical structure of a glucose molecule.

sugars: simple carbohydrates composed of monosaccharides, disaccharides, or both.

monosaccharides (mon-oh-SACK-uh-rides): carbohydrates of the general formula $C_nH_{2n}O_n$ that typically form a single ring. The monosaccharides important in nutrition are *hexoses*, sugars with six atoms of carbon and the formula $C_6H_{12}O_6$. See Appendix C for the chemical structures of the monosaccharides.

- **mono** = one
- **saccharide** = sugar
- **hex** = six

glucose (GLOO-kose): a monosaccharide; sometimes known as *blood sugar* in the body or *dextrose* in foods.

- **ose** = carbohydrate
- (blue hexagon) = glucose

*Fructose is shown as a pentagon, but like the other monosaccharides, it has six carbons (as you will see in Figure 4-3). The disaccharides are illustrated with a simple bond, but actual linkages differ (as shown in Appendix C).

> **FIGURE 4-3 The Monosaccharides**

Notice the similarities—all three monosaccharides have 6 carbons (those shown plus one in each corner), 12 hydrogens (those shown plus one at the end of each single line), and 6 oxygens (all shown). Also notice the differences compared with glucose—in fructose, the ring is five-sided and in galactose, the position of one OH group differs slightly.

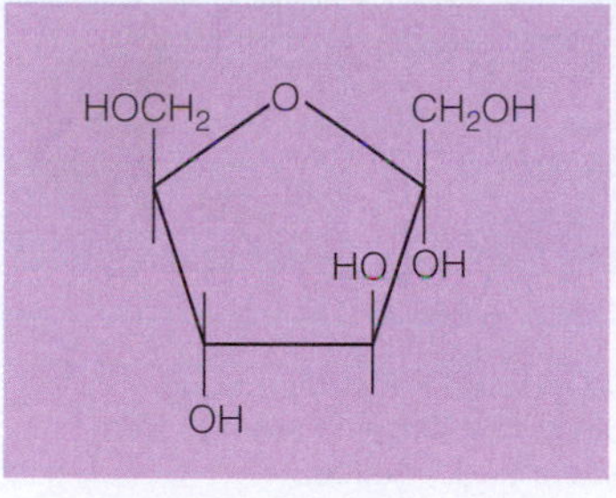

HOCH2
O
CH2OH
HO
OH
OH

Fructose

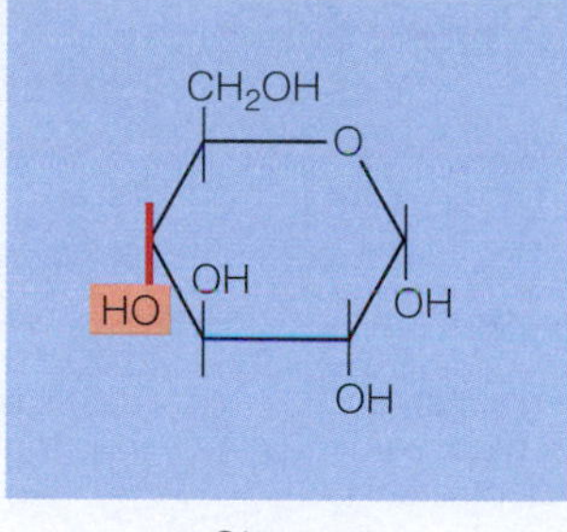

CH2OH
O
OH
HO
OH
OH

Glucose

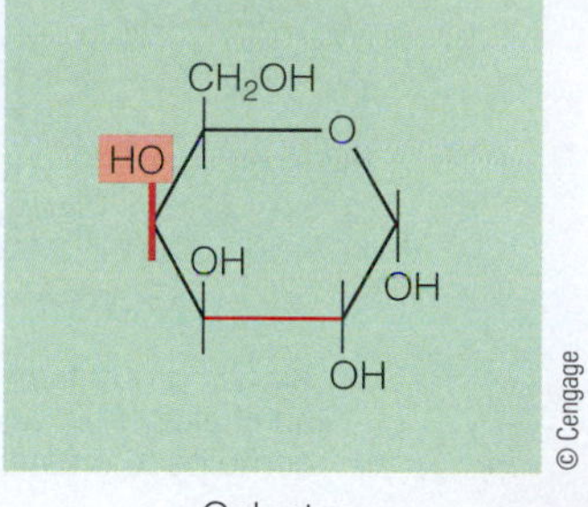

CH2OH
HO
O
OH
OH
OH

Galactose

© Cengage

Commonly known as blood sugar, glucose serves as an essential energy source for all the body's activities. Its significance to nutrition is tremendous. Later sections explain that glucose is one of the two sugars in every disaccharide and the unit from which the polysaccharides are made almost exclusively. One of these polysaccharides, starch, is the chief food source of energy for all the world's people; another, glycogen, is an important storage form of energy in the body. Glucose reappears frequently throughout this chapter and many of those that follow.

Fructose Fructose is the sweetest of the sugars. Curiously, fructose has exactly the same chemical *formula* as glucose—$C_6H_{12}O_6$—but its *structure* differs (see Figure 4-3). The arrangement of the atoms in fructose stimulates the taste buds on the tongue to produce the sweet sensation. Fructose occurs naturally in fruits (see Photo 4-1) and honey; other sources include products such as soft drinks, ready-to-eat cereals, and desserts that have been sweetened with high-fructose corn syrup (defined in Glossary 4-1, p. 110).

Galactose The monosaccharide galactose occurs naturally in foods as a single sugar only in very small amounts. Galactose has the same numbers and kinds of atoms as glucose and fructose in yet another arrangement. Figure 4-3 shows galactose beside a molecule of glucose for comparison.

Disaccharides

The disaccharides are pairs of monosaccharides. The three disaccharides most important in nutrition all contain glucose; the second member of the pair is fructose, galactose, or another glucose. These carbohydrates—and all the other energy nutrients—are put together and taken apart by similar chemical reactions: condensation and hydrolysis.

Condensation To make a disaccharide, a chemical reaction known as **condensation** links two monosaccharides together (see Figure 4-4, p. 98). A hydroxyl (OH) group from one monosaccharide and a hydrogen atom (H) from the other combine to create a molecule of water (H_2O). The two originally separate monosaccharides link together with a single oxygen (O).

Hydrolysis To break a disaccharide in two, a chemical reaction known as **hydrolysis** occurs (see Figure 4-5, p. 98). A molecule of water (H_2O) splits to provide the H and OH needed to complete the resulting monosaccharides. Hydrolysis reactions commonly occur during digestion.

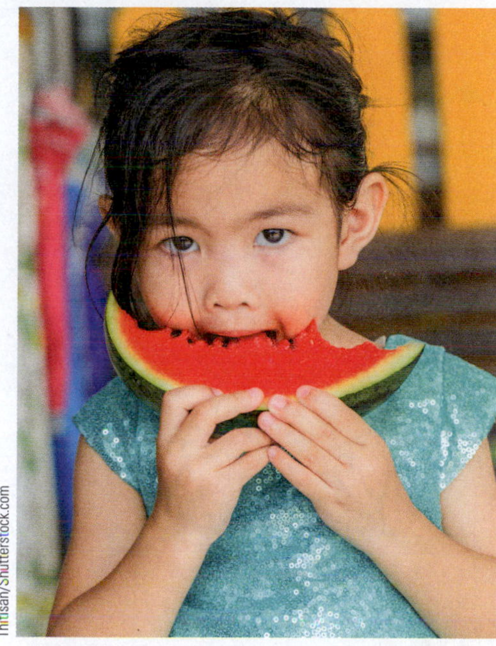

Thitisan/Shutterstock.com

> **PHOTO 4-1** Fruits package their sugars with fibers, vitamins, and minerals, making them a sweet and healthy snack.

fructose (FRUK-tose or FROOK-tose): a monosaccharide; sometimes known as *fruit sugar* or *levulose*. Fructose is found abundantly in fruits, honey, and saps.
- **fruct** = fruit
- (pentagon) = fructose

galactose (ga-LAK-tose): a monosaccharide; part of the disaccharide lactose.
- (hexagon) = galactose

disaccharides (dye-SACK-uh-rides): pairs of monosaccharides linked together.
- **di** = two

condensation: a chemical reaction in which water is released as two molecules combine to form one larger product.

hydrolysis (high-DROL-ih-sis): a chemical reaction in which one molecule is split into two molecules, with hydrogen (H) added to one and a hydroxyl group (OH) to the other (from water, H_2O). (The noun is *hydrolysis*; the verb is *hydrolyze*.)
- **hydro** = water
- **lysis** = breaking

> FIGURE 4-4 Condensation of Two Monosaccharides to Form a Disaccharide

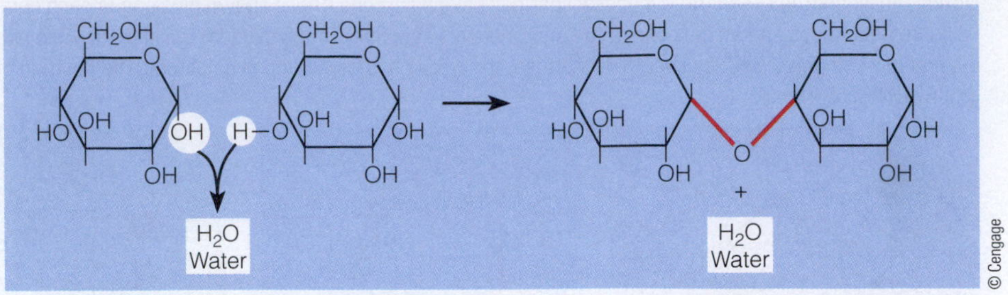

Glucose + glucose → Maltose

An OH group from one glucose and an H atom from another glucose combine to create a molecule of H_2O.

The two glucose molecules bond together with a single O atom to form the disaccharide maltose.

© Cengage

> FIGURE 4-5 Hydrolysis of a Disaccharide

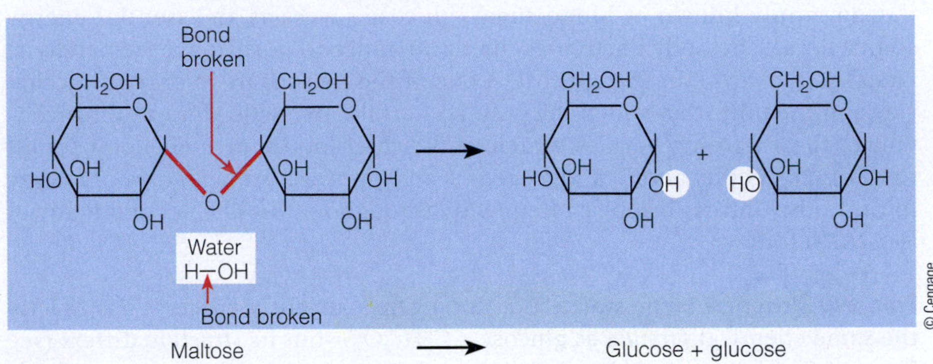

Bond broken
CH2OH
HO
OH
O
Water
H—OH
Bond broken
+
© Cengage

Maltose → Glucose + glucose

The disaccharide maltose splits into two glucose molecules with H added to one and OH to the other (from the water molecule).

maltose (MAWL-tose): a disaccharide composed of two glucose units; sometimes known as *malt sugar*. See Appendix C for the chemical structure of maltose.

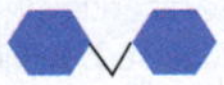

-  = maltose

sucrose (SUE-krose): a disaccharide composed of glucose and fructose; commonly known as *table sugar, beet sugar,* or *cane sugar.* Sucrose also occurs in many fruits and some vegetables and grains. See Appendix C for the chemical structure of sucrose.

- **sucro** = sugar
- = sucrose

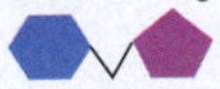

lactose (LAK-tose): a disaccharide composed of glucose and galactose; commonly known as *milk sugar.* See Appendix C for the chemical structure of lactose.

- **lac** = milk
- = lactose

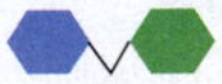

polysaccharides: compounds composed of many monosaccharides linked together. An intermediate string of 3 to 10 monosaccharides is an *oligosaccharide.*

- **poly** = many
- **oligo** = few

Maltose The disaccharide **maltose** consists of two glucose units. Maltose is produced whenever starch breaks down—as happens in human beings during carbohydrate digestion. It also occurs during the fermentation process that yields alcohol. Maltose is only a minor constituent of a few foods, most notably barley.

Sucrose Fructose and glucose together form the disaccharide **sucrose**. Sucrose is the sweetest of the disaccharides because it contains fructose, the sweetest of the monosaccharides. These sugars account for the natural sweetness of fruits, vegetables, and grains. To make table sugar, sucrose is refined from the juices of sugarcane and sugar beets, then granulated. Depending on the extent to which it is refined, the product becomes the familiar brown, white, and powdered sugars available at grocery stores.

Lactose The combination of galactose and glucose makes the disaccharide **lactose**, the principal carbohydrate of milk. Known as milk sugar, lactose contributes half of the energy (kcalories) provided by fat-free milk.

Polysaccharides

In contrast to the simple carbohydrates just mentioned—the monosaccharides glucose, fructose, and galactose and the disaccharides maltose, sucrose, and lactose—the **polysaccharides** are slightly more complex, containing many glucose units and, in some cases, a few other monosaccharides strung

> **FIGURE 4-6 Glycogen and Starch Compared**

For details of the chemical structures, see Appendix C.

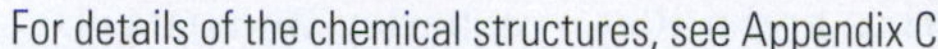

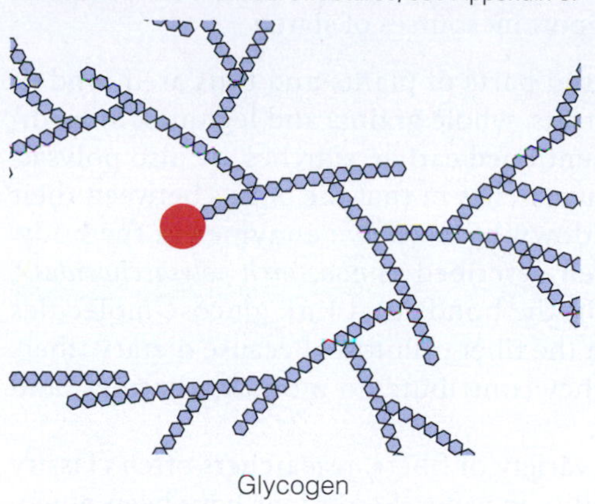

Glycogen

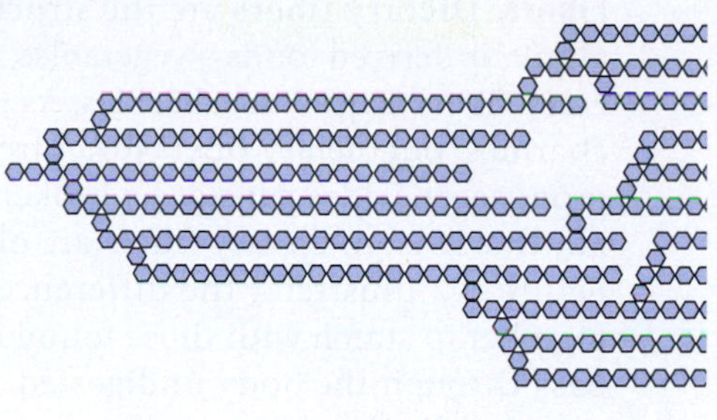

Starch (amylopectin)

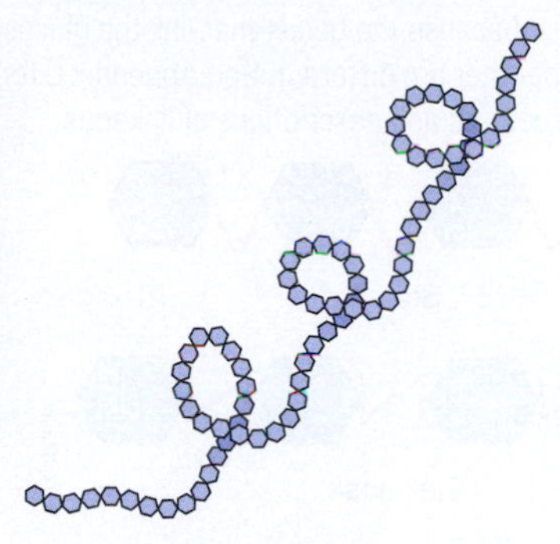

Starch (amylose)

A glycogen molecule contains hundreds of glucose units in highly branched chains. Each new glycogen molecule needs a special protein (shown here in red) for the attachment of the first glucose.

A starch molecule contains hundreds of glucose molecules in either occasionally branched chains (amylopectin) or unbranched chains (amylose).

together. Three types of polysaccharides are important in nutrition: glycogen, starches, and fibers.

Glycogen is a storage form of energy in the body; starch is the storage form of energy in plants; and fibers provide structure in stems, trunks, roots, leaves, and skins of plants. Both glycogen and starch are built of glucose units; fibers are composed of a variety of monosaccharides and other carbohydrate derivatives.

Glycogen Glycogen is found to only a limited extent in meats and not at all in plants.* For this reason, food is not a significant source of glycogen. Glycogen performs an important role in the body, however: it stores glucose for future use. Glycogen is made of many glucose molecules linked together in highly branched chains (see the left side of Figure 4-6). When the hormonal message "release energy" arrives at a liver or muscle cell, enzymes respond by attacking the many branches of glycogen simultaneously, making a surge of glucose available.**

Starches The human body stores glucose as glycogen, but plant cells store glucose as **starches**—long, branched or unbranched chains of hundreds or thousands of glucose molecules linked together (see the middle and right side of Figure 4-6). These giant starch molecules are packed side by side in grains such as wheat or rice, in root crops and tubers such as yams and potatoes, and in legumes such as peas and beans (see Photo 4-2). When you eat the plant, your body hydrolyzes the starch to glucose and uses the glucose for its own energy purposes.

All starchy foods come from plants. Grains are the richest food source of starch, providing much of the food energy for people all

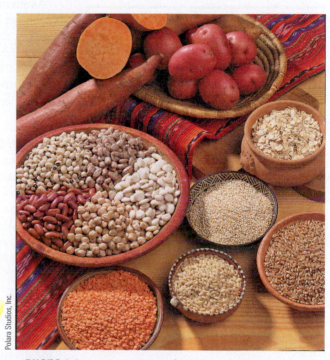

> **PHOTO 4-2** Major sources of starch include grains (such as rice, wheat, millet, rye, barley, and oats), legumes (such as kidney beans, black-eyed peas, pinto beans, navy beans, and garbanzo beans), tubers (such as potatoes), and root crops (such as yams and cassava).

glycogen (GLY-ko-jen): an animal polysaccharide composed of glucose; a storage form of glucose manufactured and stored in the liver and muscles. Glycogen is not a significant food source of carbohydrate and is not counted as a dietary carbohydrate in foods.

- **glyco** = glucose
- **gen** = gives rise to

starches: plant polysaccharides composed of many glucose molecules.

*Glycogen in animal muscles rapidly breaks down after slaughter.

**Normally, liver cells produce glucose from glycogen to be sent directly to the blood; muscle cells can also produce glucose from glycogen, but must use it themselves. Muscle cells can restore the blood glucose level indirectly, however, as Chapter 7 explains.

> FIGURE 4-7 The Bonds of Starch and Cellulose Compared

Human enzymes can digest starch but they cannot digest cellulose because the bonds that link the glucose molecules together are different. See Appendix C for chemical structures and descriptions of linkages.

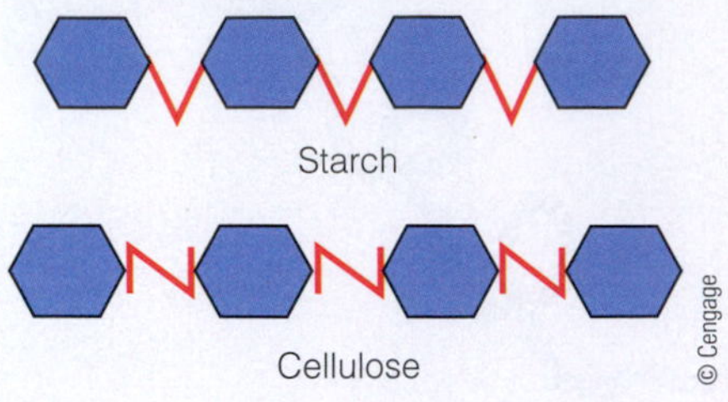
Starch
Cellulose
© Cengage

over the world—rice in Asia; wheat in Canada, the United States, and Europe; corn in much of Central and South America; and millet, rye, barley, and oats elsewhere. Legumes and tubers are also important sources of starch.

Fibers **Dietary fibers** are the structural parts of plants and thus are found in all plant-derived foods—vegetables, fruits, whole grains, and legumes. Most dietary fibers are polysaccharides. As mentioned earlier, starches are also polysaccharides, but dietary fibers differ from starches in that the bonds between their monosaccharides cannot be broken down by digestive enzymes in the body. For this reason, dietary fibers are often described as *nonstarch polysaccharides*.* Figure 4-7 illustrates the difference in the bonds that link glucose molecules together in starch with those found in the fiber cellulose. Because dietary fibers pass through the body undigested, they contribute no monosaccharides, and therefore little or no energy.

Even though most foods contain a variety of fibers, researchers often classify dietary fibers according to their solubility in water. Exceptions have been noted, but in general, **soluble fibers** benefit heart disease, diabetes, cancers, and weight management whereas **insoluble fibers** benefit GI health. Other characteristics of fibers include their viscosity and fermentability. **Viscous fibers** form gels in the GI tract and **fermentable fibers** are digested by GI bacteria.** In general, soluble fibers are more viscous and fermentable than insoluble fibers; again, exceptions have been noted.

As mentioned earlier, *dietary fibers* occur naturally in plants. When these fibers have been extracted from plants or are manufactured and then added to foods or used in supplements, they are called *functional fibers*—if they have beneficial health effects. Cellulose in cereals, for example, is a dietary fiber, but when consumed as a supplement to alleviate constipation, cellulose is considered a functional fiber. *Total fiber* refers to the sum of dietary fibers and functional fibers.

TABLE 4-1 The Carbohydrate Family

Monosaccharides	
Glucose	
Fructose	
Galactose	
Disaccharides	
Maltose (glucose + glucose)	
Sucrose (glucose + fructose)	
Lactose (glucose + galactose)	
Polysaccharides	
Glycogen[a]	
Starches (amylose and amylopectin)	
Fibers (soluble and insoluble)	

[a]Glycogen is a polysaccharide, but not a common dietary source of carbohydrate.

© Cengage

REVIEW IT Identify the monosaccharides, disaccharides, and polysaccharides common in nutrition by their chemical structures and major food sources.

The carbohydrates are made of carbon (C), oxygen (O), and hydrogen (H). Each of these atoms can form a specified number of chemical bonds: carbon forms four, oxygen forms two, and hydrogen forms one.

The three monosaccharides (glucose, fructose, and galactose) all have the same chemical formula ($C_6H_{12}O_6$), but their structures differ. The three disaccharides (maltose, sucrose, and lactose) are pairs of monosaccharides, each containing a glucose paired with one of the three monosaccharides. The sugars derive primarily from plants, except for lactose and its component galactose, which come from milk and milk products. Two monosaccharides can be linked together by a condensation reaction to form a disaccharide and water. A disaccharide, in turn, can be broken into its two monosaccharides by a hydrolysis reaction using water.

The polysaccharides are chains of monosaccharides and include glycogen, starches, and dietary fibers. Both glycogen and starch are storage forms of glucose—glycogen in the body, and starch in plants—and both yield energy for human use. The dietary fibers also contain glucose (and other monosaccharides), but their bonds cannot be broken by human digestive enzymes, so they yield little, if any, energy. Table 4-1 summarizes the carbohydrate family of compounds.

dietary fibers: in plant foods, the *nonstarch polysaccharides* that are not digested by human digestive enzymes, although some are digested by GI tract bacteria.

soluble fibers: nonstarch polysaccharides that dissolve in water to form a gel. An example is pectin from fruit, which is used to thicken jellies.

insoluble fibers: nonstarch polysaccharides that do not dissolve in water. Examples include the tough, fibrous structures found in the strings of celery and the skins of corn kernels.

viscous fibers: fibers that have gel-forming properties.

fermentable fibers: fibers that can be digested by bacteria in the GI tract.

*The nonstarch polysaccharide fibers include cellulose, hemicelluloses, pectins, gums, and mucilages. Fibers also include some *nonpolysaccharides* such as lignins, cutins, and tannins.

**Dietary fibers are fermented by bacteria in the colon to short-chain fatty acids, which are absorbed and metabolized by cells in the GI tract and liver (Chapter 5 describes fatty acids).

4.2 Digestion and Absorption of Carbohydrates

LEARN IT Summarize carbohydrate digestion and absorption.

The ultimate goal of digestion and absorption of sugars and starches is to break them into small molecules—chiefly glucose—that the body can absorb and use (see Photo 4-3). The large starch molecules require extensive breakdown; the disaccharides need be broken only once and the monosaccharides not at all. The details follow.

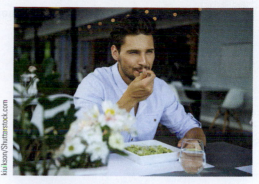

kiuikson/Shutterstock.com

> **PHOTO 4-3** When a person eats carbohydrate-rich foods, the body receives a valuable commodity—glucose.

Carbohydrate Digestion

Figure 4-8 (p. 102) traces the digestion of carbohydrates through the GI tract. When a person eats foods containing starch, enzymes hydrolyze the long chains to shorter chains, the short chains to disaccharides, and, finally, the disaccharides to monosaccharides.* This process begins in the mouth.

In the Mouth The salivary enzyme **amylase** starts to work in the mouth, hydrolyzing starch to shorter polysaccharides and to the disaccharide maltose. In fact, you can taste the change if you chew a piece of starchy food like a cracker and hold it in your mouth for a few minutes without swallowing it—the cracker begins tasting sweeter as the enzyme acts on it. Because food is in the mouth for a relatively short time, very little carbohydrate digestion takes place there.

In the Stomach Carbohydrate digestion ceases in the stomach. The activity of salivary amylase diminishes as the stomach's acid and protein-digesting enzymes inactivate the enzyme. The stomach's digestive juices contain no enzymes to break down carbohydrates. Fibers are not digested, but because they linger in the stomach, they delay gastric emptying, thereby providing a feeling of fullness and **satiety.** Carbohydrate digestion begins again in the small intestine.

In the Small Intestine The small intestine performs most of the work of carbohydrate digestion. A major carbohydrate-digesting enzyme, pancreatic amylase, enters the intestine via the pancreatic duct and continues breaking down the polysaccharides to shorter glucose chains and maltose. The final step takes place on the outer membranes of the intestinal cells. There specific enzymes break down specific disaccharides:

- **Maltase** breaks maltose into two glucose molecules.
- **Sucrase** breaks sucrose into one glucose and one fructose molecule.
- **Lactase** breaks lactose into one glucose and one galactose molecule.

At this point, all polysaccharides and disaccharides have been broken down to monosaccharides—mostly glucose molecules, with some fructose and galactose molecules as well.

In the Large Intestine Within 1 to 4 hours after a meal, all the sugars and most of the starches have been digested. Only the nondigestible carbohydrates remain in the digestive tract.

Nondigestible Carbohydrates As mentioned earlier, dietary fibers cannot be broken down by digestive enzymes; as they linger in the large intestine, they attract water, which softens the stools for passage without straining. Also, bacteria in the GI tract ferment some fibers. This process generates water, gas, and short-chain fatty acids (described in Chapter 5).** The cells of the colon use these small fat molecules for energy. Metabolism of short-chain fatty acids also occurs in the cells of the liver. Some fibers, therefore, can contribute some energy (1.5 to 2.5 kcalories per gram), depending on the extent to which they are broken down by bacteria and the fatty acids are absorbed.

*The short chains of glucose units that result from the breakdown of starch are known as *dextrins*. The word sometimes appears on food labels because dextrins can be used as thickening agents in processed foods.
**The short-chain fatty acids produced by GI bacteria are primarily acetic acid, propionic acid, and butyric acid.

amylase (AM-ih-lace): an enzyme that hydrolyzes amylose (a form of starch). Amylase is a *carbohydrase*, an enzyme that breaks down carbohydrates.

satiety (sah-TIE-eh-tee): the feeling of fullness and satisfaction that occurs after a meal and inhibits eating until the next meal. Satiety determines how much time passes between meals.

- **sate** = to fill

maltase: an enzyme that hydrolyzes maltose.

sucrase: an enzyme that hydrolyzes sucrose.

lactase: an enzyme that hydrolyzes lactose.

> **FIGURE 4-8 Carbohydrate Digestion in the GI Tract**

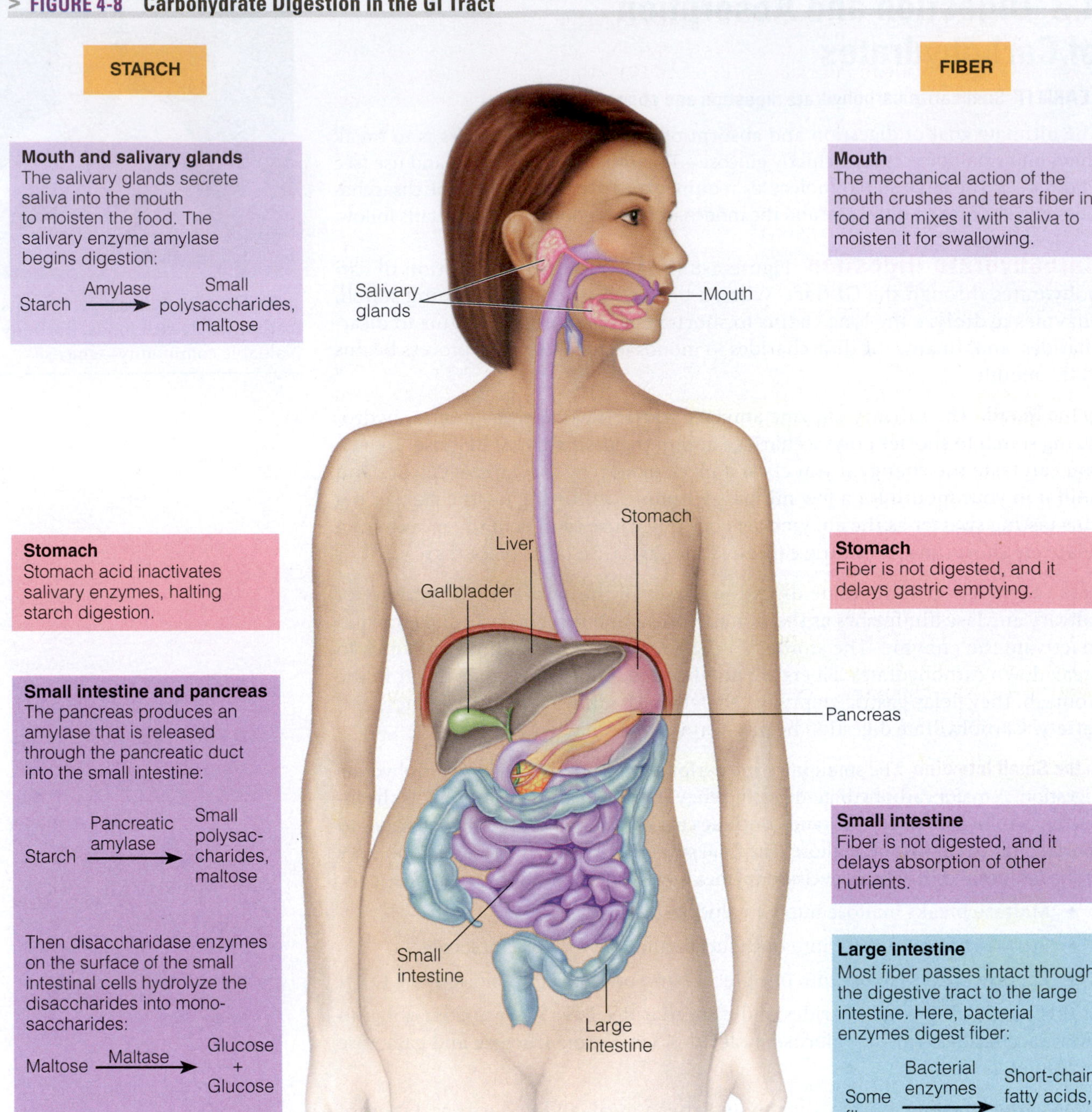

STARCH
FIBER
Mouth and salivary glands
The salivary glands secrete saliva into the mouth to moisten the food. The salivary enzyme amylase begins digestion:
Starch —Amylase→ Small polysaccharides, maltose
Mouth
The mechanical action of the mouth crushes and tears fiber in food and mixes it with saliva to moisten it for swallowing.
Salivary glands
Mouth
Stomach
Liver
Gallbladder
Pancreas
Small intestine
Large intestine
Stomach
Stomach acid inactivates salivary enzymes, halting starch digestion.
Stomach
Fiber is not digested, and it delays gastric emptying.
Small intestine and pancreas
The pancreas produces an amylase that is released through the pancreatic duct into the small intestine:
Starch —Pancreatic amylase→ Small polysaccharides, maltose
Then disaccharidase enzymes on the surface of the small intestinal cells hydrolyze the disaccharides into monosaccharides:
Maltose —Maltase→ Glucose + Glucose
Sucrose —Sucrase→ Fructose + Glucose
Lactose —Lactase→ Galactose + Glucose
Intestinal cells absorb these monosaccharides.
Small intestine
Fiber is not digested, and it delays absorption of other nutrients.
Large intestine
Most fiber passes intact through the digestive tract to the large intestine. Here, bacterial enzymes digest fiber:
Some fiber —Bacterial enzymes→ Short-chain fatty acids, gas
Fiber holds water; regulates bowel activity; and binds substances such as bile, cholesterol, and some minerals, carrying them out of the body.
© Cengage

Resistant Starches A few starches, known as **resistant starches**, also escape digestion and absorption in the small intestine. Starch may resist digestion for several reasons, including the body's digestive activities and the food's physical properties. Resistant starch is common in whole or partially milled grains, legumes, and just-ripened bananas. Cooked potatoes, pasta, and rice that have been chilled also contain resistant starch. Similar to insoluble fibers, resistant starch may prevent chronic diseases such as diabetes, colon cancer, and obesity.[1]

resistant starches: starches that escape digestion and absorption in the small intestine of healthy people.

FODMAP Other carbohydrates that are poorly digested and absorbed include the **FODMAP**—fermentable oligosaccharides, disaccharides, monosaccharides, and polyols (sugar alcohols, discussed on p. 115). Highlight 3 introduced low-FODMAP diets as part of the dietary strategy to treat irritable bowel syndrome. As FODMAP linger in the GI tract, they attract fluid, which causes abdominal bloating and pain. When FODMAP reach the large intestine, they become food for the bacteria living there. The bacterial digestion of FODMAP produces additional symptoms of irritable bowel syndrome—intestinal gas and changes in bowel habits (diarrhea, constipation, or both). Limited evidence suggests that a low-FODMAP diet may improve the diversity of the microbiota and the symptoms of irritable bowel syndrome.[2] Foods commonly restricted in a low-FODMAP diet include wheat, milk products, onions, legumes, and sugar alcohols.

Carbohydrate Absorption Glucose is unique in that it can be absorbed to some extent through the lining of the mouth, but for the most part, nutrient absorption takes place in the small intestine. Glucose and galactose enter the cells lining the small intestine by active transport (which requires energy and a specific sodium-dependent transporter); after high-carbohydrate meals, glucose and galactose may also be absorbed by facilitated transport (which requires a different transporter). Fructose is absorbed by facilitated transport (and has its own specific transporter).

As the blood from the small intestine circulates through the liver, cells there take up fructose and galactose and most often convert them to compounds within the same metabolic pathways as glucose. Figure 4-9 shows that fructose and galactose are mostly metabolized in the liver, whereas glucose is sent out to the body's cells for energy. In the end, all disaccharides provide at least one glucose molecule directly, and they can provide the equivalent of another one indirectly—through the metabolism of fructose and galactose in the liver.

Lactose Intolerance Normally, the intestinal cells produce enough of the enzyme lactase to ensure that the disaccharide lactose found in milk is both digested and absorbed efficiently. Lactase activity is highest immediately after birth, as befits an infant whose first and only food for a while will be breast milk or infant formula. In the great majority of the world's populations, lactase activity

FODMAP: a collective term used to describe **f**ermentable **o**ligosaccharides, **d**isaccharides, **m**onosaccharides, **a**nd **p**olyols that are commonly found in such foods as wheat, onions, some fruits and vegetables, sorbitol, and some dairy.

> FIGURE 4-9 **Absorption of Monosaccharides**

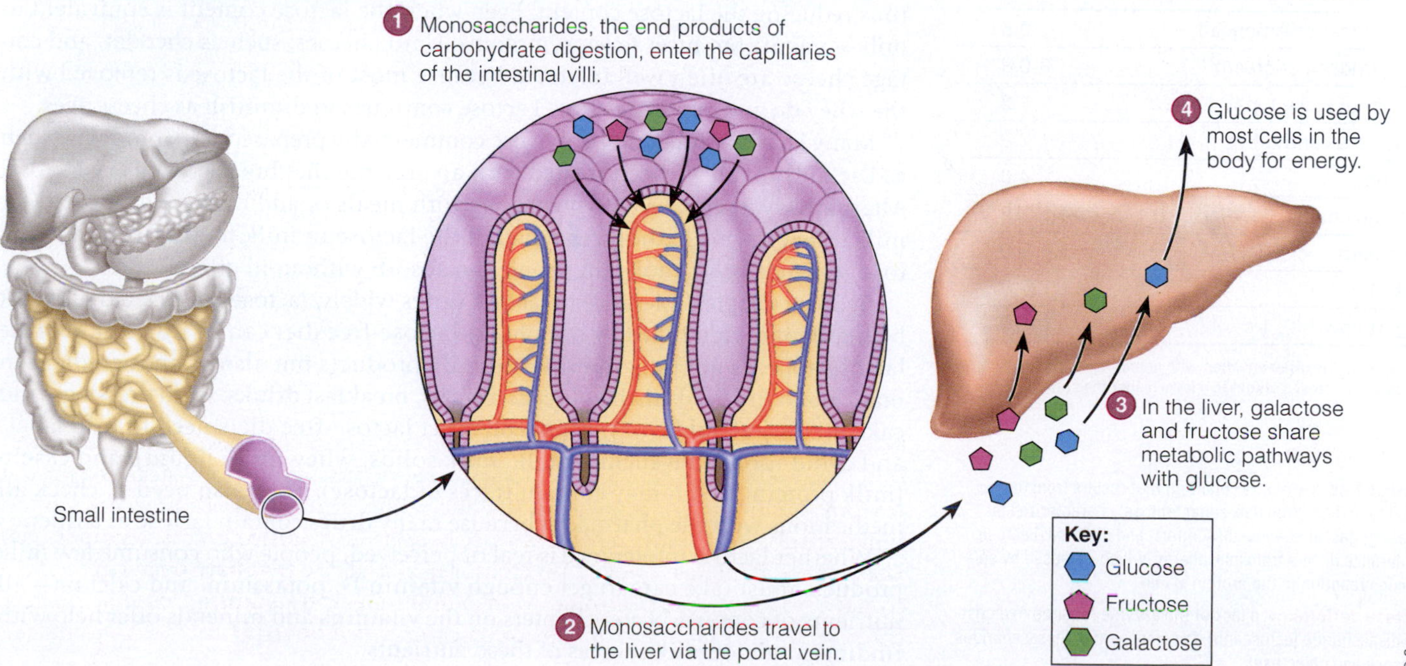
1 Monosaccharides, the end products of carbohydrate digestion, enter the capillaries of the intestinal villi.
Small intestine
2 Monosaccharides travel to the liver via the portal vein.
3 In the liver, galactose and fructose share metabolic pathways with glucose.
4 Glucose is used by most cells in the body for energy.
Key:
Glucose
Fructose
Galactose
© Cengage

declines dramatically during childhood and adolescence to about 5 to 10 percent of the activity at birth. Only a relatively small percentage (about 35 percent) of the people in the world retain enough lactase to digest and absorb lactose efficiently throughout adult life.

Symptoms When more lactose is consumed than the available lactase can handle, lactose molecules remain in the intestine undigested, attracting water and causing bloating, abdominal discomfort, and diarrhea—the symptoms of **lactose intolerance.** The undigested lactose becomes food for intestinal bacteria, which multiply and produce irritating acid and gas, further contributing to the discomfort and diarrhea.

Causes As mentioned, lactase activity commonly declines with age. **Lactase deficiency** may also develop when the intestinal villi are damaged by disease, certain medicines, prolonged diarrhea, or malnutrition. Depending on the extent of the intestinal damage, lactose malabsorption may be temporary or permanent. In extremely rare cases, an infant is born with a lactase deficiency, making feeding a challenge.

Prevalence The prevalence of lactose intolerance varies widely among ethnic groups, indicating that the trait has a genetic component. The prevalence of lactose intolerance is lowest among northern Europeans and highest among east Asians. Estimating the prevalence of lactose intolerance is difficult; many people who claim to be lactose intolerant have not be clinically diagnosed.

Dietary Changes Managing lactose intolerance requires some dietary changes, although total elimination of milk products usually is not necessary. Excluding all milk products from the diet can lead to nutrient deficiencies because these foods are a major source of several nutrients, notably the minerals calcium and potassium and vitamin D. Fortunately, many people with lactose intolerance can consume foods containing up to 6 grams of lactose (½ cup milk) without symptoms. The most successful strategies are to increase intake of milk products gradually, consume them with other foods in meals, and spread their intake throughout the day. In addition, yogurt containing live bacteria seems to improve lactose intolerance. A change in the type, number, and activity of GI bacteria—not the reappearance of the missing enzyme—accounts for the ability to adapt to milk products. Importantly, most lactose-intolerant individuals need to *manage* their dairy consumption rather than *eliminate* it.

In many cases, lactose-intolerant people can tolerate fermented milk products such as yogurt.[3] The bacteria in these products digest lactose for their own use, thus reducing the lactose content. Even when the lactose content is equivalent to milk's, yogurt produces fewer symptoms. Hard cheeses, such as cheddar, and cottage cheese are often well tolerated because most of the lactose is removed with the whey during manufacturing. Lactose continues to diminish as cheese ages.

Many lactose-intolerant people use commercially prepared milk products (such as Lactaid) that have been treated with an enzyme that breaks down the lactose. Alternatively, they take enzyme tablets with meals or add enzyme drops to their milk. The enzyme hydrolyzes much of the lactose in milk to glucose and galactose, which lactose-intolerant people can absorb without ill effects.

Because people's tolerance to lactose varies widely, lactose-restricted diets must be highly individualized. A completely lactose-free diet can be difficult because lactose appears not only in milk and milk products but also as an ingredient in many nondairy foods such as breads, cereals, breakfast drinks, salad dressings, and cake mixes (see Table 4-2). People on strict lactose-free diets need to read labels and avoid foods that include milk, milk solids, whey (milk liquid), and casein (milk protein, which may contain traces of lactose). They also need to check all medications with the pharmacist because many drugs contain lactose as a filler.

Whether lactose intolerance is real or perceived, people who consume few milk products must take care to get enough vitamin D, potassium, and calcium—all nutrients of concern.[4] Later chapters on the vitamins and minerals offer help with finding good nonmilk sources of these nutrients.

TABLE 4-2 Lactose in Selected Foods

Foods	Lactose (g)
Whole-wheat bread, 1 slice	0.5
Dinner roll, 1	0.5
Cheese, 1 oz	
Cheddar or American	0.5
Parmesan or cream	0.8
Doughnut (cake type), 1	1.2
Chocolate candy, 1 oz	2.3
Sherbet, 1 c	4.0
Cottage cheese (low-fat), 1 c	7.5
Ice cream, 1 c	9.0
Milk, 1 c	12.0
Yogurt (low-fat), 1 c	15.0

NOTE: Yogurt is often enriched with nonfat milk solids, which increase its lactose content to a level higher than milk's.

lactose intolerance: a condition that results from the inability to digest the milk sugar lactose; characterized by bloating, gas, abdominal discomfort, and diarrhea. Lactose intolerance differs from milk allergy, which is caused by an immune reaction to the protein in milk.

lactase deficiency: a lack of the enzyme required to digest the disaccharide lactose into its component monosaccharides (glucose and galactose).

REVIEW IT Summarize carbohydrate digestion and absorption.
In the digestion and absorption of carbohydrates, the body breaks down starches into disaccharides and monosaccharides, which are absorbed. The fibers help regulate the passage of food through the GI tract and slow the absorption of glucose, but they contribute little, if any, energy.

Lactose intolerance is a relatively common condition that occurs when there is insufficient lactase to digest the disaccharide lactose found in milk and milk products. Symptoms are limited to GI distress. Because treatment requires limiting milk and milk products in the diet, other sources of potassium, vitamin D, and calcium must be included.

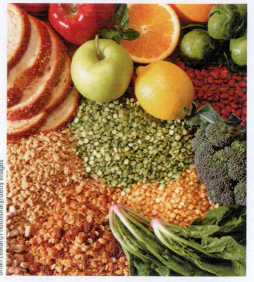
Brian Leatart/Photolibrary/Getty Images

> **PHOTO 4-4** The carbohydrates of grains, vegetables, fruits, and legumes supply most of the energy in a healthful diet.

4.3 Glucose in the Body

LEARN IT Explain how the body maintains its blood glucose concentration and what happens when blood glucose rises too high or falls too low.

The primary role of carbohydrates in the body is to supply the cells with glucose for energy. Scientists have long known that providing energy is glucose's primary role in the body, but they have also discovered additional roles that glucose and other sugars perform in the body.* When sugar molecules adhere to the body's protein and fat molecules, the consequences can be dramatic. Sugars attached to a protein change the protein's shape and function; when they bind to lipids in a cell's membranes, sugars alter the way cells recognize one another.**

A Preview of Carbohydrate Metabolism

Glucose plays the central role in carbohydrate metabolism. This brief discussion provides just enough information about carbohydrate metabolism to illustrate that the body needs and uses glucose primarily as an energy nutrient (see Photo 4-4). Chapter 7 provides a full description of energy metabolism.

Storing Glucose as Glycogen After a meal, blood glucose rises, and liver cells link excess glucose molecules by condensation reactions into long, branching chains of glycogen (review Figure 4-6, p. 99). When blood glucose falls, the liver cells break down glycogen by hydrolysis reactions into single molecules of glucose and release them into the bloodstream. Thus, glucose becomes available to supply energy to the brain and other tissues regardless of whether the person has eaten recently.

The liver stores about one-fourth of the body's total glycogen and releases glucose into the bloodstream as needed. Muscle cells also store glucose as glycogen (the other three-fourths), but muscles hoard most of their supply, using it just for themselves during exercise. The brain maintains a small amount of glycogen, which is thought to provide an emergency energy reserve during times of severe glucose deprivation.

Glycogen holds water and, therefore, is rather bulky. The liver can store only enough glycogen to provide energy for about a day. For its long-term energy reserves, for use over days or weeks of food deprivation, the body uses its abundant, water-free fuel, fat, as Chapter 5 describes.

Using Glucose for Energy Glucose fuels the work of most of the body's cells and is the preferred energy source for brain cells, other nerve cells, and developing red blood cells. Inside a cell, a series of reactions can break glucose into smaller compounds that yield energy when broken down completely to carbon dioxide and water (see Chapter 7).

Making Glucose from Protein As mentioned, the liver's glycogen stores are limited, and the brain needs glucose to fuel its activities. To keep providing glucose to meet energy needs, a person has to eat carbohydrate-rich foods frequently. Yet people who do not always attend faithfully to their bodies' carbohydrate needs still survive. How do they manage without glucose from dietary carbohydrate?

*The study of sugars and their derivatives is known as *glycobiology*.
**These combination molecules are known as *glycoproteins* and *glycolipids*, respectively.

Do they simply draw energy from the other two energy-yielding nutrients, fat and protein? They do draw energy from them, but not simply.

Fat cannot make glucose to any significant extent. The amino acids of protein can be used to make glucose to some extent, but amino acids and proteins have jobs of their own that no other nutrient can perform. Still, when a person does not replenish glucose by eating carbohydrate, body proteins are broken down to make glucose to fuel the brain and other nerve cells. These body proteins derive primarily from the liver and skeletal muscles.

The conversion of protein to glucose is called **gluconeogenesis**—literally, the making of new glucose. Only adequate dietary carbohydrate can prevent this use of protein for energy, and this role of carbohydrate is known as its **protein-sparing action.**

Making Ketone Bodies from Fat Fragments An inadequate supply of carbohydrate can shift the body's energy metabolism in a precarious direction. With less carbohydrate providing glucose to meet the brain's energy needs, fat takes an alternative metabolic pathway; instead of entering the main energy pathway, fat fragments combine with one another, forming **ketone bodies.** Ketone bodies provide an alternative fuel source during starvation, but when their production exceeds their use, they accumulate in the blood, causing **ketosis.** Because most ketone bodies are acidic, ketosis disturbs the body's normal **acid-base balance.** (Chapter 7 explores ketosis and the metabolic consequences of low-carbohydrate diets further.)

To spare body protein and prevent ketosis, the body needs 50 to 100 grams of carbohydrate a day. Dietary recommendations urge people to select abundantly from carbohydrate-rich foods to provide for considerably more.

Dean Drobot/Shutterstock.com

> **PHOTO 4-5** The brain uses glucose as its primary fuel for energy.

Using Glucose to Make Fat After meeting its immediate energy needs and filling its glycogen stores to capacity, the body must find a way to handle any extra glucose. When glucose is abundant, energy metabolism shifts to use more glucose instead of fat. If that isn't enough to restore glucose balance, the liver breaks glucose into smaller molecules and puts them together into the more permanent energy-storage compound—fat. Thus, when carbohydrate is abundant, fat is either conserved (by using more carbohydrate in the fuel mix) or created (by using excess carbohydrate to make body fat). The fat then travels to the fatty tissues of the body for storage; fat made from excess sugars may be deposited in the liver and muscles as well.[5] Unlike the liver cells, which can store only enough glycogen to meet about a day's energy needs, fat cells can store seemingly unlimited quantities of fat.

The Constancy of Blood Glucose

Every body cell depends on glucose for its fuel to some extent, and the cells of the brain and the rest of the nervous system depend almost exclusively on glucose for their energy (see Photo 4-5). The activities of these cells never cease, and they have limited ability to store glucose. Day and night, they continually draw on the supply of glucose in the fluid surrounding them. To maintain the supply, a steady stream of blood moves past these cells bringing more glucose from either the small intestine (food) or the liver (via glycogen breakdown or gluconeogenesis).

Maintaining Glucose Homeostasis To function optimally, the body must maintain blood glucose within limits that permit the cells to nourish themselves. If blood glucose falls below normal, a person may become dizzy and weak; if it rises above normal, a person may become fatigued. Left untreated, fluctuations to the extremes—either high or low—can be fatal. Among the dietary factors that most influence these fluctuations in blood glucose are carbohydrate (quality and quantity), protein, and fiber intakes.[6]

The Regulating Hormones Blood glucose homeostasis is regulated primarily by two hormones: *insulin*, which moves glucose from the blood into the cells, and *glucagon*, which brings glucose out of storage when needed. Figure 4-10 depicts these hormonal regulators at work.

gluconeogenesis (gloo-ko-nee-oh-JEN-ih-sis): the making of glucose from a noncarbohydrate source such as amino acids or glycerol (described in more detail in Chapter 7).
- **gluco** = glucose
- **neo** = new
- **genesis** = making

protein-sparing action: the action of carbohydrate (and fat) in providing energy that allows protein to be used for other purposes.

ketone (KEE-tone) **bodies:** acidic compounds produced by the liver during the breakdown of fat when carbohydrate is not available.

ketosis (kee-TOE-sis): an undesirably high concentration of ketone bodies in the blood and urine.

acid-base balance: the equilibrium in the body between acid and base concentrations (see Chapter 12).

> **FIGURE 4-10 Glucose Balance**

High blood glucose		Low blood glucose
Signals the pancreas to secrete insulin into the blood		Signals the pancreas to secrete glucagon into the blood
Insulin		**Glucagon**
Stimulates: • Uptake of glucose from the blood into cells • Storage of glycogen in the liver and muscles • Conversion of excess glucose into fat for storage	Pancreas	Stimulates: • Break down of glycogen from the liver • Release of glucose into the blood
End results		**End results**
Lower blood glucose		Raised blood glucose
Insulin secretion inhibited		Glucagon secretion inhibited

After a meal, as blood glucose rises, special cells of the pancreas respond by secreting **insulin** into the blood.* In general, the amount of insulin secreted corresponds with the rise in glucose. As the circulating insulin reaches the body's cells, receptors respond by ushering glucose from the blood into the cells. Most of the cells take only the glucose they can use for energy right away, but the liver and muscle cells can assemble the small glucose units into long, branching chains of glycogen for storage. As mentioned earlier, the liver cells also convert extra glucose to fat. Thus, elevated blood glucose returns to normal levels as excess glucose is stored as glycogen and fat.

When blood glucose falls (as occurs between meals), other special cells of the pancreas respond by secreting **glucagon** into the blood.** Glucagon raises blood glucose by signaling the liver to break down its glycogen stores and release glucose into the blood for use by all the other body cells.

Another hormone that signals the liver cells to release glucose is the "fight-or-flight" hormone, **epinephrine.** When a person experiences stress, epinephrine acts quickly to ensure that all the body cells have energy fuel in emergencies.

Balancing within the Normal Range The maintenance of normal blood glucose depends on foods and hormones. When blood glucose falls below normal, food can replenish it, or in the absence of food, glucagon can signal the liver to break down glycogen stores. When blood glucose rises above normal, insulin can signal the cells to take in glucose for energy. Eating balanced meals that provide abundant carbohydrates, including fibers, and a little fat help slow down the digestion and absorption of carbohydrate so that glucose enters the blood gradually. Eating at regular intervals also helps the body maintain a balance between the extremes.

Falling outside the Normal Range In some people, blood glucose regulation fails. When this happens, either of two conditions can result: diabetes or hypoglycemia. People with these conditions need to plan their diets and physical activities to help maintain their blood glucose within a normal range. Table 4-3 presents the blood glucose levels defining hypoglycemia, normal, prediabetes, and diabetes.

Diabetes In **diabetes,** blood glucose rises after a meal and remains above normal levels because insulin is either inadequate or ineffective. Elevated blood glucose is a characteristic of two main types of diabetes. In **type 1 diabetes,** the less common

*The *beta* (BAY-tuh) *cells,* one of several types of cells in the pancreas, secrete insulin in response to elevated blood glucose concentration.

**The *alpha cells* of the pancreas secrete glucagon in response to low blood glucose concentration.

TABLE 4-3 Fasting Blood Glucose

Hypoglycemia	<70 mg/dL
Normal	70–99 mg/dL
Prediabetes	100–125 mg/dL
Diabetes	≥126 mg/dL

NOTE: Milligrams per deciliter (mg/dL) is a unit of measure that describes the concentration of substance (glucose) in a specific amount of fluid (blood).

insulin (IN-suh-lin): a hormone secreted by special cells in the pancreas in response to (among other things) elevated blood glucose concentration. Insulin controls the transport of glucose from the bloodstream into the muscle and fat cells.

glucagon (GLOO-ka-gon): a hormone secreted by special cells in the pancreas in response to low blood glucose concentration. Glucagon elicits release of glucose from liver glycogen stores.

epinephrine (EP-ih-NEFF-rin): a hormone of the adrenal gland that modulates the stress response; formerly called *adrenaline.* When administered by injection, epinephrine counteracts anaphylactic shock by opening the airways and maintaining heartbeat and blood pressure.

diabetes (DYE-ah-BEE-teez): metabolic disorder characterized by elevated blood glucose resulting from insufficient insulin, ineffective insulin, or both; the complete medical term is *diabetes mellitus* (meh-LIE-tus). When blood glucose levels are higher than normal, but below the diagnosis of diabetes, the condition is called *prediabetes.*

type 1 diabetes: the less common type of diabetes in which the pancreas produces little or no insulin. Type 1 diabetes usually results from autoimmune destruction of pancreatic beta cells.

> **FIGURE 4-11 The Glycemic Response**

After a high-glycemic meal, blood glucose levels rise dramatically and then fall below normal. After a low-glycemic meal, blood glucose levels rise gradually and then fall to near normal.

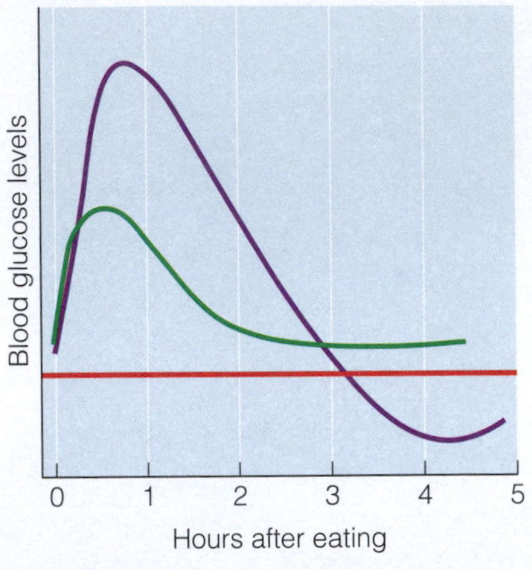

Blood glucose levels
0
1
2
3
4
5
Hours after eating

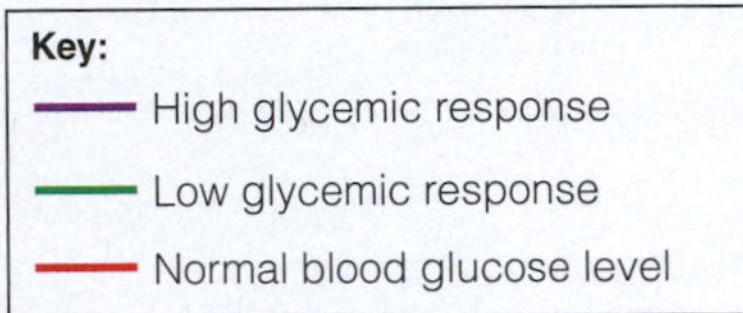

Key:
High glycemic response
Low glycemic response
Normal blood glucose level

SOURCE: Adapted from Gropper/Smith, *Advanced Nutrition and Human Metabolism*, 7th ed. (Belmont, CA: Cengage Learning, 2018), p. 76.

type, the pancreas fails to produce insulin. Although the exact cause is unclear, some research suggests that in genetically susceptible people, certain viruses activate the immune system to attack and destroy insulin-producing cells in the pancreas as if they were foreign cells. In **type 2 diabetes**, the more common type of diabetes, the cells fail to respond to insulin. This condition tends to occur as a consequence of obesity. As the incidence of obesity in the United States has risen in recent decades, so too has the incidence of diabetes. This trend is most notable among children and adolescents as obesity among the nation's youth reaches epidemic proportions. Because obesity can lead to type 2 diabetes, the best preventive measure is to maintain a healthy body weight. To manage diabetes and ensure stable blood glucose levels, food portions and choices must be balanced. It helps to eat meals and snacks at regularly scheduled times, to eat similar amounts of food at each meal and snack, and to choose nutritious foods that will support a healthy body weight. Dietitians commonly use Food Lists for Diabetes and carbohydrate counting to plan healthy meals for people with diabetes (see Appendix G). Chapter 15 describes the type of diabetes that develops in some women during pregnancy (gestational diabetes), and Chapter 18 covers type 1 and type 2 diabetes, their associated problems, and strategies to manage diet planning (including carbohydrate counting).

Hypoglycemia **Hypoglycemia** in healthy people is rare; blood glucose rises after eating and then gradually falls back into the normal range. The transition occurs without notice. Should blood glucose drop below normal, a person would experience the symptoms of hypoglycemia: weakness, rapid heartbeat, sweating, anxiety, hunger, and trembling.

Hypoglycemia is most commonly a consequence of poorly managed diabetes: too much insulin, strenuous physical activity, inadequate food intake, or illness cause blood glucose levels to plummet.[7] When caused by certain medications, pancreatic tumors, overuse of insulin, alcohol abuse, uncontrolled diabetes, or other illnesses, hypoglycemia requires medical intervention.[8]

The Glycemic Response The **glycemic response** refers to how quickly glucose is absorbed after a person eats, how high blood glucose rises, and how quickly it returns to normal. Slow absorption, a modest rise in blood glucose, and a smooth return to normal are desirable (a low glycemic response). Fast absorption, a surge in blood glucose, and an overreaction that plunges glucose below normal are less desirable (a high glycemic response). Figure 4-11 compares the response of a high-glycemic meal with a low-glycemic meal. The glycemic response may be particularly important to people with diabetes, who may benefit from limiting foods that produce too great a rise, or too sudden a fall, in blood glucose.

Different foods elicit different glycemic responses; the **glycemic index** classifies foods accordingly (see Table 4-4). Some studies have shown that selecting foods with a low glycemic index is a practical way to improve glucose control and lower the risk of diabetes.[9] Lowering the glycemic index of the diet may improve blood lipids, reduce inflammation, and lower the risk of heart disease as well, although research findings are mixed.[10] A low glycemic diet may also help with appetite regulation and weight management, although, again, research findings are mixed.[11]

Researchers debate whether selecting foods based on the glycemic index is practical or offers any real health benefits. Those opposing the use of the glycemic index argue that it is not sufficiently supported by scientific research. The glycemic index has been determined for relatively few foods, and when the glycemic index has been published, it is based on an average of multiple tests with wide variations in their results. Values vary because of differences in the physical and chemical characteristics of foods, testing methods of laboratories, and digestive processes of individuals. In fact, people can have dramatically different blood glucose responses to the same foods.[12]

Furthermore, the practical utility of the glycemic index is limited because this information is neither provided on food labels nor intuitively apparent. Indeed, a food's glycemic index is not always what one might expect. Ice cream, for example, is a high-sugar food but produces less of a glycemic response than baked potatoes,

type 2 diabetes: the more common type of diabetes in which the cells fail to respond to insulin. Type 2 diabetes usually accompanies obesity and results from insulin resistance coupled with insufficient insulin secretion.

hypoglycemia (HIGH-po-gly-SEE-me-ah): an abnormally low blood glucose concentration.

glycemic (gly-SEEM-ic) **response:** the extent to which a food raises the blood glucose concentration and elicits an insulin response.

glycemic index: a method of classifying foods according to their potential for raising blood glucose.

TABLE 4-4 Glycemic Index of Selected Common Foods

Glycemic Index	Grains	Fruits	Vegetables	Milk Products	Protein Foods[a]	Other
Low	Barley, chapati, corn tortilla, rice noodles, rolled oats, udon noodles, spaghetti	Apple, apple juice, banana, dates, mango, orange, orange juice, peaches (canned), strawberry jam	Carrots, corn	Ice cream, milk, soy milk, yogurt	Legumes	Chocolate
Medium	Brown rice, couscous	Pineapple	Potatoes (french fries), sweet potatoes			Popcorn, potato chips, soft drinks
High	Breads, breakfast cereals, white rice	Watermelon	Potatoes (boiled)			Rice crackers

NOTE: Using the glucose reference scale, foods are classified as low (55 or less), medium (56 to 69), or high (70 or greater).
[a]Protein foods that contain little or no carbohydrate (such as meats, poultry, fish, and eggs) do not raise blood glucose, and therefore do not have a glycemic index.
SOURCE: Adapted from F. S. Atkinson, K. Foster-Powell, and J. C. Brand-Miller, International tables of glycemic index and glycemic load values: 2008, *Diabetes Care* 31 (2008): 2281–2283.

a high-starch food. Perhaps most relevant to real life, a food's glycemic effect differs depending on plant variety, food processing, cooking method, time of day, and whether it is eaten alone or with other foods. White rice, for example, has a very high glycemic index, but when cooked with a little oil, vegetables, and chicken, the glycemic index of the mixed meal is reduced by about half.[13] Most people eat a variety of foods, cooked and raw, that provide different amounts of carbohydrate, fat, and protein—all of which influence the glycemic index of a meal.

Paying attention to the glycemic index may be unnecessary because current guidelines already suggest many low and moderate glycemic index choices: whole grains, legumes, vegetables, fruits, and milk and milk products. In addition, eating frequent, small meals spreads glucose absorption across the day and thus offers similar metabolic advantages to eating foods with a low glycemic response. Highlight 4 revisits the relationship of the glycemic index and body weight and explores the controversies surrounding low-carbohydrate diets.

REVIEW IT Explain how the body maintains its blood glucose concentration and what happens when blood glucose rises too high or falls too low.

Dietary carbohydrates provide glucose that can be used by the cells for energy, stored by the liver and muscles as glycogen, or converted into fat if intakes exceed needs. All of the body's cells depend on glucose; those of the brain and central nervous system are especially dependent on it. Without glucose, the body is forced to break down its protein tissues to make glucose and to alter energy metabolism to make ketone bodies from fats. Blood glucose regulation depends primarily on two pancreatic hormones: insulin to move glucose from the blood into the cells when levels are high and glucagon to free glucose from glycogen stores and release it into the blood when levels are low.

4.4 Health Effects and Recommended Intakes of Sugars

LEARN IT Describe how added sugars can contribute to health problems.

Almost everyone finds pleasure in sweet foods—after all, the taste preference for sweets is inborn. To a child, the sweeter the food, the better. In adults, this preference is somewhat diminished, but most adults still enjoy at least an occasional sweet food or beverage.

TABLE 4-5 Functions of Sugar in Foods

- Acts as a bulking agent in ice cream and baked goods
- Adds texture and color to baked goods
- Balances the acidity of tomato- and vinegar-based products such as sauces, salad dressings, and other condiments
- Enhances flavor
- Imparts a creamy consistency in frozen desserts
- Inhibits microbial growth by binding with water in jams and jellies
- Maintains the natural color and texture of preserved fruits
- Provides fuel for yeast fermentation, causing bread to rise or producing alcohol

In the United States, almost 15 percent of the average daily energy intake comes from the concentrated sugars that have been refined and added to foods for a variety of purposes (see Table 4-5). The leading source of added sugars is beverages, accounting for almost half of the added sugars consumed. An additional 25 percent of the intake comes from snacks and sweets such as cakes, ice cream, and candy (see Photo 4-6). Added sugars assume various names on food labels: sucrose, invert sugar, corn sugar, corn syrups and solids, high-fructose corn syrup, and honey. A food is likely to be high in added sugars if its ingredient list starts with any of the monosaccharides or disaccharides already defined or any of the sugars named in Glossary 4-1, or if it includes several of them.

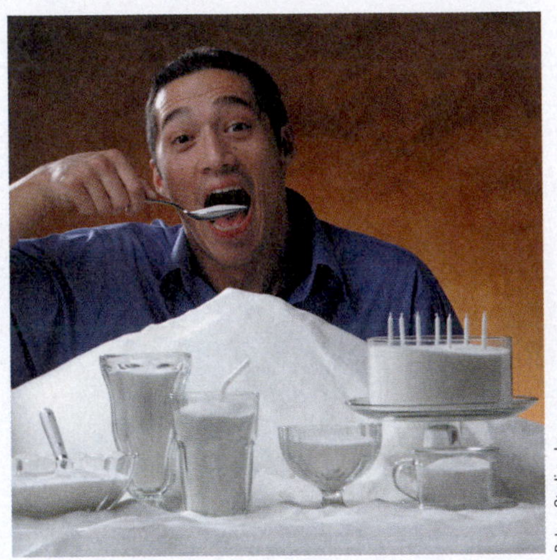

> **PHOTO 4-6** Almost half of the added sugars in our diet come from sugar-sweetened beverages, but baked goods, ice cream, candy, and breakfast cereals also make substantial contributions.

Health Effects of Sugars In moderate amounts, sugars may add pleasure to meals without harming health. In excess, however, sugars can be detrimental, and the average American diet currently delivers excessive amounts.

Obesity and Chronic Diseases Over the past several decades, as obesity rates increased sharply, consumption of added sugars reached an all-time high—much of it because of the surge in high-fructose corn syrup use, especially in beverages. High-fructose corn syrup is composed of fructose and glucose in a ratio of roughly 50:50. Compared with sucrose, high-fructose corn syrup is less expensive, easier to use, and more soluble. Manufacturers prefer high-fructose corn syrup because it retains moisture, resists drying out, controls crystallization, prevents microbial growth, and blends easily with other sweeteners, acids, and flavorings. In addition to being used in beverages, high-fructose corn syrup sweetens candies, baked goods, and hundreds of other foods.

In general, research findings tend to support an association between consuming sugary beverages and increases in energy intake and body weight.[14] Reducing

GLOSSARY 4-1 ADDED SUGAR TERMS

brown sugar: refined white sugar crystals to which manufacturers have added molasses syrup with natural flavor and color; 91 to 96 percent pure sucrose.

confectioners' sugar: finely powdered sucrose, 99.9 percent pure.

corn sweeteners: corn syrup and sugars derived from corn.

corn syrup: a syrup made from cornstarch that has been treated with acid, high temperatures, and enzymes to produce glucose, maltose, and dextrins. It may be dried and used as *corn syrup solids*. See also *high-fructose corn syrup (HFCS)*.

dextrose: the name food manufacturers use for the sugar that is chemically the same as glucose; *anhydrous dextrose* is similar, differing primarily in the temperature of crystallization.

high-fructose corn syrup (HFCS): a syrup made from cornstarch that has been treated with an enzyme that converts some of the glucose to the sweeter fructose; made especially for use in processed foods and beverages, where it is the predominant sweetener. With a chemical structure similar to sucrose, most HFCS has a fructose content of 42 or 55 percent, with glucose making up the remainder.

honey: sugar (mostly sucrose) formed from nectar gathered by bees. Composition and flavor vary, but honey always contains a mixture of sucrose, fructose, and glucose.

invert sugar: a mixture of glucose and fructose formed by the hydrolysis of sucrose in a chemical process; sold only in liquid form and sweeter than sucrose. Invert sugar is used as a food additive to help preserve freshness and prevent shrinkage.

levulose: an older name for fructose.

malt syrup: a sweetener made from sprouted barley and containing mostly maltose.

maple sugar: a sugar (mostly sucrose) purified from the concentrated sap of the sugar maple tree.

molasses: the thick brown syrup produced during sugar refining. Molasses retains residual sugar and other by-products and a few minerals; blackstrap molasses contains significant amounts of calcium and iron.

nectar: a sugary fluid secreted by plants to encourage pollination by insects.

raw sugar: the first crop of crystals harvested during sugar processing. Raw sugar cannot be sold in the United States because it contains too much filth (dirt, insect fragments, and the like). Sugar sold as "raw sugar" domestically has actually gone through more than half of the refining steps.

tagatose (TAG-ah-tose)**:** poorly absorbed monosaccharide similar in structure to fructose; naturally occurring or derived from lactose.

trehalose: a disaccharide found in organisms such as fungi and yeast that is about half as sweet as sucrose and is sometimes used as a sweetener in processed foods.

turbinado (ter-bih-NOD-oh) **sugar:** sugar produced using the same refining process as white sugar, but without the bleaching and anticaking treatment. Traces of molasses give turbinado its sandy color.

white sugar: granulated sucrose or "table sugar," produced by dissolving, concentrating, and recrystallizing raw sugar.

the consumption of sugar-sweetened beverages or replacing them with beverages such as water or milk can help support a healthy body weight.[15]

Some research suggests that added sugars in general, and fructose in particular, favor the fat-making pathways and impair the fat-clearing pathways in the liver.[16] The resulting blood lipid profile increases the risk of heart disease.[17] As the liver busily makes lipids, its handling of glucose becomes unbalanced and insulin resistance develops—an indicator of prediabetes. All in all, research is finding links between added sugars and the risk of diabetes, inflammation, hypertension, and heart disease.[18] Importantly, moderate intakes of sugars do not cause these health problems. For this reason, researchers suggest replacing sugar-sweetened beverages with water, and the American Heart Association recommends limiting added sugars to no more than 100 kcalories per day for women and 150 kcalories per day for men (which is about 5 percent of a 2000- and 2500-kcalorie diet, respectively).

Nutrient Deficiencies Foods such as whole grains, vegetables, legumes, and fruits that contain some natural sugars and lots of starches and fibers provide vitamins and minerals as well. By comparison, foods and beverages that contain lots of added sugars such as cakes, candies, and sodas provide the body with glucose and energy, but few, if any, other essential nutrients or fiber. The more added sugars (and solid fats) in the diet, the more difficult it is to meet recommendations for protein, dietary fiber, vitamins, and minerals and still stay within kcalorie limits.

A person spending 200 kcalories of a day's energy allowance on a 16-ounce soda gets little of value for those kcalories. In contrast, a person using 200 kcalories on a slice of whole-wheat bread with a tablespoon of peanut butter and a half tablespoon of jam gets 8 grams of protein, 3 grams of fiber, plus several vitamins and minerals with those kcalories. The amount of sugar a person can afford to eat depends on how many discretionary kcalories are available beyond those providing indispensable vitamins and minerals.

By following one of the USDA Food Patterns and making careful food selections, a typical adult can obtain all the needed nutrients within an allowance of about 1500 kcalories. An inactive older woman who is limited to fewer than 1500 kcalories a day can afford to eat only the most nutrient-dense foods—with few, or no, discretionary kcalories available. In contrast, an active teenage boy may need as many as 3000 kcalories a day. If he chooses wisely, then he may use discretionary kcalories for nutrient-dense foods that contain added sugars. Examples of nutrient-dense foods containing some added sugars include whole-grain breakfast cereals and vanilla yogurt.

Some people believe that because honey is a natural food, it is nutritious—or, at least, more nutritious than sugar.* A look at their chemical structures reveals the truth. Honey, like table sugar, contains glucose and fructose. The primary difference is that in table sugar the two monosaccharides are bonded together as the disaccharide sucrose, whereas in honey some of the monosaccharides are free. Whether a person eats monosaccharides individually, as in honey, or linked together, as in table sugar, they end up the same way in the body: as glucose and fructose.

Honey does contain a few vitamins and minerals, but not many. Honey is denser than crystalline sugar, too, so it provides more energy per spoonful. Table 4-6 (p. 112) shows that honey and white sugar are similar nutritionally—and both fall short of milk, legumes, fruits, grains, and vegetables.

Although the body cannot distinguish whether fructose and glucose derive from honey or table sugar, this is not to say that all sugar sources are alike. Some sugar sources are more nutritious than others. Consider a fruit, for example. The fruit may give you the same amounts of fructose and glucose and the same number of kcalories as a spoonful of sugar or honey, but the packaging is more valuable nutritionally (see Photo 4-7). The fruit's sugars arrive in the body diluted in a large volume of water, packaged in fiber, and mixed with essential vitamins, minerals, and phytochemicals.

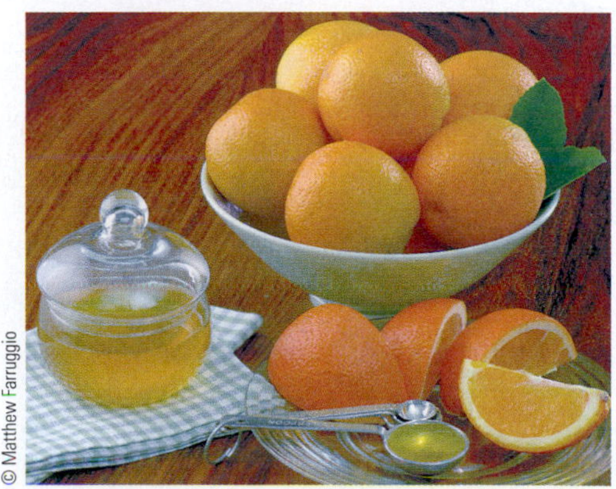

> **PHOTO 4-7** A tablespoon of honey and a large orange each provide 17 grams of sugar, but the orange also delivers valuable vitamins, minerals, and dietary fibers.

*Honey should never be fed to infants because of the risk of botulism. Chapters 16 and 19 provide more details.

TABLE 4-6 Sample Nutrients in Sugar and Other Foods

The indicated portion of any of these foods provides approximately 100 kcalories. Notice that for a similar number of kcalories and grams of carbohydrate, foods such as milk, legumes, fruits, grains, and vegetables offer more of the other nutrients than do the sugars.

	Size of 100 kcal Portion	Carbohydrate (g)	Protein (g)	Calcium (mg)	Iron (mg)	Potassium (mg)	Vitamin D (µg)
Foods							
Milk, 1% low-fat	1 c	12	8	300	0.1	397	2
Kidney beans	½ c	20	7	45	1.6	303	0
Apricots	6	24	3	30	0.8	544	0
Bread, whole-wheat	1½ slices	20	4	77	1.2	122	0
Broccoli, cooked	2 c	20	7	125	2.1	914	0
Sugars							
Sugar, white	2 tbs	24	0	0	trace	0	0
Molasses	2 tbs	28	0	82	1.9	586	0
Cola beverage	1 c	26	0	6	trace	7	0
Honey	1½ tbs	26	trace	2	0.1	16	0

As these comparisons illustrate, the significant difference between sugar sources is not between "natural" honey and "purified" sugar but between concentrated added sugars and the dilute sugars that naturally sweeten foods. You can suspect an exaggerated nutrition claim when someone asserts that one product is more nutritious than another because it contains honey.

Added sugars contribute to nutrient deficiencies by displacing nutrients. For nutrition's sake, the appropriate attitude to take is not that sugar is "bad" and must be avoided, but that nutritious foods must come first. If nutritious foods crowd sugar out of the diet, that is fine—but not the other way around. As always, balance, variety, and moderation guide healthy food choices.

> FIGURE 4-12 Dental Caries

Dental caries begins when acid dissolves the enamel that covers the tooth. If not repaired, the decay may penetrate the dentin and spread into the pulp of the tooth, causing inflammation, abscess, and possible loss of the tooth.

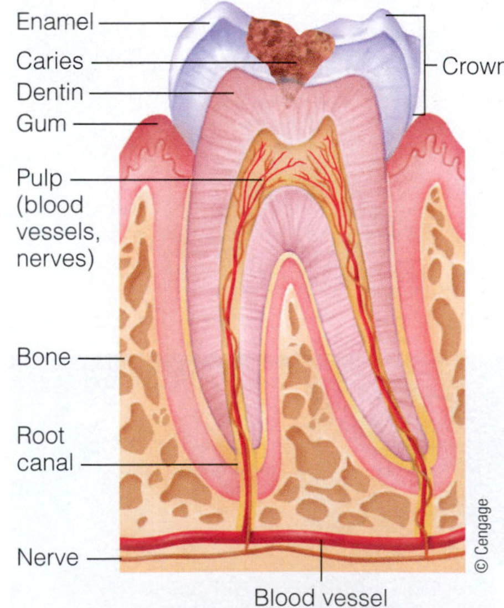

Enamel
Caries
Dentin
Gum
Crown
Pulp (blood vessels, nerves)
Bone
Root canal
Nerve
Blood vessel
© Cengage

Dental Caries Both naturally occurring and added sugars from foods and from the breakdown of starches in the mouth can contribute to tooth decay. Bacteria in the mouth ferment the sugars and, in the process, produce an acid that erodes tooth enamel (see Figure 4-12), causing **dental caries,** or tooth decay. People can eat sugar without this happening, though. Much depends on how long foods stay in the mouth. Sticky foods stay on the teeth longer and continue to yield acid longer than foods that are readily cleared from the mouth. For that reason, sugar in a juice consumed quickly, for example, is less likely to cause dental caries than sugar in a pastry. By the same token, the sugar in sticky foods such as raisins can be more detrimental than the quantity alone would suggest.

Another concern is how often people eat sugar. Bacteria produce acid for 20 to 30 minutes after each exposure. If a person eats three pieces of candy at one time, the teeth will be exposed to approximately 30 minutes of acid destruction. But, if the person eats three pieces at half-hour intervals, the time of exposure increases to 90 minutes. Likewise, slowly sipping a sugary sports beverage may be more harmful than drinking quickly and clearing the mouth of sugar. Nonsugary foods can help remove sugar from tooth surfaces; hence, it is better to eat sugar with meals than between meals. Foods such as milk and cheese may be particularly helpful in protecting against dental caries by neutralizing acids, stimulating salivary flow, inhibiting bacterial activity, and promoting remineralization of damaged enamel.

Beverages such as soft drinks, orange juice, and sports drinks not only contain sugar but also have a low pH. These acidic drinks can erode tooth enamel and may explain why the prevalence of dental erosion is growing steadily.[19]

The development of caries depends on several factors: the bacteria that reside in **dental plaque,** the saliva that cleanses the mouth, the minerals that form the

dental caries: decay of teeth.
- **caries** = rottenness

teeth, and the foods that remain after swallowing. For most people, good oral hygiene and regular dental visits will prevent dental caries (see Table 4-7).[20] In fact, regular brushing (twice a day, with a fluoride toothpaste) and flossing may be more effective in preventing dental caries than restricting sugary foods. Still, nutrition is a key component of dental health.[21] Perhaps the best advice to prevent dental caries is the combined approach of practicing good oral hygiene, drinking fluoridated water, and consuming sugar- and starch-containing foods and beverages less frequently. Reducing consumption of sugar-sweetened beverages prevents not only dental caries, but gum disease as well.[22]

TABLE 4-7 Behaviors to Prevent Dental Caries

- Limit between meal sugar-sweetened beverages (such as carbonated beverages and fruit drinks), sticky foods (such as raisins and caramels), slow-dissolving candies (such as lollipops and jaw breakers), and snacks containing sugars and starches (such as cookies and cakes).
- Brush with a fluoride toothpaste and floss teeth regularly.
- If brushing and flossing are not possible, drink some milk, rinse with water, or chew sugarless gum immediately after a meal or snack.
- Get a dental checkup regularly.
- Drink fluoridated water.

Recommended Intakes of Sugars Most of the sugars in the average American diet are added to foods and beverages by manufacturers during processing; major sources of added sugars include sugar-sweetened beverages (sodas, energy drinks, sports drinks, fruit drinks), desserts, and candy.[23] To help consumers make healthier choices, proposed food labels will include the amounts of *added sugars* in a serving. Food labels currently list the *total* grams of sugar a food provides, which reflects both added sugars and those occurring naturally in foods. To help estimate sugar and energy intakes accurately, keep in mind that 1 teaspoon of sugar—whether white sugar, brown sugar, corn syrup, honey, nectar, jam, jelly, maple syrup, or molasses—provides 4 grams of carbohydrate and *about* 20 kcalories per teaspoon. For a person who uses ketchup liberally, it may help to remember that 1 tablespoon of ketchup supplies about 1 teaspoon of sugar. And those who drink soft drinks regularly should keep in mind that a 12-ounce can of soda delivers about 10 teaspoons of sugar (see Photo 4-8).

The Dietary Reference Intakes (DRI) committee did not publish a Tolerable Upper Intake Level (UL) for sugar, but as mentioned, excessive intakes can interfere with sound nutrition and good health. Few people can eat lots of sugary treats and still meet all of their nutrient needs without exceeding their kcalorie allowance. For this reason, the *Dietary Guidelines for Americans* urge consumers to limit their daily intake of added sugars to 10 percent of total kcalories. For most people, this means reducing their intake of kcalories from added sugars (and those from solid fats as well). By reducing the intake of foods and beverages with added sugars, consumers can lower the kcalorie content of the diet without compromising the nutrient content. How To 4-1 provides strategies for reducing the intake of added sugars. People who successfully reduce their intake of added sugars seem to adapt over time, perceiving sugar more intensely

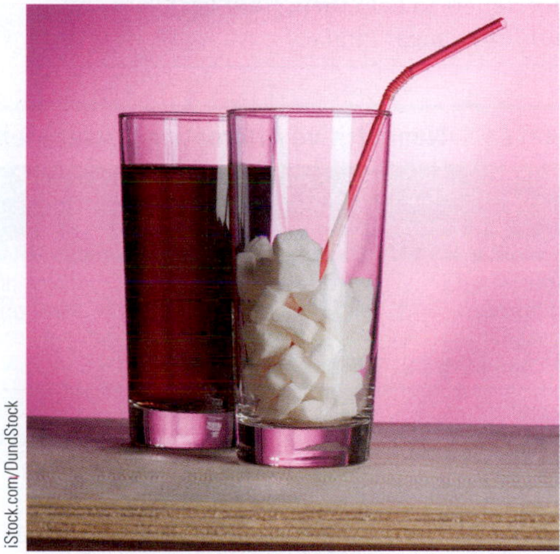

iStock.com/DundStock

> **PHOTO 4-8** Soft drinks deliver a startling amount of sugar—between 30 and 50 grams of sugar per 12-ounce can, depending on the flavor and brand.

dental plaque: a gummy mass of bacteria that grows on teeth and can lead to dental caries and gum disease.

> How To 4-1 Reduce the Intake of Added Sugars

- Use less table sugar on foods such as cereal or pancakes and in beverages such as coffee or tea.
- Use your sugar kcalories to sweeten nutrient-dense foods (such as oatmeal) instead of consuming empty kcalorie foods and beverages (such as candy and soda).
- Drink fewer regular sodas, sports drinks, energy drinks, and fruit drinks; choose water, fat-free milk, 100 percent fruit juice, or unsweetened tea or coffee instead. If you do drink sugar-sweetened beverages, have a small portion.
- Select fruit for dessert—fresh, frozen, dried, or canned in water or natural juice (not canned in syrup). Eat less cake, cookies, ice cream, other desserts, and candy. If you do eat these foods, have a small portion.
- Instead of adding sugar, add fresh fruit to cereal and dried fruit to oatmeal.
- Instead of using sugar in recipes, use unsweetened applesauce (equal amounts).
- Instead of using sugar, enhance flavors of foods with spices such as cinnamon, allspice, ginger, or nutmeg and with extracts such as almond, vanilla, orange, or lemon.
- Read the Nutrition Facts on labels to choose foods with less sugar. Select the unsweetened version of a food (such as cornflakes) instead of the sweetened version (such as frosted cornflakes) to reduce the quantity of added sugars in the diet.
- The ingredients list also helps identify foods with added sugars. A food is likely to be high in added sugars if its ingredient list starts with any of the sugars named in Glossary 4-1 (p. 110), or if it includes several of them.

> **TRY IT** Compare the energy contents, added sugars, and ingredients lists of 1 cup of the following foods: fruit-flavored yogurt and plain yogurt, sugar-frosted cornflakes and plain cornflakes, orange soda and orange juice.

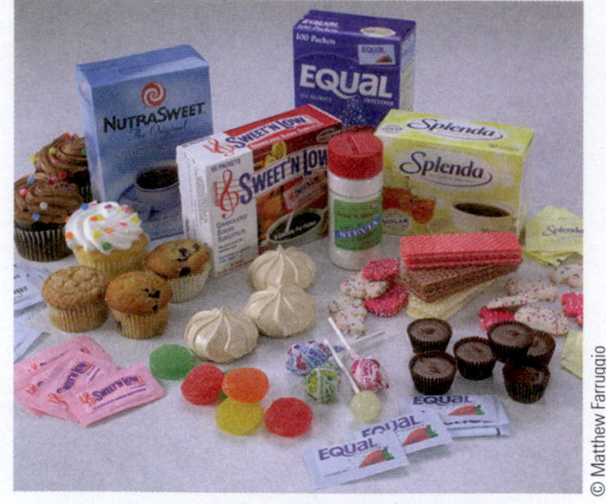

© Matthew Farruggio

> **PHOTO 4-9** Consumers use artificial sweeteners to help them limit kcalories and minimize sugar intake.

and preferring less sugar in their foods and beverages, making it a habit that is relatively easy to maintain.[24] The World Health Organization (WHO) also suggests limiting added sugars to less than 10 percent of energy intake, and notes that 5 percent or less provides additional benefits, which is in line with American Heart Association recommendations mentioned earlier.

Alternative Sweeteners To control weight gain, blood glucose, and dental caries, many consumers turn to alternative sweeteners to help them limit kcalories and minimize added sugars in the diet (see Photo 4-9). In doing so, they encounter three sets of alternative sweeteners: artificial sweeteners, other high-intensity sweeteners, and sugar alcohols. Table 4-8 provides general details about each of the sweeteners approved for use in the United States. Chapter 9 includes a discussion of their use in weight control and Chapter 19 focuses on some of the safety issues surrounding their use.

TABLE 4-8 Nonnutritive Alternative Sweeteners

Sweetener	Chemical Composition	Body's Response	Relative Sweetness[a]	Energy (kcal/g)	ADI (mg/kg body weight) and Estimated Equivalent[b]	Comments
Acesulfame potassium or AceK[c] (AY-sul-fame)	Potassium salt	Not digested or absorbed	200	0	15 (23 packets of sweetener)	Approved as a sweetener and flavor enhancer in foods (except in meat and poultry)
Advantame (ad-VAN-tame)	Aspartame derivative, similar to neotame	Rapidly, but poorly absorbed	20,000	0	32.8 (4920 packets of sweetener)	Approved as a sweetener and flavor enhancer in foods (except in meat and poultry)
Aspartame[e] (ah-SPAR-tame or ASS-par-tame)	Amino acids (phenylalanine and aspartic acid) and a methyl group	Digested and absorbed	200	4[f]	50[g] (75 packets of sweetener)	Approved as a sweetener and flavor enhancer in foods
Luo han guo[h]	Cucurbitane glycosides extracts from *Siraitia grosvenorii* swingle fruit (also known as monk fruit)	Digested and absorbed	175	1	Not determined	GRAS[i]
Neotame (NEE-oh-tame)	Aspartame with an additional side group attached	Not digested or absorbed	10,000	0	0.3 (23 packets of sweetener)	Approved as a sweetener and flavor enhancer in foods (except in meat and poultry)
Saccharin[j] (SAK-ah-ren)	Benzoic sulfimide	Rapidly absorbed and excreted	400	0	15 (45 packets of sweetener)	Approved as a sweetener only in certain special dietary foods and as an additive used for certain technological purposes
Stevia[k] (STEE-vee-ah)	Glycosides found in the leaves of the *Stevia rebaudiana* herb	Digested and absorbed	300	0	4 (9 packets of sweetener)	GRAS[i]
Sucralose[l] (SUE-kra-lose)	Sucrose with Cl atoms instead of OH groups	Not digested or absorbed	600	0	5 (23 packets of sweetener)	Approved as a sweetener in foods

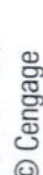

© Cengage

[a]Relative sweetness is determined by comparing the approximate sweetness of a sugar substitute with the sweetness of pure sucrose, which has been defined as 1.0. Chemical structure, temperature, acidity, and other flavors of the foods in which the substance occurs all influence relative sweetness.
[b]The Acceptable Daily Intake (ADI) is the estimated amount of a sweetener that individuals can safely consume each day over the course of a lifetime without adverse effects. The Estimated Equivalent is the number of packets of sweetener a person needs to consume to reach the ADI based on a person weighing 60 kg (132 lb).
[c]Marketed under the trade names Sunett and Sweet One.
[d]Recommendations from the WHO limit acesulfame K intake to 9 mg per kilogram of body weight per day.
[e]Marketed under the trade names NutraSweet, Equal, and Sugar Twin.
[f]Aspartame provides 4 kcal per gram, as does protein, but because so little is used, its energy contribution is negligible. In powdered form, it is sometimes mixed with lactose, however, so a 1-g packet may provide 4 kcal.
[g]Recommendations from the WHO and in Europe and Canada limit aspartame intake to 40 mg per kilogram of body weight per day.
[h]Marketed under the trade name Fruit-Sweetness.
[i]GRAS = generally recognized as safe. The GRAS list is subject to revision as new facts become known. For stevia, only one highly refined extract (known as Rebaudioside A) has been granted GRAS status; whole-leaf stevia and other extracts have not been approved.
[j]Marketed under the trade names Sweet'N Low, Sweet Twin, and Necta Sweet.
[k]Marketed under the trade names SweetLeaf, Purevia, Truvia, and Honey Leaf.
[l]Marketed under the trade name Splenda.

Artificial Sweeteners Artificial sweeteners give foods a sweet flavor without adding extra kcalories; they are sometimes called **nonnutritive sweeteners** because they provide virtually no energy or nutrients. The Food and Drug Administration (FDA) regulates all artificial sweeteners and has established an **Acceptable Daily Intake (ADI)**—the estimated amount that can be safely consumed over a lifetime without harm. Considering that all substances are toxic at some dose, it is little surprise that large doses of artificial sweeteners (or their components or metabolic by-products) may have adverse effects. The question to ask is whether their ingestion is safe for human beings in quantities people normally use (and potentially abuse).

Other High-Intensity Sweeteners Stevia leaves and monk fruit have long been used by the people of South America and China, respectively, to sweeten their foods and beverages. The FDA has approved certain extracts from these plants as **generally recognized as safe (GRAS)**; they can be used as additives in a variety of foods and beverages.

Sugar Alcohols Some "sugar-free" or reduced-kcalorie products contain **sugar alcohols.** The sugar alcohols (sometimes called polyols) occur naturally in fruits and vegetables; manufacturers also use sugar alcohols in many processed foods to add bulk and texture, to provide a cooling effect or sweet taste, to inhibit browning from heat, and to retain moisture. These products may claim to be "sugar-free" on their labels, but in this case, "sugar-free" does not mean free of kcalories. Sugar alcohols do provide kcalories (0.2 to 2.6 kcalories per gram), but fewer than the sugars. Because sugar alcohols yield energy, they are sometimes referred to as **nutritive sweeteners.**

Sugar alcohols evoke a low glycemic response. The body partially absorbs some sugar alcohols and absorbs others slowly; consequently, they are slower to enter the bloodstream than other sugars. Unabsorbed sugar alcohols may be metabolized by bacteria in the GI tract, producing side effects such as intestinal gas, abdominal discomfort, and diarrhea. For this reason, regulations require food labels to state "Excess consumption may have a laxative effect" if reasonable consumption of that food could result in the daily ingestion of 50 grams of a sugar alcohol. For perspective, a low-carbohydrate energy bar or shake may contain 10 to 15 grams of a sugar alcohol.

The real benefit of using sugar alcohols is that they do not contribute to dental caries. Bacteria in the mouth cannot metabolize sugar alcohols as rapidly as sugar. Sugar alcohols are therefore valuable in chewing gums, breath mints, and other products that people keep in their mouths for a while. Figure 4-13 (p. 116) presents labeling information for products using sugar alternatives.

For consumers choosing to use alternative sweeteners, the Academy of Nutrition and Dietetics wisely advises that they be used in moderation and only as part of a well-balanced nutritious diet.[25] When used in moderation, these sweeteners will do no harm. In fact, they may even help, by providing an alternative to sugar for people with diabetes, by inhibiting caries-causing bacteria, and by limiting energy intake.

REVIEW IT Describe how added sugars can contribute to health problems.

Sugars increase the risk of dental caries; excessive intakes displace needed nutrients and fiber and contribute to obesity when energy intake exceeds needs. Consumers are advised to limit their intake of added sugars to less than 10 percent of their daily energy intake. Alternative sweeteners may help limit kcalorie and sugar intake.

artificial sweeteners: sugar substitutes that provide negligible, if any, energy; sometimes called *nonnutritive sweeteners.*

nonnutritive sweeteners: sweeteners that yield no energy (or insignificant energy in the case of aspartame).

Acceptable Daily Intake (ADI): the estimated amount of a sweetener that individuals can safely consume each day over the course of a lifetime without adverse effect.

generally recognized as safe (GRAS): food additives that have long been in use and are believed to be safe. First established by the FDA in 1958, the GRAS list is subject to revision as new facts become known.

sugar alcohols: sugarlike compounds that can be derived from fruits or commercially produced from dextrose; also called *polyols.* Examples include *erythritol, isomalt, lactitol, maltitol, mannitol, sorbitol,* and *xylitol.*

nutritive sweeteners: sweeteners that yield energy, including both sugars and sugar alcohols.

> **FIGURE 4-13 Sugar Alternatives on Food Labels**

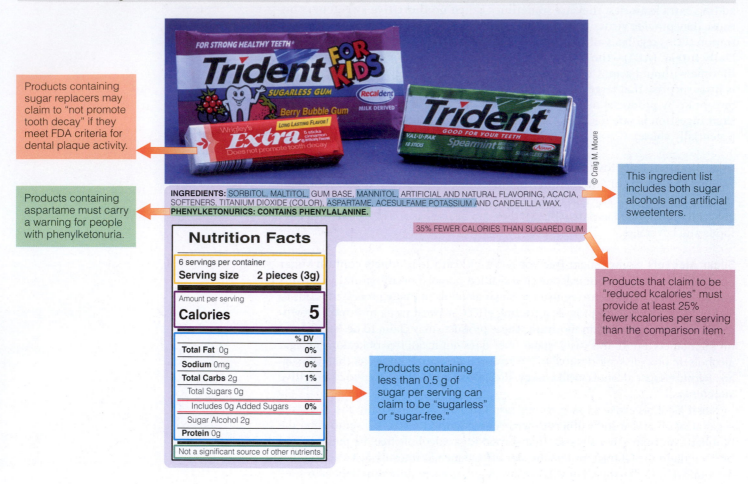

Products containing sugar replacers may claim to "not promote tooth decay" if they meet FDA criteria for dental plaque activity.

Products containing aspartame must carry a warning for people with phenylketonuria.

FOR STRONG HEALTHY TEETH*
Trident FOR KIDS
SUGARLESS GUM
Berry Bubble Gum
Recaldent
MILK DERIVED
Wrigley's
Extra
LONG LASTING FLAVOR!
5 sticks cinnamon
Does not promote tooth decay
Trident
GOOD FOR YOUR TEETH
VAL-U-PAK
18 STICKS
Spearmint

© Craig M. Moore

INGREDIENTS: SORBITOL, MALTITOL, GUM BASE, MANNITOL, ARTIFICIAL AND NATURAL FLAVORING, ACACIA, SOFTENERS, TITANIUM DIOXIDE (COLOR), ASPARTAME, ACESULFAME POTASSIUM AND CANDELILLA WAX.
PHENYLKETONURICS: CONTAINS PHENYLALANINE.

This ingredient list includes both sugar alcohols and artificial sweeteners.

35% FEWER CALORIES THAN SUGARED GUM.

Products that claim to be "reduced kcalories" must provide at least 25% fewer kcalories per serving than the comparison item.

Nutrition Facts	
6 servings per container	
Serving size	**2 pieces (3g)**
Amount per serving	
Calories	**5**
	% DV
Total Fat 0g	**0%**
Sodium 0mg	**0%**
Total Carbs 2g	**1%**
Total Sugars 0g	
Includes 0g Added Sugars	**0%**
Sugar Alcohol 2g	
Protein 0g	
Not a significant source of other nutrients.	

Products containing less than 0.5 g of sugar per serving can claim to be "sugarless" or "sugar-free."

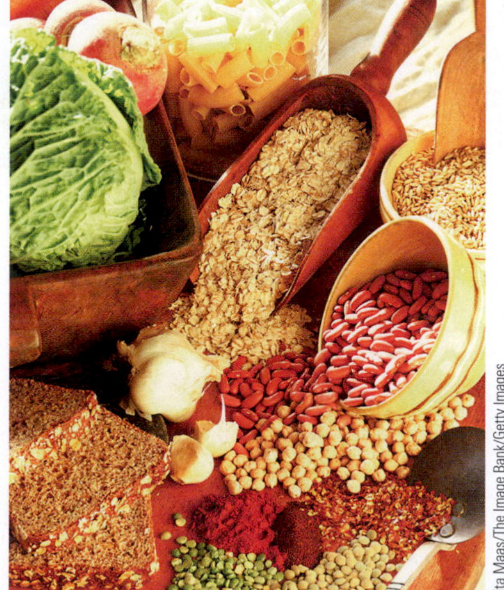

Rita Maas/The Image Bank/Getty Images

> **PHOTO 4-10** Foods rich in starch and fiber offer many health benefits.

4.5 Health Effects and Recommended Intakes of Starch and Fibers

LEARN IT Identify the health benefits of, and recommendations for, starches and fibers.

Carbohydrates and fats are the two major sources of energy in the diet. When one is high, the other is usually low—and vice versa. A diet that provides abundant carbohydrate (45 to 65 percent of energy intake) and some fat (20 to 35 percent of energy intake) within a reasonable energy allowance best supports good health. To increase carbohydrates in the diet, focus on whole grains, vegetables, legumes, and fruits—foods noted for their starch, fibers, and naturally occurring sugars.

Health Effects of Starch and Fibers

Whole grains, vegetables, legumes, and fruits provide not only starch, fibers, and natural sugars, but also valuable vitamins and minerals. The following paragraphs describe some of the health benefits of diets that include a variety of these foods daily (see Photo 4-10).

Heart Disease Unlike high-carbohydrate diets rich in added sugars that can alter blood lipids to favor heart disease, those rich in whole grains, legumes, vegetables, and fruits may protect against heart attack and stroke by lowering blood pressure, improving blood lipids, and reducing inflammation.[26] Such diets are low in animal fat and high in dietary fibers, vegetable proteins, and phytochemicals—all factors associated with a lower risk of heart disease. (The role of animal fat in heart disease is discussed in Chapter 5. The role of vegetable proteins in heart disease is presented in Chapter 6. The benefits of phytochemicals in disease prevention are featured in Highlight 13.)

Oatmeal was one of the first foods recognized for its ability to reduce blood cholesterol and the risk of heart disease. Foods rich in soluble fibers (such as oat bran, barley, and legumes) lower blood cholesterol by binding with bile acids in the GI tract and thereby increasing their excretion. Consequently, the liver must use its cholesterol to make new bile acids. In addition, the bacterial by-products of fiber fermentation in the colon inhibit cholesterol synthesis in the liver. The net result is that soluble fibers such as those found in oats lower blood cholesterol.[27]

Several researchers have speculated that fiber may also exert its effect by displacing fats in the diet. Although this is certainly helpful, even when dietary fat is low, fibers exert a separate and significant cholesterol-lowering effect. In other words, a high-fiber diet helps decrease the risk of heart disease independent of fat intake.

Diabetes High-fiber foods—especially whole grains—play a key role in managing and preventing type 2 diabetes. When soluble fibers trap nutrients and delay their transit through the GI tract, glucose absorption is slowed, which helps prevent glucose surge and rebound.

GI Health Dietary fibers also enhance the health of the large intestine. The healthier the intestinal walls, the better they can block absorption of unwanted constituents. Taken with ample fluids, insoluble fibers such as cellulose (as in cereal brans, fruits, and vegetables) increase stool weight, ease passage, and reduce transit time.

Large, soft stools ease elimination for the rectal muscles and reduce pressure in the lower bowel, preventing constipation and making it less likely that rectal veins will swell (hemorrhoids). Fiber prevents compaction of the intestinal contents, which could obstruct the appendix and permit bacteria to invade and infect it (appendicitis). In addition, fiber stimulates the GI tract muscles so that they retain their strength and resist bulging out into pouches known as diverticula (illustrated in Figure H3-3, p. 90). Recommendations typically suggest increasing fiber to protect against diverticular disease, although research findings are inconsistent.

Cancer Research studies suggest that a high-fiber diet protects against cancer of the colon and rectum.[28] Importantly, the findings support dietary fiber, not fiber supplements or additives, which lack valuable nutrients and phytochemicals that also help protect against cancer. Plant foods—vegetables, fruits, and whole-grains—reduce the risks of colon and rectal cancers.

Fibers may help prevent colon cancer by diluting, binding, and rapidly removing potential cancer-causing agents from the colon. In addition, soluble fibers stimulate bacterial fermentation of resistant starch and fiber in the colon, a process that produces short-chain fatty acids that lower the pH. These small fat molecules activate cancer-killing enzymes and inhibit inflammation in the colon.

Weight Management High-fiber and whole-grain foods may help a person to maintain a healthy body weight. Foods rich in fiber tend to be low in solid fats and added sugars and therefore prevent weight gain and promote weight loss by delivering less energy per bite. In addition, as fibers absorb water from the digestive juices, they swell, creating feelings of fullness and delaying hunger.[29]

Many weight-loss products on the market today contain bulk-inducing fibers such as methylcellulose, but using pure fiber compounds like this is neither necessary nor advisable. Instead of fiber supplements, consumers should select whole grains, legumes, fruits, and vegetables. High-fiber foods not only add bulk to the diet but are economical and nutritious as well.

TABLE 4-9 Characteristics, Sources, and Health Effects of Fibers

	Major Food Sources	Types of Fibers	Actions in the Body	Probable Health Benefits
	Viscous, Soluble, More Fermentable			
bitt24/Shutterstock.com	Barley, oats, oat bran, rye, fruits (apples, citrus), legumes (especially young green peas and black-eyed peas), seaweeds, seeds and husks, many vegetables, fibers used as food additives	Gums Pectins Psyllium[a] Some hemicellulose	Lower blood cholesterol by binding bile Slow glucose absorption Slow transit of food through upper GI tract Hold moisture in stools, softening them Yield small fat molecules after fermentation that the colon can use for energy Increase satiety	Lower risk of heart disease Lower risk of diabetes Lower risk of colon and rectal cancer Increased satiety, and may help with weight management
	Nonviscous, Insoluble, Less Fermentable			
Stockbyte/Getty Images	Brown rice, fruits, legumes, seeds, vegetables (cabbage, carrots, brussels sprouts), wheat bran, whole grains, extracted fibers used as food additives	Cellulose Lignins Resistant starch Hemicellulose	Increase fecal weight and speed fecal passage through colon Provide bulk and feelings of fullness	Alleviate constipation May lower risk of diverticulosis, hemorrhoids, and appendicitis Lower risk of colon and rectal cancer

[a]Psyllium, a soluble fiber derived from seeds, is used as a laxative and food additive.

Foods rich in dietary fiber (and especially whole grains) provide numerous health benefits and reduce the risk of death.[30] Table 4-9 summarizes fiber characteristics, food sources, actions in the body, and health benefits.

Harmful Effects of Excessive Fiber Intake Despite fibers' benefits to health, a diet excessively high in fiber also has a few drawbacks. A person who has a small capacity and eats mostly high-fiber foods may not be able to eat enough food to meet energy or nutrient needs. The malnourished, the elderly, and young children adhering to all-plant (vegan) diets are especially vulnerable to this problem.

Switching from a low-fiber diet to a high-fiber diet suddenly can cause temporary bouts of abdominal discomfort, gas, and diarrhea and, more seriously, can obstruct the GI tract. To prevent such complications, a person adopting a high-fiber diet can take the following precautions:

- Increase fiber intake gradually over several weeks to give the GI tract time to adapt.
- Drink plenty of liquids to soften the fiber as it moves through the GI tract.
- Select fiber-rich foods from a variety of sources—fruits, vegetables, legumes, and whole-grain breads and cereals.

Some fibers can limit the absorption of nutrients by speeding the transit of foods through the GI tract and by binding to minerals. When mineral intake is adequate, however, a *reasonable* intake of high-fiber foods (less than 40 grams a day) does not compromise mineral balance.

Clearly, fiber is like all nutrients in that "more" is "better" only up to a point. Again, the key dietary goals are balance, moderation, and variety. Table 4-10 presents a list of fiber sources and tips to increase fiber intake.

Recommended Intakes of Starch and Fibers

The DRI suggest that carbohydrates provide about half (45 to 65 percent) of the energy requirement.

TABLE 4-10 Fiber in Selected Foods

Food Group	Amount of Fiber (per serving)	Food Sources	Tips to Increase Fiber Intake
Grains Polara Studios, Inc.	1 to 2 g (or more)	1 slice whole-wheat, pumpernickel, rye bread 1 oz ready-to-eat cereal (100% bran cereals contain ≥10 g) ½ c cooked barley, bulgur, grits, oatmeal	Eat whole-grain breads that contain ≥3 g fiber per serving. Eat whole-grain cereals that contain ≥5 g fiber per serving.
Vegetables Polara Studios, Inc.	2 to 3 g	1 c raw bean sprouts ½ c cooked broccoli, Brussels sprouts, cabbage, carrots, cauliflower, collards, corn, eggplant, green beans, green peas, kale, mushrooms, okra, parsnips, potatoes, pumpkin, spinach, sweet potatoes, Swiss chard, winter squash ½ c chopped raw carrots, peppers	Eat raw vegetables. Eat vegetables (such as potatoes and zucchini) with their skins.
Fruits Polara Studios, Inc.	2 g	1 medium apple, banana, kiwi, nectarine, orange, pear ½ c applesauce, blackberries, blueberries, raspberries, strawberries (Fruit juices contain very little fiber)	Eat fresh and dried fruit for snacks. Eat fruits (such as apples and pears) with their skins
Legumes Polara Studios, Inc.	5 to 8 g	½ c cooked baked beans, black beans, black-eyed peas, garbanzo beans, great northern beans, kidney beans, lentils, lima beans navy beans, pinto beans, split peas	Add legumes to soups, salads, and casseroles.

(The remainder comes from fat, with 20 to 35 percent, and protein, with 10 to 35 percent.) A person consuming 2000 kcalories a day should therefore have 900 to 1300 kcalories of carbohydrate, or about 225 to 325 grams. (Appendix H explains how to calculate such math problems.) This amount is more than adequate to meet the RDA for carbohydrate, which is set at 130 grams per day, based on the average minimum amount of glucose used by the brain.

On food labels, the FDA uses the guideline of 55 percent of a 2000-kcalorie diet in setting the Daily Value for carbohydrate at 275 grams per day. To meet this goal, the *Dietary Guidelines* encourage people to choose a variety of whole grains, vegetables, fruits, and legumes daily.

Recommendations for fiber suggest a variety of plant foods: whole grains, vegetables, fruits, legumes, and nuts, which also provide minerals and vitamins.[31] Note, however, that fiber supplements do not have the same health benefits as dietary fiber from whole foods.[32] The Daily Value for fiber on food labels is set at 28 grams for a 2000-kcalorie intake and nutrient claims are allowed for "good" (2.5 grams per serving) and "excellent" (5 grams per serving) sources. The DRI recommendation is in agreement at 14 grams per 1000-kcalorie intake, or 25 grams for adult women and 38 grams for adult men. These recommendations are much higher than the average daily intake of 16 grams per day in the United States.[33] An effective way to add fiber while lowering saturated fat is to substitute plant sources of proteins (legumes) for animal sources (meats).

Because high-fiber foods are so filling, they are not likely to be eaten in excess. Too much fiber can cause GI problems for some people, but it generally does not have adverse effects in most healthy people. For these reasons, the DRI committee did not set an Upper Level for fiber.

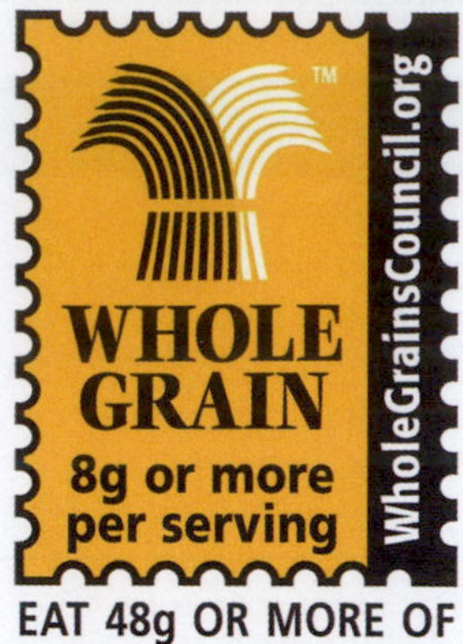
WHOLE GRAIN
8g or more per serving
WholeGrainsCouncil.org
EAT 48g OR MORE OF WHOLE GRAINS DAILY

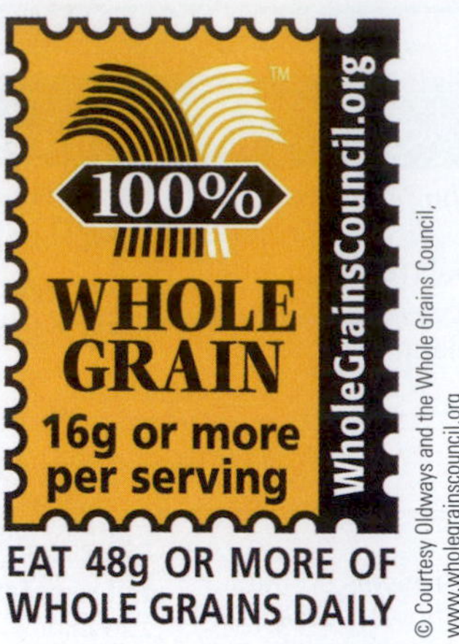
100%
WHOLE GRAIN
16g or more per serving
WholeGrainsCouncil.org
EAT 48g OR MORE OF WHOLE GRAINS DAILY

> **PHOTO 4-11** Some food labels use a "whole-grain stamp" to help consumers identify whole-grain foods.

From Guidelines to Groceries A diet following one of the USDA Food Patterns—which includes several servings of fruits, vegetables, and whole grains daily—can easily supply the recommended amount of carbohydrates and fiber. In selecting high-fiber foods, keep in mind the principle of variety. The fibers in oats lower cholesterol, whereas those in bran help promote GI tract health. (Review Table 4-9 to see the diverse health effects of various fibers.)

Grains An ounce-equivalent of most foods in the grain group (for example, one slice of bread) provides about 15 grams of carbohydrate, mostly as starch. Be aware that some foods in this group, especially snack crackers and baked goods such as biscuits, croissants, and muffins, contain added sugars, solid fats, and sodium. When selecting from the grain group, limit refined grains and be sure to include at least half as whole-grain products (see Figure 4-14). The "three are key" message may help consumers to remember to choose a whole-grain cereal for breakfast, a whole-grain bread for lunch, and a whole-grain pasta or rice for dinner (see Photo 4-11). Because whole grains are typically high in fiber, nutrients, and antioxidants, consumers who eat more whole grains tend to have healthier diets and reduced risks for heart disease, diabetes, and certain cancers.[34]

Vegetables The amount of carbohydrate a serving of vegetables provides depends primarily on its starch content. Starchy vegetables—corn, peas, or potatoes—provide about 15 grams of carbohydrate per half-cup serving. A serving of most other *nonstarchy* vegetables—such as a half-cup of broccoli, green beans, or tomatoes—provides about 5 grams.

Fruits A typical fruit serving—a small banana, apple, or orange or a half-cup of most canned or fresh fruit—contains an average of about 15 grams of carbohydrate, mostly as sugars, including the fruit sugar fructose. Fruits vary greatly in their water and fiber contents and, therefore, in their sugar concentrations.

Milks and Milk Products A serving (a cup) of milk or yogurt provides about 12 grams of carbohydrate. Cottage cheese provides about 6 grams of carbohydrate per cup, but most other cheeses contain little, if any, carbohydrate.

Protein Foods With two exceptions, protein foods deliver almost no carbohydrate to the diet. The exceptions are nuts, which provide a little starch and fiber along with their abundant fat, and legumes, which provide an abundance of both starch and fiber. Just a half-cup serving of legumes provides about 20 grams of carbohydrate, a third from fiber.

Read Food Labels Food labels list the amount, in grams, of *total* carbohydrate—including starch, fibers, and sugars—per serving (review Figure 4-14). Fiber grams are also listed separately, as are the grams of sugars (and added sugars on updated labels). With this information, you can calculate starch grams by subtracting the grams of fibers and sugars from the total carbohydrate. Using the first label in Figure 4-14 as an example, subtracting the 4 grams of fibers and sugars from the 15 grams of total carbohydrate leaves 11 grams of starch. Total carbohydrate and dietary fiber are also expressed as "% Daily Values" for a person consuming 2000 kcalories; there is no Daily Value for sugar.

> FIGURE 4-14 Bread Labels Compared

Although breads may appear similar, their ingredients vary widely. Breads made mostly from whole-grain flours provide more benefits to the body than breads made of enriched, refined, wheat flours.

Some "high-fiber" breads may contain purified cellulose or more nutritious whole grains. "Low-carbohydrate" breads may be regular white bread, thinly sliced to reduce carbohydrates per serving, or may contain soy flour, barley flour, or flaxseed to reduce starch content.

A tip for estimating a bread's content of a nutritious ingredient, such as whole-grain flour, is to read the ingredients list (ingredients are listed in order of predominance). Bread recipes generally include one teaspoon of salt per loaf. Therefore, when a bulky nutritious ingredient, such as whole grain, is listed after the salt, you'll know that less than a teaspoonful of the nutritious ingredient was added to the loaf—not enough to significantly improve the nutrient value of one slice of bread.

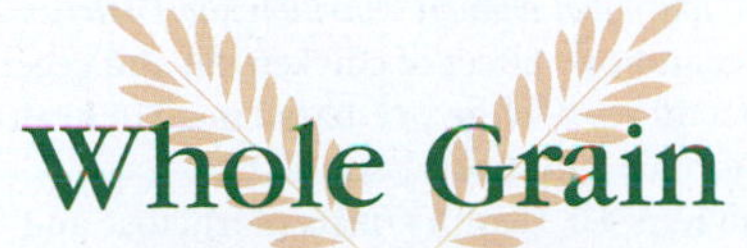
Whole Grain

WHOLE WHEAT

Nutrition Facts

18 servings per container
Serving size 1 slice (30g)

Amount per 1 slice
Calories 90

% DV	
2%	**Total Fat** 1.5g
	***Trans* Fat** 0g
6%	**Sodium** 135mg
5%	**Total Carbohydrate** 15g
7%	Dietary Fiber 2g
	Sugars 2g
	Added Sugars 2g
	Protein 4g

MADE FROM: UNBROMATED STONE GROUND 100% WHOLE WHEAT FLOUR, WATER, CRUSHED WHEAT, HIGH-FRUCTOSE CORN SYRUP, PARTIALLY HYDROGENATED VEGETABLE SHORTENING (SOYBEAN AND COTTONSEED OILS), RAISIN JUICE CONCENTRATE, WHEAT GLUTEN, YEAST, WHOLE WHEAT FLAKES, UNSULPHURED MOLASSES, SALT, HONEY, VINEGAR, ENZYME MODIFIED SOY LECITHIN, CULTURED WHEY, UNBLEACHED WHEAT FLOUR AND SOY LECITHIN.

Natural
Wheat Bread

Nutrition Facts

15 servings per container
Serving size 1 slice (30g)

Amount per 1 slice
Calories 90

% DV	
2%	**Total Fat** 1.5g
	***Trans* Fat** 0g
10%	**Sodium** 220mg
5%	**Total Carbohydrate** 15g
2%	Dietary Fiber Less than 1g
	Sugars 2g
	Added Sugars 2g
	Protein 4g

INGREDIENTS: UNBLEACHED ENRICHED WHEAT FLOUR [MALTED BARLEY FLOUR, NIACIN, REDUCED IRON, THIAMIN MONONITRATE (VITAMIN B1), RIBOFLAVIN (VITAMIN B2), FOLIC ACID], WATER, HIGH-FRUCTOSE CORN SYRUP, MOLASSES, PARTIALLY HYDROGENATED SOYBEAN OIL, YEAST, CORN FLOUR, SALT, GROUND CARAWAY, WHEAT GLUTEN, CALCIUM PROPIONATE (PRESERVATIVE), MONOGLYCERIDES, SOY LECITHIN.

Multi-fiber
Low carb

Nutrition Facts

21 servings per container
Serving size 1 slice (30g)

Amount per 1 slice
Calories 60

% DV	
2%	**Total Fat** 1.5g
	***Trans* Fat** 0g
6%	**Sodium** 135mg
3%	**Total Carbohydrate** 9g
11%	Dietary Fiber 3g
	Sugars 0g
	Added Sugars 0g
	Protein 5g

INGREDIENTS: UNBLEACHED ENRICHED WHEAT FLOUR, WATER, WHEAT GLUTEN, CELLULOSE, YEAST, SOYBEAN OIL, CRACKED WHEAT, SALT, BARLEY, NATURAL FLAVOR PRESERVATIVES, MONOCALCIUM PHOSPHATE, MILLET, CORN, OATS, SOYBEANS, BROWN RICE, FLAXSEED, SUCRALOSE.

REVIEW IT Identify the health benefits of, and recommendations for, starches and fibers.

Clearly, a diet rich in starches and fibers supports efforts to control body weight and prevent heart disease, some cancers, diabetes, and GI disorders. For these reasons, recommendations urge people to eat plenty of whole grains, vegetables, legumes, and fruits—enough to provide 45 to 65 percent of the daily energy intake from carbohydrate.

In today's world, there is one other reason why plant foods rich in complex carbohydrates and natural sugars are a better choice than animal foods or foods high in added sugars: in general, less energy and fewer resources are required to grow and process plant foods than to produce sugar or foods derived from animals. Chapter 20 takes a closer look at the environmental impacts of food production and use.

What's Online

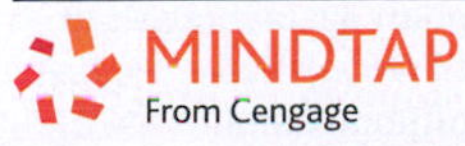
MINDTAP
From Cengage

Visit **www.cengagebrain.com** to access MindTap, a complete digital course that includes Diet & Wellness Plus, interactive quizzes, videos, and more.

REFERENCES

1. D. F. Birt and coauthors, Resistant starch: Promise for improving human health, *Advances in Nutrition* 4 (2013): 587–601.
2. L. Maagaard and coauthors, Follow-up of patients with functional bowel syndrome treated with a low FODMAP diet, *World Journal of Gastroenterology* 22 (2016): 4009–4019; F. Durchschein, W. Petritsch, and H. F. Hammer, Diet therapy for inflammatory bowel diseases: The established and the new, *World Journal of Gastroenterology* 22 (2016): 2179–2194; K. McIntosh and coauthors, FODMAPs alter symptoms and the metabolome of patients with IBS: A randomized controlled trial, *Gut* (2016): doi 10.1136/gutjnl-2015-311339; A. C. Prince and coauthors, Fermentable carbohydrate restriction (low FODMAP diet) in clinical practice improves functional gastrointestinal symptoms in patients with inflammatory bowel disease, *Inflammatory Bowel Diseases* 22 (2016): 1129–1136.
3. D. A. Savaiano, Lactose digestion from yogurt: Mechanism and relevance, *American Journal of Clinical Nutrition* 99 (2014): 1251S–1255S.
4. R. P. Heaney, Dairy intake, dietary adequacy, and lactose intolerance, *Advances in Nutrition* 4 (2013): 151–156.
5. J. Ma and coauthors, Potential link between excess added sugar intake and ectopic fat: A systematic review of randomized controlled trials, *Nutrition Reviews* 74 (2016): 18–32.
6. J. Tay, C. H. Thompson, and G. D. Brinkworth, Glycemic variability: Assessing glycemia differently and the implications for dietary management of diabetes, *Annual Review of Nutrition* 35 (2015): 389–424.
7. P. E. Cryer, Mechanisms of hypoglycemia-associated autonomic failure in diabetes, *New England Journal of Medicine* 369 (2013): 362–372.
8. Hypoglycemia, *Journal of the American Medical Association* 313 (2015): 1284.
9. M. L. Wang and coauthors, Decrease in glycemic index associated with improved glycemic control among Latinos with type 2 diabetes, *Journal of the Academy of Nutrition and Dietetics* 115 (2015): 898–906; S. N. Bhupathiraju and coauthors, Glycemic index, glycemic load, and risk of type 2 diabetes: Results from 3 large US cohorts and an updated meta-analysis, *American Journal of Clinical Nutrition* 100 (2014): 218–232; G. Livesey and coauthors, Is there a dose-response relation of dietary glycemic load to risk of type 2 diabetes? Meta-analysis of prospective cohort studies, *American Journal of Clinical Nutrition* 97 (2013): 584–596; A. G. Liu and coauthors, Reducing the glycemic index or carbohydrate content of mixed meals reduces postprandial glycemia and insulinemia over the entire day but does not affect satiety, *Diabetes Care* 35 (2012): 1633–1637.
10. F. M. Sacks and coauthors, Effects of high vs low glycemic index of dietary carbohydrate on cardiovascular disease risk factors and insulin sensitivity: The OmniCarb Randomized Clinical Trial, *Journal of the American Medical Association* 312 (2014): 2531–2541; A. Mirrahimi and coauthors, The role of glycemic index and glycemic load in cardiovascular disease and its risk factors: A review of the recent literature, *Current Atherosclerosis Reports* 16 (2014): 381; S. Sieri and coauthors, Dietary glycemic load and glycemic index and risk of cerebrovascular disease in the EPICOR cohort, *PLoS One* 8 (2013): e62625; A. S. Kristo, N. R. Matthan, and A. H. Lichtenstein, Effect of diets differing in glycemic index and glycemic load on cardiovascular risk factors: Review of randomized controlled-feeding trials, *Nutrients* 5 (2013): 1071–1080; L. M. Goff and coauthors, Low glycaemic index diets and blood lipids: A systematic review and meta-analysis of randomised controlled trials, *Nutrition, Metabolism, and Cardiovascular Diseases* 23 (2013): 1–10.
11. E. V. Pereira, J. A. Costa, and R. C. Alfenas, Effect of glycemic index on obesity control, *Archives of Endocrinology and Metabolism* 59 (2015): 245–251; J. M. Randolph and coauthors, Potatoes, glycemic index, and weight loss in free-living individuals: Practical implications, *Journal of the American College of Nutrition* 33 (2014): 375–384; M. Juanola-Falgarona and coauthors, Effect of the glycemic index of the diet on weight loss, modulation of satiety, inflammation, and other metabolic risk factors: A randomized controlled trial, *American Journal of Clinical Nutrition* 100 (2014): 27–35; A. Geliebter and coauthors, Satiety following intake of potatoes and other carbohydrate test meals, *Annals of Nutrition and Metabolism* 62 (2013): 37–43.
12. N. R. Matthan and coauthors, Estimating the reliability of glycemic index values and potential sources of methodological and biological variability, *American Journal of Clinical Nutrition* 104 (2016): 1004–1013; D. Zeevi and coauthors, Personalized nutrition by prediction of glycemic response, *Cell* 163 (2015): 1079–1094.
13. R. George, A. L. Garcia, and C. A. Edwards, Glycaemic responses of staple South Asian foods alone and combined with curried chicken as a mixed meal, *Journal of Human Nutrition and Dietetics* 28 (2015): 283–291; L. Sun and coauthors, Effect of chicken, fat and vegetable on glycaemia and insulinaemia to a white rice-based meal in healthy adults, *European Journal of Nutrition* 53 (2014): 1719–1726.
14. L. Tappy and K. A. Lê, Health effects of fructose and fructose-containing caloric sweeteners: Where do we stand 10 years after the initial whistle blowings? *Current Diabetes Reports* 15 (2015): 54; S. D. Poppitt, Beverage consumption: Are alcoholic and sugary drinks tipping the balance towards overweight and obesity? *Nutrients* 7 (2015): 6700–6718; S. C. Bundrick and coauthors, Soda consumption during ad libitum food intake predicts weight change, *Journal of the Academy of Nutrition and Dietetics* 114 (2014): 444–449; . V. S. Malik and coauthors, Sugar-sweetened beverages and weight gain in children and adults: A systematic review and meta-analysis, *American Journal of Clinical Nutrition* 98 (2013): 1084–1102; C. A. Grimes and coauthors, Dietary salt intake, sugar-sweetened beverage consumption, and obesity risk, *Pediatrics* 131 (2013): 14–21.
15. M. Zheng and coauthors, Replacing sugary drinks with milk is inversely associated with weight gain among young obesity-predisposed children, *British Journal of Nutrition* 114 (2015): 1448–1455; F. B. Hu, Resolved: There is sufficient scientific evidence that decreasing sugar-sweetened beverage consumption will reduce the prevalence of obesity and obesity-related diseases, *Obesity Reviews* 14 (2013): 606–619.
16. M. Maersk and coauthors, Sucrose-sweetener beverages increase fat storage in the liver, muscle, and visceral fat depot: A 6-mo randomized intervention study, *American Journal of Clinical Nutrition* 95 (2012): 283–289; K. Sevastianova and coauthors, Effect of short-term carbohydrate overfeeding and long-term weight loss on liver fat in overweight humans, *American Journal of Clinical Nutrition* 96 (2012): 727–734.
17. G. A. Bray, Energy and fructose from beverages sweetened with sugar or high-fructose corn syrup pose a health risk for some people, *Advances in Nutrition* 4 (2013): 220–225; K. L. Stanhope, Role of fructose-containing sugars in the epidemics of obesity and metabolic syndrome, *Annual Review of Medicine* 63 (2012): 19.1–19.15.
18. J. M. Rippe and coauthors, What is the appropriate upper limit for added sugars consumption? *Nutrition Reviews* 75 (2017): 18-36; V. S. Malik and F. B. Hu, Fructose and cardiometabolic health: What the evidence from sugar-sweetened beverages tells us, *Journal of the American College of Cardiology* 66 (2015): 1615–1624; B. Xi and coauthors, Sugar-sweetened beverages and risk of hypertension and CVD: A dose-response meta-analysis, *British Journal of Nutrition* 113 (2015): 709–717; N. V. Dhurandhar and D. Thomas, The link between dietary sugar intake and cardiovascular disease mortality: An unresolved question, *Journal of the American Medical Association* 313 (2015): 959–960; V. H. Jayalath and coauthors, Sugar-sweetened beverage consumption and incident hypertension: A systematic review and meta-analysis of prospective cohorts, *American Journal of Clinical Nutrition* 102 (2015): 914–921; K. L. Stanhope and coauthors, A dose-response study of consuming high-fructose corn syrup-sweetened beverages on lipid/lipoprotein risk factors for cardiovascular disease in young adults, *American Journal of Clinical Nutrition* 101 (2015): 1144–1154; Q. Yang and coauthors, Added sugar intake and cardiovascular diseases mortality among US adults, *JAMA Internal Medicine* 174 (2014): 516–524; B. Xi and coauthors, Intake of fruit juice and incidence of type 2 diabetes: A systematic review and meta-analysis, *PLoS One* 9 (2014): e93471; D. C. Greenwood and coauthors, Association between sugar-sweetened and artificially sweetened soft drinks and type 2 diabetes: Systematic review and dose-response meta-analysis of prospective studies, *British Journal of Nutrition* 112 (2014): 725–734; L. A. TeMorenga and coauthors, Dietary sugars and cardiometabolic risk: Systematic review and meta-analyses of randomized controlled trials of the

effects on blood pressure and lipids, *American Journal of Clinical Nutrition* 100 (2014): 65–79.

19. C. Mann and coauthors, Three-dimensional profilometric assessment of early enamel erosion simulating gastric regurgitation, *Journal of Dentistry* 42 (2014): 1411–1421.
20. Policy statement: Maintaining and improving the oral health of young children, *Pediatrics* 134 (2014): 1224–1229; B. Sen and coauthors, Effectiveness of preventive dental visits in reducing nonpreventive dental visits and expenditures, *Pediatrics* 131 (2013): 1107–1113.
21. Position of the Academy of Nutrition and Dietetics: Oral health and nutrition, *Journal of the Academy of Nutrition and Dietetics* 113 (2013): 693–701.
22. E. C. O. Lula and coauthors, Added sugars and periodontal disease in young adults: An analysis of NHANES III data, *American Journal of Clinical Nutrition* 100 (2014): 1182–1187; E. W. Evans and coauthors, Dietary intake and severe early childhood caries in low-income, young children, *Journal of the Academy of Nutrition and Dietetics* 113 (2013): 1057–1061.
23. A. Drewnowski and C. D. Rehm, Consumption of added sugars among US children and adults by food purchase location and food source, *American Journal of Clinical Nutrition* 100 (2014): 901–907.
24. P. M. Wise and coauthors, Reduced dietary intake of simple sugars alters perceived sweet taste intensity but not perceived pleasantness, *American Journal of Clinical Nutrition* 103 (2016): 50–60.
25. Position of the Academy of Nutrition and Dietetics: Use of nutritive and nonnutritive sweeteners, *Journal of the Academy of Nutrition and Dietetics* 112 (2012): 739–758.
26. D. E. Threapleton and coauthors, Dietary fibre intake and risk of cardiovascular disease systematic review and meta-analysis, *British Medical Journal* 347 (2013): f6879; K. N. Grooms and coauthors, Dietary fiber intake and cardiometabolic risks among US adults, NHANES 1999-2010, *American Journal of Medicine* 126 (2013): 1059–1067.
27. A. Whitehead and coauthors, Cholesterol-lowering effects of oat β-glucan: A meta-analysis of randomized controlled trials, *American Journal of Clinical Nutrition* 100 (2014): 1413–1421; J. Slavin, Fiber and prebiotics: Mechanisms and health benefits, *Nutrients* 5 (2013): 1417–1435.
28. N. Makarem and coauthors, Consumption of whole grains and cereal fiber in relation to cancer risk: A systematic review of longitudinal studies, *Nutrition Reviews* 74 (2016): 353–373; A. T. Kunzmann and coauthors, Dietary fiber intake and risk of colorectal cancer and incident and recurrent adenoma in the Prostate, Lung, Colorectal, and Ovarian Cancer Screening Trial, *American Journal of Clinical Nutrition* 102 (2015): 881–890; T. Norat and coauthors, Fruits and vegetables: Updating the epidemiologic evidence for the WCRF/AICR Lifestyle Recommendations for Cancer Prevention, *Cancer Treatment and Research* 159 (2014): 35–50; H. Chen and coauthors, Decreased dietary fiber intake and structural alteration of gut microbiota in patients with advanced colorectal adenoma, *American Journal of Clinical Nutrition* 97 (2013): 1044–1052; N. Murphy and coauthors, Dietary fibre intake and risks of cancers of the colon and rectum in the European Prospective Investigation into Cancer and Nutrition (EPIC), *PLoS One* 7 (2012): e39361.
29. C. J. Rebello, C. E. O'Neil, and F. L. Greenway, Dietary fiber and satiety: The effects of oats on satiety, *Nutrition Reviews* 74 (2016): 131–147; T. F. Turner and coauthors, Dietary adherence and satisfaction with a bean-based high-fiber weight loss diet: A pilot study, *ISRN Obesity* (2013): 915415.
30. G. Zong and coauthors, Whole grain intake and mortality from all causes, cardiovascular disease, and cancer, *Circulation* 133 (2016): 2370–2380; D. Aune and coauthors, Whole grain consumption and risk of cardiovascular disease, cancer, and all cause and cause specific mortality: Systematic review and dose-response meta-analysis of prospective studies, *British Medical Journal* 353 (2016): i2716; Y. Yang and coauthors, Association between dietary fiber and lower risk of all-cause mortality: A meta-analysis of cohort studies, *American Journal of Epidemiology* 181 (2015): 83–91; H. Wu and coauthors, Association between dietary whole grain intake and risk of mortality: Two large prospective studies in US men and women, *JAMA Internal Medicine* 175 (2015): 373–384.
31. Position of the Academy of Nutrition and Dietetics: Health implications of dietary fiber, *Journal of the Academy of Nutrition and Dietetics* 115 (2015): 1861–1870.
32. J. W. McRorie and coauthors, Evidence-based approach to fiber supplements and clinically meaningful health benefits, part 1, *Nutrition Today* 50 (2015): 82–89.
33. M. K. Hoy and J. D. Goldman, Fiber intake of the US population, *What We Eat in America, NHANES 2009–2010*, September 2014, www.ars.usda.gov/ba/bhnrc/fsrg.
34. C. J. Seal and I. A. Brownlee, Whole grains, dietary fibre and grain-derived phytochemicals, *Proceedings of the Nutrition Society* 74 (2015): 313–319; G. Tang and coauthors, Meta-analysis of the association between whole grain intake and coronary heart disease risk, *American Journal of Cardiology* 115 (2015): 625–629; P. L. B. Hollænder, A. B. Ross, and M. Kristensen, Whole-grain and blood lipid changes in apparently healthy adults: A systematic review and meta-analysis of randomized controlled studies, *American Journal of Clinical Nutrition* 102 (2015): 556S–572S; S. Cho and coauthors, Consumption of cereal fiber, mixtures of whole drains and bran, and whole grains and risk reduction in type 2 diabetes, obesity, and cardiovascular disease, *American Journal of Clinical Nutrition* 98 (2013): 594–619.

HIGHLIGHT > 4

LEARN IT Summarize the key scientific evidence behind some of the current controversies surrounding carbohydrates and their kcalories.

Carbs, kCalories, and Controversies

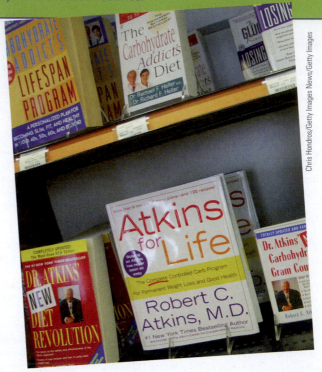

The Carbohydrate Addict's LifeSpan Program
The Carbohydrate Addicts Diet
Dr. Rachael F. Heller and Dr. Richard F. Heller
Atkins for Life
The Complete Controlled Carb Program For Permanent Weight Loss and Good Health
Robert C. Atkins, M.D.
Dr. Atkins' New Diet Revolution
Dr. Atkins' Carbohydrate Gram Counter

Chris Hondros/Getty Images News/Getty Images

Carbohydrate-rich foods are easy to like. Mashed potatoes, warm muffins, blueberry pancakes, freshly baked bread, and tasty rice and pasta dishes tempt most people's palates. In recent years, such comfort foods have been blamed for causing weight gain and harming health. Popular writers have persuaded consumers that carbohydrates are "bad." In contrast, the *Dietary Guidelines* urge people to consume plenty of fruits, vegetables, legumes, and whole grains—all carbohydrate-rich foods.

Do carbohydrate-rich foods cause obesity and related health problems? Should people "cut carbs" to lose weight and protect their health? Many popular diet books espouse a carbohydrate-restricted or carbohydrate-modified diet. Some claim that all or some types of carbohydrates are bad. Some go so far as to equate carbohydrates with toxic poisons or addictive drugs. "Bad" carbohydrates—such as sugar, white flour, and potatoes—are considered evil because they are absorbed easily and raise blood glucose. The pancreas then responds by secreting insulin—and insulin is touted as the real villain responsible for our nation's obesity epidemic. Whether restricting overall carbohydrate intake or replacing certain "bad" carbohydrates with "good" carbohydrates, many of these popular diets tend to distort the facts. This highlight examines the scientific evidence behind some of the current controversies surrounding carbohydrates and their kcalories.

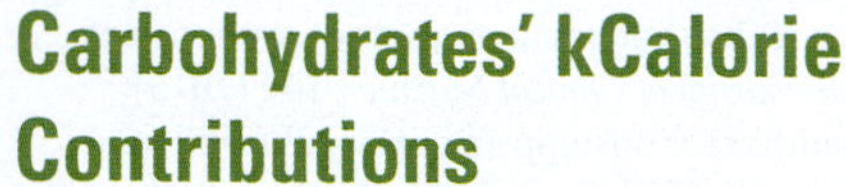

Carbohydrates' kCalorie Contributions

The incidence of obesity in the United States has risen dramatically over the past several decades (see Figure H4-1). Might too many carbohydrates in the diet be to blame for weight gains? One way researchers can explore whether the amount of carbohydrate in the diet contributes to increases in body weight over time is by reviewing national food intake survey records, such as NHANES (introduced in Chapter 1). Figure H4-2 presents a summary of energy nutrient data over the past 35 years. Since the 1970s, kcalories from carbohydrates increased from 42 percent to 51 percent.[1] At the same time, kcalories from fat dropped from 41 percent to 33 percent. The percentage of protein intake stayed about the same.

A closer look at the data reveals that, as the percentage of kcalories from the three energy nutrients shifted slightly, total daily energy intake increased significantly. In general, as food became more readily available in this nation, consumers began to eat more than they had in the past. Since the 1970s, total energy intakes have increased by almost 300 kcalories a day. All of the increase in kcalories came from an increase in carbohydrate kcalories. At the same time, most people were not active enough to use up those extra kcalories; in fact, activity levels declined.[2] Consequently, the average body weight for adults increased over these decades by about 25 to 30 pounds (review Figure H4-1).

Might a low-carbohydrate diet support weight losses? For the most part, weight loss is similar for people following either a low-carbohydrate diet or a low-fat diet. This is an important point. Weight losses reflect restricted kcalories—not the proportion of energy nutrients in the diet. Any diet can produce weight loss, at least temporarily, if energy intake is restricted. And most weight-loss diets also restrict added sugars.

> **FIGURE H4-1** Increases in Adult Body Weight over Time

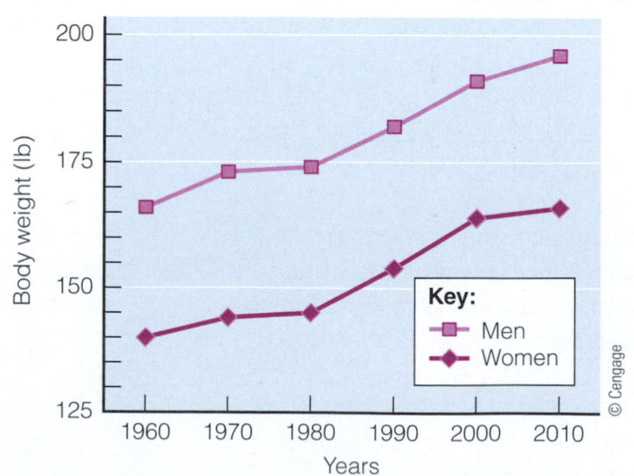

Body weight (lb)
200
175
150
125
1960
1970
1980
1990
2000
2010
Years
Key:
Men
Women
© Cengage

> FIGURE H4-2 Energy Nutrients over Time

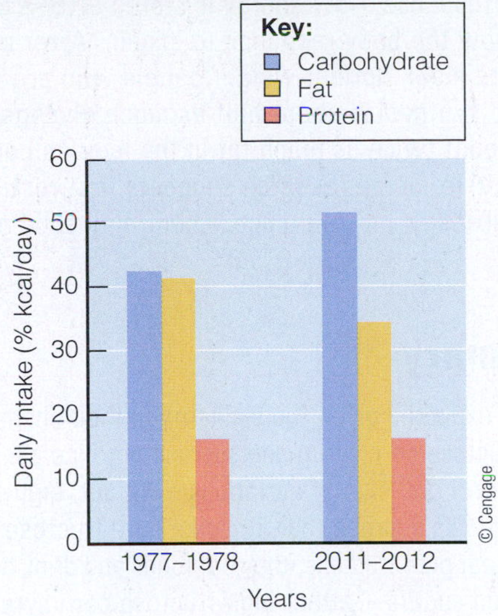
Key:
Carbohydrate
Fat
Protein
Daily intake (% kcal/day)
60
50
40
30
20
10
0
1977–1978
2011–2012
Years
© Cengage

Sugars' Share in the Problem

As Chapter 4 mentioned, the increased use of high-fructose corn syrup parallels the unprecedented increases in the incidence of obesity, but does it mean that sugar intakes are responsible for body fat and its associated health problems? When eaten in excess of need, energy from added sugars contributes to body fat stores, just as excess energy from other sources does. When total energy intake is appropriate, however, *moderate* amounts of sugar do not cause obesity. In other words, foods containing added sugars are no more likely to contribute to weight gain than any other foods.[3] Yet moderating sugar intake can be a challenge.

The liquid form of sugar in soft drinks makes it especially easy to overconsume kcalories. Swallowing liquid kcalories requires little effort. The sugar kcalories of sweet beverages also cost less than many other energy sources, and they are widely available. Also, beverages are energy-dense, providing more than 150 kcalories per 12-ounce can, and many people drink several cans a day. Drinking these beverages seems to correlate with a higher energy intake from foods as well, thus raising energy intake in two ways.[4] The convenience, economy, availability, and flavors of sugary foods and beverages make overconsumption especially likely.

Limiting selections of foods and beverages high in added sugars can be an effective weight-loss strategy, especially for people whose excess kcalories come primarily from added sugars.[5] One study reports that drinking water instead of sodas—even diet sodas—can help a person lose an additional 4 pounds in 6 months.[6] That may not sound like much, but it adds up to almost 10 pounds a year, for very little effort. Restricting sugar-sweetened beverages is also a simple strategy to reduce hypertension.[7]

Cravings and Addictions

Some people describe themselves as having "carbohydrate cravings" or being "sugar addicts." One frequently noted theory is that people seek carbohydrates as a way to increase their levels of the brain neurotransmitter serotonin, which elevates mood. Interestingly, when those with self-described carbohydrate cravings indulge, they tend to eat more of everything; the percentage of energy from carbohydrates remains unchanged.

One reasonable explanation for the carbohydrate cravings that some people experience involves the self-imposed labeling of a food as both "good" and "bad"—that is, one that is desirable but should be eaten with restraint. Restricting intake heightens the desire further (a "craving"). Then "addiction" is used to explain why resisting the food is so difficult and, sometimes, even impossible.

Carbohydrates, and sugars more specifically, are not addictive in the same ways that drugs are, but they share some of the same biological and psychological systems that are involved in rewards and self-control. Some research suggests that a meal with a high glycemic index stimulates the brain regions associated with reward and craving.[8] Other research suggests that fructose triggers feelings of hunger and desires for high-kcalorie foods by activating brain regions associated with attention and reward.[9] Highlight 8 includes more details on the concept of food addictions.

Fructose Metabolism

Unlike glucose, which is metabolized by all the body's cells, fructose is metabolized primarily in the liver. When the diet delivers high intakes of added sugars (which is half fructose), the liver handles the excess by making fat. This fat is either retained in the liver, causing fatty liver, or transported out, raising blood lipids and increasing fat stores—all risk factors for chronic diseases.[10]

Appetite Control

Recall from Chapter 4 that glucose stimulates the release of insulin from the pancreas. Insulin, in turn, sets off a sequence of hormonal actions that suppress the appetite. Fructose, in contrast, does not stimulate the release of insulin, and therefore does not suppress appetite.

Whether the meal or snack is liquid or solid may also affect appetite. Even when kcaloric intake is the same, a fresh apple suppresses appetite more than apple juice. Consequently, beverages can influence weight gains both by providing energy and by not satisfying hunger.

Insulin's Response

Several popular diet books hold insulin responsible for the obesity problem and a low-glycemic diet as the weight-loss solution. Yet, among nutrition researchers, controversy continues to surround the questions of whether insulin promotes weight gain or a low-glycemic diet fosters weight loss.

Recall that just after a meal, blood glucose rises and insulin responds. How high insulin levels surge may influence whether the body stores or uses its glucose and fat supplies. What does insulin do? Among its roles, insulin facilitates the transport of glucose into the cells, the storage of fatty acids as fat, and the synthesis of protein. It is an anabolic hormone that builds and stores. True—but there's more to the story. Insulin is only one of many factors involved in the body's metabolism of nutrients and regulation of body weight.

Most importantly, insulin is critical to maintaining health, as any person with type 1 diabetes can attest. Insulin causes problems only when a person develops insulin resistance—that is, when the body's cells do not respond to the large quantities of insulin that the pancreas continues to pump out in an effort to get a response. Insulin resistance is a major health problem—but it is not caused by dietary carbohydrate, protein, or fat. It most often results from being obese. Importantly, when a person loses weight, insulin response usually improves.

The Glycemic Index and Body Weight

As Chapter 4's discussion of the glycemic index explained, the glycemic effect of a particular food varies. The glycemic effect of a food depends on how the food is ripened, processed, and cooked; the time of day the food is eaten; the other foods eaten with it; and the presence or absence of certain diseases such as type 2 diabetes in the person eating the food. All these factors influence a food's glycemic index, yet diet books often mislead people by claiming that each food has a specific glycemic index.

Even if a true glycemic index is known, what is the relationship between a diet's glycemic index and body weight? In general, studies find that diets with a high glycemic index are positively associated with body weight.

Might a low-glycemic diet foster weight loss? A recent review suggests that low glycemic diets may help with appetite control and weight management.[11] Low-glycemic diets are also more likely to be rich in nutrients and fiber than high-glycemic diets.

The Individual's Response to Foods

The body's insulin response to carbohydrate depends not only on a food, but also on a person's metabolism. Some people react to dietary carbohydrate with a low insulin response. Others have a high insulin response. How energy is stored after a meal depends in part on how the body responds to insulin. After eating a high-carbohydrate meal, normal-weight people who are insulin resistant tend to synthesize about half as much glycogen in muscles and make about twice as much fat in the liver as people who are insulin sensitive. Some research suggests that restricting carbohydrate intake may improve glucose control, insulin response, and blood lipids.

In Summary

As might be expected given the similarity in their chemical composition, high-fructose corn syrup and sucrose produce similar effects in appetite control and energy metabolism. In fact, high-fructose corn syrup is more like sucrose than it is like pure fructose. Importantly, people don't eat pure fructose; they eat foods and drink beverages that contain added sugars—either high-fructose corn syrup or sucrose. Adverse consequences become apparent when intakes of either type of added sugars become excessive. Limiting these sugars is a helpful strategy when trying to control body weight, but restricting all carbohydrates—especially dietary fibers, vegetables, and whole grains—would be unwise.

The quality of the diet suffers when carbohydrates are restricted. Without fruits, vegetables, and whole grains, low-carbohydrate diets lack not only carbohydrate, but fiber, vitamins, minerals, and phytochemicals as well—all dietary factors protective against disease. The DRI recommends that carbohydrates contribute between 45 and 65 percent of daily energy intake. Intakes within this range can support healthy body weight and do not contribute to obesity—when added sugar intake is moderate and total energy intake is appropriate. Similarly, added sugars increase energy intake, but need not contribute to obesity—when added sugar intake is moderate and total energy intake is appropriate. When choosing carbohydrates, emphasize a variety of naturally occurring carbohydrates—such as whole grains, legumes, vegetables, and fruits—and limit foods and beverages with added sugars.

CRITICAL THINKING QUESTIONS

A. How are sugars, starches, and fibers related to weight gains and losses?

B. Your mom wants to lose 20 pounds before her high school reunion next month. She has done some research on the Internet, and has discovered an easy diet that seems to offer great success. The basis of the diet is that a person needs to eat "slow carb" foods and avoid sweets (including fruits) and starches. All white foods—such as potatoes, rice, pastas, tofu, breads, cereals, and milk—are banned and two to three workouts each week are encouraged. What evidence supports or contradicts a "slow carb" diet for weight loss?

REFERENCES

1. US Department of Agriculture, Agricultural Research Service, Beltsville Human Nutrition Research Center, Food Surveys Research Group (Beltsville, MD) and US Department of Health and Human Services, Centers for Disease Control and Prevention, National Center for Health Statistics (Hyattsville, MD), *What We Eat in America,* NHANES 2011–2012, www.ars.usda.gov/, published 2014.
2. US Department of Health and Human Services, *2008 Physical Activity Guidelines for Americans* Summary, www.health.gov/PAGuidelines /guidelines/summary.aspx.
3. L. T. Morenga, S. Mallard, J. Mann, Dietary sugars and body weight: Systematic review and meta-analyses of randomised controlled trials and cohort studies, *British Medical Journal* 346 (2013): e7492; J. L. Sievenpiper and coauthors, Effect of fructose on body weight in controlled feeding trials: A systematic review and meta-analysis, *Annals of Internal Medicine* 156(2012): 291–304.
4. A. K. Kant, B. I. Graubard, and R. D. Mattes, Association of food form with self-reported 24-h energy intake and meal patterns in US adults: NHANES 2003–2008, *American Journal of Clinical Nutrition* 96 (2012): 1369–1378.
5. G. A. Bray and B. M. Popkin, Dietary sugar and body weight: Have we reached a crisis in the epidemic of obesity and diabetes? *Diabetes Care* 37 (2014): 950–956; Obesity Society, Position statement: Reduced consumption of sugar-sweetened beverages can reduce total caloric intake, April 2014.
6. A. Madjd and coauthors, Effects on weight loss in adults of replacing diet beverages with water during a hypoenergetic diet: A randomized, 24-wk clinical trial, *American Journal of Clinical Nutrition* 102 (2015): 1305–1312.
7. A. H. Malik and coauthors, Impact of sugar-sweetened beverages on blood pressure, *American Journal of Cardiology* 113 (2014): 1574–1580.
8. B. S. Lennerz and coauthors, Effects of dietary glycemic index on brain regions related to reward and craving in men, *American Journal of Clinical Nutrition* 98 (2013): 641–647.
9. S. Luo and coauthors, Differential effects of fructose versus glucose on brain and appetitive responses to food cues and decisions for food rewards, *Proceedings of the National Academy of Sciences* 112 (2015): 6509–6514.
10. A. Kolderup and B. Svihus, Fructose metabolism and relation to atherosclerosis, type 2 diabetes, and obesity, *Journal of Nutrition and Metabolism* 2015 (2015): 823081; J. Ma and coauthors, Sugar-sweetened beverage, diet soda, and fatty liver disease in the Framingham Heart Study cohorts, *Journal of Hepatology* 63 (2015): 462–469.
11. A. Bosy-Westphal and M. J. Müller, Impact of carbohydrates on weight regain, *Current Opinions in Clinical Nutrition and Metabolic Care* 18 (2015): 389–394.

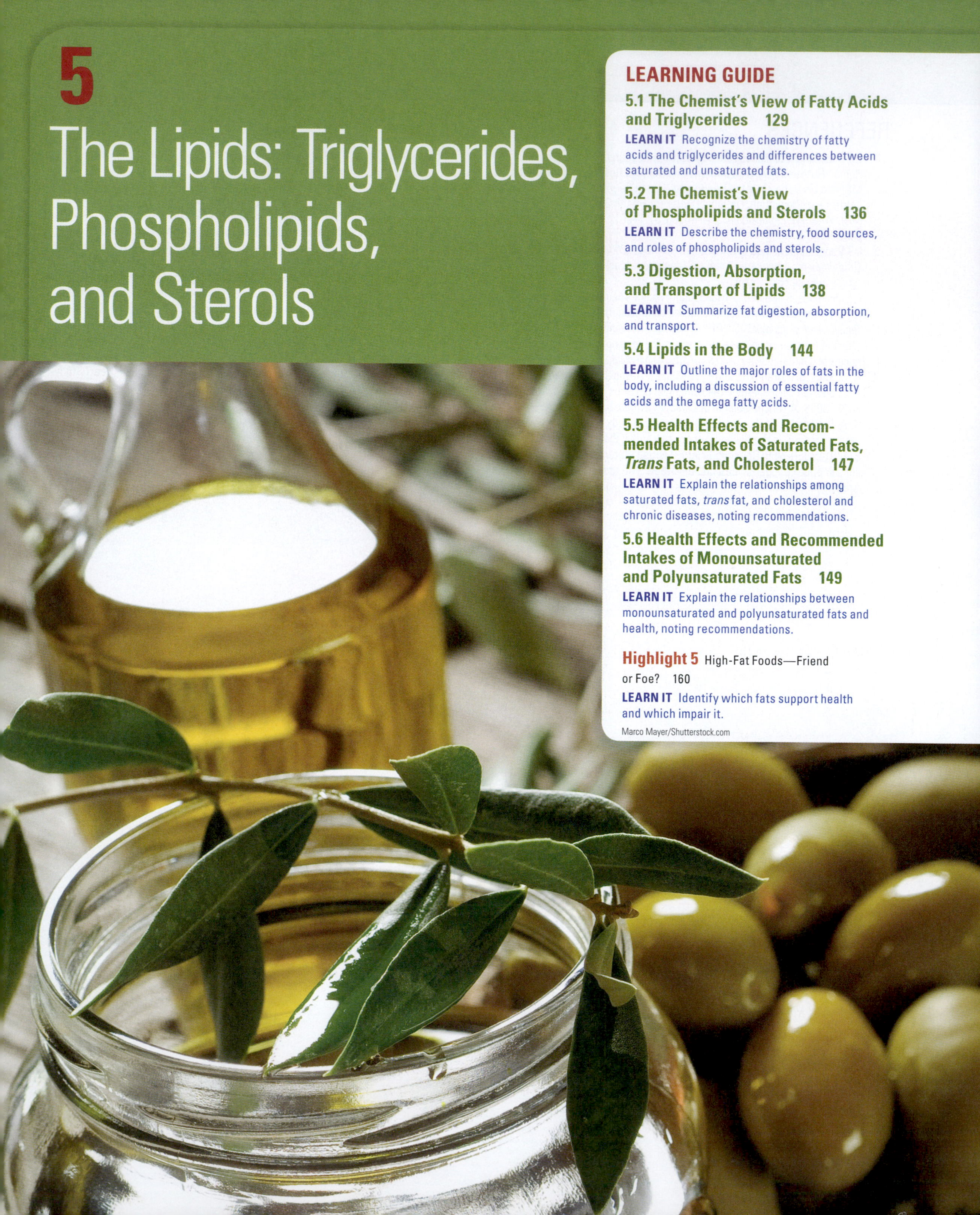

5

The Lipids: Triglycerides, Phospholipids, and Sterols

LEARNING GUIDE

Marco Mayer/Shutterstock.com

Nutrition in Your Life

Most likely, you know what you don't like about body fat, but do you appreciate how it insulates you against the cold or powers your hike around a lake? And what about food fat? You're right to credit fat for providing the delicious flavors and aromas of buttered popcorn and fried chicken—and to criticize it for contributing to the weight gain and heart disease so common today. The challenge is to strike a healthy balance of enjoying some fat, but not too much. Learning which kinds of fats are beneficial and which are most harmful will also help you make wise decisions. As you read this chapter, consider whether your current fat choices are meeting dietary goals.

No doubt you have heard that fats can contribute to the development of several chronic diseases, but did you realize that some fats are also essential to good health? Most people are surprised to learn that fat has virtues and that a well-balanced diet needs at least a little fat. Getting enough fat is rarely a problem. At least traces of fat can be found in almost all foods. In our society of abundance, people are more likely to consume too much fat, or too much of some kinds of fat—with consequent health problems. Learning which kinds of fats are harmful or helpful is key to healthy diet planning.

Fat is a type of *lipid*, but oftentimes the two terms are used interchangeably. The lipid family includes triglycerides (fats and oils), phospholipids, and sterols. Triglycerides are most abundant, both in foods and in the body. The following sections describe the similarities and differences among the remarkably diverse members of the lipid family.

5.1 The Chemist's View of Fatty Acids and Triglycerides

LEARN IT Recognize the chemistry of fatty acids and triglycerides and differences between saturated and unsaturated fats.

Like carbohydrates, **lipids** are composed of carbon (C), hydrogen (H), and oxygen (O). Because lipids have many more carbons and hydrogens in proportion to their oxygens, they can supply more energy per gram than carbohydrates can (Chapter 7 provides the metabolic details).

The many names and relationships in the lipid family can seem overwhelming—like meeting a friend's extended family for the first time. To ease the introductions, this chapter first presents each of the lipids from a chemist's point of view using both words and diagrams. Then the chapter follows the lipids through digestion and absorption and into the body to examine their roles in health and disease. For people who think more easily in words than in chemical symbols, this *preview* of the upcoming chemistry may be helpful:

1. Every triglyceride contains one molecule of glycerol and three fatty acids (basically, chains of carbon atoms).
2. Fatty acids may be 4 to 24 (even numbers of) carbons long, the 18-carbon ones being the most common in foods and especially noteworthy in nutrition.
3. Fatty acids may be saturated or unsaturated. Unsaturated fatty acids may have one or more points of unsaturation—that is, they may be *mono*unsaturated or *poly*unsaturated.
4. Of special importance in nutrition are the polyunsaturated fatty acids known as omega-3 fatty acids and omega-6 fatty acids.
5. The 18-carbon polyunsaturated fatty acids are linolenic acid (omega-3) and linoleic acid (omega-6). Both are essential fatty acids that the body cannot

lipids: a family of compounds that includes triglycerides, phospholipids, and sterols. Lipids are characterized by their insolubility in water. (Lipids also include the fat-soluble vitamins, described in Chapter 11.)

make. Each is the primary member of a family of longer-chain fatty acids that help regulate blood pressure, blood clotting, and other body functions important to health.

The paragraphs, definitions, and diagrams that follow present this information again in much more detail.

Fatty Acids All fatty acids have the same basic structure—a chain of carbon and hydrogen atoms with an acid group (COOH) at one end and a methyl group (CH_3) at the other end. Fatty acids may differ from one another, however, in the length of their carbon chains and in the number and location of their double bonds, as the following paragraphs describe. (Fatty acids and related terms are defined in Glossary 5-1.)

The Length of the Carbon Chain Most naturally occurring fatty acids contain even numbers of carbons in their chains—up to 24 carbons in length. This discussion begins with the 18-carbon fatty acids, which are abundant in our food supply. Stearic acid is the simplest of the 18-carbon fatty acids; the bonds between its carbons are all alike:

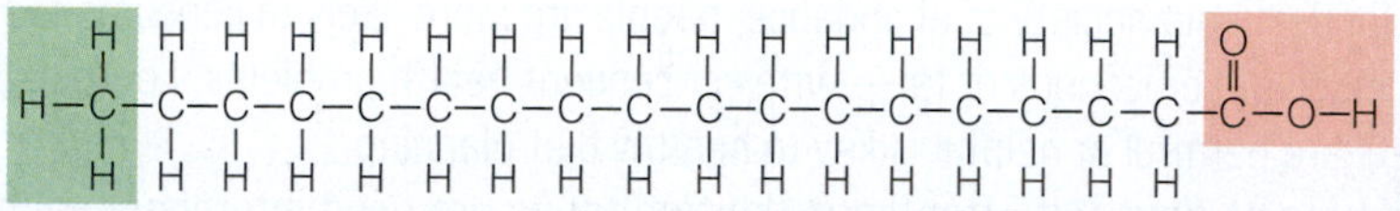

Stearic acid, an 18-carbon saturated fatty acid

© Cengage

As you can see, stearic acid is 18 carbons long, and each atom meets the rules of chemical bonding described in Figure 4-1 (p. 95). The following structure also depicts stearic acid, but in a simpler way, with each "corner" on the zigzag line representing a carbon atom with two attached hydrogens:

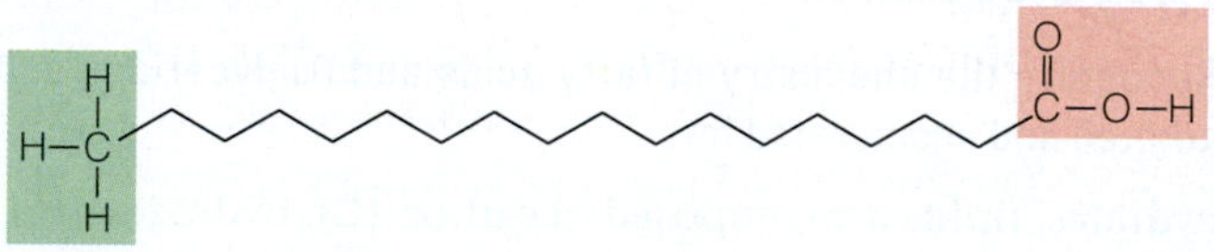

Stearic acid (simplified structure)

© Cengage

As mentioned earlier, the carbon chains of fatty acids vary in length. The long-chain (more than 12 carbons) fatty acids of meats, seafood, and vegetable oils are most common in the diet. Smaller amounts of medium-chain (8 to 12 carbons) and short-chain (up to 6 carbons) fatty acids also occur, primarily in dairy products. (Tables C-1 and C-2 in Appendix C provide the names, chain lengths, and sources of fatty acids commonly found in foods.)

GLOSSARY 5-1
FATTY ACID TERMS

fatty acids: organic compounds composed of a carbon chain with hydrogens attached and an acid group (COOH) at one end and a methyl group (CH_3) at the other end.

monounsaturated fatty acid: a fatty acid that lacks two hydrogen atoms and has one double bond between carbons; abbreviated *MUFA*. Examples include palmitoleic acid and oleic acid. A *monounsaturated fat* is composed of triglycerides in which most of the fatty acids are monounsaturated.

- **mono** = one

point of unsaturation: the double bond of a fatty acid, where hydrogen atoms can easily be added to the structure.

polyunsaturated fatty acid: a fatty acid that lacks four or more hydrogen atoms and has two or more double bonds between carbons; abbreviated *PUFA*. Examples include linoleic acid (two double bonds) and linolenic acid (three double bonds). A *polyunsaturated fat* is composed of triglycerides in which most of the fatty acids are polyunsaturated.

- **poly** = many

saturated fatty acid: a fatty acid carrying the maximum possible number of hydrogen atoms—for example, stearic acid. A *saturated fat* is composed of triglycerides in which most of the fatty acids are saturated.

unsaturated fatty acid: a fatty acid that lacks hydrogen atoms and has at least one double bond between carbons (includes monounsaturated and polyunsaturated fatty acids). An *unsaturated fat* is composed of triglycerides in which most of the fatty acids are unsaturated.

The Number of Double Bonds Stearic acid (described and shown previously) is a **saturated fatty acid.** A saturated fatty acid is fully loaded with all its hydrogen atoms and contains only single bonds between its carbon atoms. If two hydrogens were missing from the middle of the carbon chain, the remaining structure might be:

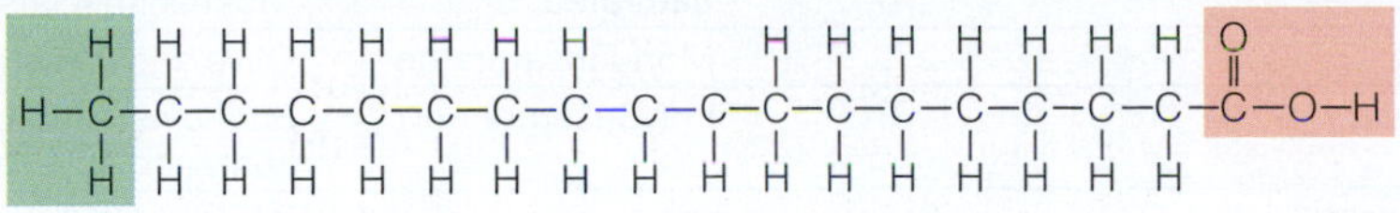

An impossible chemical structure

Notice that in the impossible chemical structure shown above, two of the carbons have only three bonds each. Such a compound cannot exist because every carbon must have four bonds. To satisfy this rule, the two carbons form a double bond:

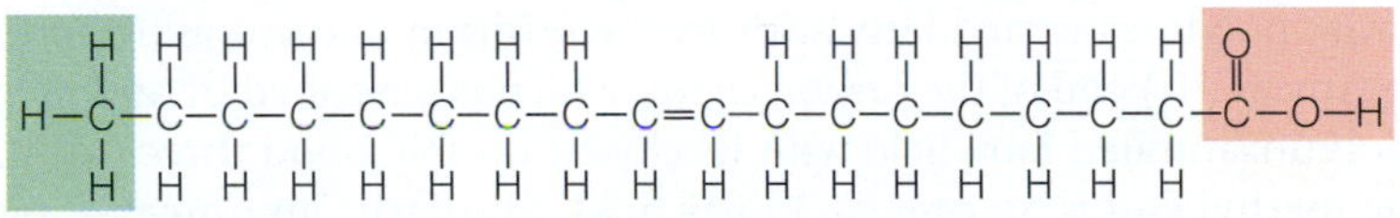

Oleic acid, an 18-carbon monounsaturated fatty acid

The same structure drawn more simply looks like this:

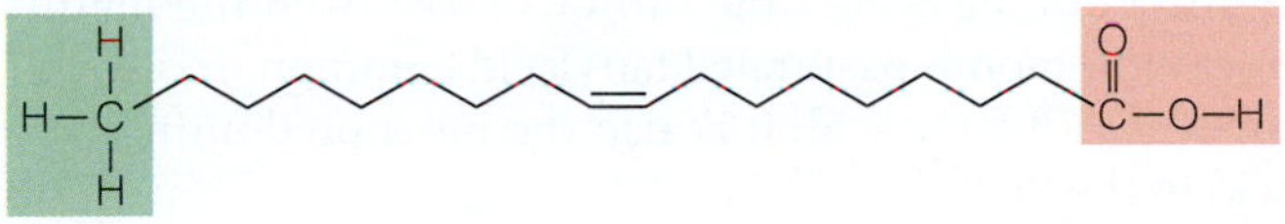

Oleic acid (simplified structure)

Although drawn straight here, the actual shape bends at the double bond. The double bond is a **point of unsaturation.** A fatty acid like this—with hydrogens missing and at least one double bond—is an **unsaturated fatty acid.** This one is the 18-carbon **monounsaturated fatty acid** oleic acid, which is abundant in olive oil and canola oil.

A **polyunsaturated fatty acid** has two or more carbon-to-carbon double bonds. **Linoleic acid,** the 18-carbon fatty acid common in vegetable oils, lacks four hydrogens and has two double bonds:

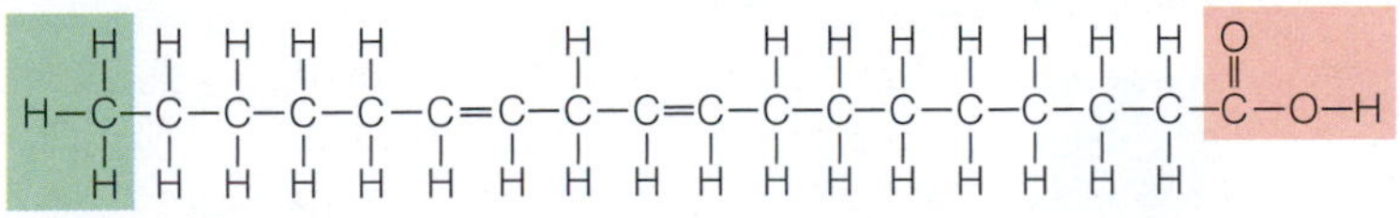

Linoleic acid, an 18-carbon polyunsaturated fatty acid

Drawn more simply, linoleic acid looks like this (though the actual shape would bend at the double bonds):

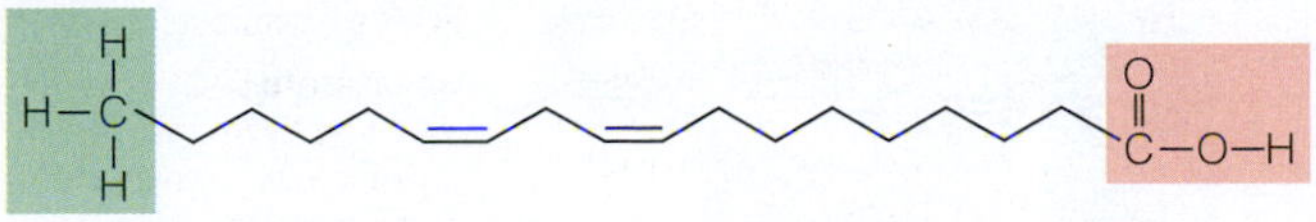

Linoleic acid (simplified structure)

A fourth 18-carbon fatty acid is **linolenic acid,** which has three double bonds. Table 5-1 (p. 132) presents the 18-carbon fatty acids.

linoleic (lin-oh-LAY-ick) **acid:** an essential fatty acid with 18 carbons and two double bonds.

linolenic (lin-oh-LEN-ick) **acid:** an essential fatty acid with 18 carbons and three double bonds.

TABLE 5-1 18-Carbon Fatty Acids

Name	Number of Carbon Atoms	Number of Double Bonds	Saturation	Common Food Sources
Stearic acid	18	0	Saturated	Most animal fats
Oleic acid	18	1	Monounsaturated	Olive and canola oils
Linoleic acid	18	2	Polyunsaturated	Sunflower, safflower, corn, and soybean oils
Linolenic acid	18	3	Polyunsaturated	Soybean and canola oils, flaxseed, walnuts

NOTE: Chemists use a shorthand notation to describe fatty acids. The first number indicates the number of carbon atoms; the second, the number of double bonds. For example, the notation for stearic acid is 18:0.

The Location of Double Bonds Fatty acids differ not only in the length of their chains and their degree of saturation, but also in the locations of their double bonds. Chemists identify polyunsaturated fatty acids by the position of the double bond closest to the methyl (CH_3) end of the carbon chain, which is described by an **omega** number. A polyunsaturated fatty acid with its closest double bond three carbons away from the methyl end is an **omega-3 fatty acid**. Similarly, an **omega-6 fatty acid** is a polyunsaturated fatty acid with its closest double bond six carbons away from the methyl end. Figure 5-1 compares two 18-carbon fatty acids—linolenic acid (an omega-3 fatty acid) and linoleic acid (an omega-6 fatty acid).

Monounsaturated fatty acids tend to belong to the omega-9 group, with their closest (and only) double bond nine carbons away from the methyl end. Oleic acid—the 18-carbon monounsaturated fatty acid common in olive oil mentioned earlier—is an omega-9 fatty acid. It is also the most predominant monounsaturated fatty acid in the diet.

Triglycerides

Few fatty acids occur free in foods or in the body. Most often, they are incorporated into **triglycerides**—lipids composed of three fatty acids attached to a **glycerol**.* Figure 5-2 presents a glycerol molecule.

> **FIGURE 5-1 Omega-3 and Omega-6 Fatty Acids Compared**

The omega number indicates the position of the double bond closest to the methyl (CH_3) end. The fatty acids of an omega family may have different lengths and different numbers of double bonds, but the location of the double bond closest to the methyl end is the same in all of them. These structures are drawn linearly here to ease counting carbons and locating double bonds, but their shapes actually bend at the double bonds.

Linolenic acid, an 18-carbon, omega-3 fatty acid

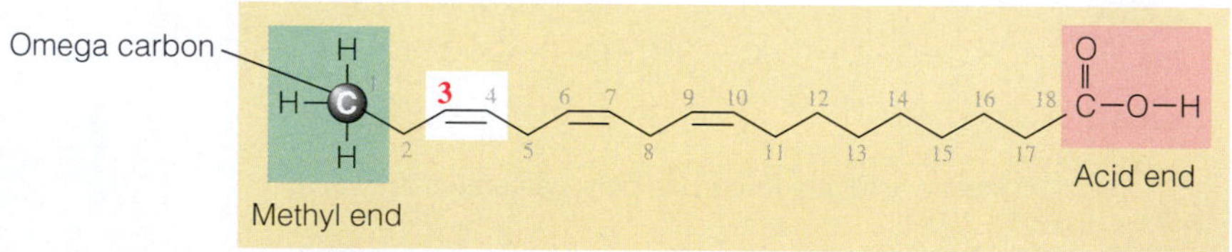

Omega carbon
H
H–C
H
1 2 3 4 5 6 7 8 9 10 11 12 13 14 15 16 17 18
C–O–H
O
Methyl end
Acid end

Linoleic acid, an 18-carbon, omega-6 fatty acid

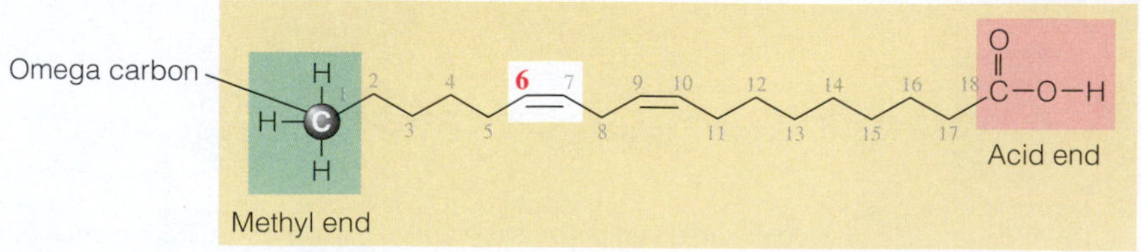

Omega carbon
H
H–C
H
1 2 3 4 5 6 7 8 9 10 11 12 13 14 15 16 17 18
C–O–H
O
Methyl end
Acid end

omega: the last letter of the Greek alphabet (ω), used by chemists to refer to the position of the closest double bond to the methyl (CH_3) end of a fatty acid.

omega-3 fatty acid: a polyunsaturated fatty acid in which the closest double bond to the methyl (CH_3) end of the carbon chain is three carbons away.

omega-6 fatty acid: a polyunsaturated fatty acid in which the closest double bond to the methyl (CH_3) end of the carbon chain is six carbons away.

triglycerides (try-GLISS-er-rides): the chief form of fat in the diet and the major storage form of fat in the body; composed of a molecule of glycerol with three fatty acids attached; also called *triacylglycerols* (try-ay-seel-GLISS-er-ols).

- **tri** = three
- **glyceride** = of glycerol

glycerol (GLISS-er-ol): an alcohol composed of a three-carbon chain, which can serve as the backbone for a triglyceride.

*Research scientists sometimes use the term *triacylglycerols*; this book continues to use the more familiar term *triglycerides*, as do many other health and nutrition books and journals.

To make a triglyceride, a series of **condensation** reactions combine a hydrogen atom (H) from the glycerol and a hydroxyl (OH) group from a fatty acid, forming a molecule of water (H_2O) and leaving a bond between the two molecules (see the left side of Figure 5-3). Most triglycerides contain a mixture of more than one type of fatty acid (as shown on the right side of Figure 5-3).

> **FIGURE 5-2 Glycerol**
>
> When glycerol is free, an OH group is attached to each carbon. When glycerol is part of a triglyceride, each carbon is attached to a fatty acid (as shown in Figure 5-3).

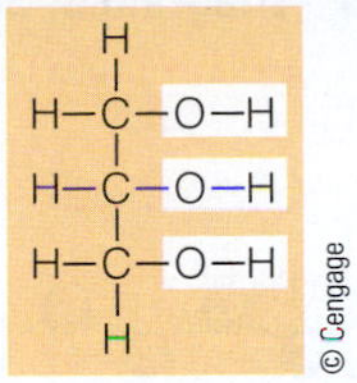

H
H–C–O–H
H–C–O–H
H–C–O–H
H

© Cengage

Characteristics of Solid Fats and Oils

The chemistry of a fatty acid—whether it is short or long, saturated or unsaturated, with its closest double bond at carbon 3 or carbon 6—influences the characteristics of foods and the health of the body. A section later in this chapter explains how these features affect health; this section describes how the chemistry influences the **fats** and **oils** in foods.

Firmness The degree of unsaturation influences the firmness of fats at room temperature (see Photo 5-1 and Figure 5-4, p. 134). Generally speaking, most polyunsaturated vegetable oils are liquid at room temperature, and the more saturated animal fats are solid. Some oils—notably, cocoa butter, palm oil, palm kernel oil, and coconut oil—are saturated; they are firmer than most vegetable oils because of their saturation, but softer than most animal fats because of their shorter carbon chains (8 to 14 carbons long). Generally, the shorter the carbon chain, the softer the fat is at room temperature. Fatty acid compositions of selected fats and oils are shown in Figure 5-5 (p. 134).

Stability The degree of unsaturation also influences stability. All fats become spoiled when exposed to oxygen. The **oxidation** of fats produces a variety of compounds that smell and taste rancid. Exposure to heat and light can also speed up rancidity. (Other types of spoilage can occur due to microbial growth.) Polyunsaturated fats spoil most readily because their double bonds are unstable; monounsaturated fats are slightly less susceptible. Saturated fats are most resistant to oxidation and thus least likely to become rancid.

Manufacturers can protect fat-containing products against rancidity in three ways—none of which is perfect. First, products may be sealed in air-tight, nonmetallic containers, protected from light, and refrigerated—an expensive and inconvenient storage system. Second, manufacturers may add **antioxidants** to compete for the oxygen and thus protect the oil (examples are the additives BHA and BHT and vitamin E).* The advantages and disadvantages of antioxidant additives in food processing are presented in Chapter 19. Third, products may undergo a process known as hydrogenation.

condensation: a chemical reaction in which water is released as two molecules combine to form one larger product.

fats: lipids that are solid at room temperature (77°F, or 25°C).

oils: lipids that are liquid at room temperature (77°F, or 25°C).

oxidation (OKS-ee-day-shun): the process of a substance combining with oxygen; oxidation reactions involve the loss of electrons.

antioxidants: as a food additive, preservatives that delay or prevent rancidity of fats in foods and other damage to food caused by oxygen.

> **FIGURE 5-3 Condensation of Glycerol and Fatty Acids to Form a Triglyceride**
>
> To make a triglyceride, three fatty acids attach to glycerol in condensation reactions.

H–C–O–H H–O–C
H–C–O–H H–O–C
H–C–O–H H–O–C
H–C–O–C
+ H_2O
+ H_2O
+ H_2O
© Cengage
Glycerol + three fatty acids
Triglyceride + three water molecules

An H atom from glycerol and an OH group from a fatty acid combine to create water, leaving the O on the glycerol and the C at the acid end of each fatty acid to form a bond.

Three fatty acids attached to a glycerol form a triglyceride and yield water. In this example, the triglyceride includes (from top to bottom) a saturated fatty acid, a monounsaturated fatty acid, and a polyunsaturated fatty acid.

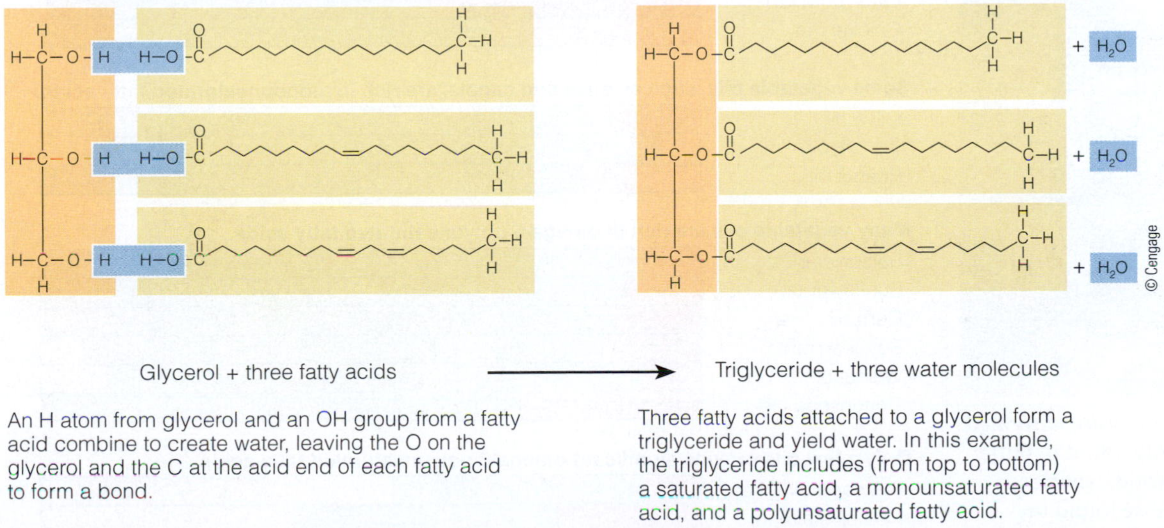

*BHA is butylated hydroxyanisole; BHT is butylated hydroxytoluene.

> FIGURE 5-4 Diagram of Saturated and Unsaturated Fatty Acids Compared

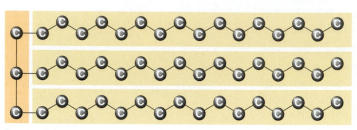

Saturated fatty acids tend to stack together. Consequently, saturated fats tend to be solid (or more firm) at room temperature.

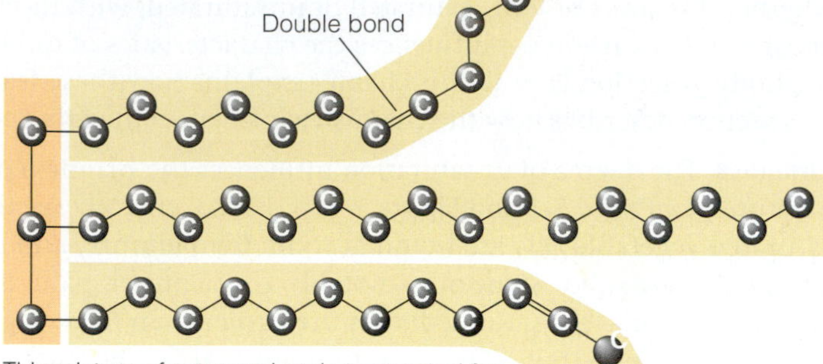

Double bond

This mixture of saturated and unsaturated fatty acids does not stack neatly because unsaturated fatty acids bend at the double bond(s). Consequently, unsaturated fats tend to be liquid (or less firm) at room temperature.

© Cengage

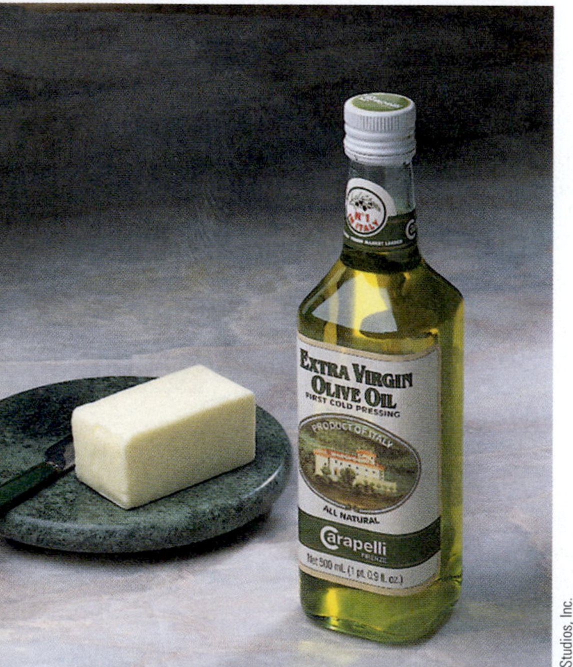

Extra Virgin
Olive Oil
First Cold Pressing
Product of Italy
All Natural
Carapelli

Polara Studios, Inc.

> **PHOTO 5-1** At room temperature, saturated fats (such as those commonly found in butter and other animal fats) are solid, whereas unsaturated fats (such as those found in vegetable oils) are usually liquid.

> FIGURE 5-5 Fatty Acid Composition of Common Food Fats

Most fats are a mixture of saturated, monounsaturated, and polyunsaturated fatty acids.

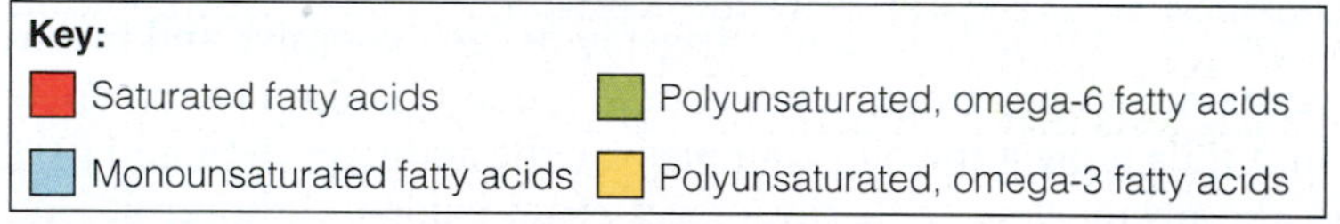

Key:
Saturated fatty acids
Polyunsaturated, omega-6 fatty acids
Monounsaturated fatty acids
Polyunsaturated, omega-3 fatty acids

Animal fats and the tropical oils of coconut and palm contain mostly saturated fatty acids.

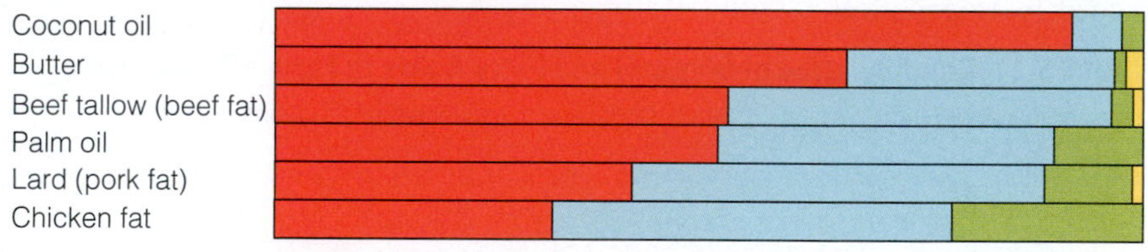

Coconut oil
Butter
Beef tallow (beef fat)
Palm oil
Lard (pork fat)
Chicken fat

Some vegetable oils, such as olive and canola, are rich in monounsaturated fatty acids.

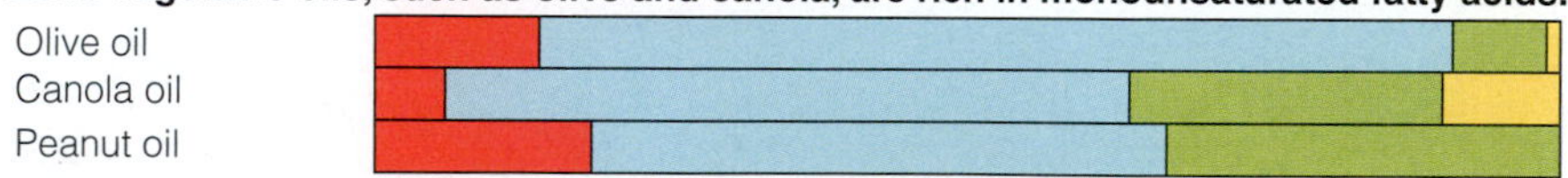

Olive oil
Canola oil
Peanut oil

Many vegetable oils are rich in omega-6 polyunsaturated fatty acids.

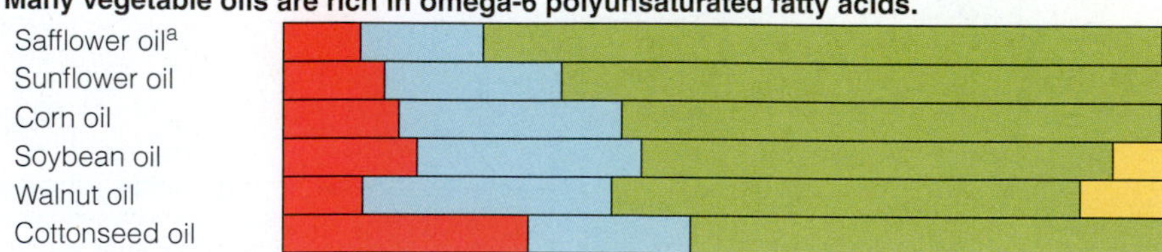

Safflower oil[a]
Sunflower oil
Corn oil
Soybean oil
Walnut oil
Cottonseed oil

Only a few oils provide significant omega-3 polyunsaturated fatty acids.

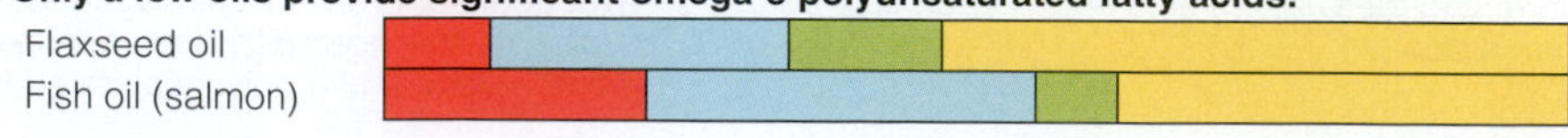

Flaxseed oil
Fish oil (salmon)

[a]*Salad or cooking type over 70% linoleic acid.*

© Cengage

> FIGURE 5-6 Hydrogenation

Double bonds in a polyunsaturated fatty acid carry a slightly negative charge and readily accept positively charged hydrogen atoms, creating a saturated fatty acid. Most often, fat is *partially* hydrogenated, creating a *trans*-fatty acid (shown in Figure 5-7).

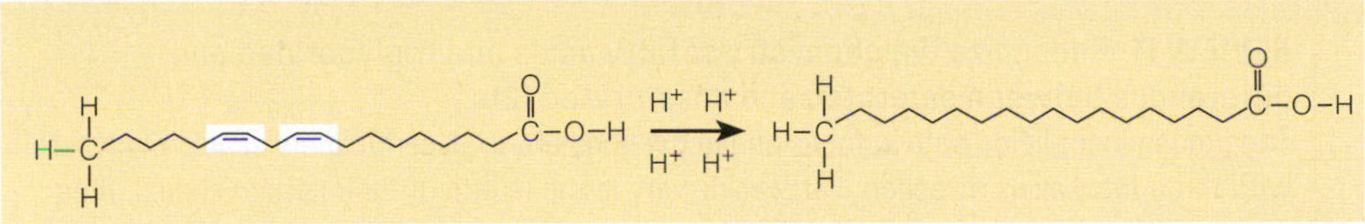

Polyunsaturated fatty acid → Hydrogenated (saturated) fatty acid

Hydrogenation During **hydrogenation**, some or all of the points of unsaturation are saturated by adding hydrogen molecules. Hydrogenation offers two food-processing advantages. First, it protects against oxidation (thereby prolonging shelf life) by making polyunsaturated fats more saturated. Second, it alters the texture of foods by making liquid vegetable oils more solid (as in margarine and shortening). Hydrogenated fats make **margarine** spreadable, pie crusts flaky, and puddings creamy.

Figure 5-6 illustrates the *total* hydrogenation of a polyunsaturated fatty acid to a saturated fatty acid. Total hydrogenation rarely occurs during food processing. Most often, a fat is *partially* hydrogenated, and some of the double bonds that remain after processing change their configuration from ***cis*** to ***trans***.

***Trans*-Fatty Acids** In nature, most double bonds are *cis*—meaning that the hydrogens next to the double bonds are on the same side of the carbon chain. Only a few fatty acids (notably a small percentage of those found in milk and meat products) naturally occur as ***trans*-fatty acids**—meaning that the hydrogens next to the double bonds are on opposite sides of the carbon chain (see Figure 5-7). In the body, *trans*-fatty acids behave more like saturated fats, increasing blood cholesterol and the risk of heart disease—a major health disadvantage.

Some research suggests that both naturally occurring and commercially created *trans* fats change blood lipids similarly; other research suggests that the negative effects are specific to only the commercial *trans* fats.[1] In any case, the important distinction is that a relatively small amount of *trans*-fat in the diet comes from natural sources.* At current levels of consumption, natural *trans*

hydrogenation (HIGH-dro-jen-AY-shun or high-DROJ-eh-NAY-shun): a chemical process by which hydrogens are added to monounsaturated or polyunsaturated fatty acids to reduce the number of double bonds, making the fats more saturated (solid) and more resistant to oxidation (protecting against rancidity). Hydrogenation produces *trans*-fatty acids.

margarine: a butter substitute made primarily of hydrogenated vegetable oils and sometimes blended with animal fats, emulsifiers, water, milk, salt, vitamins, artificial color, and other ingredients.

***cis*:** on the near side of; refers to a chemical configuration in which the hydrogen atoms are located on the same side of a double bond.

***trans*:** on the other side of; refers to a chemical configuration in which the hydrogen atoms are located on opposite sides of a double bond.

***trans*-fatty acids:** fatty acids with hydrogens on opposite sides of the double bond.

> FIGURE 5-7 *Cis*- and *Trans*-Fatty Acids Compared

This example compares the *cis* configuration for an 18-carbon monounsaturated fatty acid (oleic acid) with its corresponding *trans* configuration (elaidic acid).

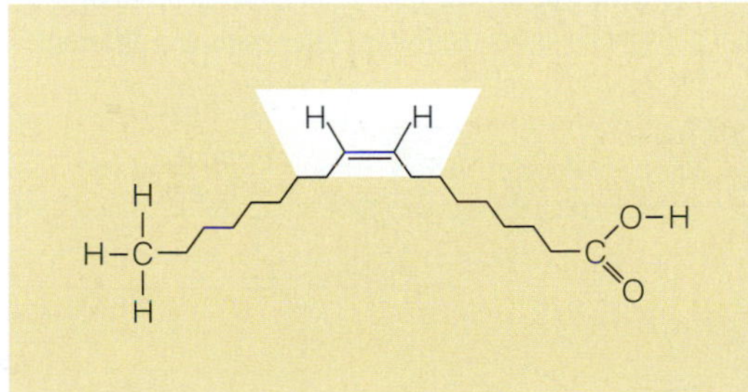

cis-fatty acid

A *cis*-fatty acid has its hydrogens on the same side of the double bond; *cis* molecules bend into a U-like formation. Most naturally occuring unsaturated fatty acids in foods are *cis*.

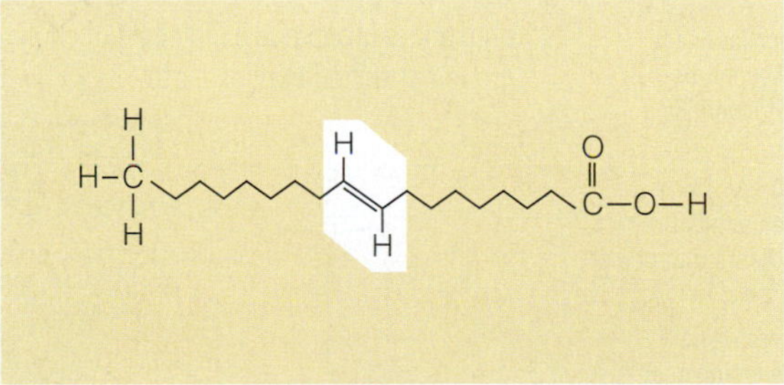

trans-fatty acid

A *trans*-fatty acid has its hydrogens on the opposite sides of the double bond; *trans* molecules are more linear. The *trans* form typically occurs in partially hydrogenated foods when hydrogen atoms shift around some double bonds and change the configuration from *cis* to *trans*.

*For example, most dairy products contain less than 0.5 gram of naturally occurring *trans* fat per serving.

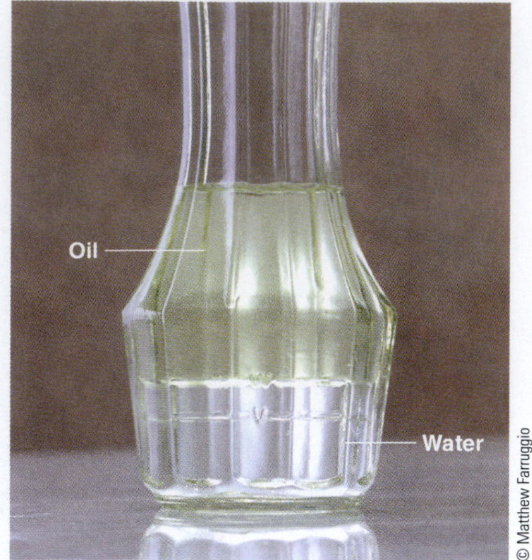
Oil
Water
© Matthew Farruggio

> **PHOTO 5-2** Without help from emulsifiers, fats and water don't mix.

fats have little, if any, effect on blood lipids. Some naturally occurring *trans*-fatty acids, known as **conjugated linoleic acids,** may even have health benefits.[2] Conjugated linoleic acids are not counted as *trans* fats on food labels.

REVIEW IT Recognize the chemistry of fatty acids and triglycerides and differences between saturated and unsaturated fats.

The predominant lipids both in foods and in the body are triglycerides: molecules of glycerol with three fatty acids attached. Fatty acids vary in the length of their carbon chains, their degrees of unsaturation (number of double bonds), and the location of their double bond(s). Those that are fully loaded with hydrogens are saturated; those that are missing hydrogens and therefore have double bonds are unsaturated (monounsaturated or polyunsaturated). The vast majority of triglycerides contain more than one type of fatty acid. Fatty acid saturation affects fats' physical characteristics and storage properties. Hydrogenation, which converts polyunsaturated fats to saturated fats, protects fats from oxidation and alters the texture by making liquid vegetable oils more solid. In the process, hydrogenation creates *trans*-fatty acids that damage health in ways similar to those of saturated fatty acids.

5.2 The Chemist's View of Phospholipids and Sterols

LEARN IT Describe the chemistry, food sources, and roles of phospholipids and sterols.

The preceding pages have been devoted to one of the classes of lipids, the triglycerides, and their component parts, glycerol and the fatty acids. The other lipids, the phospholipids and sterols, make up only 5 percent of the lipids in the diet.

Phospholipids

The best-known **phospholipid** is **lecithin** (see Figure 5-8). Notice that lecithin has one glycerol with two of its three attachment sites occupied by fatty acids like those in triglycerides. The third site is occupied by a phosphate group and a molecule of **choline**. The **hydrophobic** fatty acids make phospholipids soluble in fat; the **hydrophilic** phosphate group allows them to dissolve in water. Such versatility enables the food industry to use phospholipids as an **emulsifier** to mix fats with water in such products as mayonnaise, salad dressings, and candy bars (see Photo 5-2).

> **FIGURE 5-8 Lecithin**

Lecithin is similar to a triglyceride but contains only two fatty acids. The third position is occupied by a phosphate group and a molecule of choline. Other phospholipids have different fatty acids and different groups attached to phosphate.

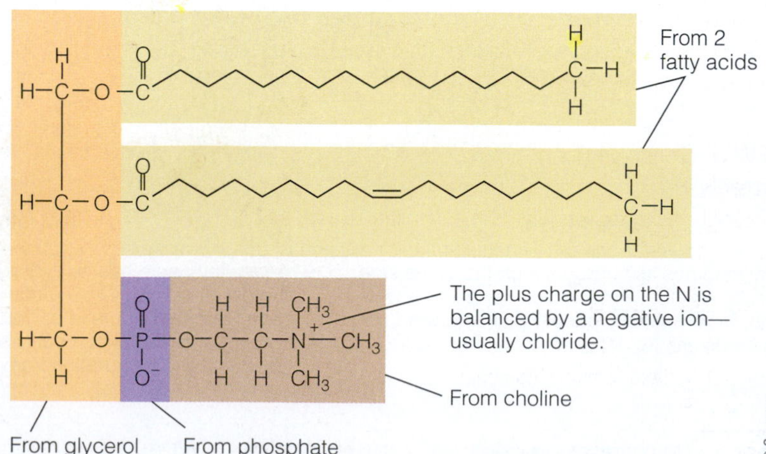
From 2 fatty acids
The plus charge on the N is balanced by a negative ion—usually chloride.
From choline
From glycerol
From phosphate
© Cengage

conjugated linoleic acids: several fatty acids that have the same chemical formula as linoleic acid (18 carbons, two double bonds) but with different configurations (the double bonds occur on adjacent carbons).

phospholipid (FOS-foe-LIP-id): a compound similar to a triglyceride but having a phosphate group (a phosphorus-containing salt) and choline (or another nitrogen-containing compound) in place of one of the fatty acids.

lecithin (LESS-uh-thin): one of the phospholipids. Both nature and the food industry use lecithin as an emulsifier to combine water-soluble and fat-soluble ingredients that do not ordinarily mix, such as water and oil.

choline (KOH-leen): a nitrogen-containing compound found in foods and made in the body from the amino acid methionine. Choline is part of the phospholipid lecithin and the neurotransmitter acetylcholine.

hydrophobic (high-dro-FOE-bick): a term referring to water-fearing, or non-water-soluble, substances; also known as *lipophilic* (fat loving).

hydrophilic (high-dro-FIL-ick): a term referring to water-loving, or water-soluble, substances.

emulsifier: a substance with both water-soluble and fat-soluble portions that promote the mixing of oils and fats in watery solutions.

Phospholipids in Foods In addition to the phospholipids used by the food industry as emulsifiers, phospholipids are also found naturally in foods. The richest food sources of lecithin are eggs, liver, soybeans, wheat germ, and peanuts.

Roles of Phospholipids Lecithin and other phospholipids are constituents of cell membranes (see Figure 5-9). Because phospholipids are soluble in both water and fat, they can help fat-soluble substances, including vitamins and hormones, to pass easily in and out of cells. Phospholipids also act as emulsifiers in the body, helping to keep fats suspended in the blood and body fluids.

Sterols

In addition to triglycerides and phospholipids, the lipids include the **sterols,** compounds with a multiple-ring structure.* The most well-known sterol is **cholesterol**; Figure 5-10 shows its chemical structure.

Sterols in Foods Foods derived from both plants and animals contain sterols, but only those from animals contain significant amounts of cholesterol—meats, eggs, seafood, poultry, and dairy products. Some people, confused about the distinction between dietary cholesterol and blood cholesterol, have asked which foods contain the "good" cholesterol. "Good" cholesterol is not a type of cholesterol found in foods, but it refers to the way the body transports cholesterol in the blood, as explained in a later section of this chapter.

Sterols other than cholesterol are naturally found in plants. Being structurally similar to cholesterol, plant sterols interfere with cholesterol absorption. By limiting cholesterol absorption, a diet rich in plant sterols lowers blood cholesterol levels.[3] Food manufacturers have fortified foods such as margarine with plant sterols, creating a functional food that helps reduce blood cholesterol.

Roles of Sterols Many vitally important body compounds are sterols. Among them are bile acids, the sex hormones (such as testosterone, androgen, and estrogen), the adrenal hormones (such as cortisol, cortisone, and aldosterone), and vitamin D, as well as cholesterol itself. Cholesterol in the body can serve as the starting material for the synthesis of these compounds or as a structural component of cell membranes; more than 90 percent of all the body's cholesterol is found in the cells. Unlike fatty acids, cholesterol cannot be used for energy.[4]

Despite common misconceptions, cholesterol is not a villain lurking in some evil foods—it is a compound the body makes and uses. The chemical structure is the same, but cholesterol that is made in the body is referred to as **endogenous**, whereas cholesterol from outside the body (from foods) is referred to as **exogenous**. Right now, as you read, your liver is manufacturing cholesterol from fragments of carbohydrate, protein, and fat. In fact, the liver makes about 800 to 1500 milligrams of cholesterol per day, thus contributing much more to the body's total than does the diet. For perspective, the Daily Value on food labels for cholesterol is 300 milligrams per day.

Cholesterol's harmful effects in the body occur when it accumulates in the artery walls and contributes to the formation of **plaque**. These plaque deposits lead to **atherosclerosis**, a disease that causes heart attacks and strokes. Chapter 18 provides many more details.

> **REVIEW IT** Describe the chemistry, food sources, and roles of phospholipids and sterols.
>
> Phospholipids, including lecithin, have a unique chemical structure that allows them to be soluble in both water and fat. The food industry uses phospholipids as emulsifiers, and in the body, phospholipids are part of cell membranes. Sterols have a multiple-ring structure that differs from the structure of other lipids. In the body, sterols include cholesterol, bile, vitamin D, and some hormones. Animal-derived foods are rich sources of cholesterol. Table 5-2 (p. 138) summarizes the lipid family of compounds.

*The four-ring core structure identifies a steroid; sterols are alcohol derivatives with a steroid ring structure.

> FIGURE 5-9 Phospholipids of a Cell Membrane

A cell membrane is made of phospholipids assembled into an orderly formation called a bilayer. The fatty acid "tails" orient themselves away from the watery fluid inside and outside the cell. The glycerol and phosphate "heads" are attracted to the watery fluid.

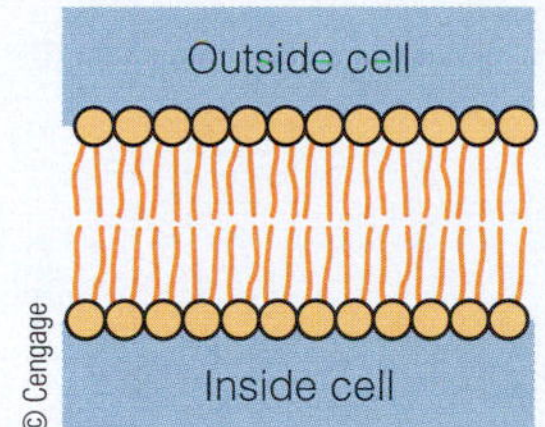
Outside cell
Watery fluid
Hydrophilic heads
Hydrophobic tails
Inside cell
Watery fluid
© Cengage

> FIGURE 5-10 Cholesterol

Notice how different cholesterol is from the triglycerides and phospholipids. The fat-soluble vitamin D is synthesized from cholesterol; notice the many structural similarities. The only difference is that cholesterol has a closed ring (highlighted in red), whereas vitamin D's is open, accounting for its vitamin activity.

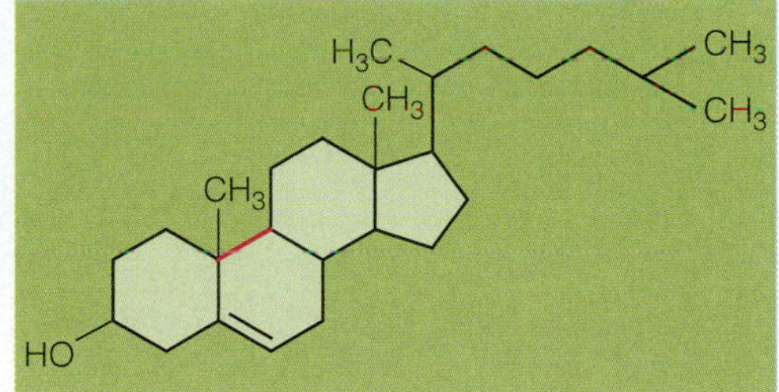
H_3C
CH_3
CH_3
CH_3
CH_3
HO

Cholesterol

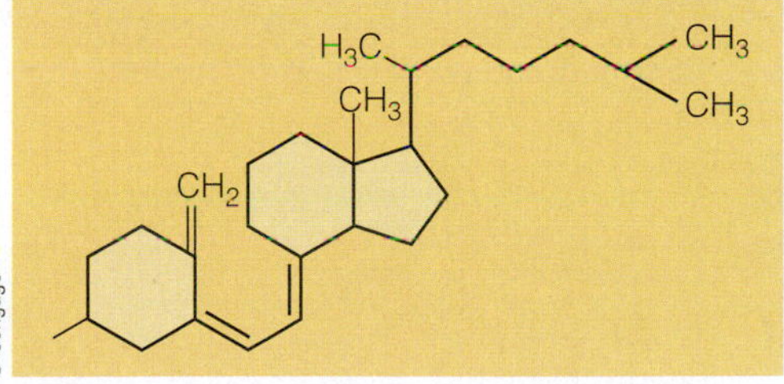
H_3C
CH_3
CH_3
CH_3
CH_2
© Cengage

Vitamin D_3

sterols (STARE-ols or STEER-ols): compounds containing a four-ring carbon structure with any of a variety of side chains attached.

cholesterol (koh-LESS-ter-ol): one of the sterols containing a four-ring carbon structure with a carbon side chain.

endogenous (en-DODGE-eh-nus): from within the body.

- **endo** = within

exogenous (eks-ODGE-eh-nus): from outside the body.

- **exo** = outside

plaque (PLACK): an accumulation of fatty deposits, smooth muscle cells, and fibrous connective tissue that develops in the artery walls in atherosclerosis; also known as *atheromatous* (ATH-er-OH-ma-tus) *plaque*.

atherosclerosis (ATH-er-oh-scler-OH-sis): a type of artery disease characterized by plaques (accumulations of lipid-containing material) on the inner walls of the arteries.

TABLE 5-2 The Lipid Family

Triglycerides

- 1 Glycerol (per triglyceride) and
- 3 Fatty acids (per triglyceride); depending on the number of double bonds, fatty acids may be:
  - Saturated (no double bonds)
  - Monounsaturated (one double bond)
  - Polyunsaturated (more than one double bond); depending on the location of the double bonds, polyunsaturated fatty acids may be:
    - Omega-3 (double bond closest to methyl end is 3 carbons away)
    - Omega-6 (double bond closest to methyl end is 6 carbons away)

Phospholipids (such as lecithin)

Sterols (such as cholesterol)

5.3 Digestion, Absorption, and Transport of Lipids

LEARN IT Summarize fat digestion, absorption, and transport.

Each day, the GI tract receives, on average from the food we eat, 50 to 100 grams of triglycerides, 4 to 8 grams of phospholipids, and 200 to 350 milligrams of cholesterol. These lipids are hydrophobic, whereas the digestive enzymes are hydrophilic. As you read, notice how the body elegantly meets the challenges of keeping the lipids mixed in the watery fluids of the GI tract and facilitating the work of the **lipases**.

Lipid Digestion

Figure 5-11 traces the digestion of fat through the GI tract. The goal of fat digestion is to dismantle triglycerides into small molecules that the body can absorb and use—namely, **monoglycerides**, fatty acids, and glycerol. The following paragraphs provide the details.

In the Mouth Fat digestion starts off slowly in the mouth, with some hard fats melting as they reach body temperature. A salivary gland at the base of the tongue releases an enzyme (lingual lipase) that plays an active role in fat digestion in infants, but a relatively minor role in adults. In infants, this enzyme efficiently digests the short- and medium-chain fatty acids found in milk.

In the Stomach In a quiet stomach, fat would float as a layer above the watery components of swallowed food. But whenever food is present, the stomach is active. The strong muscle contractions of the stomach propel its contents toward the pyloric sphincter. Some chyme passes through the pyloric sphincter periodically, but the remaining partially digested food is propelled back into the body of the stomach. This churning grinds the solid pieces to finer particles, mixes the chyme with gastric secretions, and disperses the fat into small droplets.[5] These actions help to expose the fat for attack by the gastric lipase enzyme—an enzyme that performs best in the acidic environment of the stomach. Still, little fat digestion takes place in the stomach; most of the action occurs in the small intestine.

In the Small Intestine When fat enters the small intestine, it triggers the release of the hormone cholecystokinin (CCK), which signals the gallbladder to release its stores of bile. (Remember from Chapter 3 that bile is a digestive secretion that is made by the liver, stored in the gallbladder, and released into the small intestine when needed.) Among bile's many ingredients are bile acids, which are made in the liver from cholesterol and have a similar structure. In addition, bile acids often pair up with an amino acid (a building block of protein). The amino acid end is hydrophilic, and the sterol end is hydrophobic. Having both water-soluble and fat-soluble ends enables bile to act as an emulsifier—a substance that promotes

lipases (LYE-pasez): enzymes that hydrolyze lipids (fats). *Lingual lipase* is a fat-digesting enzyme secreted from the salivary gland at the base of the tongue; *gastric lipase* is a fat-digesting enzyme secreted from the cells of the stomach.

monoglycerides: molecules of glycerol with one fatty acid attached. A molecule of glycerol with two fatty acids attached is a *diglyceride*.

- **mono** = one
- **di** = two

> FIGURE 5-11 Fat Digestion in the GI Tract

FAT

Mouth and salivary glands
Some hard fats begin to melt as they reach body temperature. The sublingual salivary gland in the base of the tongue secretes lingual lipase. The degree of hydrolysis by lingual lipase is slight for most fats but may be appreciable for milk fats.

Stomach
The stomach's churning action mixes fat with water and acid. A gastric lipase accesses and hydrolyzes (only a very small amount of) fat.

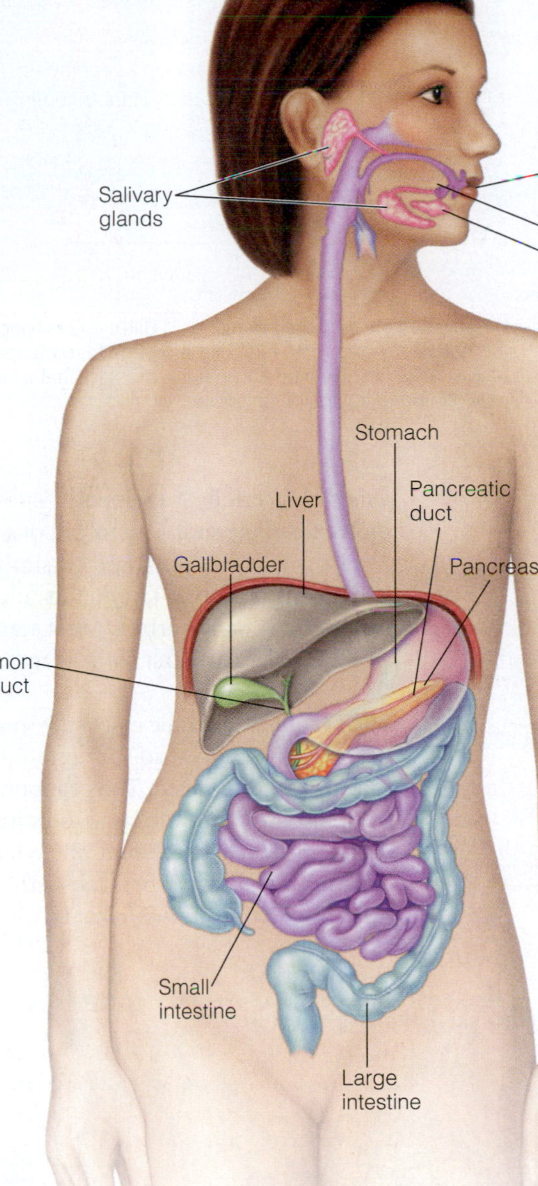

Salivary glands
Mouth
Tongue
Sublingual salivary gland
Stomach
Liver
Pancreatic duct
Gallbladder
Pancreas
Common bile duct
Small intestine
Large intestine

Small intestine
Cholecystokinin (CCK) signals the gallbladder to release bile (via the common bile duct):

Fat —Bile→ Emulsified fat

Pancreatic lipase flows in from the pancreas (via the pancreatic duct):

Emulsified fat (triglycerides) —Pancreatic (and intestinal) lipase→ Monoglycerides, glycerol, fatty acids (absorbed)

Large intestine
Some fat and cholesterol, trapped in fiber, exit in feces.

the mixing of fat molecules in the surrounding watery fluids. Note that bile is not a digestive enzyme; it is, however, essential in preparing fats for digestion by the lipase enzymes from the pancreas and small intestine. The process of emulsification is diagrammed in Figure 5-12 (p. 140).

Most of the hydrolysis of triglycerides occurs in the small intestine. The major fat-digesting enzymes are pancreatic lipases; some intestinal lipases are also active. These enzymes remove each of a triglyceride's outer fatty acids one at a time, leaving

> **FIGURE 5-12 Emulsification of Fat by Bile**

Like bile, detergents are emulsifiers and work the same way, which is why they are effective in removing grease spots from clothes. Molecule by molecule, the grease is dissolved out of the spot and suspended in the water, where it can be rinsed away.

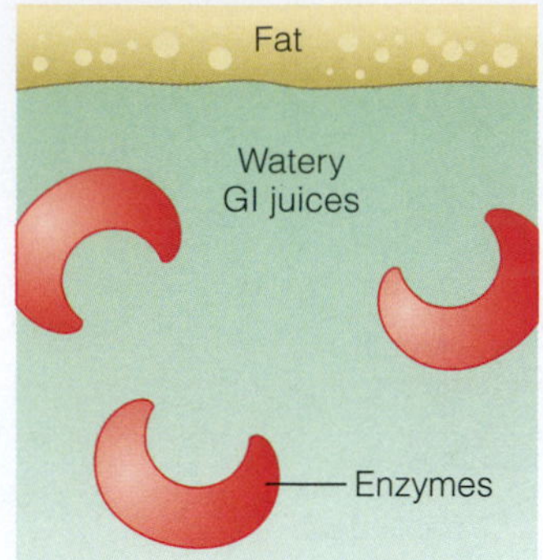

Fat
Watery GI juices
Enzymes

Fat and watery GI juices tend to separate; enzymes in the GI juices can't get at the fat.

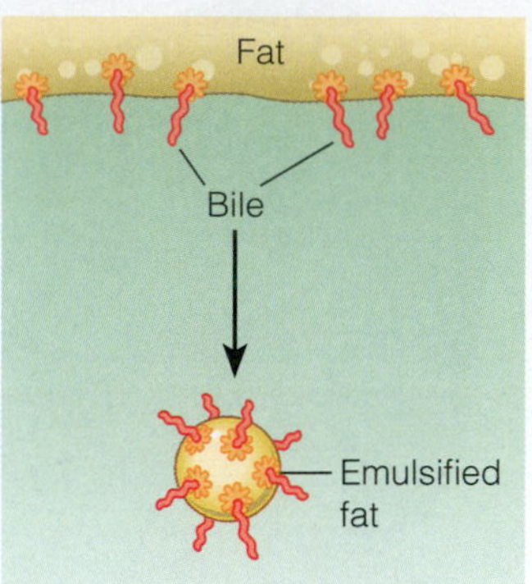

Fat
Bile
Emulsified fat

When fat enters the small intestine, the gallbladder secretes bile. Bile has an affinity for both fat and water, so it can bring the fat into the water.

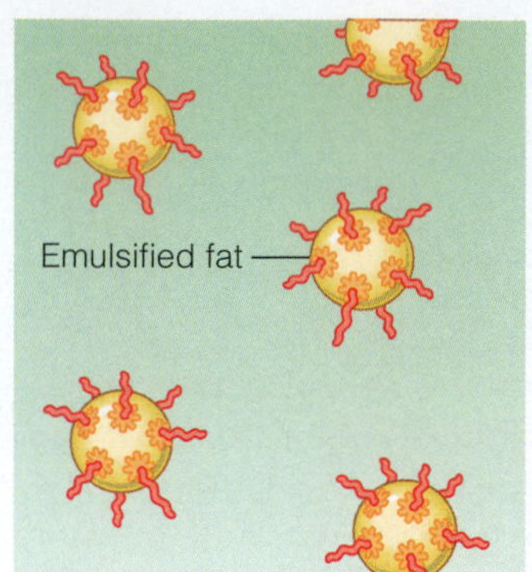

Emulsified fat

Bile's emulsifying action converts large fat globules into small droplets that repel one another.

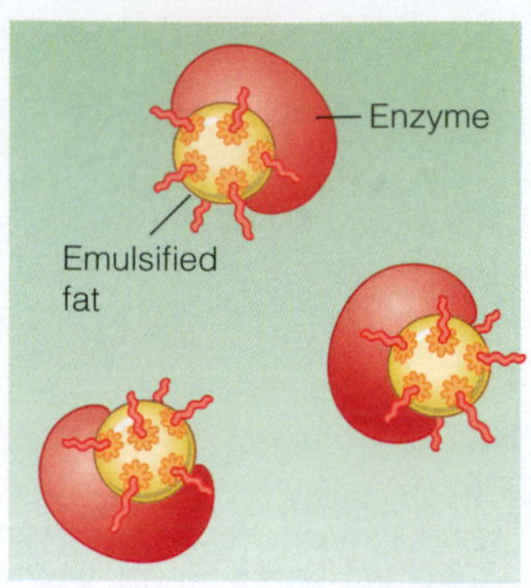

Enzyme
Emulsified fat

After emulsification, more fat is exposed to the enzymes, making fat digestion more efficient.

a monoglyceride. Occasionally, enzymes remove all three fatty acids, leaving a free molecule of glycerol. Hydrolysis of a triglyceride is shown in Figure 5-13.

Phospholipids are digested similarly—that is, their fatty acids are removed by hydrolysis. The two fatty acids and the remaining glycerol and phosphate fragments are then absorbed. Most sterols can be absorbed as is; if any fatty acids are attached, they are first hydrolyzed off.

Bile's Routes After bile enters the small intestine and emulsifies fat, it has two possible destinations, illustrated in Figure 5-14. Most of the bile is reabsorbed from the small intestine and recycled. The other possibility is that some of the bile can be trapped by dietary fibers in the large intestine and excreted. Because cholesterol is needed to make bile, the excretion of bile effectively reduces blood cholesterol. As Chapter 4 explains, the dietary fibers most effective at lowering blood cholesterol are the soluble fibers commonly found in fruits, whole grains, and legumes.

> **FIGURE 5-13 Digestion (Hydrolysis) of a Triglyceride**

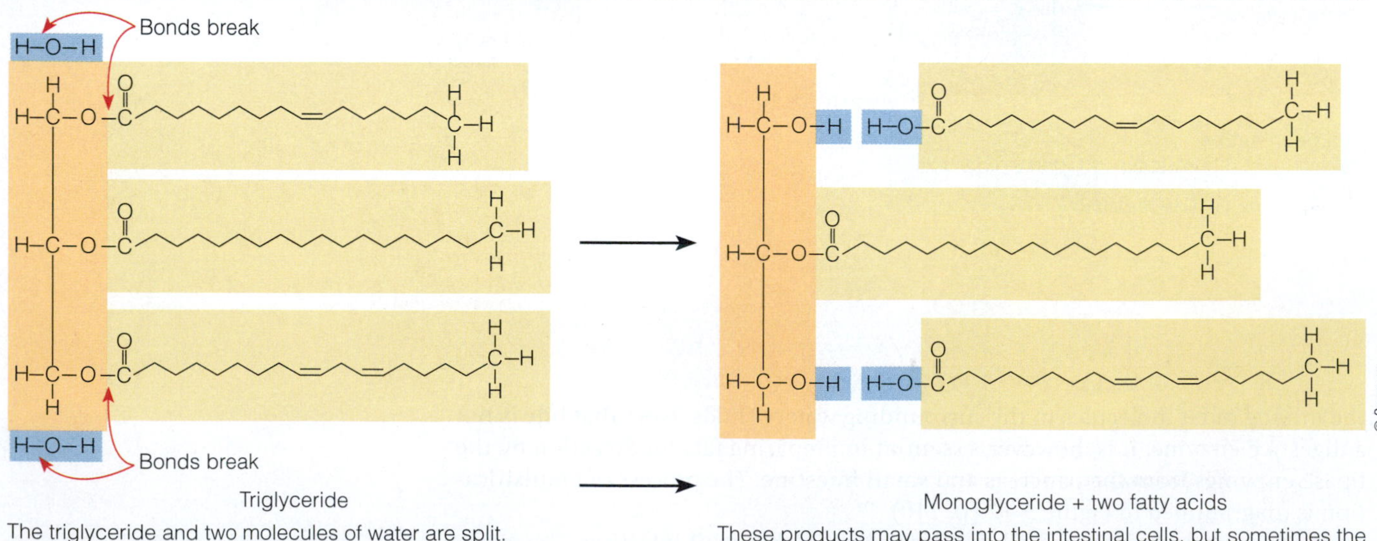

Bonds break
H–O–H
Bonds break
Triglyceride
Monoglyceride + two fatty acids

The triglyceride and two molecules of water are split. The H and OH from water complete the structures of two fatty acids and leave a monoglyceride.

These products may pass into the intestinal cells, but sometimes the monoglyceride is split with another molecule of water to give a third fatty acid and glycerol. Fatty acids, monoglycerides, and glycerol are absorbed into intestinal cells.

Lipid Absorption Figure 5-15 illustrates the absorption of lipids. Small molecules (glycerol and short- and medium-chain fatty acids) can diffuse easily into the intestinal cells; they are absorbed directly into the bloodstream. Larger molecules (monoglycerides and long-chain fatty acids) are emulsified by bile, forming spherical complexes known as **micelles**. The micelles diffuse into the intestinal cells, where the monoglycerides and long-chain fatty acids are reassembled into new triglycerides.

Within the intestinal cells, the newly made triglycerides and other lipids (cholesterol and phospholipids) are packaged with proteins to make transport vehicles known as chylomicrons. The intestinal cells carefully regulate the production and release of the chylomicrons into the lymphatic system.[6] The chylomicrons glide through the lymph until they reach a point of entry into the bloodstream at the thoracic duct near the heart. (Recall from Chapter 3 that nutrients from the GI tract that enter the lymph system initially bypass the liver.) The blood carries these lipids to the rest of the body for immediate use or storage. A look at these lipids in the body reveals the kinds of fat the diet has been delivering. The blood, fat stores, and muscle cells of people who eat a diet rich in unsaturated fats, for example, contain more unsaturated fats than those of people who select a diet high in saturated fats.

Lipid Transport The chylomicrons are one of several clusters of lipids and proteins that are used as transport vehicles for fats. As a group, these vehicles are known as **lipoproteins**, and they solve the body's challenge of transporting fat through the watery bloodstream. The body makes four main types of lipoproteins, distinguished by their size and density.* Each type of lipoprotein

> **FIGURE 5-14 Enterohepatic Circulation**

Most of the bile released into the small intestine is reabsorbed and sent back to the liver to be reused. This cycle is called the *enterohepatic circulation* of bile. Some bile is excreted.

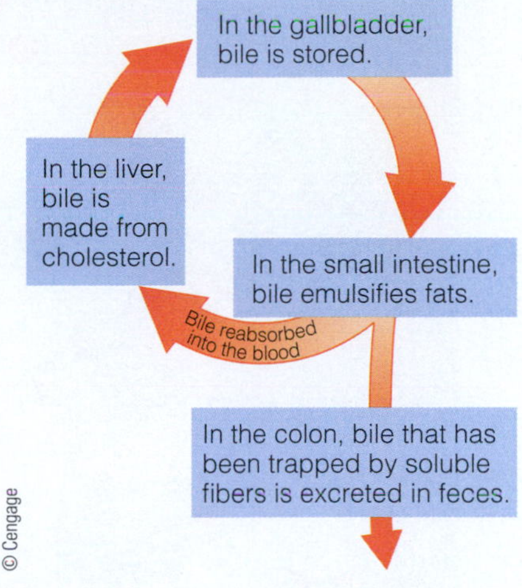
In the gallbladder, bile is stored.
In the liver, bile is made from cholesterol.
In the small intestine, bile emulsifies fats.
Bile reabsorbed into the blood
In the colon, bile that has been trapped by soluble fibers is excreted in feces.
© Cengage

> **FIGURE 5-15 Absorption of Fat**

The end products of fat digestion are mostly monoglycerides, some fatty acids, and very little glycerol. Their absorption differs depending on their size. (In reality, molecules of fatty acid are too small to see without a powerful microscope, whereas villi are visible to the naked eye.)

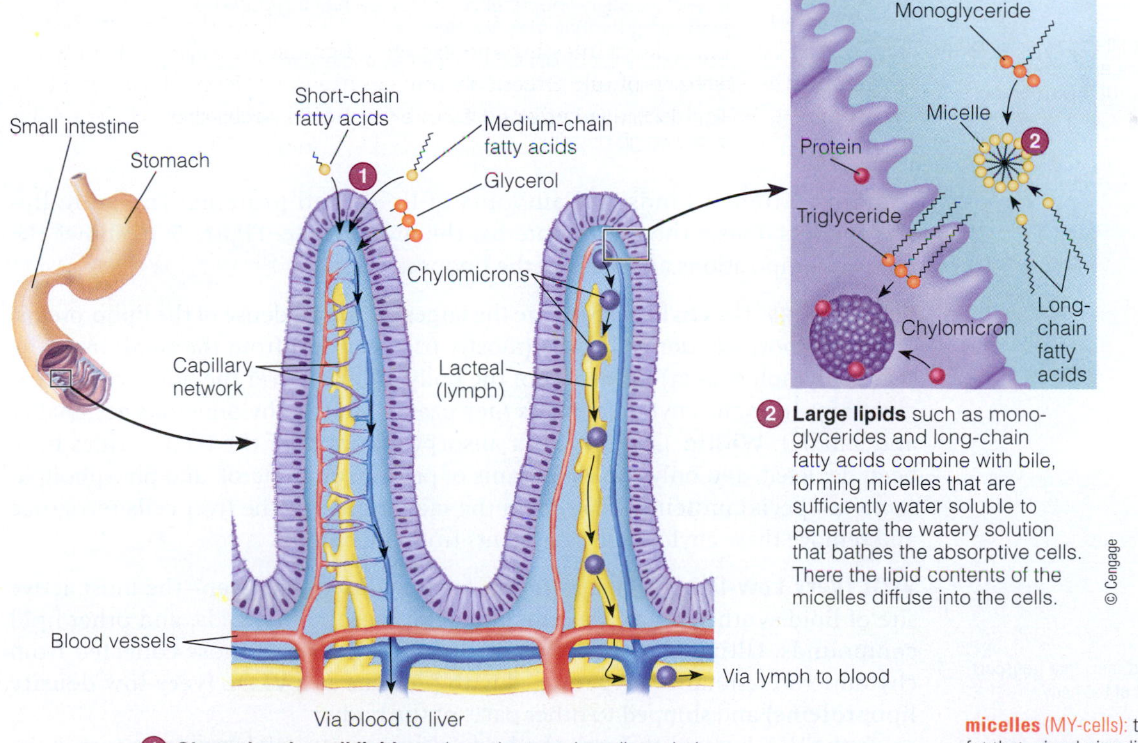
Small intestine
Stomach
Short-chain fatty acids
Medium-chain fatty acids
Glycerol
1
Chylomicrons
Capillary network
Lacteal (lymph)
Blood vessels
Via lymph to blood
Via blood to liver
Monoglyceride
Micelle
2
Protein
Triglyceride
Chylomicron
Long-chain fatty acids
© Cengage

1 **Glycerol and small lipids** such as short- and medium-chain fatty acids can move directly into the bloodstream.

2 **Large lipids** such as monoglycerides and long-chain fatty acids combine with bile, forming micelles that are sufficiently water soluble to penetrate the watery solution that bathes the absorptive cells. There the lipid contents of the micelles diffuse into the cells.

*Chemists can identify the various lipoproteins by their density. The most buoyant particles (highest in lipids) have the lowest density; the densest particles (highest in proteins) have the highest density. Others distribute themselves in between.

micelles (MY-cells): tiny spherical complexes of emulsified fat that arise during digestion; most contain bile salts and the products of lipid digestion, including fatty acids, monoglycerides, and cholesterol.

lipoproteins (LIP-oh-PRO-teenz): clusters of lipids associated with proteins that serve as transport vehicles for lipids in the lymph and blood.

> FIGURE 5-16 Sizes and Compositions of the Lipoproteins

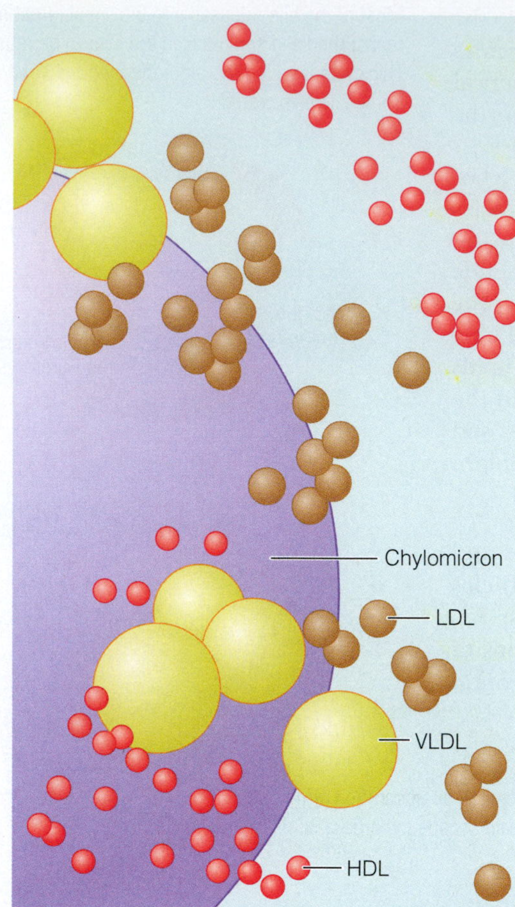
Chylomicron
LDL
VLDL
HDL

Notice how large the fat-filled chylomicron is compared with the others and how the others get progressively smaller as their proportion of fat declines and protein increases.

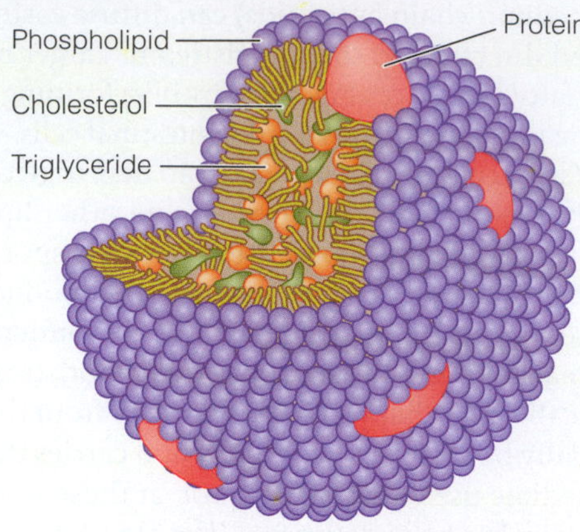
Phospholipid
Protein
Cholesterol
Triglyceride

A typical lipoprotein contains an interior of triglycerides and cholesterol surrounded by phospholipids. The phospholipids' fatty acid "tails" point toward the interior, where the lipids are. Proteins near the outer ends of the phospholipids cover the structure. This arrangement of hydrophobic molecules on the inside and hydrophilic molecules on the outside allows lipids to travel through the watery fluids of the blood.

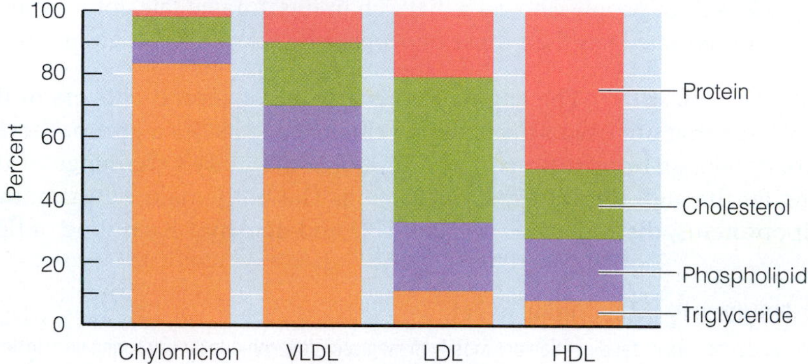
100
80
60
40
20
0
Percent
Chylomicron
VLDL
LDL
HDL
Protein
Cholesterol
Phospholipid
Triglyceride

Chylomicrons contain so little protein and so much triglyceride that they are the lowest in density.

Very-low-density lipoproteins (VLDL) are half triglycerides, accounting for their very low density.

Low-density lipoproteins (LDL) are half cholesterol, accounting for their implication in heart disease.

High-density lipoproteins (HDL) are half protein, accounting for their high density.

contains different kinds and amounts of lipids and proteins. The more lipids, the less dense; the more proteins, the more dense. Figure 5-16 shows the relative compositions and sizes of the lipoproteins.

Chylomicrons The **chylomicrons** are the largest and least dense of the lipoproteins. They transport *diet*-derived lipids (mostly triglycerides) from the small intestine (via the lymph system) to the rest of the body. Cells all over the body remove triglycerides from the chylomicrons as they pass by, so the chylomicrons get smaller and smaller. Within 14 hours after absorption, most of the triglycerides have been depleted, and only a few remnants of protein, cholesterol, and phospholipid remain. Special protein receptors on the membranes of the liver cells recognize and remove these chylomicron remnants from the blood.

VLDL (Very-Low-Density Lipoproteins) Meanwhile, in the liver—the most active site of lipid synthesis—cells are making cholesterol, fatty acids, and other lipid compounds. Ultimately, the lipids made in the liver and those collected from chylomicron remnants are packaged with proteins as a **VLDL (very-low-density lipoproteins)** and shipped to other parts of the body.

As the VLDL travel through the body, cells remove triglycerides, causing the proportion of lipids to shift. Cholesterol becomes the predominant lipid, and the lipoprotein becomes smaller and more dense. As this occurs, the VLDL become **LDL (low-density lipoproteins)**, loaded with cholesterol, but containing relatively few triglycerides.

chylomicrons (kye-lo-MY-cronz): lipoproteins that transport lipids from the intestinal cells to the rest of the body.

VLDL (very-low-density lipoproteins): lipoproteins made by the liver that transport lipids (primarily triglycerides) from the liver to other tissues.

LDL (low-density lipoproteins): lipoproteins that derive from VLDL and transport lipids (primarily cholesterol) in the blood.

LDL (Low-Density Lipoproteins) The LDL circulate throughout the body, making their contents available to the cells of all tissues—muscles (including the heart muscle), fat stores, the mammary glands, and others. The cells take triglycerides, cholesterol, and phospholipids to use for energy, make hormones or other compounds, or build new membranes. Special LDL receptors on the liver cells play a crucial role in the control of blood cholesterol concentrations by removing LDL from circulation.

HDL (High-Density Lipoproteins) The liver makes **HDL (high-density lipoproteins)** to remove cholesterol from the cells and carry it back to the liver for recycling or disposal. By efficiently clearing cholesterol, HDL help prevent plaque buildup, thereby lowering the risk of heart disease.[7] In addition, HDL have anti-inflammatory properties that seem to keep artery-clogging plaque from breaking apart and causing heart attacks.[8] Figure 5-17 summarizes lipid transport via the lipoproteins.

Health Implications The distinction between LDL and HDL has implications for the health of the heart and blood vessels. The blood lipid linked most directly to heart disease is LDL cholesterol. As mentioned, HDL also carry cholesterol, but elevated HDL represent cholesterol returning from the rest of the body to the liver for breakdown and excretion. The transport of cholesterol from the tissues back to the liver is sometimes called *reverse cholesterol transport* or the *scavenger pathway.*

High LDL and low HDL cholesterol are both associated with a high risk of heart disease. Having adequate HDL is beneficial, but having high HDL is not necessarily more beneficial. Some people think of HDL as healthy and LDL as lousy, or refer to LDL as "bad," and HDL as "good," cholesterol. Keep in mind that the cholesterol itself is the same and that the differences between LDL and HDL

HDL (high-density lipoproteins): lipoproteins that help remove cholesterol from the blood by transporting it to the liver for reuse or disposal.

> **FIGURE 5-17 Lipid Transport via Lipoproteins**

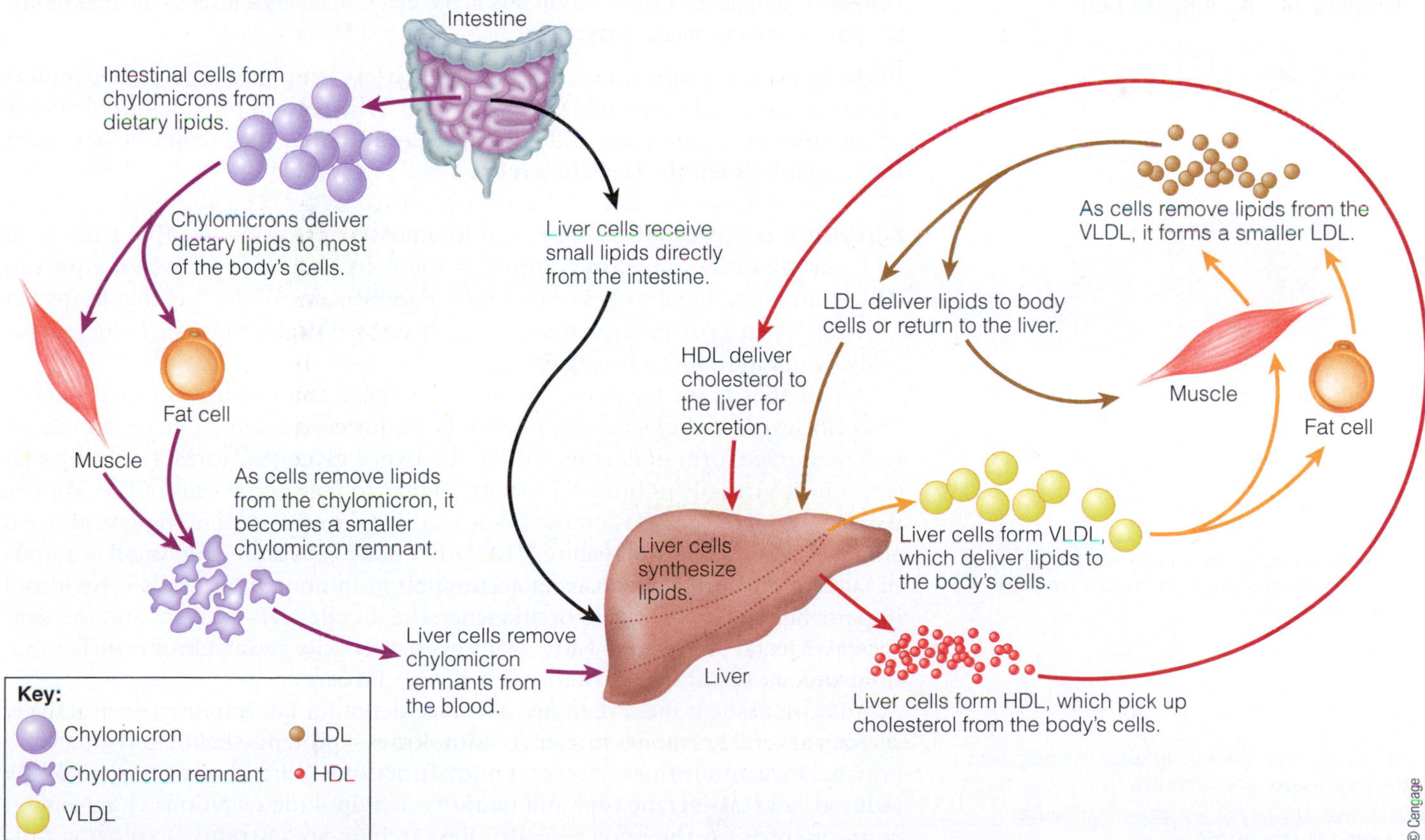

Intestine
Intestinal cells form chylomicrons from dietary lipids.
Chylomicrons deliver dietary lipids to most of the body's cells.
Liver cells receive small lipids directly from the intestine.
Muscle
Fat cell
As cells remove lipids from the chylomicron, it becomes a smaller chylomicron remnant.
Liver cells remove chylomicron remnants from the blood.
Liver cells synthesize lipids.
Liver
HDL deliver cholesterol to the liver for excretion.
LDL deliver lipids to body cells or return to the liver.
As cells remove lipids from the VLDL, it forms a smaller LDL.
Muscle
Fat cell
Liver cells form VLDL, which deliver lipids to the body's cells.
Liver cells form HDL, which pick up cholesterol from the body's cells.
Key:
Chylomicron
Chylomicron remnant
VLDL
LDL
HDL

reflect the *proportions* and *types* of lipids and proteins within them—not the type of cholesterol. The following factors help lower LDL and/or raise HDL:

- Weight control
- Monounsaturated or polyunsaturated, instead of saturated, fat in the diet
- Soluble dietary fibers
- Phytochemicals
- *Moderate* alcohol consumption
- Physical activity

Chapter 18 provides many more details.

Not too surprisingly, numerous genes influence how the body handles the synthesis, transport, and degradation of lipids and lipoproteins. Much current research is focused on how nutrient-gene interactions may direct the progression of heart disease.

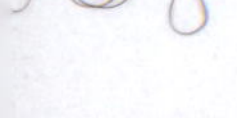

REVIEW IT Summarize fat digestion, absorption, and transport.

The body makes special arrangements to digest and absorb lipids. It provides the emulsifier bile to make them accessible to the fat-digesting lipases that dismantle triglycerides, mostly to monoglycerides and fatty acids, for absorption by the intestinal cells. Four types of lipoproteins transport all classes of lipids (triglycerides, phospholipids, and cholesterol), but the chylomicrons are the largest and contain mostly triglycerides from the diet; VLDL are smaller and are about half triglycerides; LDL are smaller still and contain mostly cholesterol; and HDL are the densest and are rich in protein. High LDL and low HDL indicate increased risk of heart disease. By clearing blood cholesterol and inhibiting inflammation, HDL have a protective effect.

5.4 Lipids in the Body

LEARN IT Outline the major roles of fats in the body, including a discussion of essential fatty acids and the omega fatty acids.

In the body, lipids provide energy, insulate against temperature extremes, protect against shock, and maintain cell membranes. This section provides an overview of the roles of triglycerides and fatty acids and then of the metabolic pathways they can follow within the body's cells.

> **FIGURE 5-18 An Adipose Cell**

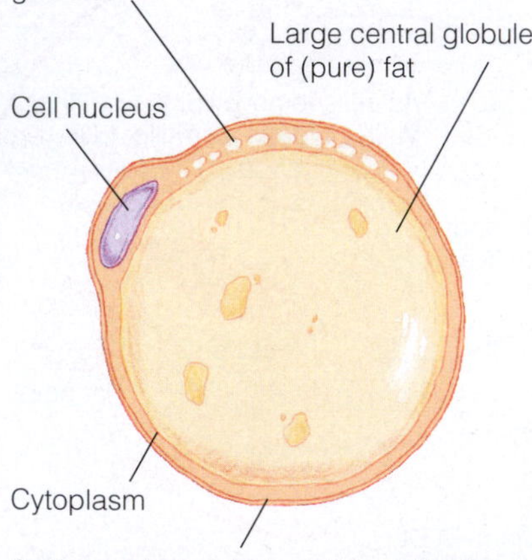
Newly imported triglycerides first form small droplets at the periphery of the cell, then merge with the large, central globule.
Large central globule of (pure) fat
Cell nucleus
Cytoplasm
As the central globule enlarges, the fat cell membrane expands to accommodate its swollen contents.

Roles of Triglycerides

First and foremost, triglycerides—either from food or from the body's fat stores—provide the cells with energy. When a person dances all night, her dinner's triglycerides provide some of the fuel that keeps her moving. When a person loses his appetite, his stored triglycerides fuel much of his body's work until he can eat again.

Recall that gram for gram, fat provides more than twice as much energy (9 kcalories) as carbohydrate or protein (4 kcalories), making it an extremely efficient storage form of energy. Unlike the liver's glycogen stores, the body's fat stores have virtually unlimited capacity, thanks to the special cells of the **adipose tissue**. The fat cells of the adipose tissue readily take up and store triglycerides. An adipose cell is depicted in Figure 5-18. Other body cells store only small amounts of fat for their immediate use; fat accumulation in nonadipose cells is toxic and impairs health. This scenario occurs when the diet delivers excesses and the liver increases its fat production. Fatty liver linked to obesity causes chronic inflammation, which can advance to fibrosis, cirrhosis, and cancer.

Adipose tissue is more than just a storage depot for fat. Adipose tissue actively secretes several hormones known as **adipokines**—proteins that help regulate energy balance and influence several body functions. When body fat is markedly reduced or excessive, the type and quantity of adipokine secretions change, with consequences for the body's health. Researchers are currently exploring how

adipose (ADD-ih-poce) **tissue:** the body's fat tissue; consists of masses of triglyceride-storing cells.

adipokines (ADD-ih-poe-kines): proteins synthesized and secreted by adipose cells.

adipokines influence the links between obesity and chronic diseases such as type 2 diabetes, hypertension, and heart disease.[9] Obesity, for example, increases the release of the adipokine **resistin** that promotes inflammation and insulin resistance—factors associated with heart disease and diabetes. Similarly, obesity decreases the release of the adipokine **adiponectin** that protects against inflammation, diabetes, and heart disease.

Fat serves other roles in the body as well. Because fat is a poor conductor of heat, the layer of fat beneath the skin insulates the body from temperature extremes. Fat pads also serve as natural shock absorbers, providing a cushion for the bones and vital organs (see Photo 5-3). Fat provides the structural material for cell membranes and participates in cell signaling pathways.

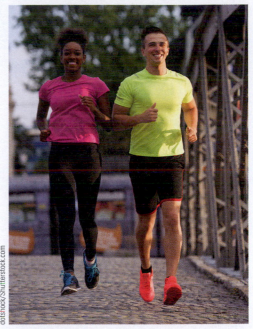

dotshock/Shutterstock.com

> **PHOTO 5-3** Double thanks: The body's fat stores provide energy for a walk, and fat pads on the heels provide cushion against the hard pavement.

Essential Fatty Acids

The human body needs fatty acids, and it can make all but two of them—linoleic acid (the 18-carbon omega-6 fatty acid) and linolenic acid (the 18-carbon omega-3 fatty acid). These two fatty acids must be supplied by the diet and are therefore **essential fatty acids**. The cells do not possess the enzymes to make any of the omega-6 or omega-3 fatty acids from scratch, nor can they convert an omega-6 fatty acid to an omega-3 fatty acid or vice versa. Cells *can*, however, use the 18-carbon member of an omega family from the diet to make the longer fatty acids of that family by forming double bonds (desaturation) and lengthening the chain two carbons at a time (elongation), as shown in Figure 5-19 (p. 146). This is a slow process because the omega-3 and omega-6 families compete for the same enzymes. Too much of a fatty acid from one family can create a deficiency of the other family's longer fatty acids, which becomes critical only when the diet fails to deliver adequate supplies. Therefore, the most effective way to maintain body supplies of all the omega-6 and omega-3 fatty acids is to obtain them directly from foods—most notably, from vegetable oils, seeds, nuts, fish, and other seafoods.

Linoleic Acid and the Omega-6 Family

Linoleic acid is an essential fatty acid and the primary member of the omega-6 fatty acid family. When the body receives linoleic acid from the diet, it can make other members of the omega-6 family—such as the 20-carbon polyunsaturated fatty acid, **arachidonic acid** (as shown in Figure 5-19). Should a linoleic acid deficiency develop, arachidonic acid, and all other omega-6 fatty acids that derive from linoleic acid, would also become essential and have to be obtained from the diet. A nonessential nutrient (such as arachidonic acid) that must be supplied by the diet in special circumstances (as in a linoleic acid deficiency) is considered a **conditionally essential nutrient**. Normally, vegetable oils and meats supply enough omega-6 fatty acids to meet the body's needs.

Linolenic Acid and the Omega-3 Family

Linolenic acid is an essential fatty acid and the primary member of the omega-3 fatty acid family.* Like linoleic acid, linolenic acid cannot be made in the body and must be supplied by foods. Given the 18-carbon linolenic acid, the body can make small amounts of the 20- and 22-carbon members of the omega-3 family, **eicosapentaenoic acid (EPA)** and **docosahexaenoic acid (DHA)**, respectively. These omega-3 fatty acids play critical roles in the optimal structure and function of cells.[10] Found abundantly in the eyes and brain, the omega-3 fatty acids are essential for normal growth, visual acuity, and cognitive development. They may also play an important role in the prevention and treatment of heart disease, as later sections explain.

Eicosanoids

The body uses the 20-carbon omega-3 and omega-6 fatty acids to make substances known as **eicosanoids**. Eicosanoids are a diverse group of more than 100 compounds. Sometimes described as "hormonelike," eicosanoids differ

*This omega-3 linolenic acid is known as alpha-linolenic acid and is the fatty acid referred to in this chapter. Another fatty acid, also with 18 carbons and three double bonds, belongs to the omega-6 family and is known as gamma-linolenic acid.

resistin (ree-ZIS-tin): a protein produced by adipose cells that promotes inflammation and causes insulin resistance.

adiponectin: a protein produced by adipose cells that inhibits inflammation and protects against insulin resistance, type 2 diabetes, and cardiovascular disease.

essential fatty acids: fatty acids that the body requires but cannot make, and so must be obtained from the diet; both linoleic acid and linolenic acid are essential fatty acids.

arachidonic (a-RACK-ih-DON-ic) **acid:** an omega-6 polyunsaturated fatty acid with 20 carbons and four double bonds; present in small amounts in meat and other animal products and synthesized in the body from linoleic acid.

conditionally essential nutrient: a nutrient that is normally nonessential, but must be supplied by the diet in special circumstances when the need for it exceeds the body's ability to produce it.

eicosapentaenoic (EYE-cossa-PENTA-ee-NO-ick) **acid (EPA):** an omega-3 polyunsaturated fatty acid with 20 carbons and five double bonds; present in fatty fish and synthesized in limited amounts in the body from linolenic acid.

docosahexaenoic (DOE-cossa-HEXA-ee-NO-ick) **acid (DHA):** an omega-3 polyunsaturated fatty acid with 22 carbons and six double bonds; present in fatty fish and synthesized in limited amounts in the body from linolenic acid.

eicosanoids (eye-COSS-uh-noyds): derivatives of 20-carbon fatty acids; biologically active compounds that help regulate blood pressure, blood clotting, and other body functions. They include *prostaglandins* (PROS-tah-GLAND-ins), *thromboxanes* (throm-BOX-ains), and *leukotrienes* (LOO-ko-TRY-eens).

> **FIGURE 5-19 The Pathway from One Omega-6 Fatty Acid to Another**

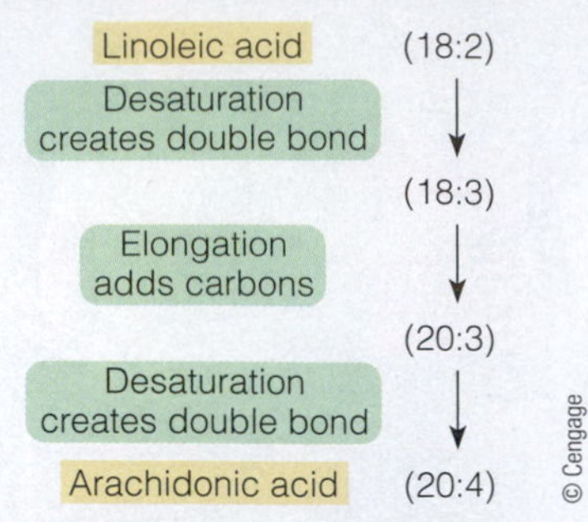
Linoleic acid (18:2)
Desaturation creates double bond
(18:3)
Elongation adds carbons
(20:3)
Desaturation creates double bond
Arachidonic acid (20:4)
© Cengage

The first number indicates the number of carbons and the second, the number of double bonds. Similar reactions occur when the body makes the omega-3 fatty acids EPA and DHA from linolenic acid.

from hormones in important ways. For one, hormones are secreted in one location and travel to affect cells all over the body, whereas eicosanoids appear to affect only the cells in which they are made or nearby cells in the same localized area. For another, hormones elicit the same response from all their target cells, whereas eicosanoids may have different effects on different cells.

The actions of various eicosanoids sometimes oppose one another. For example, one causes muscles to relax and blood vessels to dilate, whereas another causes muscles to contract and blood vessels to constrict. Certain eicosanoids participate in the immune response to injury and infection, producing fever, inflammation, and pain. One of the ways aspirin relieves these symptoms is by slowing the synthesis of these eicosanoids.

Eicosanoids that derive from omega-3 fatty acids differ from those that derive from omega-6 fatty acids, with the omega-3 family providing greater health benefits. In general, the omega-6 fatty acids have a pro-inflammatory effect and the omega-3 fatty acids have an anti-inflammatory effect—and atherosclerosis is an inflammatory disease.[11] The omega-3 eicosanoids help lower blood pressure, prevent blood clot formation, protect against irregular heartbeats, and reduce inflammation, whereas the omega-6 eicosanoids tend to promote clot formation, inflammation, and blood vessel constriction.

Omega-6 to Omega-3 Ratio Because omega-6 and omega-3 fatty acids compete for the same enzymes and their actions often oppose each other, researchers have studied whether there is an ideal ratio that best supports health.[12] Suggested ratios range from 4:1 to 10:1; while some researchers support such recommendations, others find the ratio of little value in improving health or predicting risk. Increasing the amount of omega-3 fatty acids in the diet is clearly beneficial, but reducing the amount of omega-6 fatty acids in the diet to improve the ratio may not be helpful. Omega-6 fatty acids protect heart health by lowering LDL cholesterol and improving insulin resistance.

Fatty Acid Deficiencies Most diets in the United States meet the minimum essential fatty acid requirement adequately. Historically, deficiencies have developed only in infants and young children who have been fed fat-free milk and low-fat diets or in hospital clients who have been mistakenly fed formulas that provided no polyunsaturated fatty acids for long periods of time. Classic deficiency symptoms include growth retardation, reproductive failure, skin lesions, kidney and liver disorders, and subtle neurological and visual problems.

A Preview of Lipid Metabolism

This preview of fat metabolism describes how the cells store and release energy from fat. Chapter 7 provides details.

Storing Fat as Fat When meals deliver more energy than the body needs, the excess is stored as fat in the adipose cells for later use. As Figure 5-18 (p. 144) shows, triglycerides fill the adipose cells, storing a lot of energy in a relatively small space. This accumulation of fat in adipose tissue represents a key advantage that allows humans to survive through times when food is unavailable.[13]

Using Fat for Energy After meals, the blood delivers chylomicrons and VLDL loaded with triglycerides to the body's cells. An enzyme—**lipoprotein lipase** (LPL)—hydrolyzes those triglycerides, releasing fatty acids, diglycerides, and monoglycerides into the cells for energy. Fat supplies about 60 percent of the body's ongoing energy needs during rest. During prolonged light to moderately intense exercise, fat may make a slightly greater contribution to energy needs (see Photo 5-4). As exercise intensity increases, fat contributes less (and carbohydrate contributes more) to the fuel mix.

Fat also makes a slightly greater contribution to energy needs during extended periods of food deprivation. When energy needs are not being met, several lipase enzymes (most notably **hormone-sensitive lipase**) inside the adipose cells respond by dismantling stored triglycerides and releasing the glycerol and fatty acids directly

lipoprotein lipase (LPL): an enzyme that hydrolyzes triglycerides passing by in the bloodstream and directs their parts into the cells, where they can be metabolized for energy or reassembled for storage.

hormone-sensitive lipase: an enzyme inside adipose cells that responds to the body's need for fuel by hydrolyzing triglycerides so that their parts (glycerol and fatty acids) enter the general circulation and thus become available to other cells for fuel. The signals to which this enzyme responds include epinephrine and glucagon, which oppose insulin (see Chapter 4).

solid fats: fats that are not usually liquid at room temperature; commonly found in most foods derived from animals and vegetable oils that have been hydrogenated. Solid fats typically contain more saturated and *trans* fats than most oils.

into the blood. Energy-hungry cells throughout the body can then capture these compounds and take them through a series of chemical reactions to yield energy, carbon dioxide, and water.

A person who fasts (drinking only water) will rapidly metabolize body fat. Even with abundant body fat, the person has to obtain some energy from lean protein tissue because the brain, nerves, and red blood cells need glucose—and without carbohydrate, only protein and the small glycerol molecule of a triglyceride can be converted to glucose; fatty acids cannot be. Still, in times of severe hunger and starvation, a fatter person can survive longer than a thinner person thanks to the energy reserve of adipose tissue. But as Chapter 7 explains, fasting for too long will eventually cause death, even if the person still has ample body fat.

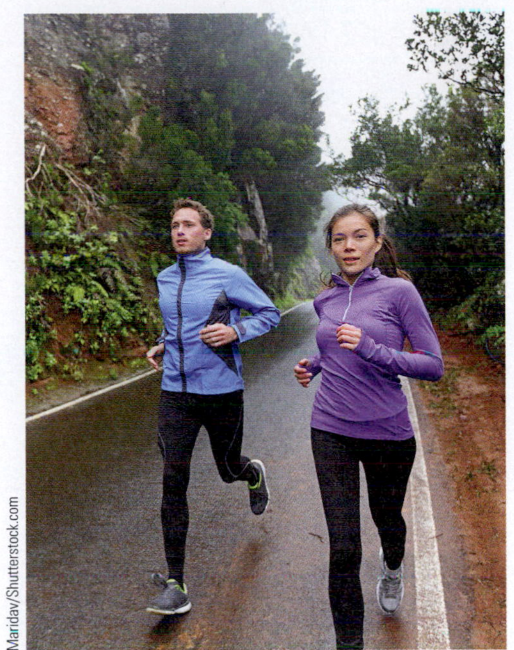

Maridav/Shutterstock.com

> **PHOTO 5-4** Fat supplies most of the energy during a long-distance run.

REVIEW IT Outline the major roles of fats in the body, including a discussion of essential fatty acids and the omega fatty acids.

In the body, triglycerides provide energy, insulate against temperature extremes, protect against shock, provide structural material for cell membranes, and participate in cell signaling pathways. Linoleic acid (18 carbons, omega-6) and linolenic acid (18 carbons, omega-3) are essential fatty acids. They serve as structural parts of cell membranes and as precursors to the longer fatty acids that can make eicosanoids—powerful compounds that participate in blood pressure regulation, blood clot formation, and the immune response to injury and infection. Because essential fatty acids are common in the diet and stored in the body, deficiencies are unlikely. The body can easily store unlimited amounts of fat if given excesses, and this body fat is used for energy when needed.

5.5 Health Effects and Recommended Intakes of Saturated Fats, *Trans* Fats, and Cholesterol

LEARN IT Explain the relationships among saturated fats, *trans* fat, and cholesterol and chronic diseases, noting recommendations.

Some fats in the diet are essential for good health, but others can be harmful.[14] For this reason, recommendations focus both on the *quantity* and the *quality* of the fat in the diet.[15] The current American diet delivers excessive amounts of **solid fats**, representing an average of almost one-fifth of the day's total kcalories. Major sources of solid fats in the American diet include desserts, pizza, cheese, and processed and fatty meats (sausages, hot dogs, bacon, ribs). Because foods made with solid fats provide abundant energy, but few if any essential nutrients, they contribute to weight gain and make it difficult to meet nutrient needs. Solid fats also provide abundant saturated fat and *trans* fat. Even without overweight or obesity, high intakes of solid fats increase the risk of some chronic diseases. One strategy to control saturated fat, *trans* fat, and kcalories is to limit solid fats in the diet.

TABLE 5-3 Desirable Blood Lipid Profile

Total cholesterol	<200 mg/dL
LDL cholesterol	<100 mg/dL
HDL cholesterol	>60 mg/dL
Triglycerides	<100 mg/dL

Health Effects of Saturated Fats, *Trans* Fats, and Cholesterol

Hearing a physician say, "Your blood lipid profile looks fine," is reassuring (see Table 5-3). The **blood lipid profile** reveals the concentrations of various lipids in the blood, notably triglycerides and cholesterol, and their lipoprotein carriers (VLDL, LDL, and HDL). This information alerts people to possible disease risks and perhaps to a need for changing their physical activity and eating habits. Both the amounts and types of fat in the diet influence the risk for disease.

Heart Disease As mentioned earlier, elevated LDL cholesterol is a major risk factor for **cardiovascular disease (CVD)**. As LDL cholesterol accumulates in the arteries, blood flow becomes restricted and blood pressure rises. The consequences are deadly; in fact, heart disease is the nation's number-one killer of adults. LDL cholesterol is often used to predict the likelihood of a person's suffering a heart

blood lipid profile: results of blood tests that reveal a person's total cholesterol, triglycerides, and various lipoproteins.

cardiovascular disease (CVD): diseases of the heart and blood vessels throughout the body. Atherosclerosis is the main cause of CVD. When the arteries that carry blood to the heart muscle become blocked, the heart suffers damage known as *coronary heart disease (CHD).*

- **cardio** = heart
- **vascular** = blood vessels

attack or stroke; the higher the LDL, the earlier and more likely the tragedy. Much of the effort to prevent and treat heart disease focuses on lowering LDL cholesterol.

Saturated fats are most often implicated in raising LDL cholesterol. In general, the more saturated fat in the diet, the more LDL cholesterol in the blood. Not all saturated fats have the same cholesterol-raising effect, however. Most notable among the saturated fatty acids that raise blood cholesterol are lauric, myristic, and palmitic acids (12, 14, and 16 carbons, respectively). In contrast, stearic acid (18 carbons) seems to have little or no effect on blood cholesterol. Making such distinctions may be impractical in diet planning, however, because these saturated fatty acids typically appear together in the same foods. In addition to raising blood cholesterol, saturated fatty acids contribute to heart disease by promoting blood clotting. Fats from animal sources (meats, milk, and milk products) are the main sources of saturated fats in most people's diets. Selecting lean cuts of meat, skinless poultry, and fat-free milk products helps lower saturated fat intake and the risk of heart disease.

Research also suggests an association between dietary *trans* fats and heart disease.[16] In the body, *trans* fats alter blood cholesterol the same way some saturated fats do: they raise LDL cholesterol and lower HDL cholesterol. Limiting the intake of *trans* fats can improve blood cholesterol and lower the risks of heart disease and all-cause mortality.[17] To that end, many restaurants and manufacturers have taken steps to eliminate or greatly reduce *trans* fats in foods.[18] The decrease in *trans* fatty acids in the food supply is apparent in a decrease in plasma concentrations of *trans* fatty acids in consumers.[19]

Unlike saturated fat and *trans* fat, dietary cholesterol raises blood cholesterol very little, if at all. Furthermore, there is no clear relationship between dietary cholesterol and heart disease, which is complicated, in part, by the influence of more than 100 gene variations.[20]

Cancer The links between dietary fats and cancer are not as evident as they are for heart disease. Dietary fat does not seem to *initiate* cancer development but, instead, may *promote* cancer once it has arisen. Stronger risk factors for cancer include smoking, alcohol, and environmental contaminants. (Chapter 18 provides many more details about these risk factors and the development of cancer.)

The relationship between dietary fat and the risk of cancer differs for various types of cancers. In the case of breast cancer, evidence has been weak and inconclusive. Some studies indicate an association between dietary fat and breast cancer; more convincing evidence indicates that body fatness contributes to the risk. In the case of colon cancer, limited evidence suggests a harmful association with foods containing animal fats.

The relationship between dietary fat and the risk of cancer differs for various types and combinations of fats as well. The increased risk in cancer from fat appears to be due primarily to saturated fats or dietary fat from meats (which is mostly saturated). Fat from milk or fish has not been implicated in cancer risk.

Obesity Remember that fat contributes more than twice as many kcalories per gram as either carbohydrate or protein. Consequently, people who eat high-fat diets regularly may exceed their energy needs and gain weight, especially if they are inactive. Because fat boosts energy intake, cutting fat from the diet can be an effective strategy in cutting kcalories. In some cases, though, choosing a fat-free food offers no kcalorie savings. Fat-free frozen desserts, for example, often have so much sugar added that the kcalorie count can be as high as in the regular-fat product. In this case, cutting fat and adding carbohydrate offers no kcalorie savings or weight-loss advantage. In fact, it may even raise energy intake and exacerbate weight problems. Later chapters revisit the role of dietary fat in the development of obesity.

Recommended Intakes of Saturated Fat, *Trans* Fat, and Cholesterol

Defining the exact amount of saturated fat or *trans* fat that begins to harm health is difficult. For this reason, no RDA or Upper Level has been set. Instead, the DRI and *Dietary Guidelines* suggest a diet that provides 20 to 35 percent of the daily energy intake from fat, less than 10 percent of daily energy intake from saturated fat, and as little *trans* fat as possible. In the 1960s, guidelines began to advise limiting dietary cholesterol to lower blood cholesterol and the risk of heart disease, but decades of research no longer support such advice.[21] For this reason, current dietary guidelines no longer limit consumption of dietary cholesterol to 300 milligrams per day, but instead suggest that individuals eat as little dietary cholesterol as possible while consuming a healthy eating pattern.[22]

These recommendations recognize that diets with up to 35 percent of kcalories from fat can be compatible with good health if energy intake is reasonable and saturated fat and *trans* fat intakes are low. When total fat exceeds 35 percent, however, saturated fat usually rises to unhealthy levels. For a 2000-kcalorie diet, 20 to 35 percent represents 400 to 700 kcalories from fat (roughly 45 to 75 grams, see Photo 5-5).

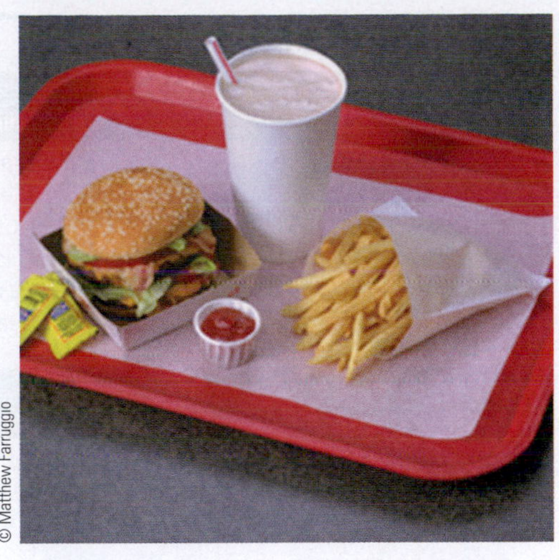

© Matthew Farruggio

> **PHOTO 5-5** Beware of fast-food meals delivering too much fat, especially saturated fat. This double bacon cheeseburger, fries, and milkshake provide more than 1600 kcalories, with almost 90 grams of fat and more than 30 grams of saturated fat—far exceeding dietary fat guidelines for the entire day.

According to surveys, diets in the United States provide about 33 percent of their total energy from fat, with saturated fat contributing about 11 percent of the total.[23] The average daily intake of *trans*-fatty acids in the United States is 1.3 grams per day—mostly from products that have been hydrogenated. Cholesterol intakes in the United States average 221 milligrams a day for women and 315 for men.

Although it is very difficult to do, some people actually manage to eat too little fat—to their detriment. Among them are people with eating disorders, described in Highlight 8, and athletes. Athletes following a diet too low in fat (less than 20 percent of total kcalories) fall short on energy, vitamins, minerals, and essential fatty acids as well as on performance.[24] As a practical guideline, it is wise to include the equivalent of at least a teaspoon of fat in every meal—a little peanut butter on toast or mayonnaise in tuna salad, for example. Dietary recommendations that limit fat are designed for healthy people older than age 2; Chapter 16 discusses the fat needs of infants and young children.

REVIEW IT Explain the relationships among saturated fats, *trans* fat, and cholesterol and chronic diseases, noting recommendations.

Although some fat in the diet is necessary, too much fat adds kcalories without nutrients, which leads to obesity and nutrient inadequacies. Too much saturated fat and *trans* fat increases the risk of heart disease and possibly cancer. For these reasons, health authorities recommend a diet moderate in total fat and low in saturated fat and *trans* fat.

5.6 Health Effects and Recommended Intakes of Monounsaturated and Polyunsaturated Fats

LEARN IT Explain the relationships between monounsaturated and polyunsaturated fats and health, noting recommendations.

Whereas saturated fats and *trans* fats are implicated in chronic diseases, monounsaturated and polyunsaturated fats seem to offer health benefits. For this reason, dietary recommendations suggest replacing sources of saturated fats and *trans* fats with foods rich in monounsaturated and polyunsaturated fats—foods such as seafood, nuts, seeds, and vegetable oils. Table 5-4 (p. 150) lists major food sources of these various lipids.

Health Effects of Monounsaturated and Polyunsaturated Fats Researchers examining eating patterns from around the world have noted that some diets support good health despite being high in fat. As Highlight 5 explains, the *type* of fat may be more important than the *amount* of fat.

TABLE 5-4 Major Sources of Various Lipids

Potentially Healthful Lipids Monounsaturated Fats	Omega-6 Polyunsaturated Fats	Omega-3 Polyunsaturated Fats
Avocado	Margarine (nonhydrogenated)	Fatty fish (herring, mackerel, salmon, sardines, tuna)
Nuts (almonds, cashews, filberts, hazelnuts, macadamia nuts, peanuts, pecans, pistachios)	Meat, poultry, eggs, mayonnaise	Flaxseed, chia seed
Oils (canola, olive, peanut, sesame)	Nuts (pine nuts, walnuts)	Marine algae
Olives	Oils (corn, cottonseed, safflower, soybean)	Nuts (walnuts)
Peanut butter	Salad dressing	Oils (canola, flaxseed)
Seeds (sesame)	Seeds (pumpkin, sunflower)	Yeast
Potentially Harmful Lipids Saturated Fats	***Trans* Fats**	**Cholesterol**
Bacon	Commercial baked goods (including doughnuts, cakes, cookies, pastries)	Eggs
Butter	Fried foods (hydrogenated shortening)	Meat, poultry, shellfish
Cheese	Frozen pizza, many fast foods	Milk and milk products
Chocolate	Many snack foods (including microwave popcorn, chips, crackers)	
Coconut	Margarines (hydrogenated or partially hydrogenated)	
Cream cheese	Nondairy coffee creamers	
Cream, half-and-half	Ready-to-eat frostings, shortening, refrigerated dough products (such as biscuits and cinnamon rolls)	
Ice cream		
Lard		
Meats (fatty cuts of pork and beef)		
Milk and milk products (whole)		
Oils (coconut, palm, palm kernel) and products containing them (such as candies, cookies, doughnuts, pastries, pies)		
Shortening		
Sour cream		

NOTE: Keep in mind that foods contain a mixture of fatty acids.

Heart Disease Replacing saturated fats with unsaturated fats reduces LDL cholesterol and lowers the risk of heart disease and related deaths.[25] To replace saturated fats with unsaturated fats, sauté foods in olive oil instead of butter, garnish salads with sunflower seeds instead of bacon, snack on mixed nuts instead of potato chips, use avocado instead of cheese on a sandwich, and eat salmon instead of steak. Table 5-5 shows how these simple substitutions can lower the saturated fat and raise the unsaturated fat in a meal. Highlight 5 provides more details about the benefits of healthy fats in the diet.

Research on the different types of fats has spotlighted the many beneficial effects of the omega-3 polyunsaturated fatty acids.[26] Regular consumption

TABLE 5-5 Replacing Saturated Fat with Unsaturated Fat

Portion sizes have been adjusted so that each of these foods provides approximately 100 kcalories. Notice that for a similar number of kcalories and total grams of fat, the second choices offer less saturated fat and more unsaturated fat.

Replace these foods . . .

	Saturated Fat (g)	Unsaturated Fat (g)	Total Fat (g)
Butter (1 tbs)	7	4	11
Bacon (2 slices)	3	6	9
Potato chips (10 chips)	2	5	7
Cheese (1 slice)	4	4	8
Steak (1½ oz)	2	3	5
Totals	**18**	**22**	**40**

. . . with these foods.

	Saturated Fat (g)	Unsaturated Fat (g)	Total Fat (g)
Olive oil (1 tbs)	2	9	11
Sunflower seeds (2 tbs)	1	7	8
Mixed nuts (2 tbs)	1	8	9
Avocado (6 slices)	2	8	10
Salmon (2 oz)	1	3	4
Totals	**7**	**35**	**42**

of omega-3 fatty acids may help prevent blood clots, protect against irregular heartbeats, improve blood lipids, and lower blood pressure, especially in people with hypertension or atherosclerosis.[27] In addition, omega-3 fatty acids lower the incidence of heart disease-related deaths, support a healthy immune system, and suppress inflammation.[28]

Cancer The omega-3 fatty acids of fatty fish may protect against some cancers as well, perhaps by suppressing inflammation.[29] Even when omega-3 fats do not protect against cancer development, there seems to be a significant reduction in cancer-related deaths. Thus, dietary advice to reduce cancer risks parallels that given to reduce heart disease risks: reduce saturated fats and increase omega-3 fatty acids. Evidence does not support omega-3 supplementation.

Other Diseases Limited research suggests that the omega-3 fatty acids of fish may protect against asthma, pancreatitis, and rheumatoid arthritis.[30] Omega-3 fats also appear to play a role in improving memory and cognition.[31]

Omega-3 Supplements Omega-3 fatty acids are available in capsules of fish oil supplements, although routine supplementation is not recommended. High intakes of omega-3 polyunsaturated fatty acids may increase bleeding time, interfere with wound healing, raise LDL cholesterol, and suppress immune function.[32] Such findings reinforce the concept that too much of a good thing can sometimes be harmful.[33] People with heart disease, however, may benefit from doses greater than can be achieved through diet alone. This paradox reminds us that dietary advice to lower the risk of heart disease may differ from dietary advice to treat patients with heart disease.[34] Because high intakes of omega-3 fatty acids can cause excessive bleeding, supplements should be used only under close medical supervision. For those who decide to use fish oil supplements, Figure 5-20 explains how to read the label.

Recommended Intakes of Monounsaturated and Polyunsaturated Fats

The 20 to 35 percent of kcalories from fat recommendation provides for the essential fatty acids—linoleic acid and linolenic acid—and Adequate Intakes (AI)

> **FIGURE 5-20 How to Read a Fish Oil Supplement Label**

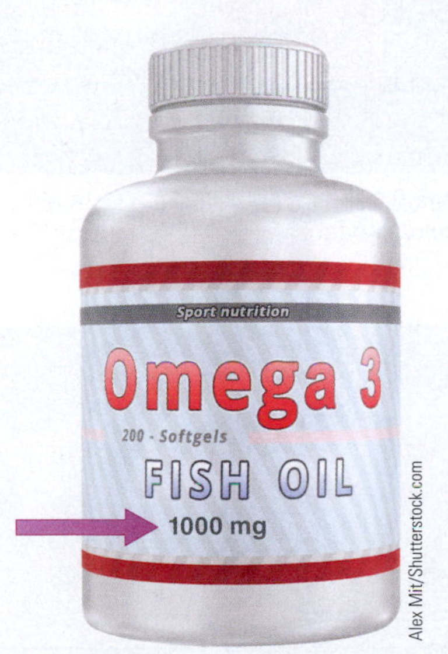

Sport nutrition
Omega 3
200 - Softgels
FISH OIL
1000 mg
Alex Mit/Shutterstock.com

Notice that this supplement offers 1000 mg of fish oil concentrate per capsule, but the oils offering the most health benefits are EPA and DHA. That information is in the Supplement Facts panel on the back.

Supplement Facts
Serving Size: 1 Softgel
Servings Per Container: 120

	Amount Per Serving	% Daily Value
Calories	10	*
Total Fat	1	2%
Saturated Fat	0.5 g	3%
Trans Fat	0g	*
Polyunsaturated Fat	0.5g	*
Monounsaturated Fat	0 g	*
Cholesterol	5 mg	2%
Omega-3 Fatty Acids	300 mg	*
EPA (Eicosapentaenoic Acid)	180 mg	*
DHA (Docosahexaenoic Acid)	120 mg	*

* Daily Value not established.

Notice that one capsule of this supplement offers 180 mg of EPA and 120 mg of DHA, for a total of 300 mg of omega-3 oils—not 1000 mg. The recommended intake for omega-3 fatty acids is 500 mg per day. For heart health, consumers may need more, perhaps 2 to 4 grams (2000 to 4000 mg) per day.

have been established for these two fatty acids (see the inside front cover for details). The DRI suggest that linoleic acid provide 5 to 10 percent of the daily energy intake and linolenic acid 0.6 to 1.2 percent. No DRI have been established for the long-chain omega-3 fatty acids EPA or DHA.[35]

From Guidelines to Groceries Fats accompany protein in foods derived from animals such as meat, seafood, poultry, milk, and eggs, and fats accompany carbohydrate in foods derived from some plants such as avocados and coconuts. Fats carry with them the four fat-soluble vitamins—A, D, E, and K—together with many of the compounds that give foods their flavor, texture, and palatability. Fat is responsible for the delicious aromas associated with sizzling bacon, hamburgers on the grill, onions being sautéed, and vegetables in a stir-fry. The essential oils of many spices are fat-soluble. Of course, these wonderful characteristics lure people into eating too much from time to time. With careful selections, a diet can support good health and still meet fat recommendations.

As the photos in Figure 5-21 show, fat accounts for much of the energy in foods, and removing the fat from foods cuts energy and saturated fat intakes dramatically. To reduce dietary fat, eliminate fat as a seasoning and in cooking; remove the fat from high-fat foods; replace high-fat foods with low-fat alternatives; and emphasize whole grains, fruits, and vegetables. How To 5-1 suggests additional heart-healthy choices by food group.

In general, except for seafood, animal fats tend to have a higher proportion of saturated fatty acids. Except for the tropical oils, plant foods tend to have a higher proportion of monounsaturated and polyunsaturated fatty acids. Consumers can find an abundant array of fresh, unprocessed foods that are naturally low in saturated fat and *trans* fat. In addition, many familiar foods have been processed to

> **FIGURE 5-21 Cutting Fat Cuts kCalories—and Saturated Fat**

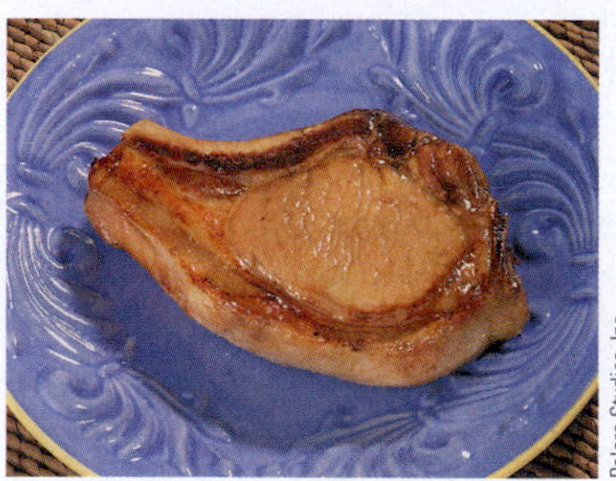
Polara Studios, Inc.

Pork chop with fat (340 kcal, 19 g fat, 7 g saturated fat)

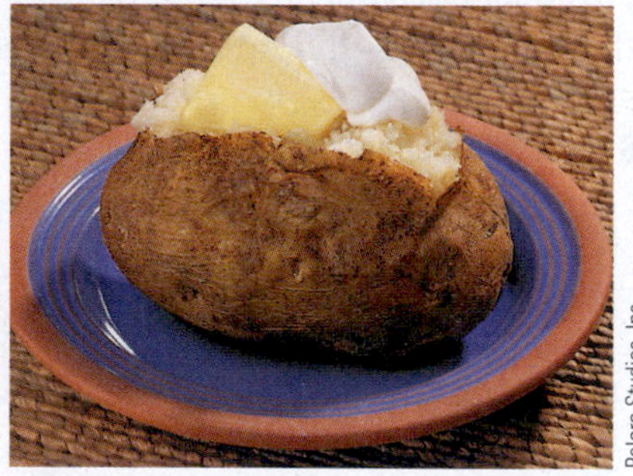
Polara Studios, Inc.

Potato with 1 tbs butter and 1 tbs sour cream (350 kcal, 14 g fat, 10 g saturated fat)

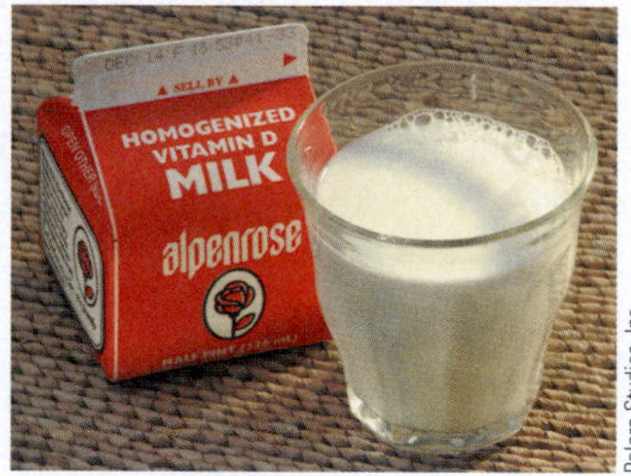
HOMOGENIZED
VITAMIN D
MILK
alpenrose
Polara Studios, Inc.

Whole milk, 1 c (150 kcal, 8 g fat, 5 g saturated fat)

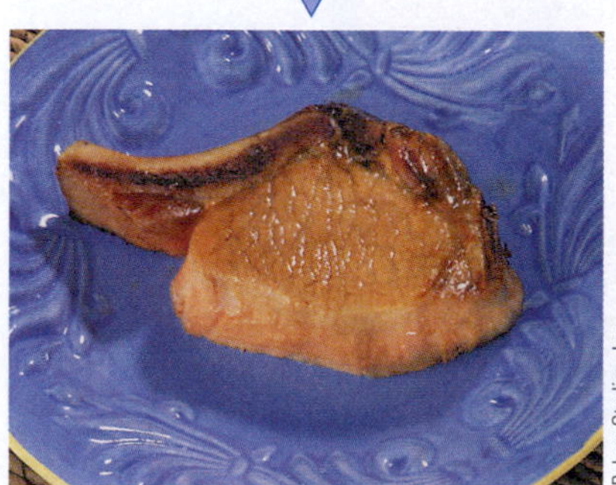
Polara Studios, Inc.

Pork chop with fat trimmed off (230 kcal, 9 g fat, 3 g saturated fat)

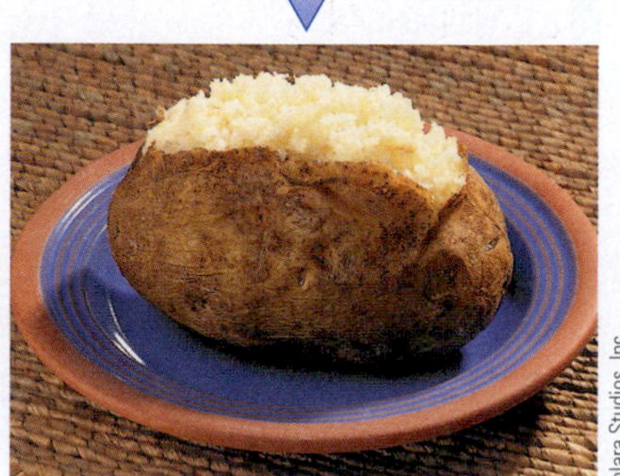

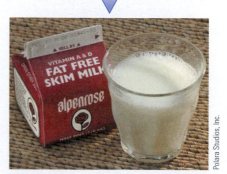
Polara Studios, Inc.

Plain potato (200 kcal, <1 g fat, 0 g saturated fat)

VITAMIN A & D
FAT FREE
SKIM MILK
alpenrose
Polara Studios, Inc.

Fat-free milk, 1 c (90 kcal, <1 g fat, <1 g saturated fat)

Savings:
110 kcal, 10 g fat, 4 g saturated fat

Savings:
150 kcal, 13 g fat, 10 g saturated fat

Savings:
60 kcal, 7 g fat, 4 g saturated fat

>How To 5-1 Make Heart-Healthy Choices—by Food Group

In General

- Select the most nutrient-dense foods from all food groups.
- Consume fewer and smaller portions of foods and beverages that contain solid fats.
- Check the Nutrition Facts label to choose foods with little or no saturated fat and no *trans* fat.

Grains

- Select breads, cereals, and crackers that are low in saturated and *trans* fat (for example, bagels instead of croissants).
- Prepare pasta with a tomato sauce instead of a cheese or cream sauce.
- Limit intake of cookies, doughnuts, pastries, and croissants.

Vegetables and Fruits

- Enjoy the natural flavor of steamed or roasted vegetables (without butter) for dinner and fruits for dessert.
- Eat at least two vegetables (in addition to a salad) with dinner.
- Snack on raw vegetables or fruits instead of high-fat items like potato chips.
- Buy frozen vegetables without sauce.

Milk and Milk Products

- Switch from whole milk to reduced-fat, from reduced-fat to low-fat, and from low-fat to fat-free (nonfat).
- Use fat-free and low-fat cheeses (such as part-skim ricotta and low-fat mozzarella) instead of regular cheeses.
- Use fat-free or low-fat yogurt or sour cream instead of regular sour cream.
- Use evaporated fat-free milk instead of cream.
- Enjoy fat-free frozen yogurt, sherbet, or ice milk instead of ice cream.

Protein Foods

- Fat adds up quickly, even with lean meat; limit intake to about 6 ounces (cooked weight) daily.
- Eat at least two servings of fish per week (particularly fish such as mackerel, lake trout, herring, sardines, and salmon).
- Choose fish, poultry, or lean cuts of pork or beef; look for unmarbled cuts named *round* or *loin* (eye of round, top round, bottom round, round tip, tenderloin, sirloin, center loin, and top loin).
- Trim the fat from pork and beef; remove the skin from poultry.
- Grill, roast, broil, bake, stir-fry, stew, or braise meats; don't fry. When possible, place food on a rack so that fat can drain.
- Use lean ground turkey or lean ground beef in recipes; brown ground meats without added fat, then drain off fat.
- Select tuna, sardines, and other canned meats packed in water; rinse oil-packed items with hot water to remove much of the fat.
- Fill kabob skewers with lots of vegetables and slivers of meat; create main dishes and casseroles by combining a little meat, fish, or poultry with some pasta or rice, and a lot of vegetables.
- Use legumes often.
- Eat a meatless meal or two daily.
- Use egg substitutes in recipes instead of whole eggs or use two egg whites in place of each whole egg.

Fats and Oils

- Use small amounts of vegetable oils in place of solid fats.
- Use butter or stick margarine sparingly; select soft margarines instead of hard margarines.
- When selecting margarine, look for soft (liquid or tub) instead of hard (stick), $\leq$2 g saturated fat, liquid vegetable oil (not hydrogenated or partially hydrogenated) as the first ingredient, and "*trans*-fat free."
- Use fruit butters, reduced-kcalorie margarines, or butter replacers instead of butter.
- Use low-fat or fat-free mayonnaise and salad dressing instead of regular.
- Limit use of lard and meat fat.
- Limit use of products made with coconut oil, palm kernel oil, and palm oil (read labels on bakery goods, processed foods, popcorn oils, and nondairy creamers).
- Reduce use of hydrogenated shortenings and stick margarines and products that contain them (read labels on crackers, cookies, and other commercially prepared baked goods); use vegetable oils instead.

Miscellaneous

- Use a nonstick pan or coat the pan lightly with vegetable oil.
- Refrigerate soups and stews; when the fat solidifies, remove it before reheating.
- Use wine; lemon, orange, or tomato juice; herbs; spices; fruits; or broth instead of butter or margarine when cooking.
- Stir-fry in a small amount of oil; add moisture and flavor with broth, tomato juice, or wine.
- Use variety to enhance enjoyment of the meal: vary colors, textures, and temperatures—hot cooked versus cool raw foods—and use garnishes to complement food.
- Omit high-fat meat gravies and cheese sauces.
- Order pizzas with lots of vegetables, a little lean meat, and half the cheese.

> TRY IT Compare the total kcalories, grams of fat, and percent kcalories from fat for 1 cup of whole milk, reduced-fat milk, low-fat milk, and nonfat milk.

TABLE 5-6 Fat Options among the Protein Foods

Very lean options	Chicken (white meat, no skin) Cod, flounder, trout, tuna (canned in water) Legumes
Lean options	Beef or pork "round" or "loin" cuts Chicken (dark meat, no skin) Herring, salmon, tuna (canned in oil)
Medium-fat options	Ground beef Eggs Tofu
High-fat options	Bacon, hot dogs, luncheon meats, sausage Peanut butter Nuts

provide less saturated and *trans* fat. For example, saturated fat is removed by skimming milk or trimming meats. Manufacturers can use fat-free milk in creamy desserts and lean meats in frozen entrées. Sometimes manufacturers simply prepare the products differently. For example, potato chips may be baked instead of fried. Such choices make healthy eating easy.

Protein Foods The fats in seafood, nuts, and seeds are considered oils, whereas the fats in meat and poultry are considered solid fats. Because these meats provide high-quality protein and valuable vitamins and minerals, however, they can be included in a healthy diet if a person makes lean choices (see Table 5-6), prepares them using the suggestions outlined in How To 5-1 (p. 153), and eats small portions. When preparing meat, fish, or poultry, consider grilling, baking, or broiling, but not frying. Fried fish does not benefit heart disease; fried fish from fast-food restaurants and frozen fried fish products are often low in omega-3 fatty acids and high in *trans*- and saturated fatty acids.

Table 5-4 (p. 150) includes sources of omega-3 and omega-6 fatty acids, and Table 5-7 sorts fish and seafood by their quantity of omega 3 fatty acids. Fatty fish are among the best sources of omega-3 fatty acids, and Highlight 5 features their role in supporting heart health. The American Heart Association recommends eating at least two servings of fish a week, with an emphasis on fatty fish (salmon, herring, and mackerel, for example). Fish provides many minerals (except iron) and vitamins. Because fish is leaner than most other animal-protein sources it can help with weight-loss efforts. The combination of losing weight and eating fish improves blood lipids even more effectively than can be explained by either the weight loss or the omega-3 fats of the fish. Chapter 19 discusses the adverse consequences of mercury, an environmental contaminant common in some fish; in general, mercury is relatively high in tilefish (also called golden snapper or golden bass), swordfish, king mackerel, and shark and relatively low in cod, haddock, pollock, salmon, sole, tilapia, and most shellfish. Most healthy

TABLE 5-7 Omega 3 Fatty Acids in Fish and Seafood

3.5-oz serving	
500 mg	European sea bass (bronzini), herring (Atlantic and Pacific), mackerel, oysters (Pacific wild), salmon (wild and farmed), sardines, toothfish (includes Chilean sea bass), trout (wild and farmed)
150–500 mg	Black bass, catfish (wild and farmed), clams, cod (Atlantic), crab (Alaskan king), croakers, flounder, haddock, hake, halibut, oysters (eastern and farmed), perch, scallops, shrimp (mixed varieties), sole, swordfish, tilapia (farmed)
<150 mg	Cod (Pacific), grouper, lobster, mahi mahi, monkfish, red snapper, skate, triggerfish, tuna, wahoo

people who eat two servings of fish a week can maximize the health benefits while incurring minimal risks. Nonfish sources of omega-3 fatty acids such as flaxseed may have less benefit.

Recall that cholesterol is found in all foods derived from animals. Consequently, eating fewer meats, eggs, and milk products helps lower dietary cholesterol intake (as well as total and saturated fat intakes). Most foods that are high in cholesterol are also high in saturated fat, but eggs are an exception. An egg contains only 1 gram of saturated fat but has a little more than 200 milligrams of cholesterol—roughly two-thirds of the previous cholesterol recommendation, which explains why people fighting heart disease were told to limit their egg consumption. For most people, however, eating eggs does not increase the risk of heart disease.[36] In fact, the *2015 Dietary Guidelines* concluded that there is no appreciable relationship between the consumption of *dietary* cholesterol and *blood* cholesterol or heart disease.

Eggs are a valuable part of the diet because they are inexpensive, useful in cooking, and a source of high-quality protein, other nutrients, and phytochemicals. To help consumers improve their omega-3 fatty acid intake, hens fed flaxseed, fish oil, or marine algae produce eggs rich in omega-3 fatty acids (up to 200 milligrams per egg). Including even one enriched egg in the diet daily can significantly increase a person's intake of omega-3 fatty acids. Food manufacturers have produced several fat-free, cholesterol-free egg substitutes.

TABLE 5-8 Fat Options among Milk and Milk Products

Fat-free and low-fat options	Fat-free (skim) or 1% (low-fat) milk or yogurt (plain)
Reduced-fat options	2% milk or yogurt (plain)
High-fat options	Whole milk, yogurt Most cheeses

Milk and Milk Products Like meats, milk and milk products should also be selected with an awareness of their saturated fat contents (see Table 5-8). Keep in mind that the fat in milk is considered a solid fat; it is apparent as butter, but less so when suspended in homogenized milk. Fat-free and low-fat milk products provide as much or more protein, calcium, and other nutrients as their whole-milk versions—but with little or no saturated fat. Selecting fermented milk products, such as yogurt, may also help to lower blood cholesterol. These foods increase the population and activity of bacteria in the colon that use cholesterol. Interestingly, cheese does not seem to raise LDL cholesterol as its saturated fat content might predict, perhaps because its calcium promotes fat excretion in the GI tract. Such findings serve as a reminder to focus more on foods and eating patterns than on individual nutrients.

Vegetables, Fruits, and Grains Most vegetables and fruits naturally contain little or no fat. Although avocados and olives are exceptions, most of their fat is unsaturated, which is not harmful to heart health; in fact, avocados can significantly improve blood lipids as can olives and their oils (see Highlight 5).[37] Most grains contain only small amounts of fat. Consumers need to read food labels carefully, though, because many refined grain products such as fried taco shells, croissants, and biscuits are high in saturated fat, and pastries, crackers, and cookies may contain *trans* fats. Similarly, many people add butter, margarine, or cheese sauce to grains and vegetables, which raises the saturated- and *trans*-fat contents. Because fruits are often eaten without added fat, a diet that includes several servings of fruit daily can help a person meet the dietary recommendations for fat.

A diet rich in vegetables, fruits, whole grains, and legumes also offers abundant vitamin C, folate, vitamin A, vitamin E, and dietary fiber—all important in supporting health. Consequently, such a diet protects against disease by reducing saturated fat as well as by increasing nutrients. It also provides valuable phytochemicals, which help defend against heart disease.

Solid Fats and Oils Solid fats include the fats in meat and poultry (as in poultry skin, luncheon meats, and sausage); the fats in whole milk, cheeses, and butter; shortening (as in fried foods and baked goods); and hard margarines. Because solid fats deliver an abundance of saturated fatty acids, they are considered discretionary kcalories. The fats of fish, nuts, and vegetable oils are *not* counted as discretionary kcalories because they provide valuable omega-3 fatty acids, essential fatty acids, and vitamin E. When discretionary kcalories are available, they may be used to add fats in cooking or at the table or to select higher fat items from the food groups.

Some solid fats, such as butter and the fat trimmed from meat, are easy to see. Others—such as the fat that "marbles" a steak or is hidden in foods such as cheese—are less apparent and can be present in foods in surprisingly high amounts. Any *fried* food contains abundant solid fats—potato chips, french fries, fried wontons, and fried fish. Many *baked* goods, too, are high in solid fats—pie crusts, pastries, crackers, biscuits, cornbread, doughnuts, sweet rolls, cookies, and cakes.

Reports on *trans*-fatty acids raise the question whether margarine or butter is a better choice for heart health. The American Heart Association has stated that because both the saturated fat of butter and the *trans* fat of hard stick margarine can raise blood cholesterol and contribute to heart disease, the best choices are soft margarines (liquid or tub). Soft margarines are less hydrogenated and relatively lower in *trans*-fatty acids; consequently, they do not raise blood cholesterol as much as the saturated fats of butter or the *trans* fats of hard (stick) margarines do. Read labels to determine how much *trans* fat a margarine contains. Many manufacturers are now offering nonhydrogenated margarines that are "*trans*-fat free." In addition, manufacturers have developed margarines fortified with plant sterols that lower blood cholesterol. (Highlight 13 explores these and other functional foods designed to support health.) Whichever you decide to use, remember to use them sparingly.

Read Food Labels Current food labels list total fat, saturated fat, *trans* fat, and cholesterol contents of foods. Because each package provides information for a single serving and because serving sizes are standardized, consumers can easily compare similar products.

Total fat, saturated fat, and cholesterol are also expressed as "% Daily Values" for a person consuming 2000 kcalories. Using 35 percent of energy intake as the guideline for fat, the Daily Value is 78 grams of fat; using 10 percent for saturated fat, the Daily Value is 20 grams of saturated fat. The Daily Value for cholesterol is 300 milligrams regardless of energy intake. There is no Daily Value for *trans* fat, but consumers should try to keep intakes as low as possible and within the 10 percent allotted for saturated fat. People who consume more or less than 2000 kcalories daily can calculate their personal Daily Value for fat as described in How To 5-2.

Be aware that the "% Daily Value" for fat is not the same as "% kcalories from fat." This important distinction is explained in How To 5-3. Because recommendations apply to average daily intakes rather than individual food items, updated food labels will no longer provide "% kcalories from fat." Still, you can get an idea of whether a particular food is high or low in fat.

Fat Replacers Some foods are made with **fat replacers**—ingredients that provide some of the taste and texture of fats, but with fewer kcalories. Because the body may digest and absorb some of these fat replacers, they may contribute energy, although significantly less energy than fat's 9 kcalories per gram.

Some fat replacers are derived from carbohydrate, protein, or fat. Carbohydrate-based fat replacers are used primarily as thickeners or stabilizers in foods such as soups and salad dressings. Protein-based fat replacers provide a creamy feeling in the mouth and are often used in foods such as ice creams and yogurts. Fat-based replacers act as emulsifiers and are heat stable, making them most versatile in shortenings used in cake mixes and cookies.

Fat replacers offering the sensory and cooking qualities of fats but none of the kcalories are called **artificial fats.** A familiar example of an artificial fat that has been approved for use in snack foods such as potato chips, crackers, and tortilla chips is **olestra.** Olestra's chemical structure is similar to that of a triglyceride but with important differences. A triglyceride is composed of a glycerol molecule with three fatty acids attached, whereas olestra is made of a sucrose molecule

fat replacers: ingredients that replace some or all of the functions of fat and may or may not provide energy.

artificial fats: zero-energy fat replacers that are chemically synthesized to mimic the sensory and cooking qualities of naturally occurring fats but are totally or partially resistant to digestion.

olestra: a synthetic fat made from sucrose and fatty acids that provides 0 kcalories per gram; also known as *sucrose polyester.*

> How To 5-2 Calculate a Personal Daily Value for Fat

The % Daily Value for fat on food labels is based on 78 grams. To know how your intake compares with this recommendation, you can either count grams until you reach 78 or add the "% Daily Values" until you reach 100 percent—if your energy intake is 2000 kcalories a day. If your energy intake is more or less, you can calculate your personal daily fat allowance in grams. Suppose your energy intake is 1800 kcalories per day and your goal is 30 percent kcalories from fat. Multiply your total energy intake by 30 percent, then divide by 9:

$$1800 \text{ total kcal} \times 0.30 \text{ from fat} = 540 \text{ fat kcal}$$
$$540 \text{ fat kcal} \div 9 \text{ kcal/g} = 60 \text{ g fat}$$

(In familiar measures, 60 grams of fat is about the same as ⅔ stick of butter or ¼ cup of oil.)

The accompanying table shows the numbers of grams of fat allowed per day for various energy intakes. With one of these numbers in mind, you can quickly evaluate the number of fat grams in foods you are considering eating.

Energy (kcal/day)	20% kCal from Fat	35% kCal from Fat	Fat (g/day)
1200	240	420	27–47
1400	280	490	31–54
1600	320	560	36–62
1800	360	630	40–70
2000	400	700	44–78
2200	440	770	49–86
2400	480	840	53–93
2600	520	910	58–101
2800	560	980	62–109
3000	600	1050	67–117

> TRY IT Calculate a personal daily fat allowance for a person with an energy intake of 2100 kcalories and a goal of 25 percent kcalories from fat.

with six to eight fatty acids attached. Enzymes in the digestive tract cannot break the bonds of olestra, so unlike sucrose or fatty acids, olestra passes through the digestive system unabsorbed.

The FDA's evaluation of olestra's safety addressed two questions. First, is olestra toxic? Research on both animals and human beings supports the safety of

> How To 5-3 Understand "% Daily Value" and "% kCalories from Fat"

The "% Daily Value" that is used on food labels to describe the amount of fat in a food is not the same as the "% kcalories from fat" that is used in dietary recommendations to describe the amount of fat in the diet. They may appear similar, but their difference is worth understanding. Consider, for example, a piece of lemon meringue pie that provides 140 kcalories and 12 grams of fat. Because the Daily Value for fat is 78 grams for a 2000-kcalorie intake, 12 grams represent about 18 percent:

$$12 \text{ g} \div 78 \text{ g} = 0.15$$
$$0.15 \times 100 = 15\%$$

The pie's "% Daily Value" is 15 percent of the day's fat allowance.

Uninformed consumers may mistakenly believe that this food meets recommendations to limit fat to "20 to 35 percent kcalories," but it doesn't—for two reasons. First, the pie's 12 grams of fat contribute 108 of the 140 kcalories, for a total of 77 percent kcalories from fat:

$$12 \text{ g fat} \times 9 \text{ kcal/g} = 108 \text{ kcal}$$
$$108 \text{ kcal} \div 140 \text{ kcal} = 77\%$$

Second, the "percent kcalories from fat" guideline applies to a day's total intake, not to an individual food. Of course, if every selection throughout the day exceeds 35 percent kcalories from fat, you can be certain that the day's total intake will, too.

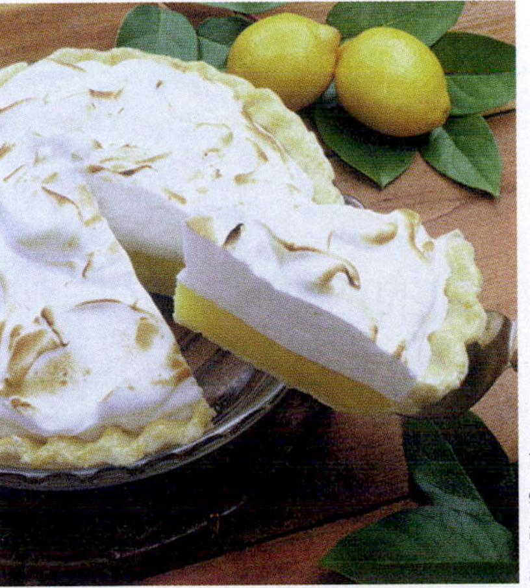
PhotoDisc/Getty Images

Whether a person's energy and fat allowance can afford a piece of a lemon meringue pie depends on the other food and activity choices made that day.

> TRY IT Calculate the percent Daily Value and the percent kcalories from fat for ½ cup frozen yogurt that provides 115 kcalories and 4 grams of fat.

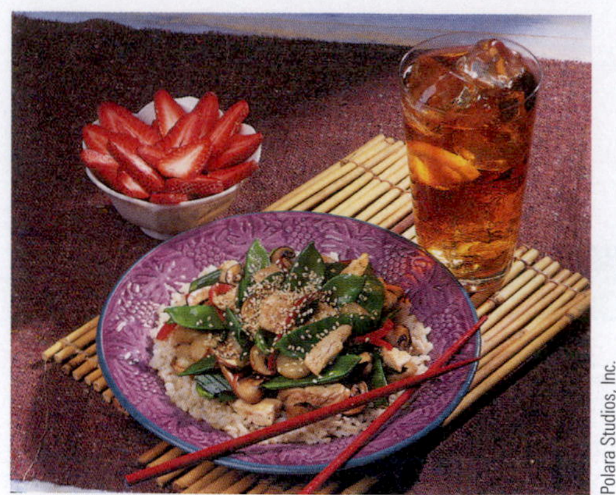

Polara Studios, Inc.

> **PHOTO 5-6** Well-balanced, healthy meals provide some fat with an emphasis on monounsaturated and polyunsaturated fats.

olestra as a partial replacement for dietary fats and oils, with no reports of cancer or birth defects. Second, does olestra affect either nutrient absorption or the health of the digestive tract? When olestra passes through the digestive tract unabsorbed, it binds with some of the fat-soluble vitamins—A, D, E, and K—and carries them out of the body, robbing the person of these valuable nutrients. To compensate for these losses, the FDA requires manufacturers to fortify olestra with vitamins A, D, E, and K. Saturating olestra with these vitamins does not make the product a good source of vitamins, but it does block olestra's ability to bind with the vitamins from other foods. An asterisk in the ingredients list informs consumers that these added vitamins are "dietarily insignificant."

Consumers need to keep in mind that low-fat and fat-free foods still deliver kcalories. Alternatives to fat can help lower energy intake and support weight loss only when they actually *replace* fat and energy in the diet.

REVIEW IT Explain the relationships between monounsaturated and polyunsaturated fats and health, noting recommendations.

Some fat in the diet has health benefits, especially the monounsaturated and polyunsaturated fats that protect against heart disease and possibly cancer. For this reason, *Dietary Guidelines* recommend replacing saturated fats with unsaturated fats, particularly the omega-3 polyunsaturated fatty acids from foods such as fatty fish, not from supplements. Many selection and preparation strategies can help bring these goals within reach, and food labels help identify foods consistent with these guidelines.

Perhaps the best advice for consumers regarding fat in the diet would be to replace saturated fat with unsaturated fat (see Photo 5-6). Sometimes these choices can be difficult, though, because fats make foods taste delicious. To maintain good health, must a person give up all high-fat foods forever—never again to eat marbled steak, hollandaise sauce, or gooey chocolate cake? Not at all. These foods bring pleasure to a meal and can be enjoyed as part of a healthy diet when eaten occasionally in small quantities; but they should not be everyday foods. The key dietary principle for fat is *moderation*, not *deprivation*. Appreciate the energy and enjoyment that fat provides, but take care not to exceed your needs.

What's Online

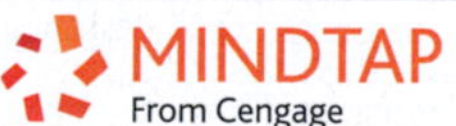
MINDTAP
From Cengage

Visit **www.cengagebrain.com** to access MindTap, a complete digital course that includes Diet & Wellness Plus, interactive quizzes, videos, and more.

REFERENCES

1. S. K. Gebauer and coauthors, Vaccenic acid and *trans* fatty acid isomers from partially hydrogenated oil both adversely affect LDL cholesterol: A double-blind, randomized controlled trial, *American Journal of Clinical Nutrition* 102 (2015): 1339–1346; R. Ganguly and G. N. Pierce, The toxicity of dietary trans fats, *Food and Chemical Toxicology* 78 (2015): 170–176; P. Nestel, Trans fatty acids: Are its cardiovascular risks fully appreciated? *Clinical Therapeutics* 36 (2014): 315–321; A. H. Lichtenstein, Dietary trans fatty acids and cardiovascular disease risk: Past and present, *Current Atherosclerosis Reports* 16 (2014): 433.
2. H. S. Moon, Biological effects of conjugated linoleic acid on obesity-related cancers, *Chemico-Biological Interactions* 224C (2014): 189–195.
3. D. S. Mackay and coauthors, Lathosterol-to-cholesterol ratio in serum predicts cholesterol-lowering response to plant sterol consumption in a dual-center, randomized single-blind placebo-controlled trial, *American Journal of Clinical Nutrition* 101 (2015): 432–439.
4. V. A. Cortes and coauthors, Physiological and pathological implications of cholesterol, *Frontiers in Bioscience* 19 (2014): 416–428.
5. A. Steingoetter and coauthors, Imaging gastric structuring of lipid emulsions and its effect on gastrointestinal function: A randomized trial in healthy subjects, *American Journal of Clinical Nutrition* 101 (2015): 714–724.
6. S. Dash and coauthors, New insights into the regulation of chylomicron production, *Annual Review of Nutrition* 35 (2015): 265–294.
7. D. Saleheen and coauthors, Association of HDL cholesterol efflux capacity with incident coronary heart disease events: A prospective case-control study, *Lancet Diabetes and Endocrinology* 3 (2015): 507–513.
8. W. Annema and A. von Eckardstein, High-density lipoproteins: Multifunctional but vulnerable protections from atherosclerosis, *Circulation* 77 (2013): 2432–2448.
9. A. Rodriguez and coauthors, Revisiting the adipocyte: A model for integration of cytokine signaling in the regulation of energy metabolism, *American Journal of Physiology: Endocrinolgy and Metabolism* 309 (2015): E691–E714.

10. S. Rajaram, Health benefits of plant-derived α-linolenic acid, *American Journal of Clinical Nutrition* 100 (2014): 443S-448S; P. C. Calder, Mechanisms of action of (n-3) fatty acids, *Journal of Nutrition* 142 (2012): 592S–599S.
11. M. Dessi and coauthors, Atherosclerosis, dyslipidemia, and inflammation: The significant role of polyunsaturated fatty acids, *ISRN Inflammation* (2013): 191823; E. Scorletti and C. D. Byrne, Omega-3 fatty acids, hepatic lipid metabolism, and nonalcoholic fatty liver disease, *Annual Review of Nutrition* 33 (2013): 231–248; W. Raphael and L. M. Sordillo, Dietary polyunsaturated fatty acids and inflammation: The role of phospholipid biosynthesis, *International Journal of Molecular Sciences* 14 (2013): 21167–21188; C. Fan, H. Zirpoli, and K. Qi, n-3 Fatty acids modulate adipose tissue inflammation and oxidative stress, *Current Opinions in Clinical Nutrition and Metabolic Care* 16 (2013): 124–132.
12. S. Marventano and coauthors, A review of recent evidence in human studies of n-3 and n-6 PUFA intake on cardiovascular disease, cancer, and depressive disorders: Does the ratio really matter? *International Journal of Food Sciences and Nutrition* 66 (2015): 611–622.
13. A. Caron, D. Richard, and M. Laplante, The roles of mTOR complexes in lipid metabolism, *Annual Review of Nutrition* 35 (2015): 321–348.
14. T. Ulven and E. Christiansen, Dietary fatty acids and their potential for controlling metabolic diseases through activation of FFA4/GPR120, *Annual Review of Nutrition* 35 (2015): 239–263.
15. Position of the Academy of Nutrition and Dietetics: Dietary fatty acids for healthy adults, *Journal of the Academy of Nutrition and Dietetics* 114 (2014): 136–153.
16. I. A. Brouwer, A. J. Wanders, and M. B. Katan, Trans fatty acids and cardiovascular health: Research completed? *European Journal of Clinical Nutrition* 67 (2013): 541–547; J. N. Kiage and coauthors, Intake of trans fat and all-cause mortality in the Reasons for Geographical and Racial Differences in Stroke (REGARDS) cohort, *American Journal of Clinical Nutrition* 97 (2013): 1121–1128; F. Imamura and coauthors, Novel circulating fatty acid patterns and risk of cardiovascular disease: The Cardiovascular Health Study, *American Journal of Clinical Nutrition* 96 (2012): 1252–1261.
17. J. N. Kiage and coauthors, Intake of trans fat and all-cause mortality in the Reasons for Geographical and Racial Differences in Stroke (REGARDS) cohort, *American Journal of Clinical Nutrition* 97 (2013): 1121–1128.
18. K. D. Brownell and J. L. Pomeranz, The trans-fat ban—Food regulation and long-term health, *New England Journal of Medicine* 370 (2014): 1773–1775; F. O. Otite and coauthors, Trends in trans fatty acids reformulations of US supermarket and brand-name foods from 2007 through 2011, *Preventing Chronic Disease* 10 (2013): 120198; W. H. Dietz and K. S. Scanlon, Eliminating the use of partially hydrogenated oil in food production and preparation, *Journal of the American Medical Association* 308 (2012): 143–144; I. Rahkovsky, S. Martinez, and F. Kuchler, *New Food Choices Free of Trans Fats Better Align US Diets with Health Recommendations*, EIB-95, US Department of Agriculture, Economic Research Service, April 2012.
19. A. Baylin, Secular trends in trans fatty acids: Decreased trans fatty acids in the food supply are reflected in decreased *trans* fatty acids in plasma, *American Journal of Clinical Nutrition* 97 (2013): 665–666.
20. M. M. H. Abdullah, P. J. H. Jones, and P. K. Eck, Nutrigenetics of cholesterol metabolism: Observational and dietary intervention studies in the postgenomic era, *Nutrition Reviews* 73 (2015): 523–543; S. Berger and coauthors, Dietary cholesterol and cardiovascular disease: A systematic review and meta-analysis, *American Journal of Clinical Nutrition* 102 (2015): 276–294.
21. D. J. McNamara, Dietary cholesterol, heart disease risk and cognitive dissonance, *Proceedings of the Nutrition Society* 73 (2014): 161–66.
22. U.S. Department of Health and Human Services and US Department of Agriculture, *2015–2020 Dietary Guidelines for Americans*, 8th ed. (2015), http://health.gov/dietaryguidelines/2015/guidelines.
23. US Department of Agriculture, Agricultural Research Service, 2014, Energy Intakes: Percentages of energy from protein, carbohydrate, fat, and alcohol, *What We Eat in American*, NHANES 2011–2012, www.ars.usda.gov.
24. Position of the American Dietetic Association, Dietitians of Canada, and the American College of Sports Medicine: Nutrition and athletic performance, *Journal of the American Dietetic Association* 100 (2000): 1543–1556.
25. U. Schwab and coauthors, Effect of the amount and type of dietary fat on cardiometabolic risk factors and risk of developing type 2 diabetes, cardiovascular diseases, and cancer: A systematic review, *Food and Nutrition Research* 58 (2014): 25145.
26. M. C. de Oliveira Otto and coauthors, Circulating and dietary omega-3 and omega-6 polyunsaturated fatty acids and incidence of CVD in the Multi-Ethnic Study of Atherosclerosis, *Journal of the American Heart Association* 2 (2013): e000506.
27. T. A. Mori, Dietary *n*-3 PUFA and CVD: A review of the evidence, *Proceedings of the Nutrition Society* 73 (2014): 57–4.
28. L. C. Del Gobbo and coauthors, ω-3 Polyunsaturated fatty acid biomarkers and coronary heart disease, *JAMA Internal Medicine* 176 (2016): 1155–1166.
29. A. Hidaka and coauthors, Fish, n-3 PUFA consumption, and pancreatic cancer risk in Japanese: A large, population-based, prospective cohort study, *American Journal of Clinical Nutrition* 102 (2015): 1490–1497; T. M. Brasky and coauthors, Long-chain ω-3 fatty acid intake and endometrial cancer risk in the Women's Health Initiative, *American Journal of Clinical Nutrition* 101 (2015): 824–834; K. Jing, T. Wu, and K. Lim, Omega-3 polyunsaturated fatty acids and cancer, *Anticancer Agents in Medicinal Chemistry* 13 (2013): 1162-1177; M. Azrad, C. Turgeon, and W. Denmark-Wahnefried, Current evidence linking polyunsaturated fatty acids with cancer risk and progression, *Frontiers in Oncology* 3 (2013): 224; K. Jing, T. Wu, and K. Lim, Omega-3 polyunsaturated fatty acids and cancer, *Anticancer Agents in Medicinal Chemistry* 13 (2013): 1162–1177; J. Zheng and coauthors, Intake of fish and marine n-3 polyunsaturated fatty acids and risk of breast cancer: Meta-analysis of data from 21 independent prospective cohort studies, *British Medical Journal* 346 (2013): f3706; K. He and coauthors, Types of fish consumed and fish preparation methods in relation to pancreatic cancer incidence: The VITAL Cohort Study, *American Journal of Epidemiology* 177 (2013): 152–160.
30. V. Oskarsson and coauthors, Fish consumption and risk of non-gallstone-related acute pancreatitis: A prospective cohort study, *American Journal of Clinical Nutrition* 101 (2015): 72–80; D. Di Giuseppe and coauthors, Long-term intake of dietary long-chain n-3 polyunsaturated fatty acids and risk of rheumatoid arthritis: A prospective cohort study of women, *Annals of Rheumatic Diseases* 73 (2014): 1949–1953.
31. K. Yurko-Mauro, D. D. Alexander, and M. E. Van Elswyk, Docosahexaenoic acid and adult memory: A systematic review and meta-analysis, *PLoS One* 10 (2015): e0120391.
32. Fish oil supplements, *Journal of the American Medical Association* 312 (2014): 839; J. I. Fenton and coauthors, Immunomodulation by dietary long chain omega-3 fatty acids and the potential for adverse health outcomes, *Prostaglandins, Leukotrienes, and Essential Fatty Acids* 89 (2013): 379–390.
33. B. S. Peskin, Why fish oil fails: A comprehensive 21st century lipids-based physiologic analysis, *Journal of Lipids* 2014 (2014): 495761.
34. B. Heydari and coauthors, Effect of omega-3 acid ethyl esters on left ventricular remodeling after acute myocardial infarction, *Circulation* 134 (2016): 378–391; M. van Bilsen and A. Planavila, Fatty acids and cardiac disease: Fuel carrying a message, *Acta Physiologica* 211 (2014): 476–490; L. G. Gao and couauthors, Influence of omega-3 polyunsaturated fatty acid-supplementation on platelet aggregation in humans: A meta-analysis of randomized controlled trials, *Atherosclerosis* 226 (2013): 328–334; B. J. McEwen and coauthors, Effects of omega-3 polyunsaturated fatty acids on platelet function in healthy subjects and subjects with cardiovascular disease, *Seminars in Thrombosis and Hemostasis* 39 (2013): 25–32.
35. M. R. Flock, W. S. Harris, and P. M. Kris-Etherton, Long-chain omega-3 fatty acids: Time to establish a dietary reference intake, *Nutrition Reviews* 71 (2013): 692–707.
36. S. C. Larsson, A. Akesson, and A. Wolk, Egg consumption and risk of heart failure, myocardial infarction, and stroke: Results from 2 prospective cohorts, *American Journal of Clinical Nutrition* 102 (2015): 1007–1013; N. R. Fuller and coauthors, The effect of a high-egg diet on cardiovascular risk factors in people with type 2 diabetes: The Diabetes and Egg (DIABEGG) study—A 3-mo randomized controlled trial, *American Journal of Clinical Nutrition* 101 (2015): 705–713.
37. S. Peou and coauthors, Impact of avocado-enriched diets on plasma lipoproteins: A meta-analysis, *Journal of Clinical Lipidology* 10 (2016): 161–171.

LEARN IT Identify which fats support health and which impair it.

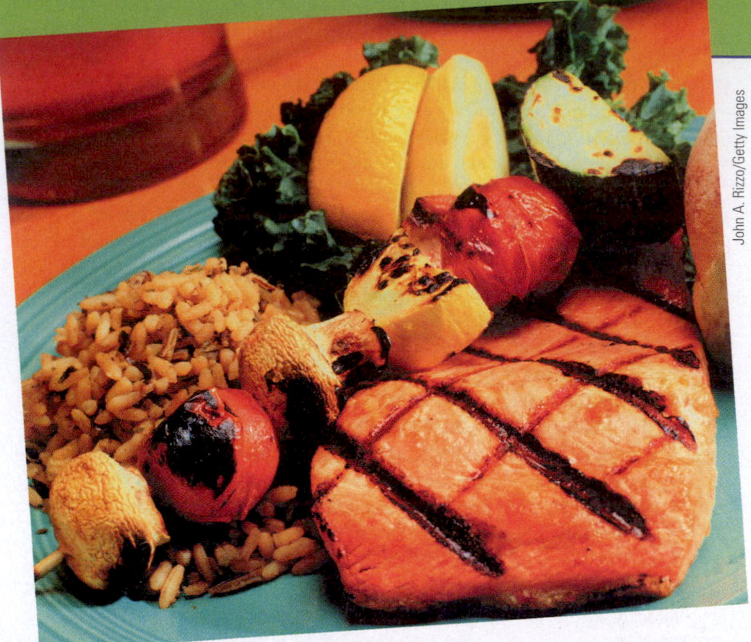
John A. Rizzo/Getty Images

High-Fat Foods—Friend or Foe?

Eat less fat. Eat more fatty fish. Give up butter. Use margarine. Give up margarine. Use olive oil. Steer clear of saturated. Seek out omega-3. Stay away from *trans*. Stick with monounsaturated and polyunsaturated. Keep fat intake moderate. Don't worry about total fat or dietary cholesterol. Today's fat messages seem to be forever multiplying and changing. No wonder some people feel confused about dietary fat. The confusion stems in part from the complexities of fat and in part from the nature of recommendations. As this chapter explains, "dietary fat" refers to several kinds of fats. Some fats support health whereas others impair it, and foods typically provide a mixture of fats in varying proportions. Researchers have spent decades sorting through the relationships among the various kinds of fat and their roles in supporting or harming health. Translating these research findings into dietary recommendations is challenging. Too little information can mislead consumers, but too much detail can overwhelm them. As research findings accumulate, recommendations slowly evolve and become more refined. Fortunately, that's where we are with fat recommendations today—refining them from the general to the specific. Though they may seem to be "forever multiplying and changing," in fact, they are becoming more meaningful.

Fat recommendations grab national headlines from time to time, especially when research studies claim that previous nutrition advice got it all wrong. For example, systematic reviews and meta-analyses recently suggested little or no association between butter and heart disease; no relationship between saturated fat and heart attacks or deaths; and no support for recommendations to increase polyunsaturated, and to decrease saturated, fats.[1] Most scientists were not surprised, nor did they toss all else aside and accept these reports as the final word. As Chapter 1 explained, all research studies are snapshots that need to be considered as part of the whole. Heart disease is complex, encompassing multiple risk factors over many decades. Diet patterns are complex, encompassing dozens of nutrients and hundreds of foods over decades of time. Research methods always need to be questioned and findings examined. How are eating patterns and nutrients measured? When saturated fats are lowered, what nutrients replace them? What endpoints are measured—blood cholesterol, inflammation, hypertension, heart attacks, or death? In the end, all researchers agree that more research is needed; that's just the way science works. Most would also agree that recommendations should focus on eating patterns more than nutrients.[2]

This highlight begins with the dietary guidelines for, and health consequences of, fat. Then it presents the Mediterranean diet, an example of an eating pattern that embraces the heart-healthy fats. It closes with strategies to help consumers choose the right amounts of the right kinds of fats for a healthy diet.

Guidelines for Fat Intake

Dietary guidelines for fat have shifted emphasis from limiting total fat, in general, to lowering saturated and *trans* fat, specifically.[3] Instead of urging people to cut back on all fats, recommendations suggest carefully replacing the "bad" saturated fats with the "good" unsaturated fats and enjoying them in moderation. The goal is to create a diet moderate in kcalories that provides enough of the fats that support good health, but not too much of those that harm health. (Turn to pp. 147–151 for a review of the health consequences of each type of fat.)

With these findings and goals in mind, the Dietary Reference Intakes (DRI) committee suggests a healthy range of 20 to 35 percent of energy intake from fat. This range appears to be compatible with low rates of heart disease, diabetes, obesity, and cancer. Heart-healthy recommendations suggest that within this range, consumers should try to minimize their intakes of saturated fat and *trans* fat and use unsaturated, especially polyunsaturated, fats instead.[4] Replacing saturated fats with monounsaturated fats or carbohydrates from whole grains also lowers the risks of heart disease some, but using carbohydrates from refined starches and added sugars increases risks.[5]

Asking consumers to limit their total fat intake is less than perfect advice, but it is straightforward—find the fat and cut back. Asking consumers to keep their intakes of saturated fats and *trans* fats low and to use monounsaturated and polyunsaturated fats instead is more on target with heart health, but it also makes diet planning a bit more challenging. To make appropriate selections, consumers must first learn which foods contain which fats.

High-Fat Foods and Heart Health

Avocados, bacon, walnuts, potato chips, and mackerel are all high-fat foods, yet some of these foods have detrimental effects on heart health when consumed in excess, whereas others seem neutral or even beneficial. This section presents some of the evidence that helps distinguish which high-fat foods belong in a healthy diet and which ones need to be kept to a minimum. As you will see, fat in the diet can be compatible with heart health, but only if most of it is unsaturated.

Cook with Olive Oil

The traditional diets of countries in the Mediterranean region offer an excellent example of eating patterns that freely use "good" fats. The primary fat in these diets is olive oil, which seems to play a key role in providing health benefits.[6] A classic study of the world's people, the Seven Countries Study, found that death rates from heart disease were strongly associated with diets high in saturated fats but only weakly linked with total fat.[7] In fact, the two regions with the highest fat intakes, Finland and the Greek island of Crete, had the highest (Finland) and lowest (Crete) rates of heart disease deaths. In both countries, the people consumed 40 percent or more of their kcalories from fat. Clearly, a high-fat diet is not the primary problem. When researchers refocused their attention on the *type* of fat, they noticed the benefits of olive oil.

A diet that uses olive oil instead of other fats, especially butter, stick margarine, and meat fats, offers numerous health benefits (see Photo H5-1). Olive oil, canola oil, and other oils rich in monounsaturated fatty acids help protect against heart disease and stroke by lowering blood-clotting factors, blood pressure, and total and LDL cholesterol (but not HDL cholesterol); reducing LDL susceptibility to oxidation; interfering with the inflammatory response; and providing antimicrobial actions.[8]

When compared with other fats, olive oil seems to be a wise choice, but it is not a magic potion; drizzling olive oil on foods does not make them healthier. Its role in a healthy diet is to *replace* the saturated fats. Other vegetable oils, such as canola or safflower oil, are also generally low in saturated fats and high in unsaturated fats. For this reason, heart-healthy diets use these unsaturated vegetable oils to replace the more saturated fats of butter, hydrogenated stick margarine, lard, or shortening. (Remember that the tropical oils—coconut, palm, and palm kernel—are too saturated to be included with the heart-healthy vegetable oils.)

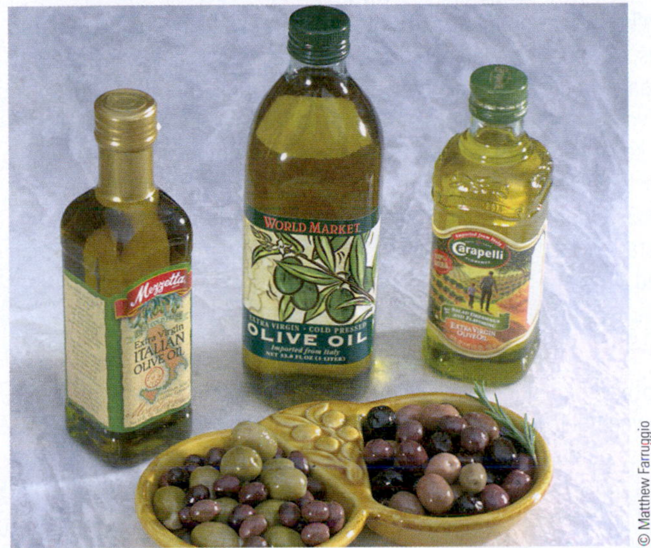
WORLD MARKET
OLIVE OIL
Carapelli
ITALIAN OLIVE OIL
© Matthew Farruggio

> **PHOTO H5-1** Olives and their oil may benefit heart health.

Nibble on Nuts

Tree nuts and peanuts are traditionally excluded from low-fat diets. Nuts provide up to 80 percent of their kcalories from fat, and a quarter cup (about an ounce) of mixed nuts provides more than 200 kcalories. Frequent nut consumption, however, correlates with lower risk of mortality and chronic diseases, such as diabetes and heart disease.[9] Benefits are seen for a variety of nuts commonly eaten in the United States: almonds, Brazil nuts, cashews, hazelnuts, macadamia nuts, pecans, pistachios, walnuts, and even peanuts. On average, these nuts contain mostly monounsaturated fat (59 percent), some polyunsaturated fat (27 percent), and little saturated fat (14 percent). Nuts also provide valuable fiber, vegetable protein, vitamin E, minerals, and phytochemicals.

Including nuts may be a wise diet strategy against heart disease (see Photo H5-2). Nuts may protect against heart disease by lowering blood cholesterol and blood pressure, and by limiting oxidative stress and inflammation. Some research suggests that a diet that includes nuts may benefit other diseases as well.

Because most of the energy nuts provide comes from fats, they deliver many kcalories per bite. Incorporating nuts in the diet, however, does not necessarily lead to weight gains and may even help with weight control by providing satiety.[10] Consumers can enjoy nuts without increasing total kcalories by using nuts *instead of, not in addition to,* other foods.

Feast on Fish

Interest in the health benefits of the long-chain omega-3 polyunsaturated fatty acids began almost 50 years ago, when researchers reported that the native peoples of Alaska, northern Canada, and Greenland—who eat a traditional diet rich in omega-3 fatty acids, notably EPA (eicosapentaenoic acid) and DHA (docosaheaenoic acid)—had a remarkably low rate of heart disease even though their diets were high in fat. More recently, a review of this early study

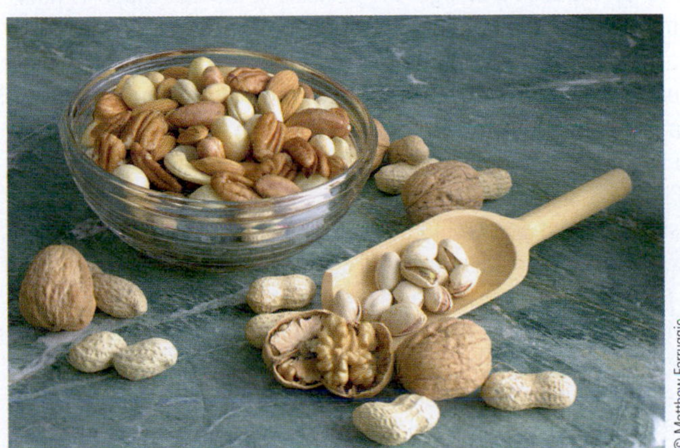
© Matthew Farruggio

> **PHOTO H5-2** For heart health, snack on a few nuts instead of potato chips.

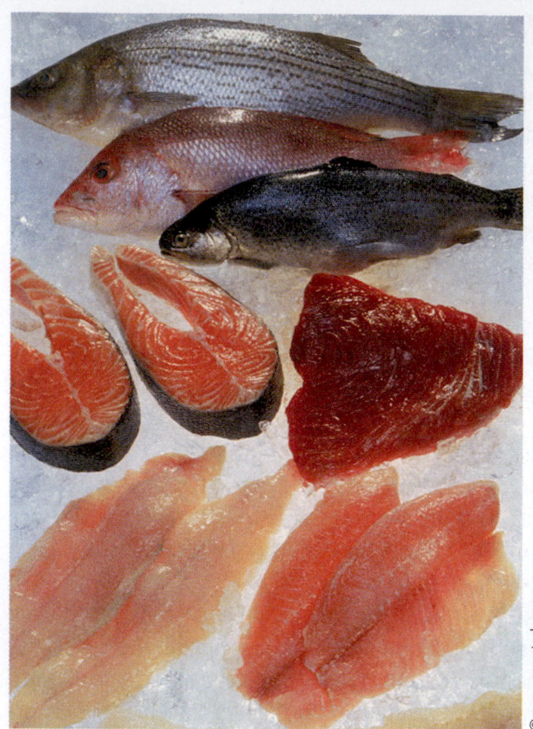
© www.comstock.com

> PHOTO H5-3 Fish is a good source of the omega-3 fatty acids.

revealed that the prevalence of heart disease among these people was not carefully investigated, and therefore the original premise was faulty.[11] The traditional dietary pattern associated with these native people may raise blood cholesterol slightly, but it is not associated with heart disease risk.[12] Decades of research has confirmed that omega-3 fatty acids help protect against heart disease by reducing blood triglycerides, blood pressure, resting heart rate, and inflammation; stabilizing plaque; and serving as precursors to eicosanoids. For people with hypertension or atherosclerosis, these actions can be lifesaving.

Because increasing omega-3 fatty acids in the diet supports heart health and lowers the rate of deaths from heart disease, the American Heart Association recommends including fish in a heart-healthy diet. Consumers in the United States currently receive only about one-third of the 8-ounce weekly recommendation of seafood. People who eat some fish each week can lower their risks of heart attack and stroke (see Photo H5-3).

Fish is the best source of EPA and DHA in the diet, but it is also a source of mercury, an environmental contaminant. Most fish contain at least trace amounts of mercury, but some have especially high levels. For this reason, the FDA advises pregnant and lactating women, women of childbearing age who may become pregnant, and young children to include fish in their diets, but to avoid tilefish (also called golden snapper or golden bass), swordfish, king mackeral, marlin, and shark. They are also advised to limit average weekly consumption of a variety of ocean fish and shellfish to 12 ounces (cooked or canned) and white (albacore) tuna to 6 ounces (cooked or canned). Commonly eaten seafood relatively low in mercury include shrimp, catfish, pollock, salmon, and canned light tuna.

In addition to the direct toxic effects of mercury, some research suggests that mercury may diminish the health benefits of omega-3 fatty acids. Such findings serve as a reminder that our health depends on a healthy environment. (Chapter 19 discusses the adverse consequences of mercury, and Chapter 20 presents the relationships between diet and the environment in more detail.)

High-Fat Foods and Heart Disease

The number-one dietary determinant of LDL cholesterol is saturated fat. Each 1 percent increase in energy from saturated fatty acids in the diet produces a 2 percent jump in heart disease risk by elevating LDL cholesterol. Conversely, reducing saturated fat intake by 1 percent can be expected to produce a 2 percent drop in heart disease risk by the same mechanism. Even a 2 percent drop in LDL represents a significant improvement for heart health. Like saturated fats, *trans* fats also raise heart disease risk by elevating LDL cholesterol. A heart-healthy diet limits foods rich in these two types of fat.

Limit Fatty Meats, Whole-Milk Products, and Tropical Oils

The major sources of saturated fats in the US diet are fatty meats, whole milk, tropical oils, and products made from any of these foods. To limit saturated fat intake, consumers must choose carefully among these high-fat foods. More than a third of the fat in most meats is saturated. Similarly, more than half of the fat is saturated in whole milk and other high-fat milk products, such as cheese, butter, cream, half-and-half, cream cheese, sour cream, and ice cream. The tropical oils of palm, palm kernel, and coconut, which are rarely used by consumers in the kitchen, are used heavily by food manufacturers, and are commonly found in many commercially prepared foods.

When choosing meats, milk products, and commercially prepared foods, look for those lowest in saturated fat. Labels help consumers to compare products.

Even with careful selections, a nutritionally adequate diet will provide some saturated fat. Zero saturated fat is not possible even when experts design menus with the mission to keep saturated fat as low as possible. Because most saturated fats come from animal foods, vegetarian diets can, and usually do, deliver fewer saturated fats than mixed diets.

Limit Hydrogenated Foods

Chapter 5 explained that solid shortening and margarine are made from vegetable oil that has been hardened through hydrogenation. This process both saturates some of the unsaturated fatty acids and introduces *trans*-fatty acids. Many convenience foods contain *trans* fats, including:

- Fried foods such as french fries, chicken, and other commercially fried foods

- Commercial baked goods such as cakes, pie crusts, frozen pizzas, biscuits, muffins, cookies, doughnuts, pastries, breads, and crackers
- Snack foods such as chips
- Imitation cheeses

To keep *trans*-fat intake low, use these foods sparingly.

Table 5-4 (p. 150) summarizes which foods provide which fats. Substituting unsaturated fats for saturated fats at each meal and snack can help protect against heart disease. Figure H5-1 compares two meals and shows how such substitutions can lower saturated fat and raise unsaturated fat—even when total fat and kcalories remain unchanged.

The Mediterranean Diet

The links between good health and traditional Mediterranean eating patterns of the mid-1900s were introduced earlier with regard to olive oil. For people who follow a Mediterranean eating pattern, the incidence of heart disease, some cancers, diabetes, and other chronic inflammatory diseases is low, and life expectancy is high.[13] The health benefits of the Mediterranean eating pattern may be partially explained by its favorable effects on body weight.[14]

Although each of the many countries that border the Mediterranean Sea has its own culture, traditions, and dietary habits, their similarities are much greater than the use of olive oil alone. In fact, no one factor alone can be credited with reducing disease risks—the association holds true only when the overall eating pattern is present. Apparently, each of the foods contributes small benefits that harmonize to produce either a substantial cumulative or synergistic effect.

The Mediterranean eating pattern features fresh, whole foods. The people select crusty breads, whole grains, potatoes, and pastas; a variety of vegetables (including wild greens) and legumes; feta and mozzarella cheeses and yogurt; nuts; and fruits (especially grapes and figs). They eat some fish, other seafood, poultry, a few eggs, and little meat. Along with olives and olive oil, their principal sources of fat are nuts and fish; they rarely use butter or encounter hydrogenated fats. They commonly use herbs and spices instead of salt. Consequently, traditional Mediterranean diets are low in saturated fat and very low in *trans* fat.

Furthermore, they are rich in monounsaturated and polyunsaturated fat, complex carbohydrate and fiber, and nutrients and phytochemicals that support good health.[15] As a result, lipid profiles improve, blood pressure lowers, plaque stabilizes, inflammation diminishes, and the risk of heart disease declines.[16]

> **FIGURE H5-1 Two Meals Compared: Replacing Saturated Fat with Unsaturated Fat**

Examples of ways to replace saturated fats with unsaturated fats include sautéing vegetables in olive oil instead of butter, garnishing salads with avocado and sunflower seeds instead of bacon and blue cheese, and eating salmon instead of steak. Each of these meals provides roughly the same number of kcalories and grams of fat, but the one on the left has almost four times as much saturated fat and only half as many omega-3 fatty acids.

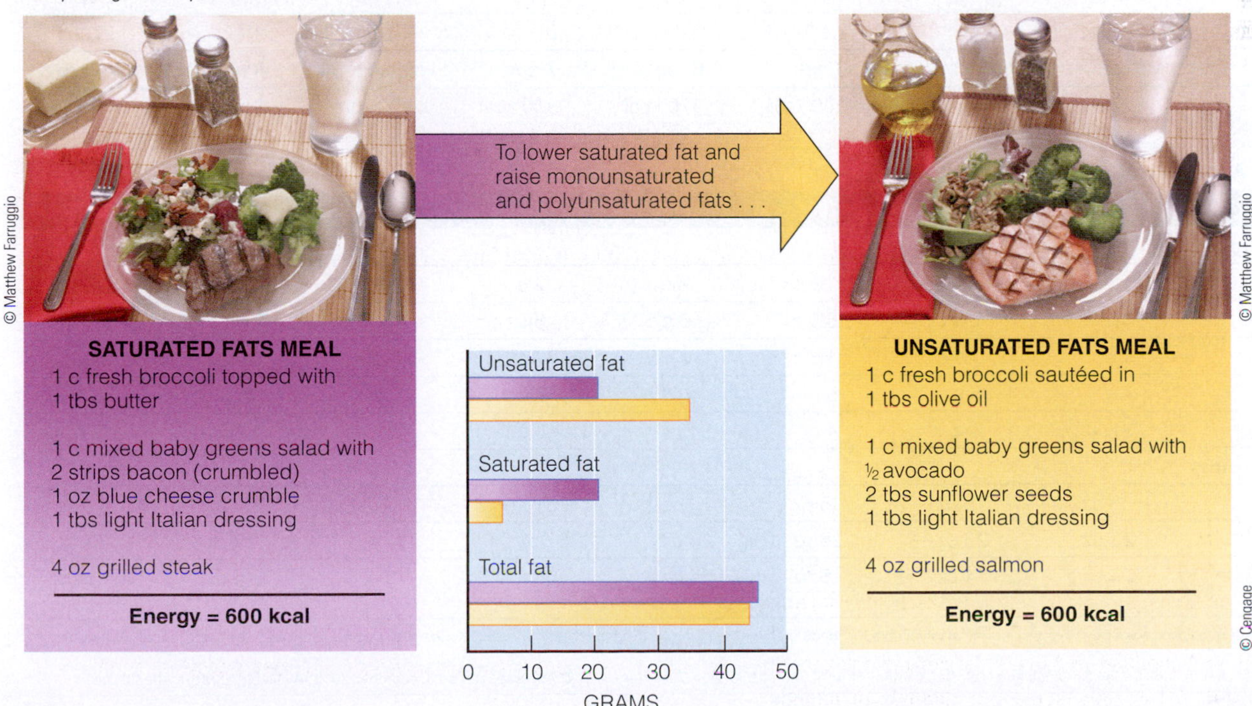
© Matthew Farruggio
To lower saturated fat and raise monounsaturated and polyunsaturated fats . . .
SATURATED FATS MEAL
1 c fresh broccoli topped with
1 tbs butter
1 c mixed baby greens salad with
2 strips bacon (crumbled)
1 oz blue cheese crumble
1 tbs light Italian dressing
4 oz grilled steak
Energy = 600 kcal
Unsaturated fat
Saturated fat
Total fat
0
10
20
30
40
50
GRAMS
UNSATURATED FATS MEAL
1 c fresh broccoli sautéed in
1 tbs olive oil
1 c mixed baby greens salad with
½ avocado
2 tbs sunflower seeds
1 tbs light Italian dressing
4 oz grilled salmon
Energy = 600 kcal
© Matthew Farruggio
© Cengage

People following the traditional Mediterranean diet can receive as much as 40 percent of a day's kcalories from fat, but their limited consumption of milk and milk products and meats provides less than 10 percent from saturated fats. In addition, because the animals in the Mediterranean region pasture-graze, the meat, milk and milk products, and eggs are richer in omega-3 fatty acids than those from animals fed grain.

Other foods typical of the Mediterranean region, such as wild plants and snails, provide omega-3 fatty acids as well. All in all, the traditional Mediterranean diet has earned a reputation for its health benefits as well as its delicious flavors. Consumers need to beware that the typical Mediterranean-style cuisine available in US restaurants, however, has been adjusted to popular tastes. Quite often, these meals are much higher in saturated fats and meats—and much lower in the polyunsaturated fats and vegetables—than the traditional fare. Unfortunately, it appears that people in the Mediterranean region who are replacing some of their traditional dietary habits with those of the United States are losing the health benefits previously enjoyed. Table H5-1 shows the USDA Healthy Mediterranean Eating Pattern, which has more fruits and seafood and fewer milk and milk products than the Healthy US-Style Eating Pattern that Chapter 2 introduced. Figure H5-2 presents a Mediterranean Diet Pyramid. Notice the emphasis on abundant plant foods.

Conclusion

Are some fats "good," and others "bad" from the body's point of view? The saturated and *trans* fats do indeed seem mostly bad for the health of the heart. Aside from providing energy, which unsaturated fats can do equally well, saturated and *trans* fats bring no benefits to the body. Furthermore, no harm can come from consuming diets low in them. Still, some foods rich in these fats are often delicious, giving them an occasional place in the diet. In contrast, the unsaturated fats are mostly good for heart health when consumed in moderation.

TABLE H5-1 USDA Food Patterns: Healthy Mediterranean Eating Pattern

The table first lists recommended amounts from each food group per *day* and then shows the amounts for vegetables and protein foods dispersed among subgroups per *week*. The highlighted rows indicate which food groups and serving sizes differ from the Healthy US-Style Eating Pattern (see Tables 2-3 and 2-4, p. 41).

Recommended Daily Amounts from Each Food Group

Food Group	1600 kcal	1800 kcal	2000 kcal	2200 kcal	2400 kcal	2600 kcal	2800 kcal	3000 kcal
Fruits	2 c	2 c	2½ c	2½ c	2½ c	2½ c	3 c	3 c
Vegetables	2 c	2½ c	2½ c	3 c	3 c	3½ c	3½ c	4 c
Grains	5 oz	6 oz	6 oz	7 oz	8 oz	9 oz	10 oz	10 oz
Protein foods	5½ oz	6 oz	6½ oz	7 oz	7½ oz	7½ oz	8 oz	8 oz
Milk and milk products	2 c	2 c	2 c	2 c	2½ c	2½ c	2½ c	2½ c
Oils	5 tsp	5 tsp	6 tsp	6 tsp	7 tsp	8 tsp	8 tsp	10 tsp
Limit on kcalories available for other uses[a]	140 kcal	160 kcal	260 kcal	270 kcal	300 kcal	330 kcal	350 kcal	430 kcal

Recommended Weekly Amounts from Subgroups

	1600 kcal	1800 kcal	2000 kcal	2200 kcal	2400 kcal	2600 kcal	2800 kcal	3000 kcal
Vegetables Subgroups								
Dark green	1½ c	1½ c	1½ c	2 c	2 c	2½ c	2½ c	2½ c
Red and orange	4 c	5½ c	5½ c	6 c	6 c	7 c	7 c	7½ c
Legumes	1 c	1½ c	1½ c	2 c	2 c	2½ c	2½ c	3 c
Starchy	4 c	5 c	5 c	6 c	6 c	7 c	7 c	8 c
Other	3½ c	4 c	4 c	5 c	5 c	5½ c	5½ c	7 c
Protein Foods Subgroups								
Seafood	11 oz	15 oz	15 oz	16 oz	16 oz	17 oz	17 oz	17 oz
Meats, poultry, eggs	23 oz	23 oz	26 oz	28 oz	31 oz	31 oz	33 oz	33 oz
Nuts, seeds, soy products	4 oz	4 oz	5 oz	5 oz	5 oz	5 oz	6 oz	6 oz

[a]The limit on kcalories for other uses describes how many kcalories are available for foods that are not in nutrient-dense forms; these kcalories may also be referred to as discretionary kcalories (discussed on p. 44).

SOURCE: U.S. Department of Health and Human Services and U.S. Department of Agriculture. *2015–2020 Dietary Guidelines for Americans*. 8th ed. December 2015. Available at https://health.gov/dietaryguidelines/2015/guidelines/.

> **FIGURE H5-2 Mediterranean Diet Pyramid**

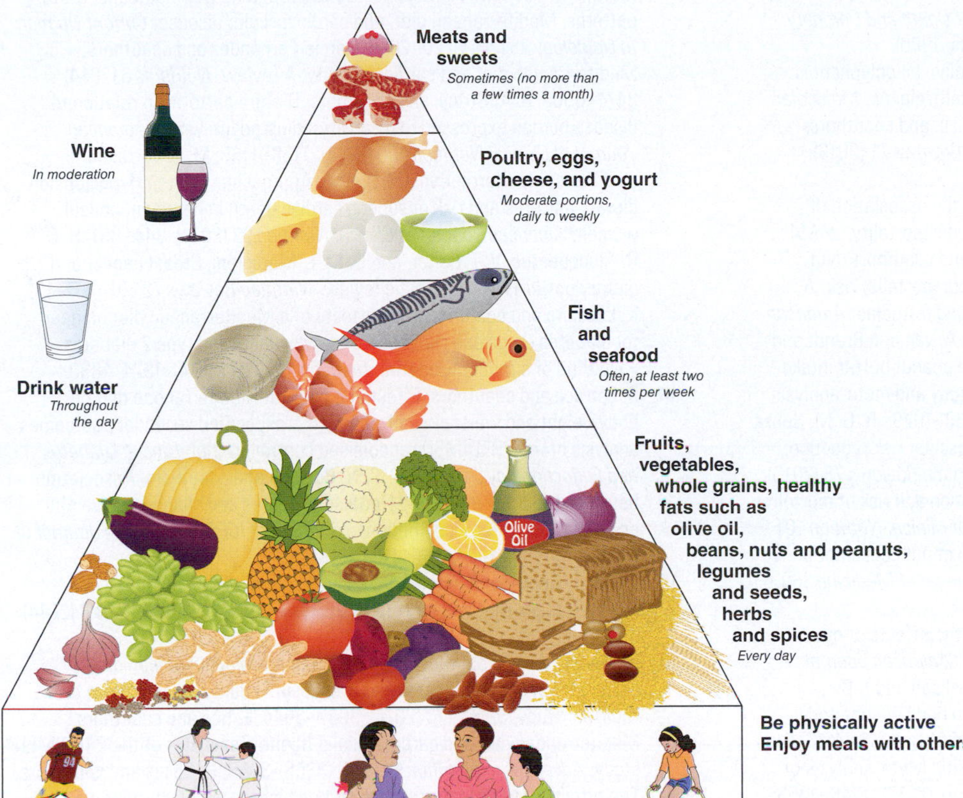
Mediterranean Diet Pyramid
A contemporary approach to delicious, healthy eating
Meats and sweets
Sometimes (no more than a few times a month)
Wine
In moderation
Poultry, eggs, cheese, and yogurt
Moderate portions, daily to weekly
Drink water
Throughout the day
Fish and seafood
Often, at least two times per week
Fruits, vegetables, whole grains, healthy fats such as olive oil, beans, nuts and peanuts, legumes and seeds, herbs and spices
Every day
Olive Oil
Be physically active
Enjoy meals with others

Clearly, different fatty acids have different actions in the body and risks of chronic diseases. When judging foods by their fatty acids, keep in mind that the fat in foods is a mixture of both unsaturated and saturated fatty acids. Even predominantly monounsaturated olive oil delivers some saturated fat. Consequently, even when a person chooses foods with mostly unsaturated fats, saturated fat can still add up if total fat is too high.

Focusing all efforts on simply lowering saturated fat in the diet may be narrow advice for heart health. Including vegetables, fruits, whole grains, and legumes as part of a balanced daily diet is a good idea, as is *replacing* saturated fats such as butter, shortening, and meat fat with unsaturated fats such as olive oil and the oils from nuts and fish.[17] These foods provide beneficial fatty acids, fiber, vitamins, minerals, and phytochemicals as well as little (or no) salt, saturated fat, and *trans* fat—all valuable in protecting the body's health. In addition, take care to select portion sizes that will best meet energy needs. And enjoy some physical activity daily. Remember that even a healthy eating pattern can be detrimental if foods are eaten in excess.

CRITICAL THINKING QUESTIONS

A. What are the features of a healthy high-fat diet?

B. Heart disease is rare among the Inuit people of Alaska who continue to eat their traditional diet of seal meat and blubber. A traditional Nordic diet of game meats, berries, root vegetables, and legumes helps lower blood cholesterol and reduce heart disease risk. People following the traditional Mediterranean diet that emphasizes fruits, vegetables, whole grains, beans, nuts and seeds, and olive oil also enjoy good heart health. How are dietary fats related to heart health? How is it that such diverse diets can have such similar health outcomes?

REFERENCES

1. L. Pimpin and coauthors, Is butter back? A systematic review and meta-analysis of butter consumption and risk of cardiovascular disease, diabetes, and total mortality, *PLoS One* 11 (2016): e0158118; N. G. Puaschitz and coauthors, Dietary intake of saturated fat is not associated with risk of coronary events or mortality in patients with established coronary artery disease, *Journal of Nutrition* 145 (2015): 299–305; R. Chowdhury and coauthors, Association of dietary, circulating, and supplement fatty acids with coronary risk: A systematic review and meta-analysis, *Annals of Internal Medicine* 160 (2014): 398–406.
2. J. A. Nettleton, P. Legrand, and R. P. Mensink, ISSFAL 2014 debate: It is time to update saturated fat recommendation, *Annals of Nutrition and Metabolism* 66 (2015): 104–108.
3. D. Mozaffarian and D. S. Ludwig, The 2015 US Dietary Guidelines lifting the ban on total dietary fat, *Journal of the American Medical Association* 313 (2015): 2421–2422.
4. M. Guasch-Ferré and coauthors, Dietary fat intake and risk of cardiovascular disease and all-cause mortality in a population at high risk of cardiovascular disease, *American Journal of Clinical Nutrition* 102 (2015): 1563–1573; D. D. Wang and coauthors, Association of specific dietary fats with total and cause-specific mortality, *JAMA Internal Medicine* (2016): doi 10.1001/2417; L. Hooper and coauthors, Reduction unsaturated fat intake for cardiovascular disease, *Cochrane Database Systematic Reviews* 6 (2015): CD011737; R. P. Mensink, Effects of saturated fatty acids on serum lipids and lipoproteins: A systematic review and regression analysis, Geneva: World Health Organization, 2016.

5. Y. Li and coauthors, Saturated fats compared with unsaturated fats and sources of carbohydrates in relation to risk of coronary heart disease, *Journal of the American College of Cardiology* 66 (2015): 1538–1548.
6. S. Bulotta and coauthors, Beneficial effects of the olive oil phenolic components oleuropein and hydroxytyrosol: Focus on protection against cardiovascular and metabolic diseases, *Journal of Translational Medicine* 12 (2014): 219.
7. A. Keys, *Seven Countries: A Multivariate Analysis of Death and Coronary Heart Disease* (Cambridge: Harvard University Press, 1980).
8. S. Martin-Paláez and coauthors, Health effects of olive oil polyphenols: Recent advances and possibilities for the use of health claims, *Molecular Nutrition and Food Research* 57 (2013): 760–761; L. Lin and coauthors, Evidence of health benefits of canola oil, *Nutrition Reviews* 71 (2013): 370–385.
9. H. N. Luu and coauthors, Prospective evaluation of the association of nut/peanut consumption with total and cause-specific mortality, *JAMA Internal Medicine* 175 (2015): 755–766; G. Grosso and coauthors, Nut consumption on all-cause, cardiovascular, and cancer mortality risk: A systematic reviewe and meta-analysis of epidemiologic studies, *American Journal of Clinical Nutrition* 101 (2015): 783–793; P. A. van den Brandt and L. J. Schouten, Relationship of tree nut, peanut and peanut butter intake with total and cause-specific mortality: A cohort study and meta-analysis, *International Journal of Epidemiology* 44 (2015): 1038–1049; R. G. M. Souza and coauthors, Nuts and legume seeds for cardiovascular risk reduction: Scientific evidence and mechanisms of action, *Nutrition Reviews* 73 (2015): 335–347; T. T. Hshieh and coauthors, Nut consumption and risk of mortality in the Physicians' Health Study, *American Journal of Clinical Nutrition* 101 (2015): 407–412; Y. Bao and coauthors, Association of nut consumption with total and cause specific mortality, *New England Journal of Medicine* 369 (2013): 2001–2011.
10. S. Y. Tan, J. Dhillion, and R. D. Mattes, A review of the effects of nuts on appetite, food intake, metabolism and body weight; *American Journal of Clinical Nutrition* 100 (2014): 412S–422S; C. L. Jackson and F. B. Hu, Long-term associations of nut consumption with body weight and obesity, *American Journal of Clinical Nutrition* 100 (2014): 408S–411S; G. Flores-Mateo and coauthors, Nut intake and adiposity: Meta-analysis of clinical trials, *American Journal of Clinical Nutrition* 97 (2013): 1346–1355; V. Vadivel, C. N. Kunyanga, and H. K. Biesalski, Health benefits of nut consumption with special reference to body weight control, *Nutrition* 28 (2012): 1089–1097; M. Fogelhom and coauthors, Dietary macronutrients and food consumption as determinants of long-term weight change in adult populations: A systematic literature review, *Food and Nutrition Research* 56 (2012): doi:10.3402.
11. J. G. Fodor and coauthors, "Fishing" for the origins of the "Eskimos and heart disease" story: Facts or wishful thinking? *Canadian Journal of Cardiology* 30 (2014): 864–868.
12. M. Labonté and coauthors, Traditional dietary pattern is associated with elevated cholesterol among the Inuit of Nunavik, *Journal of the Academy of Nutrition and Dietetics* 114 (2014): 1208–1215.
13. T. Y. N. Tong and coauthors, Prospective association of the Mediterranean diet with cardiovascular disease incidence and mortality and its population impact in a non-Mediterranean population: The EPIC-Norfolk study, *BMC Medicine* 14 (2016): 135; H. E. Bloomfield and coauthors, Effects on health outcomes of a Mediterranean diet with no restriction on fat intake: A systematic review and meta-analysis, *Annals of Internal Medicine* 165 (2016): 491–500; M. A. Martinez-Gonzalez and M. Bes-Rasteollo, Dietary patterns, Mediterranean diet, and cardiovascular disease, *Current Opinion in Lipidology* 25 (2014): 20–26; E. Garcia-Fernández and coauthors, Mediterranean diet and cardiodiabesity: A review, *Nutrients* 6 (2014): 3474–3500; E. A. Struijk and coauthors, Dietary patterns in relation to disease burden expressed in disability-adjusted life years, *American Journal of Clinical Nutrition* 100 (2014): 1158–1165; M. L. Bertoia and coauthors, Mediterranean and Dietary Approaches to Stop Hypertension dietary patterns and risk of sudden cardiac death in postmenopausal women, *American Journal of Clinical Nutrition* 99 (2014): 344–351; R. C. R. Albuquerque, V. T. Baltar, and D. M. L. Marchioni, Breast cancer and dietary patterns: A systematic review, *Nutrition Reviews* 72 (2014): 1–17; K. Esposito and coauthors, The effects of a Mediterranean diet on need for diabetes drugs and remission of newly diagnosed type 2 diabetes: Follow-up of a randomized trial, *Diabetes Care* 37 (2014): 1824–1830.
14. R. Estruch and coauthors, Effect of a high-fat Mediterranean diet on bodyweight and waist circumference: A prespecified secondary outcomes analysis of the PREDIMED randomised controlled trial, *Lancet: Diabetes and Endocrinology* (2016): S2213; N. Roswall and coauthors, Association between Mediterranean and Nordic diet scores and changes in weight and waist circumference: Influence of *FTO* and *TCF7L2*, *American Journal of Clinical Nutrition* 100 (2014): 1188–1197.
15. I. Castro-Quezada, B. Román-Viñas, and L. Serra-Majem, The Mediterranean diet and nutritional adequacy: A review, *Nutrients* 6 (2014): 231–248.
16. M. Bonaccio and coauthors, Adherence to the Mediterranean diet is associated with lower platelet and leukocyte counts: Results from the Molisani study, *Blood* 123 (2014): 3037–3044; E. Ros and coauthors, Mediterranean diet and cardiovascular health: Teachings of the PREDIMED study, *Advances in Nutrition* 5 (2014): 330S–336S, R. Casas and coauthors, The effects of the Mediterranean diet on biomarkers of vascular wall inflammation and plaque vulnerability in subjects with high risk for cardiovascular disease: A randomized trial, *PLoS One* 9 (2014): e100084; H. Gardener and coauthors, Mediterranean diet and carotid atherosclerosis in the Northern Manhattan Study, *Atherosclerosis* 234 (2014): 303–310.
17. R. J. de Souza and S. S. Anand, Saturated fat and heart disease, *British Medical Journal* 355 (2016): i6257; Position of the Academy of Nutrition and Dietetics: Dietary fatty acids for healthy adults, *Journal of the Academy of Nutrition and Dietetics* 114 (2014): 136–153.

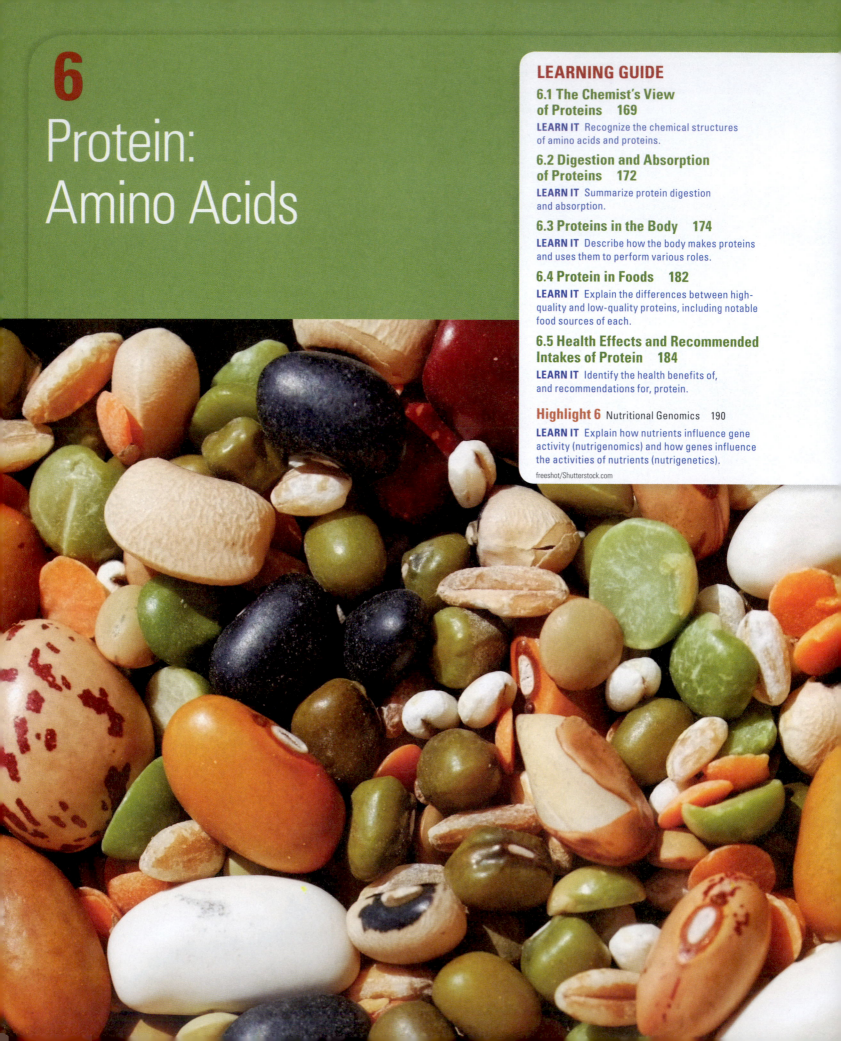

6 Protein: Amino Acids

LEARNING GUIDE

freeshot/Shutterstock.com

Nutrition in Your Life

The versatility of proteins in the body is impressive. They help your muscles contract, your blood to clot, and your eyes to see. They keep you alive and well by facilitating chemical reactions and defending against infections. Without them, your bones, skin, and hair would have no structure. No wonder they were named *proteins,* meaning "of prime importance." Does that mean proteins deserve top billing in your diet as well? Are the best sources of protein beef, beans, or broccoli? Learn which foods will supply you with enough, but not too much, high-quality protein. As you read this chapter, consider whether your diet is meeting your protein needs.

A few misconceptions surround the roles of protein in the body and the importance of protein in the diet. For example, people who associate meat with protein and protein with strength may eat steak to build muscles. Their thinking is only partly correct, however. Protein is a vital structural and working substance in all cells—not just muscle cells. To build strength, muscle cells need physical activity and all the nutrients—not just protein. Furthermore, protein is found in milk, eggs, legumes, and many grains and vegetables—not just meat. By overvaluing protein and overemphasizing meat in the diet, a person may mistakenly crowd out other, equally important nutrients and foods. As this chapter describes the various roles of protein in the body and food sources in the diet, keep in mind that protein is one of many nutrients needed to maintain good health.

6.1 The Chemist's View of Proteins

LEARN IT Recognize the chemical structures of amino acids and proteins.

Chemically, **proteins** contain nitrogen (N) atoms in addition to the same atoms as carbohydrates and lipids—carbon (C), hydrogen (H), and oxygen (O). These nitrogen atoms give the name *amino* (nitrogen-containing) to the amino acids that make the links in the chains of proteins.

Amino Acids All **amino acids** have the same basic structure—a central carbon (C) atom with a hydrogen atom (H), an amino group (NH_2), and an acid group (COOH) attached to it. Remember, however, that carbon atoms must have four bonds, so a fourth attachment is necessary. This fourth site distinguishes each amino acid from the others. Attached to the central carbon at the fourth bond is a distinct atom, or group of atoms, known as the *side group* or *side chain* (see Figure 6-1).

Unique Side Groups The side groups on the central carbon vary from one amino acid to the next, making proteins more complex than either carbohydrates or lipids. A polysaccharide (starch, for example) may be several thousand units long, but each unit is a glucose molecule just like all the others. A protein, on the other hand, is made up of about 20 different amino acids, each with a different side group. Table 6-1 (p. 170) lists the amino acids most common in proteins.

The simplest amino acid, glycine, has a hydrogen atom as its side group. A slightly more complex amino acid, alanine, has an extra carbon with three hydrogen atoms. Other amino acids have more complex side groups (see Figure 6-2, p. 170, for examples). Thus, although all amino acids share a common structure, they differ in size, shape, electrical charge, and other characteristics because of differences in these side groups.

> **FIGURE 6-1 Amino Acid Structure**

All amino acids have a central carbon with an amino group (NH_2), an acid group (COOH), a hydrogen (H), and a side group attached. The side group is a unique chemical structure that differentiates one amino acid from another.

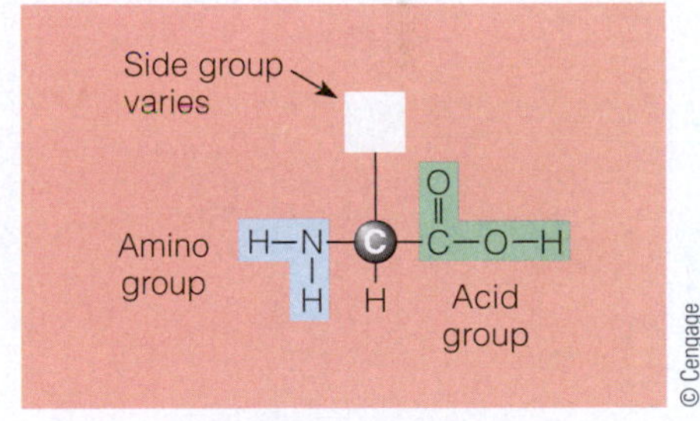
Side group varies
Amino group
H—N—C—C—O—H
H H
O
Acid group

proteins: compounds composed of carbon, hydrogen, oxygen, and nitrogen atoms, arranged into amino acids linked in a chain. Some amino acids also contain sulfur atoms.

amino (a-MEEN-oh) **acids:** building blocks of proteins. Each contains an amino group, an acid group, a hydrogen atom, and a distinctive side group, all attached to a central carbon atom.

- **amino** = containing nitrogen

TABLE 6-1 Amino Acids

Proteins are made up of about 20 common amino acids. The first column lists the *essential amino acids* for human beings (those the body cannot make—that must be provided in the diet). The second column lists the *nonessential amino acids*. In special cases, some nonessential amino acids may become *conditionally essential*. In a newborn, for example, only five amino acids are truly nonessential; the other nonessential amino acids are conditionally essential until the body's metabolic pathways are developed enough to make those amino acids in adequate amounts.

Essential Amino Acids		Nonessential Amino Acids	
Histidine	(HISS-tuh-deen)	Alanine	(AL-ah-neen)
Isoleucine	(eye-so-LOO-seen)	Arginine	(ARJ-ih-neen)
Leucine	(LOO-seen)	Asparagine	(ah-SPAR-ah-geen)
Lysine	(LYE-seen)	Aspartic acid	(ah-SPAR-tic acid)
Methionine	(meh-THIGH-oh-neen)	Cysteine	(SIS-teh-een)
Phenylalanine	(fen-il-AL-ah-neen)	Glutamic acid	(GLU-tam-ic acid)
Threonine	(THREE-oh-neen)	Glutamine	(GLU-tah-meen)
Tryptophan	(TRIP-toe-fan, TRIP-toe-fane)	Glycine	(GLY-seen)
Valine	(VAY-leen)	Proline	(PRO-leen)
		Serine	(SEER-een)
		Tyrosine	(TIE-roe-seen)

NOTE: These 20 amino acids can all be commonly found in proteins. In addition, other amino acids do not occur in proteins but can be found individually (for example, taurine and ornithine). Some amino acids occur in related forms (for example, proline can acquire an OH group to become hydroxyproline).

Nonessential Amino Acids More than half of the amino acids are *nonessential*, meaning that the body can synthesize them for itself. Proteins in foods usually deliver these amino acids, but it is not essential that they do so. The body can make all **nonessential amino acids**, given nitrogen to form the amino group and fragments from carbohydrate or fat to form the rest of the structure.

Essential Amino Acids There are nine amino acids that the human body either cannot make at all or cannot make in sufficient quantity to meet its needs. These nine amino acids must be supplied by the diet; they are *essential*. The first column in Table 6-1 presents the **essential amino acids.** Some researchers refer to essential amino acids as *indispensable* and to nonessential amino acids as *dispensable*.

Conditionally Essential Amino Acids Sometimes a nonessential amino acid becomes essential under special circumstances. For example, the body normally uses the essential amino acid phenylalanine to make tyrosine (a nonessential amino acid). But if the diet fails to supply enough phenylalanine, or if the body cannot make the conversion for some reason (as happens in the inherited disease phenylketonuria, described in Highlight 6), then tyrosine becomes a **conditionally essential amino acid.**

> **FIGURE 6-2 Examples of Amino Acids**

Note that all amino acids have a common chemical structure but that each has a different side group. Appendix C presents the chemical structures of the 20 amino acids most common in proteins.

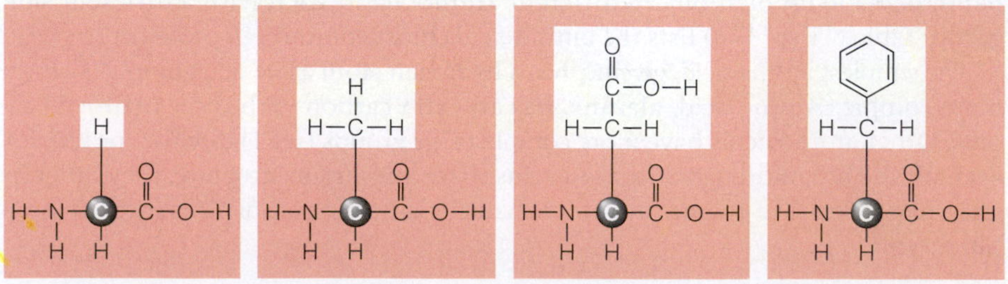

H
H–N–C–C–O–H
H H
Glycine
H
H–C–H
H–N–C–C–O–H
Alanine
O
C–O–H
H–C–H
H–N–C–C–O–H
Aspartic acid
H–C–H
H–N–C–C–O–H
Phenylalanine

nonessential amino acids: amino acids that the body can make (see Table 6-1); also called *dispensable amino acids*.

essential amino acids: amino acids that the body requires but cannot make, and so must be obtained from the diet (see Table 6-1); also called *indispensable amino acids*.

conditionally essential amino acid: an amino acid that is normally nonessential, but must be supplied by the diet in special circumstances when the need for it exceeds the body's ability to make it.

> FIGURE 6-3 Condensation of Two Amino Acids to Form a Dipeptide

H–C–H | H–N–C–C(=O)–O–H | H H — Amino acid + H–N–C–C(=O)–O–H (with H–C–H and benzene ring) — Amino acid → HOH Water → Dipeptide

Amino acid + Amino acid → Dipeptide

An OH group from the acid end of one amino acid and an H atom from the amino group of another join to form a molecule of water.

A peptide bond (highlighted in red) forms between the two amino acids, creating a dipeptide.

© Cengage

Proteins Cells link amino acids end-to-end in a variety of sequences to form thousands of different proteins. A **peptide bond** unites each amino acid to the next.

Amino Acid Chains Condensation reactions connect amino acids, just as they combine two monosaccharides to form a disaccharide and three fatty acids with a glycerol to form a triglyceride. Two amino acids bonded together form a **dipeptide** (see Figure 6-3). By another such reaction, a third amino acid can be added to the chain to form a **tripeptide.** As additional amino acids join the chain, a **polypeptide** is formed. Most proteins are a few dozen to several hundred amino acids long. Figure 6-4 illustrates the protein insulin.

> FIGURE 6-4 Amino Acid Sequence of Human Insulin

Human insulin is a relatively small protein that consists of 51 amino acids in two short polypeptide chains. (For amino acid abbreviations, see Appendix C.) Two bridges link the two chains. A third bridge spans a section within the short chain. Known as *disulfide bridges*, these links form between the cysteine (Cys) amino acids, whose side group contains sulfur (S).

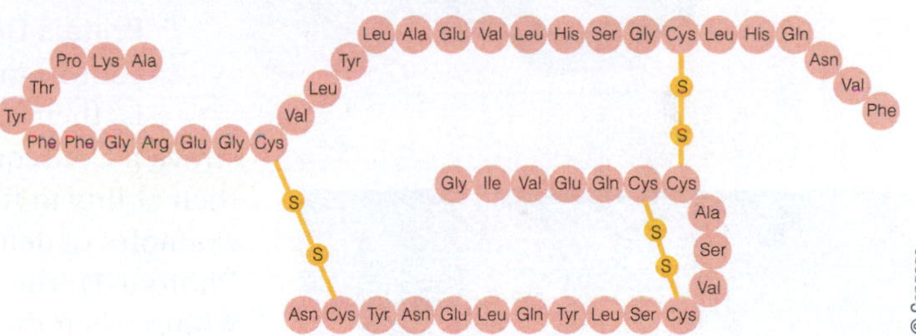

Pro Lys Ala
Thr
Tyr
Phe Phe Gly Arg Glu Gly Cys
Val
Leu
Tyr
Leu Ala Glu Val Leu His Ser Gly Cys Leu His Gln
Asn
Val
Phe
S
S
Gly Ile Val Glu Gln Cys Cys
Ala
Ser
Val
Asn Cys Tyr Asn Glu Leu Gln Tyr Leu Ser Cys
© Cengage

Primary Structure—Amino Acid Sequence The primary structure of a protein is determined by the sequence of amino acids. If a person could walk along a carbohydrate molecule like starch, the first stepping stone would be a glucose. The next stepping stone would also be a glucose, and it would be followed by a glucose, and yet another glucose. But if a person were to walk along a polypeptide chain, each stepping stone would be one of 20 different amino acids. The first stepping stone might be the amino acid methionine. The second might be an alanine. The third might be a glycine, the fourth a tryptophan, and so on. Walking along another polypeptide path, a person might step on a phenylalanine, then a valine, then a glutamine. In other words, amino acid sequences within proteins vary.

The amino acids can act somewhat like the letters in an alphabet. If you had only the letter G, all you could write would be a string of Gs: G–G–G–G–G–G–G. But with 20 different letters available, you can create poems, songs, and novels. Similarly, the 20 amino acids can be linked together in a variety of sequences—even more than are possible for letters in a word or words in a sentence. Thus, the variety of possible sequences for polypeptide chains is tremendous.

Secondary Structure—Polypeptide Shapes The secondary structure of proteins is determined not by chemical bonds as between the amino acids but by weak electrical attractions within the polypeptide chain. As positively charged hydrogens attract nearby negatively charged oxygens, sections of the polypeptide chain twist into a helix or fold into a pleated sheet, for example. These shapes give proteins strength and rigidity.

Tertiary Structure—Polypeptide Tangles The tertiary structure of proteins occurs as long polypeptide chains twist and fold into a variety of complex, tangled shapes. The unique side group of each amino acid gives it characteristics that attract it to, or repel it from, the surrounding fluids and other amino acids. Some amino acid side

peptide bond: a bond that connects the acid end of one amino acid with the amino end of another, forming a link in a protein chain.

dipeptide (dye-PEP-tide)**:** two amino acids bonded together.
- **di** = two
- **peptide** = amino acid

tripeptide: three amino acids bonded together.
- **tri** = three

polypeptide: many (10 or more) amino acids bonded together. A short peptide chain of four to nine amino acids is called an *oligopeptide* (OL-ee-go-PEP-tide).
- **poly** = many
- **oligo** = few

> **FIGURE 6-5 The Structure of Hemoglobin**

The shape of each polypeptide chain is determined by an amino acid sequence (primary structure) that twists into a helix (secondary structure) and bends itself into a ball shape (tertiary structure). Together, the four polypeptide chains make the globular hemoglobin protein (quaternary structure).

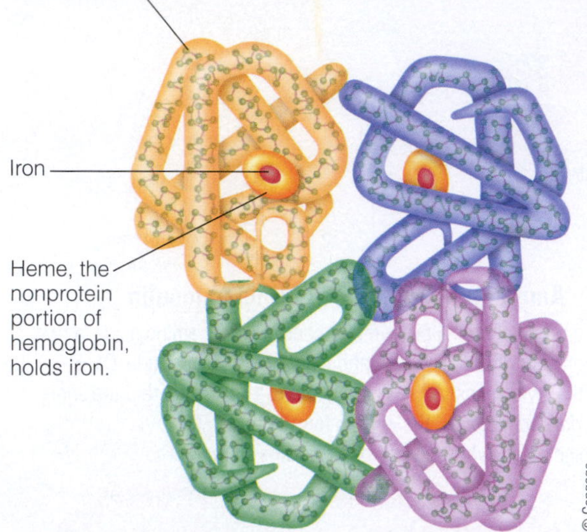
Iron
Heme, the nonprotein portion of hemoglobin, holds iron.
© Cengage

groups are attracted to water molecules; they are *hydrophilic*. Other side groups are repelled by water; they are *hydrophobic*. As amino acids are linked together to make a polypeptide, the chain folds so that its hydrophilic side groups are on the outer surface near water; the hydrophobic groups tuck themselves inside, away from water. Similarly, the disulfide bridges in insulin (see Figure 6-4) determine its tertiary structure. The extraordinary and unique shapes of proteins enable them to perform their various tasks in the body. Some form globular or spherical structures that can carry and store materials within them, and some, such as those of tendons, form linear structures that are more than 10 times as long as they are wide. The intricate shape a protein finally assumes gives it maximum stability.

Quaternary Structure—Multiple Polypeptide Interactions Some polypeptides are functioning proteins just as they are; others need to associate with other polypeptides to form larger working complexes. The quaternary structure of proteins involves the interactions between two or more polypeptides. One molecule of **hemoglobin**—the large, globular protein molecule that, by the billions, packs the red blood cells and carries oxygen—is made of four associated polypeptide chains, each holding the mineral iron. Figure 6-5 features the primary, secondary, tertiary, and quaternary structures of hemoglobin.

Protein Denaturation When proteins are subjected to heat, acid, or other conditions that disturb their stability, they undergo **denaturation**—that is, their quaternary, tertiary, and secondary structures are disrupted or destroyed. Consequently, they uncoil and lose their shapes and, as a result, also lose their ability to function. Past a certain point, denaturation is irreversible. Familiar examples of denaturation include the hardening of an egg when it is cooked (see Photo 6-1), the curdling of milk when acid is added, and the stiffening of egg whites when they are whipped. In the body, proteins are denatured during digestion when they are exposed to stomach acid.

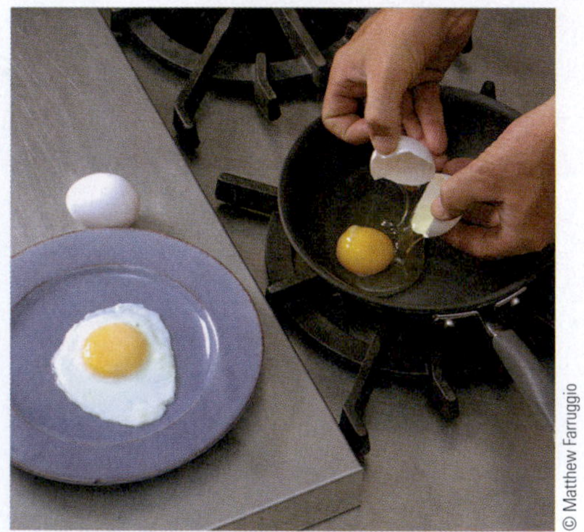
© Matthew Farruggio

> **PHOTO 6-1** Cooking an egg denatures its proteins.

REVIEW IT Recognize the chemical structures of amino acids and proteins.

Chemically speaking, proteins are more complex than carbohydrates or lipids; they are made of some 20 different amino acids, 9 of which the body cannot make (the essential amino acids). Each amino acid contains an amino group, an acid group, a hydrogen atom, and a distinctive side group, all attached to a central carbon atom. Peptide bonds link amino acids together in a series of condensation reactions to create proteins. The distinctive sequence of amino acids in each protein determines its unique shape and function.

6.2 Digestion and Absorption of Proteins

LEARN IT Summarize protein digestion and absorption.

Proteins in foods do not become body proteins directly. Instead, dietary proteins supply the amino acids from which the body makes its own proteins. When a person eats foods containing protein, enzymes break the long polypeptides into short polypeptides, the short polypeptides into tripeptides and dipeptides, and, finally, the tripeptides and dipeptides into individual amino acids.

Protein Digestion

Figure 6-6 illustrates the digestion of protein through the GI tract and includes the names and actions of protein's digestive enzymes. Proteins are crushed and moistened in the mouth, but the real action begins in the stomach.

In the Stomach The major event in the stomach is the partial breakdown (hydrolysis) of proteins. Hydrochloric acid uncoils (denatures) each protein's tangled strands so that digestive enzymes can attack the peptide bonds. The hydrochloric

hemoglobin (HE-moh-GLO-bin): the globular protein of the red blood cells that transports oxygen from the lungs to tissues throughout the body; hemoglobin accounts for 80 percent of the body's iron.
- **hemo** = blood
- **globin** = globular protein

denaturation (dee-NAY-chur-AY-shun): the change in a protein's shape and consequent loss of its function brought about by heat, agitation, acid, base, alcohol, heavy metals, or other agents.

> FIGURE 6-6 Protein Digestion in the GI Tract

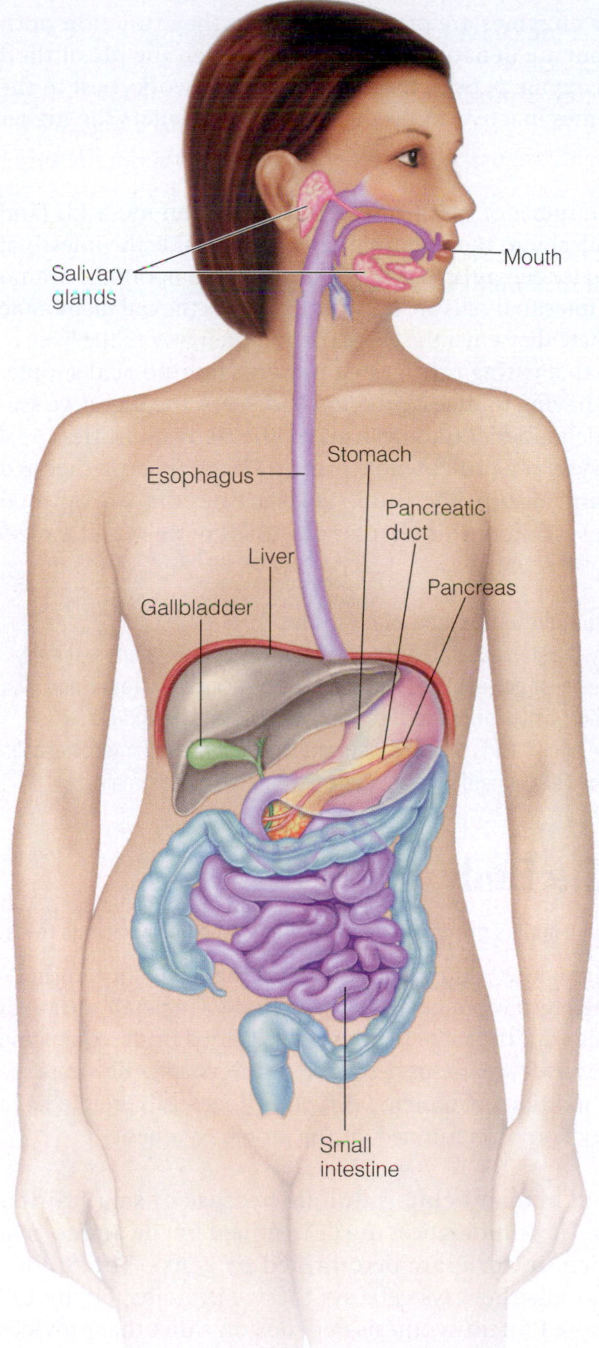
Salivary glands
Mouth
Esophagus
Stomach
Pancreatic duct
Liver
Pancreas
Gallbladder
Small intestine

PROTEIN

Mouth and salivary glands

Chewing and crushing moisten protein-rich foods and mix them with saliva to be swallowed

Stomach

Hydrochloric acid (HCl) uncoils protein strands and activates stomach enzymes:

Protein —(Pepsin, HCl)→ Smaller polypeptides

Small intestine and pancreas

Pancreatic and small intestinal enzymes split polypeptides further:

Polypeptides —(Pancreatic and intestinal proteases)→ Tripeptides, dipeptides, amino acids

Then enzymes on the surface of the small intestinal cells hydrolyze these peptides and the cells absorb them:

Peptides —(Intestinal tripeptidases and dipeptidases)→ Amino acids (absorbed)

HYDROCHLORIC ACID AND THE DIGESTIVE ENZYMES

In the stomach:

Hydrochloric acid (HCl)
- Denatures protein structure
- Activates pepsinogen to pepsin

Pepsin
- Cleaves proteins to smaller polypeptides and some free amino acids
- Inhibits pepsinogen synthesis

In the small intestine:

Enteropeptidase
- Converts pancreatic trypsinogen to trypsin

Trypsin
- Inhibits trypsinogen synthesis
- Cleaves peptide bonds next to the amino acids lysine and arginine
- Converts pancreatic procarboxypeptidases to carboxypeptidases
- Converts pancreatic chymotrypsinogen to chymotrypsin

Chymotrypsin
- Cleaves peptide bonds next to the amino acids phenylalanine, tyrosine, tryptophan, methionine, asparagine, and histidine

Carboxypeptidases
- Cleave amino acids from the acid (carboxyl) ends of polypeptides

Elastase and collagenase
- Cleave polypeptides into smaller polypeptides and tripeptides

Intestinal tripeptidases
- Cleave tripeptides to dipeptides and amino acids

Intestinal dipeptidases
- Cleave dipeptides to amino acids

Intestinal aminopeptidases
- Cleave amino acids from the amino ends of small polypeptides (oligopeptides)

acid also converts the inactive form of the enzyme pepsinogen to its active form, **pepsin.*** Pepsin cleaves proteins into small polypeptides and amino acids.

In the Small Intestine When polypeptides enter the small intestine, several pancreatic and intestinal **proteases** hydrolyze them further into short peptide chains, tripeptides, dipeptides, and amino acids. Then **peptidase** enzymes on the membrane

*The inactive form of an enzyme is called a *proenzyme* or a *zymogen* (ZYE-moh-jen).

pepsin: a gastric enzyme that hydrolyzes protein. Pepsin is secreted in an inactive form, *pepsinogen*, which is activated by hydrochloric acid in the stomach.

proteases (PRO-tee-aces): enzymes that hydrolyze protein.

peptidase: a digestive enzyme that hydrolyzes peptide bonds. *Tripeptidases* cleave tripeptides; *dipeptidases* cleave dipeptides.

- **tri** = three
- **di** = two

surfaces of the intestinal cells split most of the dipeptides and tripeptides into single amino acids. Only a few peptides escape digestion and enter the blood intact.

Remember that digestive enzymes are proteins; as such, they function optimally at their specific pH, but are denatured and digested when the pH of their environment changes. The enzyme pepsin, for example, which works best in the low pH of the stomach becomes inactive and is digested when it enters the higher pH of the small intestine.

Protein Absorption A number of specific carriers transport amino acids (and some dipeptides and tripeptides) into the intestinal cells. Once inside the intestinal cells, amino acids may be used for energy or to synthesize needed compounds. Amino acids that are not used by the intestinal cells are transported across the cell membrane into the surrounding fluid where they enter the capillaries on their way to the liver.

Some consumers believe that eating predigested proteins (amino acid supplements) saves the body from having to digest proteins and keeps the digestive system from "overworking." Such a belief underestimates the body's abilities. As a matter of fact, the digestive system handles whole proteins *better* than predigested ones because it dismantles and absorbs the amino acids at rates that are optimal for the body's use. (The last section of this chapter discusses protein and amino acid supplements further.)

REVIEW IT Summarize protein digestion and absorption.

Digestion is facilitated mostly by the stomach's acid and enzymes, which first denature dietary proteins, then cleave them into smaller polypeptides and some amino acids. Pancreatic and intestinal enzymes split these short polypeptides further, to tripeptides and dipeptides, and then split most of these to single amino acids. Then carriers in the membranes of intestinal cells transport the amino acids into the cells, where they are released into the bloodstream.

6.3 Proteins in the Body

LEARN IT Describe how the body makes proteins and uses them to perform various roles.

The human body has an estimated 20,000 to 25,000 genes that code for hundreds of thousands of proteins. Relatively few proteins have been studied in detail, although this number is growing rapidly with the surge in knowledge gained from sequencing the human genome. The relatively few proteins described in this chapter illustrate the versatility, uniqueness, and importance of proteins. As you will see, each protein has a specific function, and that function is determined during protein synthesis.

Protein Synthesis Each human being is unique because of small differences in the body's proteins. These differences are determined by the amino acid sequences of proteins, which, in turn, are determined by genes. The following paragraphs describe in words the ways cells synthesize proteins; Figure 6-7 provides a pictorial description. Protein synthesis depends on a diet that provides adequate protein and all the essential amino acids.

The instructions for making every protein in a person's body are transmitted by way of the genetic information received at conception. This body of knowledge, which is filed in the DNA (deoxyribonucleic acid) within the nucleus of every cell, never leaves the nucleus.

Delivering the Instructions Transforming the information in DNA into the appropriate sequence of amino acids needed to make a specific protein requires two major steps:

$$\text{DNA} \xrightarrow{\text{transcription}} \text{mRNA} \xrightarrow{\text{translation}} \text{protein.}$$

In the first step, known as **transcription**, a stretch of DNA is used as a template to make messenger RNA (mRNA); in other words, the genetic code is transcribed.

transcription: the process of messenger RNA being made from a template of DNA.

> **FIGURE 6-7 Protein Synthesis**

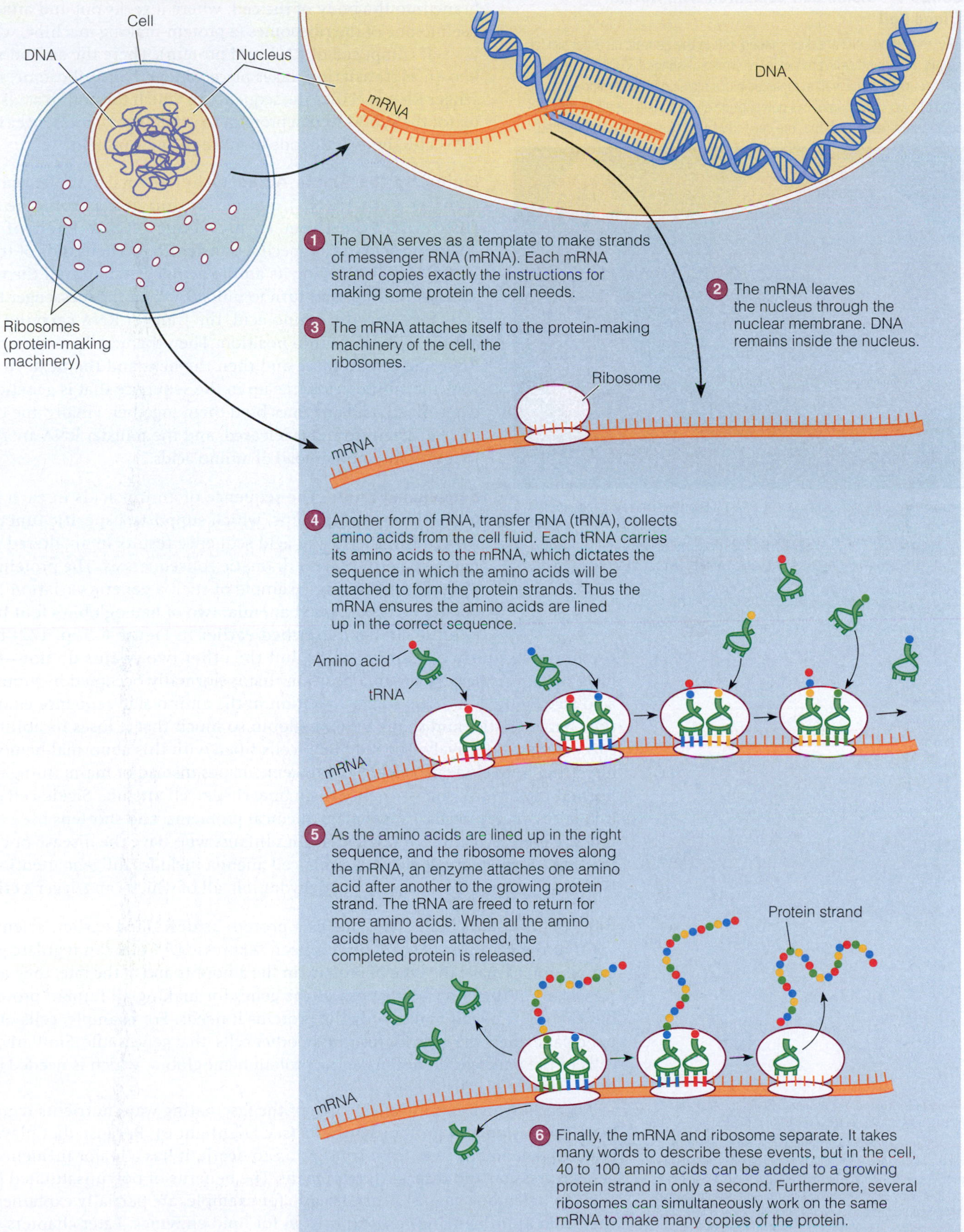
Cell
DNA
Nucleus
Ribosomes (protein-making machinery)
mRNA
DNA
1 The DNA serves as a template to make strands of messenger RNA (mRNA). Each mRNA strand copies exactly the instructions for making some protein the cell needs.
2 The mRNA leaves the nucleus through the nuclear membrane. DNA remains inside the nucleus.
3 The mRNA attaches itself to the protein-making machinery of the cell, the ribosomes.
Ribosome
mRNA
4 Another form of RNA, transfer RNA (tRNA), collects amino acids from the cell fluid. Each tRNA carries its amino acids to the mRNA, which dictates the sequence in which the amino acids will be attached to form the protein strands. Thus the mRNA ensures the amino acids are lined up in the correct sequence.
Amino acid
tRNA
mRNA
5 As the amino acids are lined up in the right sequence, and the ribosome moves along the mRNA, an enzyme attaches one amino acid after another to the growing protein strand. The tRNA are freed to return for more amino acids. When all the amino acids have been attached, the completed protein is released.
Protein strand
mRNA
6 Finally, the mRNA and ribosome separate. It takes many words to describe these events, but in the cell, 40 to 100 amino acids can be added to a growing protein strand in only a second. Furthermore, several ribosomes can simultaneously work on the same mRNA to make many copies of the protein.

> **FIGURE 6-8 Sickle Cell Compared with Normal Red Blood Cell**

Normally, red blood cells are disc-shaped, but in the genetic disorder sickle-cell anemia, red blood cells are sickle- or crescent-shaped. This difference in shape occurs because valine replaces glutamic acid in the amino acid sequence of two of hemoglobin's polypeptide chains. As a result of this difference in hemoglobin's shape, the capacity to carry oxygen is diminished.

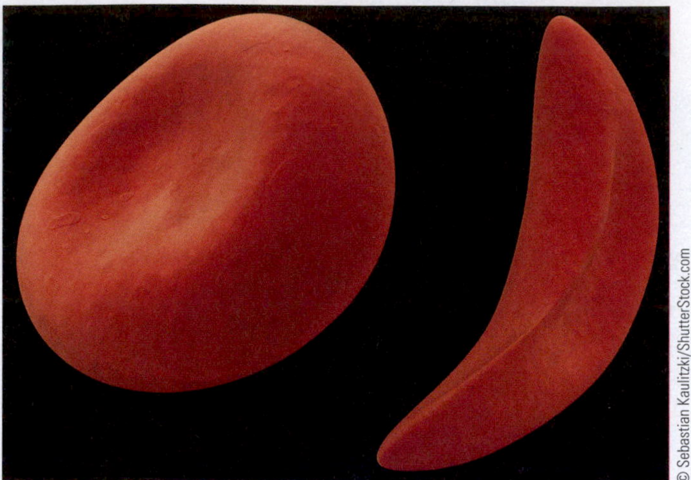

Normal red blood cell — Sickle-shaped blood cell

Amino acid sequence of normal hemoglobin:
Val–His–Leu–Thr–Pro–**Glu**–Glu

Amino acid sequence of sickle-cell hemoglobin:
Val–His–Leu–Thr–Pro–**Val**–Glu

Messenger RNA then carries the code across the nuclear membrane into the body of the cell, where it seeks out and attaches itself to one of the ribosomes (a protein-making machine, which is itself composed of RNA and protein). There the second step, known as **translation,** takes place. Situated on a ribosome, messenger RNA specifies the sequence in which the amino acids line up for the synthesis of a protein. In other words, messenger RNA translates the genetic code to make the new protein.

Lining Up the Amino Acids Other forms of RNA, called transfer RNA (tRNA), collect amino acids from the cell fluid and take them to messenger RNA. Each of the 20 amino acids has a specific transfer RNA. Thousands of transfer RNA, each carrying its amino acid, cluster around the ribosomes, awaiting their turn to unload. When the messenger RNA calls for a specific amino acid, the transfer RNA carrying that amino acid moves into position. Then the next loaded transfer RNA moves into place and then the next and the next. In this way, the amino acids line up in the sequence that is genetically determined, and enzymes bind them together. Finally, the completed protein strand is released, and the transfer RNA are freed to return for another load of amino acids.

Sequencing Errors The sequence of amino acids in each protein determines its shape, which supports a specific function. An error in the amino acid sequence results in an altered protein—sometimes with dramatic consequences. The protein hemoglobin offers one example of such a genetic variation. In a person with **sickle-cell anemia,** two of hemoglobin's four polypeptide chains (described earlier in Figure 6-5, p. 172) have the normal sequence of amino acids, but the other two chains do not—they have the amino acid valine in a position that is normally occupied by glutamic acid (see Figure 6-8). This single alteration in the amino acid sequence changes the characteristics and shape of hemoglobin so much that it loses its ability to carry oxygen effectively. The red blood cells filled with this abnormal hemoglobin stiffen into elongated sickle, or crescent, shapes instead of maintaining their normal pliable disc shape—hence the name, sickle-cell anemia. Sickle-cell anemia raises energy needs, causes many medical problems, and shortens life expectancy; genetic screening at birth identifies infants who have the disease or carry the trait.[1] Caring for people with sickle-cell anemia includes diligent attention to factors such as infection, stress, and dehydration, all of which can trigger a crisis.

Gene Expression When a cell makes a protein as described earlier, scientists say that the gene for that protein has been "expressed." Cells can regulate **gene expression** to make the type of protein, in the amounts and at the rate, they need. Nearly all of the body's cells possess the genes for making all human proteins, but each type of cell makes only the proteins it needs. For example, cells of the pancreas express the gene for insulin; in other cells, that gene is idle. Similarly, the cells of the pancreas do not make the protein hemoglobin, which is needed only by the red blood cells.

Recent research has unveiled some of the fascinating ways nutrients regulate gene expression and protein synthesis (see Highlight 6). Because diet plays an ongoing role in our lives from conception to death, it has a major influence on gene expression and disease development. The benefits of polyunsaturated fatty acids in defending against heart disease, for example, are partially explained by their role in influencing gene expression for lipid enzymes. Later chapters provide additional examples of relationships among nutrients, genes, and disease development.

translation: the process of messenger RNA directing the sequence of amino acids and synthesis of proteins.

sickle-cell anemia: a genetic form of anemia characterized by abnormal sickle- or crescent-shaped red blood cells. Sickled cells interfere with oxygen transport and blood flow. Symptoms are precipitated by dehydration and insufficient oxygen (as may occur at high altitudes) and include hemolytic anemia (red blood cells burst), fever, and severe pain in the joints and abdomen.

gene expression: the process by which a cell converts the genetic code into RNA and protein.

Roles of Proteins

Whenever the body is growing, repairing, or replacing tissue, proteins are involved. Sometimes their role is to facilitate or to regulate; other times it is to become part of a structure. Versatility is a key feature of proteins.

As Structural Materials From the moment of conception, proteins form the building blocks of muscles, blood, and skin—in fact, protein is the major structural component of all the body's cells. To build a bone or a tooth, for example, cells first lay down a **matrix** of the protein **collagen** and then fill it with crystals of calcium, phosphorus, magnesium, fluoride, and other minerals.

Collagen also provides the material of ligaments and tendons and the strengthening "glue" between the cells of the artery walls that enables the arteries to withstand the pressure of the blood surging through them with each heartbeat. Also made of collagen are scars that knit the separated parts of torn tissues together.

Proteins are also needed for replacing dead or damaged cells. The average life span of a skin cell is only about 30 days. As old skin cells are shed, new cells made largely of protein grow from underneath to replace them. Cells in the deeper skin layers synthesize new proteins to form hair and fingernails. Muscle cells make new proteins to grow larger and stronger in response to exercise. Cells of the GI tract are replaced every few days. Both inside and outside, the body continuously uses protein to create new cells that replace those that have been lost.

As Enzymes Some proteins act as **enzymes.** Digestive enzymes have appeared in every chapter since Chapter 3, but digestion is only one of the many processes facilitated by enzymes. Enzymes not only break down substances, but they also build substances (such as bone) and transform one substance into another (amino acids into glucose, for example). Breaking down reactions are *catabolic,* whereas building up reactions are *anabolic.* (Chapter 7 provides more details.) Figure 6-9 diagrams a synthesis reaction.

An analogy may help clarify the role of enzymes. Enzymes are comparable to the clergy and judges who make and dissolve marriages. When a minister marries two people, they become a couple, with a new bond between them. They are joined together—but the minister remains unchanged. The minister represents enzymes that synthesize large compounds from smaller ones. One minister can perform thousands of marriage ceremonies, just as one enzyme can expedite billions of reactions.

Similarly, a judge who lets married couples separate may decree many divorces before retiring. The judge represents enzymes that hydrolyze larger compounds to smaller ones; for example, the digestive enzymes. The point is that, like the minister and the judge, enzymes themselves are not altered by the reactions they facilitate. They are catalysts, permitting reactions to occur more quickly and efficiently than if substances depended on chance encounters alone.

As Hormones The body's many hormones are messenger molecules, and *some* hormones are proteins. (Recall from Chapter 5 that some hormones, such as estrogen and testosterone, are made from the lipid cholesterol.) Various endocrine glands in the body release hormones in response to changes that challenge the body. The blood carries the hormones from these glands to their target tissues, where they elicit the appropriate responses to restore and maintain normal conditions.

The hormone insulin provides a familiar example. After a meal, when blood glucose rises, the pancreas releases insulin. Insulin stimulates the transport proteins of the muscles and adipose tissue to pump glucose into the cells faster than it can leak out. After acting on the message, the cells destroy the insulin. As

matrix (MAY-tricks): the basic substance that gives form to a developing structure; in the body, the formative cells from which teeth and bones grow.

collagen (KOL-ah-jen): the structural protein from which connective tissues such as scars, tendons, ligaments, and the foundations of bones and teeth are made.

enzymes: proteins that facilitate chemical reactions without being changed in the process; protein catalysts.

> **FIGURE 6-9 Enzyme Action**

Each enzyme facilitates a specific chemical reaction. In this diagram, an enzyme enables two compounds to make a more complex structure, but the enzyme itself remains unchanged. Sometimes an enzyme needs to bind with a coenzyme before it can become active; coenzymes are often made from vitamins and are discussed in Chapter 10.

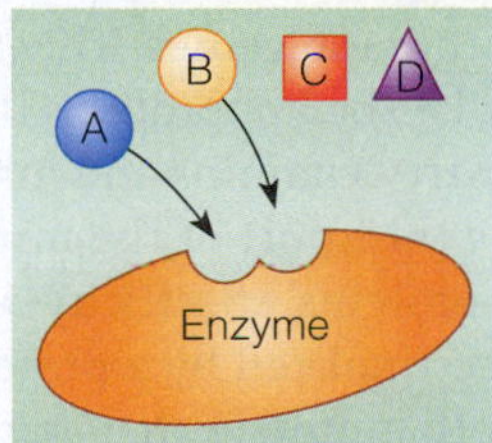
A
B
C
D
Enzyme
The separate compounds, A and B, are attracted to the enzyme's active site, making a reaction likely. Note that compounds C and D are not a good fit for the enzyme's active site and would not trigger a reaction.

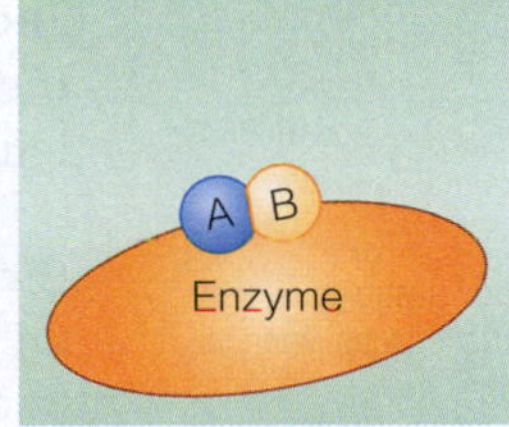
A
B
Enzyme
The enzyme forms a complex with A and B.

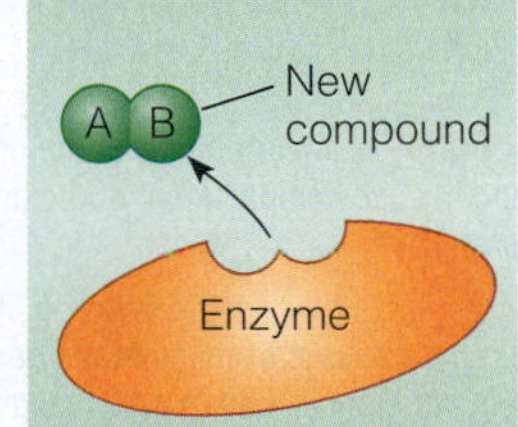
A
B
New compound
Enzyme
The enzyme is unchanged, but A and B have formed a new compound, AB.

TABLE 6-2 Examples of Hormones and Their Actions

Hormones	Actions
Oxytocin and prolactin	Support lactation (see Chapter 15)
Insulin and glucagon	Regulate blood glucose (see Chapter 4)
Thyroxine	Regulates the body's metabolic rate (see Chapter 8)
Calcitonin and parathyroid hormone	Regulate blood calcium (see Chapter 12)
Angiotensin, renin, and antidiuretic hormone	Regulate fluid and electrolyte balance (see Chapter 12)

blood glucose falls, the pancreas slows its release of insulin. Many other proteins act as hormones, regulating a variety of actions in the body (see Table 6-2 for examples).

As Regulators of Fluid Balance Proteins help maintain the body's **fluid balance**. Normally, proteins are found primarily within the cells and in the plasma (essentially blood without its red blood cells). Being large, proteins do not normally cross the walls of the blood vessels. During times of critical illness or protein malnutrition, however, plasma proteins leak out of the blood vessels into the spaces between the cells. Because proteins attract water, fluid accumulates and causes swelling. Swelling due to an excess of fluid in the tissues is known as **edema** (see Photo 6-2). The protein-related causes of edema include:

- Excessive protein losses caused by inflammation and critical illnesses
- Inadequate protein synthesis caused by liver disease
- Inadequate dietary intake of protein

Whatever the cause of edema, the result is the same: a diminished capacity to deliver nutrients and oxygen to the cells and to remove wastes from them. As a consequence, cells fail to function adequately.

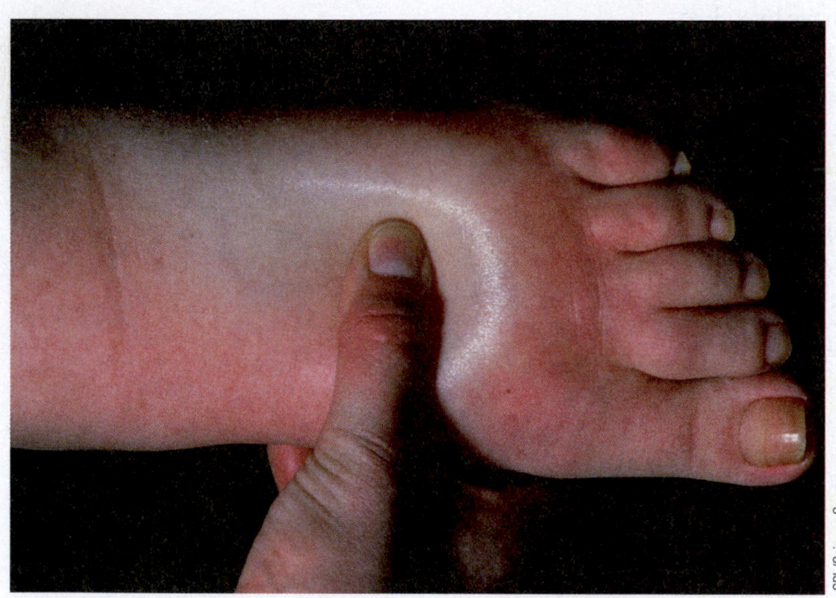

> **PHOTO 6-2** In critical illness and protein malnutrition, blood vessels become "leaky" and allow plasma proteins to move into the tissues. Because proteins attract water, the tissues swell, causing edema.

As Acid-Base Regulators Proteins also help maintain the balance between **acids** and **bases** within the body fluids. Normal body processes continuously produce acids and bases, which the blood carries to the kidneys and lungs for excretion. The challenge is to maintain acid-base balance as conditions continually change.

An acid solution contains an abundance of hydrogen ions (H^+); the greater the concentration of hydrogen ions, the more acidic the solution and the lower the pH. Proteins, which have negative charges on their surfaces, attract hydrogen ions, which have positive charges. By accepting and releasing hydrogen ions, proteins act as **buffers,** maintaining the acid-base balance of the blood and body fluids.

The blood's acid-base balance is tightly controlled to maintain pH within the narrow range of between 7.35 and 7.45. Outside this range, either **acidosis** or **alkalosis** can lead to coma and death, largely by denaturing proteins. Denaturing a protein changes its shape and renders it useless. To give just one example, denatured hemoglobin loses its capacity to carry oxygen.

As Transporters Some proteins move about in the body fluids, carrying nutrients and other molecules. The protein hemoglobin carries oxygen from the lungs to the cells. The lipoproteins transport lipids around the body. Special transport proteins carry vitamins and minerals.

The transport of the mineral iron provides an especially good illustration of these proteins' specificity and precision. When iron is absorbed, it is captured in an intestinal cell by a protein. Before leaving the intestinal cell, iron is attached to another protein that carries it through the bloodstream to the cells. Once iron enters a cell, it is attached to a storage protein that will hold the iron until it is needed. When it is needed, iron is incorporated into proteins in the red blood cells and muscles that assist in oxygen transport and use. (Chapter 13 provides more details on how these protein carriers transport and store iron.)

Some transport proteins reside in cell membranes and act as "pumps," picking up compounds on one side of the membrane and releasing them on the other as needed. Each transport protein is specific for a certain compound or group of

fluid balance: maintenance of the proper types and amounts of fluid in each compartment of the body fluids (see also Chapter 12).

edema (eh-DEEM-uh)**:** the swelling of body tissue caused by excessive amounts of fluid in the interstitial spaces; seen in protein deficiency (among other conditions).

acids: compounds that release hydrogen ions in a solution.

bases: compounds that accept hydrogen ions in a solution.

buffers: compounds that keep a solution's pH constant when acids or bases are added.

acidosis (assi-DOE-sis)**:** higher-than-normal acidity in the blood and body fluids.

alkalosis (alka-LOE-sis)**:** higher-than-normal alkalinity (base) in the blood and body fluids.

> FIGURE 6-10 An Example of a Transport Protein

This transport protein resides within a cell membrane and acts as a two-door passageway. Molecules enter on one side of the membrane and exit on the other, but the protein doesn't leave the membrane. This example shows how the transport protein moves sodium and potassium in opposite directions across the membrane to maintain a high concentration of potassium and a low concentration of sodium within the cell. This active transport system requires energy.

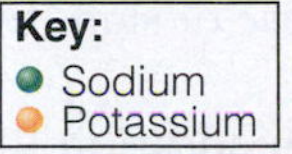
Key:
Sodium
Potassium

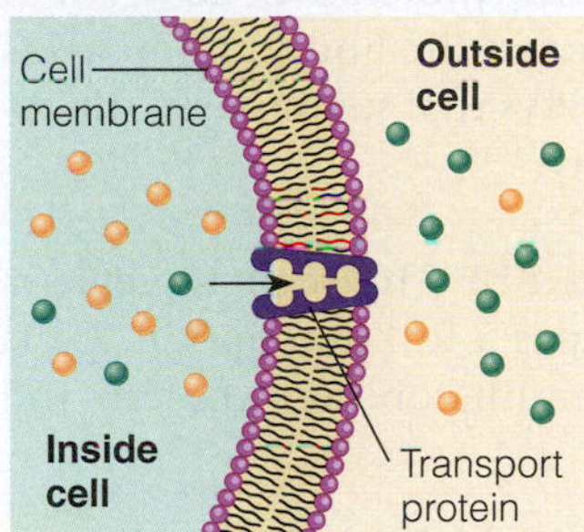
Cell membrane
Outside cell
Inside cell
Transport protein

The transport protein picks up sodium from inside the cell.

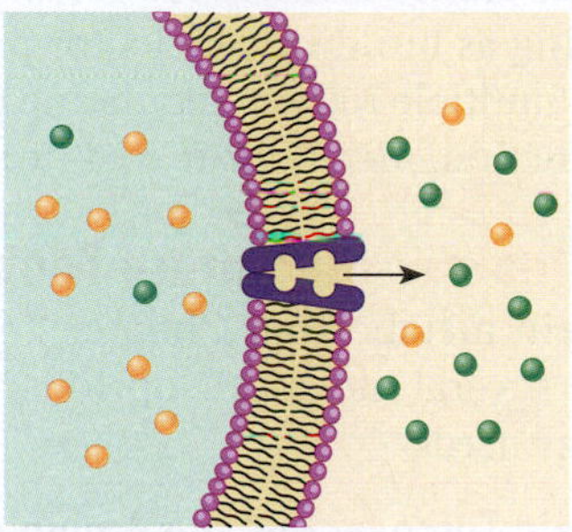

The protein changes shape and releases sodium outside the cell.

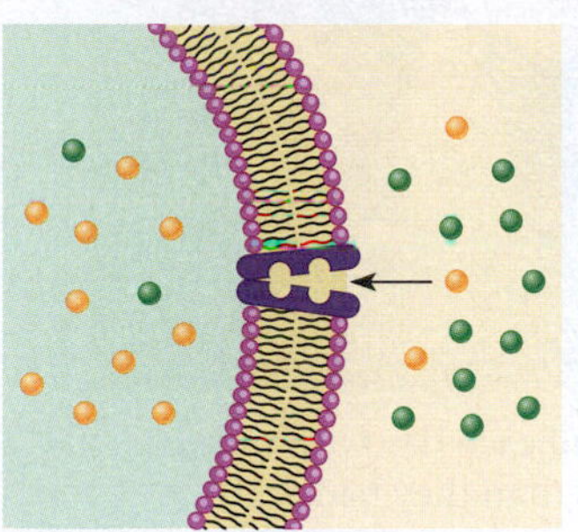

The transport protein picks up potassium from outside the cell.

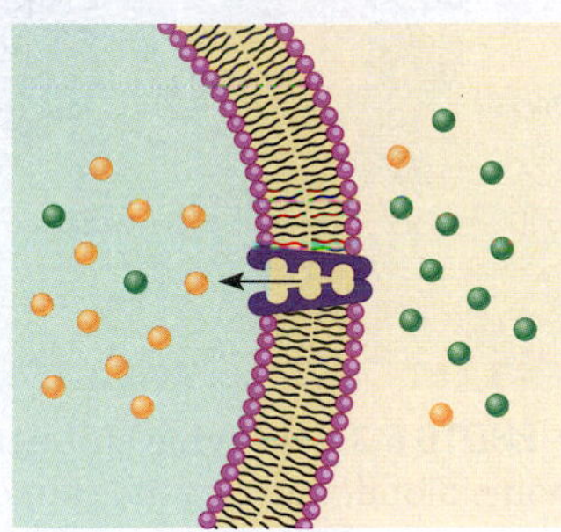

The protein changes shape and releases potassium inside the cell.

related compounds. Figure 6-10 illustrates how a membrane-bound transport protein helps maintain the sodium and potassium concentrations in the fluids inside and outside cells. The balance of these two minerals is critical to nerve transmissions and muscle contractions; imbalances can cause irregular heartbeats, muscular weakness, kidney failure, and even death.

As Antibodies Proteins also defend the body against disease. A virus—whether it is one that causes flu, smallpox, measles, or the common cold—enters the cells and multiplies there. One virus may produce 100 replicas of itself within an hour or so. Each replica can then burst out and invade 100 different cells, soon yielding 10,000 viruses, which invade 10,000 cells. Left free to do their worst, they will soon overwhelm the body with disease.

Fortunately, when the body detects these invading **antigens**, it manufactures **antibodies**, giant protein molecules designed specifically to combat them. The antibodies work so swiftly and efficiently that in a healthy individual, most diseases never get started. Without sufficient protein, though, the body cannot maintain its army of antibodies to resist infectious diseases.

Each antibody is designed to destroy a specific antigen. Once the body has manufactured antibodies against a particular antigen (such as the measles virus), it "remembers" how to make them. Consequently, the next time the body encounters that same antigen, it produces antibodies even more quickly. In other words, the body develops a molecular memory, known as **immunity**. (Chapter 16 describes food allergies—the immune system's response to food antigens.)

As a Source of Energy and Glucose Without energy, cells die; without glucose, the brain and nervous system falter. Even though proteins are needed to do the work that only they can perform, they will be sacrificed to provide energy and glucose during times of starvation or insufficient carbohydrate intake. The body will break down its tissue proteins to make amino acids available for energy or glucose production (a process known as *gluconeogenesis*). In this way, protein can maintain blood glucose levels, but at the expense of losing lean body tissue. Chapter 7 provides many more details on energy metabolism.

Other Roles As mentioned earlier, proteins form integral parts of most body structures such as skin, muscles, and bones (see Photo 6-3, p. 180). They also participate in some of the body's most amazing activities such as blood clotting and vision. When a tissue is injured, a rapid chain of events leads to the production of fibrin, a stringy, insoluble mass of protein fibers that forms a solid clot

antigens: substances that elicit the formation of antibodies or an inflammation reaction from the immune system. Examples of antigens include viruses, bacteria, and toxins.

antibodies: large proteins of the blood and body fluids, produced by the immune system in response to the invasion of the body by foreign molecules (usually proteins called *antigens*). Antibodies combine with and inactivate the foreign invaders, thus protecting the body.

immunity: the body's ability to defend itself against diseases (see also Chapter 18).

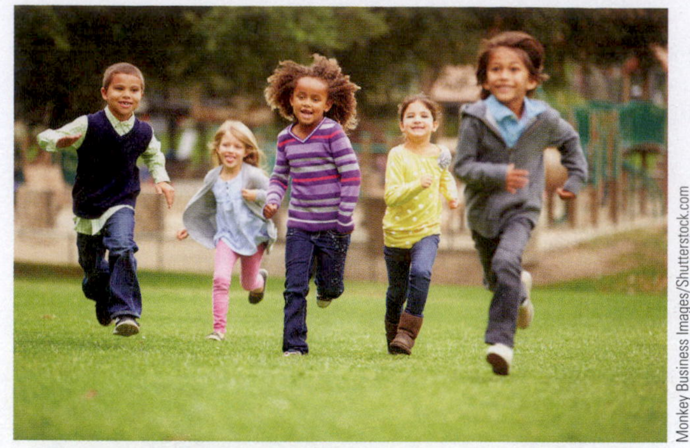

Monkey Business Images/Shutterstock.com

> **PHOTO 6-3** Growing children end each day with more bone, blood, muscle, and skin cells than they had at the beginning of the day.

from liquid blood. Later, more slowly, the protein collagen forms a scar to replace the clot and permanently heal the wound. The light-sensitive pigments in the cells of the eye's retina are molecules of the protein opsin. Opsin responds to light by changing its shape, thus initiating the nerve impulses that convey the sense of sight to the brain.

The amino acids are as versatile as the proteins. In addition to serving as building blocks for proteins in the body, amino acids have multiple roles in regulating pathways that support growth, reproduction, metabolism, and immunity.

A Preview of Protein Metabolism

This section previews protein metabolism; Chapter 7 provides a full description. Cells have several metabolic options, depending on their protein and energy needs.

Protein Turnover and the Amino Acid Pool Within each cell, proteins are continually being made and broken down, a process known as **protein turnover.** Protein breakdown releases amino acids. These amino acids mix with amino acids from the diet to form an **"amino acid pool"** within the cells and circulating blood.* The rate of protein degradation and the amount of protein intake may vary, but the *pattern* of amino acids within the pool remains fairly constant. Regardless of their source, any of these amino acids can be used to make body proteins or other nitrogen-containing compounds, or they can be stripped of their nitrogen and used for glucose or energy.

Nitrogen Balance Protein turnover and **nitrogen balance** go hand in hand. In healthy adults, protein synthesis balances with degradation, and protein intake from food balances with nitrogen excretion in the urine, feces, and sweat. When nitrogen intake equals nitrogen output, the person is in nitrogen equilibrium, or zero nitrogen balance. Researchers use nitrogen balance studies to estimate protein requirements.

If the body synthesizes more than it degrades, then protein is added and nitrogen status becomes positive. Nitrogen status is positive in growing infants, children, adolescents, pregnant women, and people recovering from protein deficiency or illness; their nitrogen intake exceeds their nitrogen excretion. They are retaining protein in new tissues as they add blood, bone, skin, and muscle cells to their bodies.

If the body degrades more than it synthesizes, then protein is being lost and nitrogen status becomes negative. Nitrogen status is negative in people who are starving or suffering other severe stresses such as burns, injuries, infections, and fever; their nitrogen excretion exceeds their nitrogen intake. During these times, the body loses nitrogen as it breaks down muscle and other body proteins for glucose or energy.

Using Amino Acids to Make Other Compounds Amino acids can be used to make compounds other than proteins. For example, the amino acid tyrosine is used to make the **neurotransmitters** norepinephrine and epinephrine, which relay nervous system messages throughout the body. Tyrosine can also be used to make the pigment melanin, which is responsible for brown hair, eye, and skin color, or the hormone thyroxine, which helps regulate the metabolic rate. For another example, the amino acid tryptophan serves as a precursor for the vitamin niacin and for **serotonin,** a neurotransmitter important in sleep regulation, appetite control, and sensory perception.

Using Amino Acids for Energy Carbohydrate and fat meet most of the body's daily energy needs, but protein usually contributes about 10 to 15 percent of these needs. This contribution may increase when energy intake is restricted. If necessary, the body

*Amino acids or proteins that derive from within the body are *endogenous* (en-DODGE-eh-nus). In contrast, those that derive from foods are *exogenous* (eks-ODGE-eh-nus).

protein turnover: the degradation and synthesis of protein.

amino acid pool: the supply of amino acids derived from either food proteins or body proteins that collect in the cells and circulating blood and stand ready to be incorporated in proteins and other compounds or used for energy.

nitrogen balance: the amount of nitrogen consumed (N in) as compared with the amount of nitrogen excreted (N out) in a given period of time.

neurotransmitters: chemicals that are released at the end of a nerve cell when a nerve impulse arrives there. They diffuse across the gap to the next cell and alter the membrane of that second cell to either inhibit or excite it.

serotonin (SER-oh-TONE-in): a neurotransmitter important in sleep regulation, appetite control, and sensory perception, among other roles. Serotonin is synthesized in the body from the amino acid tryptophan with the help of vitamin B_6.

> **FIGURE 6-11 Transamination and Synthesis of a Nonessential Amino Acid**

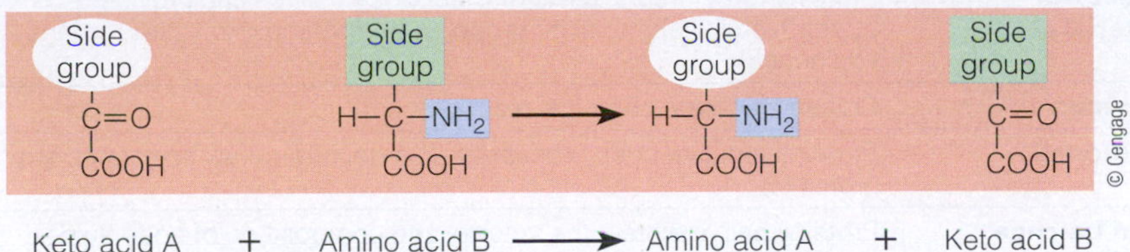
Side group
C=O
COOH
Side group
H–C–NH2
COOH
Side group
H–C–NH2
COOH
Side group
C=O
COOH
© Cengage

Keto acid A + Amino acid B ⟶ Amino acid A + Keto acid B

The body can transfer amino groups (NH_2) from an amino acid to a keto acid, forming a new *nonessential* amino acid and a new keto acid. Transamination reactions require the vitamin B_6 coenzyme.

> **FIGURE 6-12 Deamination and Synthesis of a Nonessential Amino Acid**

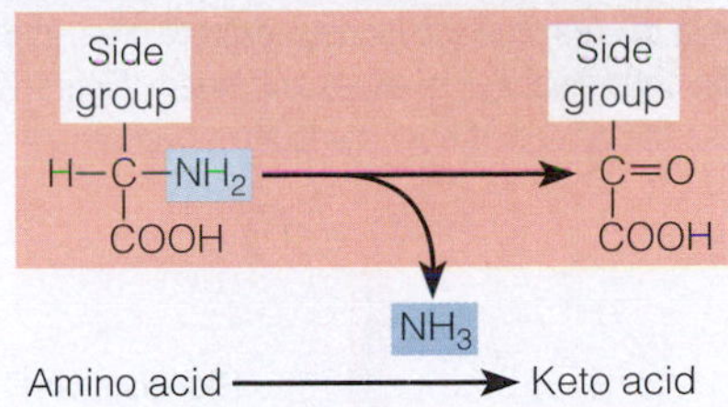
Side group
H–C–NH2
COOH
Side group
C=O
COOH
NH3

Amino acid ⟶ Keto acid

The deamination of an amino acid produces ammonia (NH_3) and a keto acid.

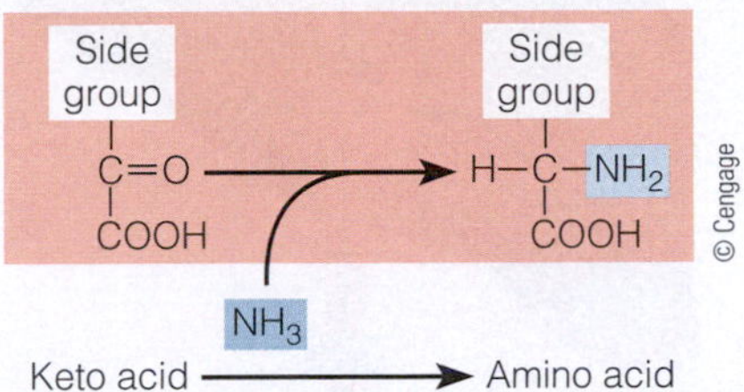
Side group
C=O
COOH
Side group
H–C–NH2
COOH
NH3
© Cengage

Keto acid ⟶ Amino acid

Given a source of NH_3, the body can make nonessential amino acids from keto acids.

will break down proteins from its lean tissue and use the amino acids to meet energy needs. Thus, over time, energy deprivation (fasting or starvation) always causes wasting of lean body tissue as well as fat loss. An adequate diet helps preserve lean tissue.

Using Amino Acids to Make Glucose As Chapter 4 explained, red blood cells and the brain depend on glucose as their primary fuel. When dietary carbohydrate is inadequate, the body can make glucose from amino acids derived from either the diet or lean tissue if necessary.

Using Amino Acids to Make Glycogen and Fat The body does not have a specialized storage site for protein as it does for carbohydrate and fat. Recall that glucose is stored as glycogen in the liver and fat as triglycerides in adipose tissue, but protein is not stored as such. When energy intake exceeds demand, excess protein is converted to glucose (via gluconeogenesis) or ketone bodies, which are stored in the body as glycogen and fat, respectively.[2]

Using Amino Acids to Make Proteins and Nonessential Amino Acids As an earlier section mentions, cells can assemble amino acids into proteins. If an essential amino acid is missing, the body may break down some of its lean tissue to obtain it. If a particular nonessential amino acid is not readily available, cells can make it from a **keto acid**—if a nitrogen source is available. Cells can also make a nonessential amino acid by transferring an amino group from one amino acid to its corresponding keto acid, as shown in Figure 6-11. Through many such **transamination** reactions, involving many different keto acids, the liver cells can synthesize the nonessential amino acids.

Deaminating Amino Acids When amino acids are broken down (as occurs when they are used for energy or to make glucose or ketone bodies), they are first deaminated—stripped of their nitrogen-containing amino groups (see Figure 6-12). Two products result from **deamination:** one is **ammonia** (NH_3); the other product is the carbon structure without its amino group—often a keto acid. Keto acids may enter a number of metabolic pathways—for example, they may be used for energy or for the production of nonessential amino acids, glucose, ketone bodies, cholesterol, or fat.*

Converting Ammonia to Urea As mentioned earlier, deamination produces ammonia. Ammonia is a toxic compound chemically identical to the strong-smelling ammonia in bottled cleaning solutions. Because ammonia is a base, excessive quantities upset the blood's critical acid-base balance. To prevent such a crisis, the liver combines ammonia with carbon dioxide to make **urea,** a much less toxic compound. Figure 6-13 provides an oversimplified diagram of urea synthesis; the details are shown in Appendix C. The production of urea increases as dietary protein increases, until production hits its maximum rate at intakes approaching 250 grams of protein per day. (For perspective, the average daily intake of protein in the United States is 80 grams.[3])

*Chemists sometimes classify amino acids according to the destinations of their carbon fragments after deamination. If the fragment leads to the production of glucose, the amino acid is called *glucogenic;* if it leads to the formation of ketone bodies, fats, and sterols, the amino acid is called *ketogenic.* There is no sharp distinction between glucogenic and ketogenic amino acids, however. A few are both, most are considered glucogenic, only leucine and lysine are clearly ketogenic.

> **FIGURE 6-13 Urea Synthesis**

Ammonia is produced when amino acids are deaminated. The liver detoxifies ammonia by combining it with another waste product, carbon dioxide, to produce urea. See Appendix C for details.

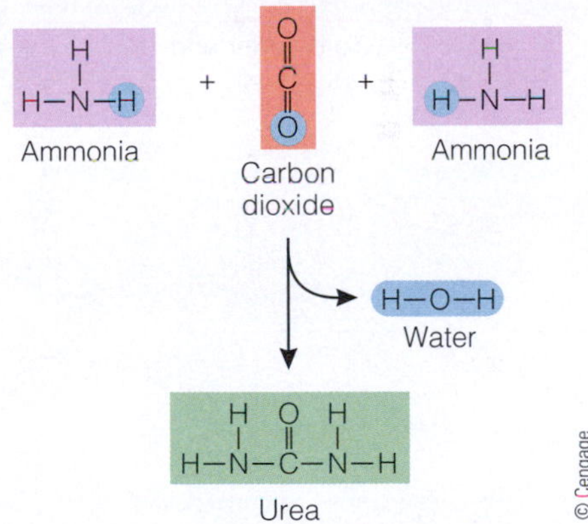
H
H–N–H
Ammonia
+
O=C=O
Carbon dioxide
+
H
H–N–H
Ammonia
H–O–H
Water
H O H
H–N–C–N–H
Urea
© Cengage

transamination (TRANS-am-ih-NAY-shun): the transfer of an amino group from one amino acid to a keto acid, producing a new nonessential amino acid and a new keto acid.

keto (KEY-toe) **acid:** an organic acid that contains a carbonyl group (C=O).

deamination (dee-AM-ih-NAY-shun): removal of the amino (NH_2) group from a compound such as an amino acid.

ammonia: a compound with the chemical formula NH_3, produced during the deamination of amino acids.

urea (you-REE-uh): the principal nitrogen-excretion product of protein metabolism. Two ammonia fragments are combined with carbon dioxide to form urea.

> **FIGURE 6-14 Urea Excretion**

When amino acids are deaminated (stripped of their nitrogen), ammonia is released. The liver converts ammonia to urea, and the kidneys excrete urea. In this way the body disposes of excess nitrogen. (Figure 12-5 provides the details of how the kidneys work.)

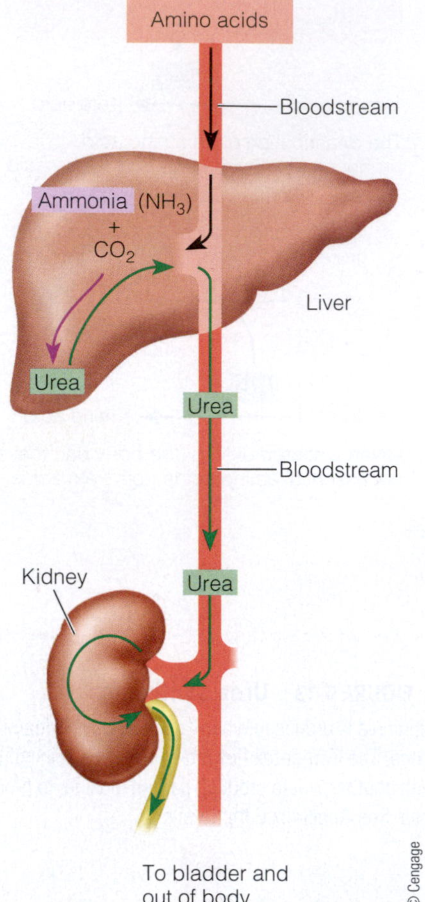

Amino acids
Bloodstream
Ammonia (NH_3)
+
CO_2
Liver
Urea
Urea
Bloodstream
Kidney
Urea
To bladder and
out of body
© Cengage

TABLE 6-3 Protein Functions in the Body

Structural materials	Proteins form integral parts of most body tissues and provide strength and shape to skin, tendons, membranes, muscles, organs, and bones.
Enzymes	Proteins facilitate chemical reactions.
Hormones	Proteins regulate body processes. (Some, but not all, hormones are proteins.)
Fluid balance	Proteins help maintain the volume and composition of body fluids.
Acid-base balance	Proteins help maintain the acid-base balance of body fluids by acting as buffers.
Transportation	Proteins transport substances, such as lipids, vitamins, minerals, and oxygen, around the body.
Antibodies	Proteins inactivate foreign invaders, thus protecting the body against diseases.
Energy and glucose	Proteins provide some fuel, and glucose if needed, for the body's energy needs.
Other	The protein fibrin creates blood clots; the protein collagen forms scars; the protein opsin participates in vision.

Excreting Urea Normally, the liver efficiently captures all the ammonia, makes urea from it, and releases the urea into the blood; then the kidneys filter out urea from the blood for excretion in the urine (see Figure 6-14). This division of labor allows easy diagnosis of diseases of both organs. In liver disease, blood ammonia is high; in kidney disease, blood urea is high.

Urea is the body's principal vehicle for excreting unused nitrogen, and the amount of urea produced increases with protein intake. To keep urea in solution, the body needs water. For this reason, a person who regularly consumes a high-protein diet (say, 100 grams a day or more) must drink plenty of water to dilute and excrete urea from the body. Without extra water, a person on a high-protein diet risks dehydration because the body uses its water to rid itself of urea. This explains some of the water loss that accompanies high-protein diets. Such losses may make high-protein diets *appear* to be effective, but water loss, of course, is of no value to the person who wants to lose body fat (as Highlight 9 explains).

REVIEW IT Describe how the body makes proteins and uses them to perform various roles.

Cells synthesize proteins according to genetic information that dictates the sequence in which amino acids are linked together. Each protein plays a specific role. Table 6-3 summarizes some of the many roles proteins play and conveys a sense of the immense variety and importance of proteins in the body. Proteins are constantly being synthesized and broken down as needed. The body's assimilation of amino acids into proteins and its release of amino acids via protein breakdown and excretion can be tracked by measuring nitrogen balance, which should be positive during growth and steady in adulthood. An energy deficit or an inadequate protein intake may force the body to use amino acids as fuel, creating a negative nitrogen balance. Protein eaten in excess of need may be deaminated and converted to glucose (and stored as glycogen) or ketone bodies (and stored as fat).

6.4 Protein in Foods

LEARN IT Explain the differences between high-quality and low-quality proteins, including notable food sources of each.

In the United States and other countries where nutritious foods are abundant, most people eat protein in large enough quantities that they receive all the amino acids they need. In countries where food is scarce and the people eat only marginal amounts of protein-rich foods, however, the *quality* of the protein becomes crucial.

Protein Quality

The protein quality of the diet determines, in large part, how well children grow and how well adults maintain their health. Put simply, **high-quality proteins** provide enough of all the essential amino acids needed to support the body's work, and low-quality proteins don't. Two factors influence protein quality—the protein's digestibility and its amino acid composition.

Digestibility As an earlier section explains, proteins must be digested before they can provide amino acids. **Protein digestibility** depends on such factors as the protein's source and the other foods eaten with it. The digestibility of most animal proteins is high (90 to 99 percent); plant proteins are less digestible (70 to 90 percent for most, but more than 90 percent for soy and other legumes).

Amino Acid Composition To make proteins, a cell must have all the needed amino acids available simultaneously. The liver can make any nonessential amino acid that may be in short supply so that the cells can continue linking amino acids into protein strands. If an essential amino acid is missing, though, a cell must dismantle its own proteins to obtain it. Therefore, to prevent protein breakdown in the body, dietary protein must supply at least the nine essential amino acids plus enough nitrogen-containing amino groups and energy for the synthesis of the nonessential ones. If the diet supplies too little of any essential amino acid, protein synthesis will be limited. The body makes whole proteins only; if one amino acid is missing, the others cannot form a "partial" protein. An essential amino acid supplied in less than the amount needed to support protein synthesis is called a **limiting amino acid.**

Reference Protein The quality of a food protein is determined by comparing its amino acid composition with the essential amino acid requirements of preschool-age children. Such a standard is called a **reference protein.** The rationale behind using the requirements of this age group is that if a protein will effectively support a young child's growth and development, then it will meet or exceed the requirements of older children and adults.

High-Quality Proteins A high-quality protein contains all the essential amino acids in relatively the same amounts and proportions that human beings require; it may or may not contain all the nonessential amino acids. Proteins that are low in an essential amino acid cannot, by themselves, support protein synthesis. Generally, foods derived from animals (meat, seafood, poultry, eggs, and milk and milk products) provide high-quality proteins, although gelatin is an exception. Gelatin lacks tryptophan and cannot support growth and health as a diet's sole protein. Proteins from plants (vegetables, nuts, seeds, grains, and legumes) have more diverse amino acid patterns and tend to be limiting in one or more essential amino acids. Some plant proteins are notoriously low quality (for example, corn protein). A few others are high quality (for example, soy protein).

Researchers have developed several methods for evaluating the quality of food proteins and identifying high-quality proteins. Appendix D provides details.

Complementary Proteins

In general, plant proteins are lower quality than animal proteins, and plants also offer less protein (per weight or measure of food). For this reason, many vegetarians improve the quality of proteins in their diets by combining plant-protein foods that have different but complementary amino acid patterns. This strategy yields **complementary proteins** that together contain all the essential amino acids in quantities sufficient to support health. The protein quality of the combination is greater than either food alone (see Figure 6-15 and Photo 6-4).

Some people have long believed that combining plant proteins at every meal is critical to protein nutrition. For most healthy vegetarians, though, it is *not* necessary to balance amino acids at each meal if protein intake is varied and energy intake is sufficient.[4] Vegetarians can receive all the amino acids they need over the course of a day by eating a variety of whole grains, legumes, seeds, nuts, and vegetables. Protein deficiency will develop, however, when fruits and certain

> **FIGURE 6-15 Complementary Proteins**

In general, legumes provide plenty of isoleucine (Ile) and lysine (Lys) but fall short in methionine (Met) and tryptophan (Trp). Grains have the opposite strengths and weaknesses, making them a perfect match for legumes.

	Ile	Lys	Met	Trp
Legumes	✓	✓		
Grains			✓	✓
Together	✓	✓	✓	✓

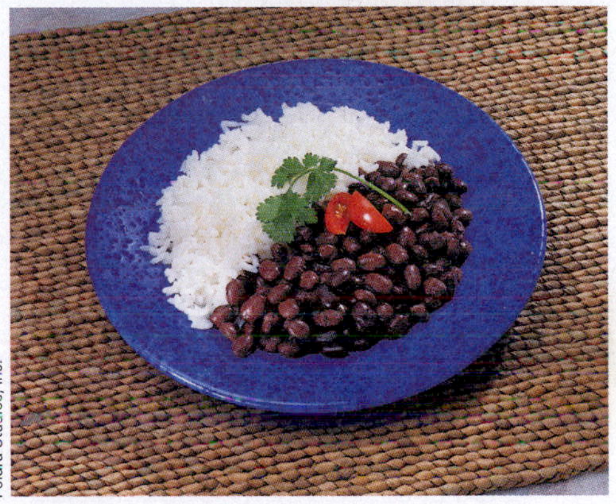

> **PHOTO 6-4** Black beans and rice, a favorite Hispanic combination, together provide a balanced array of amino acids.

high-quality proteins: dietary proteins containing all the essential amino acids in relatively the same amounts that human beings require. They may also contain nonessential amino acids.

protein digestibility: a measure of the amount of amino acids absorbed from a given protein intake.

limiting amino acid: the essential amino acid found in the shortest supply relative to the amounts needed for protein synthesis in the body. Four amino acids are most likely to be limiting:

- Lysine
- Methionine
- Threonine
- Tryptophan

reference protein: a standard against which to measure the quality of other proteins.

complementary proteins: two or more dietary proteins whose amino acid assortments complement each other in such a way that the essential amino acids missing from one are supplied by the other.

vegetables make up the core of the diet, severely limiting both the *quantity* and *quality* of protein. Highlight 2 describes how to plan a nutritious vegetarian diet.

REVIEW IT Explain the differences between high-quality and low-quality proteins, including notable food sources of each.

A diet that supplies all of the essential amino acids in adequate amounts ensures protein synthesis. The best guarantee of amino acid adequacy is to eat foods containing high-quality proteins or mixtures of foods containing complementary proteins that can each supply the amino acids missing in the other. In addition to its amino acid content, the quality of protein is measured by its digestibility and its ability to support growth. Such measures are of great importance in dealing with malnutrition worldwide, but in countries where protein deficiency is not common, the protein quality of individual foods deserves little emphasis.

6.5 Health Effects and Recommended Intakes of Protein

LEARN IT Identify the health benefits of, and recommendations for, protein.

As you know by now, protein is indispensable to life. This section examines the health effects and recommended intakes of protein.

Health Effects of Protein

It should come as no surprise that protein deficiency can have devastating effects on people's health. But like the other nutrients, protein in excess can also be harmful. High-protein diets have been implicated in several chronic diseases, including heart disease, cancer, osteoporosis, obesity, and kidney stones, but evidence is insufficient to establish an Upper Level (UL).[5]

Protein Deficiency Protein deficiency develops when the diet consistently supplies too little protein or lacks essential amino acids. When this occurs, the synthesis of body proteins decreases and degradation increases to provide cells with the amino acids they need. Without proteins to perform their critical roles, many of the body's activities come to a halt. The consequences of protein deficiency include slowed growth, impaired brain and kidney functions, poor immunity, and inadequate nutrient absorption.

The term *protein-energy malnutrition* has traditionally been used to describe the condition that develops when the diet delivers too little protein, too little energy, or both. The causes and consequences are complex, but clearly, such malnutrition reflects insufficient food intake. Importantly, not only are protein and energy inadequate, but so are many, if not all, of the vitamins and minerals. For this reason, severe malnutrition and its clinical forms—marasmus and kwashiorkor—are included in Chapter 20's discussion of world hunger.

Heart Disease In the United States and other developed countries, protein is so abundant that problems of excess are more common than deficiency. Depending on the food source, a high-protein diet may contribute to the progression of heart disease. As Chapter 5 mentioned, foods rich in animal protein also tend to be rich in saturated fats. Consequently, it is not surprising to find a correlation between animal-protein intake (red meats and milk products) and heart disease. On the other hand, substituting vegetable protein (legumes and nuts) for animal protein and using low-fat milk, poultry, and fish may improve blood pressure and blood lipids and decrease heart disease mortality.

The amino acid homocysteine is elevated in heart disease, but its role as a risk factor is unclear. Some research suggests that elevated homocysteine is a marker, describing gene activity (see Highlight 6) or free radical oxidation (see Highlight 11).[6] Lowering homocysteine by using supplements of the B vitamins (particularly folate), however, do not seem to lower the risks of heart attacks, strokes, or sudden death.

In contrast to homocysteine, the amino acid arginine may help protect against heart disease by lowering blood pressure and preventing blood clots.[7] Additional research is needed to confirm the benefits of arginine or the use of supplements.

Cancer Protein does not seem to increase the risk of cancer, but some protein-rich foods do. In fact, the World Health Organization (WHO) has classified **processed meat** as a **carcinogen**, and **red meat** as a probable carcinogen.[8] In contrast, protein-rich legumes such as soy, fish, and milk may lower the risk of some cancers. For example, soy seems to be associated with a lower risk of breast cancer, but not with endometrial cancer.[9] Chapter 18 discusses dietary links with cancer, and Chapter 19 presents food safety issues of processed meats and their additives.

Adult Bone Loss (Osteoporosis) Chapter 12 presents calcium metabolism, and Highlight 12 elaborates on the main factors that influence osteoporosis. This section briefly describes the relationships between protein intake and bone loss. When protein intake is high, calcium excretion increases. Whether excess protein depletes the bones of their chief mineral may depend upon the adequacy of calcium in the diet.[10] After all, bones need both protein and calcium for optimal growth.[11] In other words, the problem may reflect too little calcium, not too much protein. In establishing recommendations, the DRI Committee considered protein's effect on calcium metabolism and bone health, but it did not find sufficient evidence to warrant an adjustment for calcium or a UL for protein.[12]

Weight Control Research on the associations between protein intake and body weight has revealed some interesting, although often inconsistent, findings. One study examined people who were deliberately overfed by 1000 kcalories daily.[13] Not too surprisingly, they all gained weight, but those receiving a low-protein diet gained about half as much weight as those receiving an adequate- or high-protein diet. A look at their body composition revealed that the low-protein group stored almost all their excess kcalories as fat and lost a little lean body tissue. By comparison, the other protein groups stored the same amount of fat and gained some lean body tissue. Importantly, the excess kcalories increased body fat similarly for all groups; the different amounts of dietary protein affected changes in lean body mass. These findings highlight the importance of distinguishing between body weight and body fat—a point revisited in Chapters 8 and 9.

Weight-loss diets that encourage a high-protein, low-carbohydrate diet may be effective, primarily because they are low-kcalorie diets. Furthermore, including sufficient protein at each meal may help with weight loss by providing satiety; feelings of hunger are lower and feelings of fullness are higher on high-protein diets.[14]

Kidney Disease Excretion of the end products of protein metabolism depends, in part, on an adequate fluid intake and healthy kidneys. A high protein intake increases the work of the kidneys, but it does not cause kidney disease. It may, however, accelerate kidney deterioration in people with chronic kidney disease.[15] Restricting dietary protein—especially red meat—helps slow the progression of kidney disease in people who have this condition.[16]

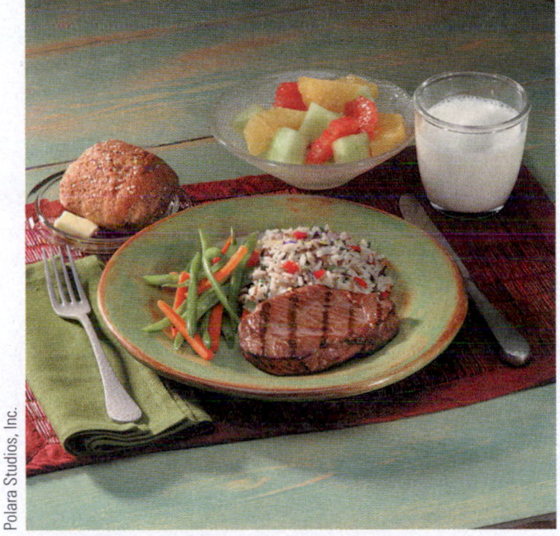
Polara Studios, Inc.

> **PHOTO 6-5** For many people, this 5-ounce steak provides almost all of the meat and much of the protein recommended for a day's intake.

Recommended Intakes of Protein

Recall that the body continuously breaks down and loses some protein and it cannot store proteins or amino acids. To replace protein, the body needs dietary protein for two reasons. First, dietary protein is the only source of the *essential* amino acids, and second, it is the only practical source of *nitrogen* with which to build the nonessential amino acids and other nitrogen-containing compounds the body needs.

Given recommendations that fat should contribute 20 to 35 percent of total food energy and carbohydrate should contribute 45 to 65 percent, that leaves 10 to 35 percent for protein. In a 2000-kcalorie diet, that represents 200 to 700 kcalories from protein, or 50 to 175 grams (see Photo 6-5). The average intake in the United States is 80 grams per day. Some research suggests that an intake slightly higher than current recommendations may be beneficial, especially for older adults.[17] Furthermore, including moderate amounts (25–35 grams) of high-quality protein at each meal may best support protein synthesis and muscle health.[18]

Protein RDA The protein RDA for adults is 0.8 gram per kilogram (0.36 gram per pound) of healthy body weight per day. For infants and children, the RDA

processed meat: meat that has been preserved or flavored by additives, curing, fermenting, salting, or smoking. Examples include bacon, ham, hot dogs, jerky, sausages, and some deli meats (such as corned beef); canned meats; and meat-based preparations and sauces.

carcinogen (CAR-sin-oh-jen or car-SIN-oh-jen): a substance that can cause cancer; the adjective is *carcinogenic.*

red meat: meat from the muscles of mammals. Examples include beef, goat, horse, lamb, mutton, pork, and veal.

> How To 6-1 Calculate Recommended Protein Intakes

To calculate your protein RDA:

- Look up the healthy weight for a person of your height (inside back cover). If your present weight falls within that range, use it for the following calculations. If your present weight falls outside the range, use the midpoint of the healthy weight range as your reference weight.
- Convert pounds to kilograms, if necessary (pounds divided by 2.2 equals kilograms).
- Multiply kilograms by 0.8 to get your RDA in grams per day. (Teens 14 to 18 years old, multiply by 0.85.) Example:

Weight = 150 lb

150 lb ÷ 2.2 lb/kg = 68 kg (rounded off)

68 kg × 0.8 g/kg = 54 g protein (rounded off)

> TRY IT Calculate your protein RDA.

is slightly higher. The table on the inside front cover lists the RDA for males and females at various ages in two ways—grams per day based on reference body weights and grams per kilogram of body weight per day.

Because the RDA meets the needs for replacing worn-out tissue, it increases for larger people; it also meets the needs for building new tissue during growth, so it increases for infants, children, adolescents, and pregnant and lactating women. How To 6-1 explains how to calculate your RDA for protein.

The protein RDA is the same for athletes as for others, even though athletes may need more protein and many fitness authorities recommend a higher range of protein intakes for athletes (see Table 14-6 in Chapter 14 for details). Most athletes in training typically don't need to actually increase their protein intakes, however, because the additional foods they eat to meet their high energy needs deliver protein as well. Importantly, these higher recommendations still fall within the 10 to 35 percent Acceptable Macronutrient Distribution Range (AMDR).

In setting the RDA, the DRI Committee assumes that people are healthy and do not have unusual metabolic needs for protein, that the protein eaten will be of mixed quality (from both high- and low-quality sources), and that the body will use the protein efficiently. In addition, the committee assumes that the protein is consumed along with sufficient carbohydrate and fat to provide adequate energy and that other nutrients in the diet are also adequate.

Adequate Energy Note the qualification "adequate energy" in the preceding statement, and consider what happens if energy intake falls short of needs. An intake of 50 grams of protein provides 200 kcalories, which represents 10 percent of the total energy from protein, if the person receives 2000 kcalories a day. But if the person cuts energy intake drastically—to, say, 800 kcalories a day—then an intake of 200 kcalories from protein is suddenly 25 percent of the total; yet it's still the same amount of protein (number of grams). The protein intake is reasonable, but the energy intake is not. The low energy intake forces the body to use the protein to meet energy needs rather than to replace lost body protein. Similarly, if the person's energy intake is high—say, 4000 kcalories—the 50-gram protein intake represents only 5 percent of the total; yet it *still* is a reasonable protein intake. Again, the energy intake is unreasonable for most people, but in this case, it permits the protein to be used to meet the body's needs.

Be careful when judging protein (or carbohydrate or fat) intake as a percentage of energy. Always consider the number of grams as well, and compare it with the RDA or another standard. A recommendation stated as a percentage of energy intake is useful only if the energy intake is within reason.

From Guidelines to Groceries A diet following the USDA Food Patterns can easily supply the recommended amount of protein. In selecting foods for protein, keep in mind the principles of variety and moderation.

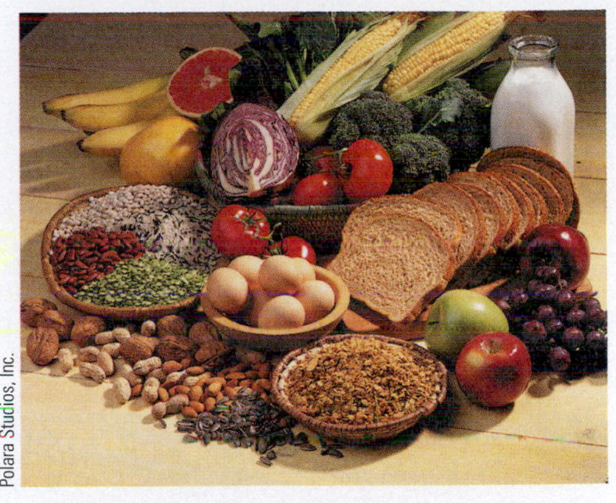

Polara Studios, Inc.

> **PHOTO 6-6** Vegetarians obtain their protein from whole grains, legumes, nuts, vegetables, and, in some cases, eggs and milk products.

Protein Foods An ounce of most protein foods delivers about 7 grams of protein. The USDA Food Patterns encourage a variety by sorting protein foods into three subgroups (review Figure 2-2, pp. 42–43, and Table 2-4, p. 41). Over a week's time, the total recommended intake of protein foods should be about 20 percent from seafood; almost 70 percent from meat, poultry, and eggs; and 10 percent from nuts, seeds, and legumes. Highlight 2 discusses protein options for vegetarians (see Photo 6-6).

Either plant or animal sources of protein can support a healthy eating pattern, but some protein foods—notably those derived from animals—may be high in saturated fat. To minimize saturated fat intake, select lean meats and poultry. Trim fat from meats before cooking and drain fat from meat after cooking. Remove skin from poultry before eating. Include plant sources of protein as well. By selecting a variety of protein foods, consumers can improve their nutrient intake and reap health benefits. Highlight 5 describes how nuts and fish can reduce the risks of heart disease when consumed in place of other protein foods.

Milk and Milk Products The only other food group to provide significant amounts of protein per serving is the milk and milk products group. A serving (a cup) of milk or yogurt provides about 8 grams of protein.

Fruits, Vegetables, and Grains Fruits do not contain protein. A serving of vegetables or grains provides 2 or 3 grams of protein, respectively.

Read Food Labels Food labels state the quantity of protein in grams. The "% Daily Value" for protein is not mandatory on all labels but is required whenever a food makes a protein claim or is intended for consumption by children younger than 4 years old. Whenever the Daily Value percentage is declared, researchers must determine the *quality* of the protein. Thus, when a % Daily Value is stated for protein, it reflects both quantity and quality.

To illustrate how easy it is to get enough protein, consider the amounts recommended by the USDA Food Pattern for a 2000-kcalorie diet. Six ounces of grains provide about 18 grams of protein; 2½ cups of vegetables deliver about 10 grams; 3 cups of milk offer 24 grams; and 5½ ounces of protein foods supply 38 grams. This totals 90 grams of protein—higher than the protein RDA for most people.

People in the United States typically get more protein than they need. If they have an adequate *food* intake, they have a more-than-adequate protein intake. The key diet-planning principle to emphasize for protein is moderation. Even though most people receive plenty of protein, some feel compelled to take supplements as well, as the next section describes.

Protein and Amino Acid Supplements Websites, health-food stores, and popular magazine articles advertise a wide variety of protein supplements, and consumers spend billions of dollars taking these supplements for many different reasons. Athletes take protein powders to build muscle. Dieters take them to spare their bodies' protein while losing weight. Women take them to strengthen their fingernails. People take individual amino acids, too—to cure herpes, to make themselves sleep better, to lose weight, and to relieve pain and depression. Like many other magic solutions to health problems, protein and amino acid supplements do not offer miracles.

Protein Powders Because the body builds muscle protein from amino acids, many athletes take protein powders soon after exercising, especially when resistance training, to promote protein synthesis and muscle strength. Whether this enhanced protein synthesis actually builds muscle or improves performance is less clear, but because protein supplements are relatively safe and inexpensive, they remain popular.[19] Athletes may prefer the convenience of protein powders and the assurance of measured quantities, but food sources of protein—lean meats, milk, eggs, and legumes—also provide an array of amino acids as well as valuable vitamins and minerals.

Whey protein appears to be particularly popular among athletes hoping to achieve greater muscle gains. A by-product of cheese manufacturing, whey protein is a high-quality protein that is commonly found in many protein powders. With a full array of essential amino acids, high leucine content, and rapid digestibility, whey supplements consumed soon after strength training exercises stimulate muscle protein synthesis.[20] Of course, muscles are also repaired and rebuilt when athletes eat balanced meals providing adequate energy and protein to support their physical activity. Chapter 14 presents additional information on the protein needs of physically active people.

Amino Acid Supplements Single amino acids do not occur naturally in foods and offer no benefit to the body; in fact, they may be harmful. The body was not designed to handle the high concentrations and unusual combinations of amino acids found in supplements. Large doses of amino acids cause diarrhea. An excess of one amino acid can create such a demand for a carrier that it limits the absorption of another amino acid, presenting the possibility of a deficiency. Those amino acids winning the competition enter in excess, creating the possibility of toxicity. Anyone considering taking amino acid supplements should be cautious not to exceed levels normally found in foods.[21]

Most healthy athletes eating well-balanced diets do not need amino acid supplements. Still, many athletes and fitness enthusiasts use dietary supplements with the hopes of increasing muscle strength, decreasing body fat, and improving performance. When combined with resistance training and taken soon after exercise, supplements of the **branched-chain amino acids** support protein synthesis. While branched-chain amino acid supplements are relatively safe, ordinary foods provide these amino acids in abundance as well.

In two cases, recommendations for single amino acid supplements have led to widespread public use—lysine to prevent or relieve the infections that cause herpes cold sores on the mouth or genital organs, and tryptophan to relieve depression and insomnia. In both cases, enthusiastic popular reports preceded careful scientific experiments and health recommendations. Research has not determined that lysine suppresses herpes infections, but it appears safe (up to 3 grams per day) when taken in divided doses with meals.[22]

Tryptophan may be effective with respect to inducing drowsiness, but caution is still advised. A review of the effects and side effects of tryptophan supplements found only modest, short-lived side effects at doses typical of use (up to 5 grams per day).[23] People taking serotonin reuptake inhibitor drugs should consult with their physicians before taking tryptophan supplements.

REVIEW IT Identify the health benefits of, and recommendations for, protein.

Protein deficiency impairs the body's ability to grow and function optimally. Excesses of protein offer no advantage; in fact, overconsumption of protein-rich foods may incur health problems as well. The optimal diet is adequate in energy from carbohydrate and fat and delivers 0.8 gram of protein per kilogram of healthy body weight each day. US diets are typically more than adequate in this respect. Normal, healthy people do not need protein or amino acid supplements.

As is true for the other nutrients as well, it is safest to obtain amino acids and protein from foods, eaten with abundant carbohydrate and some fat to facilitate their use in the body. With all that we know about science, it is hard to improve on nature.

whey protein: a by-product of cheese production; falsely promoted as increasing muscle mass. Whey is the watery part of milk that separates from the curds.

branched-chain amino acids: the essential amino acids leucine, isoleucine, and valine, which are present in large amounts in skeletal muscle tissue.

What's Online

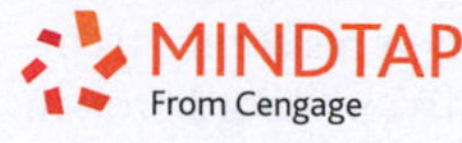
MINDTAP
From Cengage

Visit **www.cengagebrain.com** to access MindTap, a complete digital course that includes Diet & Wellness Plus, interactive quizzes, videos, and more.

REFERENCES

1. C. Taylor, P. Kavanagh, and B. Zuckerman, Sickle cell trait—neglected opportunities in the era of genomic medicine, *Journal of the American Medical Association* 311 (2014): 1495-1496; M. Brown, Managing the acutely ill adult with sickle cell disease, *British Journal of Nursing* 21 (2012): 90–96.
2. D. H. Pesta and V. T. Samuel, A high-protein diet for reducing body fat: Mechanisms and possible caveats, *Nutrition and Metabolism* 11 (2014): 53.
3. US Department of Agriculture, Agricultural Research Service, Nutrient Intakes from Food and Beverages, *What We Eat in America*, NHANES 2011-2012, published 2014.
4. Position of the Academy of Nutrition and Dietetics: Vegetarian diets, *Journal of the Academy of Nutrition and Dietetics* 116 (2016): 1970–1980.
5. Committee on Dietary Reference Intakes, *Dietary reference intakes: energy, carbohydrate, fiber, fat, fatty acids, cholesterol, protein, and amino acids* (Washington, D.C.: National Academies Press, 2005), p. 694.
6. J. E. Baggott and T. Tamura, Homocysteine, iron and cardiovascular disease: A hypothesis, *Nutrients* 7 (2015): 1108–1118; P. R. Mandaviya, L. Stolk, and S. G. Heil, Homocysteine and DNA methylation: A review of animal and human literature, *Molecular Genetics and Metabolism* 113 (2014): 243–252.
7. U. N. Das, Nutritional factors in the prevention and management of coronary artery disease and heart failure, *Nutrition* 31 (2015): 283–291.
8. Q&A on the carcinogenicity of the consumption of red meat and processed meat, October 2015, www.who.int/features/qa/cancer-red-meat.
9. S. Budhathoki and coauthors, Soy food and isoflavone intake and endometrial cancer risk: The Japan Public Health Center-based prospective study, *BJOG International Journal of Obstetrics and Gynaecology* 122 (2015): 304–311; K. P. Ko and coauthors, Dietary intake and breast cancer among carriers and noncarriers of *BRCA* mutations in the Korean Hereditary Breast Cancer Study, *American Journal of Clinical Nutrition* 98 (2013): 1493–1501.
10. J. D. Bihuniak and K. L. Insogna, The effects of dietary protein and amino acids on skeletal metabolism, *Molecular and Cellular Endocrinology* 410 (2015): 78–86; K. M. Mangano, S. Sahni, and J. E. Kerstetter, Dietary protein is beneficial to bone health under conditions of adequate calcium intake: An update on clinical research, *Current Opinion in Clinical Nutrition and Metabolic Care* 17 (2014): 69–4.
11. R. Rizzoli, Nutritional aspects of bone health, *Clinical Endocrinology and Metabolism* 28 (2014): 795–808.
12. Committee on Dietary Reference Intakes, 2005, p. 841; Committee on Dietary Reference Intakes, *Dietary Reference Intakes for Calcium and Vitamin D* (Washington, D.C.: National Academies Press, 2011).
13. G. A. Bray and coauthors, Effect of dietary protein content on weight gain, energy expenditure, and body composition during overeating: A randomized controlled trial, *Journal of the American Medical Association* 307 (2012): 47–55.
14. A. Dougkas and E. Östman, Protein-enriched liquid preloads varying in macronutrient content modulate appetite and appetite-regulating hormones in healthy adults, *Journal of Nutrition* 146 (2016): 637–645; E. A. Martens and coauthors, Protein leverage effects of beef protein on energy intake in humans, *American Journal of Clinical Nutrition* 99 (2014): 1397–1406; A. Belza and coauthors, Contribution of gastroenteropancreatic appetite hormones to protein-induced satiety, *American Journal of Clinical Nutrition* 97 (2013): 980–989.
15. M. Cuenca-Sánchez, D. Navas-Carillo, and E. Orenes-Piñero, Controversies surrounding high-protein diet intake: Satiating effect and kidney and bone health, *Advances in Nutrition* 6 (2015): 260–266.
16. Q. J. Lew and coauthors, Red meat intake and risk of ESRD, *Journal of the American Society of Nephrology* 28 (2016): 304–312.
17. M. Rafii and coauthors, Dietary protein requirement of female adults >65 years determined by the indicator amino acid oxidation technique is higher than current recommendations, *Journal of Nutrition* 145 (2015): 18–24; M. Tang and coauthors, Assessment of protein requirement in octogenarian women with use of the indicator amino acid oxidation technique, *American Journal of Clinical Nutrition* 99 (2014): 891–898.
18. E. Arentson-Lantz and coauthors, Protein: A nutrient in focus, *Applied Physiology, Nutrition, and Metabolism* 40 (2015): 755–761.
19. R. J. Maughan, Quality assurance issues in the use of dietary supplement, with special reference to protein supplements, *Journal of Nutrition* 143 (2013): 1843S–1847S.
20. M. C. Devries and S. M. Phillips, Supplemental protein in support of muscle mass and health: Advantage whey, *Journal of Food Science* 80 (2015): A8-A15; C. H. Murphy, A. J. Hector, and S. M. Phillips, Considerations for protein intake in managing weight loss in athletes, *European Journal of Sport Science* 15 (2015): 21–28.
21. Committee on Dietary Reference Intakes, *Dietary Reference Intakes: The Essential Guide to Nutrient Requirements* (Washington, D.C.: National Academies Press, 2006), p. 152.
22. C. C. Chi and coauthors, Interventions for prevention of herpes simplex labialis (cold sores on the lips), *Cochrane Database of Systematic Reviews* 8 (2015): CD010095.
23. J. D. Fernstrom, Effects and side effects associated with the nonnutritional use of tryptophan by humans, *Journal of Nutrition* 142 (2012): 2236S–2244S.

HIGHLIGHT > 6

LEARN IT Explain how nutrients influence gene activity (nutrigenomics) and how genes influence the activities of nutrients (nutrigenetics).

Nutritional Genomics

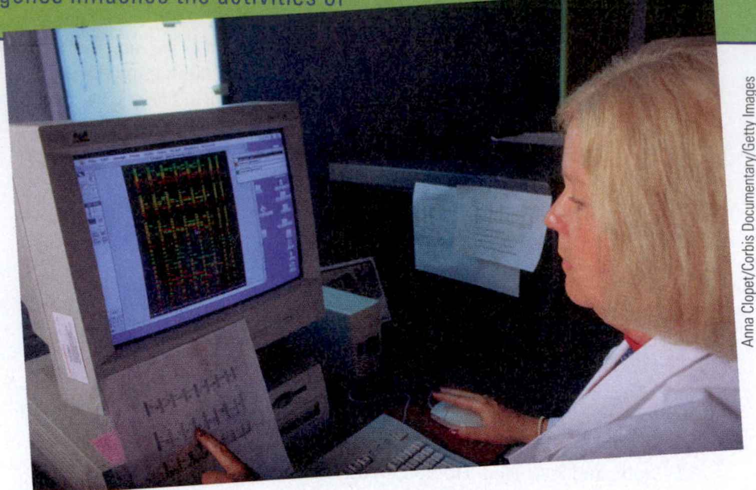
Anna Clopet/Corbis Documentary/Getty Images

Imagine this scenario: A physician scrapes a sample of cells from inside your cheek and submits it to a **genomics** lab. The lab returns a report based on your genetic profile that reveals which diseases you are most likely to develop, and your physician recommends specific lifestyle changes and medical treatments that can help you maintain good health. You may also be given a prescription for a personalized diet and dietary supplements that will best meet your unique nutrient requirements. This scenario may one day become a common reality as scientists uncover the relationships among **genetics**, diet, and disease.[1] Such genetic testing holds great promise, but consumers need to know that the FDA has yet to finalize regulations to ensure the safety and effectiveness of these tests.[2] The American Academy of Pediatrics strongly discourages direct-to-consumer testing and advises against testing children for diseases that typically develop in adulthood.[3]

Figure H6-1 introduces **nutritional genomics**, a relatively new field of study that examines how nutrients influence gene activity (nutrigenomics) and how **genes** influence the activities of nutrients (nutrigenetics). Glossary H6-1 defines related terms.

The surge in genomics research grew from the Human Genome Project, an international effort by industry and government scientists to identify and describe all of the genes in the **human genome**—that is, all the genetic information contained within a person's cells. Completed in 2003, this project developed many of the research technologies needed to study genes and genetic variation. Scientists are now working on the human **proteome** and hope to identify each of the proteins made by the genes, the genes associated with aging and diseases, and the dietary and lifestyle choices that most influence the expression of those genes. Such information will have major implications for society in general, and for health care in particular.[4]

A Genomics Primer

Figure H6-2 (p. 192) shows the relationships among the materials that comprise the genome. As Chapter 6's discussion of protein synthesis points out, genetic information is encoded in DNA molecules within the nucleus of cells. The **DNA (deoxyribonucleic acid)** molecules and associated proteins are packed within 46 **chromosomes**. The genes are segments of a DNA strand that can eventually be translated into one or more proteins. The sequence of **nucleotide bases** within each gene determines the amino acid sequence of a particular protein. Scientists currently estimate that there are between 20,000 and 25,000 protein-coding genes in the human genome.

As Figure 6-7 (p. 175) explains, when cells make proteins, a DNA sequence is used to make messenger **RNA (ribonucleic acid)**. The **nucleotide** sequence in messenger RNA then determines the amino acid sequence to make a protein. This process—from genetic information to protein synthesis—is known as **gene expression**. Gene expression can be determined by measuring the amounts of messenger

GLOSSARY H6-1

chromosomes: structures within the nucleus of a cell made of DNA and associated proteins. Human beings have 46 chromosomes in 23 pairs. Each chromosome has many genes.

DNA (deoxyribonucleic acid): the double helix molecules of which genes are made.

epigenetics: the study of heritable changes in gene function that occur without a change in the DNA sequence.

gene expression: the process by which a cell converts the genetic code into RNA and protein.

genes: sections of chromosomes that contain the instructions needed to make one or more proteins.

genetics: the study of genes and inheritance.

genomics: the study of all the genes in an organism and their interactions with environmental factors.

human genome (GEE-nome)**:** the complete set of genetic material (DNA) in a human being.

methylation: the addition of a methyl group (CH_3).

microarray technology: research tools that analyze the expression of thousands of genes simultaneously and search for particular gene changes associated with a disease. DNA microarrays are also called *DNA chips*.

mutations: permanent changes in the DNA that can be inherited.

nucleotide bases: the nitrogen-containing building blocks of DNA and RNA—cytosine (C), thymine (T), uracil (U), guanine (G), and adenine (A). In DNA, the base pairs are A–T and C–G; and in RNA, the base pairs are A–U and C–G.

nucleotides: the subunits of DNA and RNA molecules, composed of a phosphate group, a 5-carbon sugar (deoxyribose for DNA and ribose for RNA), and a nitrogen-containing base.

nutritional genomics: the science of how nutrients affect the activities of genes (*nutrigenomics*) and how genes affect the activities of nutrients (*nutrigenetics*).

phenylketonuria (FEN-il-KEY-toe-NEW-ree-ah), or **PKU:** an inherited disorder characterized by failure to metabolize the amino acid phenylalanine to tyrosine.

proteome: all proteins produced by an organism. The study of the expression, structure, and function of proteins is called *proteomics*.

RNA (ribonucleic acid): a compound similar to DNA, but RNA is a single strand with a ribose sugar instead of a deoxyribose sugar and uracil instead of thymine as one of its bases.

> **FIGURE H6-1 Nutritional Genomics**

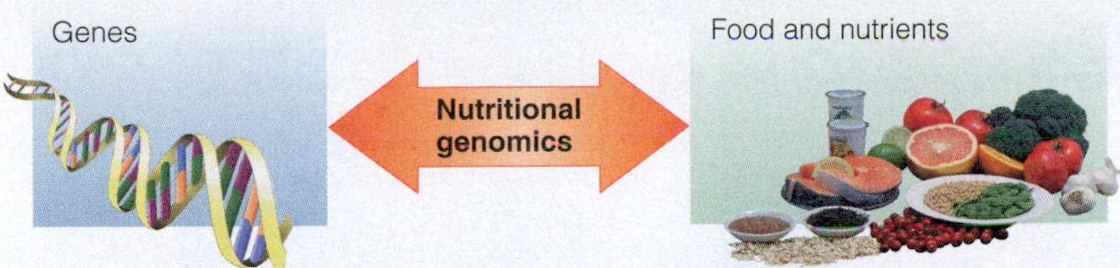
Genes
Nutritional genomics
Food and nutrients

Nutritional genomics examines the interactions of genes and nutrients. These interactions include both nutrigenetics and nutrigenomics.

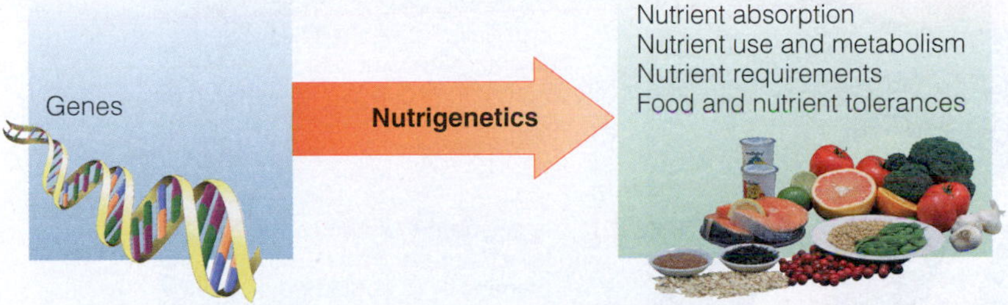
Genes
Nutrigenetics
Nutrient absorption
Nutrient use and metabolism
Nutrient requirements
Food and nutrient tolerances

Nutrigenetics (or nutritional genetics) examines how genes influence the activities of nutrients.

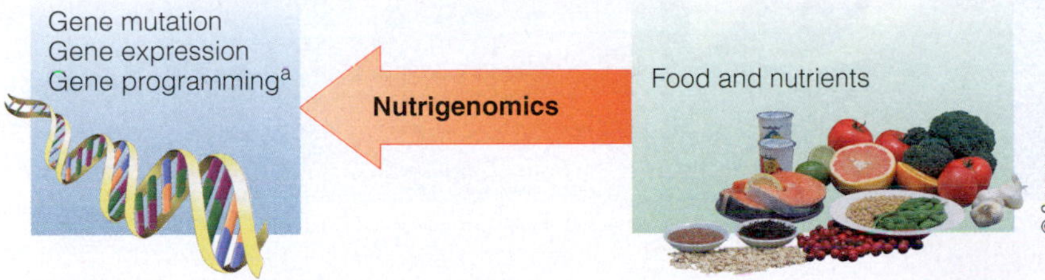
Gene mutation
Gene expression
Gene programming[a]
Nutrigenomics
Food and nutrients

Nutrigenomics, which includes epigenetics, examines how nutrients influence the activities of genes.

[a]Chapter 15 introduces fetal programming and describes how a mother's nutrition can permanently change gene expression in the fetus with consequences for future generations.

RNA in a tissue sample. **Microarray technology** (see photo on p. 190) allows researchers to detect messenger RNA and analyze the expression of thousands of genes simultaneously. These patterns of gene expression help explain the development of diseases and relationships between diet and diseases.

Simply having a certain gene does not determine that its associated trait will be expressed; the gene has to be activated. (Similarly, owning lamps does not ensure you will have light in your home unless you turn them on.) Nutrients are among many environmental factors that play key roles in either activating or silencing genes. Switching genes on and off does not change the DNA itself, but it can have dramatic consequences for a person's health.

The area of study that examines how environmental factors influence gene expression without changing the DNA is known as **epigenetics.** To turn genes on, enzymes attach proteins near the beginning of a gene. If enzymes attach a methyl group (CH_3) instead, the protein is blocked from binding to the gene and the gene remains switched off. Other factors influence gene expression as well, but **methylation** is among the most well understood. It is also known to have dietary associations.

Photo H6-1 illustrates epigenetics and how diet can influence genetic traits such as hair color and body weight. Both of the mice shown in the photo have a gene that tends to produce fat, yellow pups, but their mothers were given different diets during pregnancy. The mother of the mouse on the right was given a dietary supplement containing the B vitamins folate and vitamin B_{12}. These nutrients silenced the gene for "yellow and fat," resulting in brown pups with normal appetites. As Chapter 10 explains, one of the main roles of these B vitamins is to transfer methyl groups. In the case of the supplemented mice, methyl groups migrated onto DNA and silenced several genes, thus producing brown coats and protecting against the development of obesity (and consequently, some related diseases). Keep in mind that these changes occurred epigenetically. In other words, the DNA sequence within the genes of the mice remained the same. Maternal nutrition can influence genes in a way that creates persistent changes in the infant's metabolism and susceptibility to disease.[5] In this way, the dietary habits of parents, and even grandparents, can influence future generations.

Many nutrients and phytochemicals regulate gene expression and influence health through their involvement in DNA methylation. Some, such as folate, silence genes and protect against some cancers by increasing methylation. Others, such as a phytochemical found in green tea, activate genes and protect against some cancers by inhibiting methylation activity. Vitamin C

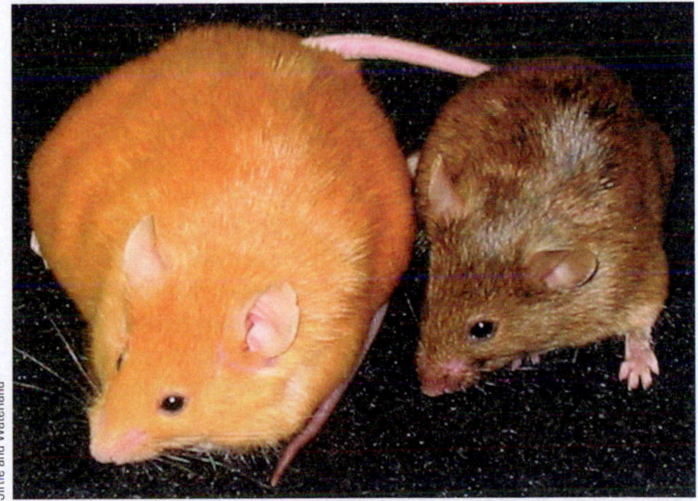

Jirtie and Waterland

> **PHOTO H6-1** Both of these mice have the gene that tends to produce fat, yellow pups, but their mothers had different diets. The mother of the mouse on the right received a dietary supplement, which silenced the gene, resulting in brown pups with normal appetites.

> FIGURE H6-2 The Human Genome

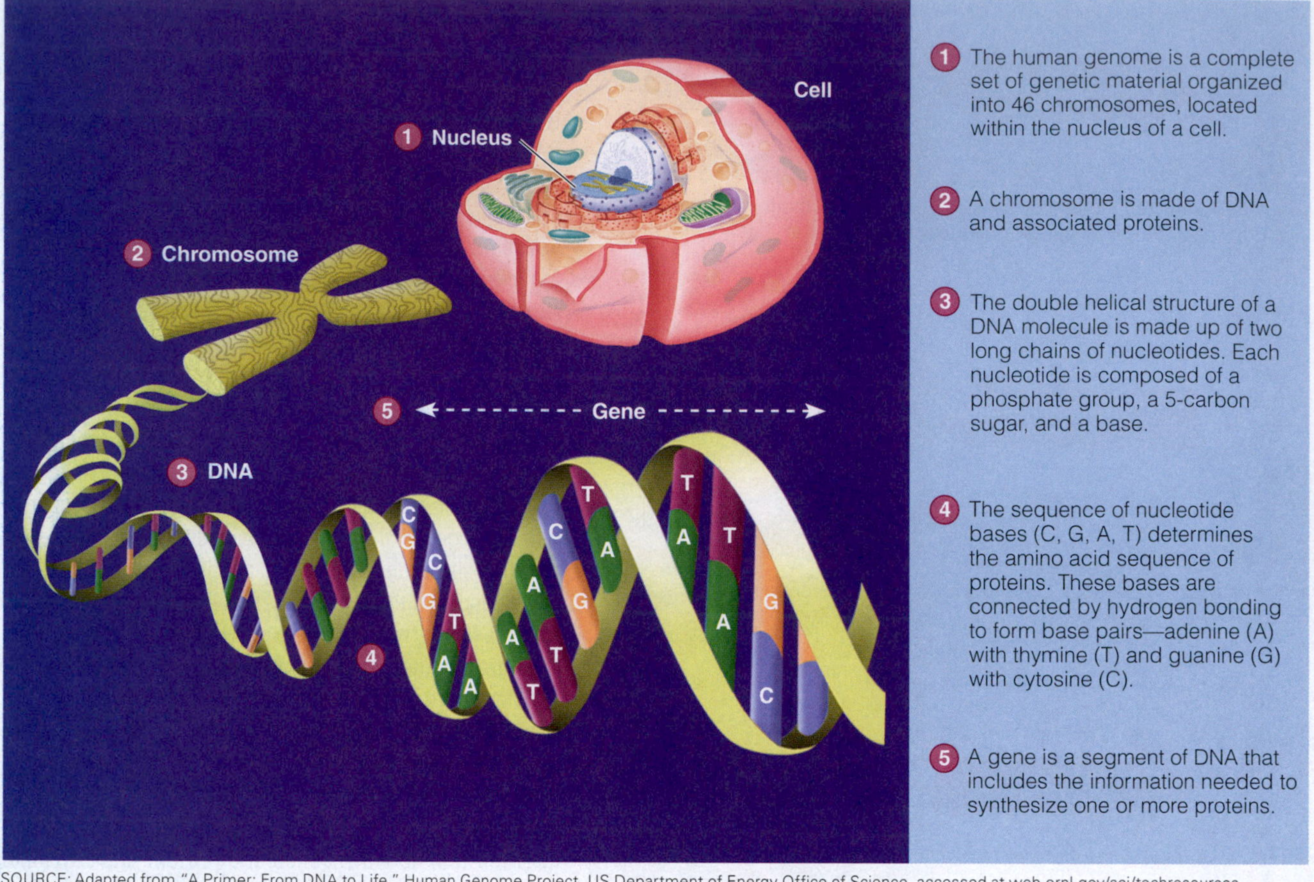
Cell
1 Nucleus
2 Chromosome
5 Gene
3 DNA
4
1 The human genome is a complete set of genetic material organized into 46 chromosomes, located within the nucleus of a cell.
2 A chromosome is made of DNA and associated proteins.
3 The double helical structure of a DNA molecule is made up of two long chains of nucleotides. Each nucleotide is composed of a phosphate group, a 5-carbon sugar, and a base.
4 The sequence of nucleotide bases (C, G, A, T) determines the amino acid sequence of proteins. These bases are connected by hydrogen bonding to form base pairs—adenine (A) with thymine (T) and guanine (G) with cytosine (C).
5 A gene is a segment of DNA that includes the information needed to synthesize one or more proteins.
© Cengage

SOURCE: Adapted from "A Primer: From DNA to Life," Human Genome Project, US Department of Energy Office of Science, accessed at web.ornl.gov/sci/techresources /Human_Genome/publicat/primer2001/primer2pager.pdf.

participates in DNA demethylation.[6] Whether silencing or activating a gene is beneficial or harmful depends on what the gene does. Silencing a gene that stimulates cancer growth, for example, would be beneficial, but silencing a gene that suppresses cancer growth would be harmful. Similarly, activating a gene that defends against obesity would be beneficial, but activating a gene that promotes obesity would be harmful. Figure H6-3 illustrates how nutrient regulation of gene expression can influence a person's health. Much research is under way to determine which nutrients activate or silence which genes. Such knowledge is expected to help researchers identify which dietary patterns might reverse the epigenetic changes that lead to cancer.[7] Similarly, researchers exploring how kcalorie-restricted diets influence DNA methylation are gaining new insights on the regulation of appetite and the metabolism of weight loss.

Genetic Variation and Disease

Except for identical twins, no two persons are genetically identical. Even then, a particular gene may become active in one twin and silenced in the other because of epigenetic changes.

The variation in the genomes of any two persons is only about 0.1 percent, a difference of only one nucleotide base in every 1000. Yet it is this incredibly small difference that makes each of us unique and explains why, given the same environmental influences, some of us develop certain diseases and others do not. Similarly, genetic variation explains why some of us respond to interventions such as diet and others do not. For example, following a diet low in saturated fats will significantly lower LDL cholesterol for most people, but the degree of change varies dramatically among individuals, with some people having only a small decrease or even a slight increase. In other words, dietary factors may be more helpful or more harmful depending on a person's particular genetic variations.[8] Such findings help explain some of the conflicting results from research studies. One of the goals of nutritional genomics is to custom design *specific* recommendations that fit the needs of *each* individual. Such personalized recommendations may present challenges, but they are also expected to provide more effective disease prevention and treatment solutions.[9]

In general, diseases characterized by a single-gene disorder are genetically predetermined, exert their effects early in life, and greatly affect those touched by them; such diseases are relatively rare. The cause and effect of single-gene disorders is clear—those with the genetic defect get the disease and those without it don't. In contrast, the more common diseases, such as heart disease and cancer, are influenced by many genes and typically develop over several decades. These chronic diseases have

> **FIGURE H6-3 Nutrient Regulation of Gene Expression**

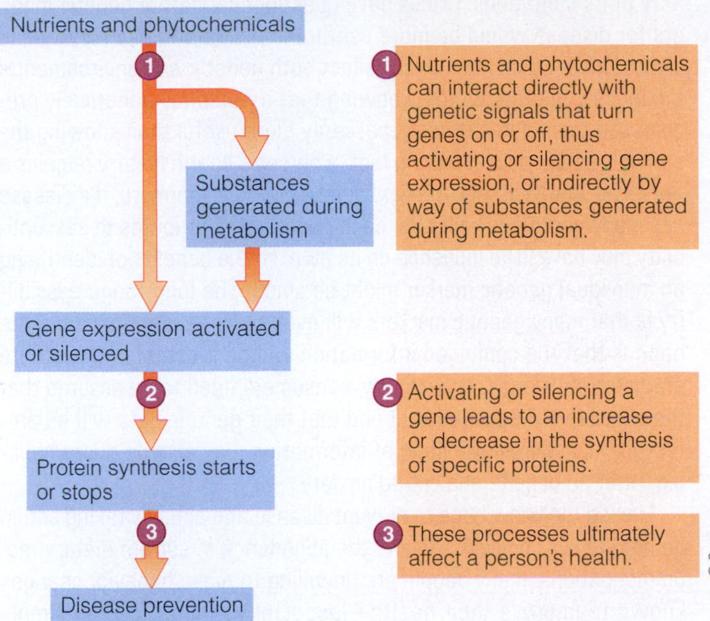
Nutrients and phytochemicals
1 Nutrients and phytochemicals can interact directly with genetic signals that turn genes on or off, thus activating or silencing gene expression, or indirectly by way of substances generated during metabolism.
Substances generated during metabolism
Gene expression activated or silenced
2 Activating or silencing a gene leads to an increase or decrease in the synthesis of specific proteins.
Protein synthesis starts or stops
3 These processes ultimately affect a person's health.
Disease prevention or progression
© Cengage

multiple genetic components that *predispose* the prevention or development of a disease, depending on a variety of environmental factors (such as smoking, diet, and physical activity). Both types of diseases are of interest to researchers studying nutritional genomics.

Single-Gene Disorders

Some disorders are caused by **mutations** in single genes that are inherited at birth. The consequences of a missing or malfunctioning protein can seriously disrupt metabolism and may require significant dietary or medical intervention. A classic example of a diet-related, single-gene disorder is **phenylketonuria**, or **PKU**.

A relatively rare disorder, PKU affects only one in 15,000 people in the United States; roughly 275 infants are born with the disease each year.[10] PKU arises from mutations in the gene that codes for the enzyme that converts the essential amino acid phenylalanine to the amino acid tyrosine. Without this enzyme, phenylalanine and its metabolites accumulate and damage the nervous system, resulting in mental retardation, seizures, and behavior abnormalities. At the same time, the body cannot make tyrosine or compounds made from it (such as the neurotransmitter epinephrine). Consequently, tyrosine becomes a conditionally essential amino acid: because the body cannot make it, the diet must supply it.

Although the most debilitating effect is on brain development, other symptoms of PKU become evident if the condition is left untreated. Infants with PKU may have poor appetites and grow slowly. They may be irritable or have tremors or seizures. Their bodies and urine may have a musty odor. Their skin coloring may be unusually pale, and they may develop skin rashes.

The effect of nutrition intervention in PKU is remarkable. In fact, the only current treatment for PKU is a diet that restricts phenylalanine and supplies tyrosine to maintain blood levels of these amino acids within safe ranges. Because all foods containing protein provide phenylalanine, the diet must depend on a special formula to supply a phenylalanine-free source of energy, amino acids, vitamins, and minerals. If the restricted diet is conscientiously followed, the symptoms of PKU can be prevented. Because phenylalanine is an essential amino acid, the diet cannot exclude it completely. Children with PKU need phenylalanine to grow, but they cannot handle excesses without detrimental effects. Therefore, their diets must provide enough phenylalanine to support normal growth and health but not enough to cause harm. The diet must also provide tyrosine. To ensure that blood concentrations of phenylalanine and tyrosine are close to normal, children and adults who have PKU must have blood tests periodically and adjust their diets as necessary.

Multigene Disorders

In multigene disorders, several genes can influence the progression of a disease, but no single gene causes the disease on its own. For this reason, genomics researchers must study the expression and interactions of *multiple* genes. Because multigene disorders are often sensitive to interactions with mulitple environmental influences, they are not as straightforward as single-gene disorders.

Heart disease provides an example of a chronic disease with multiple gene and environmental influences.[11] Consider that major risk factors for heart disease include elevated blood cholesterol levels, obesity, diabetes, and hypertension. Each of these risk factors has multiple underlying genetic and environmental causes, many of which are not completely understood. Research in nutritional genomics involves coordinating multiple findings on each of these risk factors and explaining the interactions among several genes, biochemical pathways, and nutrients. This information could then guide physicians and dietitians to prescribe the most appropriate medical and dietary interventions to reap the greatest health and economic benefits.[12] Finding the best option for each person is a major challenge given the many possible interactions between genes and environmental factors and the millions of possible gene variations in the human genome that make each individual unique.[13]

The results of genomic research are not only revealing new findings, but they also are helping to explain findings from previous research. Consider dietary fat and heart disease, for example. As Highlight 5 explains, epidemiological and clinical studies have found that a diet high in omega-3 polyunsaturated fatty acids benefits heart health. Now genetic studies offer an underlying explanation of this relationship: diets rich in omega-3 polyunsaturated fatty acids alter gene expression of immune cells to suppress inflammation and inhibit plaque build-up. Both actions support a healthy heart.

To learn more about how individuals respond to diet, researchers examine the genetic differences among people. The most common genetic differences involve a change in a single nucleotide base located in a particular region of a DNA strand—thymine replacing cytosine, for example. Such variations are called single-nucleotide polymorphisms (SNPs), and they commonly occur throughout the genome. Many SNPs (commonly pronounced "snips") have no effect on cell activity. In fact, SNPs are significant only if they affect the amino acid sequence of a protein in a way that alters its function *and* if that function is critical to the body's well-being. In these cases, SNPs may reveal fascinating answers to previously unexplained findings. Consider, for example, that people with a relatively common SNP have lower LDL when eating a diet rich in polyunsaturated fatty acids—and higher LDL with a low intake—than those without the SNP. These findings clearly show how diet (in this case, polyunsaturated fat) interacts with a gene (in this case, a lipid metabolism gene with a SNP) to influence the development of a disease (changing blood lipids implicated in heart disease).

Clinical Concerns

Because multigene, chronic diseases are common, an understanding of the human genome will have widespread ramifications for personalized medicine.[14] This new understanding of the human genome is expected to change health care by:

- Providing knowledge of an individual's genetic predisposition to specific diseases
- Allowing physicians to develop "designer" therapies—prescribing the most effective schedule of screening, behavior changes (including diet), and medical interventions based on each individual's genetic profile
- Enabling manufacturers to create new medications for each genetic variation so that physicians can prescribe the best medicine in the exact dose and frequency to enhance effectiveness and minimize the risks of side effects
- Providing a better understanding of how nutrition influences the biochemical pathways of diseases

In short, personalized dietary recommendations could be developed for each individual to achieve optimal health and minimize the risk of disease.[15] Enthusiasm surrounding genomic research needs to be put into perspective, however, given the scope of its promises and the reality of its limitations. Critics have questioned whether genetic markers for disease would be more useful than simple family history and clinical measurements, which reflect both genetic *and* environmental influences. In other words, knowing that a person is genetically predisposed to diabetes is not necessarily more useful than knowing the person's actual risk factors. In fact, a person's health history remains a powerful way to assess the risk for disease.[16] Furthermore, if a disease has many genetic risk factors, each gene that contributes to susceptibility may have little influence on its own, so the benefits of identifying an individual genetic marker might be small. The long-range possibility is that many genetic markers will eventually be identified, and the hope is that the combined information will be a useful and accurate predictor of disease. Importantly, consumers need to be assured that the benefits will be significant and that their genetic data will be protected.[17] Of course, the flood of information may also be overwhelming, offer no benefit, and create anxiety.

Having the knowledge to prevent disease and actually taking action do not always coincide. Despite the abundance of current dietary recommendations, many people are unwilling to make behavior changes known to improve their health—especially when they can simply blame their genes. For example, it has been estimated that heart disease and type 2 diabetes are 90 percent preventable when people adopt an appropriate diet, maintain a healthy body weight, and exercise regularly. Yet these two diseases remain among the leading causes of death. Given the difficulty that many people have with current general recommendations, it may be unrealistic to expect that they will enthusiastically adopt an even more detailed list of personal lifestyle modifications. Then again, compliance may be better when it is supported by information based on a personalized nutrition plan and the knowledge that the epigenetic profile can be changed.[18] Figure H6-4

> **FIGURE H6-4 Genetics and Lifestyle Factors Contribute to Health and Longevity**

Lifestyle factors such as diet, physical activity, and stress influence how genes are expressed. Given the same genetic profile, healthy choices support good health and long life better than poor choices.

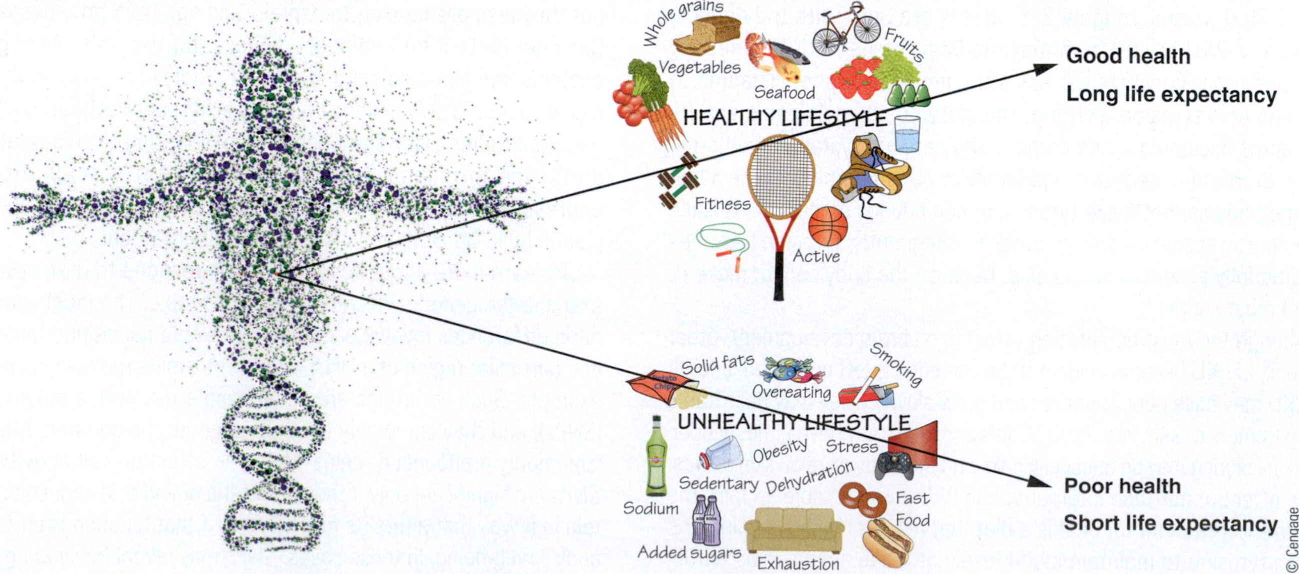
Whole grains
Vegetables
Seafood
Fruits
HEALTHY LIFESTYLE
Fitness
Active
Good health
Long life expectancy
Solid fats
Overeating
Smoking
UNHEALTHY LIFESTYLE
Obesity
Stress
Sedentary
Dehydration
Sodium
Fast Food
Added sugars
Exhaustion
Poor health
Short life expectancy
© Cengage

illustrates how the consequences of dozens of daily choices—what to eat, how active to be, when to sleep, and more—accumulate over time to affect health and longevity.

The debate over nature versus nurture—whether genes or the environment are more influential—has quieted. The focus has shifted. Scientists acknowledge the important roles of each and understand the real answers lie within the myriad interactions.[19] Current research is sorting through how nutrients and other dietary factors interact with genes to confer health benefits or risks. Answers from genomic research may not become apparent for years to come, but the opportunities and rewards may prove well worth the efforts.

CRITICAL THINKING QUESTIONS

A. How might nutritional genomics influence health care in the future?

B. You may have heard about the diet that is based on a person's blood type and claims to restore the body's natural genetic rhythms and improve health. Research may one day reveal exactly which foods might best turn on and off specific genes to defend against specific chronic diseases. No doubt marketers will rush to fill grocery shelves with foods manufactured to match genetic profiles. Why do you think these genetic approaches to diet and health might be more or less appealing than eating patterns that include a variety of fruits, vegetables, whole grains, milk products, and meats?

REFERENCES

1. Position of the Academy of Nutrition and Dietetics: Nutritional genomics, *Journal of the Academy of Nutrition and Dietetics* 114 (2014): 299–312; G. S. Ginsburg, Realizing the opportunities of genomics in health care, *Journal of the American Medical Association* 309 (2013): 1463–1464.
2. B. J. Evans, W. Burke, and G. P. Jarvik, The FDA and genomic tests: Getting regulation right, *New England Journal of Medicine* 372 (2015): 2258–2264.
3. American Academy of Pediatrics, Policy statement: Ethical and policy issues in genetic testing and screening of children, *Pediatrics* 131 (2013): 620–622.
4. G. S. Ginsburg, Realizing the opportunities of genomics in health care, *Journal of the American Medical Association* 309 (2013): 1463–1464.
5. J. Zheng and coauthors, DNA methylation: The pivotal interaction between early-life nutrition and glucose metabolism in later life, *British Journal of Nutrition* 112 (2014): 1850–1857; P. Dominguez-Salas and coauthors, Maternal nutrition at conception modulates DNA methylation of human metastable epialleles, *Nature Communications* 5 (2014): 3746.
6. J. I. Young, S. Züchner, and G. Wang, Regulation of the epigenome by vitamin C, *Annual Review of Nutrition* 35 (2015): 545–564.
7. G. Supic, M. Jagodic, and Z. Magic, Epigenetics: A new link between nutrition and cancer, *Nutrition and Cancer* 65 (2013): 781–792.
8. M. M. H. Abdullah, P. J. H. Jones, and P. K. Eck, Nutrigenetics of cholesterol metabolism: Observational and dietary intervention studies in the postgenomic era, *Nutrition Reviews* 73 (2015): 523–543.
9. R. San-Cristobal and coauthors, Future challenges and present ethical considerations in the use of personalized nutrition based on genetic advice, *Journal of the Academy of Nutrition and Dietetics* 113 (2013): 1447–1464.
10. J. P. Brosco and D. B. Paul, The political history of PKU: Reflections on 50 years of newborn screening, *Pediatrics* 132 (2013): 987–989.
11. E. Incalcaterra and coauthors, Pro-inflammatory genetic markers of atherosclerosis, *Current Atherosclerosis Reports* 15 (2013): 329–335.
12. M. M. Byrne, R. T. Murphy, and A. W. Ryan, Epigenetic modulation in the treatment of atherosclerotic disease, *Frontiers in Genetics* 5 (2014): 364.
13. T. I. Pollin and M. Quartuccio, What we know about diet, genes, and dyslipidemia: Is there potential for translation? *Current Nutrition Reports* 2 (2013): 236–242.
14. J. A. Doudna, Genomic engineering and the future of medicine, *Journal of the American Medical Association* 314 (2015): 791–792; M. J. Joyner and N. Paneth, Seven questions for personalized medicine, *Journal of the American Medical Association* 314 (2015): 999–1000.
15. G. Astarita and J. Langridge, An emerging role for metabolomics in nutrition science, *Journal of Nutrigenetics and Nutrigenomics*, 6 (2013): 181–200.
16. B. M. Welch, W. Dere, and J. D. Schiffman, Family health history: The case for better tools, *Journal of the American Medical Association* 313 (2015): 1711–1712.
17. R. Poinhos and coauthors, Psychological determinants of consumer acceptance of personalised nutrition in 9 European countries, *PLoS One* 9 (2014): e110614.
18. C. Celis-Morales and coauthors, Effect of personalized nutrition on health-related behaviour change: Evidence from the Food4me European randomized controlled trial, *International Journal of Epidemiology* (2016): pii: dyw186.
19. A. P. Feinberg and M. D. Fallin, Epigenetics at the crossroads of genes and the environment, *Journal of the American Medical Association* 314 (2015): 1129–1130.

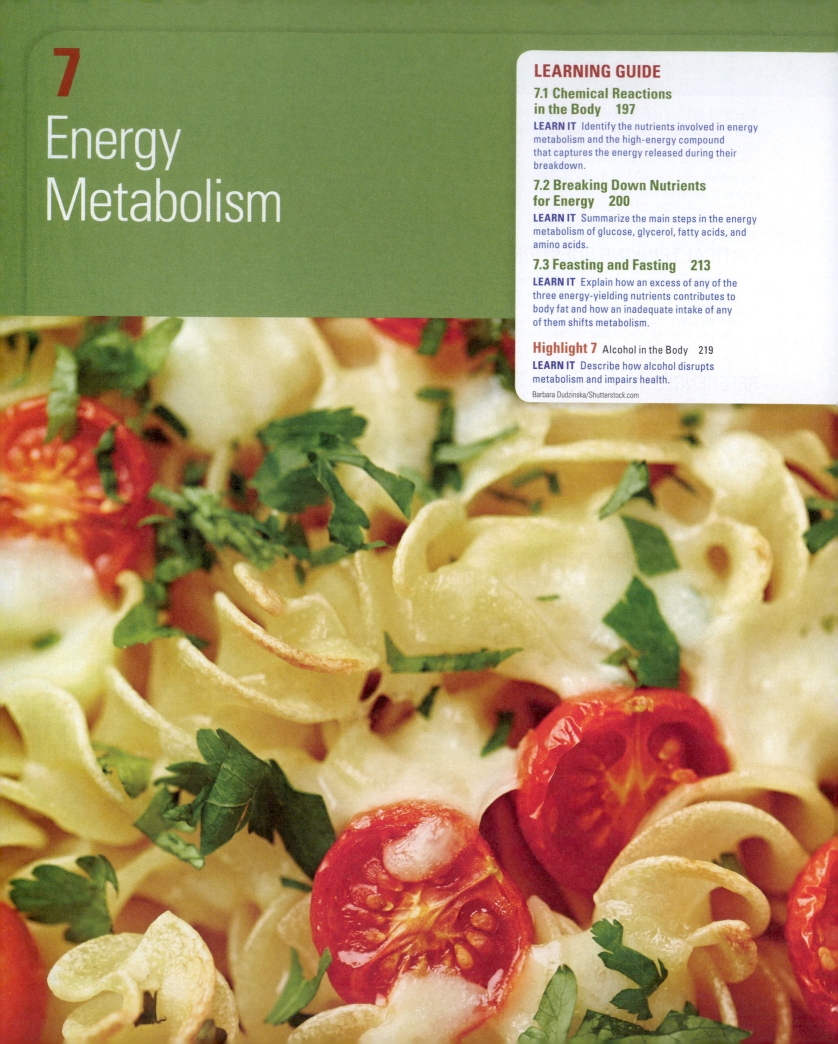

7 Energy Metabolism

LEARNING GUIDE

Barbara Dudzinska/Shutterstock.com

Nutrition in Your Life

You eat breakfast and hustle off to class. After lunch, you study for tomorrow's exam. Dinner is followed by an evening of dancing. Do you ever think about how the food you eat powers the activities of your life? What happens when you don't eat—or when you eat too much? Learn how the cells of your body transform carbohydrates, fats, and proteins into energy—and what happens when you give your cells too much or too little of any of these nutrients. Discover the metabolic pathways that lead to body fat and those that support physical activity. It's really quite fascinating. As you read this chapter, consider whether your diet provides a healthy balance of the energy nutrients.

Energy makes it possible for people to breathe, ride bicycles, compose music, and do everything else they do. As Chapter 1 explained, *energy* is the capacity to do work. Although every aspect of our lives depends on energy, the concept of energy can be difficult to grasp because it cannot be seen or touched, and it manifests in various forms, including heat, mechanical, electrical, and chemical energy. In the body, heat energy maintains a constant body temperature, mechanical energy moves muscles, and electrical energy sends nerve impulses. Energy is stored in foods and in the body as chemical energy. This chemical energy powers the myriad activities of all cells.

By studying metabolism, you will understand how the body uses foods to meet its needs and why some foods meet those needs better than others. Readers who are interested in weight control will discover which foods contribute most to body fat and which to select when trying to gain or lose weight safely. Readers who are physically active will discover which foods best support endurance activities and which to select when trying to build lean body mass.

7.1 Chemical Reactions in the Body

LEARN IT Identify the nutrients involved in energy metabolism and the high-energy compound that captures the energy released during their breakdown.

Earlier chapters introduced some of the body's chemical reactions: the making and breaking of the bonds in carbohydrates, fats, and proteins. Metabolism is the sum of these and all the other chemical reactions that go on in living cells; *energy metabolism* includes all the ways the body obtains and uses energy from food.

All the energy that sustains human life initially comes from the sun—the ultimate source of energy. During **photosynthesis,** plants make simple sugars from carbon dioxide and capture the sun's light energy in the chemical bonds of those sugars. Then human beings eat either the plants or the animals that have eaten the plants. These foods provide energy, but how does the body obtain that energy from foods? This chapter answers that question by following the nutrients that provide the body with **fuel** through a series of reactions that release energy from their chemical bonds. As the bonds break, they release energy in a controlled version of the same process by which wood burns in a fire. Both wood and food have the potential to provide energy. When wood burns in the presence of oxygen, it generates heat and light (energy), steam (water), and some carbon dioxide and ash (waste). Similarly, during **metabolism,** the body releases energy, water, and carbon dioxide (and other waste products).

The Site of Metabolic Reactions—Cells The human body is made up of trillions of cells, and each cell busily conducts its metabolic work all the time. (Appendix A presents a brief summary of the structure and function of the cell.) Figure 7-1 (p. 198) depicts a typical cell and shows where the major reactions of energy

photosynthesis: the process in which green plants use the sun's energy to make carbohydrates from carbon dioxide and water.

- **photo** = light
- **synthesis** = put together (making)

fuel: compounds that cells can use for energy. The major fuels include glucose, fatty acids, and amino acids; other fuels include ketone bodies, lactate, glycerol, and alcohol.

metabolism: the sum total of all the chemical reactions that go on in living cells. *Energy metabolism* includes all the reactions by which the body obtains and expends the energy from food.

- **metaballein** = change

> **FIGURE 7-1 A Typical Cell (Simplified Diagram)**

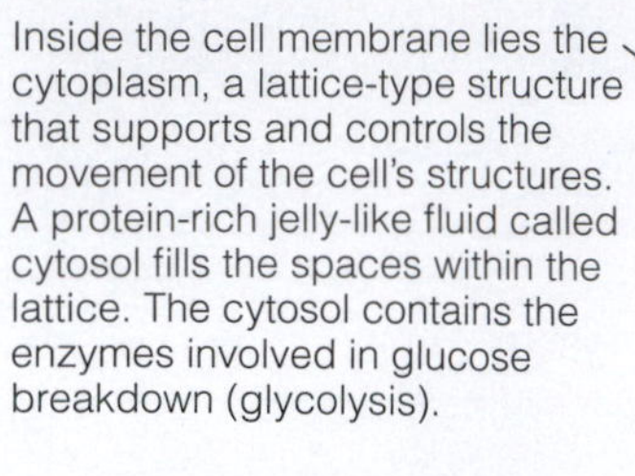

Inside the cell membrane lies the cytoplasm, a lattice-type structure that supports and controls the movement of the cell's structures. A protein-rich jelly-like fluid called cytosol fills the spaces within the lattice. The cytosol contains the enzymes involved in glucose breakdown (glycolysis).
A separate inner membrane encloses the cell's nucleus.
Inside the nucleus are the chromosomes, which contain the genetic material DNA.
Known as the "powerhouses" of the cells, the mitochondria are intricately folded membranes that house all the enzymes involved in the conversion of pyruvate to acetyl CoA, fatty acid oxidation, the TCA cycle, and the electron transport chain (described later in the chapter).
This network of membranes is known as smooth endoplasmic reticulum—the site of lipid synthesis.
A membrane encloses each cell's contents and regulates the passage of molecules in and out of the cell.
Rough endoplasmic reticulum is dotted with ribosomes—the site of protein synthesis (described in Chapter 6).

metabolism take place. The type and extent of metabolic activities vary depending on the type of cell, but of all the body's cells, the liver cells are the most versatile and metabolically active. Table 7-1 offers insights into the liver's work.

The Building Reactions—Anabolism Earlier chapters described how condensation reactions combine molecules to build body compounds. Glucose molecules may be joined together to make glycogen chains. Glycerol and fatty acids may be assembled into triglycerides. Amino acids may be linked together to make proteins. Each

TABLE 7-1 Metabolic Work of the Liver

The liver is the most active processing center in the body. When nutrients enter the body from the digestive tract, the liver receives them first; then it metabolizes, packages, stores, or ships them out for use by other tissues. When alcohol, drugs, or poisons enter the body, they are also sent directly to the liver, where they are detoxified and their by-products shipped out for excretion. An enthusiastic anatomy and physiology professor once remarked that given the many vital activities of the liver, we should express our feelings for others by saying, "I love you with all my liver" instead of "with all my heart." Granted, this declaration lacks romance, but it makes a valid point. Here are just some of the many jobs performed by the liver. To renew your appreciation for this remarkable organ, review Figure 3-11 (p. 81).

Carbohydrates

- Metabolizes fructose, galactose, and glucose
- Makes and stores glycogen
- Breaks down glycogen and releases glucose
- Breaks down glucose for energy when needed
- Makes glucose from some amino acids and glycerol when needed
- Converts excess glucose and fructose to fatty acids

Lipids

- Builds and breaks down triglycerides, phospholipids, and cholesterol as needed
- Breaks down fatty acids for energy when needed
- Packages lipids in lipoproteins for transport to other body tissues
- Manufactures bile to send to the gallbladder for use in fat digestion
- Makes ketone bodies when necessary

Proteins

- Manufactures nonessential amino acids that are in short supply
- Removes from circulation amino acids that are present in excess of need and converts them to other amino acids or deaminates them and converts them to glucose or fatty acids
- Removes ammonia from the blood and converts it to urea to be sent to the kidneys for excretion
- Makes other nitrogen-containing compounds the body needs (such as bases used in DNA and RNA)
- Makes many proteins

Other

- Detoxifies alcohol, other drugs, and poisons; prepares waste products for excretion
- Helps dismantle old red blood cells and captures the iron for recycling
- Stores most vitamins and many minerals
- Activates vitamin D

> **FIGURE 7-2 Anabolic and Catabolic Reactions Compared**

ANABOLIC REACTIONS

Anabolic reactions include the making of glycogen, triglycerides, and protein; these reactions require differing amounts of energy.

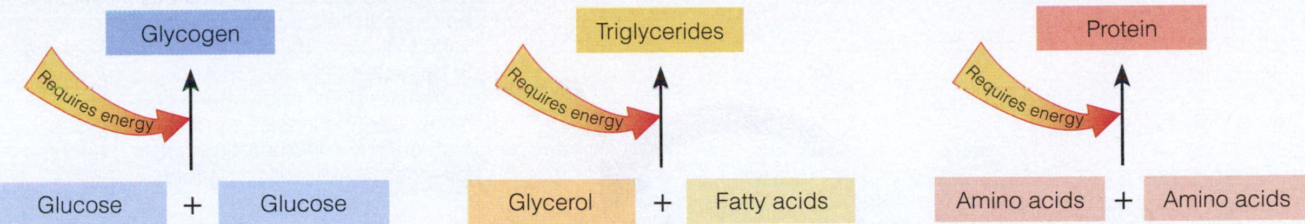

Glycogen
Requires energy
Glucose + Glucose
Triglycerides
Requires energy
Glycerol + Fatty acids
Protein
Requires energy
Amino acids + Amino acids

CATABOLIC REACTIONS

Catabolic reactions include the breakdown of glycogen, triglycerides, and protein; the further catabolism of glucose, glycerol, fatty acids, and amino acids releases differing amounts of energy. Much of the energy released is captured in the bonds of adenosine triphosphate (ATP).

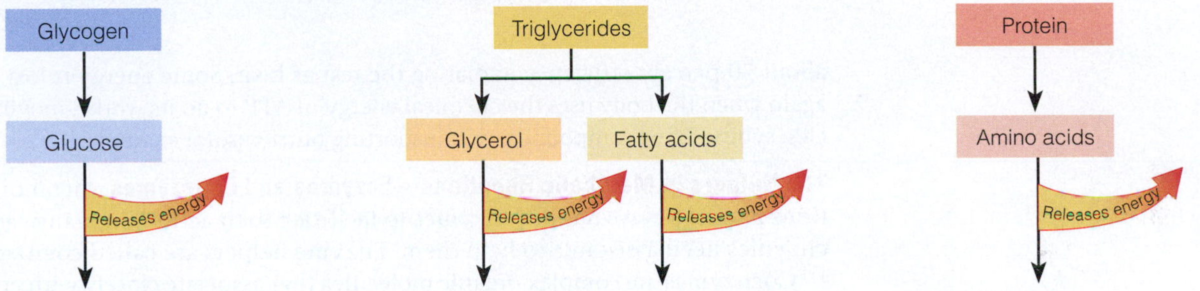

Glycogen
Glucose
Releases energy
Triglycerides
Glycerol
Fatty acids
Releases energy
Releases energy
Protein
Amino acids
Releases energy

NOTE: You need not memorize a color code to understand the figures in this chapter, but you may find it helpful to know that blue is used for carbohydrates, yellow for fats, and red for proteins.

of these reactions starts with small, simple compounds and uses them as building blocks to form larger, more complex structures. Because such reactions involve doing work, they require energy. The building up of body compounds is known as **anabolism.** Anabolic reactions are represented in this book, wherever possible, with "up" arrows in chemical diagrams (such as those shown at the top of Figure 7-2).

The Breakdown Reactions—Catabolism The breaking down of body compounds is known as **catabolism;** catabolic reactions release energy and are represented, wherever possible, by "down" arrows in chemical diagrams (as in the bottom of Figure 7-2). Earlier chapters described how hydrolysis reactions break down glycogen to glucose, triglycerides to fatty acids and glycerol, and proteins to amino acids. When the body needs energy, it breaks down these molecules further.

The Transfer of Energy in Reactions—ATP Some of the energy released during the breakdown of glucose, glycerol, fatty acids, and amino acids is captured in the high-energy compound **ATP (adenosine triphosphate).** ATP, as its name indicates, contains three phosphate groups (see Figure 7-3). The negative charges on the phosphate groups make ATP vulnerable to hydrolysis. During hydrolysis, the bonds between the phosphate groups readily break, splitting off one or two phosphate groups and releasing energy. In this way, ATP provides the energy that powers all the activities of living cells. Figure 7-4 (p. 200) describes how the body captures and releases energy in the bonds of ATP.

Quite often, the hydrolysis of ATP occurs simultaneously with reactions that will use that energy—a metabolic duet known as **coupled reactions.** In essence, the body uses ATP to transfer the energy released during catabolic reactions to power anabolic reactions that require energy. The body converts the chemical energy of food to the chemical energy of ATP with

anabolism (an-AB-o-lism): reactions in which small molecules are put together to build larger ones. Anabolic reactions require energy.

- **ana** = (build) up

catabolism (ca-TAB-o-lism): reactions in which large molecules are broken down to smaller ones. Catabolic reactions release energy.

- **kata** = (break) down

ATP, or **adenosine** (ah-DEN-oh-seen) **triphosphate** (try-FOS-fate): a common high-energy compound composed of a purine (adenine), a sugar (ribose), and three phosphate groups. ATP = A–P~P~P, with each ~ denoting a "high-energy" bond.

coupled reactions: pairs of chemical reactions in which some of the energy released from the breakdown of one compound is used to create a bond in the formation of another compound.

> **FIGURE 7-3 ATP (Adenosine Triphosphate)**

Notice that the bonds connecting the three phosphate groups have been drawn as wavy lines, indicating a high-energy bond. When these bonds are broken, energy is released.

NH_2 … CH_2–O–P–O~P–O~P–O⁻

Adenosine + 3 phosphate groups

> **FIGURE 7-4 The Capture and Release of Energy by ATP**

It may help to think of ATP as a rechargeable battery—capturing and releasing energy as it does the body's work.

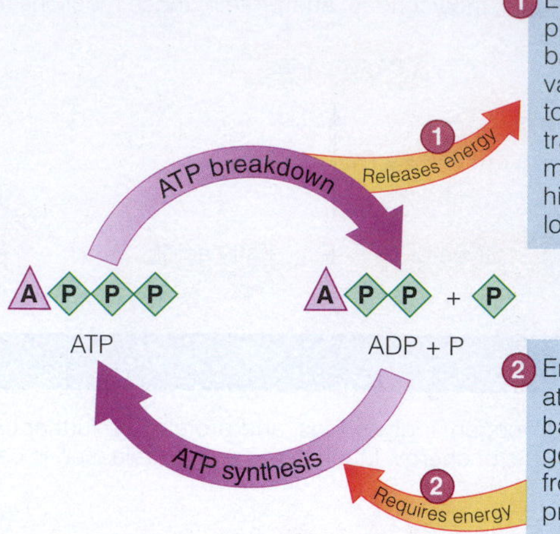

ATP breakdown
1 Releases energy
A P P P
ATP
A P P + P
ADP + P
ATP synthesis
2 Requires energy

1 Energy is released when a high-energy phosphate bond in ATP is broken. Just as a battery can be used to provide energy for a variety of uses, the energy from ATP can be used to do most of the body's work—contract muscles, transport compounds, make new molecules, and more. With the loss of a phosphate group, high-energy ATP (charged battery) becomes low-energy ADP (used battery).

2 Energy is required when a phosphate group is attached to ADP, making ATP. Just as a used battery needs energy from an electrical outlet to get recharged, ADP (used battery) needs energy from the breakdown of carbohydrate, fat, and protein to make ATP (recharged battery).

about 50 percent efficiency, radiating the rest as heat. Some energy is lost as heat again when the body uses the chemical energy of ATP to do its work—moving muscles, synthesizing compounds, or transporting nutrients, for example.

The Helpers in Metabolic Reactions—Enzymes and Coenzymes Metabolic reactions almost always require **enzymes** to facilitate their action. In many cases, the enzymes need assistants to help them. Enzyme helpers are called **coenzymes.***

Coenzymes are complex organic molecules that associate closely with enzymes but are not proteins themselves. The relationships between various coenzymes and their respective enzymes may differ in detail, but one thing is true of all: without its coenzyme, an enzyme cannot function. Some of the B vitamins serve as coenzymes that participate in the energy metabolism of glucose, glycerol, fatty acids, and amino acids. (Chapter 10 provides more details.)

REVIEW IT Identify the nutrients involved in energy metabolism and the high-energy compound that captures the energy released during their breakdown.

During digestion the energy-yielding nutrients—carbohydrates, fats, and proteins—are broken down to glucose (and other monosaccharides), glycerol, fatty acids, and amino acids. With the help of enzymes and coenzymes, the cells use these molecules to build more complex compounds (anabolism) or break them down further to release energy (catabolism). High-energy compounds such as ATP may capture the energy released during catabolism and provide the energy needed for anabolism.

7.2 Breaking Down Nutrients for Energy

LEARN IT Summarize the main steps in the energy metabolism of glucose, glycerol, fatty acids, and amino acids.

Chapters 4, 5, and 6 provided previews of metabolism; a brief review may be helpful. During digestion, the body breaks down the three energy-yielding nutrients—carbohydrates, fats, and proteins—into smaller molecules that can be absorbed:

- From carbohydrates—glucose (and other monosaccharides)
- From fats (triglycerides)—glycerol and fatty acids
- From proteins—amino acids

Each molecule of glucose, glycerol, fatty acids, and amino acids is composed of atoms—carbons, nitrogens, oxygens, and hydrogens. During catabolism, the

*The general term for substances that facilitate enzyme action is *cofactors;* they include both organic coenzymes made from vitamins and inorganic substances such as minerals.

enzymes: proteins that facilitate chemical reactions without being changed in the process; protein catalysts.

coenzymes: complex organic molecules that work with enzymes to facilitate the enzymes' activity. Many coenzymes have B vitamins as part of their structures. (Figure 10-2, p. 297 illustrates coenzyme action.)

- **co** = with

bonds between these atoms break, releasing energy. To follow this action, recall how many carbons are in each of these molecules:

- Glucose has 6 carbons:

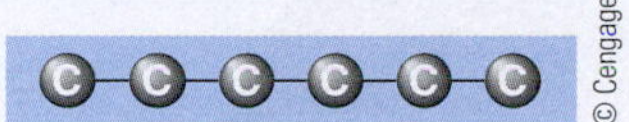

C C C C C C
© Cengage

- Glycerol has 3 carbons:

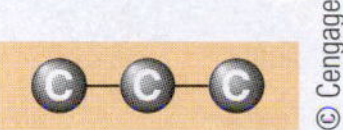

C C C
© Cengage

- A fatty acid may have 4 to 20 or more, usually an even number, of carbons, with 16 or 18 carbons most prevalent:

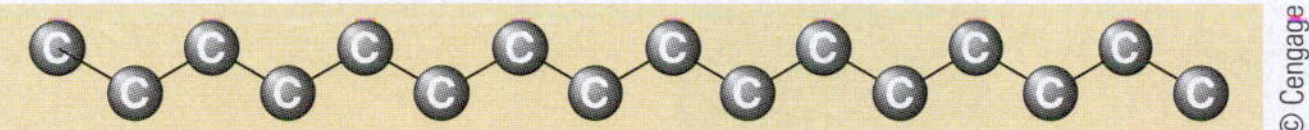

C C C C C C C C C C C C C C C C
© Cengage

- An amino acid may contain more carbons and assume other structural shapes, but this chapter commonly shows amino acids as having 2, 3, or 5 carbons with a nitrogen attached:

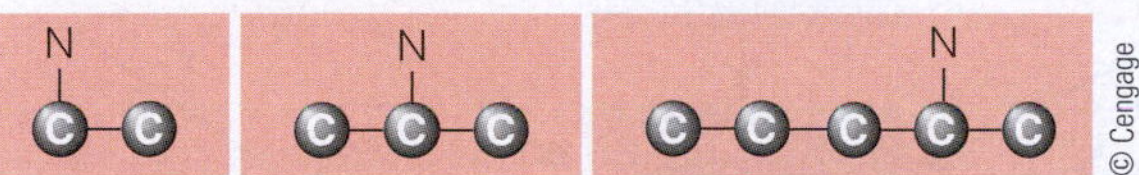

N
C C
N
C C C
N
C C C C C
© Cengage

Full chemical structures and reactions appear both in the earlier chapters and in Appendix C. This chapter diagrams the reactions using just the compounds' carbon and nitrogen atoms.

As you will see, each of these molecules—glucose, glycerol, fatty acids, and amino acids—starts down a different path, but they all can end up in the same place. (Similarly, three people entering an interstate highway at three different locations can all travel to the same destination.) Along the way, two new names appear—**pyruvate** (a 3-carbon structure) and **acetyl CoA** (a 2-carbon structure with a coenzyme, **CoA,** attached)—and the rest of the story falls into place around them.* Two major points to notice in the following discussion:

- Pyruvate can be used to make glucose.
- Acetyl CoA cannot be used to make glucose.

The body uses carbohydrates, fats, and proteins to fuel all its activities (see Photo 7-1). Learning which fuels can be used to make glucose and which cannot is a major key to understanding energy metabolism. Amino acids and glycerol can be converted to pyruvate and therefore *can* provide glucose for the body. Fatty acids are converted to acetyl CoA and therefore *cannot* make glucose. Acetyl CoA can readily make fat. Whereas most of the body's cells can use glucose, fat, or both for energy, the body *must* have glucose to fuel the activities of the central nervous system and red blood cells. Without glucose from food, the body will break down its own lean (protein-containing) tissue to get the amino acids needed to make glucose. To protect this protein tissue, the body needs foods that provide glucose—primarily carbohydrate. Eating only fat provides abundant acetyl CoA, but forces the body to break down protein tissue to make glucose. Eating only protein requires the body to convert protein to glucose. Clearly, the best diet provides ample carbohydrate (45 to 65 percent of kcalories), adequate protein (10 to 35 percent of kcalories), and some fat (20 to 35 percent of kcalories).

Figure 7-5 (p. 202) provides a simplified overview of the energy-yielding pathways. Upcoming sections of the chapter describe how each of the energy-yielding nutrients follows its pathway as it is broken down to acetyl CoA. Their paths merge at acetyl CoA, where the real action begins. Acetyl CoA enters the **TCA cycle,** and energy is harnessed through the **electron transport chain.** The TCA cycle and electron transport chain have central roles in energy metabolism and receive full attention later in the chapter—after following each of the energy nutrient pathways to acetyl CoA.

*The term *pyruvate* means a salt of *pyruvic acid*. (Throughout this book, the ending *-ate* is used interchangeably with *-ic acid*; for our purposes they mean the same thing.)

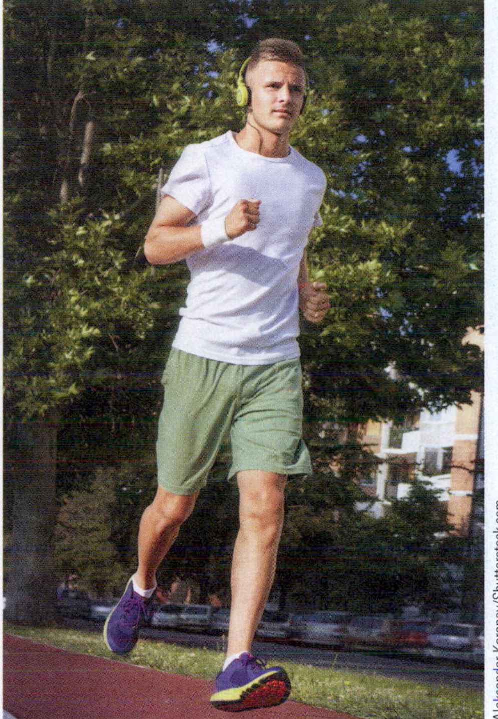

Aleksandar Karanov/Shutterstock.com

> **PHOTO 7-1** All the energy used to keep the heart beating, the brain thinking, and the body moving comes from the carbohydrates, fats, and proteins in foods.

pyruvate (PIE-roo-vate): a 3-carbon compound that plays a key role in energy metabolism.

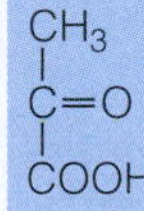

CH_3
C=O
COOH

acetyl CoA (ASS-eh-teel or ah-SEET-il, coh-AY): a 2-carbon compound (acetate or acetic acid) to which a molecule of CoA is attached.

CoA (coh-AY): coenzyme A; the coenzyme derived from the B vitamin pantothenic acid and central to energy metabolism.

TCA cycle or **tricarboxylic** (try-car-box-ILL-ick) **acid cycle:** a series of metabolic reactions that break down molecules of acetyl CoA to carbon dioxide and hydrogen atoms; also called the *citric acid cycle* or the *Krebs cycle* after the biochemist who elucidated its reactions.

electron transport chain: the final pathway in energy metabolism that transports electrons from hydrogen to oxygen and captures the energy released in the bonds of ATP; also called the *respiratory chain.*

> **FIGURE 7-5** Simplified Overview of Energy-Yielding Pathways

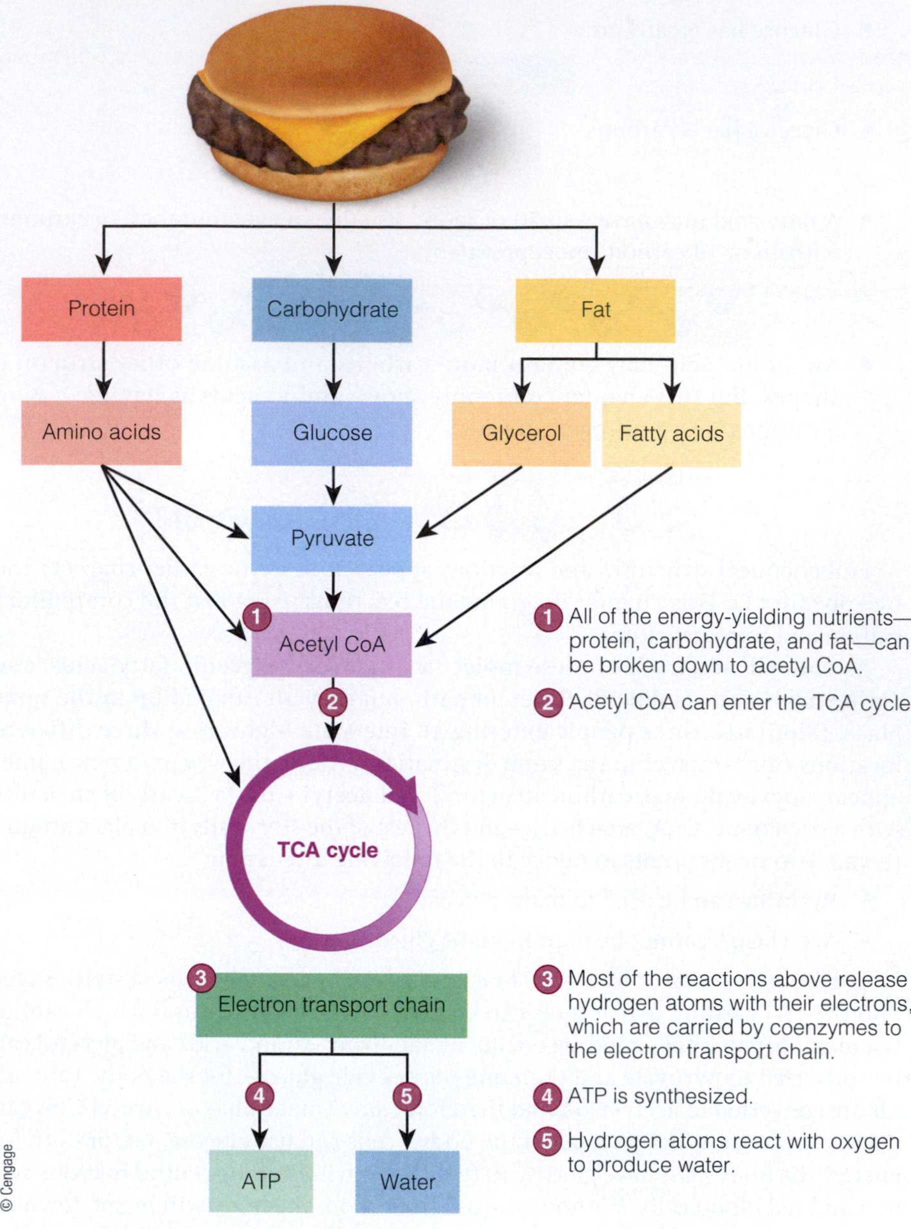

Protein
Carbohydrate
Fat
Amino acids
Glucose
Glycerol
Fatty acids
Pyruvate
Acetyl CoA
TCA cycle
Electron transport chain
ATP
Water
1 All of the energy-yielding nutrients—protein, carbohydrate, and fat—can be broken down to acetyl CoA.
2 Acetyl CoA can enter the TCA cycle.
3 Most of the reactions above release hydrogen atoms with their electrons, which are carried by coenzymes to the electron transport chain.
4 ATP is synthesized.
5 Hydrogen atoms react with oxygen to produce water.
© Cengage

Glucose

What happens to glucose, glycerol, fatty acids, and amino acids during energy metabolism can best be understood by starting with glucose. This discussion features glucose because of its central role in all cells' metabolism and because liver cells can convert the monosaccharides fructose and galactose to compounds that can enter the same energy pathways.

Glucose-to-Pyruvate The first pathway glucose takes on its way to yield energy is called **glycolysis** (glucose splitting).* Figure 7-6 shows a simplified drawing of glycolysis. (This pathway actually involves several more steps and several enzymes, which are detailed in Appendix C.) In a series of reactions, the 6-carbon glucose is converted to similar 6-carbon compounds before being split in half, forming two 3-carbon compounds. These 3-carbon compounds continue along the pathway until they are converted to pyruvate. Thus the net yield of one glucose molecule is two pyruvate molecules.

glycolysis (gly-COLL-ih-sis): the metabolic breakdown of glucose to pyruvate. Glycolysis does not require oxygen (anaerobic).

- **glyco** = glucose
- **lysis** = breakdown

*Glycolysis takes place in the cytosol of the cell (see Figure 7-1, p. 198).

> **FIGURE 7-6 Glycolysis: Glucose-to-Pyruvate**

This simplified overview of glycolysis illustrates the steps in the process of converting glucose to pyruvate. (Appendix C provides more details.) Notice that these arrows point down, indicating the breakdown of glucose to pyruvate during energy metabolism. (Alternatively, the arrows could point up, indicating the making of glucose from pyruvate, but that is not the focus of this discussion.)

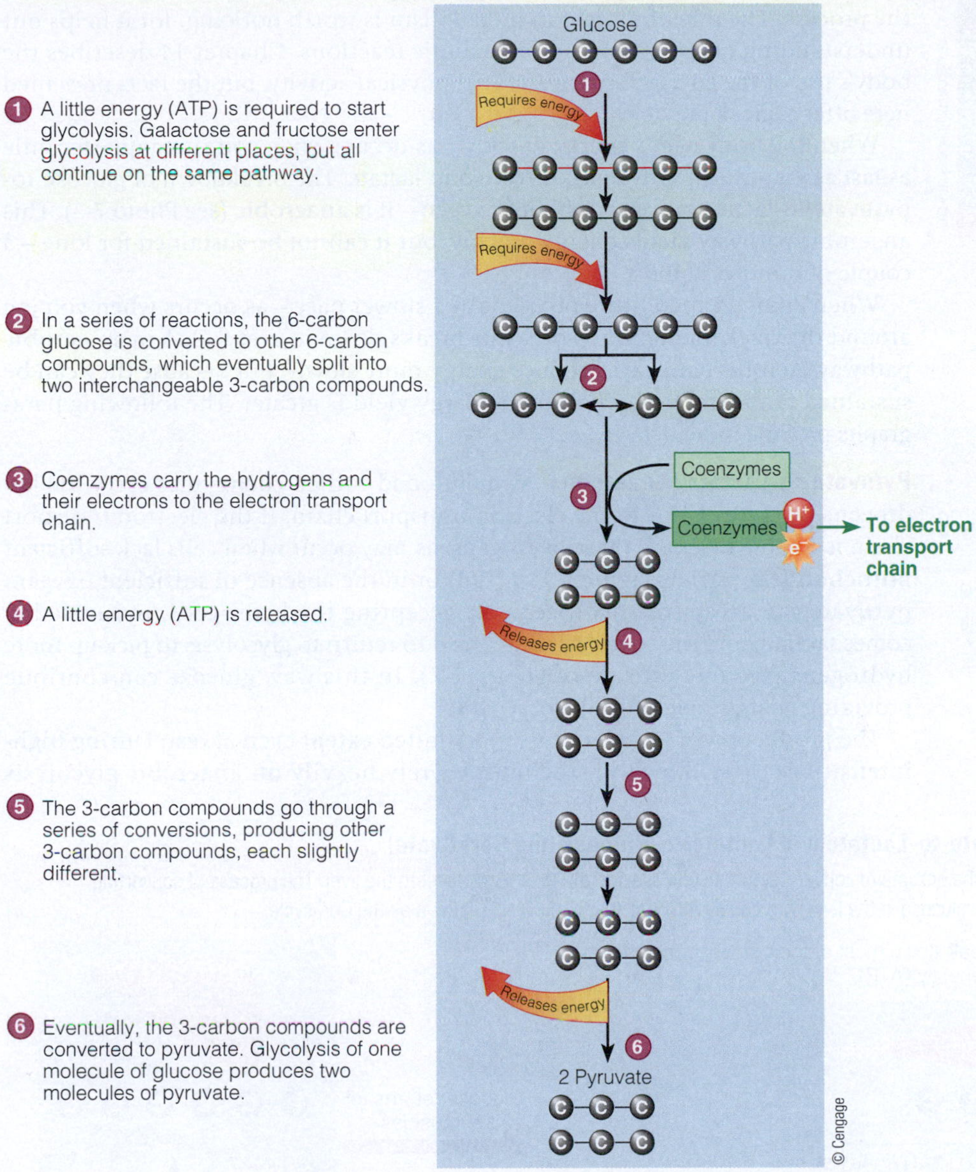

Glucose
C-C-C-C-C-C
1
Requires energy
Requires energy
2
Coenzymes
Coenzymes
3
H+
e-
To electron transport chain
Releases energy
4
5
Releases energy
6
2 Pyruvate
© Cengage

1 A little energy (ATP) is required to start glycolysis. Galactose and fructose enter glycolysis at different places, but all continue on the same pathway.

2 In a series of reactions, the 6-carbon glucose is converted to other 6-carbon compounds, which eventually split into two interchangeable 3-carbon compounds.

3 Coenzymes carry the hydrogens and their electrons to the electron transport chain.

4 A little energy (ATP) is released.

5 The 3-carbon compounds go through a series of conversions, producing other 3-carbon compounds, each slightly different.

6 Eventually, the 3-carbon compounds are converted to pyruvate. Glycolysis of one molecule of glucose produces two molecules of pyruvate.

NOTE: The cell uses a little energy (–2 ATP) to begin the breakdown of glucose to pyruvate, but then it gains a little more energy (+4 ATP), for a small net gain (of 2 ATP).

The net yield of energy at this point is small; to start glycolysis, the cell needs a little energy and then releases only a little more than it invested initially.* In addition, as glucose breaks down to pyruvate, hydrogen atoms with their electrons are released and carried to the electron transport chain by coenzymes made from the B vitamin niacin. A later section of the chapter explains how oxygen accepts the electrons and combines with the hydrogens to form water and how the process captures energy in the bonds of ATP.

This discussion focuses primarily on the breakdown of glucose for energy, but if needed, cells in the liver (and to some extent, the kidneys) can make glucose again from pyruvate in a process similar to the reversal of glycolysis. For this reason, the

*The cell uses two ATP to begin the breakdown of glucose to pyruvate, but it then gains four ATP, for a net gain of two ATP.

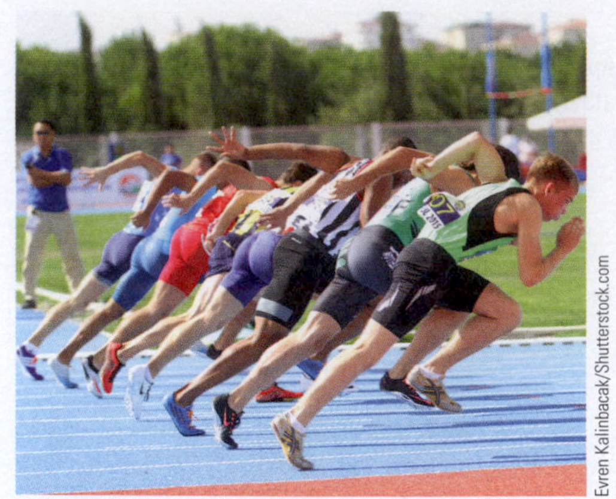
Evren Kalinbacak/Shutterstock.com

> **PHOTO 7-2** The anaerobic breakdown of glucose-to-pyruvate-to-lactate is the major source of energy for short, intense exercise.

anaerobic (AN-air-ROE-bic): not requiring oxygen.
- **an** = not

aerobic (air-ROE-bic): requiring oxygen.

mitochondria (my-toh-KON-dree-uh): the cellular organelles responsible for producing ATP aerobically; made of membranes with enzymes mounted on them. (The singular is *mitochondrion.*)
- **mitos** = thread (referring to their slender shape)
- **chondros** = cartilage (referring to their external appearance)

lactate: a 3-carbon compound produced from pyruvate during anaerobic metabolism.

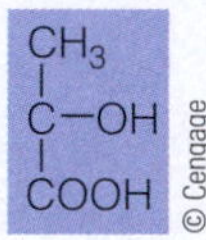
CH3
C—OH
COOH
© Cengage

arrows between glucose and pyruvate could point up as well as down. Making glucose requires energy, however, and different enzymes. Still, depending on the cell's needs, glucose may go "down" to make pyruvate, or pyruvate may go "up" to make glucose.

Pyruvate's Options—Anaerobic or Aerobic Whenever carbohydrates, fats, or proteins are broken down to provide energy, oxygen is always ultimately involved in the process. The role of oxygen in metabolism is worth noticing, for it helps our understanding of physiology and metabolic reactions. Chapter 14 describes the body's use of the energy nutrients to fuel physical activity, but the facts presented here offer a sneak preview.

When the body needs energy quickly—as occurs when you run a quarter mile as fast as you can—pyruvate is converted to lactate. The breakdown of glucose-to-pyruvate-to-lactate proceeds without oxygen—it is **anaerobic** (see Photo 7-2). This anaerobic pathway yields energy quickly, but it cannot be sustained for long—a couple of minutes at most.

When energy expenditure proceeds at a slower pace—as occurs when you jog around the track for an hour—pyruvate breaks down to acetyl CoA in an **aerobic** pathway. Aerobic pathways produce energy more slowly, but because they can be sustained for a long time, their total energy yield is greater. The following paragraphs provide more details.

Pyruvate-to-Lactate (Anaerobic) As mentioned earlier, coenzymes carry the hydrogens from glycolysis to the electron transport chain. If the electron transport chain is unable to accept these hydrogens, as may occur when cells lack sufficient **mitochondria** (review Figure 7-1, p. 198) or in the absence of sufficient oxygen, pyruvate can accept the hydrogens. By accepting the hydrogens, pyruvate becomes **lactate,** and the coenzymes are freed to return to glycolysis to pick up more hydrogens (see the left side of Figure 7-7). In this way, glucose can continue providing energy anaerobically for a while.

The production of lactate occurs to a limited extent even at rest. During high-intensity exercise, however, the muscles rely heavily on anaerobic glycolysis

> **FIGURE 7-7 Pyruvate-to-Lactate and Lactate-to-Glucose (the Cori Cycle)**

Because muscle cells lack the enzyme to convert lactate to glucose, lactate must first travel to the liver. The process of converting lactate from the muscles to glucose in the liver that can be returned to the muscles is known as the Cori cycle.

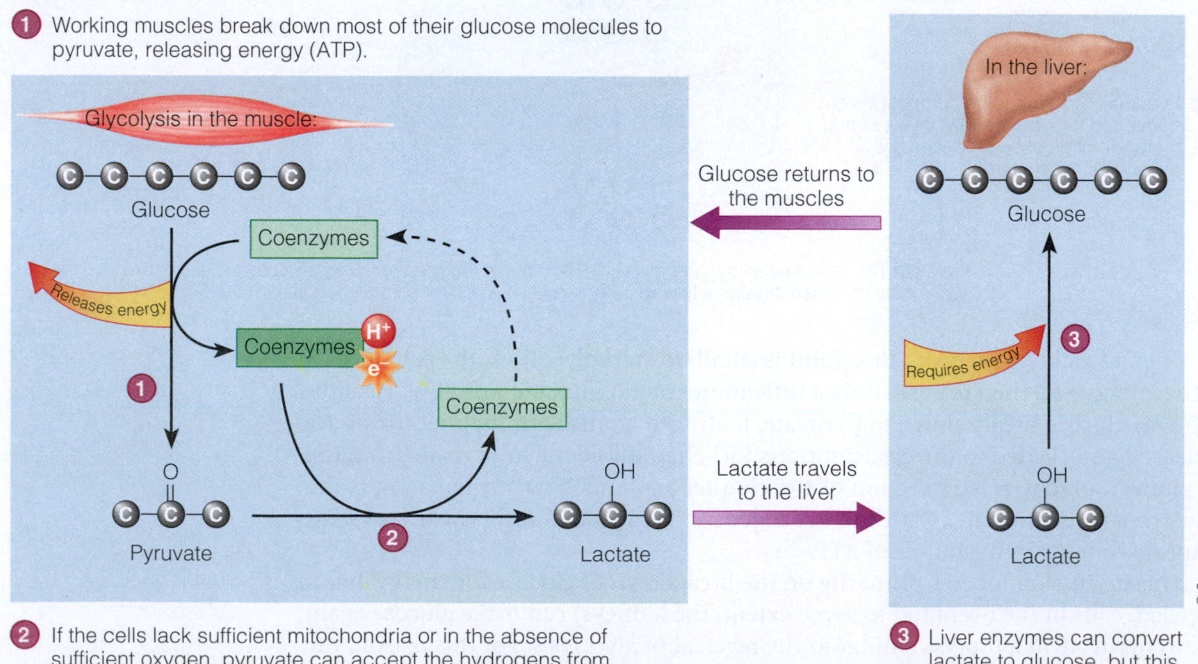
1 Working muscles break down most of their glucose molecules to pyruvate, releasing energy (ATP).
Glycolysis in the muscle:
C-C-C-C-C-C
Glucose
Coenzymes
Releases energy
Coenzymes
H+
e
1
Coenzymes
O
C-C-C
Pyruvate
2
OH
C-C-C
Lactate
Glucose returns to the muscles
Lactate travels to the liver
In the liver:
C-C-C-C-C-C
Glucose
Requires energy
3
OH
C-C-C
Lactate
© Cengage
2 If the cells lack sufficient mitochondria or in the absence of sufficient oxygen, pyruvate can accept the hydrogens from glucose breakdown and become lactate. This conversion frees the coenzymes so that glycolysis can continue.
3 Liver enzymes can convert lactate to glucose, but this reaction requires energy (ATP).

to produce ATP quickly, and the concentration of lactate increases dramatically. The rapid rate of glycolysis produces abundant pyruvate and releases hydrogen-carrying coenzymes more rapidly than the mitochondria can handle. To enable exercise to continue at this intensity, pyruvate is converted to lactate and coenzymes are released, which allows glycolysis to continue. The accumulation of lactate in the muscles coincides with—but does not seem to be the cause of—the subsequent drop in blood pH, burning pain, and fatigue that are commonly associated with intense exercise. In fact, making lactate from pyruvate removes two hydrogen ions, which actually diminishes acidity and improves the performance of tired muscles. A person performing the same exercise following endurance training actually experiences less discomfort—in part because the number of mitochondria in the muscle cells has increased. This adaptation improves the mitochondria's ability to keep pace with the muscles' demand for energy.

One possible fate of lactate is to be transported from the muscles to the liver. The liver can convert the lactate produced in muscles to glucose, which can then be returned to the muscles. (Muscle cells cannot convert lactate to glucose because they lack the necessary enzyme.) This recycling process is called the **Cori cycle** (see the right side of Figure 7-7).

Pyruvate-to-Acetyl CoA (Aerobic) If a cell needs energy and oxygen is available, pyruvate molecules enter the mitochondria of the cell. There a carbon group (COOH) from the 3-carbon pyruvate is removed to produce a 2-carbon compound that bonds with a molecule of CoA, becoming acetyl CoA. The carbon group from pyruvate becomes carbon dioxide (CO_2), which is released into the blood, circulated to the lungs, and breathed out. Figure 7-8 diagrams the pyruvate-to-acetyl CoA reaction.

Figure 7-9 shows that many of the body's metabolic pathways are reversible, but the step from pyruvate to acetyl CoA is not one of them. A cell cannot retrieve the carbons from carbon dioxide to remake pyruvate and then glucose. The pyruvate to acetyl CoA pathway is one way only.

The story of acetyl CoA continues on p. 207 after a discussion of how fat and protein arrive at the same crossroads. For now, know that when acetyl CoA continues on its energy-yielding pathway, much more ATP is produced than during glycolysis.

> FIGURE 7-8 Pyruvate-to-Acetyl CoA

The pyruvate-to-acetyl CoA reaction is not reversible.

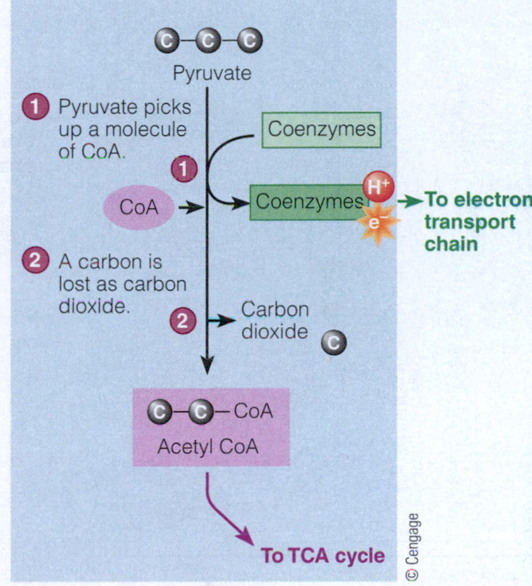

C–C–C
Pyruvate
1 Pyruvate picks up a molecule of CoA.
Coenzymes
CoA
Coenzymes
H+
e-
To electron transport chain
2 A carbon is lost as carbon dioxide.
Carbon dioxide
C
C–C–CoA
Acetyl CoA
To TCA cycle
© Cengage

REVIEW IT

The glucose-to-energy pathway begins with glycolysis—the breakdown of glucose to pyruvate. Pyruvate may be converted to lactate anaerobically or to acetyl CoA aerobically. The pathway from pyruvate to acetyl CoA is irreversible. Once the commitment to acetyl CoA is made, glucose is not retrievable; acetyl CoA cannot go back to glucose. Glucose can be synthesized only from pyruvate or compounds earlier in the pathway. Figure 7-10 (p. 206) summarizes the metabolism of glucose for energy.

> FIGURE 7-9 The Paths of Pyruvate and Acetyl CoA

Pyruvate may follow several reversible paths, but the path from pyruvate to acetyl CoA is irreversible. Notice that fatty acids cannot be used to make glucose.

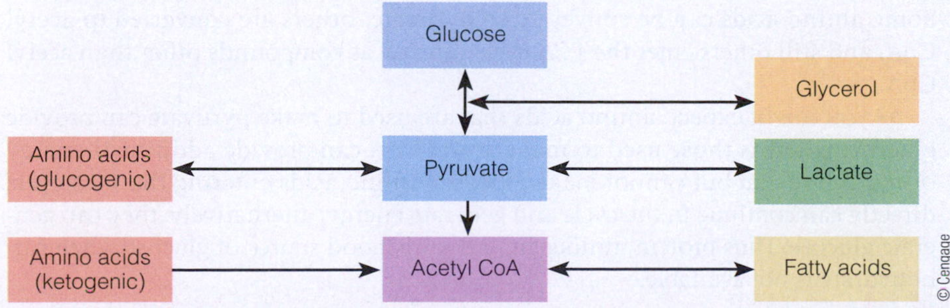

Glucose
Glycerol
Amino acids (glucogenic)
Pyruvate
Lactate
Amino acids (ketogenic)
Acetyl CoA
Fatty acids
© Cengage

NOTE: Amino acids that can be used to make glucose are called *glucogenic;* amino acids that are converted to acetyl CoA are called *ketogenic*.

Cori cycle: the pathway in which glucose is metabolized to lactate (by anaerobic glycolysis) in the muscle, lactate is converted back to glucose in the liver, and then glucose is returned to the muscle; named after the scientist who elucidated this pathway.

FIGURE 7-10 Glucose Enters the Energy Pathway

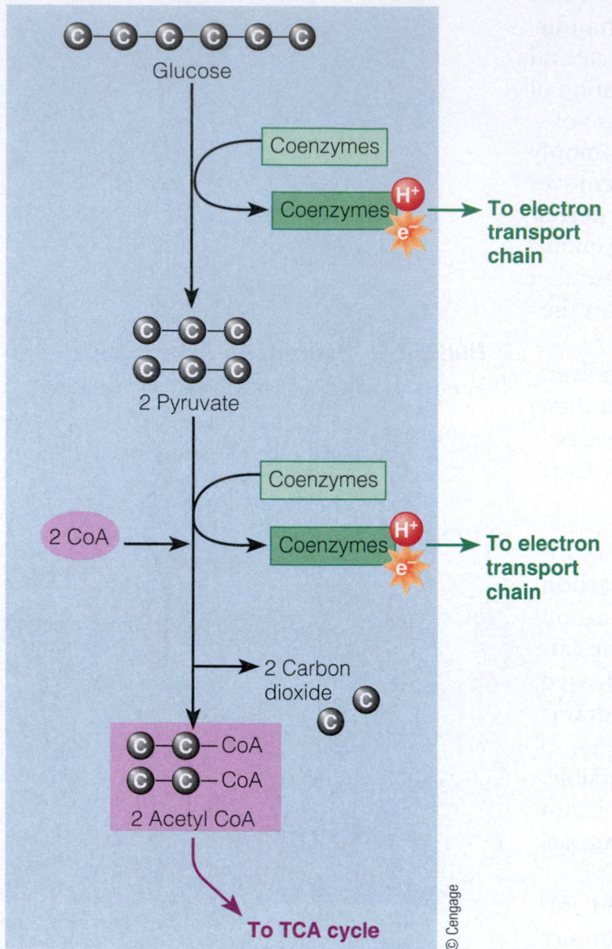
C C C C C C
Glucose
Coenzymes
Coenzymes
H+
e-
To electron transport chain
C C C
C C C
2 Pyruvate
Coenzymes
2 CoA
Coenzymes
H+
e-
To electron transport chain
2 Carbon dioxide
C
C
C C CoA
C C CoA
2 Acetyl CoA
To TCA cycle
© Cengage

REVIEW IT
1 glucose yields 2 pyruvate, which yield 2 acetyl CoA.

Glycerol and Fatty Acids

Recall that triglycerides can break down to glycerol and fatty acids. They enter energy metabolism via different pathways.

Glycerol-to-Pyruvate Glycerol is a 3-carbon compound like pyruvate but with a different arrangement of H and OH on the C. As such, glycerol can easily be converted to another 3-carbon compound that can go either "up" to glucose or "down" to pyruvate and then to acetyl CoA (review Figure 7-9, p. 205).

Fatty Acids-to-Acetyl CoA Fatty acids are taken apart two carbons at a time in a series of reactions known as **fatty acid oxidation.*** Figure 7-11 illustrates fatty acid oxidation and shows that in the process, each 2-carbon fragment splits off and combines with a molecule of CoA to make acetyl CoA. As each 2-carbon fragment breaks off, hydrogens and their electrons are released and carried to the electron transport chain by coenzymes made from the B vitamins riboflavin and niacin.

Fatty Acids Cannot Make Glucose As mentioned earlier, red blood cells and the brain and nervous system depend primarily on glucose as fuel. When carbohydrate is unavailable, liver cells can make glucose from pyruvate and other 3-carbon compounds, such as glycerol. Importantly, cells cannot make glucose from the 2-carbon fragments of fatty acids.

Remember that almost all dietary fats are triglycerides and that triglycerides contain only one small molecule of glycerol with three fatty acids. The glycerol can yield glucose, but that represents only 3 of the 50 or so carbons in a triglyceride—about 5 percent of its weight. The other 95 percent cannot be used to make glucose.

REVIEW IT
The body can convert the small glycerol portion of a triglyceride to either pyruvate (and then glucose) or acetyl CoA. The fatty acids of a triglyceride, on the other hand, cannot make glucose, but they can provide abundant acetyl CoA. Acetyl CoA may then enter the TCA cycle to release energy or combine with other molecules of acetyl CoA to make body fat. Figure 7-12 (p. 208) summarizes the metabolism of fats for energy.

Amino Acids

The preceding two sections described how the breakdown of carbohydrate and fat produces acetyl CoA. One energy-yielding nutrient remains: protein or, rather, the amino acids of protein.

Amino Acid Deamination Before entering the metabolic pathways, amino acids are deaminated (that is, they lose their nitrogen-containing amino group). Chapter 6 described how deamination produces ammonia (NH_3), which provides the nitrogen needed to make nonessential amino acids and other nitrogen-containing compounds. Any remaining ammonia is cleared from the body via urea synthesis in the liver and excretion in the kidneys.

Amino Acid Pathways Amino acids can enter the energy pathway several ways. Some amino acids can be converted to pyruvate, others are converted to acetyl CoA, and still others enter the TCA cycle directly as compounds other than acetyl CoA.

As you might expect, amino acids that are used to make pyruvate can provide glucose, whereas those used to make acetyl CoA can provide additional energy or make body fat but cannot make glucose. Amino acids entering the TCA cycle directly can continue in the cycle and generate energy; alternatively, they can generate glucose. Thus protein, unlike fat, is a fairly good source of glucose when carbohydrate is not available.

*Oxidation of fatty acids occurs in the mitochondria of the cells (review Figure 7-1, p. 198).

> **FIGURE 7-11 Fatty Acid-to-Acetyl CoA**

Fatty acids are broken apart into 2-carbon fragments that combine with CoA to make acetyl CoA.

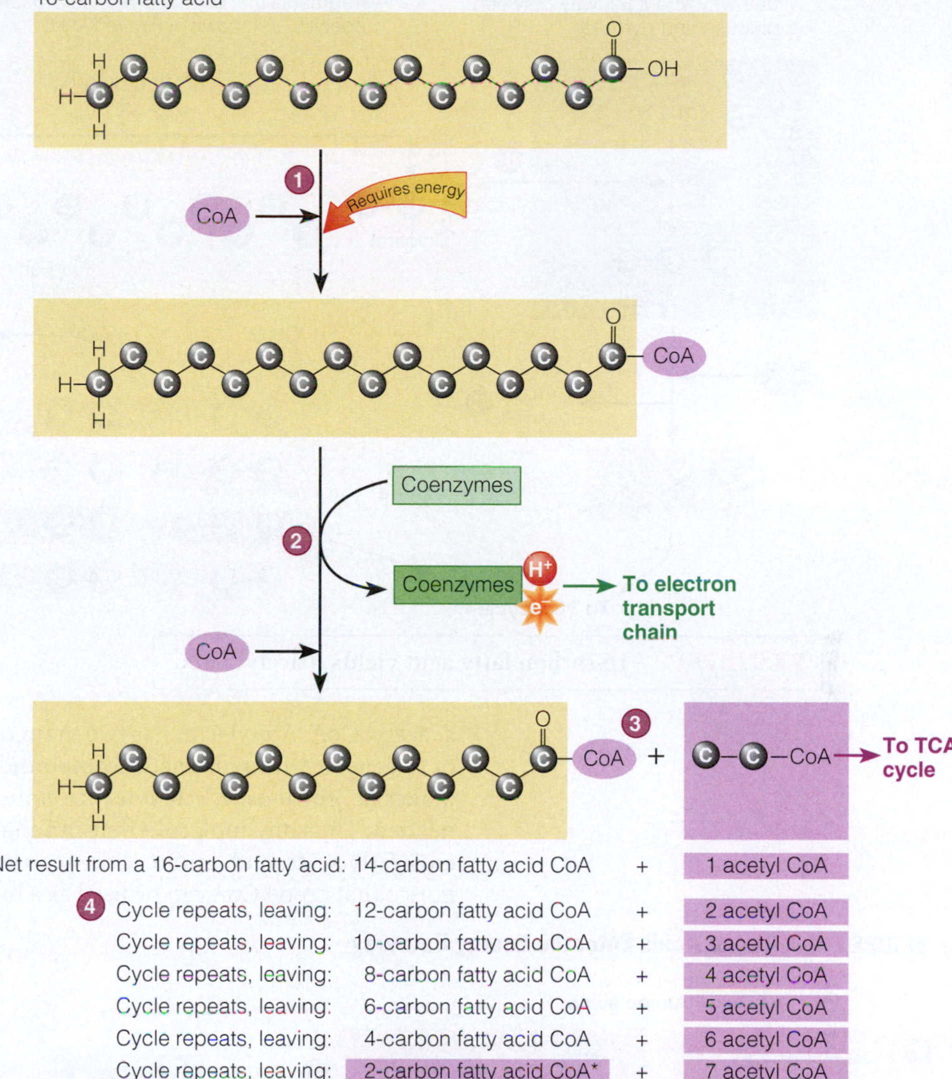

16-carbon fatty acid
H
H–C
H
O
C–OH
CoA
Requires energy
1 The fatty acid is first activated by coenzyme A, which requires energy.
CoA
Coenzymes
Coenzymes
H+
e
To electron transport chain
2 As each carbon-carbon bond is broken, hydrogens and their electrons are released, and coenzymes pick them up.
CoA
3 Another CoA joins the chain, and the bond at the second carbon (the beta-carbon) weakens. Acetyl CoA splits off, leaving a fatty acid that is two carbons shorter.
CoA
C–C–CoA
To TCA cycle
Net result from a 16-carbon fatty acid: 14-carbon fatty acid CoA + 1 acetyl CoA
4 Cycle repeats, leaving: 12-carbon fatty acid CoA + 2 acetyl CoA
Cycle repeats, leaving: 10-carbon fatty acid CoA + 3 acetyl CoA
Cycle repeats, leaving: 8-carbon fatty acid CoA + 4 acetyl CoA
Cycle repeats, leaving: 6-carbon fatty acid CoA + 5 acetyl CoA
Cycle repeats, leaving: 4-carbon fatty acid CoA + 6 acetyl CoA
Cycle repeats, leaving: 2-carbon fatty acid CoA* + 7 acetyl CoA
4 The shorter fatty acid enters the pathway and the cycle repeats, releasing more hydrogens with their electrons to coenzymes and producing more acetyl CoA. The molecules of acetyl CoA enter the TCA cycle, and the coenzymes carry the hydrogens and their electrons to the electron transport chain.
*Notice that 2-carbon fatty acid CoA = acetyl CoA, so that the final yield from a 16-carbon fatty acid is 8 acetyl CoA.

REVIEW IT

The body can use some amino acids to make glucose, whereas others can be used either to provide energy or to make fat. Before an amino acid enters any of these metabolic pathways, its nitrogen-containing amino group must be removed through deamination. Figure 7-13 (p. 208) summarizes how amino acids enter the energy pathway.

Table 7-2 (p. 209) reviews the ways the body can use the energy-yielding nutrients. To obtain energy, the body uses glucose and fatty acids as its primary fuels and amino acids to a lesser extent. To make glucose, the body can use all carbohydrates, most amino acids, and the glycerol portion of a triglyceride. Fatty acids cannot make glucose. To make proteins, the body needs amino acids. It can use glucose and glycerol to make some nonessential amino acids when nitrogen is available; it cannot use fatty acids to make proteins. Finally, when energy intake exceeds the body's needs, all three energy-yielding nutrients can make fat.

The Final Steps of Energy Metabolism Thus far the discussion has followed each of the energy-yielding nutrients down different pathways, all arriving

> **FIGURE 7-12 Fats Enter the Energy Pathway**

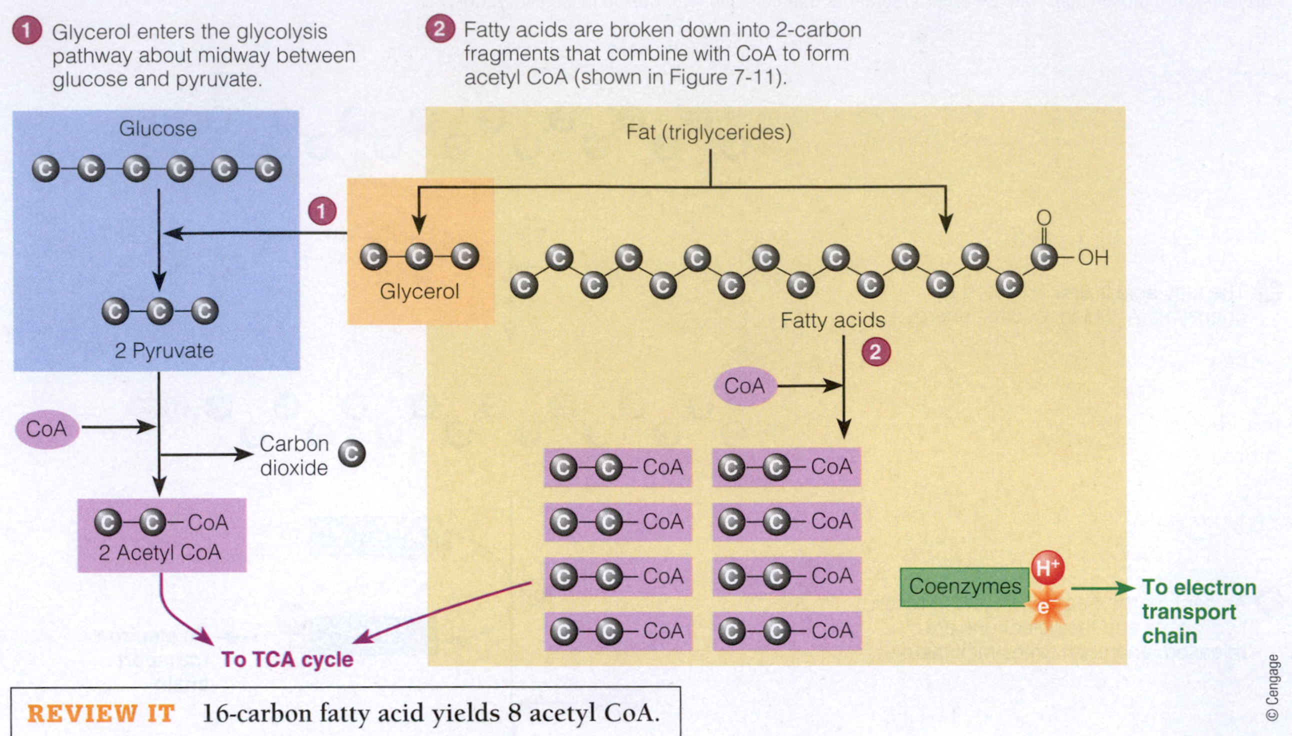

1 Glycerol enters the glycolysis pathway about midway between glucose and pyruvate.
2 Fatty acids are broken down into 2-carbon fragments that combine with CoA to form acetyl CoA (shown in Figure 7-11).
Glucose
Fat (triglycerides)
Glycerol
Fatty acids
2 Pyruvate
CoA
Carbon dioxide
2 Acetyl CoA
Coenzymes
To electron transport chain
To TCA cycle
© Cengage

REVIEW IT 16-carbon fatty acid yields 8 acetyl CoA.

at acetyl CoA. Acetyl CoA has two main options—it may be used to synthesize fats or to generate the high-energy compound ATP. When ATP is abundant, acetyl CoA makes fat, the most efficient way to store energy for later use when energy may be needed. Thus any molecule that can make acetyl CoA—including glucose, glycerol, fatty acids, and amino acids—can make fat. In reviewing Figure 7-9 (p. 205), notice that acetyl CoA can be used as a building block for fatty acids, but it cannot

> **FIGURE 7-13 Amino Acids Enter the Energy Pathway**

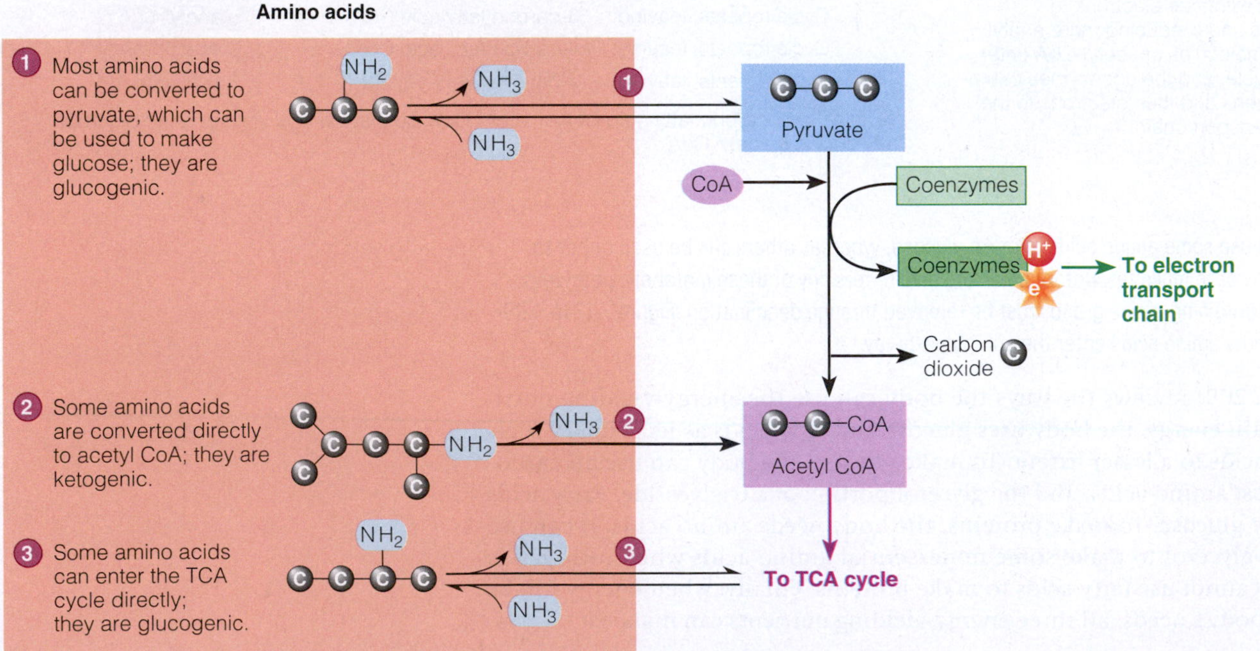

Amino acids
1 Most amino acids can be converted to pyruvate, which can be used to make glucose; they are glucogenic.
2 Some amino acids are converted directly to acetyl CoA; they are ketogenic.
3 Some amino acids can enter the TCA cycle directly; they are glucogenic.
NH_2
NH_3
Pyruvate
CoA
Coenzymes
To electron transport chain
Carbon dioxide
Acetyl CoA
To TCA cycle
© Cengage

NOTE: Deamination and the synthesis of urea were discussed and illustrated in Chapter 6, Figures 6-12 and 6-13 (p. 181). The arrows from pyruvate and the TCA cycle to amino acids are possible only for *nonessential* amino acids; remember, the body cannot make essential amino acids.

be used to make glucose or amino acids. When ATP is low and the cells need energy, acetyl CoA may proceed through the TCA cycle, releasing hydrogens with their electrons to the electron transport chain.

The TCA Cycle The TCA cycle is the final common metabolic pathway for carbohydrates, fats, and amino acids.[1] Its reactions take place in the inner compartment of the mitochondria. Examine the structure of the mitochondria shown in Figure 7-14. The significance of its structure will become evident as details unfold.

TABLE 7-2 Review of Energy-Yielding Nutrient End Points

Nutrient	Yields energy?	Yields glucose?	Yields amino acids and body proteins?	Yields fat stores?
Carbohydrates (glucose)	Yes	Yes	Yes—when nitrogen is available, can yield *nonessential* amino acids	Yes
Lipids (fatty acids)	Yes	No	No	Yes
Lipids (glycerol)	Yes	Yes—when carbohydrate is unavailable	Yes—when nitrogen is available, can yield *nonessential* amino acids	Yes
Proteins (amino acids)	Yes	Yes—when carbohydrate is unavailable	Yes	Yes

When cells need energy, acetyl CoA enters the TCA cycle, a busy metabolic traffic center. The TCA cycle is a circular path, but that doesn't mean it regenerates acetyl CoA. Acetyl CoA goes one way only—down to two carbon dioxide molecules and a coenzyme (CoA). The TCA cycle is a circular path because a 4-carbon compound known as **oxaloacetate** is needed in the first step and it is synthesized in the last step.

Oxaloacetate's role in replenishing the TCA cycle is critical. When oxaloacetate is insufficient, the TCA cycle slows down, and the cells face an energy crisis. Oxaloacetate is made primarily from pyruvate, although it can also be made from certain amino acids when pyruvate is unavailable. Importantly, oxaloacetate cannot be made from fat. That oxaloacetate must be available for acetyl CoA to enter the TCA cycle underscores the importance of carbohydrates in the diet. A diet that provides ample carbohydrate ensures an adequate supply of oxaloacetate—because glucose produces pyruvate during glycolysis. (This chapter closes with a discussion of the consequences of low-carbohydrate diets.)

As Figure 7-15 (p. 210) shows, oxaloacetate is the first 4-carbon compound to enter the TCA cycle. It picks up acetyl CoA, becomes a 6-carbon compound, drops off one carbon (as carbon dioxide), then another carbon (as carbon dioxide), and returns as 4-carbon oxaloacetate to pick up another acetyl CoA. As for acetyl CoA, its carbons go to carbon dioxide (see Appendix C for details).*

As compounds in the TCA cycle lose a carbon to carbon dioxide, hydrogen atoms with their electrons are carried off by coenzymes made from the B vitamins niacin and riboflavin to the electron transport chain—much like a taxicab that picks up passengers in one location and drops them off in another. Each turn of the TCA cycle releases a total of eight electrons.

The Electron Transport Chain The electron transport chain captures energy in the high-energy bonds of ATP. The electron transport chain consists of a series of proteins that serve as electron "carriers." These carriers are mounted in sequence on the inner membrane of a mitochondion (as shown in Figure 7-14). As the coenzymes deliver their electrons from the TCA cycle, glycolysis, and fatty acid oxidation to the

> FIGURE 7-14 A Mitochondrion

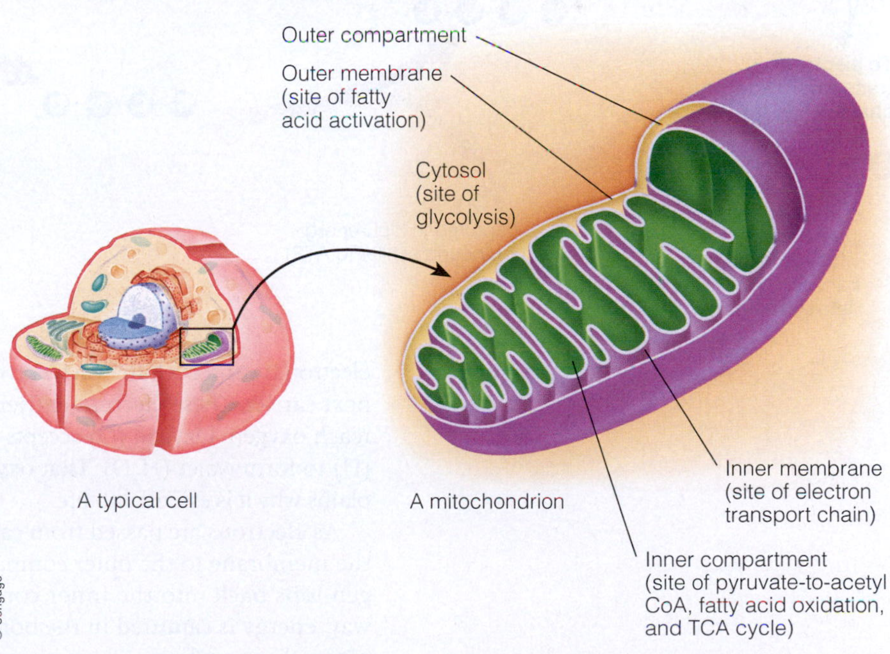
Outer compartment
Outer membrane (site of fatty acid activation)
Cytosol (site of glycolysis)
A typical cell
A mitochondrion
Inner membrane (site of electron transport chain)
Inner compartment (site of pyruvate-to-acetyl CoA, fatty acid oxidation, and TCA cycle)

*Actually, the carbons that enter the cycle in acetyl CoA may not be the exact ones that are given off as carbon dioxide. In one of the steps of the cycle, a 6-carbon compound of the cycle becomes symmetrical, both ends being identical. Thereafter it loses carbons to carbon dioxide at one end or the other. Thus only half of the carbons from acetyl CoA are given off as carbon dioxide in any one turn of the cycle; the other half become part of the compound that returns to pick up another acetyl CoA. It is true to say, though, that for each acetyl CoA that enters the TCA cycle, two carbons are given off as carbon dioxide. It is also true that with each turn of the cycle, the energy equivalent of one acetyl CoA is released.

oxaloacetate (OKS-ah-low-AS-eh-tate): a carbohydrate intermediate of the TCA cycle.

> FIGURE 7-15 The TCA Cycle

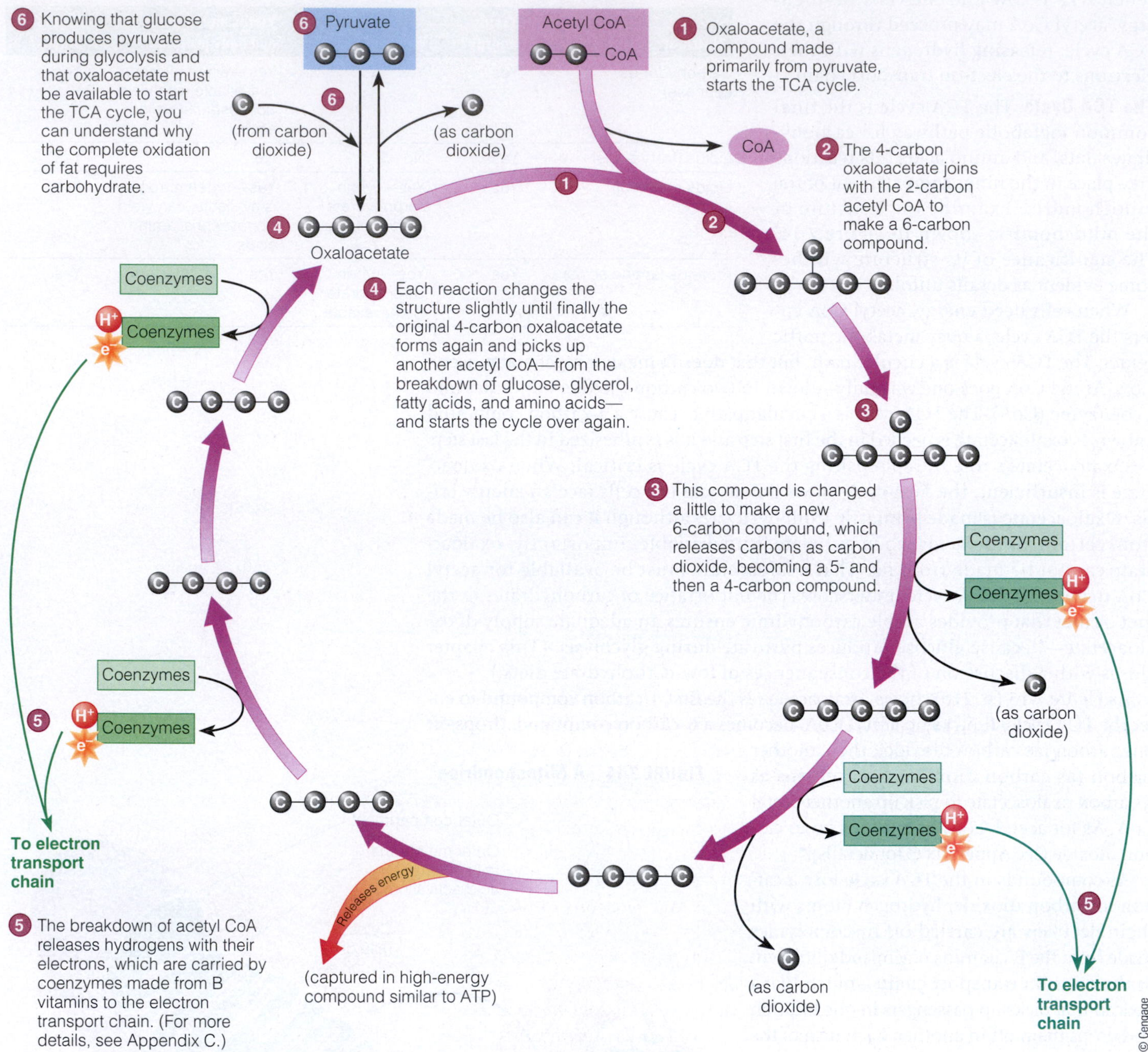

6 Knowing that glucose produces pyruvate during glycolysis and that oxaloacetate must be available to start the TCA cycle, you can understand why the complete oxidation of fat requires carbohydrate.
6 Pyruvate
C C C
Acetyl CoA
C C CoA
1 Oxaloacetate, a compound made primarily from pyruvate, starts the TCA cycle.
C
(from carbon dioxide)
6
C
(as carbon dioxide)
CoA
2 The 4-carbon oxaloacetate joins with the 2-carbon acetyl CoA to make a 6-carbon compound.
1
2
4
Oxaloacetate
Coenzymes
H+
e
Coenzymes
4 Each reaction changes the structure slightly until finally the original 4-carbon oxaloacetate forms again and picks up another acetyl CoA—from the breakdown of glucose, glycerol, fatty acids, and amino acids—and starts the cycle over again.
3
3 This compound is changed a little to make a new 6-carbon compound, which releases carbons as carbon dioxide, becoming a 5- and then a 4-carbon compound.
Coenzymes
H+
e
Coenzymes
Coenzymes
H+
e
Coenzymes
5
C
(as carbon dioxide)
Coenzymes
H+
e
Coenzymes
To electron transport chain
Releases energy
5 The breakdown of acetyl CoA releases hydrogens with their electrons, which are carried by coenzymes made from B vitamins to the electron transport chain. (For more details, see Appendix C.)
(captured in high-energy compound similar to ATP)
C
(as carbon dioxide)
5
To electron transport chain
© Cengage

electron transport chain, each carrier receives the electrons and passes them on to the next carrier. These electron carriers continue passing the electrons down until they reach oxygen. Oxygen (O) accepts the electrons and combines with hydrogen atoms (H) to form water (H_2O). That oxygen must be available for energy metabolism explains why it is essential to life.

As electrons are passed from carrier to carrier, hydrogen ions are pumped across the membrane to the outer compartment of the mitochondria. The rush of hydrogen ions back into the inner compartment powers the synthesis of ATP. In this way, energy is captured in the bonds of ATP. The ATP leaves the mitochondria and enters the cytoplasm, where it can be used for energy. Figure 7-16 provides a simple diagram of the electron transport chain (see Appendix C for details).

The kCalories-per-Gram Secret Revealed Of the three energy-yielding nutrients, fat provides the most energy per gram. The reason may be apparent in

> **FIGURE 7-16 Electron Transport Chain and ATP Synthesis**

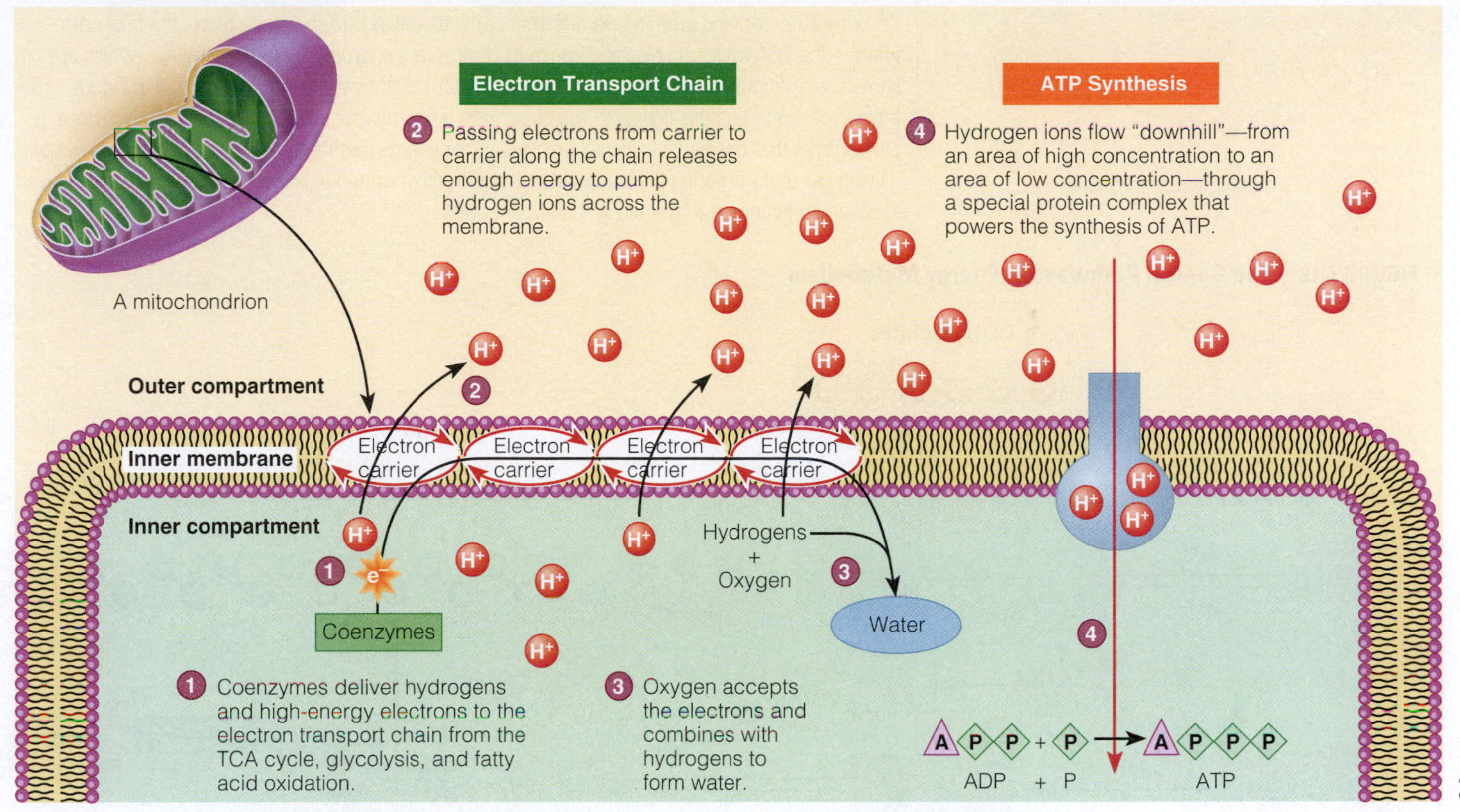

Electron Transport Chain
ATP Synthesis
2 Passing electrons from carrier to carrier along the chain releases enough energy to pump hydrogen ions across the membrane.
4 Hydrogen ions flow "downhill"—from an area of high concentration to an area of low concentration—through a special protein complex that powers the synthesis of ATP.
A mitochondrion
Outer compartment
Inner membrane
Inner compartment
Electron carrier
Electron carrier
Electron carrier
Electron carrier
Hydrogens + Oxygen
Coenzymes
Water
1 Coenzymes deliver hydrogens and high-energy electrons to the electron transport chain from the TCA cycle, glycolysis, and fatty acid oxidation.
3 Oxygen accepts the electrons and combines with hydrogens to form water.
ADP + P
ATP
© Cengage

Figure 7-17, which compares a fatty acid with a glucose molecule. Notice that nearly all the bonds in the fatty acid are between carbons and hydrogens. Oxygen can be added to all of them—forming carbon dioxide (CO_2) with the carbons and water (H_2O) with the hydrogens. As this happens, hydrogens are released to coenzymes heading for the electron transport chain. In glucose, on the other hand, an oxygen is already bonded to each carbon. Thus there is less potential for oxidation, and fewer hydrogens are released when the remaining bonds are broken.

Because fat contains many carbon-hydrogen bonds that can be readily oxidized, it sends numerous coenzymes with their hydrogens and electrons to the electron transport chain, where that energy can be captured in the bonds of ATP. This explains why fat yields more kcalories per gram than carbohydrate or protein. (Remember that each ATP holds energy and that kcalories measure energy; thus the more ATP, the more kcalories.) For example, one glucose molecule will yield 30 to 32 ATP when completely oxidized. In comparison, one 16-carbon fatty acid molecule will yield 129 ATP when completely oxidized. Fat is a more efficient fuel source. Gram for gram, fat can provide much more energy than either of the other two energy-yielding nutrients, making it the body's preferred form of energy storage. (Similarly, you might prefer to fill your car with a fuel that provides 130 miles per gallon versus one that provides 30 miles per gallon.)

> **FIGURE 7-17 Chemical Structures of a Fatty Acid and Glucose Compared**

To ease comparison, the structure shown here for glucose is not the ring structure shown in Chapter 4, but an alternative way of drawing its chemical structure.

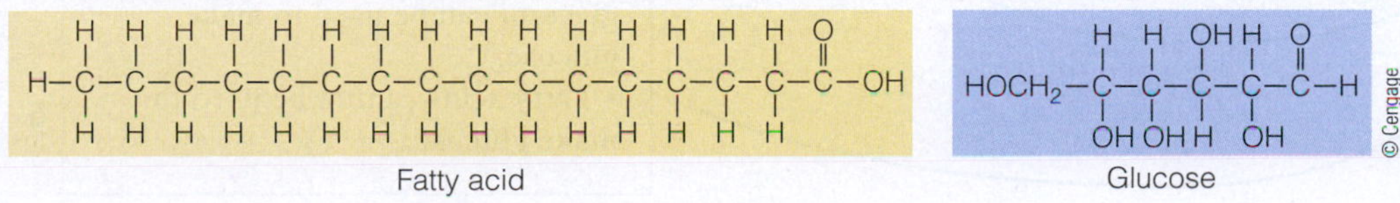

Fatty acid
Glucose
© Cengage

REVIEW IT **Summarize the main steps in the energy metabolism of glucose, glycerol, fatty acids, and amino acids.**

Carbohydrate, fat, and protein take different paths to acetyl CoA, but once there, the final pathways—the TCA cycle and electron transport chain—are shared. All of the pathways, which are shown as a simplified overview in Figure 7-5 (p. 202), are shown again in more detail in Figure 7-18. Instead of dismissing this figure as "too busy," take a few moments to appreciate the busyness of it all. Consider that this figure is merely an overview of energy metabolism, and then imagine how busy a living cell really is during the metabolism of hundreds of compounds, each of which may be involved in several reactions, each requiring specific enzymes.

> **FIGURE 7-18** **The Central Pathways of Energy Metabolism**

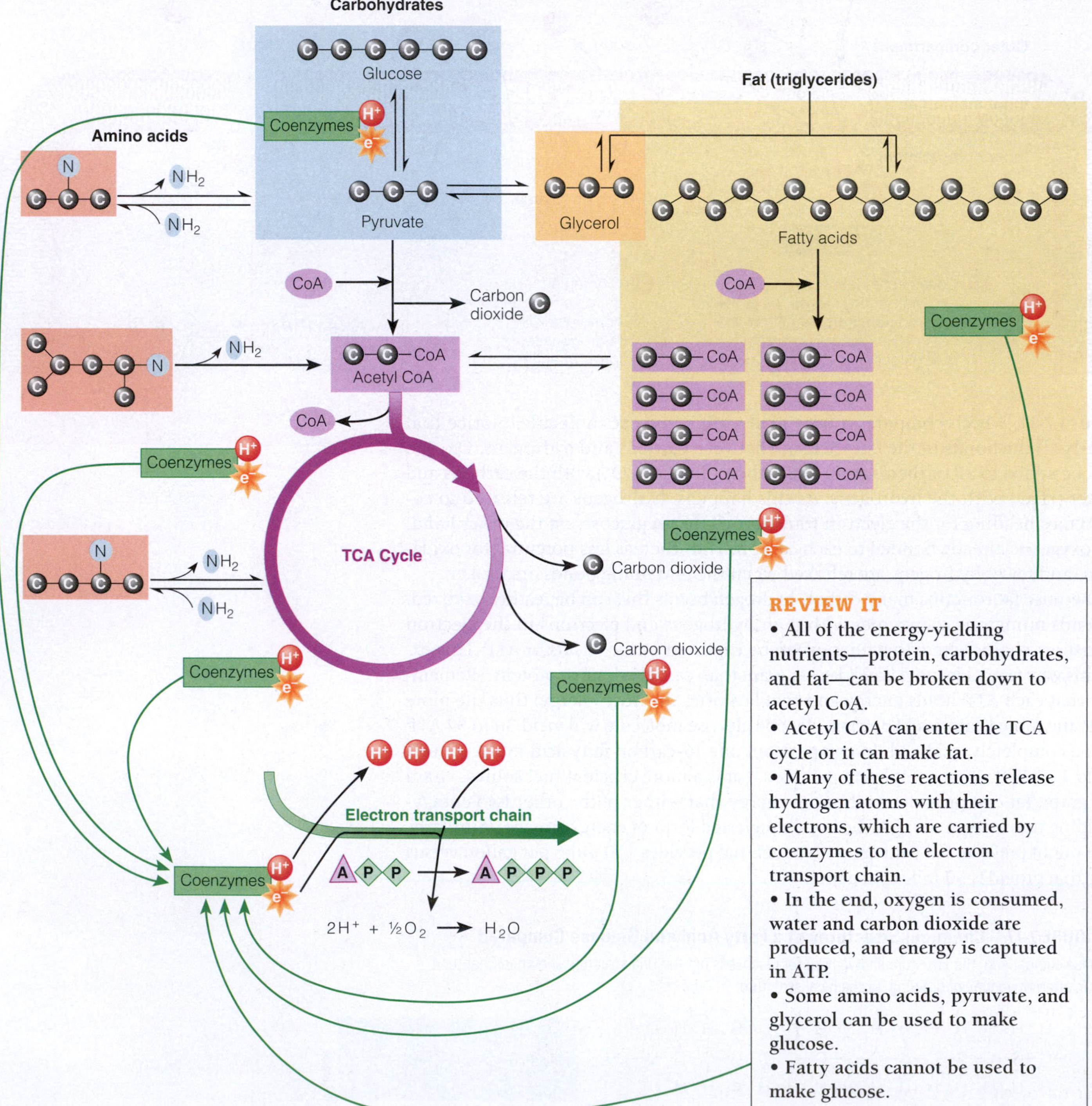
Carbohydrates
Glucose
Coenzymes
H+
e-
Pyruvate
Amino acids
N
NH2
NH2
Fat (triglycerides)
Glycerol
Fatty acids
CoA
Carbon dioxide
Acetyl CoA
CoA
TCA Cycle
Carbon dioxide
Carbon dioxide
Electron transport chain
A P P
A P P P
2H+ + ½O2 → H2O
REVIEW IT
• All of the energy-yielding nutrients—protein, carbohydrates, and fat—can be broken down to acetyl CoA.
• Acetyl CoA can enter the TCA cycle or it can make fat.
• Many of these reactions release hydrogen atoms with their electrons, which are carried by coenzymes to the electron transport chain.
• In the end, oxygen is consumed, water and carbon dioxide are produced, and energy is captured in ATP.
• Some amino acids, pyruvate, and glycerol can be used to make glucose.
• Fatty acids cannot be used to make glucose.
© Cengage

7.3 Feasting and Fasting

LEARN IT Explain how an excess of any of the three energy-yielding nutrients contributes to body fat and how an inadequate intake of any of them shifts metabolism.

Every day, a healthy diet delivers more than a thousand kcalories of energy—from carbohydrate, fat, and protein—to fuel the physical activity and metabolic work of the body. The details of energy metabolism have already been described; this discussion examines what happens when energy intake is excessive or inadequate and how metabolism shifts when the three energy-yielding nutrients are out of balance.

Feasting—Excess Energy When a person eats too much, metabolism favors fat formation. Fat cells enlarge regardless of whether the excess in kcalories derives from protein, carbohydrate, or fat. The pathway from dietary fat to body fat, however, is the most direct (requiring only a few metabolic steps) and the most efficient (costing only a few kcalories). To convert a dietary triglyceride to a triglyceride in adipose tissue, the body removes two of the fatty acids from the glycerol, absorbs the parts, and puts them (and others) together again. By comparison, to convert a molecule of sucrose, the body has to split glucose from fructose, absorb them, dismantle them to pyruvate and acetyl CoA, assemble many acetyl CoA molecules into fatty acid chains, and finally attach fatty acids to a glycerol molecule to make a triglyceride for storage in adipose tissue. Quite simply, the body uses much less energy to convert dietary fat to body fat than it does to convert dietary carbohydrate to body fat. On average, storing excess energy from dietary fat as body fat uses only 5 percent of the ingested energy intake, but storing excess energy from dietary carbohydrate as body fat requires 25 percent of the ingested energy intake.

The pathways from excess protein and excess carbohydrate to body fat are not only indirect and inefficient, but they are also less preferred by the body (having other priorities for using these nutrients). Before entering fat storage, protein must first tend to its many roles in the body's lean tissues, and carbohydrate must fill the glycogen stores. Simply put, using these two nutrients to make fat is a low priority for the body. Still, if eaten in abundance, any of the energy-yielding nutrients can be converted to fat for storage (see Photo 7-3).

This chapter has described each of the energy-yielding nutrients individually, but cells use a mixture of these fuels. How much of which nutrient is in the fuel mix depends, in part, on its availability from the diet. (The proportion of each fuel also depends on physical activity, as Chapter 14 explains.) Usually, protein's contribution to the fuel mix is relatively minor and fairly constant, but protein oxidation does increase when protein is eaten in excess. Similarly, carbohydrate eaten in excess significantly enhances carbohydrate oxidation. In contrast, fat oxidation does *not* respond to dietary fat intake. Instead of being oxidized, fat accumulates in storage. The details follow.

Excess Protein Recall from Chapter 6 that the body cannot store excess amino acids as such; it has to convert them to other compounds. Contrary to popular opinion, a person cannot grow muscle simply by overeating protein. Lean tissue such as muscle develops in response to a stimulus such as hormones or physical activity. When a person overeats protein, the body uses the surplus first by replacing normal daily losses and then by increasing protein oxidation. If excess protein is still available, the amino acids are deaminated and the remaining carbons are converted to ketone bodies, which are stored as fat in adipose tissue. Thus, a person can grow fat by eating too much protein.

Excess Carbohydrate Compared with protein, the proportion of carbohydrate in the fuel mix changes more dramatically when a person overeats. The body handles

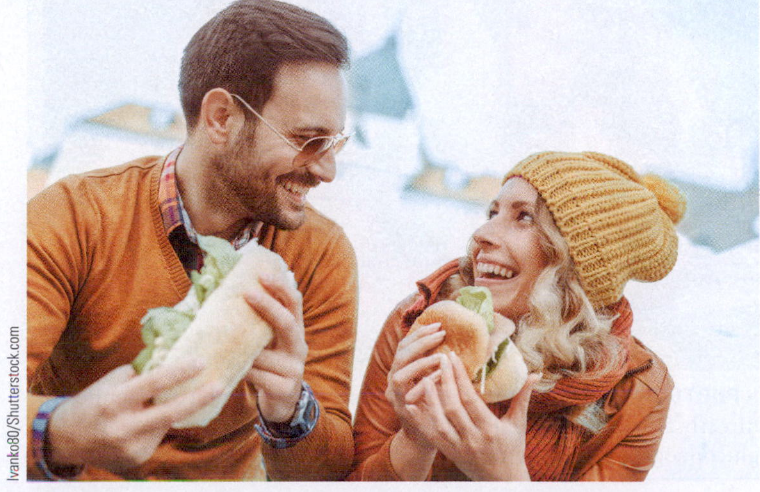
Ivanko80/Shutterstock.com

> **PHOTO 7-3** People can enjoy bountiful meals such as this without storing body fat, provided they expend as much energy as they take in.

abundant carbohydrate by first storing it as glycogen, but glycogen storage areas are limited and fill quickly. Because maintaining glucose balance is critical, the body uses glucose frugally when the diet provides only small amounts and freely when supplies are abundant. In other words, glucose oxidation rapidly adjusts to the dietary intake of carbohydrate.

Like protein, excess glucose can also be converted to fat. This pathway is relatively minor, however. As mentioned earlier, converting glucose to fat is energetically expensive and does not occur until after glycogen stores have been filled. Still, new body fat is made whenever carbohydrate intake is excessive.

Excess dietary carbohydrate can also displace fat in the fuel mix. When this occurs, carbohydrate spares both dietary fat and body fat from oxidation—an effect that may be more pronounced in overweight people than in lean people. The net result: excess carbohydrate contributes to obesity or at least to the maintenance of an overweight body.

Excess Fat Unlike excess protein and carbohydrate, which both increase oxidation, eating too much fat does not promote fat oxidation. Instead, excess dietary fat moves efficiently into the body's fat stores; almost all of the excess is stored.

The Transition from Feasting to Fasting

Figure 7-19 shows the metabolic pathways operating in the body as it shifts from feasting (part A) to fasting (parts B and C). After a meal, glucose, glycerol, and fatty acids from foods are used as needed and then stored. Later, as the body shifts from a fed state to a fasting one, it begins drawing on these stores. Glycogen and fat are released from storage to provide more glucose, glycerol, and fatty acids for energy.

Energy is needed all the time. Even when a person is asleep and totally relaxed, the cells are hard at work. In fact, this work—the cells' work that maintains all life processes without any conscious effort—represents about two-thirds of the total energy a person expends in a day.* The relatively small remainder is the work that a person's muscles perform voluntarily during waking hours.

The body's top priority is to meet the cells' needs for energy, and it normally does this by periodic refueling—that is, by eating several times a day. When food is not available, the body turns to its own tissues for fuel. If people choose not to eat, we say they are fasting; if they have no choice, we say they are starving. The body makes no such distinction. In either case, the body must draw on its reserves of carbohydrate and fat and, within a day or so, on its vital protein tissues as well.

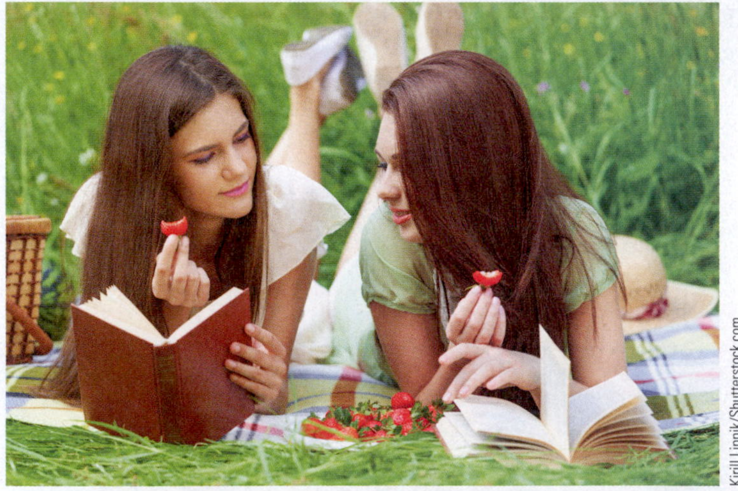
Kirill Linnik/Shutterstock.com

> **PHOTO 7-4** The brain and nerve cells depend on glucose—either directly from carbohydrates or indirectly from proteins (through gluconeogenesis). Importantly, fatty acids cannot provide glucose.

Fasting—Inadequate Energy

During fasting, carbohydrate, fat, and protein are all eventually used for energy—fuel must be delivered to every cell. As the fast begins, glucose from the liver's stored glycogen and fatty acids from the adipose tissue's stored fat travel to the cells. As described earlier, these molecules are broken down to acetyl CoA, which enters the energy pathways that power the cells' work. Several hours later, however, liver glycogen is depleted and blood glucose begins to fall. The body must adjust its normal metabolism to survive without food. Starvation demands that cells degrade their components for fuel.

Adaptation: Making Glucose At this point, most cells are using fatty acids for their fuel. But, as mentioned earlier, red blood cells and the cells of the nervous system need glucose. Glucose is their primary energy fuel (see Photo 7-4). Normally, the brain and nerve cells—which weigh only

*The cells' work that maintains all life processes refers to the body's *basal metabolism*, which is described in Chapter 8.

FIGURE 7-19 Feasting and Fasting

A Feasting: When a person eats in excess of energy needs, the body stores a small amount of glycogen and much larger quantities of fat.

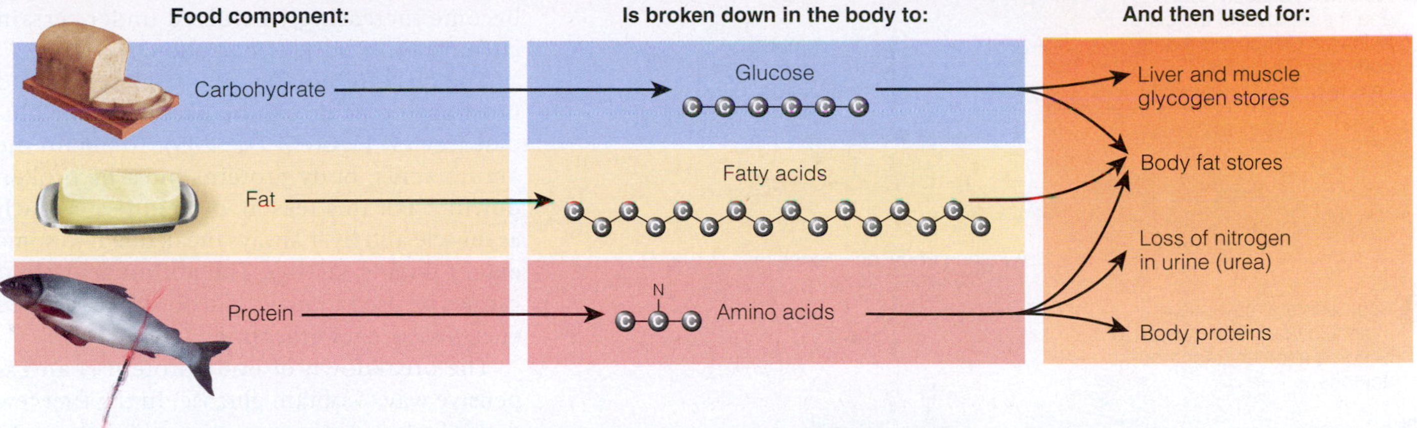
Food component:
Is broken down in the body to:
And then used for:
Carbohydrate
Glucose
Liver and muscle glycogen stores
Body fat stores
Fat
Fatty acids
Loss of nitrogen in urine (urea)
Protein
N
Amino acids
Body proteins

B Fasting: When nutrients from a meal are no longer available to provide energy (about 2 to 3 hours after a meal), the body draws on its glycogen and fat stores for energy.

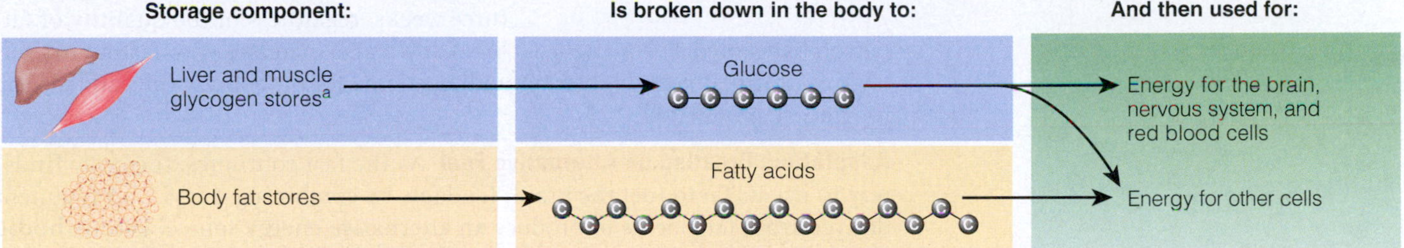
Storage component:
Is broken down in the body to:
And then used for:
Liver and muscle glycogen stores[a]
Glucose
Energy for the brain, nervous system, and red blood cells
Body fat stores
Fatty acids
Energy for other cells

C Fasting beyond glycogen depletion: As glycogen stores dwindle (after about 24 hours of starvation), the body begins to break down its protein (muscle and lean tissue) to amino acids to synthesize glucose needed for brain and nervous system energy. In addition, the liver converts fats to ketone bodies, which serve as an alternative energy source for the brain, thus slowing the breakdown of body protein.

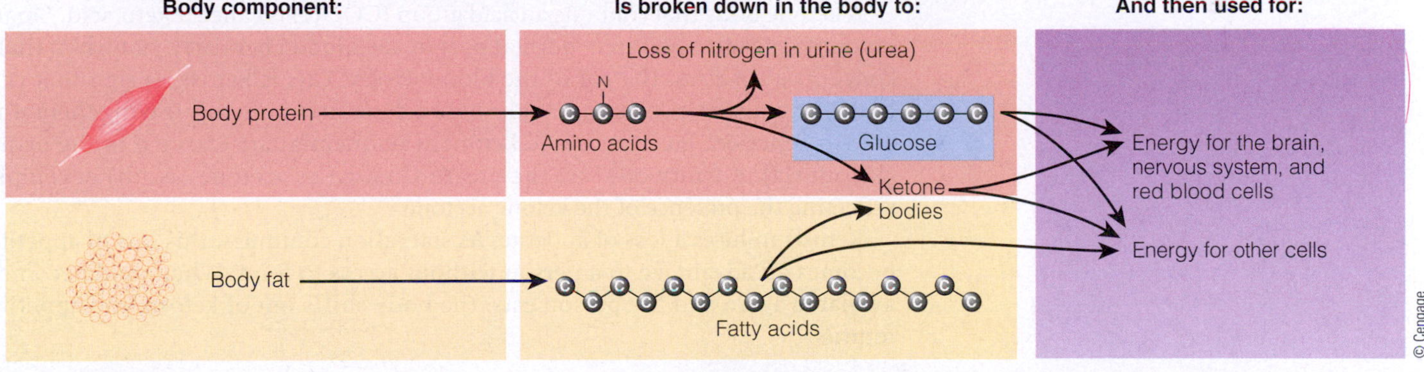
Body component:
Is broken down in the body to:
And then used for:
Loss of nitrogen in urine (urea)
Body protein
N
Amino acids
Glucose
Ketone bodies
Energy for the brain, nervous system, and red blood cells
Energy for other cells
Body fat
Fatty acids
© Cengage

NOTE: Alcohol is not included because it is a toxin and not a nutrient, but it does contribute energy to the body. After detoxifying the alcohol, the body uses the remaining two carbon fragments to build fatty acids and stores them as fat.

[a]The muscles' stored glycogen provides glucose only for the muscle in which the glycogen is stored.

about three pounds—consume about half of the total *glucose* used each day (about 500 kcalories' worth). About one-fourth of the *energy* the adult body uses when it is at rest is spent by the brain.

During a fast, the need for glucose poses a major problem. The body can use its stores of fat, which may be quite generous, to furnish most of its cells with energy, but the red blood cells are completely dependent on glucose, and the brain and

> **FIGURE 7-20 Ketone Body Formation**

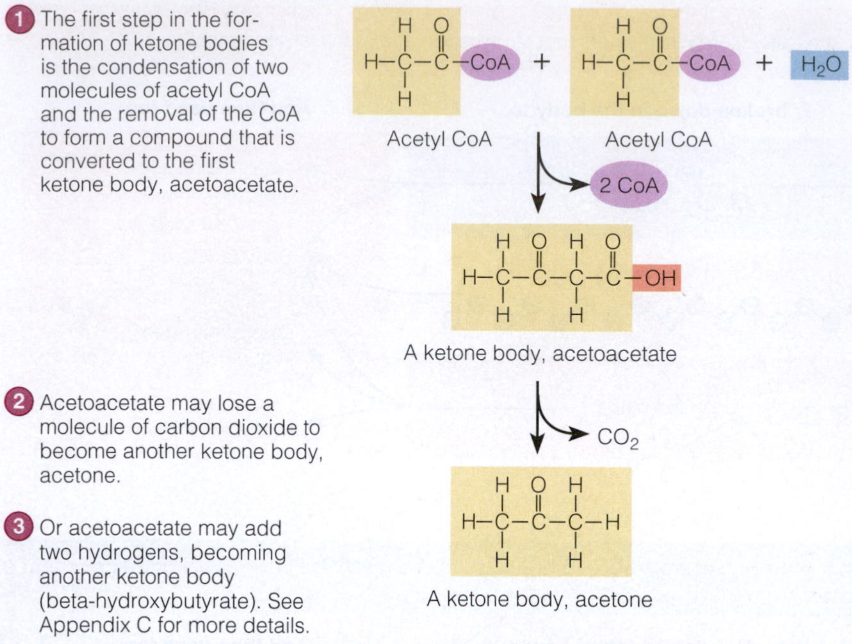

1 The first step in the formation of ketone bodies is the condensation of two molecules of acetyl CoA and the removal of the CoA to form a compound that is converted to the first ketone body, acetoacetate.
Acetyl CoA
Acetyl CoA
H_2O
2 CoA
A ketone body, acetoacetate
2 Acetoacetate may lose a molecule of carbon dioxide to become another ketone body, acetone.
CO_2
3 Or acetoacetate may add two hydrogens, becoming another ketone body (beta-hydroxybutyrate). See Appendix C for more details.
A ketone body, acetone
© Cengage

nerves prefer energy in the form of glucose.* Amino acids that yield pyruvate can be used for **gluconeogenesis**—the making of glucose from noncarbohydrate sources. The liver is the major site of gluconeogenesis, but the kidneys become increasingly involved under certain circumstances, such as starvation.

The glycerol portion of a triglyceride and most amino acids can be used to make glucose (review Figure 7-9, p. 205). To obtain the amino acids, body proteins must be broken down.** For this reason, protein tissues such as muscle and liver always break down to some extent during fasting. The amino acids that cannot be used to make glucose are used as an energy source for other body cells.

The breakdown of body protein is an expensive way to obtain glucose. In the first few days of a fast, body protein provides about 90 percent of the needed glucose; glycerol, about 10 percent. If body protein losses were to continue at this rate, death would follow within three weeks, regardless of the quantity of fat a person had stored. Fortunately, fat breakdown also increases with fasting—in fact, fat breakdown almost doubles, providing energy for other body cells and glycerol for glucose production.

Adaptation: Creating an Alternative Fuel As the fast continues, the body finds a way to use its fat to fuel the brain. It adapts by combining acetyl CoA fragments derived from fatty acids to produce an alternative energy source, **ketone bodies** (see Figure 7-20). Normally produced and used only in small quantities, ketone bodies can efficiently provide fuel for brain cells. Ketone body production rises until, after about 10 days of fasting, it is meeting much of the nervous system's energy needs. Still, many areas of the brain rely exclusively on glucose, and to produce it, the body continues to sacrifice protein—albeit at a slower rate than in the early days of fasting.

A ketone body that contains an acid group (COOH) is called a **keto acid.** Small amounts of keto acids are a normal part of the blood chemistry, but when their concentration rises, the pH of the blood drops. This is ketosis, a sign that the body's chemistry is shifting.[2] Acidic blood denatures proteins, leaving them unable to function. Elevated blood ketones (ketonemia) are excreted in the urine (ketonuria). A fruity odor on the breath (known as acetone breath) develops, reflecting the presence of the ketone acetone.

Ketosis induces a loss of appetite. As starvation continues, this loss of appetite becomes an advantage to a person without access to food. When food becomes available again and the person eats, the body shifts out of ketosis and appetite returns.

Adaptation: Conserving Energy In an effort to conserve body tissues for as long as possible, the hormones of fasting slow metabolism. As the body shifts to the use of ketone bodies, it simultaneously reduces its energy output and conserves both its fat and its lean tissue. Still the lean protein tissues diminish and perform less metabolic work, reducing energy expenditures. As the muscles waste, they can do less work and so demand less energy, reducing expenditures further. Although

gluconeogenesis (gloo-ko-nee-oh-JEN-ih-sis): the making of glucose from a noncarbohydrate source such as amino acids or glycerol.

- **gluco** = glucose
- **neo** = new
- **genesis** = making

ketone (KEE-tone) **bodies:** acidic compounds produced by the liver during the incomplete breakdown of fat when carbohydrate is not available.

keto (KEY-toe) **acid:** an organic acid that contains a carbonyl group (C=O).

*Red blood cells contain no mitochondria. Review Figure 7-1 (p. 198) to fully appreciate why red blood cells must depend on glucose for energy.

**An estimated 1 gram of protein can make ½ gram of glucose.

fasting may promote dramatic *weight* loss, a low-kcalorie diet and physical activity better support *fat* loss while retaining lean tissue.

These adaptations of fasting—slowing of energy output and reduction in fat loss—occur in the starving child, the hungry homeless adult, the adolescent with anorexia nervosa, and the malnourished hospital patient. Such adaptations help prolong their lives and explain the physical symptoms of starvation: wasting; slowed heart rate, respiration, and metabolism; lowered body temperature; impaired vision; organ failure; and reduced resistance to disease. Psychological effects of food deprivation include depression, anxiety, and food-related dreams.

The body's adaptations to fasting are sufficient to maintain life for a long time—up to 2 months. Mental alertness need not be diminished, and even some physical energy may remain unimpaired for a surprisingly long time. These remarkable adaptations, however, should not prevent anyone from recognizing the very real hazards that extensive fasting presents.

Intermittent Fasting Intermittent fasting has gained renewed interest in recent years. Some people practice alternate-day fasting, in which they alternate days of consuming no energy-containing foods or beverages with days of eating and drinking whatever they like. Others practice modified fasting in which they consume only 20 to 25 percent of their energy needs a couple of nonconsecutive days each week. These eating patterns result in some weight loss, although no more than typically occurs with standard energy-restricted weight-loss diet plans.[3] Little evidence suggests that intermittent fasting is harmful physically or mentally, and a few studies even suggest some health benefits.[4]

Time-restricted feeding is an alternative form of intermittent fasting that defines a time frame for eating. For example, a person might eat freely for 8 hours a day, but then fast for the remaining 16. Limited research suggests that time-restricted feeding may improve body weight, blood lipids, and blood glucose.[5]

Low-Carbohydrate Diets

When a person consumes a low-carbohydrate diet, a metabolism similar to that of fasting prevails (see Photo 7-5). With little dietary carbohydrate coming in, the body uses its glycogen stores to provide glucose for the cells of the brain, nerves, and blood. Once the body depletes its glycogen reserves, it begins making glucose from the amino acids of protein (gluconeogenesis). A low-carbohydrate diet may provide abundant protein from food, but the body still uses some protein from body tissues.

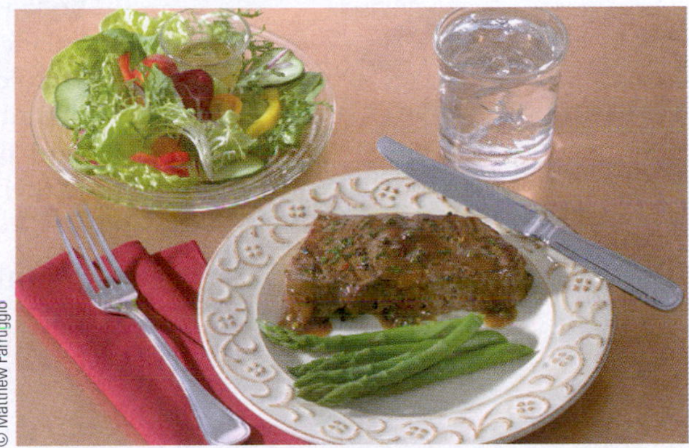

© Matthew Farruggio

> **PHOTO 7-5** Low-carbohydrate meals overemphasize meat, fish, poultry, eggs, and cheeses, and shun breads, pastas, fruits, and starchy vegetables.

Dieters can know glycogen depletion has occurred and gluconeogenesis has begun by monitoring their urine. Whenever glycogen or protein is broken down, water is released and urine production increases. Low-carbohydrate diets also induce ketosis, and ketones can be detected in the urine. Ketones form whenever glucose is lacking and fat breakdown is incomplete.

Many fad diets regard ketosis as the key to losing weight, but studies comparing weight-loss diets find no relation between ketosis and weight loss. People in ketosis may experience a loss of appetite and a dramatic weight loss within the first few days. They should know that much of this weight loss reflects the loss of glycogen and protein together with large quantities of body fluids and important minerals. They need to appreciate the difference between loss of *fat* and loss of *weight*. Fat losses on ketogenic diets are no greater than on other diets providing the same number of kcalories. Once the dieter returns to well-balanced meals that provide adequate energy, carbohydrate, fat, protein, vitamins, and minerals, the body avidly retains these needed nutrients. The weight will return, quite often to a level higher than the starting point. In addition to weight loss, ketogenic diets are often used in the treatment of several diseases, most notably epilepsy.[6] Table 7-3 lists some of the consequences of a ketogenic diet.

TABLE 7-3 Adverse Side Effects of Low-Carbohydrate, Ketogenic Diets

- Nausea
- Fatigue (especially if physically active)
- Constipation
- Low blood pressure
- Elevated uric acid (which may exacerbate kidney disease and cause inflammation of the joints in those predisposed to gout)
- Stale, foul taste in the mouth (bad breath)
- In pregnant women, fetal harm and stillbirth

This chapter has described how the cells use carbohydrate, fat, and protein from the diet to fuel the body's metabolic activities. For optimal health, the following balance is recommended:

- Carbohydrate: 45 to 65 percent
- Fat: 20 to 35 percent
- Protein: 10 to 35 percent

At any given level of energy intake, if one of these nutrients increases, one or both of the others decrease in proportion. Carbohydrate and fat typically contribute the most to a person's daily energy intake; protein makes a smaller and less varied contribution. Consequently, high-carbohydrate diets tend to be low-fat diets and low-carbohydrate diets tend to be high-fat diets. Balanced diets best support optimal metabolic activity.

REVIEW IT Explain how an excess of any of the three energy-yielding nutrients contributes to body fat and how an inadequate intake of any of them shifts metabolism.

When energy intake exceeds energy needs, the body makes fat—regardless of whether the excess intake is from protein, carbohydrate, or fat. The only difference is that the body is much more efficient at storing energy when the excess derives from dietary fat.

When fasting, the body makes a number of adaptations: increasing the breakdown of fat to provide energy for most of the cells, using glycerol and amino acids to make glucose for the red blood cells and central nervous system, producing ketones to fuel the brain, suppressing the appetite, and slowing metabolism. All of these measures conserve energy and minimize losses. Low-carbohydrate diets incur similar changes in metabolism.

This chapter has probed the intricate details of metabolism at the level of the cells. Several upcoming chapters and highlights build on this information. The highlight that follows this chapter focuses on how alcohol disrupts metabolism. Chapter 8 describes how a person's intake and expenditure of energy are reflected in body weight and body composition. Chapter 9 examines the consequences of unbalanced energy budgets—overweight and underweight. Chapter 10 shows the vital roles the B vitamins play as coenzymes assisting in all the metabolic pathways described here. And Chapter 14 revisits metabolism to show how it supports the work of physically active people and how athletes can best apply that information in their choices of foods to eat.

What's Online

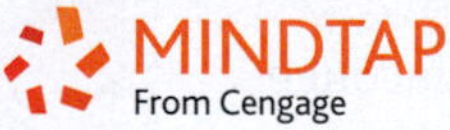
MINDTAP
From Cengage

Visit **www.cengagebrain.com** to access MindTap, a complete digital course that includes Diet & Wellness Plus, interactive quizzes, videos, and more.

REFERENCES

1. M. Akram, Citric acid cycle and role of its intermediates in metabolism, *Cell Biochemistry and Biophysics* 68 (2014): 475–478.
2. J. C. Newman and E. Verdin, Ketone bodies as signaling metabolites, *Trends in Endocrinology and Metabolism* 25 (2014): 42–52.
3. R. E. Patterson and coauthors, Intermittent fasting and human metabolic health, *Journal of the Academy of Nutrition and Dietetics* 115 (2015): 1203–1212.
4. B. D. Horne, J. B. Muhlestein, and J. L. Anderson, Health effects of intermittent fasting: Hormesis or harm? A systematic review, *American Journal of Clinical Nutrition* 102 (2015): 464–470; G. M. Tinsley and P. M. LaBounty, Effects of intermittent fasting on body composition and clinical health markers in humans, *Nutrition Reviews* 73 (2015): 661–674.
5. J. Rothschild and coauthors, Time restricted feeding and risk of metabolic disease: A review of human and animal studies, *Nutrition Reviews* 72 (2014): 308–318.
6. P. Klein, I. Tyrlikova, and G. C. Mathews, Dietary treatment in adults with refractory epilepsy: A review, *Neurology* 83 (2014): 1978–1985; A. Paoli and coauthors, Beyond weight loss: A review of the therapeutic uses of very-low-carbohydrate (ketogenic) diets, *European Journal of Clinical Nutrition* 67 (2013): 789–796.

LEARN IT Describe how alcohol disrupts metabolism and impairs health.

Alcohol in the Body

With the understanding of metabolism gained from Chapter 7, you are in a position to understand how the body handles alcohol, how alcohol interferes with metabolism, and how alcohol impairs health and nutrition. Before examining alcohol's damaging effects, it may be appropriate to mention that drinking alcohol in *moderation* may have some health benefits, including reduced risks of heart disease, diabetes, and osteoporosis.[1] Moderate alcohol consumption may lower mortality from all causes, but only in older adults. For people between the ages of 15 and 49, alcohol is the leading risk factor for premature death and disability.[2] Importantly, health care professionals do not recommend alcohol to nondrinkers because any benefits of moderate alcohol use outweigh the many harmful effects of excessive alcohol use, including an elevated risk of mortality.[3]

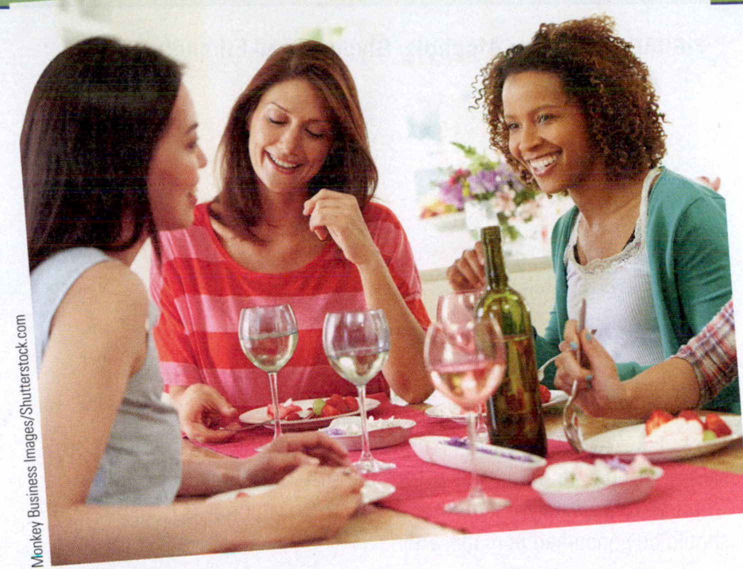

Monkey Business Images/Shutterstock.com

Alcohol in Beverages

To the chemist, **alcohol** refers to a class of organic compounds containing hydroxyl (OH) groups (Glossary H7-1 defines *alcohol* and related terms). The glycerol to which fatty acids are attached in triglycerides is an example of an alcohol to a chemist. To most people, though, *alcohol* refers to the intoxicating ingredient in **beer, wine,** and **liquor (distilled spirits).** The chemist's name for this particular alcohol is *ethyl alcohol,* or **ethanol.** Glycerol has three carbons with three hydroxyl groups attached; ethanol has only two carbons and one hydroxyl group (see Figure H7-1, p. 220). The remainder of this highlight features the particular alcohol ethanol but refers to it simply as *alcohol.*

Alcohols affect living things profoundly, partly because they act as lipid solvents. Their ability to dissolve lipids out of cell membranes allows alcohols to penetrate rapidly into cells, destroying cell structures and thereby killing the cells. For this reason, most alcohols are toxic in relatively small amounts; by the same token, because they kill microbial cells, they are useful as disinfectants.

Ethanol is less toxic than other alcohols. Sufficiently diluted and taken in small enough doses, its action in the brain produces an effect that people seek—not with zero risk, but with a low enough risk (if the doses are low enough) to be tolerable. Used in this way,

GLOSSARY H7-1

acetaldehyde (ass-et-AL-duh-hide)**:** an intermediate in alcohol metabolism.

alcohol: a class of organic compounds containing hydroxyl (OH) groups.

- **ol** = alcohol

alcohol abuse: a pattern of drinking that includes failure to fulfill work, school, or home responsibilities; drinking in situations that are physically dangerous (as in driving while intoxicated); recurring alcohol-related legal problems (as in aggravated assault charges); or continued drinking despite ongoing social problems that are caused by or worsened by alcohol.

alcohol dehydrogenase (dee-high-DROJ-eh-nayz)**:** an enzyme active in the stomach and the liver that converts ethanol to acetaldehyde.

alcoholism: a pattern of drinking that includes a strong craving for alcohol, a loss of control and an inability to stop drinking once begun, withdrawal symptoms (nausea, sweating, shakiness, and anxiety) after heavy drinking, and the need for increasing amounts of alcohol to feel "high."

antidiuretic hormone (ADH): a hormone produced by the pituitary gland in response to dehydration (or a high sodium concentration in the blood) that stimulates the kidneys to reabsorb more water and therefore to excrete less. In addition to its antidiuretic effect, ADH elevates blood pressure and so is also called *vasopressin* (VAS-oh-PRES-in).

beer: an alcoholic beverage traditionally brewed by fermenting malted barley and adding hops for flavor.

binge drinking: pattern of drinking that raises blood alcohol concentration to 0.08 percent or higher; usually corresponds to four or more drinks for women and five or more drinks for men on a single occasion, generally within a couple of hours.

cirrhosis (seer-OH-sis)**:** advanced liver disease in which liver cells turn orange, die, and harden, permanently losing their function; often associated with alcoholism.

- **cirrhos** = an orange

drink: a dose of any alcoholic beverage that delivers ½ ounce of pure ethanol:

- 5 ounces of wine
- 10 ounces of wine cooler
- 12 ounces of beer
- 1½ ounces of liquor (80 proof whiskey, scotch, rum, or vodka)

drug: a substance that can modify one or more of the body's functions.

ethanol: a particular type of alcohol found in beer, wine, and liquor; also called *ethyl alcohol* (see Figure H7-1, p. 220).

excessive drinking: heavy drinking, binge drinking, or both.

fatty liver: an early stage of liver deterioration seen in several diseases, including obesity and alcoholic liver disease. Fatty liver is characterized by an accumulation of fat in the liver cells.

fibrosis (fye-BROH-sis)**:** an intermediate stage of liver deterioration seen in several diseases, including viral hepatitis and alcoholic liver disease. In fibrosis, the liver cells lose their function and assume the characteristics of connective tissue cells (fibers).

heavy drinking: more than three drinks on any day for women and more than four drinks on any day for men.

liquor or **distilled spirits:** an alcoholic beverage traditionally made by fermenting and distilling a carbohydrate source such as molasses, potatoes, rye, beets, barley, or corn.

MEOS or **microsomal** (my-krow-SO-mal) **ethanol-oxidizing system:** a system of enzymes in the liver that oxidize not only alcohol but also several classes of drugs.

moderation (alcohol): up to one drink per day for women and up to two drinks per day for men.

narcotic (nar-KOT-ic)**:** a drug that dulls the senses, induces sleep, and becomes addictive with prolonged use.

proof: a way of stating the percentage of alcohol in distilled liquor. Liquor that is 100 proof is 50 percent alcohol; 90 proof is 45 percent, and so forth.

Wernicke-Korsakoff (VER-nee-key KORE-sah-kof) **syndrome:** a neurological disorder typically associated with chronic alcoholism and caused by a deficiency of the B vitamin thiamin; also called *alcohol-related dementia.*

wine: an alcoholic beverage traditionally made by fermenting a sugar source such as grape juice.

> **FIGURE H7-1 Two Alcohols: Glycerol and Ethanol**

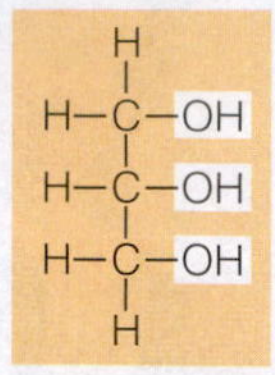
H
H—C—OH
H—C—OH
H—C—OH
H

Glycerol is the alcohol used to make triglycerides.

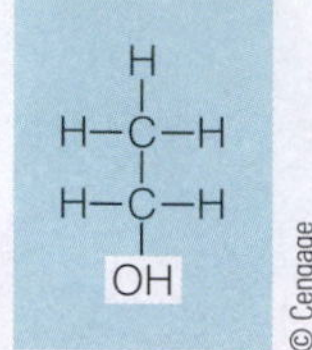
H
H—C—H
H—C—H
OH

Ethanol is the alcohol in beer, wine, and liquor.

© Cengage

alcohol is a **drug**—that is, a substance that modifies body functions. Like all drugs, alcohol both offers benefits and poses hazards. The *Dietary Guidelines for Americans* advise "if alcohol is consumed, it should be consumed in moderation."

The term **moderation** is important when describing alcohol use. How many drinks constitute moderate use, and how much is "a drink"? First, a **drink** is any alcoholic beverage that delivers ½ ounce of *pure ethanol* (see Figure H7-2):

- 5 ounces of wine
- 10 ounces of wine cooler
- 12 ounces of beer
- 1½ ounces of liquor (80 proof whiskey, scotch, rum, or vodka)

As a practical tip, prevent overpouring by measuring liquids and using small glasses.[4]

Beer, wine, and liquor deliver different amounts of alcohol. The amount of alcohol in liquor is stated as **proof:** 100 proof liquor is 50 percent alcohol, 80 proof is 40 percent alcohol, and so forth. Wine and beer have less alcohol than liquor, although some fortified wines and beers have more alcohol than the regular varieties. Figure H7-3 presents examples of labels for beer, wine, and liquor.

Second, because people have different tolerances for alcohol, it is impossible to name an exact daily amount of alcohol that is appropriate for everyone. Authorities have attempted to identify amounts that are acceptable for most healthy people. An accepted definition of *moderation* is up to two drinks per day for men and up to one drink per day for women. (Pregnant women are advised to abstain from alcohol, as Highlight 15 explains.) Notice that this advice is stated as a maximum, not as an average; seven drinks one night a week would not be considered moderate, even though one a day would be. Doubtless, some people could consume slightly more; others could not handle nearly so much without risk. The amount a person can drink safely is highly individual, depending on genetics, health, gender, body composition, age, and family history. A recent study of adult drinkers in the United States reports that two out of three consume more than moderate amounts at least once a month.[5]

> **FIGURE H7-2**

Each of these servings equals one drink. Moderation is up to one drink per day for women and two drinks per day for men.

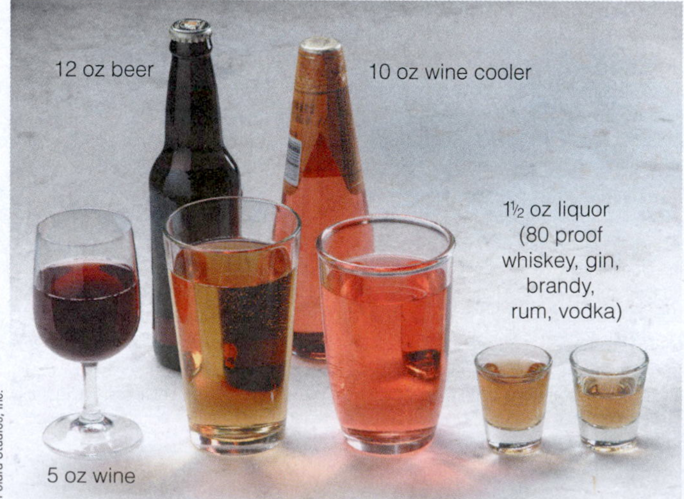
12 oz beer
10 oz wine cooler
1½ oz liquor (80 proof whiskey, gin, brandy, rum, vodka)
5 oz wine

Polara Studios, Inc.

Alcohol's Influence

From the moment an alcoholic beverage enters the body, alcohol is treated as if it has special privileges. Its influence is most apparent in the GI tract, the liver, and the brain.

In the GI Tract

Unlike foods, which require time for digestion, alcohol needs no digestion and is quickly absorbed across the walls of an empty stomach, reaching the brain within a few minutes. Consequently, a person can immediately feel euphoric when drinking, especially on an empty stomach.

When the stomach is full of food, alcohol has less chance of touching the walls and diffusing through, so its influence on the brain is slightly delayed. This information leads to another practical tip: eat snacks when drinking alcoholic beverages. Carbohydrate snacks slow alcohol absorption and high-fat snacks slow peristalsis, keeping the alcohol in the stomach longer. Salty snacks make a person thirsty; to quench thirst, drink water instead of more alcohol.

The stomach begins to break down alcohol with its **alcohol dehydrogenase** enzyme. Women produce less of this stomach enzyme than men; consequently, more alcohol reaches the intestine for absorption into the bloodstream. As a result, women absorb more alcohol than men of the same size who drink the same amount of alcohol. For this reason, women are more likely to become intoxicated on less alcohol than men. Such differences between men and women help explain why women have a lower alcohol tolerance and a lower guideline for moderate intake.

In the small intestine, alcohol is rapidly absorbed. From this point on, alcohol receives priority treatment: it gets absorbed and metabolized before most nutrients. Alcohol's priority status helps ensure a speedy disposal and reflects two facts: alcohol cannot be stored in the body, and it is potentially toxic.

> **FIGURE H7-3** **Example of Alcohol Beverage Labels**

All alcohol beverage labels provide the brand name, which identifies and markets the product; the name and address, which identifies the bottler or importer; and a health warning, which provides a government warning of health issues associated with alcohol beverages containing >0.5 percent alcohol by volume. Additional information is provided depending on whether the beverage is beer, wine, or liquor.

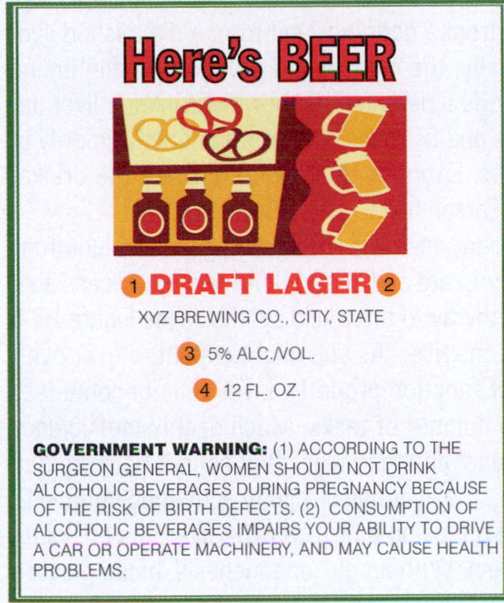
Here's BEER
1 DRAFT LAGER 2
XYZ BREWING CO., CITY, STATE
3 5% ALC./VOL.
4 12 FL. OZ.
GOVERNMENT WARNING: (1) ACCORDING TO THE SURGEON GENERAL, WOMEN SHOULD NOT DRINK ALCOHOLIC BEVERAGES DURING PREGNANCY BECAUSE OF THE RISK OF BIRTH DEFECTS. (2) CONSUMPTION OF ALCOHOLIC BEVERAGES IMPAIRS YOUR ABILITY TO DRIVE A CAR OR OPERATE MACHINERY, AND MAY CAUSE HEALTH PROBLEMS.

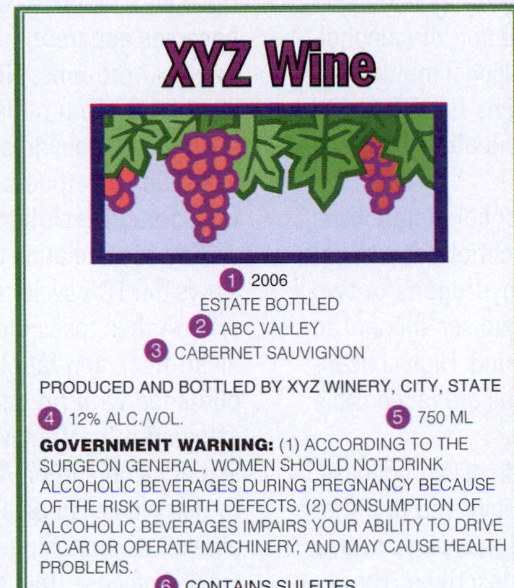
XYZ Wine
1 2006
ESTATE BOTTLED
2 ABC VALLEY
3 CABERNET SAUVIGNON
PRODUCED AND BOTTLED BY XYZ WINERY, CITY, STATE
4 12% ALC./VOL.
5 750 ML
GOVERNMENT WARNING: (1) ACCORDING TO THE SURGEON GENERAL, WOMEN SHOULD NOT DRINK ALCOHOLIC BEVERAGES DURING PREGNANCY BECAUSE OF THE RISK OF BIRTH DEFECTS. (2) CONSUMPTION OF ALCOHOLIC BEVERAGES IMPAIRS YOUR ABILITY TO DRIVE A CAR OR OPERATE MACHINERY, AND MAY CAUSE HEALTH PROBLEMS.
6 CONTAINS SULFITES

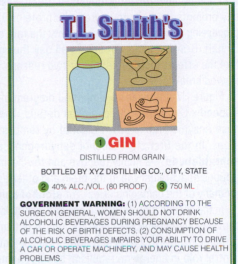
T.L. Smith's
1 GIN
DISTILLED FROM GRAIN
BOTTLED BY XYZ DISTILLING CO., CITY, STATE
2 40% ALC./VOL. (80 PROOF)
3 750 ML
GOVERNMENT WARNING: (1) ACCORDING TO THE SURGEON GENERAL, WOMEN SHOULD NOT DRINK ALCOHOLIC BEVERAGES DURING PREGNANCY BECAUSE OF THE RISK OF BIRTH DEFECTS. (2) CONSUMPTION OF ALCOHOLIC BEVERAGES IMPAIRS YOUR ABILITY TO DRIVE A CAR OR OPERATE MACHINERY, AND MAY CAUSE HEALTH PROBLEMS.

1. **DRAFT/DRAUGHT**
   Means the product has not been pasteurized and another method of controlling bacteria has been used; also used to describe beer packaged in large containers and drawn off through a tap
2. **CLASS DESIGNATION**
   Identifies the product based on the ingredients and processes used (for example, ales, stouts, and porters are fermented at relatively high temperatures and wheat beer is made from a fermentable base that is $\geq$ 25 percent malted wheat)
3. **ALCOHOL CONTENT**
   Beers typically contain <5 percent alcohol by volume and malt liquors 5 to 8 percent; regulations vary, with some states requiring alcohol content on beer labels and others prohibiting such statements
4. **NET CONTENTS**
   States the bottle quantity in English units (for example, pints or fluid ounces)

1. **VINTAGE DATE**
   Indicates year of grape harvest
2. **APPELLATION OF ORIGIN**
   Locates where most of the grapes were grown
3. **VARIETAL DESIGNATION**
   Names the dominant grapes in the wine (for example, chardonnay, merlot, or zinfandel)
4. **ALCOHOL CONTENT**
   Wines contain 7 to 24 percent alcohol by volume; wines with <14 percent may simply state "table wine" or "light wine"
5. **NET CONTENTS**
   States the bottle quantity in metric units
6. **DECLARATION OF SULFITES**
   Contains $\geq$10 ppm of sulfur dioxide

1. **CLASS/TYPE DESIGNATION**
   Identifies the product based on the ingredients and processes used (for example, gin's flavor derives from juniper berries, rum derives from fermented juice of sugar cane products, and tequila derives from the agave plant)
2. **ALCOHOL CONTENT**
   Most common liquors contain about 40 percent alcohol (80 proof), but this varies; alcohol content is stated as a percent by volume and by proof
3. **NET CONTENTS**
   States the bottle quantity in metric units

In the Liver

As Chapter 3 explained, the capillaries of the digestive tract merge into veins that carry blood first to the liver. These veins branch and rebranch into a capillary network that touches every liver cell. Consequently, liver cells are the first to receive alcohol-laden blood. Liver cells are also the only other cells in the body that can make enough of the alcohol dehydrogenase enzyme to oxidize alcohol at an appreciable rate. The routing of blood through the liver cells gives them the chance to dispose of some alcohol before it moves on.

Alcohol affects every organ of the body, but the most dramatic evidence of its disruptive behavior appears in the liver. If liver cells could talk, they would describe alcohol as demanding, egocentric, and disruptive of the liver's efficient way of running its business. For example, liver cells normally prefer fatty acids as their fuel, and they like to package excess fatty acids into triglycerides and ship them out to other tissues. When alcohol is present, however, the liver cells metabolize alcohol first and let the fatty acids accumulate, sometimes in huge stockpiles. Alcohol metabolism can also permanently change liver cell structure, impairing the liver's ability to metabolize fats. As a result, heavy drinkers develop **fatty livers**.

The liver is the primary site of alcohol metabolism. It can process about ½ ounce of *ethanol* per hour (the amount defined as a drink), depending on the person's body size, previous drinking experience, food intake, and general health. This maximum rate of alcohol breakdown is determined by the amount of alcohol dehydrogenase available. If more alcohol arrives at the liver than the enzymes can handle, the extra alcohol travels around the body, circulating again and again until liver enzymes are finally available to process it. Another practical tip derives from this information: drink slowly enough to allow the liver to keep up—no more than one drink per hour.

The amount of alcohol dehydrogenase enzyme present in the liver varies with individuals, depending on the genes they have inherited and on how recently they have eaten. Fasting for as little as a day prompts the body to degrade its proteins, including the alcohol-processing enzymes, and this can slow the rate of alcohol metabolism by half. Drinking after not eating all day thus causes the drinker to feel the effects more promptly for two reasons: rapid absorption and slowed breakdown.

Figure H7-4 provides a simplified diagram of alcohol metabolism; Appendix C provides the chemical details. The alcohol dehydrogenase enzyme breaks down alcohol by removing hydrogens in two steps. In the first step, alcohol dehydrogenase oxidizes alcohol to **acetaldehyde**—a highly reactive and toxic compound. High concentrations of acetaldehyde in the brain and other tissues are responsible for many of the damaging effects of **alcohol abuse.**

In the second step, a related enzyme, acetaldehyde dehydrogenase, converts acetaldehyde to acetate, which is then converted to either carbon dioxide (CO_2) or acetyl CoA—the compound that plays such a central role in energy metabolism, as this chapter describes. The reactions from alcohol to acetaldehyde to acetate produce hydrogens (H^+) and electrons. The B vitamin niacin, in its role as a coenzyme, helpfully picks up these hydrogens and electrons and escorts them to the electron transport chain. (Chapter 10 presents information on the coenzyme roles of the B vitamins.)

During alcohol metabolism, the multitude of other metabolic processes for which the niacin coenzyme is required, including glycolysis, the TCA cycle, and the electron transport chain, falter. Its presence is sorely missed in these energy pathways because it is the chief carrier of the hydrogens that travel with their electrons along the electron transport chain. Without adequate coenzymes, these energy pathways cannot function. Traffic either backs up or an alternate route is taken.

Such changes in the normal flow of energy pathways have striking metabolic consequences. For one, the accumulation of hydrogen ions during alcohol metabolism shifts the body's acid-base balance toward acid. For another, alcohol's interference with energy metabolism promotes the making of lactate from pyruvate. The conversion of pyruvate to lactate uses some of the excess hydrogens, but a lactate build-up has serious consequences of its own—it adds still further to the body's acid burden and interferes with the excretion of another acid, uric acid, causing inflammation of the joints.

Alcohol alters both amino acid and protein metabolism. Synthesis of proteins important in the immune system slows down, weakening the body's defenses against infections. Evidence of protein deficiency becomes apparent, both from a poor diet and from a diminished synthesis of proteins. Normally, the cells would at least use the amino acids from the protein foods a person eats, but the drinker's liver deaminates the amino acids and uses the carbon fragments primarily to make fat or ketone bodies. Eating well does not protect the drinker from protein depletion; a person has to stop drinking alcohol.

The accumulation of coenzymes with their hydrogens and electrons slows the TCA cycle, so pyruvate and acetyl CoA build up. Excess acetyl CoA then takes the pathway to fatty acid synthesis (as Figure H7-5 illustrates), and fat clogs the liver. As you might expect, a liver overburdened with fat cannot function properly. Liver cells become less efficient at performing a number of tasks. Much of this inefficiency impairs a person's nutritional health in ways that cannot be corrected by diet alone. For example, the liver has difficulty activating vitamin D, as well as producing and releasing bile. The fatty liver has difficulty making glucose from protein. Without gluconeogenesis, blood glucose can plummet, leading to irreversible damage to the central nervous system. The lack of glucose together with the overabundance of acetyl CoA sets the stage for ketosis. The body uses excess acetyl CoA to make ketone bodies; their acidity pushes the acid-base balance further toward acid and suppresses nervous system activity. To overcome such problems, a person needs to stop drinking alcohol.

The synthesis of fatty acids accelerates with exposure to alcohol. Fat accumulation can be seen in the liver after a single night of heavy drinking. Fatty liver, the first stage of liver deterioration seen in heavy drinkers, interferes with the distribution of nutrients and oxygen to the liver cells. Fatty liver is reversible with abstinence from alcohol. If fatty liver lasts long enough, however, the liver cells will die and form fibrous scar tissue. This second stage of liver deterioration is called **fibrosis.** Some liver cells can regenerate with good nutrition and abstinence from alcohol, but in the most advanced stage, **cirrhosis,** damage is the least reversible.

The liver's priority treatment of alcohol affects its handling of drugs as well as nutrients. In addition to the dehydrogenase enzymes already described, the liver possesses an enzyme system that

> **FIGURE H7-4 Alcohol Metabolism**

The conversion of alcohol to acetyl CoA requires the B vitamin niacin in its role as a coenzyme. When the enzymes oxidize alcohol, they remove H atoms and attach them to the niacin coenzyme.

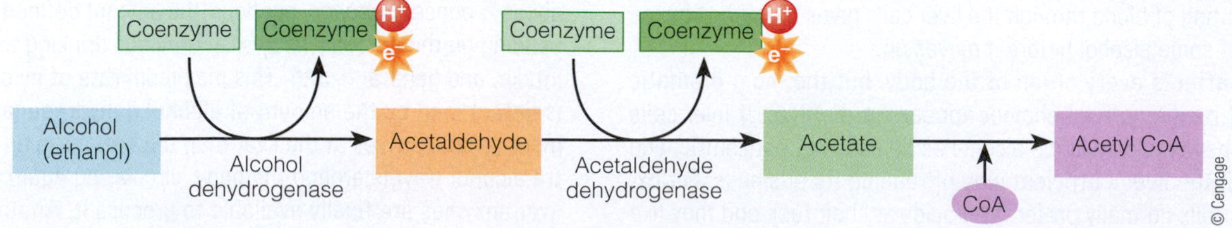

Coenzyme
Coenzyme
H+
e-
Coenzyme
Coenzyme
H+
e-
Alcohol (ethanol)
Alcohol dehydrogenase
Acetaldehyde
Acetaldehyde dehydrogenase
Acetate
CoA
Acetyl CoA
© Cengage

> **FIGURE H7-5 Alternate Route for Acetyl CoA: To Fat**

Acetyl CoA molecules are blocked from getting into the TCA cycle by the low level of coenzymes. Instead of being used for energy, the acetyl CoA molecules become building blocks for fatty acids.

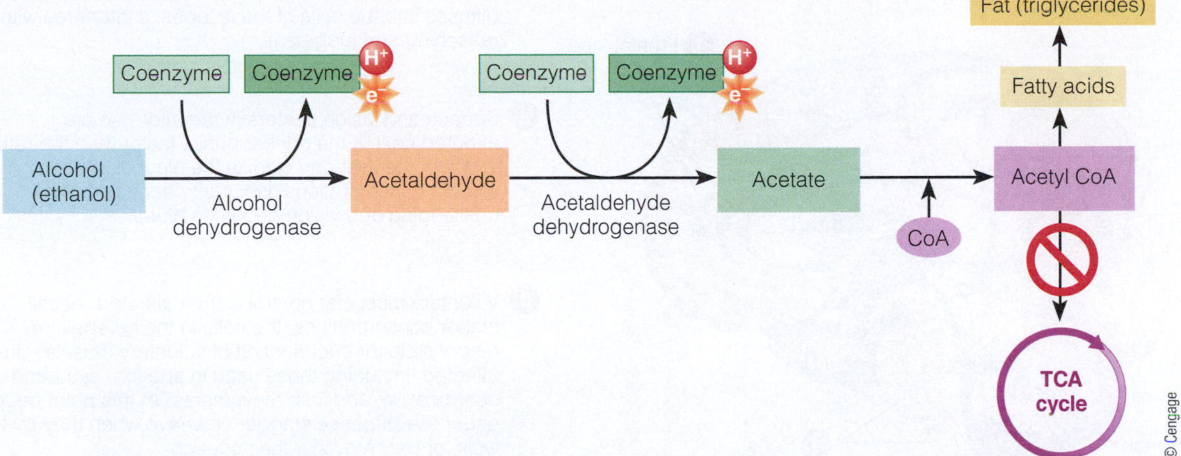

Coenzyme
Coenzyme
H+
e−
Coenzyme
Coenzyme
H+
e−
Fat (triglycerides)
Fatty acids
Alcohol (ethanol)
Alcohol dehydrogenase
Acetaldehyde
Acetaldehyde dehydrogenase
Acetate
CoA
Acetyl CoA
TCA cycle
© Cengage

metabolizes *both* alcohol and several other types of drugs. Called the **MEOS (microsomal ethanol-oxidizing system),** this system handles about one-fifth of the total alcohol a person consumes. At high blood concentrations or with repeated exposures, alcohol stimulates the synthesis of enzymes in the MEOS. The result is a more efficient metabolism of alcohol and tolerance to its effects.

As a person's blood alcohol rises, alcohol competes with—and wins out over—other drugs whose metabolism also relies on the MEOS. If a person drinks and uses another drug at the same time, the MEOS will dispose of alcohol first and metabolize the drug more slowly. While the drug waits to be handled later, the dose may build up so that its effects are greatly amplified—sometimes to the point of being fatal. Many drug labels provide warnings to avoid alcohol while taking the drug.

In contrast, once a heavy drinker stops drinking and alcohol is no longer competing with other drugs, the enhanced MEOS metabolizes drugs much faster than before. As a result, determining the correct dosages of medications can be challenging.

This discussion has emphasized the major way that the blood is cleared of alcohol—metabolism by the liver—but there is another way. About 10 percent of the alcohol leaves the body through the breath and in the urine. This is the basis for the breath and urine tests to determine blood alcohol concentrations. The amounts of alcohol in the breath and in the urine are in proportion to the amount still in the bloodstream and brain. In all states, legal drunkenness is set at 0.08 percent or less, reflecting the relationship between alcohol use and traffic and other accidents.

In the Brain

Figure H7-6 (p. 224) describes alcohol's effects on the brain. Alcohol is a **narcotic.** People used it for centuries as an anesthetic because it can deaden pain. But alcohol was a poor anesthetic because one could never be sure how much a person would need and how much would be a fatal dose. Today's anesthetics provide a more predictable response. Alcohol continues to be used socially to help people relax or to relieve anxiety. People think that alcohol is a stimulant because it seems to relieve inhibitions. Actually, though, it accomplishes this by sedating *inhibitory* nerves, which are more numerous than excitatory nerves. Ultimately, alcohol acts as a depressant and affects all the nerve cells.

It is lucky that the brain centers respond to a rising blood alcohol concentration in the order described in Figure H7-6, because a person usually passes out before managing to drink a lethal dose. It is possible, though, to drink so fast that the effects of alcohol continue to accelerate after the person has passed out. Occasionally, a person drinks so much as to stop breathing and die. Table H7-1 (p. 224) shows the blood alcohol concentrations that correspond to progressively greater intoxication, and Table H7-2 (p. 225) shows the brain responses that occur at these blood levels.

Like liver cells, brain cells die with excessive exposure to alcohol. Liver cells may be replaced, but not all brain cells can regenerate. Thus some heavy drinkers suffer permanent brain damage. Whether alcohol impairs cognition in moderate drinkers is unclear.

Alcohol's Damage

As alcohol busily disrupts cellular activities, the physical consequences become apparent. People become dehydrated and malnourished; their alcohol use brings both short- and long-term effects.

Dehydration

People who drink alcoholic beverages may notice that they urinate more, but they may be unaware of the vicious cycle that results. Alcohol depresses production of **antidiuretic hormone (ADH),** a hormone produced by the pituitary gland that retains water—consequently, with less ADH, more water is lost. Loss of body water

> **FIGURE H7-6 Alcohol's Effects on the Brain**

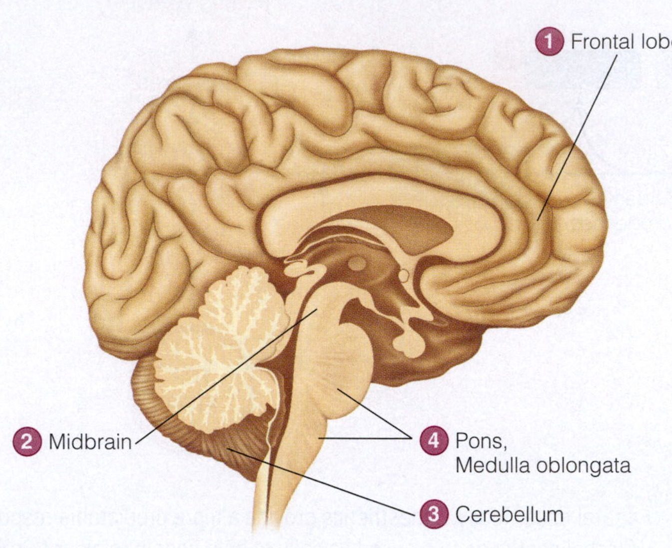
1 Frontal lobe
2 Midbrain
4 Pons,
Medulla oblongata
3 Cerebellum

1. Judgment and reasoning centers are most sensitive to alcohol. When alcohol flows to the brain, it first sedates the frontal lobe, the center of all conscious activity. As alcohol diffuses into the cells of these lobes, it interferes with reasoning and judgment.

2. Speech and vision centers in the midbrain are affected next. If the drinker drinks faster than the rate at which the liver can oxidize the alcohol, blood alcohol concentrations rise: the speech becomes challenging and vision becomes blurry.

3. Voluntary muscular control is then affected. At still higher concentrations, the cells in the cerebellum responsible for coordination of voluntary muscles are affected, including those used in speech, eye-hand coordination, and limb movements. At this point people under the influence stagger or weave when they try to walk, or they may slur their speech.

4. Respiration and heart action are the last to be affected. Finally, the conscious brain is completely subdued, and the person passes out. Now the person can drink no more; this is fortunate because higher doses would anesthetize the deepest brain centers that control breathing and heartbeat, causing death.

leads to thirst, and thirst leads to more drinking. Water will relieve dehydration, but the thirsty drinker may drink alcohol instead, which only worsens the problem. Such information provides another practical tip: drink water when thirsty and before each alcoholic drink. Drink an extra glass or two before going to bed. This strategy will help lessen the effects of a hangover.

Water loss is accompanied by the loss of important minerals. As Chapters 12 and 13 explain, these minerals are vital to the body's fluid balance and to many chemical reactions in the cells, including muscle action. Detoxification treatment includes restoration of mineral balance as quickly as possible.

TABLE H7-1 Alcohol Doses and Approximate Blood Level Percentages for Men and Women

Drinks[a]	Body Weight in Pounds—Men								
	100	120	140	160	180	200	220	240	
	00	00	00	00	00	00	00	00	ONLY SAFE DRIVING LIMIT
1	.04	.03	.03	.02	.02	.02	.02	.02	IMPAIRMENT BEGINS
2	.08	.06	.05	.05	.04	.04	.03	.03	
3	.11	.09	.08	.07	.06	.06	.05	.05	DRIVING SKILLS SIGNIFICANTLY AFFECTED
4	.15	.12	.11	.09	.08	.08	.07	.06	
5	.19	.16	.13	.12	.11	.09	.09	.08	
6	.23	.19	.16	.14	.13	.11	.10	.09	
7	.26	.22	.19	.16	.15	.13	.12	.11	LEGALLY INTOXICATED
8	.30	.25	.21	.19	.17	.15	.14	.13	
9	.34	.28	.24	.21	.19	.17	.15	.14	
10	.38	.31	.27	.23	.21	.19	.17	.16	

Drinks[a]	Body Weight in Pounds—Women									
	90	100	120	140	160	180	200	220	240	
	00	00	00	00	00	00	00	00	00	ONLY SAFE DRIVING LIMIT
1	.05	.05	.04	.03	.03	.03	.02	.02	.02	IMPAIRMENT BEGINS
2	.10	.09	.08	.07	.06	.05	.05	.04	.04	DRIVING SKILLS SIGNIFICANTLY AFFECTED
3	.15	.14	.11	.10	.09	.08	.07	.06	.06	
4	.20	.18	.15	.13	.11	.10	.09	.08	.08	
5	.25	.23	.19	.16	.14	.13	.11	.10	.09	
6	.30	.27	.23	.19	.17	.15	.14	.12	.11	LEGALLY INTOXICATED
7	.35	.32	.27	.23	.20	.18	.16	.14	.13	
8	.40	.36	.30	.26	.23	.20	.18	.17	.15	
9	.45	.41	.34	.29	.26	.23	.20	.19	.17	
10	.51	.45	.38	.32	.28	.25	.23	.21	.19	

NOTE: Driving under the influence is proved when an adult's blood contains 0.08 percent alcohol. Many states have adopted a "zero-tolerance" policy for drivers under age 21, using 0.00 to 0.02 percent as the limit.
[a]Taken within an hour or so; each drink equivalent to ½ ounce of pure ethanol.
SOURCE: National Clearinghouse for Alcohol and Drug Information.

TABLE H7-2 Effects of Blood Alcohol

Blood Alcohol Concentration (%)	Typical Effects
.02	Loss of judgment, altered mood
.05	Exaggerated behavior, loss of small muscle control, impaired judgment, lowered alertness
.08	Poor muscle coordination; impaired self-control, reasoning, and memory
.10	Deterioration of reaction time and control, slurred speech, poor coordination, slowed thinking
.15	Minimal muscle control, loss of balance
.20	Confusion, disorientation, possible blackouts
.30	Stupor, minimal comprehension
.40	Lethal dose (heart beat and respiration slow down dramatically and may stop)

NOTE: Blood alcohol concentration depends on a number of factors, including alcohol in the beverage, the number and rate of consumption, the person's gender, and body weight.
SOURCE: Centers for Disease Control and Prevention (www.cdc.gov).

TABLE H7-3 kCalories in Alcoholic Beverages and Mixers

Beverage	Amount (oz)	Energy (kcal)	Alcohol (g)
Beer			
Regular	12	153	14
Light	12	103	11
Nonalcoholic	12	32	0
Cocktails			
Daiquiri, canned	6.8	259	20
Daiquiri, from recipe	4.5	223	28
Piña colada, canned	6.8	526	20
Piña colada, from recipe	4.5	245	14
Tequila sunrise, canned	6.8	232	20
Whiskey sour, canned	6.8	249	20
Liquor (gin, rum, vodka, whiskey)			
80 proof	1.5	97	14
86 proof	1.5	105	15
90 proof	1.5	110	16
94 proof	1.5	116	17
100 proof	1.5	124	18
Sake	1.5	58	7
Liqueurs			
Coffee and cream liqueur, 34 proof	1.5	154	7
Coffee liqueur, 53 proof	1.5	170	11
Coffee liqueur, 63 proof	1.5	160	14
Crème de menthe, 72 proof	1.5	186	15
Mixers			
Club soda	12	0	0
Cola	12	136	0
Cranberry juice cocktail	4	72	0
Ginger ale or tonic water	12	124	0
Grapefruit juice	4	48	0
Orange juice	4	56	0
Tomato or vegetable juice	4	21	0
Wine			
Champagne	5	105	13
Cooking	5	72	5
Dessert, dry	5	224	23
Dessert, sweet	5	236	23
Red or rosé	5	125	16
White	5	121	15
Wine cooler	10	150	11

Malnutrition

For some light-to-moderate drinkers, alcohol may suppress food intake and prevent weight gains. For others, however, alcohol may actually stimulate appetite. Moderate drinkers usually consume alcohol as an *addition*—on top of their normal food intake. In moderate doses, the alcohol is efficiently metabolized. Consequently, alcohol can contribute to body fat and weight gain—either by inhibiting oxidation or by being converted to fat. Metabolically, alcohol is almost as efficient as fat in promoting obesity; each ounce of alcohol represents about a half-ounce of fat. Alcohol's contribution to body fat is most evident in the abdominal obesity that commonly accompanies alcohol consumption, popularly known as the "beer belly."[6] Although not required, some beer, wine, and liquor labels provide information on the serving size, servings per container, kcalories, carbohydrates, protein, and fat per serving.

Alcohol in heavy doses, though, is not efficiently metabolized, generating more heat than fat. Heavy drinkers usually consume alcohol as a *substitution*—instead of their normal food intake. Diet quality declines as alcohol consumption increases. Consequently, many heavy drinkers suffer malnutrition.[7] Even moderate drinkers tend to have poorer diets on drinking days.[8]

On average, adults in the United States consume almost 100 kcalories from alcohol daily.[9] Alcohol is rich in energy (7 kcalories per gram), but as with pure sugar or fat, the kcalories are empty of nutrients. The more alcohol people drink, the less likely that they will eat enough food to obtain adequate nutrients. The more kcalories used for alcohol, the fewer kcalories available to use from nutritious foods. Table H7-3 shows the kcalorie amounts of typical alcoholic beverages.

Chronic alcohol abuse not only displaces nutrients from the diet, but it also interferes with the body's metabolism of nutrients. Most dramatic is alcohol's effect on the B vitamin folate. The liver loses its ability to retain folate, and the kidneys increase their excretion of it. Alcohol abuse creates a folate deficiency that devastates digestive system function. The small intestine normally releases and retrieves folate continuously, but it becomes damaged by folate deficiency and alcohol toxicity, so it fails to retrieve its own folate and misses any available from food as well. Alcohol also interferes with the action of folate in converting the amino acid homocysteine to methionine. The result is an excess of homocysteine, which has been linked to heart disease, and an inadequate supply of methionine, which slows the production of new cells, especially the rapidly dividing cells of the intestine and the blood. The combination of poor folate status and alcohol consumption has also been implicated in promoting colorectal cancer.[10]

The inadequate food intake and impaired nutrient absorption that accompany chronic alcohol abuse frequently lead to a deficiency of another B vitamin—thiamin. In fact, the cluster of thiamin-deficiency symptoms commonly seen in chronic **alcoholism** has its own name—**Wernicke-Korsakoff syndrome.** This syndrome is characterized by paralysis of the eye muscles, poor muscle coordination, impaired memory, and damaged nerves; it and other alcohol-related memory problems may respond to thiamin supplements.

Acetaldehyde, an intermediate in alcohol metabolism (review Figure H7-4, p. 222), interferes with nutrient use, too. For example, acetaldehyde dislodges vitamin B_6 from its protective binding protein so that it is destroyed, causing a vitamin B_6 deficiency and, thereby, lowered production of red blood cells.

Malnutrition occurs not only because of lack of intake and altered metabolism but also because of direct toxic effects as well. Alcohol causes stomach cells to oversecrete both gastric acid and histamine, an immune system agent that produces inflammation. Beer in particular stimulates gastric acid secretion, irritating the linings of the stomach and esophagus and making them vulnerable to ulcer formation.

Overall, nutrient deficiencies are virtually inevitable in alcohol abuse, not only because alcohol displaces food but also because alcohol directly interferes with the body's use of nutrients, making them ineffective even if they are present. Intestinal cells fail to absorb B vitamins, notably, thiamin, folate, and vitamin B_{12}. Liver cells lose efficiency in activating vitamin D. Cells in the retina of the eye, which normally process the alcohol form of vitamin A (retinol) to the aldehyde form needed in vision (retinal), find themselves processing ethanol to acetaldehyde instead. Likewise, the liver cannot convert the aldehyde form of vitamin A to its acid form (retinoic acid), which is needed to support the growth of its (and all) cells. Regardless of dietary intake, excessive drinking over a lifetime creates deficits of all the nutrients mentioned in this discussion and more. No diet can compensate for the damage caused by heavy alcohol consumption.

Short-Term Effects

The effects of abusing alcohol may be apparent immediately, or they may not become evident for years to come. Among the immediate consequences, all of the following involve alcohol use:

- 14 percent of all boating fatalities
- 22 percent of all suicides
- 31 percent of all traffic fatalities
- 28 percent of all residential fire fatalities
- 86 percent of all homicides
- 61 percent of all domestic violence incidents

These statistics are sobering. The consequences of heavy drinking touch all races and all segments of society—men and women, young and old, rich and poor. One group particularly hard hit by heavy drinking is college students—not because they are prone to alcoholism, but because they live in an environment and are in a developmental stage of life in which risk-taking behaviors are common and heavy drinking is acceptable.

Excessive drinking—including both **heavy drinking** and **binge drinking**—is widespread on college campuses and poses serious health and social consequences to drinkers and nondrinkers alike. In fact, binge drinking can kill; on average, 6 alcohol poisoning deaths occur every day.[11] Excessive alcohol can shut down the respiratory center of the brain and stop breathing. Alcohol can also cause coronary artery spasms, leading to a heart attack and death.

Binge drinking is relatively common among college students, especially males. Compared with nondrinkers or moderate drinkers, people who frequently binge drink (at least three times within two weeks) are more likely to engage in unprotected sex, have multiple sex partners, damage property, and perform poorly in school. Binge drinking poses serious health and safety risks.[12] On average, *every day* alcohol is involved in the:

- Death of 5 college students
- Sexual assault of 266 college students
- Assault of 1907 college students

The dangers of binge drinking have been amplified by the use of beverages that contain caffeine as an additive. The caffeine seems to mask the sensory cues that an individual normally relies on to determine intoxication. Consequently, individuals drinking these beverages typically consume more alcohol and become more intoxicated than they realize. The Food and Drug Administration (FDA) has warned manufacturers of packaged caffeinated alcoholic beverages to stop sales. The combination of alcohol and added caffeine has not been approved because these products are associated with risky behaviors that may lead to hazardous and life-threatening situations.[13] For the same reasons, individuals should not mix alcohol with high-energy drinks.

Another phenomenon closely related to binge drinking is "drunkorexia," a popular term used to describe the restrictive eating, excessive exercising, and abusive drinking patterns of some college students.[14] In an effort to compensate for the kcalories of an evening's drinking binge and to amplify the high, these students skip meals and exercise vigorously during the day; they might also drink excessively in an effort to vomit any food previously eaten. These students may perceive themselves to be "weight conscious" drinkers, but in reality, their restrictive eating, excessive exercising, and abusive drinking patterns are not supportive of healthy weight loss.

Binge drinking is not limited to college campuses, of course, but it is most common among 18 to 34 year olds.[15] That age group and campus environment seem most accepting of such "party" behavior despite its problems. Social acceptance may make it difficult for binge drinkers to recognize themselves as problem drinkers. For this reason, interventions must focus both on educating individuals and on changing the campus social environment. The damage alcohol causes becomes worse if the pattern is not broken. Alcohol abuse sets in much more quickly in young people than in older adults. Those who start drinking at an early age more often suffer from alcoholism than others. Table H7-4 lists the key signs of alcoholism.

TABLE H7-4 Signs of Alcoholism

- Tolerance: the person needs higher and higher intakes of alcohol to achieve intoxication.
- Withdrawal: the person who stops drinking experiences anxiety, agitation, increased blood pressure, or seizures, or seeks alcohol to relieve these symptoms.
- Impaired control: the person intends to have 1 or 2 drinks, but has many more instead, or the person tries to control or quit drinking, but efforts are unsuccessful.
- Disinterest: the person neglects important social, family, job, or school activities because of drinking.
- Time: the person spends a great deal of time obtaining and drinking alcohol or recovering from excessive drinking.
- Cravings: the person has strong urges to use alcohol.
- Impaired ability: the person's intoxication or withdrawal symptoms interfere with work, school, or home.
- Problems: the person continues drinking despite physical hazards or medical, legal, psychological, family, employment, or school problems caused or exacerbated by alcohol.

These conditions suggest that a person may have an alcohol problem and might benefit from an abstinence program or professional help.

SOURCE: Adapted from *Diagnostic and Statistical Manual of Mental Disorders*, 5th ed. (Washington, D.C.: American Psychiatric Association, 2013).

Long-Term Effects

The most devastating long-term effect of alcohol is the damage done to a child whose mother drinks alcohol during pregnancy. The effects of alcohol on the unborn and the message that pregnant women should not drink alcohol are presented in Highlight 15. Quite simply, there is no safe amount of drinking during pregnancy.[16]

For nonpregnant adults, a drink or two sets in motion many destructive processes in the body, but the next day's abstinence reverses them. As long as the doses are moderate, the time between them is ample, and nutrition is adequate, recovery is probably complete.

If the doses of alcohol are heavy and the time between them short, complete recovery cannot take place. Repeated onslaughts of alcohol gradually take a toll on all parts of the body and increase the risks of several chronic diseases (see Table H7-5). Compared with nondrinkers and moderate drinkers, heavy drinkers have significantly greater risks of dying from all causes. Excessive alcohol consumption is the third leading preventable cause of death in the United States. Worldwide, alcohol contributes to 1 out of 15 deaths.[17]

TABLE H7-5 Health Effects of Heavy Alcohol Consumption

Health Problem	Effects of Alcohol
Arthritis	Increases the risk of inflamed joints.
Bone loss	Decreases bone mass and strength.
Cancer	Increases the risk of cancer of the liver, breast, mouth, pharynx, larynx, esophagus, colon, and rectum.
Fetal alcohol syndrome	Causes physical and behavioral abnormalities in the fetus (see Highlight 15).
Heart disease	In heavy drinkers, raises blood pressure, blood lipids, and the risk of stroke and heart disease; when compared with those who abstain, heart disease risk is generally lower in light-to-moderate drinkers.
Hyperglycemia	Raises blood glucose.
Hypoglycemia	Lowers blood glucose, especially in people with diabetes.
Infertility	Increases the risks of menstrual disorders and spontaneous abortions (in women); suppresses luteinizing hormone (in women) and testosterone (in men).
Kidney disease	Enlarges the kidneys, alters hormone functions, and increases the risk of kidney failure.
Liver disease	Causes fatty liver, alcoholic hepatitis, and cirrhosis.
Lung disease	Damages lung tissue
Malnutrition	Increases the risk of malnutrition; low intakes of protein, calcium, iron, vitamin A, vitamin C, thiamin, vitamin B_6, and riboflavin; and impaired absorption of calcium, phosphorus, vitamin D, and zinc.
Nerve disorders	Causes neuropathy and dementia; impairs balance and memory.
Obesity	Increases energy intake, but is not a primary cause of obesity.
Psychological disturbances	Causes depression, anxiety, and insomnia.

NOTE: This list is by no means all-inclusive. Alcohol has direct toxic effects on all body systems.

Personal Strategies

One obvious option available to people attending social gatherings is to enjoy the conversation, eat the food, and drink nonalcoholic beverages. Several nonalcoholic beverages are available that mimic the look and taste of their alcoholic counterparts. For those who enjoy champagne or beer, sparkling ciders and beers without alcohol are available. Instead of drinking a cocktail, a person can sip tomato juice with a slice of lime and a stalk of celery or just a plain cola beverage. The person who chooses to drink alcohol should sip each drink slowly accompanied by food and water.

If you want to help sober up a friend who has had too much to drink, don't bother walking arm in arm around the block. Walking muscles have to work harder, but muscle cells don't have the enzymes to metabolize alcohol; only liver cells can clear alcohol from the blood. Remember that each person has a limited amount of the alcohol dehydrogenase enzyme, which clears the blood at a steady rate. Time alone will do the job. Nor will it help give your friend a cup of coffee. Caffeine is a stimulant, but it won't speed up alcohol metabolism. Table H7-6 (p. 228) presents other alcohol myths.

People who have passed out from drinking need 24 hours to sober up completely. Let them sleep, but watch over them. Encourage them to lie on their sides, instead of their backs. That way, if they vomit, they won't choke.

Don't drive after drinking. Every day, an estimated 28 people in the United States die in traffic accidents that involve an alcohol-impaired driver; said another way, an alcohol-related auto accident kills someone every 53 minutes.[18] The lack of glucose for the brain to function and the length of time to clear the blood of alcohol make alcohol's

TABLE H7-6 Myths and Truths Concerning Alcohol

Myth	Truth
Liquors such as rum, vodka, and tequila are more harmful than wine and beer.	The damage caused by alcohol depends largely on the *amount* consumed. Compared with liquor, beer and wine have relatively low percentages of alcohol, but they are often consumed in larger quantities.
Consuming alcohol with raw seafood diminishes the likelihood of getting hepatitis.	People have eaten contaminated oysters while drinking alcoholic beverages and not gotten as sick as those who were not drinking. But do not be misled: hepatitis is too serious an illness for anyone to depend on alcohol for protection.
Alcohol stimulates the appetite.	For some people, alcohol may stimulate appetite, but it seems to have the opposite effect in heavy drinkers. Heavy drinkers tend to eat poorly and suffer malnutrition.
Drinking alcohol is healthy.	Moderate alcohol consumption is associated with a lower risk for heart disease. Higher intakes, however, raise the risks for high blood pressure, stroke, heart disease, some cancers, accidents, violence, suicide, birth defects, and deaths in general. Furthermore, excessive alcohol consumption damages the liver, pancreas, brain, and heart. No authority recommends that nondrinkers begin drinking alcoholic beverages to obtain health benefits.
Wine increases the body's absorption of minerals.	Wine may increase the body's absorption of potassium, calcium, phosphorus, magnesium, and zinc, but the alcohol in wine also promotes the body's excretion of these minerals, so no benefit is gained.
Alcohol is legal and, therefore, not a drug.	Alcohol is legal for adults 21 years old and older, but it is also a drug—a substance that alters one or more of the body's functions.
A shot of alcohol warms you up.	Alcohol diverts blood flow to the skin making you *feel* warmer, but it actually cools the body.
Wine and beer are mild; they do not lead to alcoholism.	Alcoholism is not related to the kind of beverage, but rather to the quantity and frequency of consumption.
Mixing different types of drinks gives you a hangover.	Too much alcohol in any form produces a hangover.
Alcohol is a stimulant.	People think alcohol is a stimulant because it seems to relieve inhibitions, but it does so by depressing the activity of the brain. Alcohol is medically defined as a depressant drug.
Beer is a great source of carbohydrate, vitamins, minerals, and fluids.	Beer does provide some carbohydrate, but most of its kcalories come from alcohol. The few vitamins and minerals in beer cannot compete with rich food sources. And the diuretic effect of alcohol causes the body to lose more fluid in urine than is provided by the beer.

adverse effects linger long after its blood concentration has fallen. Driving coordination is still impaired the morning after a night of drinking, even if the drinking was moderate. Responsible aircraft pilots know that they must allow 24 hours for their bodies to clear alcohol completely, and they do not fly any sooner. The Federal Aviation Administration and major airlines enforce this rule.

Look again at the drawing of the brain in Figure H7-6 (p. 224), and note that when someone drinks, judgment fails first. Judgment might tell a person to limit alcohol consumption to two drinks at a party, but if the first drink takes judgment away, many more drinks may follow. The failure to stop drinking as planned, on repeated occasions, is a warning sign that the person may have an alcohol abuse problem.

Ethanol interferes with a multitude of metabolic reactions in the body—many more than have been enumerated here. With heavy alcohol consumption, the potential for harm is great. If you drink alcoholic beverages, do so with care, and in moderation.

CRITICAL THINKING QUESTIONS

A. If body organs could talk, what might some of them say to alcohol about its role in metabolism and disease development?

B. Some people choose to abstain from drinking alcoholic beverages. Others overindulge, to the detriment of their health and safety. Moderation lies somewhere between the two ends of the spectrum. How would you plan a social gathering that would ensure that guests of legal age could enjoy an evening that includes alcoholic beverages in a safe and responsible way?

REFERENCES

1. A. Gonçalves and coauthors, Alcohol consumption and risk of heart failure: The Atherosclerosis Risk in Communities Study, *European Heart Journal* 36 (2015): 939–945.
2. National Institute on Alcohol Abuse and Alcoholism, Alcohol facts and statistics, www.niaaa.nih.gov/alcohol-health/overview-alcohol-consumption/alcohol-facts-and-statistics, June 2016.
3. A. D. Plunk and coauthors, Alcohol consumption, heavy drinking, and mortality: Rethinking the j-shaped curve, *Alcoholism, Clinical and Experimental Research* 38 (2014): 471–478; J. H. O'Keefe and coauthors, Alcohol and cardiovascular health: The dose makes the poison . . . or the remedy, *Mayo Clinic Proceedings* 89 (2014): 382–393.

4. R. Pechey and coauthors, Does wine glass size influence sales for on-site consumption? A multiple treatment reversal design, *BMC Public Health* 16 (2016): 390.
5. S. J. Henley and coauthors, Alcohol control efforts in comprehensive cancer control plans and alcohol use among adults in the United States, *Alcohol* 49 (2014): 661–667.
6. T. Kondoh and coauthors, Association of dietary factors with abdominal subcutaneous and visceral adiposity in Japanese men, *Obesity Research and Clinical Practice* 8 (2014): e16–e25; N. T. Bendsen and coauthors, Is beer consumption related to measures of abdominal and general obesity? A systematic review and meta-analysis, *Nutrition Reviews* 71 (2013): 67–87.
7. P. S. Ge and B. A. Runyon, Treatment of patients with cirrhosis, *New England Journal of Medicine* 375 (2016): 767–777.
8. R. A. Breslow and coauthors, Diets of drinkers on drinking and nondrinking days: NHANES 2003–2008, *American Journal of Clinical Nutrition* 97 (2013): 1068–1075.
9. S. J. Nielsen and coauthors, Calories consumed from alcoholic beverages by US adults, 2007–2010, www.cdc.gov/nchs/data/databriefs/db110.htm, published November 2012.
10. M. Varela-Rey and coauthors, Alcohol, DNA methylation, and cancer, *Alcohol Research* 35 (2013): 25–35.
11. D. Kanny and coauthors, Vital signs: Alcohol poisoning deaths—United States, 2010-2012, *Morbidity and Mortality Weekly Report* 63 (2015): 1238–242.
12. National Institute on Alcohol Abuse and Alcoholism, College drinking, http://pubs.niaaa.nih.gov/publications/CollegeFactSheet/CollegeFactSheet.pdf, published December 2015.
13. J. Howland and D. J. Rohsenow, Risks of energy drinks mixed with alcohol, *Journal of the American Medical Association* 309 (2013): 245–246.
14. Research Society on Alcoholism, Drunkorexia 101: Increasing alcohol's effects through diet and exercise behaviors, *Science Daily*, 27 June 2016; A. E. Barry and A. K. Piazza-Gardner, Drunkorexia: Understanding the co-occurrence of alcohol consumption and eating/exercise weight management behaviors, *Journal of American College Health* 60 (2012): 236–243.
15. Centers for Disease Control and Prevention, Vital signs: Binge drinking prevalence, frequency, and intensity among adults—the United States, 2010, *Morbidity and Mortality Weekly Report* 61 (2012): 14–19.
16. S. Feldman, Prenatal alcohol exposure patterns and alcohol-related birth defects and growth deficiencies: A prospective study, *Alcoholism: Clinical and Experimental Research* 36 (2012): 670–676.
17. World Health Organization, Management of substance abuse: Alcohol, www.who.int/substance_abuse/facts/alcohol/en, 2016.
18. Traffic safety facts 2014 data: Alcohol-impaired driving (Washington, DC: NHTSA), 2015, www-nrd.nhtsa.dot.gov/Pubs/812231.pdf.

8 Energy Balance and Body Composition

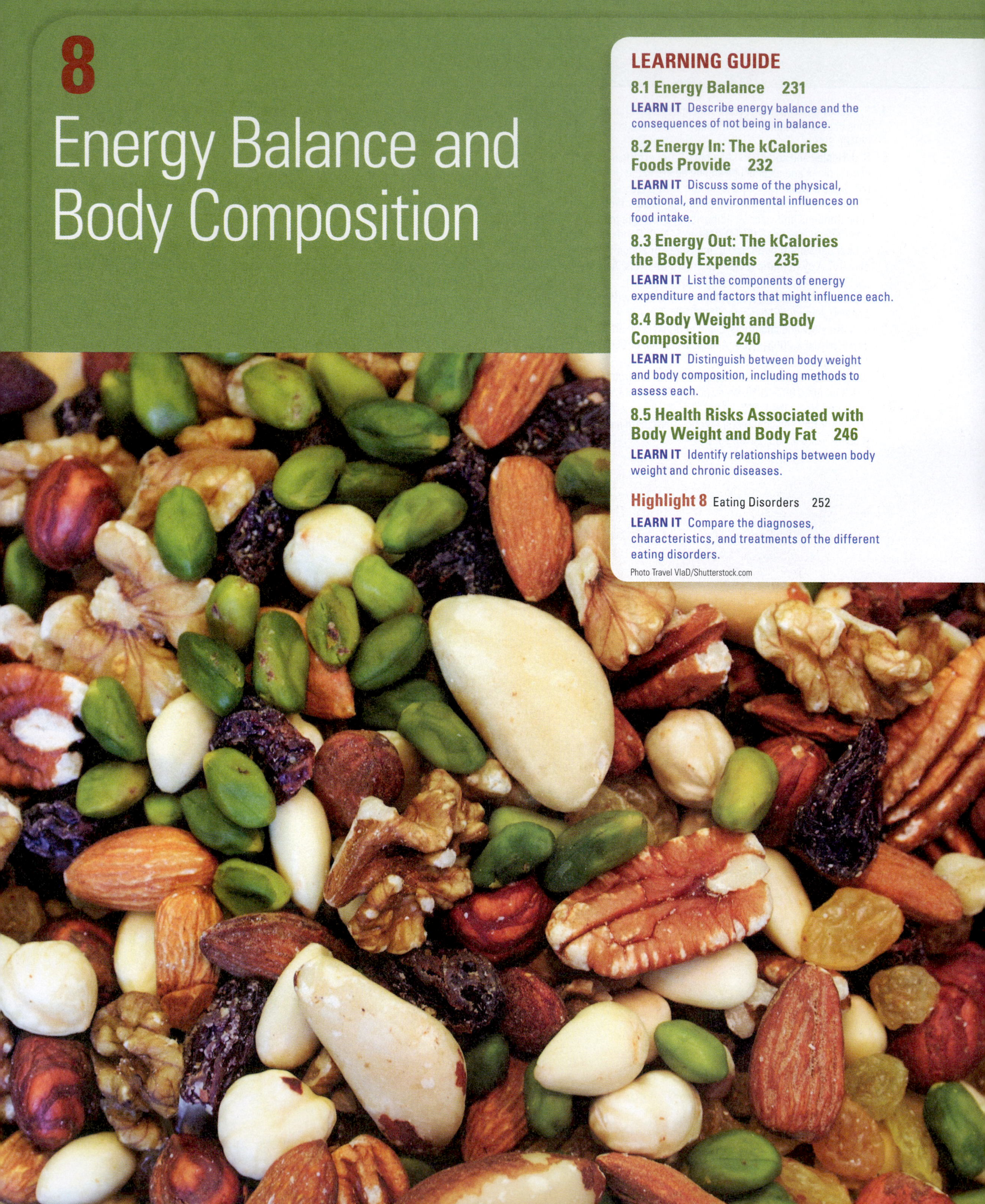

LEARNING GUIDE

Photo Travel VlaD/Shutterstock.com

Nutrition in Your Life

It's simple: energy balance occurs when energy in = energy out. The reality, of course, is much more complex. One day you may devour a dozen doughnuts at midnight and sleep through your morning workout—tipping the scales toward weight gain. Another day you may snack on veggies and train for this weekend's 10K race—shifting the balance toward weight loss. Your body weight—especially as it relates to your body fat—and your level of fitness have consequences for your health. So, how are you doing? As you read this chapter, consider how your "energy in" and "energy out" balance and whether your body weight and fat measures are consistent with good health.

As Chapter 7 explained, the body's remarkable metabolism can cope with variations in the diet. When the diet delivers too little energy, carbohydrate, or protein, the body uses its glycogen and fat stores to meet glucose and energy needs and degrades its lean tissue to meet protein (and glucose) needs. When the diet delivers too much energy—whether from excess carbohydrate, excess protein, or excess fat—the body stores fat.

The simple picture is as follows. People who consume more food energy than they expend store the surplus as body fat. To reduce body fat, they need to expend more energy than they take in from food. In contrast, people who consume too little food energy to support their bodies' activities must rely on their bodies' fat stores and possibly some of their lean tissues as well. To gain weight, these people need to take in more food energy than they expend. As you will see, though, the details of energy balance and weight regulation are quite complex. This chapter describes energy balance and body composition and examines the health problems associated with having too much or too little body fat. The next chapter presents strategies to alleviate these problems.

8.1 Energy Balance

LEARN IT Describe energy balance and the consequences of not being in balance.

People expend energy continuously and eat periodically to refuel. Ideally, their energy intakes cover their energy expenditures with little, or no, excess. Excess energy is stored as fat, and stored fat is used for energy between meals. The fat stores of even a healthy-weight adult represent an ample reserve of energy—50,000 to 200,000 kcalories.

The amount of body fat a person deposits in, or withdraws from, storage on any given day depends on the **energy balance** for that day—the amount consumed (energy in) versus the amount expended (energy out). When a person is maintaining weight, "energy in" equals "energy out " (see Figure 8-1). When the balance shifts, weight changes.

A classic rule states that for each 3500 kcalories eaten in excess, a pound of body fat is stored; similarly, a pound of fat is lost for each 3500 kcalories expended beyond those consumed.* To that end, many diet plans recommend lowering energy intake by 500 kcalories a day to incur a weight loss of 1 pound per week. This "3500 kcalorie rule" has been used for more than 50 years, but it has several limitations.[1] For one, as a person loses weight, the deficit in energy needed to continue losing weight shifts; in general, the kcalorie deficit is relatively low and weight loss is relatively rapid in the early phase but then it is followed by a markedly slower weight loss that plateaus as the kcalorie deficit needed to continue

> FIGURE 8-1 Energy Balance

When "energy in" balances with "energy out", a person's body weight is stable.

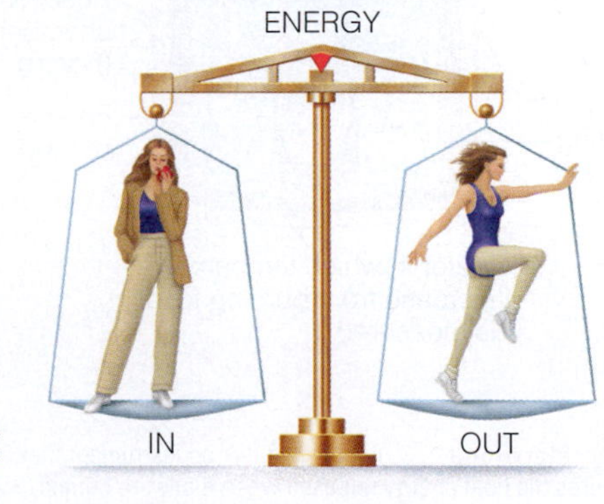
ENERGY
IN
OUT
© Cengage

energy balance: the energy (kcalories) consumed from foods and beverages compared with the energy expended through metabolic processes and physical activities.

*Body fat, or adipose tissue, is composed of a mixture of mostly fat, some protein, and water. A pound of body fat (454 g) is approximately 87 percent fat, or (454 × 0.87) 395 g, and 395 g × 9 kcal/g = 3555 kcal.

losing weight gradually increases. For another, body composition differs dramatically for men and women and for obese and lean people; in general, the kcalorie deficit needed for weight loss is relatively larger for women than for men and for obese than for lean people. Understanding the dynamic nature of weight loss may help people adopt more realistic expectations than those provided by a fixed 3500-kcalorie rule.

Quick changes in body weight are not simple changes in fat stores. Weight gained or lost rapidly includes some fat, large amounts of fluid, and some lean tissues such as muscle proteins and bone minerals. Because water constitutes about 60 percent of an adult's body weight, retention or loss of water can greatly influence body weight. Even over the long term, the composition of weight gained or lost is normally about 75 percent fat and 25 percent lean. During starvation, losses of fat and lean are about equal. (Recall from Chapter 7 that without adequate carbohydrate, protein-rich lean tissues break down to provide glucose.) Invariably, though, *fat* gains and losses are gradual. The next two sections examine the two sides of the energy-balance equation—energy in and energy out. As you read, keep in mind that this simple equation falls short of fully explaining the many metabolic changes that cause obesity.

REVIEW IT Describe energy balance and the consequences of not being in balance.

When energy consumed equals energy expended, a person is in energy balance and body weight is stable. If more energy is taken in than is expended, a person gains weight. If more energy is expended than is taken in, a person loses weight.

8.2 Energy In: The kCalories Foods Provide

LEARN IT Discuss some of the physical, emotional, and environmental influences on food intake.

Foods and beverages provide the "energy in" part of the energy-balance equation. How much energy a person receives depends on the composition of the foods and beverages and on the amount the person eats and drinks.

Food Composition To find out how many kcalories a food provides, a scientist can burn the food in a **bomb calorimeter** (see Figure 8-2). When the food burns, energy is released in the form of heat. The amount of heat given off provides a *direct* measure of the food's energy value (remember that kcalories are units of heat energy).* In addition to releasing heat, these reactions generate carbon dioxide and water—just as the body's cells do when they metabolize the energy-yielding nutrients from foods. Details of the chemical reactions in a calorimeter and in the body differ, but the overall process is similar: when the food burns and the chemical bonds break, the carbons (C) and hydrogens (H) combine with oxygens (O) to form carbon dioxide (CO_2) and water (H_2O). The amount of oxygen consumed gives an *indirect* measure of the amount of energy released.

> FIGURE 8-2 Bomb Calorimeter

When food is burned, energy is released in the form of heat. Heat energy is measured in kcalories.

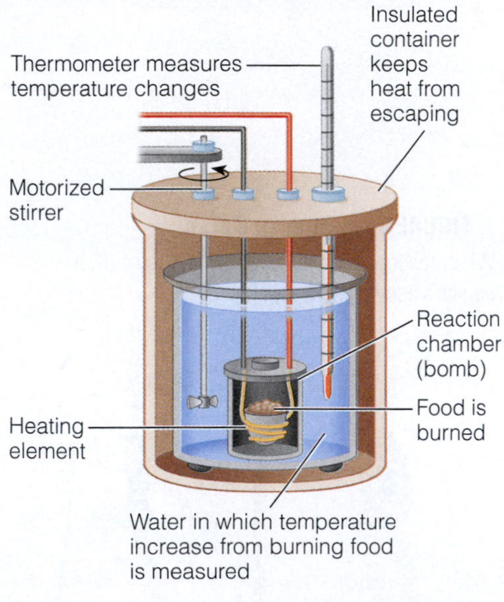
Insulated container keeps heat from escaping
Thermometer measures temperature changes
Motorized stirrer
Reaction chamber (bomb)
Food is burned
Heating element
Water in which temperature increase from burning food is measured
© Cengage

A bomb calorimeter measures the available energy in foods but overstates the **physiological fuel value**—the amount of energy that the human body derives from foods. The body is less efficient than a calorimeter and cannot metabolize all of the energy-yielding nutrients in a food completely. Researchers can correct for this discrepancy mathematically to create useful tables of the energy values of foods such as the USDA Food Composition Database (https://ndb.nal.usda.gov/). These values provide reasonable estimates, but they do not reflect the *precise* amount of energy a person will derive from the foods consumed.

The energy values of foods can also be computed from the amounts of carbohydrate, fat, and protein (and alcohol, if present) in the foods. For example, a food

bomb calorimeter (KAL-oh-RIM-eh-ter): an instrument that measures the heat energy released when foods are burned, thus providing an estimate of the potential energy of the foods.
- **calor** = heat
- **metron** = measure

physiological fuel value: the number of kcalories that the body derives from a food, in contrast to the number of kcalories determined by calorimetry.

*As Chapter 1 mentioned, many scientists measure food energy in *kilojoules* (a measure of work energy). Conversion factors for these and other measures can be found in Appendix H.

containing 12 grams of carbohydrate, 5 grams of fat, and 8 grams of protein will provide 48 carbohydrate kcalories, 45 fat kcalories, and 32 protein kcalories, for a total of 125 kcalories. (To review how to calculate the energy foods provide, turn to How To 1-2, p. 10.)

Food Intake

To achieve energy balance, the body must meet its needs without taking in too much or too little energy. **Appetite** prompts a person to eat—or not to eat. Somehow the body decides how much and how often to eat—when to start eating and when to stop. As you will see, many signals—from both the environment and genetics—initiate or delay eating.

Hunger People eat for a variety of reasons, most obviously (although not necessarily most commonly) because they are hungry. Most people recognize **hunger** as an irritating feeling that prompts thoughts of food and motivates them to start eating. In the body, hunger is the physiological response to a need for food triggered by nerve signals and chemical messengers originating and acting in the brain, primarily in the **hypothalamus**. Hunger can be influenced by such factors as the presence or absence of nutrients in the bloodstream, the size and composition of the preceding meal, customary eating patterns, climate (heat reduces food intake; cold increases it), physical activity, hormones, and illnesses. Hunger determines what to eat, when to eat, and how much to eat.

The stomach is ideally designed to handle periodic batches of food, and people typically eat meals at roughly 4-hour intervals. Four hours after a meal, most, if not all, of the food has left the stomach. Most people do not feel like eating again until the stomach is either empty or almost so. Even then, a person may not feel hungry for quite a while.

Satiation During the course of a meal, as food enters the GI tract and hunger diminishes, **satiation** occurs. As receptors in the stomach stretch and hormones such as cholecystokinin become active, the person begins to feel full. The response: satiation, which prompts the person to stop eating.

Satiety After a meal, the feeling of **satiety** continues to suppress hunger and allows a person to not eat again for a while. Whereas *satiation* tells us to "stop eating," *satiety* reminds us to "not start eating again." Figure 8-3 (p. 234) summarizes the relationships among hunger, satiation, and satiety. Of course, people can override these signals, especially when presented with stressful situations or favorite foods.

Overriding Hunger and Satiety Not surprisingly, eating can be triggered by signals other than hunger, even when the body does not need food. Some people experience food cravings when they are bored or anxious. In fact, they may eat in response to any kind of stress, negative or positive. ("What do I do when I'm grieving? Eat. What do I do when I'm celebrating? Eat!") Eating to relieve stress can easily lead to overeating (making especially poor food choices) and weight gain.[2]

Many people respond to external cues such as the time of day ("It's time to eat") or the availability, sight, and taste of food ("I'd love a piece of chocolate even though I'm full"). Environmental influences such as large portion sizes, favorite foods, or an abundance or variety of foods stimulate eating and increase energy intake (see Photo 8-1, p. 234). Cognitive influences—such as perceptions, memories, intellect, and social interactions—can easily lead to weight gain. Those who are overweight or obese may be especially susceptible to external cues that trigger hunger and the desire to eat.

Eating can also be suppressed by signals other than satiety, even when a person is hungry. People with the eating disorder anorexia nervosa, for example, use tremendous discipline to ignore the pangs of hunger. (Highlight 8 features anorexia nervosa and other eating disorders.) Some people simply cannot eat during times of stress, negative or positive. ("I'm too sad to eat." "I'm too excited to eat!") Why some people overeat in response to stress and others cannot eat at all remains a bit of a mystery, although researchers are beginning to understand the connections

appetite: the integrated response to the sight, smell, thought, or taste of food that initiates or delays eating.

hunger: the painful sensation caused by a lack of food that initiates food-seeking behavior.

hypothalamus (high-po-THAL-ah-mus): a brain center that controls activities such as maintenance of water balance, regulation of body temperature, and control of appetite.

satiation (say-she-AY-shun): the feeling of satisfaction and fullness that occurs during a meal and halts eating. Satiation determines how much food is consumed during a meal.

satiety (sah-TIE-eh-tee): the feeling of fullness and satisfaction that occurs after a meal and inhibits eating until the next meal. Satiety determines how much time passes between meals.

> **FIGURE 8-3 Hunger, Satiation, and Satiety**

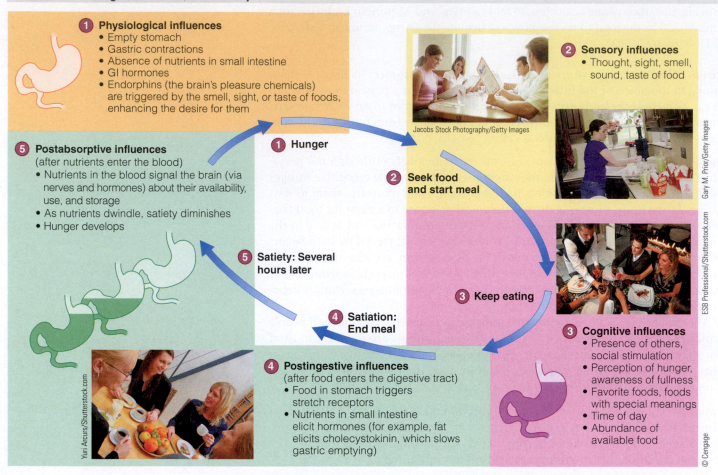

1 Physiological influences
- Empty stomach
- Gastric contractions
- Absence of nutrients in small intestine
- GI hormones
- Endorphins (the brain's pleasure chemicals) are triggered by the smell, sight, or taste of foods, enhancing the desire for them

2 Sensory influences
- Thought, sight, smell, sound, taste of food

Jacobs Stock Photography/Getty Images

Gary M. Prior/Getty Images

1 Hunger

2 Seek food and start meal

3 Keep eating

4 Satiation: End meal

5 Satiety: Several hours later

5 Postabsorptive influences
(after nutrients enter the blood)
- Nutrients in the blood signal the brain (via nerves and hormones) about their availability, use, and storage
- As nutrients dwindle, satiety diminishes
- Hunger develops

ESB Professional/Shutterstock.com

3 Cognitive influences
- Presence of others, social stimulation
- Perception of hunger, awareness of fullness
- Favorite foods, foods with special meanings
- Time of day
- Abundance of available food

Yuri Arcurs/Shutterstock.com

4 Postingestive influences
(after food enters the digestive tract)
- Food in stomach triggers stretch receptors
- Nutrients in small intestine elicit hormones (for example, fat elicits cholecystokinin, which slows gastric emptying)

between hormones, brain activity, mood, and "comfort foods."[3] Interestingly, one study reports that when hungry, both lean and obese women have increased brain activity in response to images of food, whereas after eating, brain activity quickly diminishes in lean women, but remains elevated in obese women—even though both groups report feeling full.[4]

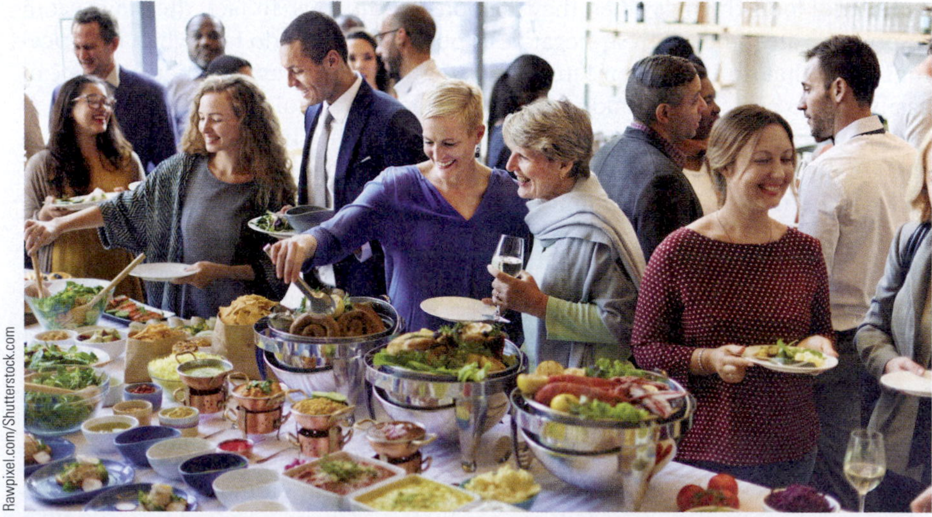

Rawpixel.com/Shutterstock.com

> **PHOTO 8-1** Regardless of hunger, people typically overeat when offered the abundance and variety of a buffet. To limit unhealthy weight gains, listen to hunger and satiety signals.

Sustaining Satiation and Satiety The extent to which foods produce satiation and sustain satiety depends in part on the nutrient composition of a meal. Of the three energy-yielding nutrients, protein is considered the most **satiating.** In fact, too little protein in the diet can leave a person feeling hungry. Including some protein—such as drinking milk—provides feelings of fullness and satiety, which may help decrease energy intake at the next meal.[5] In contrast, fructose in a sugary fruit drink seems to stimulate appetite and increase food intake.

Chapter 1 explained that energy density is a measure of the energy a food provides relative to the amount of food (kcalories per gram). Foods with a high energy density provide more kcalories, and those with low energy density provide fewer kcalories, for the same amount of food. Foods low in energy density are also more satiating. High-fiber foods effectively provide satiation by filling the stomach and delaying the absorption of nutrients.[6] For this reason, eating a large salad as a first course helps a person eat less during the meal. In contrast, fat has a weak effect on satiation; consequently, eating high-fat foods may lead to passive overconsumption. High-fat foods are flavorful, which stimulates the appetite and entices people to eat more. High-fat foods are also energy dense; consequently, they deliver more kcalories per bite. (Chapter 9 describes how considering a food's energy density can help with weight management.) Although fat provides little satiation during a meal, it produces strong satiety signals once it enters the intestine. Fat in the intestine triggers the release of cholecystokinin—a hormone that signals satiety and inhibits food intake.

Message Central—The Hypothalamus As you can see, eating is a complex behavior controlled by a variety of genetic, psychological, social, metabolic, and physiological factors. The hypothalamus appears to be the control center, integrating a variety of nerve and hormone messages about energy intake, expenditure, and storage from other parts of the body.[7] Some of these messages influence satiation, which helps control the size of a meal; others influence satiety, which helps determine the frequency of meals.

By understanding the action of hormones that influence appetite control and energy balance, researchers may one day be able to develop obesity treatments. An added challenge is to sort out the many actions of related brain chemicals. For example, one brain chemical, **neuropeptide Y,** causes carbohydrate cravings, initiates eating, decreases energy expenditure, and increases fat storage—all factors favoring a positive energy balance and weight gain.

REVIEW IT Discuss some of the physical, emotional, and environmental influences on food intake.

A mixture of signals governs a person's eating behaviors. Hunger and appetite initiate eating, whereas satiation and satiety stop and delay eating, respectively. Each responds to messages from the nervous and hormonal systems. Superimposed on these signals are complex factors involving emotions, habits, and other aspects of human behavior.

8.3 Energy Out: The kCalories the Body Expends

LEARN IT List the components of energy expenditure and factors that might influence each.

Chapter 7 explained that heat is released whenever the body breaks down carbohydrate, fat, or protein for energy and again when that energy is used to do work. The generation of heat, known as **thermogenesis,** can be measured to determine the amount of energy expended. The total energy a body expends reflects three main categories of thermogenesis:

- Energy expended for basal metabolism
- Energy expended for physical activity
- Energy expended for food consumption

A fourth category is sometimes involved:

- Energy expended for adaptation

satiating: having the power to suppress hunger and inhibit eating.

neuropeptide Y: a chemical produced in the brain that stimulates appetite, diminishes energy expenditure, and increases fat storage.

thermogenesis: the generation of heat; used in physiology and nutrition studies as an index of how much energy the body is expending.

> **FIGURE 8-4 Components of Energy Expenditure**

The amount of energy expended in a day differs for each individual, but in general, basal metabolism is the largest component of energy expenditure and thermic effect of food is the smallest.

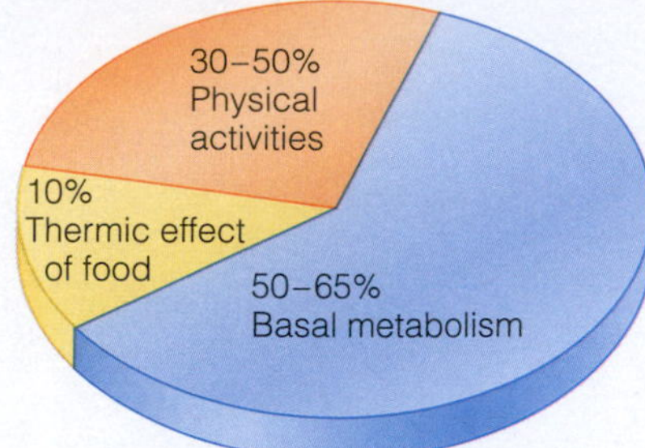
30–50%
Physical
activities
10%
Thermic effect
of food
50–65%
Basal metabolism

The amount of energy expended in voluntary physical activities has the greatest variability, depending on a person's activity patterns. For a sedentary person, physical activities may account for less than half as much energy as basal metabolism, whereas an extremely active person may expend as much on physical activity as for basal metabolism.

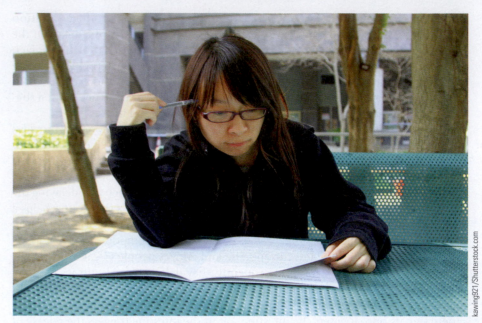

> **PHOTO 8-2** It feels like work and it may make you tired, but studying requires only one or two kcalories per minute.

Components of Energy Expenditure People expend energy when they are physically active, of course, but they also expend energy when they are resting quietly (see Photo 8-2). In fact, quiet metabolic activities account for the largest share of most people's energy expenditures, as Figure 8-4 shows.

Basal Metabolism About two-thirds of the energy the average person expends in a day supports the body's **basal metabolism.** Metabolic activities include the lungs inhaling and exhaling air, the bone marrow making new red blood cells, the heart beating 100,000 times a day, and the kidneys filtering wastes—in short, they support all the basic processes of life.

The **basal metabolic rate (BMR)** is the rate at which the body expends energy for these life-sustaining activities. The rate varies from person to person and may vary for the same individual with a change in circumstance or physical condition.[8] The rate is slowest when a person is sleeping undisturbed, but it is usually measured in a room with a comfortable temperature when the person is awake, but lying still, after a restful sleep and an overnight (12 to 14 hours) fast. A similar measure of energy output—called the **resting metabolic rate (RMR)**—is slightly higher than the BMR because its criteria for recent food intake and physical activity are not as strict. When energy needs cannot be measured, equations can provide reasonably accurate estimates (see Table 8-1).

basal metabolism: the energy needed to maintain life when a body is at complete digestive, physical, and emotional rest.

basal metabolic rate (BMR): the rate of energy use for metabolism under specified conditions: after a 12-hour fast and restful sleep, without any physical activity or emotional excitement, and in a comfortable setting. It is usually expressed as kcalories per kilogram of body weight per hour.

resting metabolic rate (RMR): similar to the basal metabolic rate (BMR), a measure of energy use for a person at rest in a comfortable setting, but with less stringent criteria for recent food intake and physical activity. Consequently, the RMR is easier to determine, but slightly higher than the BMR.

TABLE 8-1 Estimating Energy Expended on Basal Metabolism

	BMR Estimates[a]	BMR Equations[b]
Men	Slightly >1 kcal/min (1.1 to 1.3 kcal/min) or 24 kcal/kg/day	(10 × wt) + (6.25 × ht) − (5 × age) + 5
Women	Slightly <1 kcal/min (0.8 to 1.0 kcal/min) or 23 kcal/kg/day	(10 × wt) + (6.25 × ht) − (5 × age) − 161

[a]For perspective, a burning candle or a 75-watt light bulb releases about 1 kcal/min.
[b]Use actual weight in kilograms, height in centimeters, and age in years.

In general, the more a person weighs, the more *total* energy is expended on basal metabolism, but the amount of energy *per pound* of body weight may be lower. For example, an adult's BMR might be 1500 kcalories per day and an infant's only 500, but compared to body weight, the infant's BMR is more than twice as fast. Similarly, a normal-weight adult may have a metabolic rate one and a half times that of an obese adult when compared to body weight because lean tissue is metabolically more active than body fat.

Table 8-2 summarizes the factors that raise and lower the BMR. For the most part, the BMR is highest in people who are growing (children, adolescents, and pregnant women) and in those with considerable **lean body mass** (physically fit people and males). One way to increase the BMR, then, is to participate in endurance and strength-training activities regularly to maximize lean body mass. The BMR is also high in people with fever or under stress and in people with highly active thyroid glands. The BMR slows down with a loss of lean body mass and during fasting and malnutrition.

Physical Activity The second component of a person's energy output is physical activity: voluntary movement of the skeletal muscles and support systems. Physical activity is the most variable—and the most changeable—component of energy expenditure. Consequently, its influence on both weight gain and weight loss can be significant.

During physical activity, the muscles need extra energy to move, and the heart and lungs need extra energy to deliver nutrients and oxygen and dispose of wastes. The amount of energy needed for any activity, whether playing tennis or studying for an exam, depends on three factors: muscle mass, body weight, and activity. The larger the muscle mass and the heavier the weight of the body part being moved, the more energy is expended. Table 8-3 (p. 238) gives average energy expenditures for various activities. The activity's duration, frequency, and

TABLE 8-2 Factors That Affect the BMR

Factor	Effect on BMR
Age	Lean body mass diminishes with age, slowing the BMR.[a]
Height	In tall, thin people, the BMR is higher.[b]
Growth	In children, adolescents, and pregnant women, the BMR is higher.
Body composition (gender)	The more lean tissue, the higher the BMR (which is why males usually have a higher BMR than females). The more fat tissue, the lower the BMR.
Fever	Fever raises the BMR.[c]
Stresses	Stresses (including many diseases and certain drugs) raise the BMR.
Environmental temperature	Both heat and cold raise the BMR.
Fasting/starvation	Fasting/starvation lowers the BMR.[d]
Malnutrition	Malnutrition lowers the BMR.
Hormones	The thyroid hormone thyroxine, for example, can speed up or slow down the BMR.[e] Premenstrual hormones slightly raise the BMR.
Smoking	Nicotine increases energy expenditure.
Caffeine	Caffeine increases energy expenditure.
Sleep	BMR is lowest when sleeping.

[a]The BMR begins to decrease in early adulthood (after growth and development cease) at a rate of about 2 percent/decade. A reduction in voluntary activity as well brings the total decline in energy expenditure to about 5 percent/decade.
[b]If two people weigh the same, the taller, thinner person will have the faster metabolic rate, reflecting the greater skin surface, through which heat is lost by radiation, in proportion to the body's volume (see Figure 8-5, p. 239).
[c]Fever raises the BMR by 7 percent for each degree Fahrenheit.
[d]Prolonged starvation reduces the total amount of metabolically active lean tissue in the body, although the decline occurs sooner and to a greater extent than body losses alone can explain. More likely, the neural and hormonal changes that accompany fasting are responsible for changes in the BMR.
[e]The thyroid gland releases hormones that travel to the cells and influence cellular metabolism. Thyroid hormone activity can speed up or slow down the rate of metabolism by as much as 50 percent.

lean body mass: the body minus its fat.

TABLE 8-3 Estimating Energy Expended on Physical Activities

The values listed in this table reflect both the energy expended in physical activity and the amount used for BMR. To calculate kcalories spent per minute of activity for your own body weight, multiply kcal/lb/min (or kcal/kg/min) by your exact weight and then multiply that number by the number of minutes spent in the activity. For example, if you weigh 142 pounds, and you want to know how many kcalories you spent doing 30 minutes of vigorous aerobic dance: 0.062 × 142 = 8.8 kcalories per minute; 8.8 × 30 minutes = 264 total kcalories expended.

Activity	kCal/lb min	kCal/kg min
Aerobic dance (vigorous)	.062	.136
Basketball (vigorous, full court)	.097	.213
Bicycling		
13 mph	.045	.099
15 mph	.049	.108
17 mph	.057	.125
19 mph	.076	.167
21 mph	.090	.198
23 mph	.109	.240
25 mph	.139	.306
Canoeing, flat water, moderate pace	.045	.099
Cross-country skiing 8 mph	.104	.229
Gardening	.045	.099
Golf (carrying clubs)	.045	.099
Handball	.078	.172
Horseback riding (trot)	.052	.114
Rowing (vigorous)	.097	.213
Running		
5 mph	.061	.134
6 mph	.074	.163
7.5 mph	.094	.207
9 mph	.103	.227
10 mph	.114	.251
11 mph	.131	.288
Soccer (vigorous)	.097	.213
Studying	.011	.024
Swimming		
20 yd/min	.032	.070
45 yd/min	.058	.128
50 yd/min	.070	.154
Table tennis (skilled)	.045	.099
Tennis (beginner)	.032	.070
Vacuuming and other household tasks	.030	.066
Walking		
3.5 mph	.035	.077
4.5 mph	.048	.106
Weight lifting		
light-to-moderate	.024	.053
vigorous	.048	.106
Wheelchair basketball	.084	.185
Wheeling self in wheelchair	.030	.066
Wii games		
bowling	.021	.046
boxing	.021	.047
tennis	.022	.048

intensity also influence energy expenditure: the longer, the more frequent, and the more intense the activity, the more kcalories expended. (Chapter 14 describes how an activity's duration, frequency, and intensity also influence the body's use of the energy-yielding nutrients.)

Thermic Effect of Food When a person eats, the GI tract muscles speed up their rhythmic contractions, the cells that manufacture and secrete digestive juices become active, and some nutrients require energy to be absorbed. This acceleration of activity requires energy and produces heat; it is known as the **thermic effect of food (TEF).**

The thermic effect of food is proportional to the food energy taken in and is usually estimated at 10 percent of energy intake. Thus a person who ingests 2000 kcalories probably expends about 200 kcalories on the thermic effect of food. The proportions vary for different foods, however, and are also influenced by factors such as meal size and frequency. In general, the thermic effect of food is greater for high-protein foods than for high-fat foods (see Table 8-4)

TABLE 8-4 Thermic Effect of Foods

Food Component	Energy Expended
Carbohydrate	5–10%
Fat	0–5%
Protein	20–30%
Alcohol	15–20%

NOTE: Percentages are calculated by dividing the energy expended during digestion and absorption (above basal) by the energy content of the food.

thermic effect of food (TEF): an estimation of the energy required to process food (digest, absorb, transport, metabolize, and store ingested nutrients); also called the *specific dynamic effect (SDE)* of food or the *specific dynamic activity (SDA)* of food. The sum of the TEF and any increase in the metabolic rate due to overeating is known as *diet-induced thermogenesis (DIT).*

and for a meal eaten all at once rather than spread out over a couple of hours. For most purposes, however, the thermic effect of food can be ignored when estimating energy expenditure because its contribution to total energy output is smaller than the probable errors involved in estimating overall energy intake and output.

Adaptive Thermogenesis Additional energy is expended when circumstances in the body are dramatically changed. A body challenged by physical conditioning, extreme cold, overfeeding, starvation, trauma, or other types of stress must adapt; it has extra work to do and uses extra energy to build the tissues and produce the enzymes and hormones necessary to cope with the demand. This energy is known as **adaptive thermogenesis,** and in some circumstances (for example, in burn victims), it makes a considerable difference in the total energy expended. Because this component of energy expenditure is so variable and specific to individuals, it is not included when estimating energy requirements for most healthy people.

> **FIGURE 8-5 How Body Size Influences BMR**

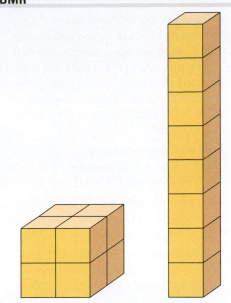

Each of these structures is made of eight blocks. They weigh the same, but they are arranged differently. The short, wide structure has 24 sides exposed and the tall, thin one has 34. Because the tall, thin structure has a greater surface area, it will lose more heat (expend more energy) than the short, wide one. Similarly, two people of different heights might weigh the same, but the taller, thin one will have a higher BMR (expending more energy) because of the greater skin surface.

Estimating Energy Requirements

In estimating energy requirements, the DRI Committee developed equations based on research measuring total daily energy expenditure. These equations consider how the following factors influence BMR and consequently energy expenditure:

- *Gender.* In general, women have lower energy requirements than men, in large part because men typically have more lean body mass. Two sets of energy equations—one for men and one for women—were developed to accommodate the influence of gender on energy expenditure (provided in How To 8-1, p. 240).
- *Growth.* Energy needs are high in people who are growing. For this reason, pregnant and lactating women, infants, children, and adolescents have their own sets of energy equations.
- *Age.* Energy needs decline during adulthood as lean body mass diminishes. This change in body composition occurs, in part, because some hormones that influence appetite, body weight, and metabolism become more, or less, active with age. Physical activities tend to decline as well, bringing the average reduction in energy expenditure to about 5 percent per decade. Because age influences energy expenditure, it is also factored into the energy equations.
- *Physical activity.* Using individual values for various physical activities (as in Table 8-3) is time-consuming and impractical for estimating the energy needs of a population. Instead, various activities are clustered according to the typical intensity of a day's efforts. Energy equations include a physical activity factor for various levels of intensity for each gender.
- *Body composition and body size.* Energy needs are high in people who are tall and so have a large surface area, as illustrated in Figure 8-5. Similarly, the more a person weighs, the more energy is expended on basal metabolism. For these reasons, energy equations include a factor for both height and weight.

As just explained, energy needs vary between individuals depending on such factors as gender, growth, age, physical activity, and body size and composition. Even when two people are similarly matched, however, their energy needs still differ because of genetic differences. Perhaps one day genetic research will reveal how to estimate requirements for each individual. For now, How To 8-1 (p. 240) provides instructions on estimating energy requirements using the DRI equations and physical activity factors. Appendix F presents a table of estimated daily energy needs by age, gender, and activity level, based on the DRI equations using reference heights and weights.

adaptive thermogenesis: adjustments in energy expenditure related to changes in environment such as extreme cold and to physiological events such as overfeeding, trauma, and changes in hormone status.

>How To 8-1 Estimate Energy Requirements

To determine your estimated energy requirement (EER), use the appropriate equation, inserting your age in years, weight (wt) in kilograms, height (ht) in meters, and physical activity (PA) factor from the accompanying table. (To convert pounds to kilograms, divide by 2.2; to convert inches to meters, divide by 39.37.)

- For men 19 years and older:
  EER = [662 − (9.53 × age)] + PA × [(15.91 × wt) + (539.6 × ht)]
- For women 19 years and older:
  EER = [354 − (6.91 × age)] + PA × [(9.36 × wt) + (726 × ht)]

For example, consider an active 30-year-old male who is 5 feet 11 inches tall and weighs 178 pounds. First, he converts his weight from pounds to kilograms and his height from inches to meters, if necessary:

$$178 \text{ lb} \div 2.2 = 80.9 \text{ kg}$$

$$71 \text{ in} \div 39.37 = 1.8 \text{ m}$$

Next, he considers his level of daily physical activity and selects the appropriate PA factor from the accompanying table. (In this example, 1.25 for an active male.) Then, he inserts his age, PA factor, weight, and height into the appropriate equation:

$$\text{EER} = [662 - (9.53 \times 30)] + 1.25 \times [(15.91 \times 80.9) + (539.6 \times 1.8)]$$

(A reminder: Do calculations within the parentheses first.) He calculates:

$$\text{EER} = [662 - 286] + 1.25 \times [1287 + 971]$$

(Another reminder: Do calculations within the brackets next.)

$$\text{EER} = 376 + 1.25 \times 2258$$

(One more reminder: Do multiplication before addition.)

$$\text{EER} = 376 + 2823$$

$$\text{EER} = 3199$$

The estimated energy requirement for an active 30-year-old male who is 5 feet 11 inches tall and weighs 178 pounds is about 3200 kcalories/day. His actual requirement probably falls within a range of 200 kcalories above and below this estimate.

NOTE: Appendix F provides estimates of energy needs based on EER equations, using reference heights and weights for each age-gender group.

Physical Activity (PA) Factors for EER Equations

	Men	Women	Physical Activity
Sedentary	1.0	1.0	Typical daily living activities
Low active	1.11	1.12	plus 30–60 min moderate activity
Active	1.25	1.27	plus ≥ 60 min moderate activity
Very active	1.48	1.45	plus ≥ 60 min moderate activity and 60 min vigorous or 120 min moderate activity

NOTE: Moderate activity is equivalent to walking at 3 to 4½ mph.

> TRY IT Estimate your energy requirement based on your current age, weight, height, and activity level.

REVIEW IT List the components of energy expenditure and factors that might influence each.

A person in energy balance takes in energy from food and expends much of it on basal metabolism, some of it on physical activities, and a little on the thermic effect of food. Energy requirements vary from person to person, depending on such factors as gender, age, weight, and height as well as the intensity and duration of physical activity. All of these factors must be considered when estimating energy requirements.

8.4 Body Weight and Body Composition

LEARN IT Distinguish between body weight and body composition, including methods to assess each.

A person 5 feet 10 inches tall who weighs 150 pounds may carry only about 30 of those pounds as fat.* The rest is mostly water and lean tissues—muscles, organs such as the heart and liver, and the bones of the skeleton. Direct measures of

*In metric terms, a person 1.78 meters tall who weights 68 kilograms may carry only about 14 of those kilograms as fat.

body composition are impossible in living human beings; instead, researchers assess body composition indirectly based on the following assumption:

Body weight = fat + lean tissue (including water)

Weight gains and losses tell us nothing about how the body's composition may have changed, yet weight is the measure most people use to judge "fatness." For many people, overweight is overfat, but this is not always the case. Athletes with dense bones and well-developed muscles may be overweight by some standards but have little body fat. Conversely, inactive people may seem to have acceptable weights, when, in fact, they may have too much body fat.

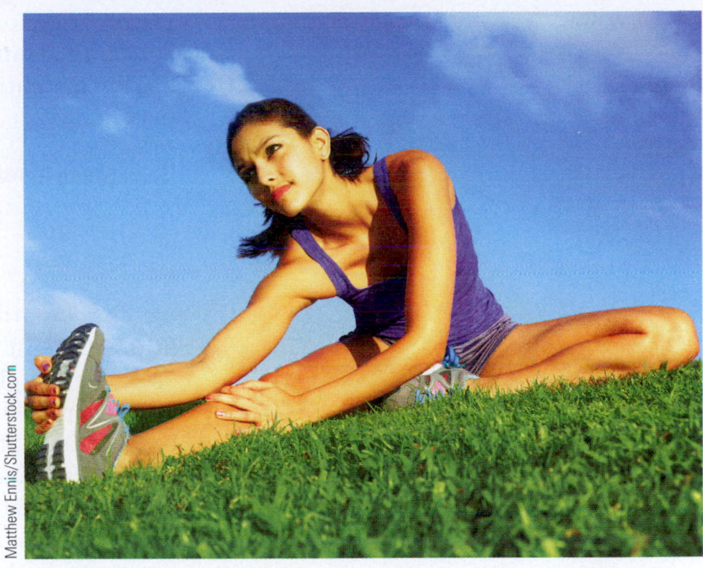
Matthew Ennis/Shutterstock.com

> **PHOTO 8-3** A healthy body contains enough lean tissue to support health and the right amount of fat to meet body needs.

Defining Healthy Body Weight

How much should a person weigh? How can a person know if her weight is appropriate for her height? How can a person know if his weight is jeopardizing his health? Such questions seem so simple, yet the answers can be complex—and quite different depending on whom you ask.

The Criterion of Fashion In asking what is ideal, people often mistakenly turn to friends and fashion for the answer and judge body weight by appearances. Our society sets unrealistic ideals for body weight, especially for women. Magazines, movies, and television all convey the message that to be thin is to be beautiful and happy. As a result, the media have a great influence on the weight concerns and dieting patterns of people of all ages, but most tragically on young, impressionable children and adolescents.

Importantly, perceived body image may have little to do with actual body weight or size. People of all shapes, sizes, and ages—including extremely thin fashion models with anorexia nervosa and fitness instructors with ideal body composition—have learned to be unhappy with their "overweight" bodies. Such dissatisfaction can lead to damaging behaviors, such as starvation diets, diet pill abuse, and health-care avoidance. The first step toward making healthy changes may be self-acceptance. Keep in mind that fashion is fickle; the body shapes valued by society change with time. Furthermore, body shapes valued by one society differ from those of other societies. The standards defining "ideal" are subjective and may have little in common with health. Table 8-5 offers some tips for adopting health as an ideal.

The Criterion of Health People of all shapes and sizes may be beautiful, but they may not be healthy. Ideally, a person weighs enough and has enough body fat to meet basic needs but not so much as to incur health risks (see Photo 8-3). Too much body fat is a major risk factor for several life-threatening diseases, including heart disease, type 2 diabetes, and some cancers. For this

body composition: the proportions of muscle, bone, fat, and other tissue that make up a person's total body weight.

body mass index (BMI): a measure of a person's weight relative to height; determined by dividing the weight (in kilograms) by the square of the height (in meters).

underweight: body weight lower than the weight range that is considered healthy; BMI less than 18.5.

overweight: body weight greater than the weight range that is considered healthy; BMI 25 to 29.9.

obese: too much body fat with adverse health effects; BMI 30 or more.

TABLE 8-5 Tips for Accepting a Healthy Body Weight

- Value yourself and others for human attributes other than body weight. Realize that prejudging people by weight is as harmful as prejudging them by race, religion, or gender.
- Use positive, nonjudgmental descriptions of your body.
- Accept positive comments from others.
- Focus on your whole self, including your intelligence, social grace, and professional and scholastic achievements.
- Accept that no magic diet exists.
- Stop dieting to lose weight. Adopt a lifestyle of healthy eating and physical activity permanently.
- Follow the USDA Food Patterns. Never restrict food intake below the minimum levels that meet nutrient needs.
- Become physically active, not because it will help you get thin but because it will make you feel good and improve your health.
- Seek support from loved ones. Tell them of your plan for a healthy life in the body you have been given.
- Seek professional counseling from someone who can help you make gains in self-esteem without weight as the primary focus.
- Appreciate body weight for its influence on health, not appearance.

reason, the most important criterion for determining ideal body weight is not appearance but good health and longevity. A range of healthy body weights has been identified using a common measure of weight and height—the body mass index.

Body Mass Index The **body mass index (BMI)** describes relative weight for height:

$$\text{BMI} = \frac{\text{weight (kg)}}{\text{height (m)}^2} \quad \text{or} \quad \frac{\text{weight (lb)}}{\text{height (in.)}^2} \times 703$$

Weight classifications based on BMI are presented in Table 8-6. Notice that healthy weight falls between a BMI of 18.5 and 24.9, with **underweight** below 18.5, **overweight** above 25, and **obese** above 30. Figure 8-6 shows examples of body shapes with different BMI. The prevalence of obesity in the United States has increased steadily in recent decades.[9] More than two-thirds of adults in the United States have a BMI greater than 25, as Figure 8-7 shows.

Obesity-related diseases become evident beyond a BMI of 25. For this reason, a BMI of 25 for adults represents a healthy goal for overweight people and an upper limit for others. The lower end of the healthy range may be a reasonable target for severely underweight people. BMI values slightly below the healthy range may be compatible with good health if food intake is adequate, but signs of illness, reduced work capacity, and poor reproductive function become apparent when BMI

TABLE 8-6 Body Mass Index (BMI)

	Underweight	Healthy Weight						Overweight					Obese										
	(<18.5)	(18.5–24.9)						(25–29.9)					(≥30)										
	18	19	20	21	22	23	24	25	26	27	28	29	30	31	32	33	34	35	36	37	38	39	40
Height	***Body weight (pounds)***																						
4′10″	86	91	96	100	105	110	115	119	124	129	134	138	143	148	153	158	162	167	172	177	181	186	191
4′11″	89	94	99	104	109	114	119	124	128	133	138	143	148	153	158	163	168	173	178	183	188	193	198
5′0″	92	97	102	107	112	118	123	128	133	138	143	148	153	158	163	168	174	179	184	189	194	199	204
5′1″	95	100	106	111	116	122	127	132	137	143	148	153	158	164	169	174	180	185	190	195	201	206	211
5′2″	98	104	109	115	120	126	131	136	142	147	153	158	164	169	175	180	186	191	196	202	207	213	218
5′3″	102	107	113	118	124	130	135	141	146	152	158	163	169	175	180	186	191	197	203	208	214	220	225
5′4″	105	110	116	122	128	134	140	145	151	157	163	169	174	180	186	192	197	204	209	215	221	227	232
5′5″	108	114	120	126	132	138	144	150	156	162	168	174	180	186	192	198	204	210	216	222	228	234	240
5′6″	112	118	124	130	136	142	148	155	161	167	173	179	186	192	198	204	210	216	223	229	235	241	247
5′7″	115	121	127	134	140	146	153	159	166	172	178	185	191	198	204	211	217	223	230	236	242	249	255
5′8″	118	125	131	138	144	151	158	164	171	177	184	190	197	203	210	216	223	230	236	243	249	256	262
5′9″	122	128	135	142	149	155	162	169	176	182	189	196	203	209	216	223	230	236	243	250	257	263	270
5′10″	126	132	139	146	153	160	167	174	181	188	195	202	209	216	222	229	236	243	250	257	264	271	278
5′11″	129	136	143	150	157	165	172	179	186	193	200	208	215	222	229	236	243	250	257	265	272	279	286
6′0″	132	140	147	154	162	169	177	184	191	199	206	213	221	228	235	242	250	258	265	272	279	287	294
6′1″	136	144	151	159	166	174	182	189	197	204	212	219	227	235	242	250	257	265	272	280	288	295	302
6′2″	141	148	155	163	171	179	186	194	202	210	218	225	233	241	249	256	264	272	280	287	295	303	311
6′3″	144	152	160	168	176	184	192	200	208	216	224	232	240	248	256	264	272	279	287	295	303	311	319
6′4″	148	156	164	172	180	189	197	205	213	221	230	238	246	254	263	271	279	287	295	304	312	320	328
6′5″	151	160	168	176	185	193	202	210	218	227	235	244	252	261	269	277	286	294	303	311	319	328	336
6′6″	155	164	172	181	190	198	207	216	224	233	241	250	259	267	276	284	293	302	310	319	328	336	345

> **FIGURE 8-6 BMI and Body Shapes**

Standard silhouette figures such as those shown below are commonly used in research studies (without the BMI numbers) to determine how accurately people perceive their body size.

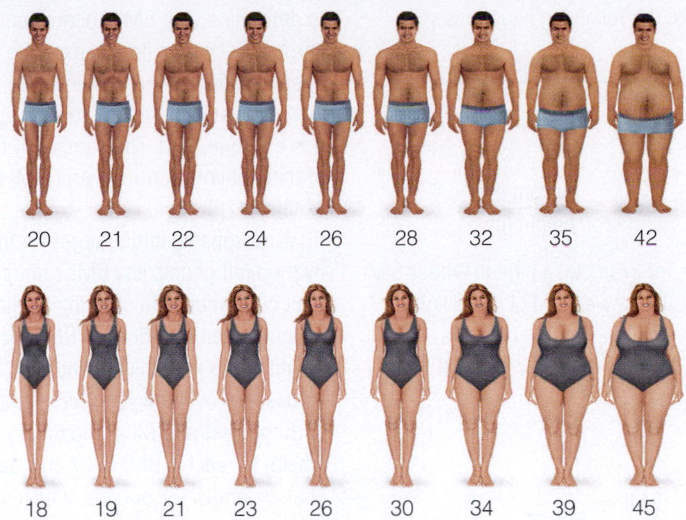

20 21 22 24 26 28 32 35 42
18 19 21 23 26 30 34 39 45

SOURCE: A. J. Stunkard, T. Sorensen, and F. Schulsinger, Use of the Danish Adoption Register for the study of obesity and thinness, *Research Publications: Association for Research in Nervous and Mental Disorders* 60 (1983): 115–120.

> **FIGURE 8-7 Distribution of Body Weights in US Adults**

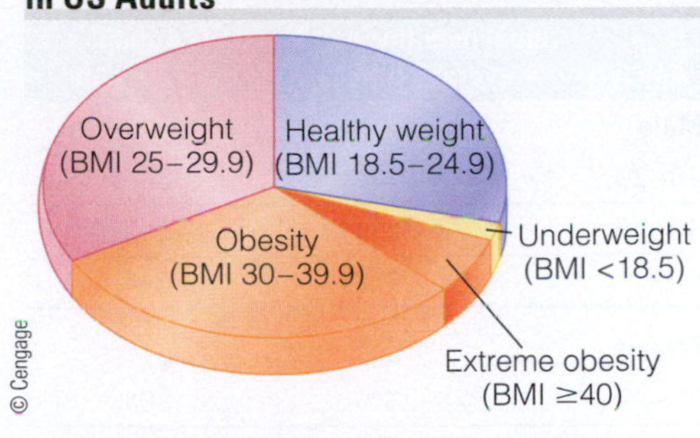

Overweight (BMI 25–29.9)
Healthy weight (BMI 18.5–24.9)
Obesity (BMI 30–39.9)
Underweight (BMI <18.5)
Extreme obesity (BMI ≥40)
© Cengage

is below 17. How To 8-2 (p. 244) describes how to determine your BMI and how to find a goal weight based on a desired BMI.

Keep in mind that BMI reflects height and weight measures and not body composition. Consequently, muscular athletes may be classified as over*weight* by BMI standards and not be over*fat*. At the peak of his bodybuilding career, Arnold Schwarzenegger won the Mr. Olympia competition with a BMI of 31, the same BMI as the man running in Photo 8-4. Yet neither would be considered obese. Striking differences in body composition are also apparent among people of different ages and various ethnic and racial groups, making standard BMI guidelines inappropriate for some populations. For example, blacks tend to have a greater bone density and protein content than whites; consequently, using BMI as the standard may overestimate the prevalence of overweight and obesity among blacks.

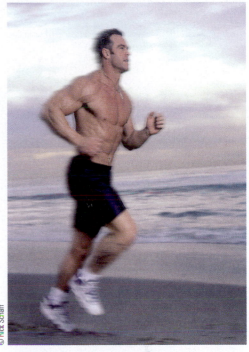

© Rick Schaff

> **PHOTO 8-4** At 6 feet 4 inches tall and 250 pounds (1.93 meters and 113 kilograms), this runner would be considered over*weight* by BMI standards. Yet he is clearly not over*fat*.

Body Fat and Its Distribution

Although weight measures are inexpensive, easy to take, and highly accurate, they fail to reveal two valuable pieces of information in assessing disease risk: how much of the weight is fat and where the fat is located. The ideal amount of body fat depends partly on the person. Table 8-7 shows the percent body fat in the US population at various BMI.

TABLE 8-7 Percent Body Fat at Various BMI

BMI	Men	Women
18.5	12–19%	25–32%
25	23–28%	35–40%
30	27–32%	40–44%
35	31–35%	43–47%
40	34–38%	46–49%

NOTE: In general, women have roughly 12% more body fat than men at the same BMI.

SOURCE: Adapted from M. Heo and coauthors, Percentage of body fat cutoffs by sex, age, and race-ethnicity in the US adult population from NHANES 1999–2004, *American Journal of Clinical Nutrition* 95 (2012): 594–602.

Some People Need Less Body Fat For many athletes, a lower percentage of body fat may be ideal—just enough fat to provide fuel, insulate and protect the body, assist in nerve impulse transmissions, and support normal hormone activity, but not so much as to burden the body with excess bulk. Percent body fat for athletes, then, might be 7 to 16 percent for young men and 15 to 22 percent for young women. (Review Photo 8-4 to appreciate what 8 percent body fat looks like—even with a BMI greater than 30.) Table 8-8 (p. 244) compares percent body fat values of healthy weight, average fitness individuals with averages from national surveys.

Some People Need More Body Fat For an Alaska fisherman, a higher percentage of body fat is probably beneficial because fat provides an insulating blanket to prevent excessive loss of body heat in cold climates. A woman starting a pregnancy needs sufficient body fat to support conception and fetal growth. Below a certain threshold for body fat, hormone synthesis falters, and individuals may become infertile, develop depression, experience abnormal hunger regulation, or

TABLE 8-8 Percent Body Fat: Ideal vs Actual

Age (yr)	Ideal (healthy weight, average fitness)	Actual (US average)
Male		
20–39	18–21%	26%
40–59	22–25%	29%
60+	24–27%	31%
Female		
20–39	23–26%	38%
40–59	28–32%	41%
60+	31–34%	42%

SOURCE: L. G. Borrud and coauthors, Body composition data for individuals 8 years of age and older: US population, 1999–2004, *Vital and Health Statistics* 11 (2010): 1–87; *ACSM's Health-Related Physical Fitness Assessment Manual*, 2nd ed. (Baltimore, MD: Lippincott Williams & Wilkins, 2008), p. 59.

> How To 8-2 Determine BMI

To calculate your body mass index (BMI), use one of the following equations:

$$\text{BMI} = \frac{\text{weight (lb)}}{\text{height (in.)}^2} \times 703$$

or

$$\text{BMI} = \frac{\text{weight (kg)}}{\text{height (m)}^2}$$

Consider, for example, a person who is 5′5″ (1.65 m) tall and weighs 174 lb (79 kg):

$$\text{BMI} = \frac{174 \text{ lb}}{65 \text{ in.}^2} \times 703 = 29$$

or

$$\text{BMI} = \frac{79 \text{ kg}}{1.65 \text{ m}^2} = 29$$

This person has a BMI of 29 and is considered overweight.

You could also use Table 8-6 (p. 242) to determine your BMI. Locate your height in the first column (in this example, 5′5″). Then look across the row until you find the number that is closest to your weight (in this example, 174). The number at the top of that column identifies your BMI (in this example, 29).

A reasonable initial target for most overweight people is a BMI 2 units below their current one. To determine a goal weight based on a desired BMI, locate your height in the first column and then look across the row until you reach the column with the desired BMI at the top. In this example, to reach a BMI of 27, this person's goal weight is 162 pounds, which represents a 12-pound weight loss. Such a determination can help a person set realistic weight goals using health risk as a guide.

> TRY IT Calculate your BMI and determine whether you are underweight, healthy weight, overweight, or obese. If your BMI is less than 18.5 or greater than 25, identify a weight that takes your BMI 2 units closer to the healthy weight range.

become unable to keep warm. These thresholds differ for each function and for each individual; much remains to be learned about them.

Fat Distribution The location of fat on the body may influence health as much, or more than, total fat alone. Excessive **visceral fat** stored around the organs of the abdomen is referred to as **central obesity** or upper-body fat (see Figure 8-8). Central obesity—significantly and independently of BMI—contributes to heart disease, cancers, diabetes, and related deaths.[10] **Subcutaneous fat** stored directly under the skin does not.

Visceral fat is most common in men and to a lesser extent in women past menopause. Even when total body fat is similar, men have more visceral fat than women. Lower body fat around the hips and thighs is most common in women during their reproductive years, and is associated with fewer heart disease risks.[11] Figure 8-9 compares the body shapes of people with upper-body fat and lower-body fat.

Waist Circumference A person's **waist circumference** is a good indicator of central obesity and its associated health risks.[12] In general, women with a waist circumference of greater than 35 inches (88 centimeters) and men with a waist circumference of greater than 40 inches (102 centimeters) have a high risk of central obesity–related health problems; the average waist circumference among US adults is 38 inches for women and 40 inches for men. To simplify the message, waist circumference should be less than half of a person's height; the waist-to-height ratio is also a useful measure of disease risks. As waist circumference increases, disease risks increase. Appendix E includes instructions for measuring waist circumference and assessing central obesity.

Some researchers use the waist-to-hip ratio as an indicator of disease risks. The ratio requires another step or two (measuring the hips and comparing that measurement to the waist measurement), but it does not provide any additional

visceral fat: fat stored within the abdominal cavity in association with the internal abdominal organs; also called *intra-abdominal fat*.

central obesity: excess fat around the trunk of the body; also called *abdominal fat* or *upper-body fat*.

subcutaneous fat: fat stored directly under the skin.
- **sub** = beneath
- **cutaneous** = skin

waist circumference: an anthropometric measurement used to assess a person's abdominal fat.

> **FIGURE 8-8 Central Obesity**

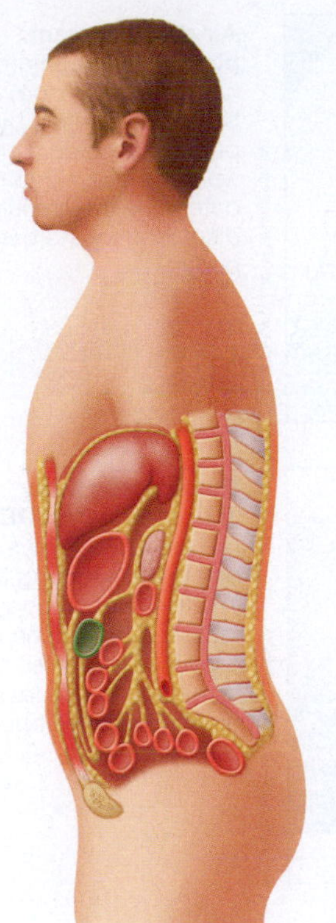

In healthy-weight people, some visceral fat protects the organs of the abdomen.

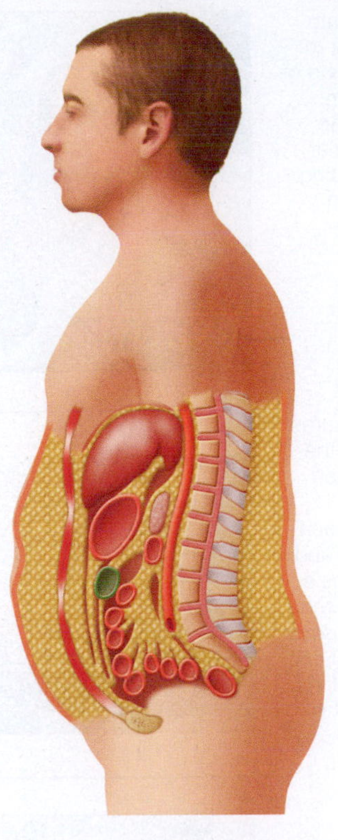

In overweight people, excess visceral fat increases the risks of diseases.

© Cengage

> **FIGURE 8-9 "Apple" and "Pear" Body Shapes Compared**

Popular articles sometimes call bodies with upper-body fat "apples" and those with lower-body fat, "pears." Researchers sometimes refer to upper-body fat as "android" (manlike) obesity and to lower-body fat as "gynoid" (womanlike) obesity.

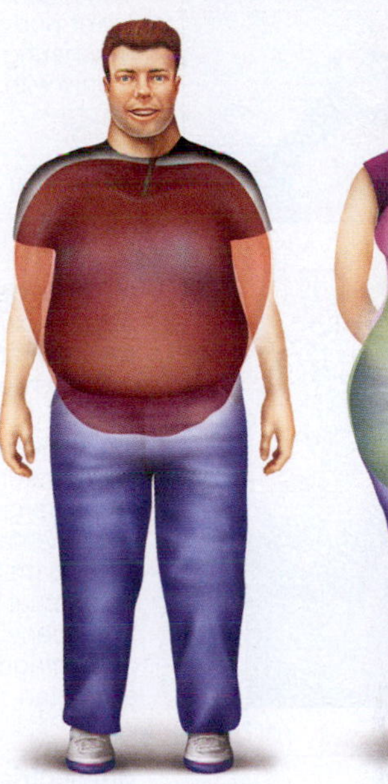

Upper-body fat is more common in men than in women and may be more closely associated with chronic diseases.

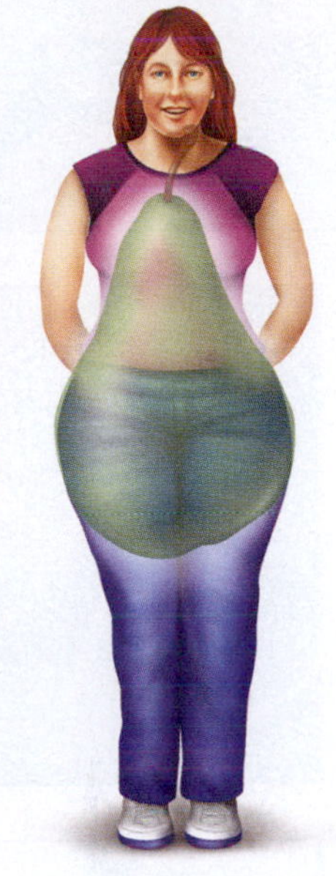

Lower-body fat is more common in women than in men and is not usually associated with chronic diseases.

© Cengage

SOURCE: R.E.C. Wildman and D. M. Medeiros, *Advanced Human Nutrition* (Boca Raton, FL: CRC Press, 2000), pp. 321–323. Copyright © 2000 Taylor and Francis Books LLC. Reprinted with permission.

information. Therefore, waist circumference alone is the preferred method for assessing central obesity in a clinical setting.

Other Measures of Body Composition Health-care professionals commonly use BMI and waist circumference measurements because they are relatively easy and inexpensive. Together, these two measurements prove most valuable in assessing a person's health risks and monitoring changes over time. Researchers needing more precise measures of body composition may choose any of several other techniques to estimate body fat and its distribution (see Figure 8-10, p. 246). Mastering these techniques requires proper instruction and practice to ensure reliability. In addition to the methods shown in Figure 8-10, researchers sometimes estimate body composition using these methods: total body water, radioactive potassium count, near-infrared spectrophotometry, ultrasound, computed tomography, and magnetic resonance imaging. Each method has advantages and disadvantages with respect to cost, technical difficulty, and precision of estimating body fat. Appendix E provides additional details and includes many of the tables and charts routinely used in assessment procedures.

REVIEW IT Distinguish between body weight and body composition, including methods to assess each.

The BMI is based on weight relative to height and serves as a reliable indicator of chronic disease risks, but it says little about body composition. The ideal amount of body fat varies from person to person, but researchers have found that body fat in excess of 22 percent for young men and 27 percent for young women (the levels rise slightly with age) poses health risks. Central obesity is measured by waist circumference and indicates excess abdominal fat distributed around the trunk of the body. Central obesity contributes to chronic diseases and related deaths.

> **FIGURE 8-10** Common Methods Used to Assess Body Fat

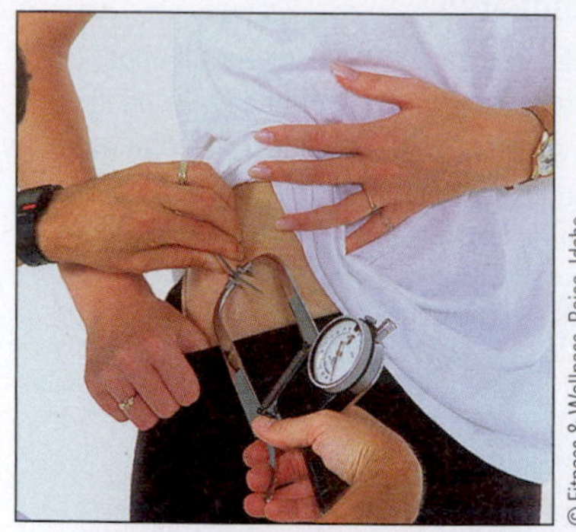

© Fitness & Wellness, Boise, Idaho

Skinfold measures estimate body fat by using a caliper to gauge the thickness of a fold of skin on the back of the arm (over the triceps), below the shoulder blade (subscapular), and in other places (including lower-body sites), and then comparing these measurements with standards.

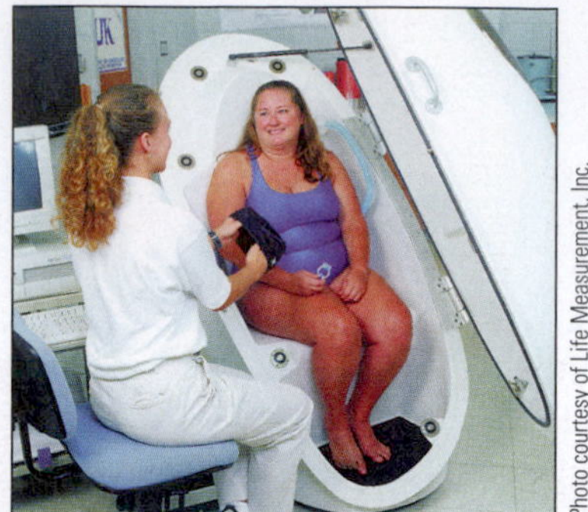

Photo courtesy of Life Measurement, Inc.

Air-displacement plethysmography (commonly called the *bod pod*) estimates body composition by having a person sit inside a chamber while computerized sensors determine the amount of air displaced by the person's body.

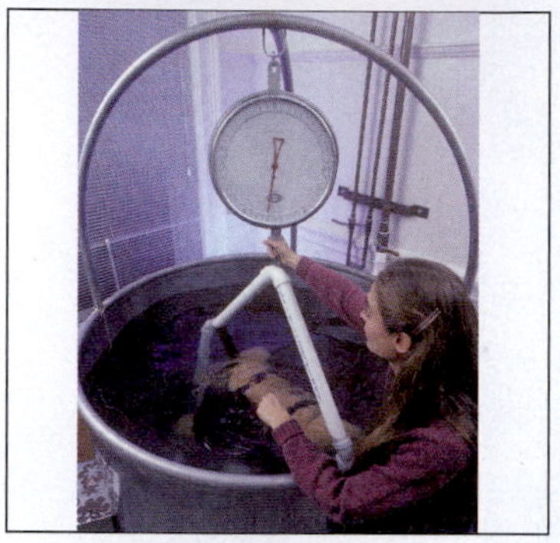

Yoav Levy/Phototake

Hydrodensitometry measures body density by weighing the person first on land and then again while submerged in water. The difference between the person's actual weight and underwater weight provides a measure of the body's volume. A mathematical equation using the two measurements (volume and actual weight) determines body density, from which the percentage of body fat can be estimated.

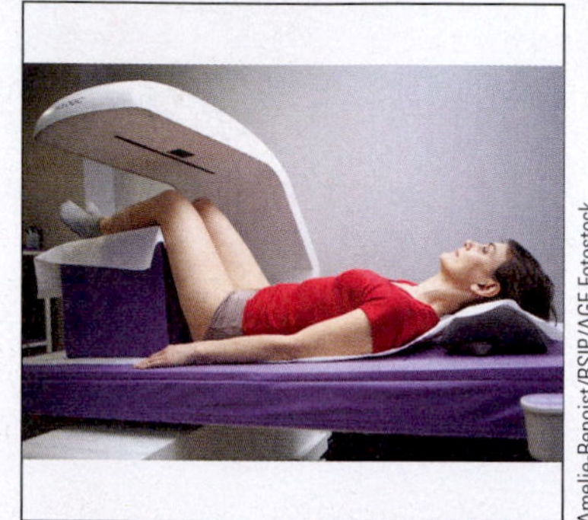

Amelie-Benoist/BSIP/AGE Fotostock

Dual-energy X-ray absorptiometry (DEXA) uses two low-dose X-rays that differentiate among fat-free soft tissue (lean body mass), fat tissue, and bone tissue, providing a precise measurement of total fat and its distribution in all but extremely obese subjects.

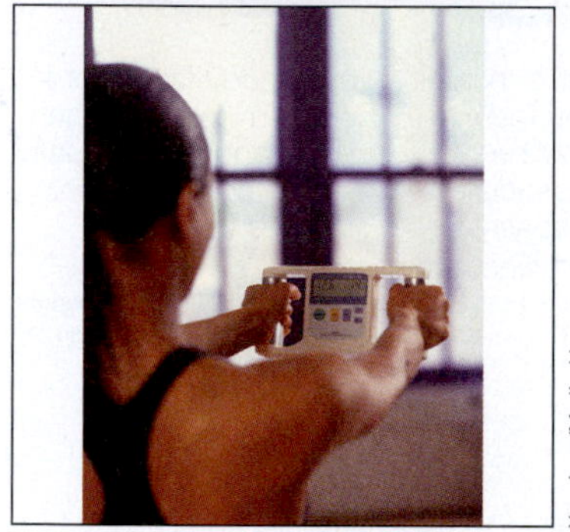

Yoav Levy/Medical Images

Bioelectrical impedance measures body fat by using a low-intensity electrical current. Because electrolyte-containing fluids, which readily conduct an electrical current, are found primarily in lean body tissues, the leaner the person, the less resistance to the current. The measurement of electrical resistance is then used in a mathematical equation to estimate the percentage of body fat.

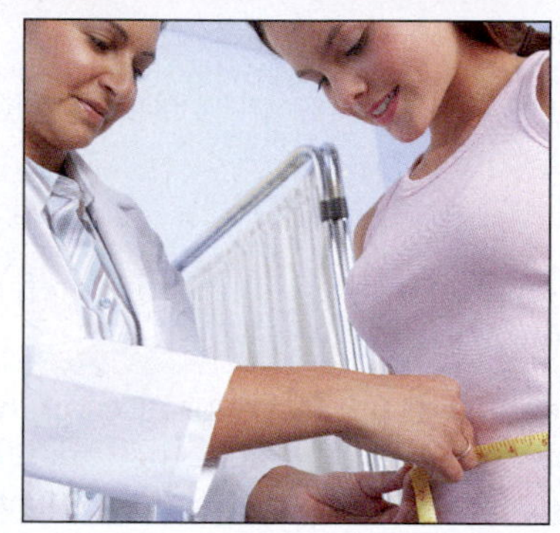

Adam Gault/SPL/Getty Images

Waist circumference measures central obesity by placing a nonstretchable measuring tape around the waist just above the bony crest of the hip. The tape runs parallel to the floor and is snug, but does not compress the skin.

> **FIGURE 8-11** BMI and Mortality

This J-shaped curve describes the relationship between body mass index (BMI) and mortality and shows that both underweight and overweight present risks of a premature death.

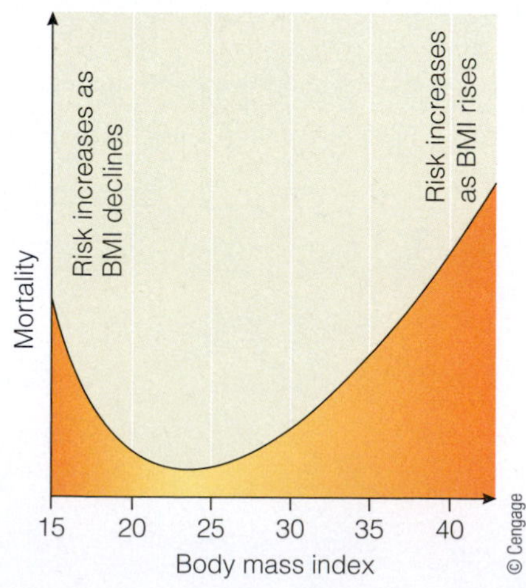
Mortality
Risk increases as BMI declines
Risk increases as BMI rises
15
20
25
30
35
40
Body mass index

© Cengage

8.5 Health Risks Associated with Body Weight and Body Fat

LEARN IT Identify relationships between body weight and chronic diseases.

Body weight and body fat correlate with disease risks and life expectancy. The correlation suggests a greater *likelihood* of developing chronic diseases and shortening life expectancy for those with a higher BMI and waist circumference.[13] Not all overweight and underweight people will get sick and die before their time nor will all normal-weight people live long healthy lives. *Correlations* are not *causes.* For the most part though, people with a BMI between 18.5 and 24.9 have relatively few weight-related health risks; risks increase as BMI falls below or rises above this range, indicating that both underweight and overweight impair health.[14] Epidemiological data show a J- or U-shaped relationship between body weights and mortality (see Figure 8-11). People who are extremely underweight or extremely obese carry higher risks of early deaths than those whose weights fall within the healthy or even the slightly overweight range.[15] These mortality risks decline with age and shift with a person's state of health.[16] In cancer, for example, a higher weight is associated with a survival advantage.[17]

Independently of BMI, factors such as smoking habits raise health risks, and physical fitness lowers them. A man with a BMI of 22 who smokes two packs of cigarettes a day is jeopardizing his health, whereas a woman with a BMI of 32 who walks briskly for an hour a day is improving her health.

Health Risks of Underweight Fewer than 2 percent of US adults are underweight.[18] Some underweight people enjoy an active, healthy life, but others are underweight because of malnutrition, smoking habits, substance abuse, or illnesses. Weight and fat measures alone would not reveal these underlying causes, but a complete assessment that includes a diet and medical history, physical examination, and laboratory tests would.

An underweight person, especially an older adult, may be unable to preserve lean tissue during the fight against a wasting disease such as cancer or a digestive disorder, especially when the disease is accompanied by malnutrition. Without adequate nutrient and energy reserves, an underweight person will have a particularly tough battle against such medical stresses and face increased risks of mortality.[19] Underweight women develop menstrual irregularities and become infertile. Those who do conceive may give birth to unhealthy infants. An underweight woman can improve her chances of having a healthy infant by gaining weight prior to conception, during pregnancy, or both. Underweight and significant weight loss are also associated with osteoporosis and bone fractures. For all these reasons, underweight people may benefit from enough of a weight gain to provide an energy reserve and protective amounts of all the nutrients.

Health Risks of Overweight and Obesity As for excessive body fat, the health risks are so many that it has been designated a disease—obesity. Among the health risks associated with obesity are diabetes, hypertension, cardiovascular disease, sleep apnea (abnormal cessation of breathing during sleep), osteoarthritis, some cancers, gallbladder disease, kidney stones, respiratory problems (including Pickwickian syndrome, a breathing blockage linked with sudden death), infertility, and complications in pregnancy and surgery. Obese people are more likely to be disabled in their later years.[20] Each year, these obesity-related illnesses cost our nation $147 billion—in fact, as much as, or more than, the medical costs of smoking. Billions more are lost each year in workplace productivity.

The cost in terms of lives is also great.[21] In fact, obesity is second only to tobacco in causing heart attacks and premature deaths (see Photo 8-5, p. 248).[22]

Cardiovascular Disease The relationship between obesity and cardiovascular disease risk is strong, with links to both elevated blood cholesterol and hypertension.[23] Central obesity may raise the risk of heart attack and stroke as much as the three leading risk factors (high LDL cholesterol, hypertension, and smoking) do. In addition to body fat, weight gain also increases the risk of cardiovascular disease. Weight loss, on the other hand, can effectively reverse atherosclerosis and lower both blood cholesterol and blood pressure in overweight and obese people.[24] Of course, lean and normal-weight people may also have high blood cholesterol and blood pressure, and these factors are just as dangerous in lean people as in obese people.

Type 2 Diabetes The incidence of diabetes has risen dramatically in recent decades, as the nation's population has grown more obese.[25] Type 2 diabetes is far more likely to develop in an obese person than in a nonobese person.[26] Furthermore, the person with type 2 diabetes often has central obesity. Central-body fat cells appear to be larger and more insulin-resistant than lower-body fat cells. The association between **insulin resistance** and obesity is strong, and both are major risk factors for the development of type 2 diabetes.

Diabetes appears to be influenced by weight gains as well as by body weight. A weight gain of more than 10 pounds (4.5 kilograms) after the age of 18 doubles the risk of developing diabetes, even in adults of average weight. In contrast, weight loss is effective in improving glucose tolerance and insulin resistance.

insulin resistance: the condition in which a normal amount of insulin produces a subnormal effect in muscle, adipose, and liver cells, resulting in an elevated fasting glucose; a metabolic consequence of obesity that precedes type 2 diabetes.

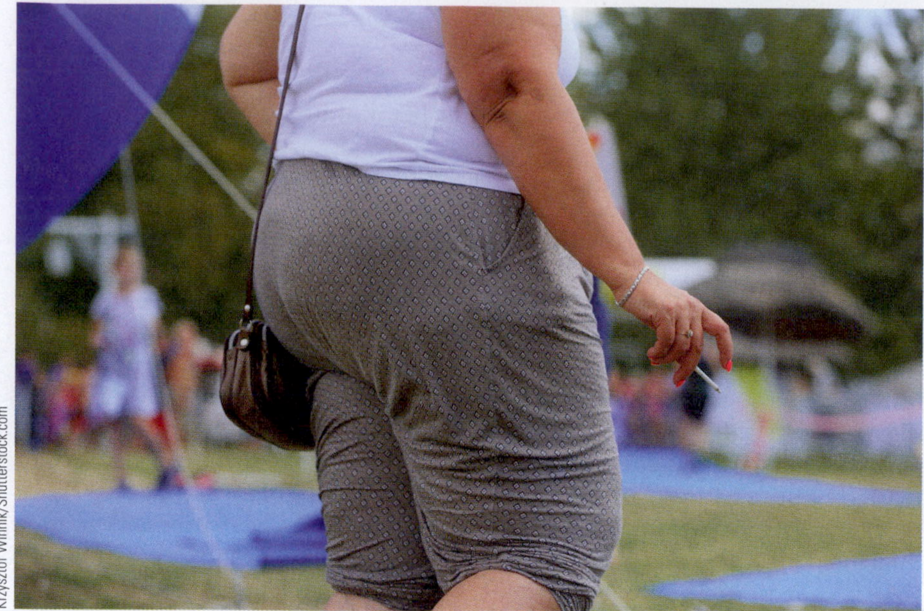
Krzysztof Winnik/Shutterstock.com

> **PHOTO 8-5** Smoking is the leading cause of preventable illnesses and early deaths. Obesity is a close second. A BMI of 40 or greater is equivalent to a lifetime of smoking, representing 10 years' loss of life.

Inflammation and the Metabolic Syndrome Chronic **inflammation** accompanies obesity, and inflammation contributes to chronic diseases.[27] As a person grows fatter, lipids first fill the adipose tissue and then migrate into other tissues such as the muscles and liver. This fat that accumulates outside of adipose tissue—called **ectopic fat**—disrupts normal metabolism and contributes to the many diseases associated with obesity.[28] The combination of inflammation and ectopic fat results in insulin resistance (and high blood glucose), abnormal blood lipids, and high blood pressure.[29] This cluster of symptoms—collectively known as the **metabolic syndrome**—increases the risks for diabetes, hypertension, and atherosclerosis.[30]

Fat accumulation activates genes that code for proteins (adipokines) involved in inflammation.[31] Furthermore, although relatively few immune cells are commonly found in adipose tissue, weight gain significantly increases their number and their role in inflammation. Elevated blood lipids—whether due to obesity or to a high-fat diet—also promote inflammation. Together, these factors help to explain why chronic inflammation accompanies obesity and how obesity contributes to the metabolic syndrome and the progression of chronic diseases. Interestingly, the combination of inflammation and insulin resistance predict how likely a person is to lose weight initially or regain weight after weight loss.[32] As might be expected, physical activity and weight loss improves inflammation and the metabolic syndrome.[33]

Cancer Both the duration and the severity of overweight or obesity increases the risk of developing some cancers and interferes with some treatments.[34] One possible explanation may be that obese people have elevated levels of hormones that could influence cancer development. For example, adipose tissue is the major site of estrogen synthesis in women, obese women have elevated levels of estrogen, and estrogen has been implicated in the development of cancers of the female reproductive system—cancers that account for half of all cancers in women. Another possible explanation may be that the chronic inflammation that accompanies obesity is a risk factor for several cancers; restricting energy intake may not only induce weight loss, but may also inhibit cancer by reducing inflammation.[35]

inflammation: an immunological response to cellular injury characterized by an increase in white blood cells.

ectopic fat: excess fat in locations other than adipose tissue.
- **ektopos** = out of place

metabolic syndrome: a combination of risk factors—elevated fasting blood glucose, hypertension, abnormal blood lipids, and abdominal obesity—that greatly increase a person's risk of developing heart disease.

Other Considerations Importantly, BMI and weight gains and losses do not tell the whole story. A low BMI with a high percent body fat, for example, increases health risks.[36] Physical activity and fitness play major roles in health and longevity, as Chapter 14 confirms. Normal-weight people who are physically active have fewer health risks than normal-weight people who are inactive (see Photo 8-6). Similarly, physically active obese people have fewer health problems than inactive obese people.[37]

Some obese people have been described as "healthy obese" or "metabolically normal obese;" they have normal blood pressure, blood glucose, and blood lipids.[38] Most notable is that they maintain their sensitivity to insulin.[39] Compared with insulin-resistant obese people, insulin-sensitive obese people tend to have less central obesity, fatty liver, and inflammation and more adiponectin. Their higher adiponectin levels help protect against insulin resistance and inflammation, thus defending against type 2 diabetes and heart disease—at least for a short while. Healthy obesity appears to be a relatively unstable condition, with a transition to unhealthy over time.[40] Healthy obesity is an area of active research.[41] Similarly, normal weight with excessive body fat is another area of active research that falls outside the classic model of health being based on BMI. People with **normal-weight obesity syndrome** have a BMI within the "healthy" range (18.5 to 24.9), but their excessive body fat raises the risks of heart disease, insulin resistance, hypertension, and abnormal blood lipids.[42] Clearly, good health depends on much more than a person's BMI.

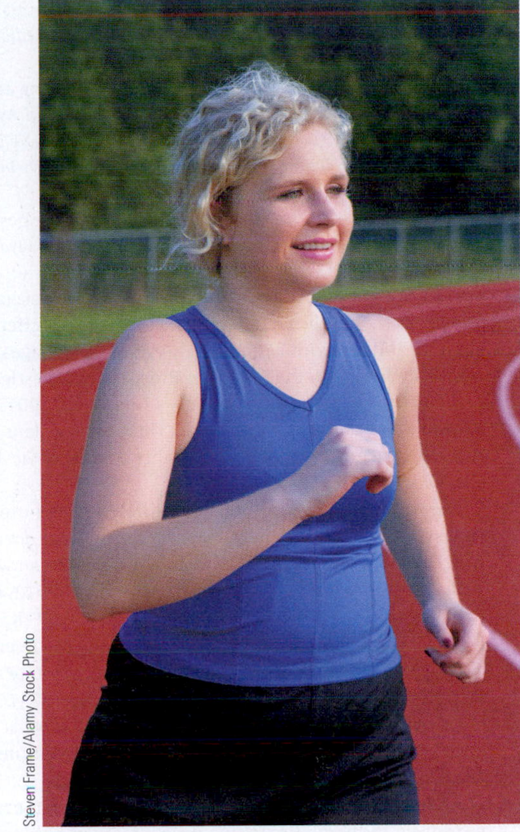

Steven Frame/Alamy Stock Photo

> **PHOTO 8-6** Regardless of body weight, being active is healthier than being sedentary.

normal-weight obesity syndrome: a condition characterized by excess body fat, an adequate BMI, and increased risk factors for chronic diseases.

REVIEW IT Identify relationships between body weight and chronic diseases.
The weight appropriate for an individual depends largely on factors specific to that individual, including body fat distribution, family health history, and current health status. At the extremes, both overweight and underweight carry clear risks to health.

This chapter has described energy balance and body composition with a focus on the health problems associated with too much or too little body weight and body fat. Highlight 8 examines the health problems that arise when efforts to control body weight become eating disorders. The next chapter continues the discussion with a look at weight management and the benefits of choosing nutritious foods and being physically active.

What's Online

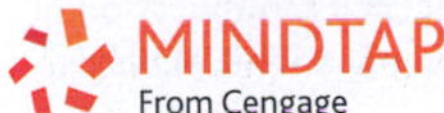
MINDTAP
From Cengage

Visit **www.cengagebrain.com** to access MindTap, a complete digital course that includes Diet & Wellness Plus, interactive quizzes, videos, and more.

REFERENCES

1. D. M. Thomas and coauthors, Time to correctly predict the amount of weight loss with dieting, *Journal of the Academy of Nutrition and Dietetics* 114 (2014): 857–861.
2. J. K. Kiecolt-Glaser and coauthors, Daily stressors, past depression, and metabolic responses to high-fat meals: A novel path to obesity, *Biological Psychiatry* 77 (2015): 653–660; E. Manzato and coauthors, Risk factors for weight gain: A longitudinal study in non-weight loss treatment-seeking overweight adults, *Eating and Weight Disorders* 20 (2015): 371–378.
3. L. Sominsky and S. J. Spencer, Eating behavior and stress: A pathway to obesity, *Frontiers in Psychology* 5 (2014): doi:10.3389/fpsyg.2014.00434; M. R. Parker and coauthors, Expression and nuclear translocation of glucocorticoid receptors in type 2 taste receptor cells, *Neuroscience Letters* 571 (2014): 72–77; B. Wagner and coauthors, The myth of comfort food, *Health Psychology* 33 (2014): 1552–1557.
4. N. Puzziferri and coauthors, Brain imaging demonstrates a reduced neural impact of eating in obesity, *Obesity* 24 (2016): 829–836.
5. J. Dhillon and coauthors, The effects of increased protein intake on fullness: A meta-analysis and its limitations, *Journal of the Academy of Nutrition and Dietetics* 116 (2016): 968–983.
6. C. J. Rebello, C. E. O'Neil, and F. L. Greenway, Dietary fiber and satiety: The effects of oats on satiety, *Nutrition Reviews* 74 (2016): 131–147.
7. G. J. Schwartz and L. M. Zeltser, Functional organization of neuronal and humoral signals regulating feeding behavior, *Annual Review of Nutrition* 33 (2013): 1–21; J. A. Parker and S. R. Bloom, Hypothalamic neuropeptides and the regulation of appetite, *Neuropharmacology* 63 (2012): 18–30.

8. R. G. McMurray and coauthors, Examining variations of resting metabolic rate of adults: A public health perspective, *Medicine and Science in Sports and Exercise* 46 (2014): 1352–1358.
9. K. M Flegal and coauthors, Trends in obesity among adults in the United States, 2005 to 2014, *Journal of the American Medical Association* 315 (2016): 2284–2291; J. W. Zylke and H. Bauchner, The unrelenting challenge of obesity, *Journal of the American Medical Association* 315 (2016): 2277–2278.
10. S. Sharma and coauthors, Normal-weight central obesity and mortality risk in older adults with coronary artery disease, *Mayo Clinic Proceedings* 91 (2016): 343–351; K. R. Sahakyan and coauthors, Normal-weight central obesity: Implications for total and cardiovascular mortality, *Annals of Internal Medicine* 163 (2015): 827-835; A. Steffen and coauthors, General and abdominal obesity and risk of esophageal and gastric adenocarcinoma in the European Prospective Investigation into Cancer and Nutrition, *International Journal of Cancer* 137 (2015): 646–657; K. A. Britton and coauthors, Body fat distribution, incident cardiovascular disease, cancer, and all-cause mortality, *Journal of the American College of Cardiology* 62 (2013): 921–925.
11. K. Karastergiou and coauthors, Sex differences in human adipose tissues—The biology of pear shape, *Biology of Sex Differences* 3 (2012): 13.
12. E. S. Ford, L. M. Maynard, and C. Li, Trends in mean waist circumference and abdominal obesity among US adults, 1999-2012, *Journal of the American Medical Association* 312 (2014): 1151–1153; P. T. Katzmarzyk, S. B. Heymsfield, and C. Bouchard, Clinical utility of visceral adipose tissue for the identification of cardiometabolic risk in white and African American adults, *American Journal of Clinical Nutrition* 97 (2013): 480–486.
13. J. R. Cerhan and coauthors, A pooled analysis of waist circumference and mortality in 650,000 adults, *Mayo Clinic Proceedings* 89 (2014): 335–345.
14. The Global BMI Mortality Collaboration, Body-mass index and all-cause mortality: Individual-participant-data meta-analysis of 239 prospective studies in four continents, *Lancet* 388 (2016): 776–786; A. V. Patel, J. S. Hildebrand, and S. M. Gapstur, Body mass index and all-cause mortality in a large prospective cohort of white and black US adults, *PLoS One* 9 (2014): e109153.
15. D. K. Tobias and coauthors, Body-mass index and mortality among adults with incident type 2 diabetes, *New England Journal of Medicine* 370 (2014): 233–244; K. M. Flegal and coauthors, Association of all-cause mortality with overweight and obesity using standard body mass index categories: A systematic review and meta-analysis, *Journal of the American Medical Association* 309 (2013): 71–82.
16. J. E. Winter and coauthors, BMI and all-cause mortality in older adults: A meta-analysis, *American Journal of Clinical Nutrition* 99 (2014): 875–890; J. B. Dixon and G. J. Egger, A narrow view of optimal weight for health generates the obesity paradox, *American Journal of Clinical Nutrition* 99 (2014): 969–970; D. W. Ford and coauthors, Body mass index, poor diet quality, and health-related quality of life are associated with mortality in rural older adults, *Journal of Nutrition in Gerontology and Geriatrics* 33 (2014): 23–34.
17. M. C. Gonzalez and coauthors, Obesity paradox in cancer: New insights provided by body composition, *American Journal of Clinical Nutrition* 99 (2014): 999–1005.
18. C. D. Fryar and C. L. Ogden, Prevalence of underweight among adults aged 20 years and over: the United States, 1960–1962 through 2011-2012, *NCHS Health E-Stat*, November 2015.
19. L. A. Renfro and coauthors, Body mass index is prognostic in metastatic colorectal cancer: Pooled analysis of patients from first-line clinical trials in the ARCAD database, *Journal of Clinical Oncology* 34 (2016): 144–150.
20. R. A. Murphy and coauthors, Associations of BMI and adipose tissue area and density with incident mobility limitation and poor performance in older adults, *American Journal of Clinical Nutrition* 99 (2014): 1059–1065.
21. S. A. Grover and coauthors, Years of life lost and healthy life-years lost from diabetes and cardiovascular disease in overweight and obese people: A modeling study, *Lancet: Diabetes and Endocrinology* 3 (2015): 114–22.
22. D. Dicker and coauthors, Obesity or smoking: Which factor contributes more to the incidence of myocardial infarction? *European Journal of Internal Medicine* 32 (2016): 43–46.
23. H. E. Bays and coauthors, Obesity, adiposity, and dyslipidemia: A consensus statement from the *National Lipid Association* 7 (2013): 304–383; L. Landsberg and coauthors, Obesity-related hypertension: Pathogenesis, cardiovascular risk, and treatment, *Journal of Clinical Hypertension* 15 (2013): 14–33.
24. L. Flores and coauthors, Longitudinal changes of blood pressure after weight loss: Factors involved, *Surgery for Obesity and Related Diseases* 11 (2015): 215–221.
25. F. Guo and T. Garvey, Trends in cardiovascular health metrics in obese adults: National Health and Nutrition Examination Survey (NHANES), 1988-2014, *Journal of the American Heart Association* 5 (2016): e003619.
26. P. Nordström and coauthors, Risks of myocardial infarction, death, and diabetes in identical twin pairs with different body mass indexes, *JAMA Internal Medicine* (2016): doi:10.1001.
27. S. B. Heymsfield and T. A. Wadden, Mechanisms, pathophysiology, and management of obesity, *New England Journal of Medicine* 376 (2017): 254–266; N. Esser and coauthors, Inflammation as a link between obesity, metabolic syndrome and type 2 diabetes, *Diabetes Research and Clinical Practice* 105 (2014): 141–150; M. Exley and coauthors, The interplay between the immune system and adipose in obesity, *Journal of Endocrinology* 223 (2014): 41–48; G. Martinez-Santibañez and C. Lumeng, Macrophages and the regulation of adipose tissue remodeling, *Annual Review of Nutrition* 34 (2014): 57–76.
28. S. Sookoian and coauthors, Serum aminotransferases in nonalcoholic fatty liver disease are a signature of liver metabolic perturbations at the amino acid and Krebs cycle level, *American Journal of Clinical Nutrition* 103 (2016): 422–434.
29. M. Bastien and coauthors, Overview of epidemiology and contribution of obesity to cardiovascular disease, *Progress in Cardiovascular Disease* 56 (2014): 369–381; G. I. Shulman, Ectopic fat in insulin resistance, dyslipidemia, and cardiometabolic disease, *New England Journal of Medicine* 371 (2014): 1131–1141; A. R. Aroor and coauthors, Maladaptive immune and inflammatory pathways lead to cardiovascular insulin resistance, *Metabolism* 62 (2013): 1543–1552.
30. M. Santaniemi and coauthors, Metabolic syndrome in the prediction of cardiovascular events: The potential additive role of hsCRP and adiponectin, *European Journal of Preventive Cardiology* 21 (2014): 1242–1248.
31. H. Cao, Adipocytokines in obesity and metabolic disease, *Journal of Endocrinology* 8 (2014): T47–T59; V. G. Giby and T. A. Ajith, Role of adipokines and peroxisome proliferator-activated receptors in nonalcoholic fatty liver disease, *World Journal of Hepatology* 6 (2014): 570–579; M. J. Lee, Y. Wu, and S. K. Fried, Adipose tissue heterogeneity: Implication of depot differences in adipose tissue for obesity complications, *Molecular Aspects of Medicine* 34 (2013): 1–11.
32. L. C. Kong and coauthors, Insulin resistance and inflammation predict kinetic body weight changes in response to dietary weight loss and maintenance in overweight and obese subjects by using a Bayesian network approach, *American Journal of Clinical Nutrition* 98 (2013): 1385–1394.
33. A. M. Hill and coauthors, Type and amount of dietary protein in the treatment of metabolic syndrome: A randomized controlled trial, *American Journal of Clinical Nutrition* 102 (2015): 757–770; F. M. Schmidt and coauthors, Inflammatory cytokines in general and central obesity and modulating effects of physical activity, *PLoS One* 10 (2015): e0121971.
34. M. Arnold and coauthors, Duration of adulthood overweight, obesity, and cancer risk in the Women's Health Initiative: A longitudinal study from the United States, *PLoS Med* 13 (2016): e1002081; M. Arnold and coauthors, Global burden of cancer attributable to high body-mass index in 2012: A population-based study, *Lancet Oncology* 36 (2015): 36–46; J. A. Ligibel and coauthors, American Society of Clinical Oncology position statement on obesity and cancer, *Journal of Clinical Oncology* 32 (2014): 3568–3574; K. Bhaskaran and coauthors, Body-mass index

and risk of 22 specific cancers: A population-based cohort study of 5.24 million UK adults, *Lancet* 384 (2014): 755–765; C. N. S. Bisschop and coauthors, Weight change later in life and colon and rectal cancer risk in participants in the EPIC-PANACEA study, *American Journal of Clinical Nutrition* 99 (2014): 139–147; R. Z. Stolzenberg-Solomon and coauthors, Lifetime adiposity and risk of pancreatic cancer in the NIH-AARP Diet and Health Study cohort, *American Journal of Clinical Nutrition* 98 (2013): 1057–1065.

35. S. D. Hursting and coauthors, Calorie restriction and cancer prevention: A mechanistic perspective, *Cancer and Metabolism* 1 (2013): 10.
36. R. Padwal and coauthors, Relationship among body fat percentage, body mass index, and all-cause mortality: A cohort study, *Annals of Internal Medicine* 164 (2016): 532–541.
37. J. A. Bell and coauthors, Healthy obesity and objective physical activity, *American Journal of Clinical Nutrition* 102 (2015): 268–275.
38. E. Fabbrini and coauthors, metabolically normal obese people are protected from adverse effects following weight gain, *Journal of Clinical Investigation* 125 (2015): 787–795; E. Navarro and coauthors, Can metabolically healthy obesity be explained by diet, genetics, and inflammation? *Molecular Nutrition and Food Research* 59 (2015): 75–93.
39. T. F. S. Teixeira and coauthors, Main characteristics of metabolically obese normal weight and metabolically healthy obese phenotypes, *Nutrition Reviews* 73 (2015): 175–190.
40. M. Hamer and coauthors, Stability of metabolically healthy obesity over 8 years: The English Longitudinal Study of Ageing, *European Journal of Endocrinology* 173 (2015): 703–708; C. K. Kramer, B. Zinman, and R. Retnakaran, Are metabolically healthy overweight and obesity benign conditions? A systematic review and meta-analysis, *Annals of Internal Medicine* 159 (2013): 758–769.
41. E. Lopez-Garcia and coauthors, Metabolically healthy obesity and health-related quality of life: A prospective cohort study, *Clinical Nutrition* 16 (2016): doi:10.1016/j.clnu.2016.04.028; M. Rydén and coauthors, The adipose transcriptional response to insulin is determined by obesity, not insulin sensitivity, *Cell Reports* 16 (2016): 1–10; R. W. Kimokoti and coauthors, Metabolically healthy obesity is not associated with food intake in white or black men, *Journal of Nutrition* 145 (2015): 2551–2561.
42. L. P. Franco, C. C. Morais, and C. Cominetti, Normal-weight obesity syndrome: Diagnosis, prevalence, and clinical implications, *Nutrition Reviews* 74 (2016): 558–570.

HIGHLIGHT > 8

LEARN IT Compare the diagnoses, characteristics, and treatments of the different eating disorders.

Eating Disorders

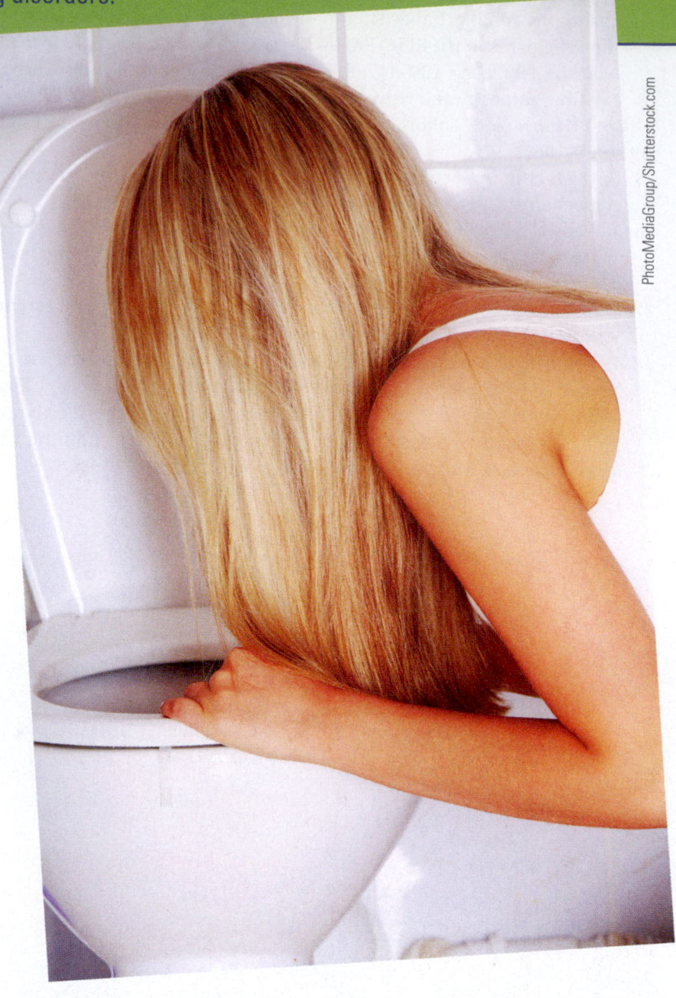

PhotoMediaGroup/Shutterstock.com

For some people, the struggle with body weight manifests itself as an **eating disorder**. (Glossary H8-1 defines this and related terms.) Three eating disorders—anorexia nervosa, bulimia nervosa, and binge eating disorder—are relatively uncommon, but present real concerns because of their health consequences. Findings from large national surveys suggest that 0.9 percent of women and 0.3 percent of men suffer from anorexia nervosa at some time in their lives.[1] Lifetime prevalence for bulimia nervosa is slightly lower, with 0.5 percent of women and 0.1 percent of men. Binge eating disorder is somewhat higher, with 3.5 percent of women and 2 percent of men. Many more suffer from other unspecified eating disorders that do not meet the strict diagnostic criteria but still imperil a person's well-being.

Why do so many people in our society suffer from eating disorders? Most experts agree that the causes include multiple factors: sociocultural, psychological, and perhaps neurochemical. Excessive pressure to be thin is at least partly to blame. Family attitudes concerning body shape and eating habits can have profound effects. Young people may have learned to identify discomforts such as anger, jealousy, or disappointment with "feeling fat." They often have other psychological issues such as depression, anxiety, or substance abuse. As weight issues become more of a focus, psychological problems worsen, and the likelihood of developing eating disorders intensifies. Unfortunately, few seek health care for eating disorders. Athletes and dancers are among those most likely to develop eating disorders.

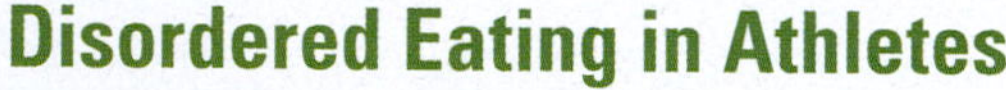

Disordered Eating in Athletes

At age 14, Suzanne was a top contender for a spot on the state gymnastics team. Each day her coach reminded team members that they must weigh no more than their assigned weights to qualify for competition. The coach chastised gymnasts who gained weight, and Suzanne was terrified of being singled out. Convinced that the less she weighed the better she would perform, Suzanne weighed herself several times a day to confirm that she had not exceeded her 80-pound limit. Driven to excel in her sport, Suzanne kept her weight down by eating very little and training very hard. Unlike many of her friends, Suzanne never began to menstruate. A few months before her fifteenth birthday, Suzanne's coach dropped her back to the second-level team. Suzanne blamed her poor performance on a slow-healing stress fracture. Mentally stressed and physically exhausted, she quit gymnastics and began overeating between periods of self-starvation. Suzanne had developed

GLOSSARY H8-1

amenorrhea (ay-MEN-oh-REE-ah): the absence of or cessation of menstruation. *Primary amenorrhea* is menarche delayed beyond 15 years of age. *Secondary amenorrhea* is the absence of three consecutive menstrual cycles.

anorexia (an-oh-RECK-see-ah) **nervosa:** an eating disorder characterized by a refusal to maintain a minimally normal body weight and a distortion in perception of body shape and weight.

- **an** = without
- **orex** = mouth
- **nervos** = of nervous origin

binge-eating disorder: an eating disorder characterized by recurring episodes of eating a significant amount of food in a short period of time with marked feelings of lack of control.

bulimia (byoo-LEEM-ee-ah) **nervosa:** an eating disorder characterized by repeated episodes of binge eating usually followed by self-induced vomiting, misuse of laxatives or diuretics, fasting, or excessive exercise.

cathartic (ka-THAR-tik): a strong laxative.

disordered eating: eating behaviors that are neither normal nor healthy, including restrained eating, fasting, binge eating, and purging.

eating disorder: disturbances in eating behavior that jeopardize a person's physical or psychological health.

emetic (em-ETT-ic): an agent that causes vomiting.

female athlete triad: a potentially fatal combination of three medical problems—disordered eating, amenorrhea, and osteoporosis.

muscle dysmorphia (dis-MORE-fee-ah): a psychiatric disorder characterized by a preoccupation with building body mass.

orthorexia nervosa: an obsession with good nutrition to improve health that is characterized by restrictive diets, ritualized patterns of eating, and rigid avoidance of foods believed to be unhealthy.

relative energy deficiency in sport (RED-S): a syndrome of impaired physiological functions caused by relative energy deficiency (too little energy intake for the energy expended).

stress fractures: bone damage or breaks caused by stress on bone surfaces during exercise.

the dangerous combination of problems known as the **female athlete triad**—disordered eating, amenorrhea, and osteoporosis.[2] Because the problems reach beyond these three components and male athletes are also affected, some, but not all, researchers use a more comprehensive term: **relative energy deficiency in sport (RED-S).**[3]

Relative Energy Deficiency

An energy deficiency develops when an athlete's diet provides too little energy given the amount of energy expended to support health, activities of daily living, growth, and sports. Sometimes this occurs as the result of mismanaged athletic programs to quickly reduce body weight. Consider David, for example. Each week throughout the season, David drastically restricts his food and fluid intake before a wrestling match in an effort to "make weight." He believes that competing in a lower weight class will give him a competitive advantage over smaller opponents. To make weight, athletes often intensify exercise, skip meals, restrict fluids, and use laxatives and diuretics.[4] David hopes to replenish the lost fluids, glycogen, and lean tissue during the hours between weigh-in and competition, but the body needs days to correct this metabolic mayhem. Reestablishing fluid and electrolyte balances may take 1 to 2 days, replenishing glycogen stores may take 2 to 3 days, and replacing lean tissue may take even longer.

Ironically, the combination of food deprivation and dehydration impairs physical performance by reducing muscle strength, decreasing anaerobic power, and reducing endurance capacity. For optimal performance, athletes need to first achieve their competitive weight during the off-season and then eat well-balanced meals and drink plenty of fluids during the competitive season.

Disordered Eating

One reason many athletes engage in **disordered eating** is that they and their coaches have embraced unsuitable weight standards. An athlete's body must be heavier for a given height than a nonathlete's body because the athlete's body is dense, containing more healthy bone and muscle and less fat. When athletes rely only on the scales, they may mistakenly believe they are too fat because weight standards, such as the BMI, do not provide adequate information about body composition.

Many young athletes severely restrict energy intakes to improve performance, enhance appearance, or meet the weight guidelines of a specific sport. They fail to realize that the loss of lean tissue that accompanies energy restriction actually impairs their physical performance. Risk factors for eating disorders among athletes include:

- Young age (adolescence)
- Pressure to excel at a chosen sport
- Focus on achieving or maintaining an "ideal" body weight or body fat percentage
- Participation in sports or competitions that emphasize a lean appearance or judge performance on aesthetic appeal such as gymnastics, wrestling, figure skating, or dance
- Weight-loss dieting at an early age
- Unsupervised dieting

Disordered eating among athletes usually involves energy deficits and weight loss, but some athletes, usually males, go to extreme measures to bulk up and *gain* weight. People afflicted with **muscle dysmorphia** eat high-protein diets, take dietary supplements, weight train for hours at a time, and often abuse steroids in an attempt to increase muscle mass. Their bodies are large and muscular, yet they see themselves as puny 90-pound weaklings. They are preoccupied with the idea that their bodies are too small or inadequately muscular. Like others with distorted body images, people with muscle dysmorphia weigh themselves frequently and center their lives on diet and exercise.

Sometimes efforts to improve health become obsessive behaviors that take eating and exercising to extremes.[5] Ironically, these obsessions are often characterized by such restrictive diets, ritualized eating patterns, and rigid food avoidance that nutrient deficiencies and medical problems arise.[6] Disordered eating in the name of health is known as **orthorexia nervosa**, a relatively new food practice that allows some people to hide behind their eating disorders.[7] Paying attention to diet and exercise for fitness is admirable, but obsessing over it can cause serious social, occupational, and physical problems.

Adverse Consequences

A prolonged, inadequate energy intake has numerous adverse consequences, as outlined in Table H8-1. It leads to nutrient deficiencies (including anemia), chronic fatigue, and increased risk of infections and illnesses. Protein synthesis decreases and blood lipids increase, favoring heart disease. All of these consequences harm health and impair performance.

As mentioned earlier, females commonly develop **amenorrhea.** The prevalence of amenorrhea among premenopausal women in the United States is about 2 to 5 percent overall, but among female athletes, it may be as high as 65 to 70 percent. Body fat stores and hormone levels are too inadequate to support normal menstruation. Amenorrhea is often accompanied by bone losses.

TABLE H8-1 Consequences of Relative Energy Deficiency

Physiological functions	Psychological problems	Physical performance
Altered hormone activities	Decreased concentration	Decreased coordination
Anemia	Depression	Decreased endurance
Bone loss	Impaired judgment	Decreased muscle strength
Decreased glycogen stores	Irritability	Decreased training response
Decreased protein synthesis		Increased injuries
Impaired metabolism		
Menstrual dysfunction		
Poor growth		

SOURCE: Adapted from M. Mountjoy and coauthors, The IOC statement: Beyond the Female Athlete Triad—Relative Energy Deficiency in Sport (RED-S), *British Journal of Sports Medicine* 48 (2014): 491–497.

In general, physical activity increases bone density, but for women with amenorrhea, physical activity increases bone losses and **stress fractures**.[8] To grow strong bones, athletes should be encouraged to consume 1300 milligrams of calcium each day, to eat nutrient-dense foods, and to obtain enough energy to support both a healthy body weight and the energy expended in physical activity. Nutrition is critical to bone recovery.

Preventing Eating Disorders in Athletes

To prevent eating disorders in athletes and dancers, the performers, their coaches, and their parents must learn about inappropriate body weight ideals, improper weight-loss techniques, eating disorder development, proper nutrition, and safe weight-management strategies.[9] Young people naturally search for identity and will often follow the advice of a person in authority without question. Therefore, coaches and dance instructors should never encourage unhealthy weight loss to qualify for competition or to conform to distorted artistic ideals. Athletes who need to lose weight for health's sake should try to do so during the off-season and under the supervision of a health-care professional.

Table H8-2 includes suggestions to help athletes and dancers protect themselves against developing eating disorders. The remaining sections describe eating disorders that anyone, athlete or nonathlete, may experience.

Anorexia Nervosa

Julie, 18 years old, is a superachiever in school. She watches her diet with great care, and she exercises daily, maintaining a rigorous schedule of self-discipline. She is thin, but she is determined to lose more weight. She is 5 feet 6 inches tall and weighs 104 pounds (roughly 1.68 meters and 47 kilograms). Her BMI is less than 17. She has **anorexia nervosa.**

TABLE H8-2 Tips for Combating Eating Disorders

General Guidelines

- Never restrict food amounts to below those suggested for adequacy by the USDA Food Patterns (see Table 2-3, p. 41).
- Eat frequently. Include healthy snacks between meals. The person who eats frequently never gets so hungry as to allow hunger to dictate food choices.
- If not at a healthy weight, establish a reasonable weight goal based on a healthy body composition.
- Allow a reasonable time to achieve the goal. A reasonable loss of excess fat can be achieved at the rate of about 10 percent of body weight in 6 months.
- Establish a weight-maintenance support group with people who share interests.

Specific Guidelines for Athletes and Dancers

- Adopt realistic and health-promoting goals related to weight and body composition instead of weight-restrictive guidelines.
- Disregard critical comments about weight and body composition.
- Recognize that eating disorders impair health and physical performance. Seek professional treatment if needed.
- Emphasize nutrition as an important key to optimal performance.

Characteristics of Anorexia Nervosa

Julie is unaware that she is undernourished, and she sees no need to obtain treatment. She developed amenorrhea several months ago and has become moody and chronically depressed. She views normal healthy body weight as too fat and insists that she needs to lose weight. Julie denies that she is ever tired, although she is close to physical exhaustion and no longer sleeps easily. Her family is concerned, and though reluctant to push her, they have finally insisted that she see a psychiatrist. Julie's psychiatrist has diagnosed anorexia nervosa using specific criteria that describe such characteristics as a significantly low body weight caused by persistent restriction of energy intake; an intense fear of gaining weight or becoming fat, or persistent behaviors that interfere with weight gains; and a disturbance in self-perceived weight or shape.[10] She is prescribed group therapy as a start and if she does not begin to gain weight soon, she may need to enter a residential program or be hospitalized.

Central to the diagnosis of anorexia nervosa is a distorted body image that overestimates personal body fatness (see Photo H8-1). When Julie looks at herself in the mirror, she sees a "fat" 104-pound body. The more Julie overestimates her body size, the more resistant she is to treatment, and the more unwilling she is to examine her faulty values and misconceptions. In fact, she finds value in her condition. Malnutrition and weight loss affect brain functioning and judgment in this way,

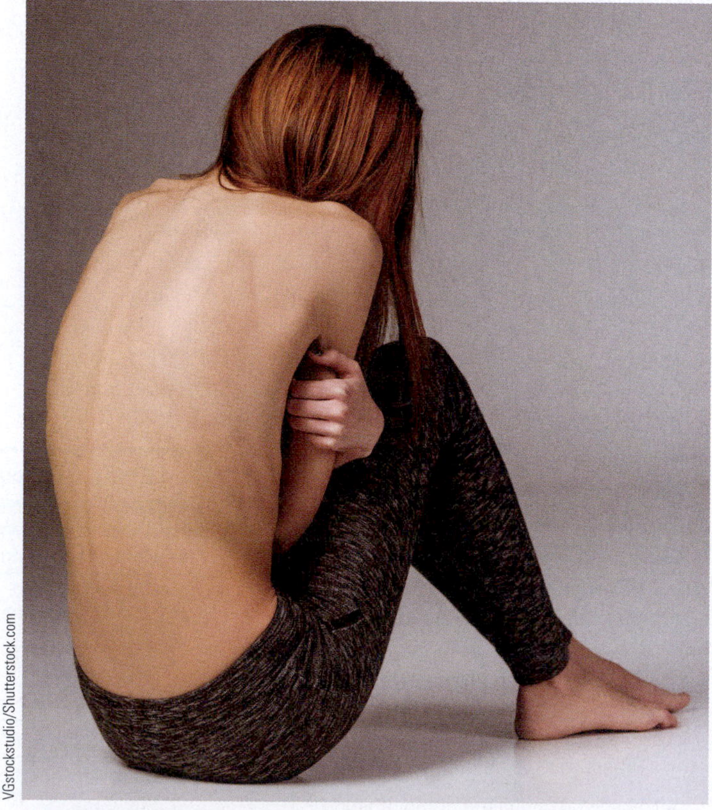

VGstockstudio/Shutterstock.com

> PHOTO H8-1 People with anorexia nervosa see themselves as fat, even when they are dangerously underweight.

causing lethargy, confusion, and delirium and influencing mood, anxiety, and emotions.

Anorexia nervosa cannot be self-diagnosed. Many people in our society are engaged in the pursuit of thinness, and denial runs high among people with anorexia nervosa. Some women have all the attitudes and behaviors associated with the condition, but without the dramatic weight loss.

How can a person as thin as Julie continue to starve herself? Julie uses tremendous discipline against her hunger to strictly limit her portions of low-kcalorie foods. She will deny her hunger, and having adapted to eating so little food, she feels full after nibbling on a few carrot sticks. She knows the kcalorie intake of various foods and the kcalorie expenditure of different physical activities. If she feels that she has gained an ounce of weight, she runs or jumps rope until she is sure she has exercised it off. If she fears that the food she has eaten outweighs her physical activity, she may take laxatives to hasten the passage of food from her system. She drinks water incessantly to fill her stomach, risking dangerous mineral imbalances. She is desperately hungry. In fact, she is starving, but she doesn't eat because her need for self-control dominates.

Many people, on learning of this disorder, say they wish they had "a touch" of it to get thin. They mistakenly think that people with anorexia nervosa feel no hunger. They also fail to recognize the pain of the associated psychological and physical trauma.

The starvation of anorexia nervosa damages the body just as the starvation of war and poverty does. In fact, most people with anorexia nervosa are malnourished. Their bodies have been depleted of both body fat and lean protein. Victims are dying to be thin—quite literally. In young people, growth ceases and normal development falters. They lose so much lean tissue that their basal metabolic rate slows. In addition, the heart pumps inefficiently and irregularly, the heart muscle becomes weak and thin, the chambers diminish in size, and the blood pressure falls. Minerals that help regulate heartbeat become unbalanced. Many deaths occur because of multiple organ system failure when the heart, kidneys, and liver cease to function.

Starvation brings other physical consequences as well, such as loss of brain tissue, impaired immune response, anemia, and a loss of digestive functions that worsen malnutrition. Peristalsis becomes sluggish, the stomach empties slowly, and the lining of the intestinal tract atrophies. The pancreas slows its production of digestive enzymes. The deteriorated GI tract fails to provide sufficient digestive enzymes and absorptive surfaces for handling any food that is eaten. The person may suffer from diarrhea, further worsening malnutrition.

Other effects of starvation include altered blood lipids, high blood vitamin A and vitamin E, low blood proteins, dry thin skin, abnormal nerve functioning, reduced bone density, low body temperature, low blood pressure, and the development of fine body hair (the body's attempt to keep warm). The electrical activity of the brain becomes abnormal, and insomnia is common. Both women and men lose their sex drives. In short, the metabolic mayhem of anorexia nervosa results in numerous physical complications, many of them life-threatening.

Women with anorexia nervosa commonly develop amenorrhea. In young girls, the onset of menstruation is delayed. Menstrual periods typically resume with recovery, although some women never restart even after they have gained weight. Should an underweight woman with anorexia nervosa become pregnant, she is likely to give birth to an underweight baby—and low-birthweight babies face many health problems (as Chapter 15 explains). Mothers with anorexia nervosa may underfeed their children, who then fail to grow and may also suffer the other consequences of starvation.

Treatment of Anorexia Nervosa

Treatment of eating disorders requires a multidisciplinary approach.[11] Teams of physicians, nurses, psychiatrists, family therapists, and dietitians work together to resolve two sets of issues and behaviors: those relating to food and body weight and those involving relationships with oneself and others.

The first dietary objective is to stop weight loss while establishing regular eating patterns. Appropriate diet is crucial to recovery and must be tailored to each individual's needs. Because body weight is low and fear of weight gain is high, initial food intake may be small—perhaps only 1200 kcalories per day. A variety of foods and foods with a higher energy density help ensure greater success. As eating becomes more comfortable, clients should gradually increase energy intake. Initially, clients may be unwilling to eat for themselves. Those who do eat will have a good chance of recovering without additional interventions. Even after recovery, however, energy intakes and eating behaviors may not fully return to normal. Furthermore, weight gains may be slow because energy needs may be slightly elevated because of anxiety, abdominal pain, and cigarette smoking.

Because anorexia nervosa is like starvation physically, health-care professionals classify clients based on indicators of malnutrition. Low-risk clients need dietary counseling. Intermediate-risk clients may need supplements such as high-kcalorie, high-protein formulas in addition to regular meals. High-risk clients may require hospitalization and may need to be fed by tube at first to prevent death. Residential programs that provide intensive behavioral treatment may be most appropriate for those who do not respond to less intensive approaches.

Denial runs high among those with anorexia nervosa. Few seek treatment on their own. Habits are well entrenched, creating a persistent problem that resists solutions.[12] About half of the women who are treated can maintain their body weight at 85 percent or more of a healthy weight, and at that weight, many of them may begin menstruating again. The other half have poor to fair treatment outcomes, relapse into abnormal eating behaviors, or die. Anorexia nervosa has the highest premature mortality rate of any psychiatric disorder—most commonly from cardiac complications or by suicide.[13] Much like treatment for drug addictions, treatment for eating disorders engages family members. Therapists help family members to understand how their past interactions have enabled the client to continue destructive behaviors and how new ways of interacting can support change.

Before drawing conclusions about someone who is extremely thin or who eats very little, remember that diagnosis requires professional assessment. Several national organizations offer information for people who are seeking help with anorexia nervosa, either for themselves or for others.

Bulimia Nervosa

Kelly is a charming, intelligent, 30-year-old flight attendant of normal weight who thinks constantly about food. She alternates between starving herself and secretly bingeing, and when she has eaten too much, she makes herself vomit. Most readers recognize these symptoms as those of **bulimia nervosa**.

Characteristics of Bulimia Nervosa

Bulimia nervosa is not as physically apparent as anorexia nervosa. The secretive nature of bulimic behaviors makes recognition of the problem difficult, but once it is recognized, diagnosis is based on such criteria as number and frequency of binge-eating episodes, inappropriate compensatory behaviors to prevent weight gain (such as self-induced vomiting or misuse of laxatives), and self-evaluation unduly influenced by body shape and weight.[14]

Like the typical person with bulimia nervosa, Kelly is single, female, and white. She is well educated and close to her ideal body weight, although her weight fluctuates over a range of 10 pounds or so every few weeks. She prefers to weigh less than the weight that her body maintains naturally.

Kelly seldom lets her eating disorder interfere with work or other activities, although a third of all bulimics do. From early childhood, she has been a high achiever and emotionally dependent on her parents. As a young teen, Kelly frequently followed severely restricted diets but could never maintain the weight loss. Kelly feels anxious at social events and cannot easily establish close personal relationships. She is usually depressed, is often impulsive, and has low self-esteem.[15] When crisis hits, Kelly responds by replaying events, worrying excessively, and blaming herself but never asking for help—behaviors that interfere with effective coping.

Like the person with anorexia nervosa, the person with bulimia nervosa spends much time thinking about body image and food. The preoccupation with food manifests itself in secret binge-eating episodes, which usually progress through several emotional stages: anticipation and planning, anxiety, urgency to begin, rapid and uncontrollable consumption of food, relief and relaxation, disappointment, and finally shame or disgust.

A bulimic binge is characterized by a sense of no control over eating. During a binge, the person consumes food for its emotional comfort and cannot stop eating or control what or how much is eaten. A typical binge occurs periodically, in secret, usually at night, and lasts an hour or more. Because a binge frequently follows a period of restrictive dieting, eating is accelerated by intense hunger. Energy restriction followed by bingeing can set in motion a pattern of weight cycling, which may make weight loss and maintenance more difficult over time.

During a binge, Kelly consumes thousands of kcalories of easy-to-eat, low-fiber, high-fat, and, especially, high-carbohydrate foods. Typically, she chooses cookies, cakes, and ice cream—and she eats the entire bag of cookies, the whole cake, and every last spoonful in a carton of ice cream. After the binge, Kelly pays the price with swollen hands and feet, bloating, fatigue, headache, nausea, and pain.

To purge the food from her body, Kelly may use a **cathartic**—a strong laxative that can injure the lower intestinal tract. Or she may induce vomiting, with or without the use of an **emetic**—a drug intended as first aid for poisoning. These purging behaviors are often accompanied by feelings of shame or guilt. Hence a vicious cycle develops: negative self-perceptions followed by dieting, bingeing, and purging, which in turn lead to negative self-perceptions (see Figure H8-1).

On first glance, purging seems to offer a quick and easy solution to the problems of unwanted kcalories and body weight. Many people perceive such behavior as neutral or even positive, when, in fact, binge eating and purging have serious physical consequences. Signs of subclinical malnutrition are evident in a compromised immune system. Fluid and mineral imbalances caused by vomiting or diarrhea can lead to abnormal heart rhythms and injury to the kidneys. Urinary tract infections can lead to kidney failure. Vomiting causes irritation and infection of the pharynx, esophagus, and salivary glands; painful sores in the mouth; erosion of the teeth; and dental caries. The esophagus may rupture or tear, as may the stomach. Sometimes the eyes become red from pressure during vomiting. The hands may be calloused or cut by the teeth while inducing vomiting. Overuse of emetics depletes potassium concentrations and can lead to death by heart failure.

Unlike Julie, Kelly is aware that her behavior is abnormal, and she is deeply ashamed of it. She wants to recover, and this makes recovery more likely for her than for Julie, who clings to denial. Feeling inadequate ("I can't even control my eating"), Kelly tends to be passive and to look to others for confirmation of her sense of worth. When she experiences rejection, either in reality or in her imagination, her bulimia nervosa becomes worse. If Kelly's depression deepens, she may seek solace in drug or alcohol abuse or in other addictive behaviors. Clinical depression is common in people with bulimia nervosa, and the rates of substance abuse are high.

> **FIGURE H8-1 The Vicious Cycle of Restrictive Dieting and Binge Eating**

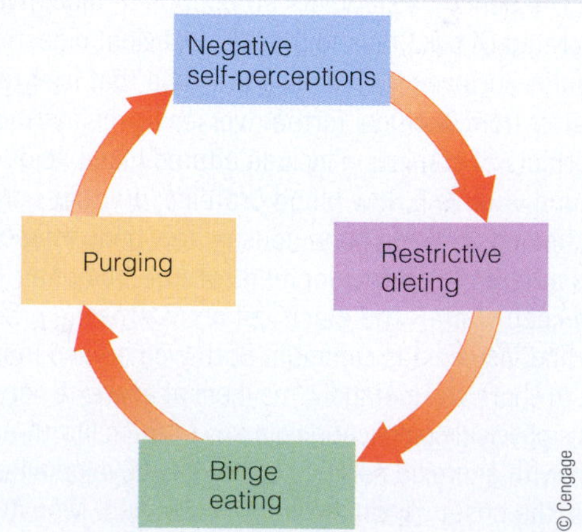
Negative self-perceptions
Restrictive dieting
Binge eating
Purging
© Cengage

Treatment of Bulimia Nervosa

Kelly needs to establish regular eating patterns. She may also benefit from a regular exercise program. Weight maintenance, rather than cyclic weight gains and losses, is the treatment goal. Major steps toward recovery include discontinuing purging and restrictive dieting habits and learning to eat three meals a day plus snacks. Initially, energy intake should provide enough food to satisfy hunger and maintain body weight. Table H8-3 offers diet strategies to correct the eating problems of bulimia nervosa. A mental health professional should be on the treatment team to help clients with their depression and addictive behaviors.

Anorexia nervosa and bulimia nervosa are distinct eating disorders, yet they sometimes overlap in important ways. Anorexia victims may purge, and victims of both disorders are overly concerned with body image and have a tendency to drastically undereat. Many perceive foods as "forbidden" and "give in" to an eating binge. The two disorders can also appear in the same person, or one can lead to the other. Treatment is challenging and relapses are common. Another common eating disorder is **binge-eating disorder**.

TABLE H8-3 Diet Strategies for Combating Bulimia Nervosa

Planning Principles

- Plan meals and snacks; record plans in a food diary prior to eating.
- Plan meals and snacks that require eating at the table and using utensils.
- Refrain from eating finger foods.
- Refrain from "dieting" or skipping meals.

Nutrition Principles

- Eat a well-balanced diet and regularly timed meals consisting of a variety of foods.
- Include raw vegetables, salad, or raw fruit at meals to prolong eating times.
- Choose whole-grain, high-fiber breads, pasta, rice, and cereals to increase bulk.
- Consume adequate fluid, particularly water.

Other Tips

- Choose foods that provide protein and fat for satiety and bulky, fiber-rich carbohydrates for immediate feelings of fullness.
- Try including soups and other water-rich foods for satiety.
- Choose portions that meet the definition of "a serving" according to the USDA Food Patterns (pp. 40–43).
- For convenience (and to reduce temptation) select foods that naturally divide into portions. Select one potato, rather than rice or pasta that can be overloaded onto the plate; purchase yogurt and cottage cheese in individual containers; look for small packages of precut steak or chicken; choose frozen dinners with measured portions.
- Include 30 minutes of physical activity every day—exercise may be an important tool in defeating bulimia.

Binge-Eating Disorder

Charlie is a 40-year-old schoolteacher who has been overweight all his life. His friends and family are forever encouraging him to lose weight, and he has come to believe that if he only had more willpower, dieting would work. He periodically gives dieting his best shot—restricting energy intake for a day or two only to succumb to uncontrollable cravings, especially for high-fat foods. Like Charlie, up to half of the obese people who try to lose weight periodically binge; unlike people with bulimia nervosa, however, they typically do not purge. Binge-eating disorder has its own specific diagnostic criteria based on recurring episodes of binge eating, with a marked sense of lack of control. It can occur in people of normal weight as well as those who are severely overweight. Obesity alone is not an eating disorder.

Clinicians note differences between people with bulimia nervosa and those with binge-eating disorder. People with binge-eating disorder typically consume less during a binge, rarely purge, and exert less restraint during times of dieting. Similarities also exist, including feeling out of control, disgusted, depressed, embarrassed, guilty, or distressed because of their self-perceived gluttony.

There are also differences between obese binge eaters and obese people who do not binge. Those with binge-eating disorder report higher rates of self-loathing, disgust about body size, depression, and anxiety. Their eating habits differ as well. Obese binge eaters tend to consume more kcalories and more dessert and snack-type foods during regular meals and binges than obese people who do not binge. Binge eating may incur health risks greater than those of obesity alone.

Some of the characteristics seen in people with bulimia nervosa and binge-eating disorder are similar to those seen in people with substance-use disorders: strong cravings, poor self-control, a diminished sensitivity to pleasure, and patterns of compulsive use.[16] These resemblances have given rise to the concept of *food addictions* and may reflect the same biological and psychological systems that are involved in rewards and self-control.[17] When the reward of delicious foods tempts a person, the ability to resist depends on self-control.[18] Neural images show that certain foods (especially those with added sugars and solid fats) have effects on the brain similar to those seen with addictive drugs. Dopamine activity—which helps regulate emotional and motivational behavior—is also similarly altered in both drug addicts and those with compulsive eating behaviors.[19] Some researchers suggest that the term *eating addiction* is a better descriptor than food addiction, focusing more on the behavior than on the substance.[20]

Binge eating can be resolved with treatment that combines behavioral and drug therapies.[21] Reducing binge eating makes participation in weight-control programs easier. It also improves physical health, mental health, and the chances of success in breaking the cycle of rapid weight losses and gains.

Eating Disorders in Society

Society plays a central role in eating disorders. Consider that the average height and weight of US women is 5 feet 4 inches tall and 166 pounds, whereas the average model is 6 inches taller and weighs 50 pounds less. Similarly, the average height and weight of US men is 5 feet 9 inches tall and 196 pounds, and the average male model is at least that tall and weighs between 120 and 170 pounds. Teens and adults who obsess over weight loss and accept these models as beauty ideals are likely to harbor negative feelings about their own bodies and engage in unhealthy eating habits.[22]

Further proof of society's influence is found in the demographic distribution of eating disorders—historically, they were once known only in developed nations, but they have become more prevalent in developing countries as wealth increases, global fashion and beauty infiltrate, and food becomes plentiful.[23] Some people point to the vomitoriums of ancient times and claim that bulimia nervosa is not new, but the two are actually distinct. Ancient people were eating for pleasure, without guilt, and in the company of others; they vomited so that they could rejoin the feast. Bulimia nervosa is a disorder of isolation and is often accompanied by low self-esteem.

Our society sets unrealistic, underweight ideals for body weight, especially for women, although eating disorders are also relatively common, but overlooked, among men.[24] Anorexia nervosa and bulimia nervosa are not a form of rebellion against these unreasonable expectations, but rather an exaggerated acceptance of them. In fact, some people fail to recognize the health dangers and endorse eating disorders as a lifestyle choice. Hundreds of websites encourage, support, and motivate users to continue their lives with anorexia and bulimia. These eating disorders thrive in the social media world of photos, friendships, and affirmations. Young adults who are most active on social media are most likely to express eating concerns.[25]

The prevalence of eating disorders in young people continues to increase.[26] Most alarming is the rising prevalence at progressively younger ages. Restrained eating, fasting, binge eating, purging, fear of fatness, and distortion of body image are extraordinarily common among children and adolescents. Those who are teased about being overweight are particularly vulnerable.[27] Most are "on diets," and many are poorly nourished. Some eat too little food to support normal growth, thus they miss out on their adolescent growth spurts and may never catch up. Many eat so little that hunger propels them into binge-purge cycles. Disordered eating behaviors set a pattern that likely continues into young adulthood.

Prevention and treatment of eating disorders present numerous challenges.[28] Perhaps a person's best defense against these disorders is to learn to appreciate his or her own uniqueness. Focus should be on a healthy lifestyle rather than on body weight.[29] When people discover and honor their body's real physical needs, they become unwilling to sacrifice health. To value and care for oneself may be lifesaving.

CRITICAL THINKING QUESTIONS

A. How do eating disorders affect health?

B. You overheard someone saying that eating disorders aren't really diseases and that if people who have anorexia or bulimia would just eat normally, they'd be cured. What is your opinion of this position? How can you make a distinction between someone with an eating disorder and others who are concerned with managing their body weight?

REFERENCES

1. National Institutes of Health, *Eating disorders*, www.nimh.nih.gov/health/topics/eating-disorders, February 2016.
2. A. K. W. Kelly and S. Hecht, The female athlete triad, *Pediatrics* 138 (2016): 80–89; M. J. DeSouza and coauthors, 2014 Female Athlete Triad Coalition consensus statement on treatment and return to play of the female athlete triad, *Clinical Journal of Sport Medicine* 24 (2014): 96–119; J. C. Gibbs, N. I. Williams, and M. J. deSouza, Prevalence of individual and combined components of the female athlete triad, *Medicine and Science in Sports and Exercise* 45 (2013): 985–996.
3. M. Mountjoy and coauthors, The IOC statement: Beyond the female athlete triad—relative energy deficiency in sport (RED-S), *British Journal of Sports Medicine* 48 (2014): 491–497; M. J. deSouza and coauthors, Misunderstanding the female athlete triad: Refuting the IOC consensus statement on relative energy deficiency in sport (RED-S), *British Medical Journal* 48 (2014): 1461–1465.
4. G. Wilson and coauthors, Weight-making strategies in professional jockeys: Implications for physical and mental health and well-beings, *Sports Medicine* 44 (2014): 785–796.
5. L. Håman and coauthors, Orthorexia nervosa: An integrative literature review of a lifestyle syndrome, *International Journal of Qualitative Studies on Health and Well-being* 10 (2015): 26799.
6. N. S. Koven and A. W. Abry, The clinical basis of orthorexia nervosa: Emerging perspectives, *Neuropsychiatric Disease and Treatment* 11 (2015): 385–394.
7. C. Musolino and coauthors, "Healthy anorexia": The complexity of care in disordered eating, *Social Science in Medicine* 139 (2015): 18–25.
8. K. E. Ackerman and coauthors, Fractures in relation to menstrual status and bone parameters in young athletes, *Medicine and Science in Sports and Exercise* 47 (2015): 1577–1586; M. T. Barrack and coauthors, Higher incidence of bone stress injuries with increasing female athlete triad-related risk factors: A prospective multisite study of exercising girls and women, *American Journal of Sports Medicine* 42 (2014): 949–958.
9. G. M. de Oliveira Coelho and coauthors, Prevention of eating disorders in female athletes, *Journal of Sports Medicine* 5 (2014): 105–113.
10. American Psychiatric Association, *Diagnostic and Statistical Manual of Mental Disorders* (Washington, D.C.: American Psychiatric Publishing, 2013).
11. Position of the American Dietetic Association: Nutrition intervention in the treatment of eating disorders, *Journal of the American Dietetic Association* 111 (2011): 1236–1241.
12. B. T. Walsh, The enigmatic persistence of anorexia nervosa, *American Journal of Psychiatry* 170 (2013): 477–484.
13. A. Keshaviah and coauthors, Re-examining premature mortality in anorexia nervosa: A meta-analysis redux, *Comprehensive Psychiatry* 55 (2014): 1773–1784; G. DiCola and coauthors, Cardiovascular disorders in anorexia nervosa and potential therapeutic targets, *Internal and Emergency Medicine* 9 (2014): 717–721.
14. American Psychiatric Association, *Diagnostic and Statistical Manual of Mental Disorders*.
15. I. Brechan and I. L. Kvalem, Relationship between body dissatisfaction and disordered eating: Mediating role of self-esteem and depression, *Eating Behaviors* 17 (2015): 49–58; S. E. Racine and coauthors, Examining

associations between negative urgency and key components of objective binge episodes, *International Journal of Eating Disorders* 48 (2015): 527–531.

16. A. Meule, V. vonRezori, and J. Blechert, Food addiction and bulimia nervosa, *European Eating Disorders Review* 22 (2014): 331–337; N. A. Hadad and L. A. Knackstedt, Addicted to palatable foods: Comparing the neurobiology of bulimia nervosa to that of drug addiction, *Psychopharmacology* 231 (2014): 1897–1912; American Psychiatric Association, *Diagnostic and Statistical Manual of Mental Disorders*.
17. A. Carter and coauthors, The neurobiology of "food addiction" and its implications for obesity treatment and policy, *Annual Review of Nutrition* 36 (2016): 105-128; M. Alonso-Alonso and coauthors, Food reward system: Current perspectives and future research needs, *Nutrition Reviews* 73 (2015): 296–307; N. Carlier and coauthors, Genetic similarities between compulsive overeating and addiction phenotypes: A case for "food addiction"? *Current Psychiatry Reports* 17 (2015): 96; A. Meule and A. N. Gearhardt, Food addiction in the light of DSM-5, *Nutrients* 6 (2014): 3653–3671; K. Blum, P. K. Thanos, and M. S. Gold, dopamine and glucose, obesity, and reward deficiency syndrome, *Frontiers in Psychology* 5 (2014): 1–11; D. G. Smith and T. W. Robbins, The neurobiological underpinnings of obesity and binge eating: A rationale for adopting the food addiction model, *Biological Psychiatry* 73 (2013): 804–810; N. D. Volkow and coauthors, Obesity and addiction: Neurobiological overlaps, *Obesity Reviews* 14 (2013): 2–18.
18. N. D. Volkow and coauthors, The addictive dimensionality of obesity, *Biological Psychiatry* 73 (2013): 811–818.
19. J. H. Baik, Dopamine signaling in food addiction: Role of Dopamine D2 receptors, *BMB Reports* 46 (2013): 519–526.
20. J. Hebebrand and coauthors, "Eating addiction," rather than "food addiction," better captures addictive-like eating behavior, *Neuroscience and Biobehavioral Reviews* 47 (2014): 295–306.
21. K. A. Brownley and coauthors, Binge-eating disorder in adults: A systematic review and meta-analysis, *Annals of Internal Medicine* 165 (2016): 409–420.
22. A. Dakanalis and coauthors, The developmental effects of media-ideal internalization and self-objectification on adolescents' negative body-feelings, dietary restraint, and binge-eating, *European Child and Adolescent Psychiatry* 24 (2015): 997–1010.
23. K. M. Pike, H. W. Hoek, and P. E. Dunne, Cultural trends and eating disorders, *Current Opinion in Psychiatry* 27 (2014): 436–442.
24. L. P. MacNeill and L. A. Best, Perceived current and ideal body size in female undergraduates, *Eating Behaviors* 18 (2015): 71–75; A. E. Field and coauthors, Prospective associations of concerns about physique and the development of obesity, binge drinking, and drug use among adolescent boys and young adult men, *JAMA Pediatrics* 168 (2014): 34–39; U. Räisänen and K. Hunt, The role of gendered constructions of eating disorders in delayed help-seeking in men: A qualitative interview study, *BMJ Open* 4 (2014): e004342.
25. J. E. Sidani and coauthors, The association between social media use and eating concerns among US young adults, *Journal of the Academy of Nutrition and Dietetics* 116 (2016): 1465–1472; A. G. Mabe and coauthors, Do you "like" my photo? Facebook use maintains eating disorder risk, *International Journal of Eating Disorders* 47 (2014): 516–523.
26. B. Herpertz-Dahlmann, Adolescent eating disorders: Update on definitions, symptomatology, epidemiology, and comorbidity, *Child and Adolescent Psychiatric Clinics of North America* 24 (2015): 177–196.
27. N. Olvera and coauthors, Pathways for disordered eating behaviors in minority girls: The role of adiposity, peer weight-related teasing, and desire to be thinner, *Journal of Early Adolescence* (2015): doi:10.1177/0272431615609155.
28. A. P. Bailey and coauthors, Mapping the evidence for the prevention and treatment of eating disorders in young people, *Journal of Eating Disorders* 2 (2014): 5; A. E. Kass, R. P. Kolko, and D. E. Wilfley, Psychological treatments for eating disorders, *Current Opinions in Psychiatry* 26 (2013): 549–555.
29. N. H. Golden, M. Schneider, and C. Wood, Preventing obesity and eating disorders in adolescents, *Pediatrics* 138 (2016): 114–123.

9

Weight Management: Overweight, Obesity, and Underweight

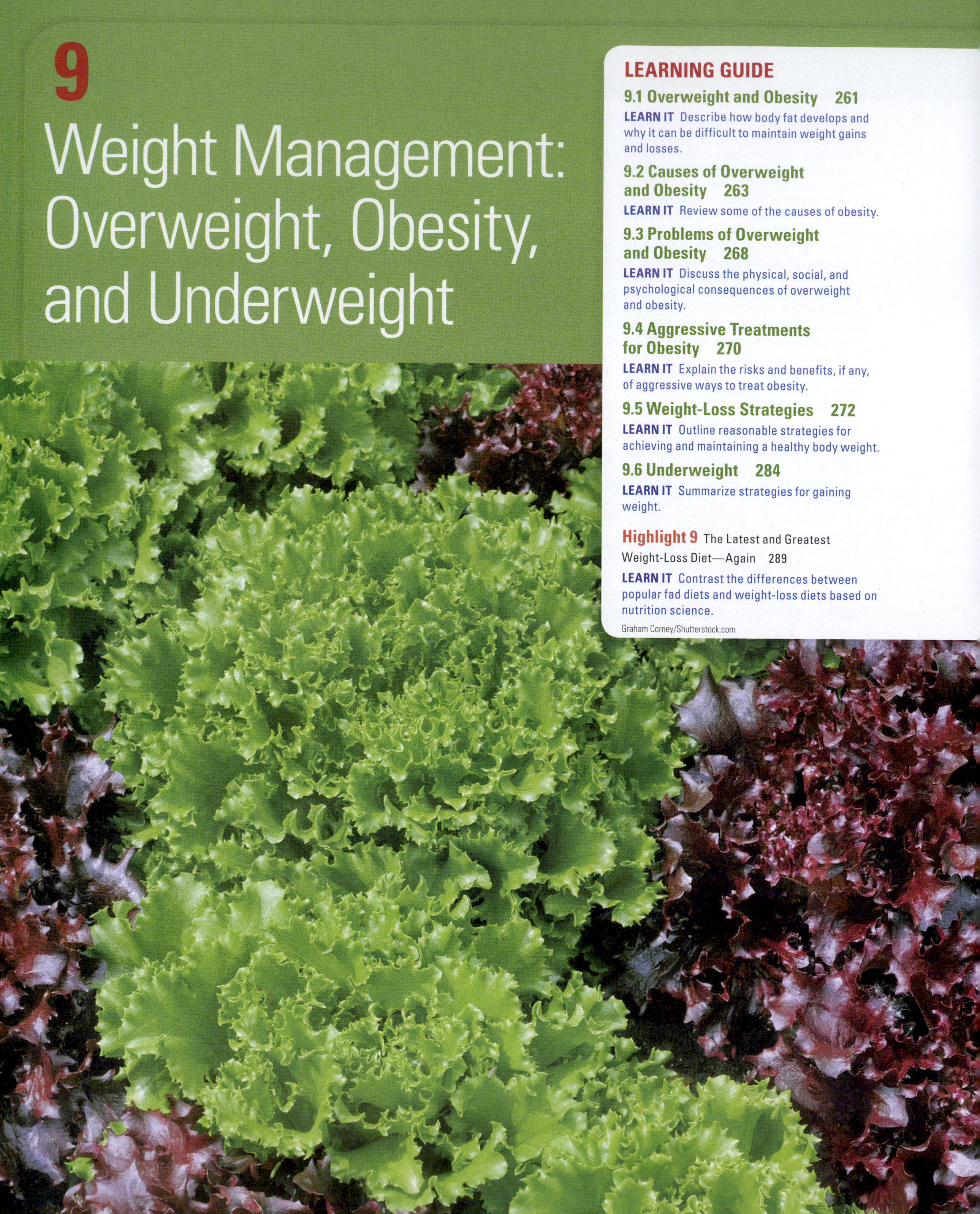

LEARNING GUIDE

Graham Corney/Shutterstock.com

Nutrition in Your Life

Are you pleased with your body weight? If so, you are a rare individual. Most people in our society think they should weigh more or less (mostly less) than they do. Usually, their primary concern is appearance, but they often understand that physical health is also somehow related to body weight. One does not necessarily cause the other—that is, an ideal body weight does not ensure good health. Instead, both depend on diet and physical activity. A well-balanced diet and active lifestyle support good health—and help maintain body weight within a reasonable range. As you read this chapter, consider whether your eating habits and physical activities are supporting good health and a reasonable body weight.

Chapter 8 described how body weight is stable when "energy in" equals "energy out." Weight gains occur when energy intake exceeds energy expended, and conversely, weight losses occur when energy expended exceeds energy intake. At the extremes, both overweight and underweight present health risks. **Weight management** is a key component of good health. To that end, this chapter offers strategies to help achieve and maintain a healthy body weight. It also explores overweight and obesity by examining some of the causes, consequences, and treatments.

This chapter emphasizes overweight (BMI 25 to 29.9) and obesity (BMI ≥30), partly because they have been more intensively studied and partly because they represent a major health problem in the United States and a growing concern worldwide. Underweight (BMI <18.5) is a far less prevalent problem. Information on underweight is presented at the end of the chapter. Highlight 9 examines fad diets.

> **FIGURE 9-1 Increasing Prevalence of Obesity (BMI ≥30) among US Adults**

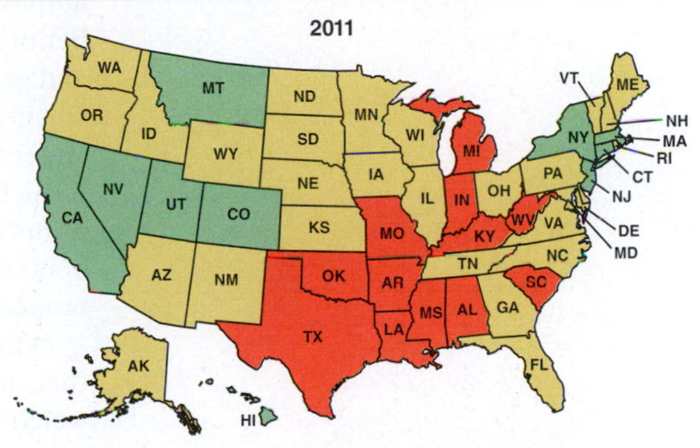
2011
WA
OR
CA
MT
ID
NV
WY
UT
CO
AZ
NM
ND
SD
NE
KS
OK
TX
MN
IA
MO
AR
LA
WI
IL
MI
IN
OH
KY
TN
MS
AL
GA
FL
SC
NC
VA
WV
PA
NY
VT
ME
NH
MA
RI
CT
NJ
DE
MD
AK
HI

<20%	20% to 24.9%	25% to 29.9%	30% to 34.9%	≥35%
0 states	11 states	27 states	12 states	0 states

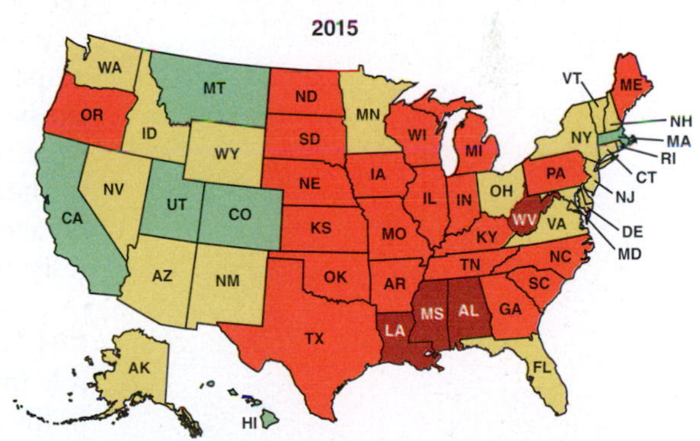
2015
WA
OR
CA
MT
ID
NV
WY
UT
CO
AZ
NM
ND
SD
NE
KS
OK
TX
MN
IA
MO
AR
LA
WI
IL
MI
IN
OH
KY
TN
MS
AL
GA
FL
SC
NC
VA
WV
PA
NY
VT
ME
NH
MA
RI
CT
NJ
DE
MD
AK
HI

<20%	20% to 24.9%	25% to 29.9%	30% to 34.9%	≥35%
0 states	6 states	19 states	21 states	4 states

SOURCE: http://www.cdc.gov/obesity/data/prevalence-maps.html, September 2016.

9.1 Overweight and Obesity

LEARN IT Describe how body fat develops and why it can be difficult to maintain weight gains and losses.

Despite our preoccupation with body image and weight loss, the prevalence of overweight and obesity in the United States continues to be high.[1] The maps in Figure 9-1 offer a glimpse of the dramatic increases in the prevalence of obesity over the past five years alone. Because of changes in methods, estimates of obesity prevalence prior to 2011 cannot be compared to estimates from subsequent years, but trends clearly indicate that over the past five decades, obesity increased in every state, in both genders, and across all ages, races, and educational levels. An estimated 70 percent of the adults in the United States are now considered overweight or obese, as defined by a BMI of 25 to 29.9, or 30 and greater, respectively.[2]

The prevalence of overweight among children in the United States has also risen at an alarming rate. Chapter 16 presents information on overweight during childhood and adolescence.

Obesity has spread worldwide, affecting 1.9 billion adults and 41 million children younger than age 5.[3] Increasing rates of obesity in countries around the world reflect a global food system that delivers an abundance of energy-dense, processed, affordable, and effectively marketed products. Before examining the suspected causes of obesity and the various strategies used to treat it, it is helpful to understand the development and metabolism of body fat.

weight management: maintaining body weight in a healthy range by preventing gradual weight gains over time and losing weight if overweight, and by preventing weight losses and gaining weight if underweight.

> **FIGURE 9-2 Fat Cell Development**

Fat cells are capable of increasing their size by 20-fold and their number by several thousandfold.

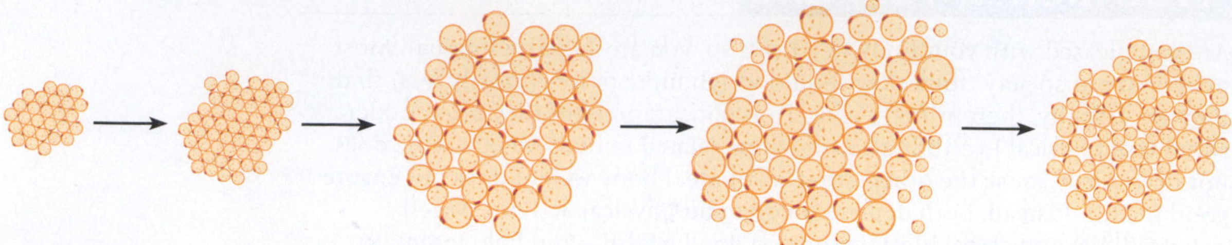
During growth, fat cells increase in number.
When energy intake exceeds expenditure, fat cells increase in size.
When fat cells have enlarged and energy intake continues to exceed energy expenditure, fat cells may increase in number again.
With fat loss, the size of the fat cells shrinks but not the number.
© Cengage

Fat Cell Development When "energy in" exceeds "energy out," much of the excess energy is stored in the fat cells of adipose tissue. The amount of fat in adipose tissue reflects both the number and the size of the fat cells.* The number of fat cells increases most rapidly during the growing years of late childhood and early puberty. After growth ceases, fat cell numbers may continue to increase whenever energy balance is positive. Obese people have more fat cells—as well as larger fat cells—than healthy-weight people.

As fat cells accumulate triglycerides, they expand in size (review Figure 5-18, p. 144). When the cells enlarge, they stimulate cell proliferation so that their numbers increase again. Thus obesity develops when a person's fat cells increase in number, in size, or quite often both. Figure 9-2 illustrates fat cell development.

When "energy out" exceeds "energy in," the size of fat cells dwindles, but not their number. People with extra fat cells tend to regain lost weight rapidly; with weight gain, their many fat cells readily fill. In contrast, people with an average number of enlarged fat cells may be more successful in maintaining weight losses; when their cells shrink, both cell size and number are normal. Prevention of obesity is most critical, then, during the growing years of childhood and adolescence, when fat cells increase in number. Researchers are exploring ways to induce fat cell death—which would decrease the number.[4]**

As mentioned earlier, excess fat first fills the body's natural storage site—adipose tissue. If fat is still abundant, the excess is deposited in organs such as the heart and liver. As Chapter 8 mentioned, fat that accumulates outside of adipose tissue—called ectopic fat—disrupts normal metabolism and contributes to the development of diseases such as heart failure and fatty liver. As ectopic fat accumulates, metabolic changes that indicate disease risk—such as insulin resistance—become apparent and chronic inflammation develops.

Fat Cell Metabolism The enzyme **lipoprotein lipase (LPL)** plays a major role in the metabolism and transport of lipids and consequently is a participant in the development of obesity. One of its roles is to remove triglycerides from the blood for storage in both adipose tissue and muscle cells. Obese people generally have much more LPL activity in their adipose cells than lean people do (their muscle cell LPL activity is similar, though). This high LPL activity makes fat storage especially efficient. Consequently, even modest excesses in energy intake have a more dramatic impact on obese people than on lean people.

The activity of LPL in different regions of the body is partially influenced by gender. In women, fat cells in the breasts, hips, and thighs produce abundant LPL, storing fat in those body sites; in men, fat cells in the abdomen produce

lipoprotein lipase (LPL): an enzyme that hydrolyzes triglycerides passing by in the bloodstream and directs their parts into the cells, where they can be metabolized or reassembled for storage.

*Obesity due to an increase in the *number* of fat cells is *hyperplastic obesity.* Obesity due to an increase in the *size* of fat cells is *hypertrophic obesity.*

**Cell death is known as as *apoptosis.*

abundant LPL. This enzyme activity explains why men tend to develop central obesity around the abdomen (apple-shaped) whereas women more readily develop lower-body fat around the hips and thighs (pear-shaped).

Gender differences are also apparent in the activity of the lipase enzymes controlling the release and breakdown of fat in various parts of the body. The release of lower-body fat is less active in women than in men, whereas the release of upper-body fat is similar. Furthermore, the rate of fat breakdown is lower in women than in men. Consequently, women may have a more difficult time losing fat in general, and from the hips and thighs in particular.

Enzyme activity may also explain why some people who lose weight regain it so easily.[5] After weight loss, adipose tissue LPL activity increases. It's as if the LPL enzyme gene is saying "Make more fat-storing enzymes." The activities of LPL and other proteins provide an explanation for the observation that some biological mechanism seems to set a person's body weight at a fixed point; the body will make adjustments to restore that **set point** if the person tries to change it.

Set-Point Theory

Many physiological variables, such as blood glucose, blood pH, and body temperature, remain fairly stable under a variety of conditions. The hypothalamus and other regulatory centers constantly monitor and delicately adjust conditions to maintain homeostasis. The stability of such complex systems may depend on set-point regulators that maintain variables within specified limits.

Researchers have confirmed that after weight losses, the body adjusts its metabolism to favor weight regain.[6] The decrease in the metabolic rate after weight loss is greater than would be expected based on body composition alone.[7] This adaptation helps explain why it can be difficult to maintain weight losses.

REVIEW IT Describe how body fat develops and why it can be difficult to maintain weight gains and losses.

Fat cells develop by increasing in number and size. Obesity prevention depends on maintaining a reasonable number of fat cells. With weight gains or losses, the body adjusts in an attempt to return to its set-point weight.

9.2 Causes of Overweight and Obesity

LEARN IT Review some of the causes of obesity.

Why do people accumulate excess body fat? The obvious answer is that they take in more energy from foods and beverages than they expend in physical activity and metabolic processes. But that answer falls short of explaining why they do this. Is it genetic? Environmental? Cultural? Behavioral? Socioeconomic? Psychological? Metabolic? All of these? Most likely the latter. Many factors contribute to the development of obesity and most are interrelated. This section reviews the two major contributing and interacting factors—genetics and the environment.[8]

Genetics and Epigenetics

Genetics plays a clear causative role in relatively few cases of obesity, for example, in Prader-Willi syndrome—a genetic disorder characterized by excessive appetite, massive obesity, short stature, and often intellectual disability.[9] Most cases of obesity, however, do not stem from a single gene; more than 100 sites in the human genome are associated with obesity and fat distribution.[10] Highlight 6 describes epigenetics—the influence of environmental factors, such as diet and physical activity, on gene expression. Obesity provides a classic example of epigenetic regulation.[11]

Researchers have found that adopted children tend to be more similar in weight to their biological parents than to their adoptive parents. Studies of twins yield similar findings: compared with fraternal twins, identical twins are far more likely to weigh the same. These findings suggest an important role for genetics

set point: the point at which controls are set (for example, on a thermostat). The set-point theory that relates to body weight proposes that the body tends to maintain a certain weight by means of its own internal controls.

> **FIGURE 9-3 Mice with and without Leptin Compared**

Both of these mice have a defective *ob* gene. Consequently, they do not produce leptin. They both became obese, but the one on the right received daily injections of leptin, which suppressed food intake and increased energy expenditure, resulting in weight loss.

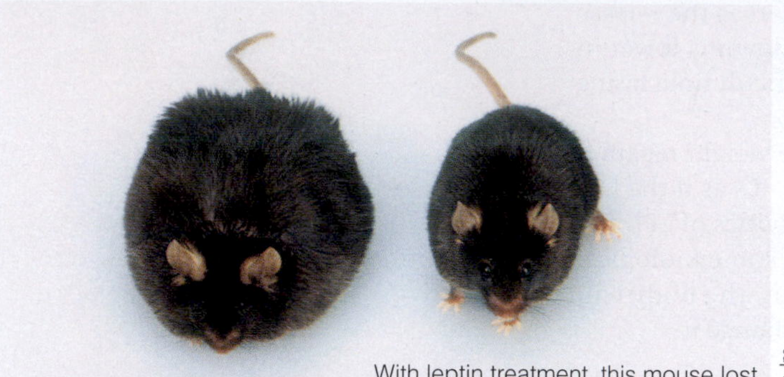

Without leptin, this mouse weighs almost three times as much as a normal mouse.

With leptin treatment, this mouse lost a significant amount of weight but still weighs almost one and a half times as much as a normal mouse.

in determining a person's *susceptibility* to obesity. In other words, genes interact with the diet and activity patterns that lead to obesity and the metabolic pathways that influence satiety and energy balance. Even identical twins with identical genes become different over the years as epigenetic changes accumulate. This raises an important point: you cannot change the genome you inherit, but you can influence the epigenome. Physical activity, for example, can minimize the genetic influences on body fat. Likewise, solid fats, added sugars, and physical inactivity can accentuate the genetic influences on obesity.

Clearly, something genetic makes a person more or less likely to gain or lose weight when overeating or undereating. Some people gain more weight than others on comparable energy intakes. Given an extra 1000 kcalories a day for 100 days, some pairs of identical twins gain less than 10 pounds while others gain up to 30 pounds. Within each pair, the amounts of weight gained, percentages of body fat, and locations of fat deposits are similar. Also, some people lose more weight than others following comparable exercise routines.

Researchers have been examining the human genome in search of genetic and epigenetic answers to obesity questions. As the section on protein synthesis in Chapter 6 described, each cell expresses only the genes for the proteins it needs, and each protein performs a unique function. The following paragraphs describe only a couple of the proteins that help explain appetite control, energy regulation, and obesity development.

Leptin An obesity gene, called *ob*, is expressed primarily in the adipose tissue and codes for the protein **leptin**. Leptin acts as a hormone, primarily in the hypothalamus. Leptin maintains homeostasis by regulating food intake and energy expenditure in response to adipose tissue. When body fat increases, leptin increases—which suppresses appetite. When body fat decreases, leptin decreases—which stimulates appetite and suppresses energy expenditure. In short, leptin promotes a negative energy balance and a decrease in body weight and fatness.[12]

Mice with a defective *ob* gene do not produce leptin and can weigh up to three times as much as normal mice and have five times as much body fat (see Figure 9-3). When injected with leptin, the mice rapidly lose body fat. (Because leptin is a protein, it would be destroyed during digestion if given orally; consequently, it must be given by injection.) The fat cells not only lose fat, but they self-destruct (reducing cell number), which may explain why weight gains are delayed when the mice are fed again.

Although extremely rare, a genetic deficiency of leptin or genetic mutation of its receptor has been identified in human beings as well. Extremely obese children with barely detectable blood levels of leptin have little appetite control; they are constantly hungry and eat considerably more than their siblings or peers.[13] Given daily injections of leptin, these children lose a substantial amount of weight, confirming leptin's role in regulating appetite and body weight.

Very few obese people have a leptin deficiency, however. As mentioned earlier, leptin levels increase as body fat increases. Leptin sensitivity, however, decreases—a condition researchers describe as **leptin resistance**.[14] Researchers are exploring ways to increase leptin levels and enhance leptin sensitivity as possible obesity treatment options.[15]

Ghrelin Another protein, known as **ghrelin**, also acts as a hormone primarily in the hypothalamus. In contrast to leptin, ghrelin is secreted mainly by the stomach cells and promotes a positive energy balance and an increase in body weight and fatness.[16]

Ghrelin stimulates appetite and triggers the desire to eat. Blood levels of ghrelin typically rise before a meal and decline afterward—reflecting the hunger and satiety that precede and follow eating. On average, ghrelin levels are high

leptin: a protein produced by fat cells under direction of the *ob* gene that decreases appetite and increases energy expenditure.

- **leptos** = thin

leptin resistance: a condition in which leptin levels are increased and leptin sensitivity is decreased.

ghrelin (GRELL-in): a protein produced by the stomach cells that stimulates appetite and decreases energy expenditure.

- **ghre** = growth

TABLE 9-1 Characteristics of Ghrelin and Leptin

	Nickname	Secreted primarily by	Action	Production
Ghrelin	Hunger hormone	Stomach cells	Stimulates appetite Increases food intake Decreases energy expenditure	Increases with fasting, hunger, starvation Decreases with food intake
Leptin	Satiety hormone	Adipose cells	Suppresses appetite Enhances satiety Increases energy expenditure	Increases with increased body fat

whenever the body is in negative energy balance, as occurs during low-kcalorie diets, for example. Ghrelin levels are low whenever the body is in positive energy balance, as occurs with weight gains.

Findings from an interesting research study suggest that a person's mindset also influences ghrelin's response to a meal.[17] Young adults were given beverages on two separate occasions—either a beverage labeled as a high-fat, 620-kcalorie "indulgent" milkshake or one labeled as a low-fat, 140-kcalorie "sensible" milkshake. Ghrelin's rise in anticipation of drinking the indulgent milkshake and its decline afterward was much steeper than for the sensible milkshake. In reality, though, the two milkshakes were identical (380 kcalories). Not only was the ghrelin response different, but the participants' satiety differed, reflecting their perceptions of the products. Drinking the sensible milkshake was not as satisfying, despite having the exact same nutrient contents as the indulgent milkshake. The sensible mindset with its relatively flat ghrelin response leaves a person with an increased appetite. These researchers suggest there may be a physiological benefit to adopting a psychological mindset of indulgence when eating low-energy-density, healthy foods.

Some research indicates that ghrelin also promotes sleep. Interestingly, a lack of sleep increases the hunger hormone ghrelin and decreases the satiety hormone leptin—which may help explain some of the association between inadequate sleep and increases in the desire for high-kcalorie foods, energy intake, and weight gains.[18]

Table 9-1 summarizes key characteristics of leptin and ghrelin. Together, these two proteins illustrate some of the complex factors involved in the regulation of food intake and energy homeostasis. Scientists have identified numerous proteins expressed by dozens of genes linked to food intake, obesity, and fat distribution in the body.[19] Each of these genes has slight variations that differ among individuals. Furthermore, these genes interact with one another and with the environment. The complexity of it all creates a multitude of possible genetic explanations.

Uncoupling Proteins Genes also code for proteins involved in energy metabolism. These proteins may influence the storing or expending of energy with different efficiencies or in different types of fat. The body has different types of adipose tissue and the quantities of each is determined by genes.[20] White adipose tissue stores fat for other cells to use for energy; **brown adipose tissue** releases stored energy as heat, thus defending against cold and preventing obesity. Recall from Chapter 7 that in *coupled reactions*, the energy released from the breakdown of one compound is used to create a bond in the formation of another compound. For example, when fat is oxidized, some of the energy is released in heat and some is captured in the formation of ATP. Metabolism in brown adipose tissue differs; oxidation is uncoupled from ATP formation. In *uncoupled reactions*, all of the energy is released as heat. By radiating energy away as heat, the body expends, rather than stores, energy. In contrast, efficient coupling facilitates synthesis reactions, including the making of fat for storage. In other words, weight gains or losses may depend on whether the body dissipates the energy from an ice cream sundae as heat or stores it in body fat.

brown adipose tissue: masses of specialized fat cells packed with pigmented mitochondria that produce heat instead of ATP.

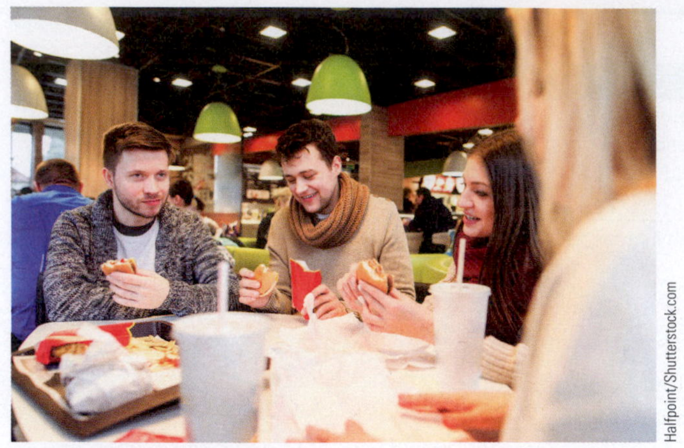
Halfpoint/Shutterstock.com

> **PHOTO 9-1** The food industry spends billions of dollars a year on advertising. The message? "Eat more."

Brown fat and heat production is particularly important in newborn infants and in animals exposed to cold weather, especially those that hibernate. They have plenty of brown adipose tissue. In contrast, human adults have little brown fat, stored primarily around the neck and clavicle. Brown fat is most metabolically active during exposure to cold. Importantly, brown fat activity declines with age and with obesity; overweight and obese individuals have less brown fat activity than others. The role of brown fat in body weight regulation is not yet fully understood, but such an understanding may prove most useful in developing obesity treatments.[21]

Some white fat cells can undergo a process known as browning as they take on characteristics of brown fat, most notably the activity of uncoupled proteins; these fat cells are called **brite adipocytes.**[22] Brite fat cells are far more abundant than brown fat cells in adults. By learning how browning is regulated, researchers hope to tilt energy balance from storage to expenditure in the effort to fight obesity. Interestingly, among the factors that trigger browning is physical activity. During exercise, muscle cells release a protein (the myokine irisin) that triggers the transformation of white fat cells into brite fat cells. Such findings help explain one of the many ways physical activity expends energy and supports weight management. Another factor gaining attention for its influence on the browning of white fat cells is the GI microbiota; the GI microbiota in people who are obese tend to be more limited in diversity and in activity than those in people who are not overweight.[23]

Environment With obesity rates rising and the **gene pool** remaining relatively unchanged, environment must also play a role in obesity. Obesity reflects the interactions between genes and the environment. An **obesogenic environment** includes all of the circumstances that we encounter daily that push us toward fatness (see Photo 9-1). Over the past several decades, the demand for physical activity has decreased as the abundance of food has increased, challenging the human body's ability to defend against weight gains.

Keep in mind that genetic and environmental factors are not mutually exclusive; in fact, their *interactions* create the epigenetics that provide a greater understanding of obesity and related diseases. Genes can influence eating behaviors, for example, and food and activity behaviors influence the genes that regulate body weight.[24] Interestingly, even social relationships can influence food choices and the development of obesity.[25] The likelihood that a person will become obese increases when a friend, sibling, or spouse becomes obese.

Overeating One explanation for obesity is that overweight people overeat, although diet histories may not always reflect high intakes. Diet histories are not always accurate records of actual intakes; both normal-weight and obese people commonly misreport their dietary intakes. Most importantly, current dietary intakes may not reflect the eating habits that led to obesity. Obese people who had a positive energy balance for years and accumulated excess body fat may not currently have a positive energy balance. This reality highlights an important point: the energy-balance equation must consider time. Both present *and* past eating and activity patterns influence current body weight.

We live in an environment that exposes us to an abundance of high-kcalorie foods that are readily available, relatively inexpensive, heavily advertised, and reasonably tasty. No hunger necessary. Food is available everywhere, all the time—thanks largely to fast food. Our highways are lined with fast-food restaurants. Convenience stores and service stations offer fast food and snacks as well. Fast food is available in our schools, malls, and airports. The mere proximity of fast food increases the risk of obesity. Restaurants automatically send mobile coupons to phones as potential customers approach. Food is convenient and it's available morning, noon, and night—and all times in between. Consequently, we

brite adipocytes: white fat cells with brown fat cell characteristics; also called *beige adipocytes.*

gene pool: all the genetic information of a population at a given time.

obesogenic (oh-BES-oh-JEN-ick) **environment:** all the factors surrounding a person that promote weight gain, such as increased food intake, especially of unhealthy choices, and decreased physical activity.

are eating more meals more frequently than in decades past—and energy intake has risen accordingly. By comparison, simply eating meals at regularly scheduled times can be helpful in managing weight.[26]

Most alarming are the extraordinarily large portions and ready-to-go combo-meals (see Photo 9-2). Eating large portion sizes multiple times a day accounts for much of the weight increase seen over the decades. People buy the large portions and combinations, perceiving them to be a good value, but then they eat more than they need—a bad deal.

Simply put, large portion sizes deliver more kcalories. And portion sizes of virtually all foods and beverages have increased markedly in the past several decades, most notably at fast-food restaurants. Not only have portion sizes increased over time, but they are now two to eight times larger than standard serving sizes. The trend toward large portion sizes parallels the increasing prevalence of overweight and obesity in the United States, beginning in the 1970s, increasing sharply in the 1980s, and continuing today.

Restaurant food, especially fast food, contributes significantly to the development of obesity. Fast food is often energy-dense food, which increases energy intake, BMI, and body fatness. The combination of large portions and energy-dense foods is a double whammy. Reducing portion sizes is somewhat helpful, but the real kcalorie savings come from lowering the energy density. Low-energy-density foods such as fruits and vegetables can help with weight loss.

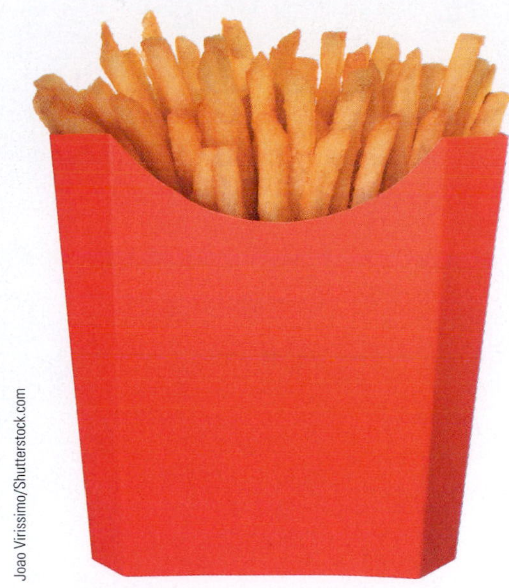

Joao Virissimo/Shutterstock.com

> **PHOTO 9-2** "Want fries with that?" A supersize portion delivers more than 600 kcalories.

Physical Inactivity Our environment fosters physical inactivity as well. Life requires little exertion. Modern technology has replaced physical activity at home, at work, and in transportation. Inactivity contributes to weight gain and poor health. Most physical inactivity occurs when watching television, playing video games, and using the computer. The more time people spend in these sedentary activities, the more likely they are to be overweight—and to incur the metabolic risk factors of chronic diseases (high blood lipids, high blood pressure, and high blood glucose).[27]

Sedentary activities contribute to weight gain in several ways. First, they require little energy beyond the resting metabolic rate. Second, they replace time spent in more vigorous activities. Third, watching television influences food purchases and correlates with between-meal snacking on the high-kcalorie, solid fat and added sugars foods and beverages most heavily advertised.

Some obese people are so extraordinarily inactive that even when they eat less than lean people, they still have an energy surplus. Reducing their food intake further would incur nutrient deficiencies and jeopardize health. Physical activity is a necessary component of nutritional health. People must be physically active if they are to eat enough food to deliver all the nutrients they need without unhealthy weight gain. In fact, *to prevent weight gain,* the DRI suggests an accumulation of 60 minutes of moderately intense physical activities every day in addition to the less intense activities of daily living. Recommendations *to lose weight* encourage even greater duration, intensity, or frequency of physical activity (as a later section of the chapter discusses).

People may be obese, therefore, not because they eat too much, but because they move too little, not only in purposeful exercise, but also in the activities of daily life (see Photo 9-3).[28] Studies report that the differences in the time obese and lean people spend lying, sitting, standing, and moving accounts for about 350 kcalories a day. In general, lean people tend to be more spontaneously active in their occupations and their leisure time. The energy expended in these everyday spontaneous activities—called *nonexercise activity thermogenesis (NEAT)*—plays a pivotal role in energy balance and weight management.

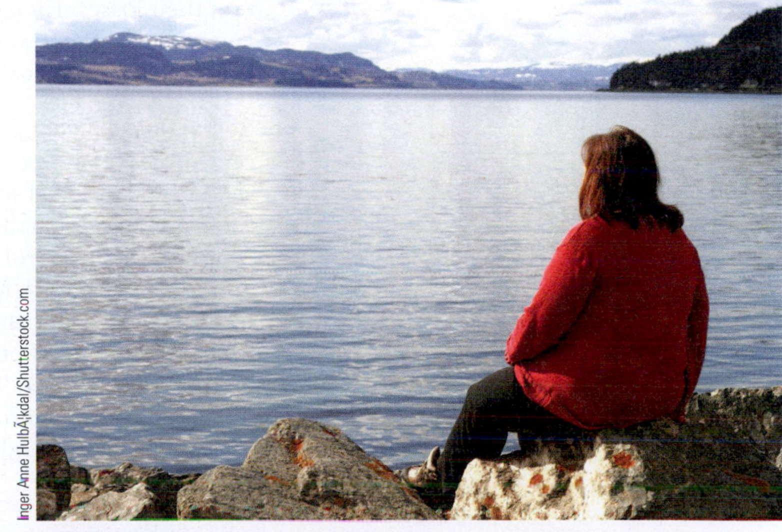

Inger Anne HulbÃ¦kdal/Shutterstock.com

> **PHOTO 9-3** Lack of physical activity fosters obesity.

REVIEW IT Review some of the causes of obesity.
Obesity has many causes and most interact, creating a complex scenario. Environmental factors, such as overeating and physical inactivity, may influence a person's genetic susceptibility to obesity.

9.3 Problems of Overweight and Obesity

LEARN IT Discuss the physical, social, and psychological consequences of overweight and obesity.

Millions of US adults are trying to lose weight on any given day. Some of these people may not even need to lose weight. Others may benefit from weight loss, but they will not be successful. Relatively few people succeed in losing weight, and even fewer succeed permanently. For many, improving diet and activity habits to simply prevent further weight gains may be sufficient. Whether a person will benefit from weight loss is a question of health.

Health Risks

Chapter 8 described some of the health problems that commonly accompany obesity. To determine the potential health risks of obesity, health-care professionals use BMI and waist circumference. The higher the BMI and the greater the waist circumference, the greater the risk of heart disease, type 2 diabetes, and all-cause mortality.

Weight loss is recommended for people who are obese (BMI ≥30) and for those who are overweight (BMI 25 to 29.9) with one or more of the following obesity-related risk factors:

- Hypertension
- Fatty liver disease
- Abnormal blood lipids
- Diabetes or prediabetes
- Sleep apnea

Even modest, sustained weight loss can improve blood lipids, blood glucose, and blood pressure; greater weight loss may produce greater benefits and even reduce the need for medications.[29]

Perceptions and Prejudices

Many people assume that every obese person can achieve slenderness and should pursue that goal. First consider that most obese people do not—for whatever reason—successfully lose weight and maintain their losses. Then consider the prejudice involved in that assumption. People come with varying weight tendencies, just as they come with varying potentials for height and physical talents.

Social Consequences Large segments of our society place such enormous value on thinness that obese people face prejudice and discrimination on the job, at school, and in social situations: they are judged on their appearance more than on their character. Socially, obese people may be negatively stereotyped as lazy and lacking in self-control. Such discrimination may actually exacerbate overeating and increase the risk for obesity.[30] This critical view of overweight is not prevalent in many other cultures, including segments of our own society. Instead, overweight is simply accepted or even embraced as a sign of robust health and beauty. To free society of its obsession with body weight and prejudice against obesity, people must first learn to judge others—and themselves—for who they are and not for what they weigh.

Psychological Problems Psychologically, obese people may suffer embarrassment when others treat them with hostility and contempt, and many have come to view their own bodies as flawed. Feelings of rejection, shame, and depression are common among obese people. Anxiety and depression, in turn, may contribute to the development of obesity, which perpetuates the problem.

Most weight-loss programs assume that the problem can be solved simply by applying willpower and hard work. If determination were the only factor involved, though, the success rate would be far greater than it is. Overweight people may readily assume blame for failure to lose weight and maintain the losses when, in fact, it is the programs that have failed. Ineffective treatment and its associated sense of failure add to a person's psychological burden. Figure 9-4 illustrates how the devastating psychological effects of obesity and dieting perpetuate themselves.

> **FIGURE 9-4 The Psychology of Weight Cycling**

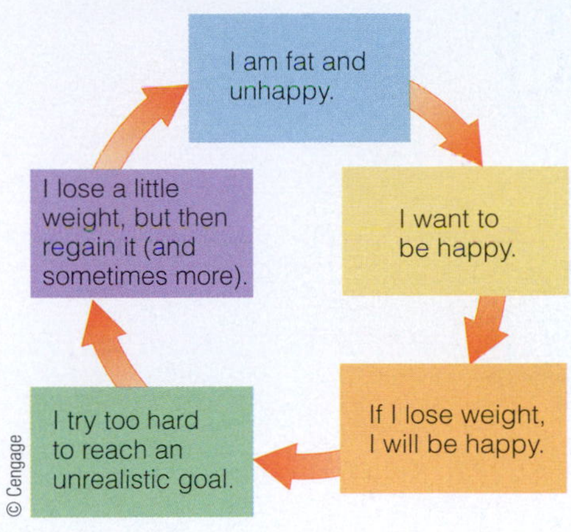
I am fat and unhappy.
I want to be happy.
If I lose weight, I will be happy.
I try too hard to reach an unrealistic goal.
I lose a little weight, but then regain it (and sometimes more).
© Cengage

Dangerous Interventions Some people attach so many dreams of happiness to weight loss that they willingly risk huge sums of money for the slightest chance of success. As a result, weight-loss schemes flourish. Of the tens of thousands of claims, treatments, and theories for losing weight, few are effective—and many are downright dangerous. The negative consequences must be carefully considered before embarking on any weight-loss program. Some interventions entail greater dangers than the risk of being overweight. Physical, metabolic, and psychosocial problems may arise from fad diets and **weight cycling**.[31] Wise consumers scrutinize fad diets, magic potions, and wonder gizmos with a healthy dose of skepticism.

Some of the nation's most popular diet books and weight-loss programs have misled consumers with unsubstantiated claims and deceptive testimonials. Furthermore, they fail to provide an assessment of the short- and long-term results of their treatment plans, even though such evaluations are possible and would permit consumers to make informed decisions. Of course, some weight-loss programs are better than others in terms of cost, approach, and customer satisfaction. Reputable weight-loss programs will explain the risks associated with their plans and provide honest predictions of success.

Fad Diets **Fad diets** often sound good, but they typically fall short of delivering on their promises. They espouse exaggerated or false theories of weight loss and advise consumers to follow inadequate diets. Some fad diets are hazardous to health as Highlight 9 explains. Adverse reactions can be as minor as headaches, nausea, and dizziness or as serious as death. How To H9-1 (p. 291) offers guidelines for identifying unsound weight-loss schemes and fad diets.

Weight-Loss Products In their search for weight-loss magic, some consumers turn to "natural" herbal products and dietary supplements, even though few have proved to be effective and many have proved to be harmful (see Photo 9-4).

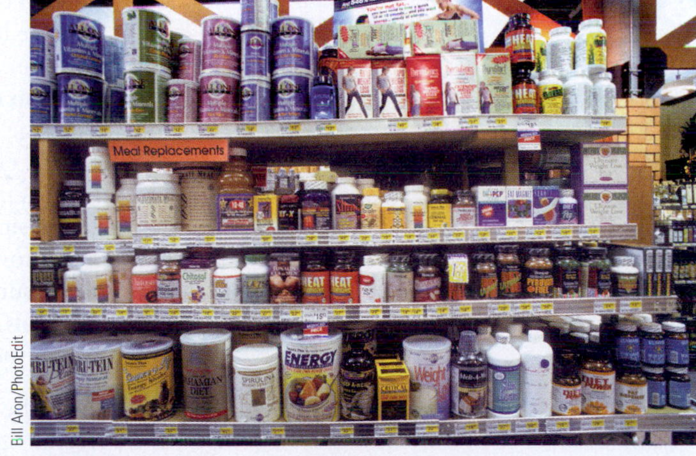
Meal Replacements
Bill Aron/PhotoEdit

> **PHOTO 9-4** So many promises, so little success.

Highlight 18 explores the possible benefits and potential dangers of herbal products and other alternative therapies. As it explains, dietary supplements do not need to be approved by the FDA, and manufacturers do not need to test the safety or effectiveness of any product. In other words, consumers cannot assume that an herbal product or dietary supplement is safe or effective just because it is available on the market. In fact, the FDA has identified hundreds of products that contain undeclared, active pharmaceutical ingredients that can have serious consequences such as seizures and heart attacks.[32] These ingredients are not listed on the labels, and consumers have no way of knowing what the products actually contain. Thousands of young adults seek help from an emergency room each year for symptoms such as chest pain and heart palpitations caused by herbal and complementary nutritional products used for weight loss.[33] Anyone considering whether to use dietary supplements for weight loss should consult with a physician and research the product with the FDA (www.fda.gov).

Other Gimmicks Other gimmicks don't help with weight loss either. Hot baths do not speed up metabolism so that pounds can be lost in hours. Steam and sauna

weight cycling: repeated loss and regain of body weight; sometimes called *yo-yo* dieting when weight cycling results from sporadic restrictive dieting.

fad diets: popular eating plans that promise quick weight loss. Most fad diets severely limit certain foods or overemphasize others (for example, never eat potatoes or pasta, or eat cabbage soup daily).

baths do not melt the fat off the body, although they may dehydrate people so that they lose water weight. Brushes, sponges, wraps, creams, and massages intended to move, burn, or break up fat do nothing of the kind.

REVIEW IT Discuss the physical, social, and psychological consequences of overweight and obesity.

The question of whether a person should lose weight depends on many factors: among them are the extent of overweight, age, health, and genetic makeup. Not all obesity will cause disease or shorten life expectancy. Just as there are unhealthy, normal-weight people, there are healthy, overweight people. Some people may risk more in the process of losing weight than in remaining overweight. Fad diets and weight-loss supplements can be as physically and psychologically damaging as excess body weight.

9.4 Aggressive Treatments for Obesity

LEARN IT Explain the risks and benefits, if any, of aggressive ways to treat obesity.

The appropriate strategies for weight loss depend on the degree of obesity and the risk of disease. An overweight person in good health may need only to improve eating habits and increase physical activity, but someone with **clinically severe obesity** may need more aggressive treatment options—drugs or surgery. Drugs appear to be modestly effective and safe, at least in the short term; surgery appears to be dramatically effective but can have severe complications, at least for some people.

Drugs

Based on new understandings of obesity's genetic component and its classification as a chronic disease, much research effort has focused on drug treatments for obesity. Experts reason that if obesity is a chronic disease, it should be treated as such—and the treatment of most chronic diseases includes drugs. The challenge, then, is to develop an effective drug—or more likely, a combination of drugs—that can be used over time without adverse side effects or the potential for abuse. Weight-loss drugs should be prescribed only to those with medical risks—not for cosmetic reasons—and in tandem with a healthy diet and activity program.

Several drugs for weight loss have been tried over the years, with varying degrees of effectiveness and safety. When used as part of a long-term, comprehensive weight-loss program, drugs can help with meaningful weight loss.[34] Because weight regain commonly occurs with the discontinuation of drug therapy, treatment must be long term. Yet the long-term use of drugs poses risks. We don't yet know whether a person would be harmed more from maintaining a 100-pound excess or from taking a drug for a decade to keep the 100 pounds off. Physicians must prescribe drugs appropriately, inform consumers of the potential risks, and monitor side effects carefully. Table 9-2 presents the drugs to treat obesity that meet the FDA mandate that "benefits must exceed risks."[35]

Some physicians prescribe drugs that have not been approved for weight loss, a practice known as "off-label" use. These drugs have been approved for other conditions (such as seizures) and incidentally cause modest weight loss. Physicians using off-label drugs must be well-informed of the drugs' use and effects and monitor their patients' responses closely.

Surgery

The US prevalence of clinically severe obesity (BMI ≥40) is estimated at 8 percent.[36] At this level of obesity, lifestyle changes and modest weight losses can improve disease risks a little, but the most effective treatment is **bariatric** surgery.[37] Surgery may be an option for people with all of the following conditions:

- Unable to achieve adequate weight loss with diet and exercise
- BMI ≥40 or BMI ≥35 with obesity-related health problems (such as diabetes or hypertension)
- No medical or psychological contraindications
- Understanding of risks and strong motivation to comply with post-surgery treatment plan

clinically severe obesity: a BMI of 40 or greater or a BMI of 35 or greater with additional medical problems. A less preferred term used to describe the same condition is *morbid obesity*.

bariatric: pertaining to the field of medicine that specializes in treating obesity.

TABLE 9-2 FDA-Approved Drugs for Weight Loss

Drugs	Actions	Side Effects
Bupropion (an antidepressant and smoking cessation drug) and naltrexone (an opioid receptor antagonist used for alcohol and drug abuse) combination, trade name: Contrave	Increases metabolism, suppresses appetite	Nausea, increased heart rate and blood pressure, suicidal thoughts
Liraglutide, trade name: Saxenda	Acts like a hormone to control blood glucose, suppresses appetite	Nausea, diarrhea, constipation, vomiting, low blood glucose, increased heart rate, pancreatitis, gallbladder disease, suicidal thoughts
Lorcaserin (lor-ka-SER-in) hydrochloride, trade name: Belviq (BELL-veek)	Interacts with brain serotonin receptors to increase satiety and reduce food intake	Headache, dizziness, fatigue, nausea, dry mouth, and constipation; low blood glucose in people with diabetes; serotonin syndrome, including agitation, confusion, fever, loss of coordination, rapid or irregular heart rate, shivering, seizures, and unconsciousness; cannot be safely used by pregnant or lactating women or people with heart-valve problems; high doses cause hallucinations
Orlistat (OR-leh-stat), trade names: Alli, Xenical	Inhibits pancreatic lipase activity in the GI tract, thus blocking digestion and absorption of dietary fat and limiting energy intake	GI cramping, diarrhea, gas, frequent bowel movements, reduced absorption of fat-soluble vitamins; rare cases of liver injury
Phentermine (an appetite suppressant) and topiramate (a seizure/migraine medication) combination, trade name: Qsymia (kyoo-sim-EE-uh)	Enhances the release of the neurotransmitter norepinephrine, which suppresses appetite, and increases the feeling of being full, making foods taste less appealing	Increased heart rate; can cause birth defects if taken in the first weeks or months of pregnancy; suicidal thoughts; may worsen glaucoma and other eye problems

NOTE: Weight-loss drugs are most effective when taken as directed and used in combination with reduced-kcalorie diet and increased physical activity.

Almost 200,000 such surgeries are performed in the United States annually. Figure 9-5 shows how common surgical procedures effectively limit food intake by reducing the capacity of the stomach. In addition, bariatric surgery suppresses hunger and alters metabolism by changing production of hormones.[38] Changes in appetite, food preferences, and GI microbiota may also influence weight losses.[39] The results are significant: depending on the type of surgery, 20 to 30 percent of the excess weight remains lost after 10 years.[40] Importantly, most people experience dramatic and lasting improvements in their diabetes,

> FIGURE 9-5 Surgical Procedures for Severe Obesity

All of these surgical procedures limit the amount of food that can be comfortably eaten. The dark pink area shows the altered flow of food through the GI tract. The pale pink area indicates the bypassed sections.

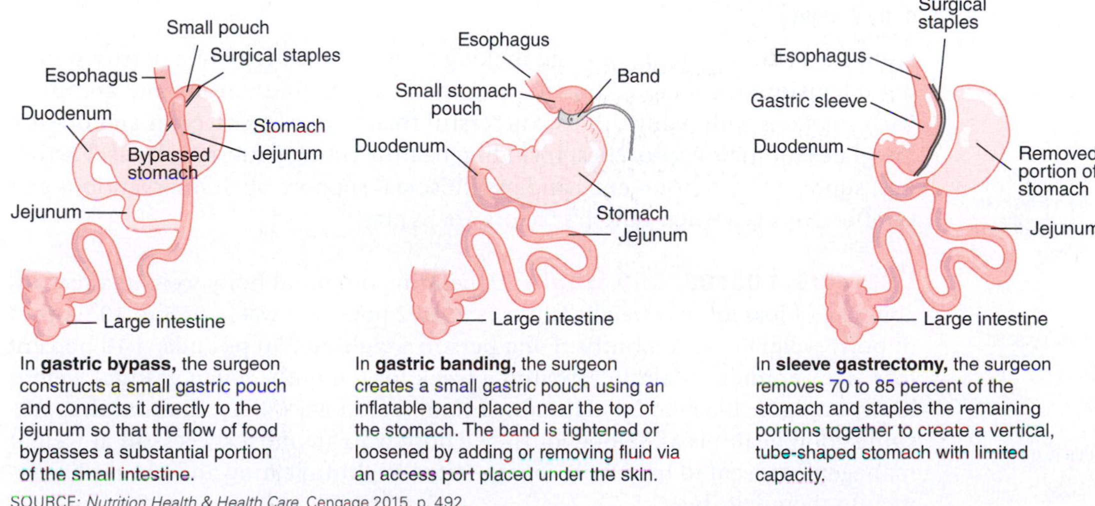
Small pouch
Surgical staples
Esophagus
Duodenum
Stomach
Bypassed stomach
Jejunum
Jejunum
Large intestine
Esophagus
Small stomach pouch
Band
Duodenum
Stomach
Jejunum
Large intestine
Surgical staples
Esophagus
Gastric sleeve
Duodenum
Removed portion of stomach
Jejunum
Large intestine

In **gastric bypass,** the surgeon constructs a small gastric pouch and connects it directly to the jejunum so that the flow of food bypasses a substantial portion of the small intestine.

In **gastric banding,** the surgeon creates a small gastric pouch using an inflatable band placed near the top of the stomach. The band is tightened or loosened by adding or removing fluid via an access port placed under the skin.

In **sleeve gastrectomy,** the surgeon removes 70 to 85 percent of the stomach and staples the remaining portions together to create a vertical, tube-shaped stomach with limited capacity.

SOURCE: *Nutrition Health & Health Care*, Cengage 2015, p. 492.

blood lipids, and blood pressure; the risk of heart attacks, strokes, and cancer is also reduced.[41] Some evidence suggests improvements in depression and anxiety as well.[42] Overall, bariatric surgery provides clear advantages for greater weight loss and long-term survival over nonsurgical options for obese adults.[43]

The long-term safety and effectiveness of surgery depend, in large part, on compliance with dietary instructions, making nutrition care plans essential in follow-up treatment.[44] With limited food intake and reduced absorptive surfaces, vitamin and mineral deficiencies are common, and have been linked to problems such as periodontal disease.[45] Care plans include instructions to improve food selections as well as prescriptions for dietary supplements.[46] Weight regain may occur and psychological problems—such as disordered eating behaviors—may also develop. Lifelong medical supervision is necessary, but the possible health benefits of weight loss—improved blood lipds, blood pressure, and insulin sensitivity—may outweigh the risks. Overall risk of death and heart disease is lower for obese people after successful surgery than for obese people who do not undergo surgery.

Other Medical Procedures Several **endoscopic procedures** have recently been approved for weight loss. One such effective procedure involves the insertion of an **intragastric balloon**, which occupies space in the stomach, thus enhancing feelings of fullness and diminishing food intake.[47] Another safe and effective procedure uses **gastric aspiration** to empty the contents of the stomach 20 to 30 minutes after each meal.[48] Compared with drugs and surgery, these endoscopic procedures are less invasive, less expensive, and easily reversible.[49]

A different type of medical procedure removes some fat deposits by liposuction. This cosmetic procedure has little effect on body weight (less than 10 pounds), but can alter body shape in specific areas. Liposuction is a popular procedure in part because of its perceived safety, but immediate and delayed complications can arise. Furthermore, removing adipose tissue by way of liposuction does not provide the health benefits that typically accompany weight loss.

REVIEW IT Explain the risks and benefits, if any, of aggressive ways to treat obesity.

Overweight and obese people may benefit most from improving eating and activity habits. Those with clinically severe obesity and high risks of medical problems may need more aggressive treatment, including drugs or surgery. Such treatments may offer benefits, but also incur some risks.

9.5 Weight-Loss Strategies

LEARN IT Outline reasonable strategies for achieving and maintaining a healthy body weight.

From the bustling activity of a cell making fat to the inactivity of a person watching television, the factors contributing to obesity are numerous and complex. Each interacts with many others. Successful treatment of overweight and obesity integrates multiple approaches, including healthy eating patterns, physical activities, supportive environments, and psychosocial support; such interventions can be effective, even when genetics factors are in play.[50]

Changes, Losses, and Goals Depending on initial body weight, a reasonable rate of loss for overweight adults is ½ to 2 pounds a week, or 5 to 10 percent of body weight over 6 months. For a person weighing 250 pounds, a 10 percent loss is 25 pounds, or about 1 pound a week for 6 months. Such gradual weight losses are more likely to be maintained than rapid losses. Keep in mind that pursuing good health is a lifelong journey. Those who are most successful at weight management seem to have fully incorporated healthful eating and physical activity into their daily lives.

endoscopic procedures: practices that require a physician to insert a medical device into the body (in this case, the gastrointestinal tract) to examine or treat a disorder.
- **endo** = within
- **scope** = examine

intragastric balloon: a saline-filled silicone device placed in the stomach to limit food intake.
- **intra** = within
- **gastric** = stomach

gastric aspiration: a technique that uses a tube to empty the contents of the stomach after every meal.
- **aspire** = drawing something in or out

Even modest weight loss can improve blood glucose and reduce the risks of heart disease by lowering blood pressure and blood lipds, especially for those with central obesity. Improvements in physical capabilities and quality of life become evident with even a 5-percent weight loss.[51] For these reasons, parameters such as blood pressure, blood lipds, or even vitality are more useful than body weight in marking success. People less concerned with disease risks may prefer to set goals for personal fitness, such as being able to play with children or climb stairs without becoming short of breath. Importantly, they can focus on healthy eating and activity habits instead of weight loss.

Eating Patterns

Contrary to the claims of fad diets, no single food plan is magical, and no specific food must be included or avoided in a weight-management program. In designing an eating pattern, people need only consider foods that they like or can learn to like, that are available, and that are within their means. Instead of focusing on unhealthy foods to avoid (such as french fries), successful dieters embrace healthy foods (such as spinach) that they are willing to eat.[52] Creating a healthful eating pattern is the first step. The important next step is following it for the rest of one's life. Achieving and maintaining a healthy weight requires permanent lifestyle changes.

Be Realistic about Energy Intake The main characteristic of a weight-loss diet is that it provides less energy than the person needs to maintain present body weight. If food energy is restricted too severely, dieters may not receive sufficient nutrients. Rapid weight loss usually means excessive loss of lean tissue, a lower BMR, and rapid weight regains to follow. The composition of regained weight is more fat and less lean than the composition of the originally lost weight. In addition, restrictive eating may create stress or foster the unhealthy behaviors of eating disorders, as Highlight 8 describes.

Energy intake should provide nutritional adequacy without excess—that is, somewhere between deprivation and complete freedom to eat whatever, whenever. A reasonable suggestion for overweight and obese adults is to increase activity and reduce food intake enough to create a deficit of 500 to 750 kcalories per day. Such a deficit produces a weight loss of about 1 to 2 pounds per week—a rate that supports the loss of fat efficiently while retaining lean tissue. In general, weight-loss diets need to provide about 1200 to 1500 kcalories per day for women and 1500 to 1800 kcalories a day for men.

Some people skip meals, typically breakfast, in an effort to reduce energy intake and lose weight. Research does not support such a causal relationship between breakfast and weight loss, but it does suggest some interesting associations.[53] Breakfast frequency is inversely associated with obesity and its associated risk factors—that is, people who regularly eat breakfast have a lower BMI, blood pressure, and blood lipds than those who tend to skip breakfast.[54] Furthermore, eating breakfast, especially a protein-rich breakfast, improves satiety and diet quality—two factors that support healthy body weight.[55] One study found that even when total kcalories were the same on two weight-loss diets, the "breakfast diet" (big breakfast, medium lunch, and small dinner) had better results than the "dinner diet" (small breakfast, medium lunch, and big dinner).[56] After three months, the women on the breakfast diet lost 10 more pounds than the others; had better triglycerides, HDL, blood glucose, and waist circumference measures; and were less hungry.

Emphasize Nutritional Adequacy Healthy eating patterns make nutritional adequacy a priority. Nutritional adequacy is difficult to achieve on fewer than 1200 kcalories a day, and most healthy adults need never consume any less. A plan that provides an adequate intake supports a healthier and more successful weight loss than a restrictive plan that creates feelings of starvation and deprivation, which can lead to an irresistible urge to binge.

Table 9-3 (p. 274) specifies the amounts of foods from each food group for diets providing 1200 to 1800 kcalories. Such an intake would allow most

TABLE 9-3 Daily Amounts from Each Food Group for 1200- to 1800-kCalorie Diets

Food Group	1200 kCalories	1400 kCalories	1600 kCalories	1800 kCalories
Fruit	1 c	1½ c	1½ c	1½ c
Vegetables	1½ c	1½ c	2 c	2½ c
Grains	4 oz	5 oz	5 oz	6 oz
Protein foods	3 oz	4 oz	5 oz	5 oz
Milk and milk products	2½ c	2½ c	3 c	3 c
Oils	4 tsp	4 tsp	5 tsp	5 tsp

people to lose weight and still meet their nutrient needs with careful selections of low-kcalorie, nutrient-dense foods. Keep in mind, too, that well-balanced diets that emphasize fruits, vegetables, whole grains, lean protein foods, and low-fat milk products offer many health rewards even when they don't result in weight loss.[57] A dietary supplement providing vitamins and minerals—especially iron and calcium for women—at or below 100 percent of the Daily Values can help people following low-kcalorie diets to achieve nutrient adequacy.

Eat Small Portions As mentioned earlier, portion sizes at markets, at restaurants, and even at home have increased dramatically over the years, contributing significantly to energy intake and weight gains. We have come to expect large portions, and we have learned to clean our plates. Many of us pay more attention to these external cues defining how much to eat than to our internal cues of hunger and satiety. For health's sake, we may need to learn to eat less food at each meal—one piece of chicken for dinner instead of two, a teaspoon of butter on vegetables instead of a tablespoon, and one cookie for dessert instead of six. Single-serve packages may be helpful in limiting portions.[58] The goal is to eat enough food for adequate energy, abundant vitamins and minerals, and some pleasure, but not more. This amount should leave a person feeling satisfied—not stuffed. A saying credited to Confucius captures this concept—*hara hachi bu*—which translates to "eat until you are 80 percent full."

People who have difficulty making low-kcalorie selections or controlling portion sizes may find it easier to use prepared meal plans. Prepared meals that provide low-kcalorie, nutritious meals or snacks can support weight loss, lower the risk of type 2 diabetes, and ease the task of diet planning.[59] Ideally, those using a prepared meal plan will also receive counseling from a registered dietitian nutritionist to learn how to select appropriately from conventional food choices as well.

Slow Down Eating can be a pleasurable experience, and taking the time to savor the flavors can help with weight management. Eating slowly, taking small bites, and chewing thoroughly all help to decrease food intake.[60] A person who slows down and savors each bite eats less before hormones signal satiety and the end of a meal. Consequently, energy intake is lower when meals are eaten slowly. Savoring each bite also activates the pleasure centers of the brain. Some research suggests that people may overeat when the brain doesn't sense enough gratification from food. Faster eating correlates with lower diet-induced thermogenesis, greater energy intake, and higher BMI.[61]

Lower Energy Density Most people take their cues about how much to eat based on portion sizes, and the larger the portion size, the more they eat. To lower energy intake, a person can either reduce the portion size or reduce the energy density. Reducing energy density while maintaining or even increasing food viscosity or quantity seems to be a successful strategy to control hunger and manage weight.[62] This concept of using large quantities of low-energy-density foods is

> FIGURE 9-6 Energy Density

Decreasing the energy density (kcal/g) of foods allows a person to eat satisfying portions while still reducing energy intake. To lower energy density, select foods high in water or fiber and low in fat.

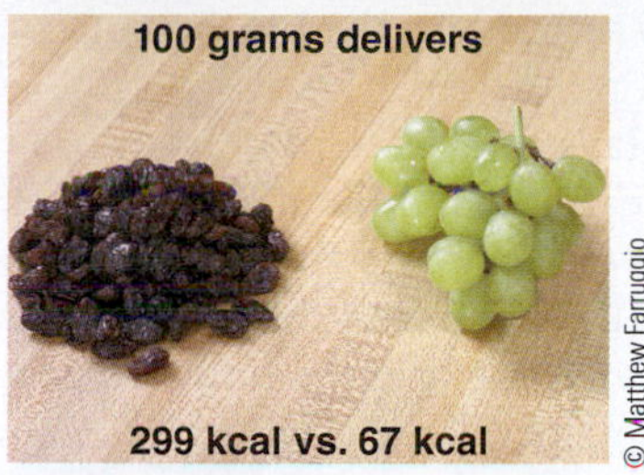
100 grams delivers
299 kcal vs. 67 kcal
© Matthew Farruggio

Selecting grapes with their high water content instead of raisins increases the volume and cuts the energy intake.

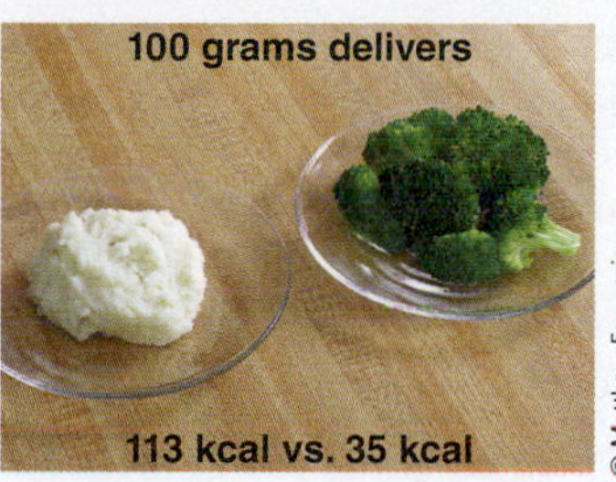
100 grams delivers
113 kcal vs. 35 kcal
© Matthew Farruggio

Even at the same weight and similar serving sizes, the fiber-rich broccoli delivers twice the fiber for about one-third the energy of mashed potatoes.

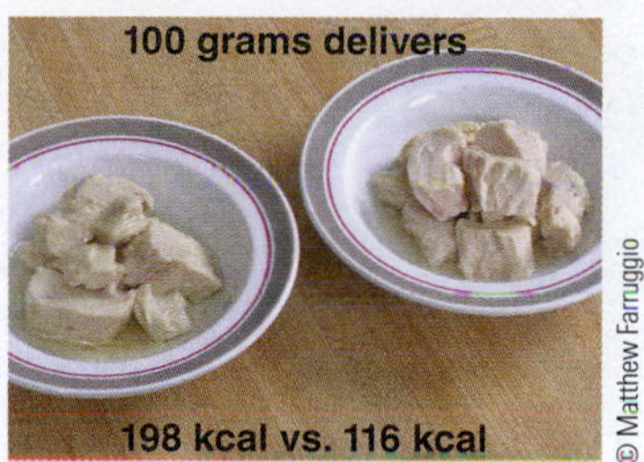
100 grams delivers
198 kcal vs. 116 kcal
© Matthew Farruggio

By selecting the water-packed tuna (on the right) instead of the oil-packed tuna (on the left), a person can enjoy the same amount for fewer kcalories.

sometimes referred to as *volumetrics*. Figure 9-6 illustrates how water, fiber, and fat influence energy density, and How To 9-1 compares foods based on their energy density. Foods containing water, those rich in fiber, and those low in fat help to lower energy density, providing more satiety for fewer kcalories. Because a low-energy-density diet is a low-fat, high-fiber diet rich in many vitamins and minerals, it supports good health in addition to weight loss.

Remember Water In addition to lowering the energy density of foods, water seems to help those who are trying to lose or maintain weight.[63] For one, foods with high water content (such as broth-based soups) increase fullness, reduce hunger, and consequently reduce energy intake. For another, drinking a large glass of water before a meal eases hunger, fills the stomach, and consequently reduces energy intake. Importantly, water adds no kcalories. On average, sugar-sweetened beverages contribute about 135 kcalories a day. Simply replacing nutrient-poor, energy-dense soda with water can help a person lower energy intake by at least 5 percent.[64] Water also helps the GI tract adapt to a high-fiber diet.

Focus on Plant-Based Foods Plant-based foods such as fresh fruits, vegetables, legumes, and whole grains and vegetarian eating patterns may help with weight management and improve the inflammation that accompanies obesity.[65] These foods offer abundant vitamins, minerals, and fiber. Eating high-fiber foods also takes time, which eases hunger and promotes satiety.

> How To 9-1 Compare Foods Based on Energy Density

Chapter 2 described how to evaluate foods based on their nutrient density—their nutrient contribution per kcalorie. Another way to evaluate foods is to consider their energy density—their energy contribution per gram. This example compares carrot sticks with french fries. The conclusion is no surprise, but understanding the mathematics may offer valuable insight into the concept of energy density. A carrot weighing 72 grams delivers 31 kcalories. To calculate the energy density, divide kcalories by grams:

$$\frac{31\text{ kcal}}{72\text{ g}} = 0.43\text{ kcal/g}$$

Do the same for french fries weighing 50 grams and contributing 167 kcalories:

$$\frac{167\text{ kcal}}{50\text{ g}} = 3.34\text{ kcal/g}$$

The more kcalories per gram, the greater the energy density. French fries are more energy dense than carrots. They provide more energy per gram—and per bite. Considering a food's energy density is especially useful in planning diets for weight management. Foods with a high energy density help with weight gain, whereas foods with a low energy density help with weight loss.

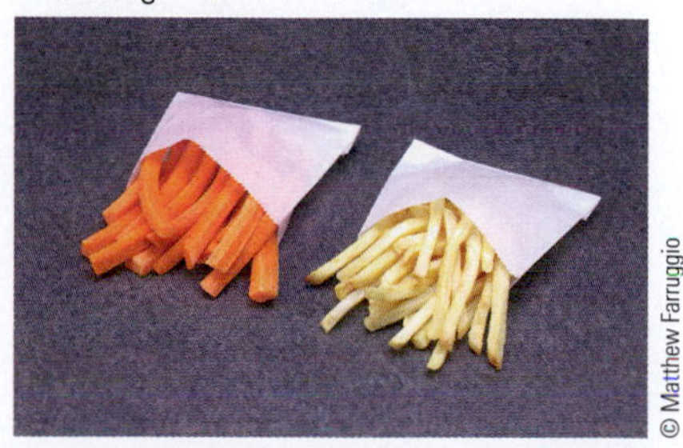
© Matthew Farruggio

> TRY IT Compare the energy density of a hard-boiled egg (50 grams and 78 kcalories) with light tuna canned in water (57 grams and 66 kcalories).

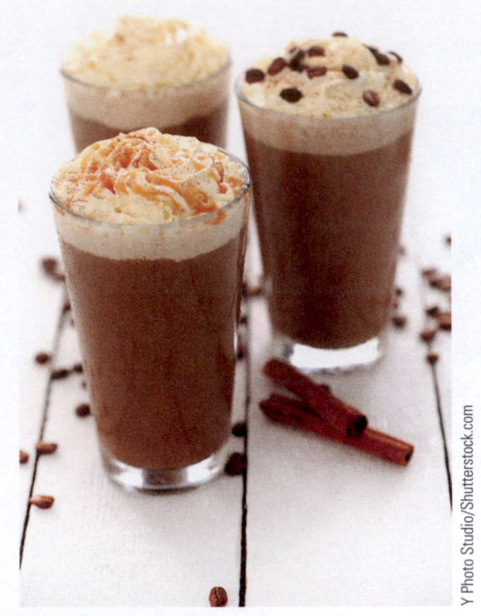

Y Photo Studio/Shutterstock.com

> **PHOTO 9-5** If you want to lose weight, steer clear of the empty kcalories in fancy coffee drinks. A 16-ounce caffè mocha delivers 400 kcalories—half of them from fat and the other half from sugar.

Choose Fats Sensibly One way to lower energy intake is to lower fat intake. Lowering the fat content of a food lowers its energy density—for example, selecting fat-free milk instead of whole milk. That way, a person can consume the usual amount (say, a cup of milk) at a lower energy intake (85 instead of 150 kcalories).

Fat has a weak satiating effect, and satiation plays a key role in determining food intake during a meal. Consequently, a person eating a high-fat meal increases energy intake in two ways—more food and more fat kcalories (see Photo 9-5). For these reasons, measure fat with extra caution. (Review p. 153 for strategies to lower fat in the diet.) Be careful not to take this advice to extremes, however; too little fat incurs health risks as well, as Chapter 5 explained.

A low-fat diet can lead to weight loss, but no more so than other plans.[66] An important point to notice in any discussion on weight-loss diets is total energy intake. A low-fat diet supports weight loss only when energy intake is less than energy expenditure.

Select Carbohydrates Carefully Another popular way to lower energy intake is to lower carbohydrate intake. Highlight 4's discussion of carbohydrate-restricted and carbohydrate-modified diets reaches the same conclusion as the previous paragraph on low-fat diets: they work only when energy intake is less than energy expenditure.

Chapter 4 described how foods with added sugars increase energy intake and contribute to weight gain. Limiting consumption of foods with added sugars can help with weight management. One way people try to control weight is to use foods and beverages sweetened with artificial sweeteners. Using artificial sweeteners instead of sugars can lower energy intake and may support modest weight loss, or at least prevent weight gain, although evidence is inconsistent.[67] In fact, some research indicates that artificial sweeteners may stimulate appetite by diminishing brain activity that signals reward and controls food intake, thus making it more likely that people drinking diet sodas would eat more later in the day. Artificial sweeteners may also induce glucose intolerance by changing the diversity and activity of GI microbiota, thus making it more likely that people drinking diet sodas would have higher blood glucose levels.[68]

To what extent artificial sweeteners can help someone lose weight depends in part on the person's motivations and actions. For example, one person might drink an artificially sweetened beverage now so as to be able to eat a high-kcalorie food later. This person's energy intake might stay the same or increase. A person trying to control energy intake might drink an artificially sweetened beverage now and choose a low-kcalorie food later. This plan would help reduce the person's total energy intake. Findings from a national survey reveal that among overweight and obese consumers, those who drink diet beverages end up with the same total energy intake as those who drink sugar-sweetened beverages because they consume more kcalories from their meals and snacks.[69] Clearly, using artificial sweeteners will not automatically lower energy intake. To control energy intake successfully, a person needs to make informed diet and activity decisions throughout the day.

Watch for Other Empty kCalories A person trying to achieve or maintain a healthy weight needs to pay attention not only to fat and sugar, but to alcohol too. Not only does alcohol add kcalories, but it disproportionately contributes to visceral fat.[70] Accompanying mixers can also add both kcalories and fat, especially in creamy drinks such as piña coladas (review Table H7-3, p. 225). Furthermore, drinking alcohol reduces a person's inhibitions, which can lead to excessive eating.

Physical Activity

Whether trying to minimize weight gains or support weight losses, the best approach includes physical activity.[71] To prevent weight gains and support weight losses, current recommendations advise 200 to 300 minutes of moderately intense physical activity a week in addition to activities of daily living.[72]

People who combine diet and exercise typically lose more fat, retain more muscle, and regain less weight than those who only follow a weight-loss diet. Even when they do not lose more weight, they seem to follow their diet plans more closely and maintain their losses better than those who do not exercise. Consequently, they benefit from taking in a little less energy from the diet as well as from expending a little more energy in physical activity. Importantly, those who exercise reap important health benefits—reduced abdominal obesity and improved blood pressure, insulin resistance, and cardiorespiratory fitness—regardless of weight loss.[73] Fitness benefits—such as strength and balance—also improve when exercise is part of a weight-loss program. Chapter 14 presents the many benefits of physical activity; the focus here is on its role in weight management.

Activity and Energy Expenditure Table 8-3 (p. 238) shows how much energy each of several activities uses. The number of kcalories spent in an activity depends on body weight, intensity, and duration. For example, a person who weighs 150 pounds and walks 3½ miles in 60 minutes expends about 315 kcalories. That same person running 3 miles in 30 minutes uses a similar amount. By comparison, a 200-pound person running 3 miles in 30 minutes expends an additional 100 kcalories or so. The goal is to expend as much energy as your time allows. The greater the energy deficit created by exercise, the greater the fat loss. And be careful not to compensate for the energy expended in exercise by eating more food. Otherwise, energy balance won't shift, and fat loss will be less significant.

Activity and Discretionary kCalories Chapter 2 introduced the concept of discretionary kcalories as the difference between the kcalories needed to supply nutrients and those needed to maintain energy balance. Because exercise expends energy, the energy allowance to maintain weight increases with increased physical activity—yet the energy needed to deliver needed nutrients remains about the same. In this way, physical activity increases discretionary kcalories (see Figure 9-7). Having more discretionary kcalories puts a little wiggle room in a weight-loss diet for such options as second helpings, sweet treats, or alcoholic beverages on occasion. Of course, selecting nutrient-dense foods and *not* using discretionary kcalories will maximize weight loss.

Activity and Metabolism Activity also contributes to energy expenditure in an indirect way—by speeding up metabolism for hours or even days.[74] This postexercise effect may raise the energy expenditure of exercise up to 15 percent. Over the long term, a person who engages in daily vigorous activity gradually develops more lean tissue. Metabolic rate rises accordingly, and this supports continued weight loss or maintenance.

Activity and Body Composition Physically active people have less body fat than sedentary people do—even if they have the same BMI. Physical activity, even without weight loss, changes body composition: body fat decreases and lean body mass increases; high-intensity intermittent exercises may be even more effective at reducing body fat than other types of exercise. Furthermore, physical activity reduces abdominal fat even without weight loss.

Activity and Appetite Control Some people think that being active will increase hunger, but research does not show that exercise causes overeating; in fact, when sedentary people participate in an ongoing activity program, they reduce their energy intake. Active people do have healthy appetites, but appetite is suppressed after exercise.[75] The body has released fuels from storage to support the exercise, so glucose and fatty acids are abundant in the blood. At the same time, the body has suppressed its digestive

> FIGURE 9-7 Influence of Physical Activity on Discretionary kCalories

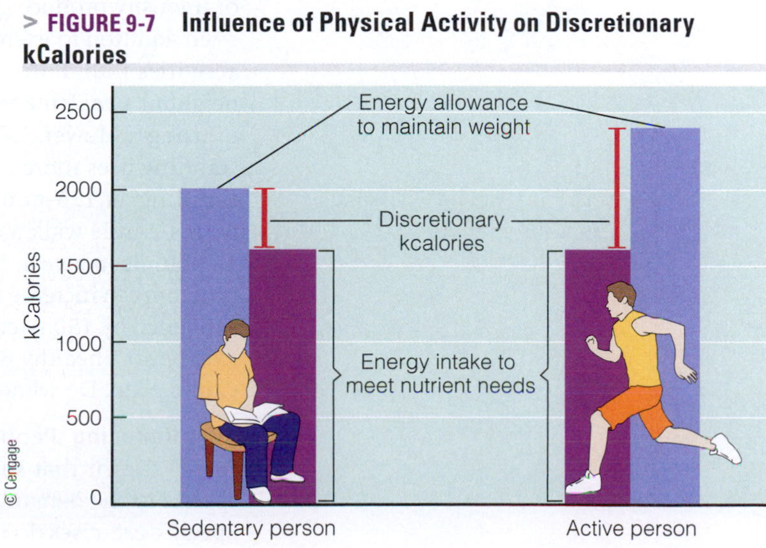
2500
2000
1500
1000
500
0
kCalories
Energy allowance to maintain weight
Discretionary kcalories
Energy intake to meet nutrient needs
Sedentary person
Active person
© Cengage

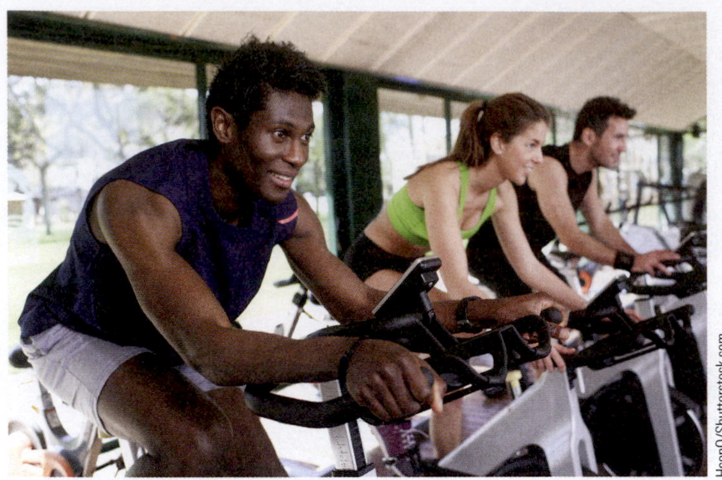
HconQ/Shutterstock.com

> **PHOTO 9-6** The key to good health is to combine sensible eating with regular exercise.

functions. Hard physical work and eating are not compatible. A person must calm down, put energy fuels back in storage, and relax before eating. At that time, a physically active person may eat more than a sedentary person, but not so much as to fully compensate for the energy expended in exercise.

Exercise may also help curb the inappropriate appetite that accompanies boredom, anxiety, or depression. Weight-management programs encourage people who feel the urge to eat when not particularly hungry to exercise instead. The activity passes time, relieves anxiety, and prevents inappropriate eating.

Activity and Psychological Benefits Activity also helps reduce stress, which is especially helpful for people who respond to stress with inappropriate eating. In addition, physical activity helps improve body image and separate the connections between body weight and self-worth. A physically active person begins to look and feel healthy and, as a result, gains self-esteem. High self-esteem motivates a person to continue seeking good health and fitness, which keeps the beneficial cycle going.

Choosing Activities Clearly, physical activity is a plus in a weight-management program (see Photo 9-6). What kind of physical activity is best? Any number of physical activity programs may be equally effective at reducing body weight and improving body composition when combined with a low-kcalorie eating pattern.[76] People should choose activities that they enjoy and are willing to do regularly. What schedule of physical activity is best? It doesn't matter; a person can benefit from either several short bouts of exercise or one continuous workout. Any activity is better than being sedentary. For an active life, limit sedentary activities, engage in strength and flexibility activities, enjoy leisure activities often, engage in vigorous activities regularly, and be as active as possible every day.

Health-care professionals frequently advise people to engage in activities of low-to-moderate intensity for a long duration, such as an hour-long, fast-paced walk. The reasoning behind such advice is that walking offers the health benefits of aerobic physical activity with low risk of injury. It can be done almost anywhere at any time. A person who stays with an activity routine long enough to enjoy the rewards will be less inclined to give it up and will, over the long term, reap many health benefits. A regular walking program can prevent or slow the weight gain that commonly occurs in most adults. An average of 60 minutes a day of moderate-intensity activity or an expenditure of at least 2000 kcalories per week is especially helpful for weight management. Higher levels of duration, frequency, or intensity produce greater losses.

In addition to exercise, a person can incorporate hundreds of energy-expending activities into daily routines: take the stairs instead of the elevator, walk to the neighbor's apartment instead of making a phone call, and rake the leaves instead of using a blower. Remember that sitting uses more kcalories than lying down, standing uses more kcalories than sitting, and moving uses more kcalories than standing. A 175-pound person who replaces a 30-minute television program with a 2-mile walk a day can expend enough energy to lose (or at least not gain) 18 pounds in a year. Even walking in place during the commercials of a one-hour program can increase activity time by 25 minutes, steps taken by 2100, and kcalories expended by 150. Meeting an activity goal of 10,000 steps a day is an excellent way to support a healthy BMI. The point is to be active. Walk. Run. Swim. Dance. Cycle. Climb. Skip. Do whatever you enjoy doing—and do it often.

Spot Reducing People sometimes ask about "spot reducing." Muscles do not "own" the fat that surrounds them. Fat cells all over the body release fat in response to the demand of physical activity for use by whatever muscles are active. Specific exercises do not influence the site of adipose tissue loss.

Exercise can help with trouble spots in another way, though. The "trouble spot" for most men is the abdomen, their primary site of fat storage. During aerobic exercise, abdominal fat readily releases its stores, providing fuel to the physically active body. With regular exercise and weight loss, men will deplete these abdominal fat stores before those in the lower body. Women may also deplete abdominal fat with exercise, but their "trouble spots" are more likely to be their hips and thighs.

In addition to aerobic activity, strength training can help improve the tone of muscles in a trouble area, and stretching to gain flexibility can help with associated posture problems. A combination of aerobic, strength, and flexibility workouts best improves fitness and physical appearance.

Environmental Influences Chapter 8 described how hormones regulate hunger, satiety, and satiation, but people don't always pay close attention to such internal signals. Instead, their eating behaviors are often dictated by environmental factors—those surrounding the eating experience as well as those pertaining to the food itself. Changing any of these factors can influence how much a person eats.

Atmosphere The environment surrounding a meal or snack influences its duration. When the lighting, décor, aromas, and sounds of an environment are pleasant and comfortable, people tend to spend more time eating and thus eat more. A person needn't eat under neon lights with offensive music to eat less, of course. Instead, after completing a meal, remove food from the table and enjoy the ambience—without the presence of visual cues to stimulate additional eating.

Accessibility Among the strongest influences on how much we eat are the accessibility, ease, and convenience of obtaining food. In general, the less effort needed to obtain food, the more likely food will be eaten. Think about it. Are you more likely to eat if half a leftover pizza is in your refrigerator or if you have to drive to the grocery store, buy a frozen pizza, and bake it for 45 minutes? Similarly you are more likely to reach for a second helping of potatoes or another piece of chicken if they are on the dining table in front of you than if the leftovers have already been wrapped and refrigerated. Having food nearby and visible encourages eating—regardless of hunger. The message is clear. For people wanting to eat fewer empty-kcalorie or high-kcalorie foods, keep them out of sight in an inconvenient place, or better yet, don't even bring them home. In contrast, a bowl of fruit on the counter and vegetables in the refrigerator promote healthy eating options.

Socializing People tend to eat more when socializing with others. Pleasant conversations extend the duration of a meal, allowing a person more time to eat more, and the longer the meal, the greater the consumption. In addition, by taking a visual cue from companions, a person might eat more when others at the table eat large portions or go to the buffet line for seconds. One way to eat less is to pace yourself with the person who seems to be eating the least and slowest.

Social interactions also distract a person from paying attention to how much has been eaten. In some cases, socializing with friends during a meal may provide comfort and lower a person's motivation to limit consumption. In other cases, socializing with unfamiliar people during a meal—during a job interview or blind date, for example—may create stress and reduce food consumption. To eat less while socializing, pay attention to portion size.

Distractions Distractions influence food intake by initiating eating, interfering with internal controls to stop eating, and extending the duration of eating. Some people start eating dinner when a favorite television program comes on, regardless of hunger. Other people continue eating breakfast until they finish reading the news. Such mindless eating can easily become overeating. Distractions interfere with a person's ability to perceive and regulate how much is consumed. Not only do people tend to eat more and feel less full after eating a meal while distracted, they tend to eat more at the next meal or snack.[77]

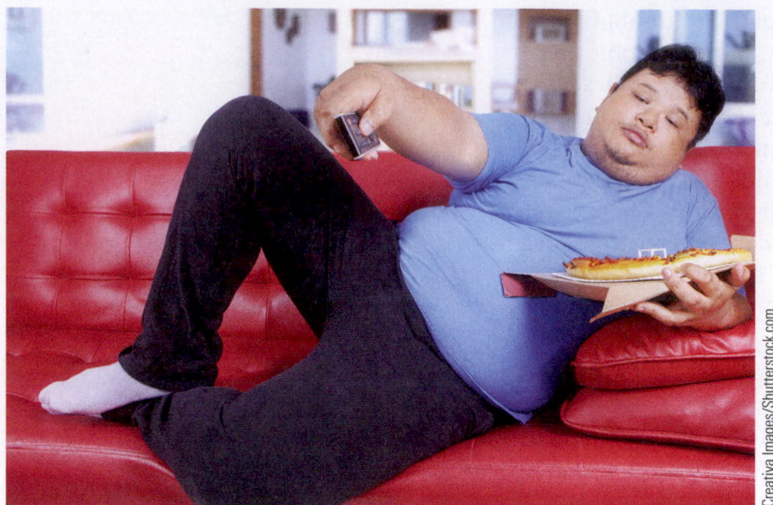

Creativa Images/Shutterstock.com

> **PHOTO 9-7** Eating large portions from the package while distracted by television is a weight-gaining combination.

If distractions are a part of the eating experience, extra care is needed to control portion sizes (see Photo 9-7).

Multiple Choices When offered a large assortment of foods, or several flavors of the same food, people tend to eat more. To limit intake, then, focus on a limited number of foods per meal; be careful, however, not to abandon variety in diet planning. Eating a variety of nutrient-dense foods from each of the food groups helps ensure adequacy.

Package and Portion Sizes As noted earlier, the sizes of packages in grocery stores as well as portion sizes at restaurants and at home have increased dramatically in recent decades, contributing to the increase in obesity in the United States. Put simply, we tend to clean our plates and finish the package. The larger the bag of potato chips, the greater the intake. To keep from overeating, repackage snacks into smaller containers or eat a measured portion from a plate, not directly from the package.

Serving Containers We often use plates, utensils, and glasses as visual cues to guide our decisions on how much to eat and drink. If you plan to eat a bowl of ice cream, it matters whether the bowl you select holds 8 ounces or 24 ounces. Large dinner plates and wide glasses create illusions and misperceptions about quantities consumed. A scoop of mashed potatoes on a small plate looks larger than the same-size scoop on a large plate, leading a person to underestimate the amount of food eaten when eating from a large plate. To control portion sizes, use small bowls and plates, small serving spoons, and tall, narrow glasses. Of course, using a small plate will not result in less food eaten if multiple servings are taken.

Behavior and Attitude

Changes in behavior and attitude can be very effective in supporting efforts to achieve and maintain appropriate body weight and composition. **Behavior modification** focuses on how to change behaviors to increase energy expenditure and decrease energy intake. A person must commit to taking action. Adopting a positive, matter-of-fact attitude helps to ensure success. Healthy eating and activity choices are an essential part of healthy living and should simply be incorporated into the day—much like brushing one's teeth or wearing a safety belt.

Become Aware of Behaviors To solve a problem, a person must first identify all the behaviors that created the problem. Keeping a record will help identify eating and exercise behaviors that may need changing. Such self-monitoring raises awareness, establishes a baseline against which to measure future progress, and improves compliance.[78]

In this era of technology, many companies have developed weight-loss applications for smartphones to help users manage their daily food and physical activity behaviors.* Applications include diet analysis tools that can track eating habits, scanning devices that can quickly enter food data, customized activity and meal plans that can be sent to users, and support programs that deliver encouraging messages and helpful tips (see Photo 9-8). Social media sites allow users to upload progress reports and receive texts. Using these applications can help a person become more aware of behaviors that lead to weight gains and losses.

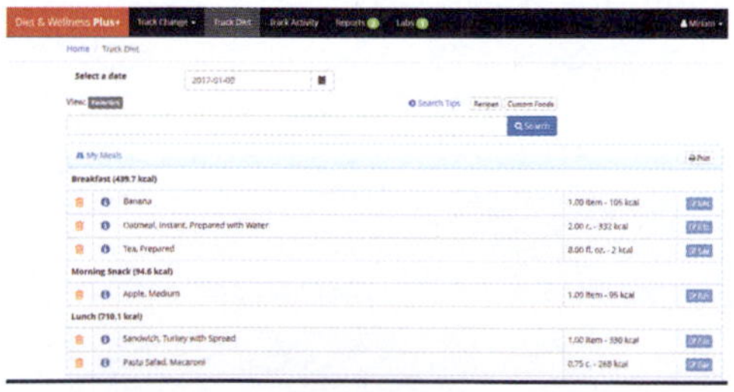

© Cengage

> **PHOTO 9-8** Diet analysis programs help people identify high-kcalorie foods and monitor their eating habits.

Change Behaviors Behavior modification strategies focus on learning desired eating and activity behaviors and eliminating unwanted behaviors. Examples include not grocery shopping when hungry and exercising when watching television. With so many possible behavior changes, a person can feel overwhelmed. To help

behavior modification: the changing of behavior by the manipulation of antecedents (cues or environmental factors that trigger behavior), the behavior itself, and consequences (the penalties or rewards attached to behavior).

*Reliable reviews of food and nutrition apps are available at www.eatright.org.

TABLE 9-4 SMART Goals

	Too Broad	SMART
Specific—define goal clearly	I want to get healthy.	I will lose 10 pounds and lower my blood pressure to within the normal range.
Measurable—track progress and measure outcomes	I want to eat better and exercise more.	I will eat 5 servings of fruits and vegetables each day and run 30 or more minutes at least 4 days a week.
Attainable—set a goal that is challenging, but still realistically achievable	I want to run a marathon next month.	I will complete a 10K race by the end of the year.
Relevant—confirm that goal is meaningful and fits lifestyle	I want to have a long and active life.	I will keep mindful of eating and activity patterns that lower blood pressure and improve blood lipids.
Time based—create a time frame with specific dates for beginning actions and accomplishing goals	I want to get started soon and be healthy by my next doctor's visit.	I will start my new behaviors today, measure my weight and blood pressure weekly, and check my overall success at the end of the semester.

ensure success, health care professionals suggest setting SMART goals, as described in Table 9-4. Start with small time-specific, measurable, and achievable goals for each behavior—for example, "I'm going to take a 30-minute walk after dinner every evening" instead of "I'm going to run in a marathon someday." Practice desired behaviors until they become routine. Addressing multiple behaviors that focus on a common goal simultaneously may better support changes than taking on one at a time. Using a reward system also seems to effectively support weight-loss efforts.

Cognitive Skills Successful behavior changes depend in part on two cognitive skills—problem solving and cognitive restructuring. Problem-solving skills enable a person to identify the problem, generate potential solutions, list the pros and cons of each, implement the most feasible solution, and evaluate whether behaviors should be continued or abandoned. Cognitive restructuring requires a person to replace negative thoughts that derail success with positive thoughts that support behavior change. In general, people who believe they can complete tasks and reach goals are more likely to follow a diet plan and achieve success than those lacking that confidence.

The effectiveness of cognitive behavioral treatment in weight loss extends to other health behaviors as well. Overweight smokers who participate in a cognitive program for weight management lose weight, make healthy food choices, increase their confidence in managing their eating and smoking habits, decrease the number of cigarettes smoked, and increase their readiness to quit smoking. Such findings highlight the need to include dietary strategies in smoking cessation programs. Smoking a cigarette overrides feelings of hunger. When smokers receive a hunger signal, they can quiet it with cigarettes instead of food. In fact, smokers may smoke, in part, to control their weight.[79] Such behavior ignores body signals and postpones energy and nutrient intake. Indeed, smokers tend to weigh less than nonsmokers and to gain weight when they stop smoking. People contemplating giving up cigarettes should know that the average weight gain is about 10 pounds in the first year. Smokers wanting to quit should prepare for the possibility of weight gain and adjust their diet and activity habits so as to maintain weight during and after quitting.

Personal Attitude For many people, overeating and being overweight have become an integral part of their identity. Those who fully understand their personal relationships with food are best prepared to make healthful changes in eating and activity behaviors.

Sometimes people overeat to cope with the stresses of life. Weight gains, in turn, contribute to psychosocial stress, thus creating an unhealthy cycle. To break out of that pattern, they must first identify the particular stressors that trigger the urge to overeat. Then, when faced with these situations, they must learn and practice problem-solving skills that will help them respond appropriately. Learning to reduce episodes of emotional eating can help lead to weight loss.

All this is not to imply that psychotherapy holds the magic answer to a weight problem. Still, efforts to improve one's general well-being may result in healthy eating and activity habits even when weight loss is not the primary goal or result. When the problems that trigger the urge to overeat are resolved in alternative ways, people may find they eat less. They may begin to respond appropriately to internal cues of hunger rather than inappropriately to external cues of stress. Sound emotional health supports a person's ability to take care of physical health in all ways—including nutrition, weight management, and fitness.

Support Groups Group support can prove helpful when making life changes. Some people find success in structured programs such as Take Off Pounds Sensibly (TOPS), Weight Watchers (WW), Overeaters Anonymous (OA), and others.[80] Some dieters prefer to form their own self-help groups or find support online. The Internet offers numerous opportunities for weight-loss education and counseling that may be effective alternatives to face-to-face or telephone counseling programs. As always, consumers need to choose wisely and avoid rip-offs.

Weight Maintenance

The prevalence of **successful weight-loss maintenance** is difficult to determine, in part because researchers have used different criteria. Some look at success after 1 year and others after 5 years; some quantify success as 10 or more pounds lost and others as 5 or 10 percent of initial body weight lost.

Those who are successful in maintaining their weight loss continue to follow regular exercise regimens and careful eating patterns, taking in less energy than the national average.[81] Because formerly overweight people are more efficient at storing fat, they do not have the same flexibility in their food and activity habits as their friends who have never been overweight. With weight loss, hormones involved in appetite regulation shift in a way that encourages weight gain, and metabolism shifts downward so that formerly overweight people require less energy than might be expected given their current body weight and body composition. These hormonal and metabolic changes persist over time.[82] Consequently, to keep weight off, they must either eat less or exercise more than people the same size who have never been obese. Put simply, it takes more effort to prevent weight regain than to prevent weight gain.

Physical activity plays a key role in preventing weight gains and maintaining weight losses (see Photo 9-9). Those who consistently exercise are far more successful than those who are inactive. Weight maintenance may require a person to

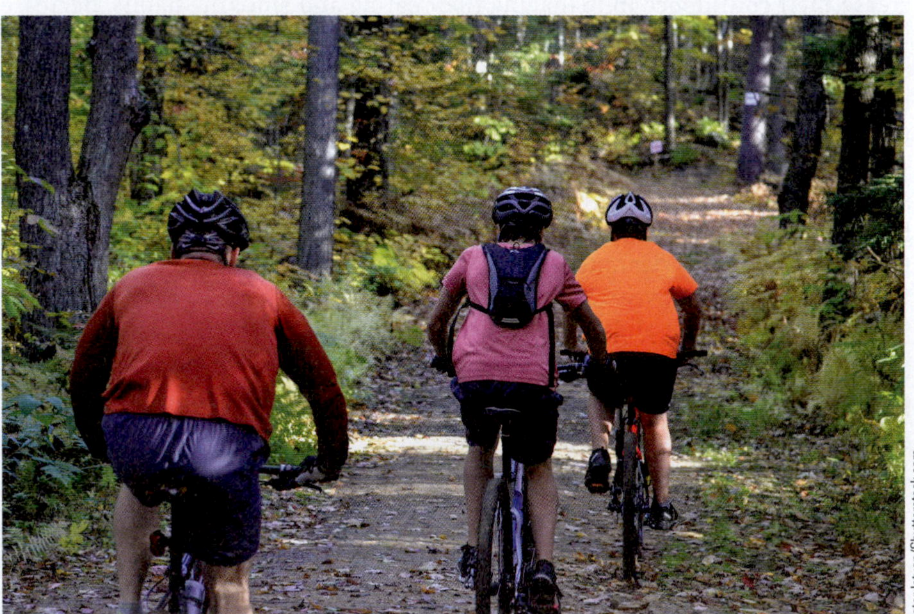
Peter Istvan/Shutterstock.com

> **PHOTO 9-9** Maintaining a healthy body weight requires maintaining the vigorous physical activities and careful eating habits that supported weight loss.

successful weight-loss maintenance: achieving a weight loss of at least 5 to 10 percent of initial body weight and maintaining the loss for at least 1 year.

expend at least 2500 kcalories in physical activity per week. To accomplish this, a person might exercise either moderately (such as brisk walking at 4 miles per hour) for 60 minutes a day or vigorously (such as fast bicycling at 18 miles per hour) for 30 minutes a day, for example. Being active during both work hours and leisure time also helps a person expend more energy and maintain weight loss.

In addition to limiting energy intake and exercising regularly, one other strategy helps with weight maintenance: frequent self-monitoring. People who weigh themselves periodically and monitor their eating and exercise habits regularly can detect weight gains in the early stages and promptly initiate changes to prevent relapse.[83] Quite simply, weighing daily helps a person stay on track.[84]

Losing weight and maintaining the loss may not be easy, but it is possible with sustained behavior change.[85] The National Weight Control Registry tracks over 10,000 individuals who have maintained a significant weight loss over time. Strategies of those who have been successful may differ in the details, but in general, most do the following:

- Eat a low-kcalorie diet (usually small portions four to five times a day).
- Follow a diet that is high in nutrient density and low in energy density.
- Eat breakfast (curbs hunger).
- Engage in physical activity regularly (at least 60 minutes of moderate activity daily).
- Monitor weight frequently (at least weekly) and take prompt action with small gains.
- Use productive problem-solving skills and positive self-talk.
- Limit television time (less than 10 hours a week).
- Consult a registered dietitian nutritionist, physician, or other support person (or group).

Importantly, people who are successful in losing weight find that it gets easier with time—the changes in diet and activity patterns become permanent.

Prevention Given the information presented up to this point in the chapter, the adage "An ounce of prevention is worth a pound of cure" seems particularly apropos. Obesity is a major risk factor for numerous diseases, and losing weight is challenging and often temporary.[86] Many of the strategies for preventing weight gain are very similar to those for losing weight, with one exception: they begin early. Over the years, these strategies become an integral part of a person's life:

- Eat regular meals and limit snacking
- Drink water instead of high-kcalorie beverages
- Select sensible portion sizes and limit daily energy intake to no more than energy expended
- Be physically active and limit sedentary activities

It is much easier for a person to resist doughnuts for breakfast if he rarely eats them. Similarly, a person will have little trouble walking each morning if she has always been active.

Community Programs Reversing the US obesity epidemic is a challenge in an environment of abundant food and physical inactivity. Success may depend on community actions to promote healthy lifestyle choices. Table 9-5 lists health strategies to speed the progress in obesity prevention in the United States. Whether changes in public policy—such as providing pedestrian-friendly streets or taxing sugar-sweetened beverages and empty-kcalorie snacks—will influence activity or diet habits remains to be seen.[87] Clearly, effective strategies will need to reach beyond individuals to address social networks, community institutions, and government policies.

TABLE 9-5 National Strategies to Prevent Obesity

- Provide a variety of opportunities to help make physical activity an integral and routine part of life.
- Create environments that ensure healthy foods and beverages are visible, attractive, and easy-to-obtain.
- Encourage media messages that promote physically active lifestyles and nutritionally healthy diets.
- Support health care providers in offering information on weight management and employers in offering wellness programs.
- Make schools centers for health and wellness.

SOURCE: *Accelerating Progress in Obesity Prevention: Solving the Weight of the Nation*, (Washington, DC: Institute of Medicine of the National Academies), 2012.

REVIEW IT Outline reasonable strategies for achieving and maintaining a healthy body weight.

A surefire remedy for obesity has yet to be found, although many people find a combination of approaches to be most effective. Diet and exercise shift energy balance so that more energy is expended than is taken in. Behavior modification and cognitive restructuring retrain habits to support a healthy eating and activity plan. Such a plan requires time, individualization, and sometimes the assistance of a registered dietitian nutritionist or support group.

9.6 Underweight

LEARN IT Summarize strategies for gaining weight.

Underweight is a far less prevalent problem than overweight in the United States, affecting no more than 2 percent of adults (review Figure 8-7, p. 243). Whether an underweight person needs to gain weight is a question of health and, like weight loss, a highly individual matter. There are no compelling reasons for people who are healthy at their present weight to try to gain weight. Those who are thin because of malnourishment or illness, however, might benefit from a diet that supports weight gain. Medical advice can help make the distinction.

Thin people may find gaining weight difficult. Unlike the genes expressed in obesity, the genes in lean people protect against energy excesses. Those who wish to gain weight for appearance's sake or to improve their athletic performance need to be aware that healthful weight gains can be achieved only by physical conditioning combined with high energy intakes. On a high-kcalorie diet alone, a person may gain weight, but it will be mostly fat. Even if the gain improves appearance, it can be detrimental to health and might impair athletic performance. Therefore, in weight gain, as in weight loss, physical activity and energy intake are essential components of a sound plan.

Problems of Underweight

The causes of underweight may be as diverse as those of overweight—genetic tendencies; hunger, appetite, and satiety irregularities; psychological traits; and metabolic factors. Habits learned early in childhood, especially food aversions, may perpetuate themselves.

The high demand for energy to support physical activity and growth may contribute to underweight. An active, growing boy may need more than 4000 kcalories a day to maintain his weight and may be too busy to take time to eat adequately. In addition, underweight people may find it hard to gain weight because they are expending energy in adaptive thermogenesis. So much energy may be expended adapting to a higher food intake that at first as many as 750 to 800 extra kcalories a day may be needed to gain a pound a week. Like those who want to lose weight, people who want to gain must learn new habits and learn to like new foods. They are also similarly vulnerable to potentially harmful schemes.

As Highlight 8 described, the underweight condition anorexia nervosa sometimes develops in people who employ self-denial to control their weight. They go to such extremes that they become severely undernourished, achieving final body weights of 70 pounds or even less. One difference between a person with anorexia nervosa and other underweight people is that starvation is intentional. (See Highlight 8 for a review of anorexia nervosa and other eating disorders.)

Weight-Gain Strategies

Adequacy and balance are the key diet-planning strategies for weight gain. Meals focus on energy-dense foods to provide many kcalories in a small volume and exercise to build muscle. By using the USDA Food Pattern recommendations for the higher kcalorie levels (see Table 2-3, p. 41), a person can gain weight while meeting nutrient needs.

Energy-Dense Foods

Energy-dense foods (the very ones eliminated from a successful weight-loss diet) hold the key to weight gain. Pick the highest-kcalorie items from each food group—that is, milk shakes instead of fat-free milk, salmon

underweight: body weight lower than the weight range that is considered healthy; BMI less than 18.5.

instead of snapper, avocados instead of cucumbers, a cup of grape juice instead of a small apple, and whole-wheat muffins instead of whole-wheat bread. Because fat provides more than twice as many kcalories per teaspoon as sugar does, fat adds kcalories without adding much bulk.

Although eating high-kcalorie, high-fat foods is not healthy for most people, it may be essential for an underweight individual who needs to gain weight. An underweight person who is physically active and eating a nutritionally adequate diet can afford a few extra kcalories from fat. For health's sake, it is wise to select foods with monounsaturated and polyunsaturated fats instead of those with saturated or *trans* fats: for example, sautéing vegetables in olive oil instead of butter or hydrogenated margarine.

Regular Meals Daily People who are underweight need to make meals a priority and take the time to plan, prepare, and eat each meal. They should eat at least three healthy meals every day. Another suggestion is to eat meaty appetizers or the main course first and leave the soup or salad until later.

Large Portions Underweight people need to learn to eat more food at each meal. For example, they can add extra slices of ham and cheese on a sandwich for lunch, drink a larger glass of milk, and eat a larger bowl of cereal.

The person should expect to feel full. Most underweight individuals are accustomed to small quantities of food. When they begin eating significantly more, they feel uncomfortable. This is normal and passes with time.

Extra Snacks Because a substantially higher energy intake is needed each day, in addition to eating more food at each meal, it is necessary to eat more frequently. Between-meal snacks can readily add to weight gains. For example, a student might make three sandwiches in the morning and eat them between classes in addition to the day's three regular meals. Snacking on dried fruit, nuts, and seeds is also an easy way to add kcalories.

Juice and Milk Beverages provide an easy way to increase energy intake. Consider that 6 cups of cranberry juice add almost 1000 kcalories to the day's intake. kCalories can be added to milk by mixing in powdered milk or packets of instant breakfast.

For people who are underweight because of illness, liquid dietary supplements are often recommended because a weak person can swallow them easily. Used in addition to regular meals, these high-protein, high-kcalorie formulas can help an underweight person maintain or gain weight easily.

Exercising to Build Muscles To gain weight, use strength training primarily, and increase energy intake to support that exercise. Eating extra food to provide an additional 500 to 1000 kcalories a day above normal energy needs can support the exercise as well as build muscle.

REVIEW IT Summarize strategies for gaining weight.

Both the incidence of underweight and the health problems associated with it are less prevalent than overweight and its associated problems. To gain weight, a person must train physically and increase energy intake by selecting energy-dense foods, eating regular meals, taking larger portions, and consuming extra snacks and beverages.

Achieving and maintaining a healthy weight requires vigilant attention to diet and physical activity. Taking care of oneself is a lifelong responsibility.

What's Online

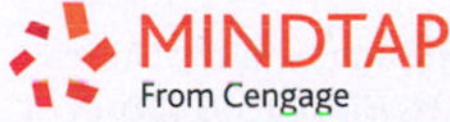
MINDTAP
From Cengage

Visit **www.cengagebrain.com** to access MindTap, a complete digital course that includes Diet & Wellness Plus, interactive quizzes, videos, and more.

REFERENCES

1. C. L. Ogden and coauthors, Prevalence of childhood and adult obesity in the United States, 2011–2012, *Journal of the American Medical Association* 311 (2014): 806–814.
2. National Center for Health Statistics, *Health, United States, 2015: With Special Feature on Racial and Ethnic Health Disparities* (Hyattsville, MD: 2016).
3. World Health Organization, Obesity and overweight fact sheet, June 2016, www.who.int/mediacentre/factsheets/fs311/en.
4. M. Colitti and S. Grasso, Nutraceuticals and regulation of adipocyte life: Premises or promises, *Biofactors* 40 (2014): 398–418.
5. P. Mauriège and coauthors, Weight loss and regain in obese individuals: A link with adipose tissue metabolism indices? *Journal of Physiology and Biochemistry* 69 (2013): 497–505.
6. F. Magkos and coauthors, The battle of the bulge: Defense versus offense, *American Journal of Clinical Nutrition* 100 (2014): 991–992.
7. S. Camps, S. Verhoef, and K. R. Westerterp, Weight loss, weight maintenance, and adaptive thermogenesis, *American Journal of Clinical Nutrition* 97 (2013): 990–994.
8. T. Huang and F. B. Hu, Gene-environment interactions and obesity: Recent developments and future directions, *BMC Medical Genomics* 8 (2015): 1; J. R. Speakman, Evolutionary perspectives on the obesity epidemic: Adaptive, maladaptive, and neutral viewpoints, *Annual Review of Nutrition* 33 (2013): 289–317.
9. M. A. Angulo, M. G. Butler, and M. E. Cataletto, Prader-Willi syndrome: A review of clinical, genetic, and endocrine findings, *Journal of Endocrinological Investigation* 38 (2015): 1249–1263.
10. A. E. Locke and coauthors, Genetic studies of body mass index yield new insights for obesity biology, *Nature* 518 (2015): 197–206; D. Shungin and coauthors, New genetic loci link adipose and insulin biology to body fat distribution, *Nature* 518 (2015): 187–196.
11. R. A. Waterland, Epigenetic mechanisms affecting regulation of energy balance: Many questions, few answers, *Annual Review of Nutrition* 34 (2014): 337–355; L. Goni and coauthors, Single-nucleotide polymorphisms and DNA methylation markers associated with central obesity and regulation of body weight, *Nutrition Reviews* 72 (2014): 673–690.
12. M. B. Allison and M. G. Myers Jr., Connecting leptin signaling to biological function, *Journal of Endocrinology* 223 (2014): T25–T35.
13. M. Wabitsch and coauthors, Biologically inactive leptin and early-onset extreme obesity, *New England Journal of Medicine* 372 (2015): 48–54.
14. H. Pan, J. Guo, and Z. Su, Advances in understanding the interrelations between leptin resistance and obesity, *Physiology and Behavior* 130 (2014): 157–169; H. K. Park and R. S. Ahima, Physiology of leptin: Energy homeostasis, neuroendocrine function and metabolism, *Metabolism* 64 (2014): 24–34.
15. S. Ramirez and M. Claret, Hypothalamic ER stress: A bridge between leptin resistance and obesity, *FEBS Letters* 589 (2015): 1678–1687.
16. O. A. Massadi and coauthors, What is the real relevance of endogenous ghrelin? *Peptides* 70 (2015): 1–6.
17. A. J. Crum and coauthors, Mind over milkshakes: Mindsets, not just nutrients, determine ghrelin response, *Health Psychology* 30 (2011): 424–429.
18. H. K. Al Khatib and coauthors, The effects of partial sleep deprivation on energy balance: A systematic review and meta-analysis, *European Journal of Clinical Nutrition* (2016): doi:10.1038/ejcn.2016.201; H. S. Dashti and coauthors, Habitual sleep duration is associated with BMI and macronutrient intake and may be modified by *CLOCK* genetic variants, *American Journal of Clinical Nutrition* 101 (2015): 135–143; E. Tasali and coauthors, The effects of extended bedtimes on sleep duration and food desire in overweight young adults: A home-based intervention, *Appetite* 80 (2014): 220–224; A. M. Spaeth, D. F. Dinges, and N. Goel, Sex and race differences in caloric intake during sleep restriction in healthy adults, *American Journal of Clinical Nutrition* 100 (2014): 559–566.
19. C. S. Crespo and coauthors, Peptides and food intake, *Frontiers in Endocrinology* 5 (2014): e58.
20. M. Claussnitzer and coauthors, *FTO* obesity variant circuitry and adipocyte browning in humans, *New England Journal of Medicine* 373 (2015): 895–907; M. E. Symonds, M. Pope, and H. Budge, The ontogeny of brown adipose tissue, *Annual Review of Nutrition* 35 (2015): 295–320.
21. P. Lee, Wasting energy to treat obesity, *New England Journal of Medicine* 375 (2016): 2298–2300; S. Kajimura and M. Saito, A new era in brown adipose tissue biology: Molecular control of brown fat development and energy homeostasis, *Annual Review of Physiology* 76 (2014): 225–249; T. J. Schulz and Y. H. Tseng, Brown adipose tissue: Development, metabolism and beyond, *Biochemical Journal* 453 (2013): 167–178.
22. H. B. Ruan and coauthors, O-GlcNAc transferase enable AgRP neurons to suppress browning of white fat, *Cell* 159 (2014): 306–317; K. A. Lo and L. Sun, Turning WAT into BAT: A review on regulators controlling the browning of white adipocytes, *Bioscience Reports* 33 (2013): 711–719; G. E. Beranger, In vitro brown and "brite"/"beige"adipogenesis: Human cellular models and molecular aspects, *Biochimica et Biophysica Acta* 1831 (2013): 905–914; M. L. Bonet, P. Oliver, and A. Palou, Pharmacological and nutritional agents promoting browning of white adipose tissue, *Biochimica et Biophysica Acta* 1831 (2013): n969–n985.
23. E. D. Rosen, Burning fat by bugging the system, *New England Journal of Medicine* 374 (2016): 885–887; C. Graham, A. Mullen, and K. Whelan, Obesity and the gastrointestinal microbiota: A review of associations and mechanisms, *Nutrition Reviews* 73 (2015): 376–385; J. Shen, M. S. Obin, and L. Zhao, The gut microbiota, obesity and insulin resistance, *Molecular Aspects of Medicine* 34 (2013): 39–58; E. Le Chatelier and coauthors, Richness of human gut microbiome correlates with metabolic markers, *Nature* 500 (2013): 541–546.
24. S. Walter and coauthors, Association of a genetic risk score with body mass index across different birth cohorts, *Journal of the American Medical Association* 316 (2016): 63–69.
25. E. Robinson and coauthors, What everyone else is eating: A systematic review and meta-analysis of the effect of informational eating norms on eating behavior, *Journal of the Academy of Nutrition and Dietetics* 114 (2014): 414–429.
26. M. H. Alhussain, I. A. Macdonald, and M. A. Taylor, Irregular meal-pattern effects on energy expenditure, metabolism, and appetite regulation: A randomized controlled trial in healthy normal-weight women, *American College of Clinical Nutrition* 104 (2016): 21–32.
27. J. A. Mitchell and coauthors, A prospective study of sedentary behavior and changes in the body mass index distribution, *Medicine and Science in Sports and Exercise* 46 (2014): 2244–2252.
28. U. Ladabaum and coauthors, Obesity, abdominal obesity, physical activity, and caloric intake in US adults: 1988-2010, *American Journal of Medicine* 127 (2014): 717–727.
29. C. F. Rueda-Clausen, A. A. Ogunleye, and A. M. Sharma, Health benefits of long-term weight-loss maintenance, *Annual Review of Nutrition* 35 (2015): 475–516; M. D. Jensen and D. H. Ryan, New obesity guidelines: Promise and potential, *Journal of the American Medical Association* 311 (2014): 23–24.
30. A. R. Sutin and A. Terracciano, Perceived weight discrimination and obesity, *PLoS One* 8 (2013): e70048.
31. J. P. Montani, Y. Schutz, and A. G. Dulloo, Dieting and weight cycling as risk factors for cardiometabolic diseases: Who is really at risk? *Obesity Reviews* 16 (2015): 7–18; D. P. Beavers and coauthors, Cardiometabolic risk after weight loss and subsequent weight regain in overweight and obese postmenopausal women, *Journals of Gerontology Series A: Biological Sciences and Medical Sciences* 68 (2013): 691–698.
32. FDA, Tainted weight loss products, http://www.fda.gov/drugs/resourcesforyou/consumers/buyingusingmedicinesafely/medicationhealthfraud/ucm234592.htm, November 2016.
33. A. I. Geller and coauthors, Emergency department visits for adverse events related to dietary supplements, *New England Journal of Medicine* 373 (2015): 1531–1540.
34. S. Z. Yanovski and J. A. Yanovski, Long-term drug treatment for obesity: A systematic and clinical review, *Journal of the American Medical Association* 311 (2014): 74–86.
35. Two drugs for weight loss, *Journal of the American Medical Association* 312 (2014): 955–957.
36. K. M. Flegal and coauthors, Trends in obesity among adults in the United States, 2005–2014, *Journal of the American Medical Association* 315 (2016): 2284–2291.

37. S. H. Chang and coauthors, Effectiveness and risks of bariatric surgery: An updated systematic review and meta-analysis, 2003-2012, *JAMA Surgery* 19 (2014): 275–287.
38. N. Abrahamsson and coauthors, Gastric bypass reduces symptoms and hormonal responses in hypoglycemia, *Diabetes* 65 (2016): 2667–2675; S. Barja-Fernández and coauthors, Peripheral signals mediate the beneficial effects of gastric surgery in obesity, *Gastroenterology Research and Practice* (2015): 560938; J. B. Dixon, E. A. Lambert, and G. W. Lambert, Neuroendocrine adaptations to bariatric surgery, *Molecular and Cellular Endocrinology* 418 (2015): 143–152; E. Mans and coauthors, Sleeve gastrectomy effects on hunger, satiation, and gastrointestinal hormone and motility responses after a liquid meal test, *American Journal of Clinical Nutrition* 102 (2015): 540–547.
39. V. Tremaroli and coauthors, Roux-en-Y gastric bypass and vertical banded gastroplasty induce long-term changes on the human gut microbiome contributing to fat mass regulation, *Cell Metabolism* 22 (2015): 228–238; L. Graham, G. Murty, and D. J. Bowrey, Taste, smell and appetite change after Roux-en-Y gastric bypass surgery, *Obesity Surgery* 24 (2014): 1463–1468.
40. M. L. Maciejewski and coauthors, Bariatric surgery and long-term durability of weight loss, *JAMA Surgery* (2016): doi:10.1001/jamasurg.2016.2317.
41. J. Hoffstedt and coauthors, Long-term protective changes in adipose tissue after gastric bypass, *Diabetes Care* 40 (2017): 77–84; D. Arterburn and D. McCulloch, Bariatric surgery for type 2 diabetes getting closer to the long-term goal, *JAMA Surgery* 150 (2015): 931–940; L. Sjöström and coauthors, Association of bariatric surgery with long-term remission of type 2 diabetes and with microvascular and macrovascular complications, *Journal of the American Medical Association* 311 (2014): 2297–2304; C. S. Kwok and coauthors, Bariatric surgery and its impact on cardiovascular disease and mortality: A systematic review and meta-analysis, *International Journal of Cardiology* 173 (2014): 20–28; P. R. Schauer and coauthors, Bariatric surgery versus intensive medical therapy for diabetes—3-year outcomes, *New England Journal of Medicine* 370 (2014): 2002–2013; B. M. Wolfe and S. H. Belle, Long-term risks and benefits of bariatric surgery: A research challenge, *Journal of the American Medical Association* 312 (2014): 1792–1793; D. S. Casagrande and coauthors, Incidence of cancer following bariatric surgery: Systematic review and meta-analysis, *Obesity Surgery* 24 (2014): 1499–1509.
42. A. J. Dawes and coauthors, Mental health conditions among patients seeking and undergoing bariatric surgery: A meta-analysis, *Journal of the American Medical Association* 315 (2016): 150–163.
43. C. A. Guidry and coauthors, Gastric bypass improves survival compared with propensity-matched controls: A cohort study with over 10-year follow-up, *American Journal of Surgery* 209 (2015): 463–467; D. E. Arterburn and coauthors, Association between bariatric surgery and long-term survival, *Journal of the American Medical Association* 313 (2015): 62–70.
44. M. Shah and coauthors, The effect of dietary counseling on nutrient intakes in gastric banding surgery patients, *Journal of Investigative Medicine* 61 (2013): 1165–1172.
45. P. G. de Moura-Grec and coauthors, Impact of bariatric surgery on oral health conditions: 6-months cohort study, *International Dental Journal* 64 (2014): 144–149; T. Weideman and R. Heuberger, The nutritional status of the bariatric patient and its effect on periodontal disease, *Bariatric Surgical Practice and Patient Care* 8 (2013): 161–165; L. Beckman and C. Earthman, Nutritional implications of bariatric surgery and the role of registered dietitians, *Journal of the Academy of Nutrition and Dietetics* 113 (2013): 398–399.
46. E. Saltzman and J. P. Karl, Nutrient deficiencies after gastric bypass surgery, *Annual Review of Nutrition* 33 (2013): 183–203.
47. V. B. Popov and coauthors, The impact of intragastric balloons on obesity-related co-morbidities: A systematic review and meta-analysis, *American Journal of Gastroenterology* (2017) : doi 10.1038/ajg.2016.530; C. J. Neylan and coauthors, Endoscopic treatments of obesity: A comprehensive review, *Surgery for Obesity and Related Diseases* 12 (2016): 1108–1115; E. Caglar, A. Dobrucali, and K. Bal, Gastric balloon to treat obesity: Filled with air or fluid? *Digestive Endoscopy* 25 (2013): 502–507.
48. H. Forssell and E. Norén, A novel endoscopic weight loss therapy using gastric aspiration: Results after 6 months, *Endoscopy* 47 (2015): 68–71; S. Sullivan and coauthors, Aspiration therapy leads to weight loss in obese subjects: A pilot study, *Gastroenterology* 145 (2013): 1245–1252.
49. N. Kumar, Endoscopic therapy for weight loss: Gastroplasty, duodenal sleeves, intragastric balloons, and aspiration, *World Journal of Gastrointestinal Endoscopy* 7 (2015): 847–859.
50. B. Y. Lee and coauthors, A systems approach to obesity, *Nutrition Reviews* 75 (2017): 94–106; Position of the Academy of Nutrition and Dietetics: Interventions for the treatment of overweight and obesity in adults, *Journal of the Academy of Nutrition and Dietetics* 116 (2016): 129–147; K. M. Livingstone and coauthors, FTO genotype and weight loss: Systematic review and meta-analysis of 9563 individual participant data from eight randomised controlled trials, *British Medical Journal* 354 (2016): i4707.
51. US Department of Health and Human Services, *Managing Overweight and Obesity in Adults: Systematic Evidence Review from the Obesity Expert Panel, 2013*, http://www.nhlbi.nih.gov/guidelines.
52. M. E. David and K. L. Haws, Saying "no" to cake or "yes" to kale: Approach and avoidance strategies in pursuit of health goals, *Psychology and Marketing* 33 (2016): 588–594.
53. E. J. Dhurandhar and coauthors, The effectiveness of breakfast recommendations on weight loss: A randomized controlled trial, *American Journal of Clinical Nutrition* 100 (2014): 507–513; A. W. Brown, M. M. B. Brown, and D. B. Allison, Belief beyond the evidence: Using the proposed effect of breakfast on obesity to show 2 practices that distort scientific evidence, *American Journal of Clinical Nutrition* 98 (2013): 1298–1308.
54. P. G. Williams, The benefits of breakfast cereal consumption: A systematic review of the evidence base, *Advances in Nutrition* 5 (2014): 636S–673S; C. E. O'Neil, T. A. Nicklas, and V. L. Fulgoni III, Nutrient intake, diet quality, and weight/adiposity parameters in breakfast patterns compared with no breakfast in adults: National Health and Nutrition Examination Survey 2001–2008, *Journal of the Academy of Nutrition and Dietetics* 114 (2014): S27–S43; A. de la Hunty, S. Gibson, and M. Ashwell, Does regular breakfast cereal consumption help children and adolescents stay slimmer? A systematic review and meta-analysis, *Obesity Facts* 6 (2013): 70–85; P. Deshmukh-Taskar and coauthors, The relationship of breakfast skipping and type of breakfast consumed with overweight/obesity, abdominal obesity, other cardiometabolic risk factors and the metabolic syndrome in young adults. The National Health and Nutrition Examination Survey (NHANES): 1999–2006, *Public Health Nutrition* 16 (2013): 2073–2082.
55. H. J. Leidy and coauthors, Beneficial effects of a higher-protein breakfast on the appetitive, hormonal, and neural signals controlling energy intake regulation in overweight/obese, "breakfast skipping," late-adolescent girls, *American Journal of Clinical Nutrition* 97 (2013): 677–688.
56. D. Jakubowicz and coauthors, High caloric intake at breakfast vs. dinner differentially influences weight loss of overweight and obese women, *Obesity* 21 (2013): 2504–2512.
57. L. C. Kong and coauthors, Dietary patterns differently associate with inflammation and gut microbiota in overweight and obese subjects, *PLoS One* 9 (2014): e109434.
58. C. Haire and H. A. Raynor, Weight status moderates the relationship between package size and food intake, *Journal of the Academy of Nutrition and Dietetics* 114 (2014): 1251–1256.
59. G. Zong and coauthors, Consumption of meals prepared at home and risk of type 2 diabetes: An analysis of two prospective cohort studies, *PLoS Medicine* 13 (2016): e1002052.
60. M. Shah and coauthors, Slower eating speed lowers energy intake in normal-weight but not overweight/obese subjects, *Journal of the Academy of Nutrition and Dietetics* 114 (2014): 393–402; Y. Zhu and J. H. Hollis, Increasing the number of chews before swallowing reduces meal size in normal-weight, overweight, and obese adults, *Journal of the Academy of Nutrition and Dietetics* 114 (2014): 926–931.
61. E. Robinson and coauthors, A systematic review and meta-analysis examining the effect of eating rate on energy intake and hunger, *American Journal of Clinical Nutrition* 100 (2014): 123–151; Y. Hamada, H. Kashima, and N. Hayashi, The number of chews and meal duration affect diet-induced thermogenesis and splanchnic circulation, *Obesity* 22 (2014): E62–E69.
62. G. Camps and coauthors, Empty calories and phantom fullness: A randomized trial studying the relative effects of energy density and viscosity

on gastric emptying determined by MRI and satiety, *American Journal of Clinical Nutrition* 104 (2016): 73B–80B. J. Rolls, What is the role of portion control in weight management? *International Journal of Obesity* 38 (2014): S1–S8; R. A. Williams, L. S. Roe, and B. J. Rolls, Comparison of three methods to reduce energy density: Effects on daily energy intake, *Appetite* 66 (2013): 75–83.

63. R. Muckelbauer and coauthors, Association between water consumption and body weight outcomes: A systematic review, *American Journal of Clinical Nutrition* 98 (2013): 282–299.
64. K. J. Duffey and J. Poti, Modeling the effect of replacing sugar-sweetened beverage consumption with water on energy intake, HBI score, and obesity prevalence, *Nutrients* 8 (2016): e395.
65. F. Eichelmann and coauthors, Effect of plant-based diets on obesity-related inflammatory profiles: A systematic review and meta-analysis of intervention trials, *Obesity Reviews* 17 (2016): 1067–1079; N. D. Barnard, S. M. Levin, and Y. Yokoyama, A systematic review and meta-analysis of changes in body weight in clinical trials of vegetarian diets, *Journal of the Academy of Nutrition and Dietetics* 115 (2015): 954–969; G. M. Turner-McGrievy and coauthors, Comparative effectiveness of plant-based diets for weight loss: A randomized controlled trial of five different diets, *Nutrition* 31 (2015): 350–358; B. Farmer, Nutritional adequacy of plant-based diets for weight management: Observations from the NHANES, *American Journal of Clinical Nutrition* 100 (2014): 365S–368S.
66. D. K. Tobias and coauthors, Effect of low-fat diet interventions versus other diet interventions on long-term weight change in adults: A systematic review and meta-analysis, *Lancet Diabetes and Endocrinology* 3 (2015): 968–979.
67. P. E. Miller and V. Perez, Low-calorie sweeteners and body weight and composition: A meta-analysis of randomized controlled trials and prospective cohort studies, *American Journal of Clinical Nutrition* 100 (2014): 765–777.
68. J. Suez and coauthors, Artificial sweeteners induce glucose intolerance by altering the gut microbiota, *Nature* 514 (2014): 181–186.
69. S. N. Bleich and coauthors, Diet-beverage consumption and caloric intake among US adults, overall and by body weight, *American Journal of Public Health* 104 (2014): e72–e78.
70. T. Kondoh and coauthors, Association of dietary factors with abdominal subcutaneous and visceral adiposity in Japanese men, *Obesity Research and Clinical Practice* 8 (2014): e16–e25.
71. D. J. Johns and coauthors, Diet or exercise interventions vs combined behavioral weight management programs: A systematic review and meta-analysis of direct comparisons, *Journal of the Academy of Nutrition and Dietetics* 114 (2014): 1557–1568.
72. J. E. Donnelly and coauthors, American College of Sports Medicine Position Stand: Appropriate physical activity intervention strategies for weight loss and prevention of weight regain for adults, *Medicine and Science in Sports and Exercise* 41 (2009): 459–471; Committee on Dietary Reference Intakes, *Dietary Reference Intakes for Energy, Carbohydrate, Fiber, Fat, Fatty Acids, Cholesterol, Protein, and Amino Acids* (Washington, D.C.: National Academies Press, 2005).
73. R. J. Verheggen and coauthors, A systematic review and meta-analysis on the effects of exercise training versus hypocaloric diet: Distinct effects on body weight and visceral adipose tissue, *Obesity Reviews* 17 (2016): 664–690; D. L. Swift and coauthors, The role of exercise and physical activity in weight loss and maintenance, *Progress in Cardiovascular Diseases* 56 (2014): 441–447.
74. G. C. Henderson and B. L. Alderman, Determinants of resting lipid oxidation in response to a prior bout of endurance exercise, *Journal of Applied Physiology* 116 (2014): 95–103.
75. M. M. Schubert and coauthors, Acute exercise and hormones related to appetite regulation: A meta-analysis, *Sports Medicine* 44 (2014): 387–403; K. J. Guelfi, C. E. Conges, and R. Duffield, Beneficial effects of 12 weeks of aerobic compared with resistance exercise training on perceived appetite in previously sedentary overweight and obese men, *Metabolism: Clinical and Experimental* 62 (2013): 235–243.
76. P. J. Benito and coauthors, Change in weight and body composition in obese subjects following a hypocaloric diet plus different training programs or physical activity recommendation, *Journal of Applied Physiology* 118 (2015): 1006–1013.
77. S. Higgs, Manipulations of attention during eating and their effects on later snack intake, *Appetite* 92 (2015): 287–294; E. Robinson and coauthors, Eating attentively: A systematic review and meta-analysis of the effect of food intake memory and awareness on eating, *American Journal of Clinical Nutrition* 97 (2013): 728–742.
78. A. Kong and coauthors, Self-monitoring and eating-related behaviors are associated with 12-month weight loss in postmenopausal overweight-to-obese women, *Journal of the Academy of Nutrition and Dietetics* 112 (2012): 1428–1435.
79. J. Cawley, D. Dragone, and H. K. Scholder, The demand for cigarettes as derived from the demand for weight loss: A theoretical and empirical investigation, *Health Economics* 25 (2016): 8–23.
80. K. A. Gudzune and coauthors, Efficacy of commercial weight-loss programs: An updated systematic review, *Annals of Internal Medicine* 162 (2015): 501–512.
81. N. J. Davis and coauthors, Predictors of sustained reduction in energy and fat intake in the diabetes prevention program outcomes study intensive lifestyle intervention, *Academy of Nutrition and Dietetics* 113 (2013): 1455–1464.
82. E. Fothergill and coauthors, Persistent metabolic adaptation 6 years after "The Biggest Loser" competition, *Obesity* 24 (2016): 1612–1619.
83. Z. Yu, C. Sealey-Potts, and J. Rodriguez, Dietary self-monitoring in weight management: Current evidence on efficacy and adherence, *Journal of the Academy of Nutrition and Dietetics* 115 (2015): 1931–1938.
84. D. M. Steinberg and coauthors, Weighing every day matters: Daily weighing improves weight loss and adoption of weight control behaviors, *Journal of the Academy of Nutrition and Dietetics* 115 (2015): 511–518; C. R. Pacanowski and D. A. Levitsky, Frequent self-weighing and visual feedback for weight loss in overweight adults, *Journal of Obesity* (2015): 763680; E. E. Helander and coauthors, Are breaks in daily self-weighing associated with weight gain? *PLoS One* 9 (2014): e113164.
85. P. Wilson, Physical activity and dietary determinants of weight loss success in the US general population, *American Journal of Public Health* 106 (2016): 321–326; J. G. Thomas and coauthors, Weight-loss maintenance for 10 years in the National Weight Control Registry, *American Journal of Preventive Medicine* 46 (2014): 17–23.
86. A. Fildes and coauthors, Probability of an obese person attaining normal body weight: Cohort study using electronic health records, *American Journal of Public Health* 105 (2015): e54–e59.
87. M. I. Creatore and coauthors, Association of neighborhood walkability with change in overweight, obesity, and diabetes, *Journal of the American Medical Association* 315 (2016): 2211–2220; Centers for Disease Control and Prevention, Community efforts, www.cdc.gov/obesity/strategies/community.html, October 27, 2015; S. Sarlio-Lähteenkorva and J. Winkler, Could a sugar tax help combat obesity? *British Medical Journal* 351 (2015): h4047; A. M. Thow, S. Downs, and S. Jan, A systematic review of the effectiveness of food taxes and subsidies to improve diets: Understanding the recent evidence, *Nutrition Reviews* 72 (2014): 551–565; D. Mozaffarian, K. S. Rogoff, and D. S. Ludwig, The real cost of food: Can taxes and subsidies improve public health? *Journal of the American Medical Association* 312 (2014): 889–890; R. Sturm and R. An, Obesity and economic environments, *Cancer Journal for Clinicians* 64 (2014): 337–350; E. Cerin and coauthors, Neighborhood environments and objectively measured physical activity in 11 countries, *Medicine and Science in Sports and Exercise* 46 (2014): 2253–2264.

HIGHLIGHT > 9

LEARN IT Contrast the differences between popular fad diets and weight-loss diets based on nutrition science.

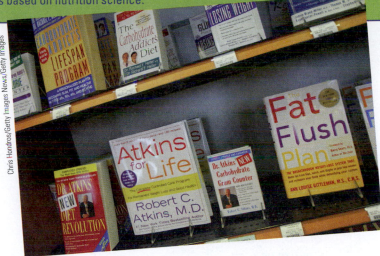

Atkins for Life
Robert C. Atkins, M.D.
Fat Flush Plan
The Carbohydrate Addict's Diet
Dr. Atkins New Carbohydrate Gram Counter
Dr. Atkins New Diet Revolution

Chris Hondros/Getty Images News/Getty Images

The Latest and Greatest Weight-Loss Diet—Again

To paraphrase William Shakespeare, "A fad diet by any other name would still be a fad diet." Year after year, "new and improved" diets appear on bookstore shelves, pop up on websites, and circulate among friends. People of all sizes eagerly try the best diet ever on the market, hoping that this one will really work. Sometimes these diets seem to work for a while, but more often than not, their success is short-lived. Then another diet takes the spotlight. Here's how Dr. K. Brownell, an obesity researcher and dean at Duke University's Sanford School of Public Policy, describes this phenomenon: "When I get calls about the latest diet fad, I imagine a trick birthday cake candle that keeps lighting up and we have to keep blowing it out."

Realizing that fad diets do not offer a safe and effective long-term plan for weight loss, health professionals speak out, but they never get the candle blown out permanently. New fad diets can keep making outrageous claims because no one requires their advocates to prove what they say. Fad diet gurus do not have to conduct credible research on the benefits or dangers of their diets. They can simply make recommendations and then later, if questioned, search for bits and pieces of research that support the conclusions they have already reached. That's backward. Diet and health recommendations should *follow* years of sound scientific research *before* being offered to the public.

Because anyone can publish anything—in books or on the Internet—peddlers of fad diets can make unsubstantiated statements that fall far short of the truth but sound impressive to the uninformed. They often offer distorted bits of legitimate research. They may start with one or more actual facts but then leap from one erroneous conclusion to the next. Anyone who wants to believe these claims has to wonder how the thousands of scientists working on obesity research over the past century could possibly have missed such obvious connections.

Fad diets come in almost as many shapes and sizes as the people who search them out. Some restrict fats or carbohydrates, some limit portion sizes, some focus on food combinations, and some claim that a person's genetic type or blood type determines the foods best suited to manage weight and prevent disease. A lack of scientific evidence just doesn't seem to stop diets from making claims.[1] Research on the effectiveness of popular diets in supporting weight loss and improving health does not find any one as being more beneficial than the others.[2] The Academy of Nutrition and Dietetics offers evaluations of popular diets; look for reviews of popular diets at their website, www.eatright.org/dietreviews.

Fad Diets' Appeal

With more than half of our nation's adults overweight and many more concerned about their weight, the market for a weight-loss book, product, or program is huge (no pun intended). Americans spend an estimated $60 billion a year on weight-loss services and products.[3] Even a plan that offers only minimal weight-loss success easily attracts a following.

Perhaps the greatest appeal of fad diets is that they tend to ignore dietary recommendations. Foods such as meats and milk products that need to be selected carefully to limit saturated fat can be eaten with abandon. Whole grains, legumes, vegetables, and fruits that should be eaten in abundance can now be bypassed. For some people, this is a dream come true: steaks without the potatoes, ribs without the baked beans, and meatballs without the pasta. Who can resist the promise of weight loss while eating freely from a list of favorite foods?

Dieters are also lured into fad diets by sophisticated—yet often erroneous—explanations of the metabolic consequences of eating certain foods. Terms such as *eicosanoids* and *de novo lipogenesis* are scattered about, often intimidating readers into believing that the authors must be right given their brilliance in understanding nutrition.

If fad diets were as successful as some people claim, then consumers who tried them would lose weight, and their obesity problems would be solved. But this is not the case. Similarly, if fad diets were as worthless as others claim, then consumers would eventually stop pursuing them. Clearly, this is not happening either. Most fad diets have enough going for them that they work for some people at least for a short time, but they fail to produce long-lasting results for most people.

Don't Count kCalories

Who wants to count kcalories? Even experienced dieters find counting kcalories burdensome, not to mention timeworn. They want a new, easy way to lose weight, and fad diet plans seem to offer this boon. But, though fad diets often claim to disregard kcalories, their design typically ensures a low energy intake. Most of the sample menu plans, especially in the early stages, are designed to deliver an average of 1200 kcalories a day.

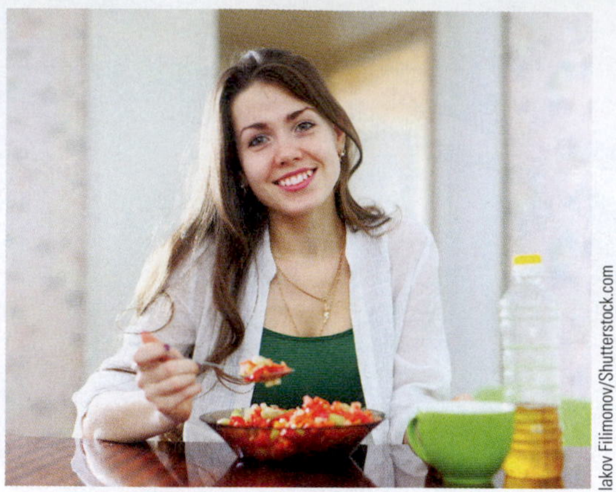

Iakov Filimonov/Shutterstock.com

> **PHOTO H9-1** The wise consumer seeks a diet that supports not only weight loss, but also health gains.

Even when counting kcalories is truly not necessary, total kcalories tend to be low simply because food intake is so limited. Diets that omit hundreds of foods and several food groups limit a person's options and lack variety. Chapter 2 praised variety as a valuable way to ensure an adequate intake of nutrients, but variety also entices people to eat more food and gain more weight. Without variety, some people lose interest in eating, which further reduces energy intake. Even if the allowed foods are favorites, eating the same foods day after day can become monotonous.

Without its refried beans, tortilla wrapping, and chopped vegetables, a burrito is reduced to a pile of ground beef. Without the baked potato, there's no need for butter and sour cream. Weight loss occurs because of the low energy intake. This is an important point. Any diet can produce weight loss, at least temporarily, if intake is restricted. The real value of a diet is determined by its ability to maintain weight loss and support good health over the long term. The goal is not simply weight loss, but health gains—and most fad diets cannot support optimal health over time. In fact, some weight-loss diets can create or exacerbate health problems.

When food choices are limited, nutrient intakes may be inadequate. To help shore up some of these inadequacies, fad diets often recommend a dietary supplement. Conveniently, many of the companies selling fad diets also peddle these supplements. But as Highlights 10 and 11 explain, foods offer many more health benefits than any supplement can provide. Quite simply, if the diet is inadequate, it needs to be improved.

Follow a Plan

Most people need specific instructions and examples to make dietary changes. Popular diets offer dieters a plan. The user doesn't have to decide what foods to eat, how to prepare them, or how much to eat. Unfortunately, these instructions typically serve only short-term weight-loss needs. They do not provide for long-term changes in lifestyle that will support weight maintenance or health goals (see Photo H9-1).

The success of any weight-loss diet depends on the person adopting the plan and sticking with it. People who prefer a high-protein, low-carbohydrate diet over a high-carbohydrate, low-fat diet, for example, may have more success at sticking with it, perhaps because of protein's role in providing satiety.[4] Too much protein, however, may increase the likelihood of weight gain and early death for some people with obesity-related risk factors.[5] Keep in mind that weight loss occurs because of the duration of a low-kcalorie plan—not the proportion of energy nutrients.[6]

The Real Deal

Fad diets attribute magical powers to their weight-loss plans, but in reality, the magic is in tipping the energy balance so that metabolic and physical activities expend more kcalories than foods bring in. Because new diets emerge in the market regularly, it can be challenging to sort the fad diets from the healthy options. Furthermore, it can be difficult determining how a diet's overall quality rates and how it compares with others.

Keep in mind that healthy weight loss requires long-term lifestyle changes in eating and activity habits—not quick, short-term fixes. A healthy plan may not be quick, but it allows for flexibility and a variety of foods, including some favorite treats on occasion.

Some currently popular diet plans offer a sensible approach to weight loss and healthy eating. The challenge is sorting through "the good, the bad, and the ugly." How To H9-1 offers tips for identifying fad diets and other weight-loss scams and includes guidelines from the Federal Trade Commission (FTC).[7] Fad diets may not harm healthy people if used for only a little while, but they cannot support optimal health for the long term. Chapter 9 includes reasonable approaches to weight management and concludes that the ideal diet is one you can live with for the rest of your life. Keep that criterion in mind when you evaluate the next "latest and greatest weight-loss diet" that comes along.

> How To H9-1 Identify a Fad Diet or Weight-Loss Scam

It may be a fad diet or weight-loss scam if it:

- Sounds too good to be true.
- Recommends using a single food consistently as the key to the program's success.
- Promises quick and easy weight loss with no change in diet or activity. "Lose weight while you sleep!"
- Eliminates an entire food group such as grains or milk and milk products.
- Guarantees an unrealistic outcome in an unreasonable time period. "Lose 10 pounds in 2 days!"
- Bases evidence for its effectiveness solely on anecdotal stories.
- Requires you to buy special products that are not readily available in the marketplace at affordable prices.
- Specifies a proportion for the energy nutrients that falls outside the recommended ranges—carbohydrate (45 to 65 percent), fat (20 to 35 percent), and protein (10 to 35 percent).
- Claims to alter your genetic code or reset your metabolism.
- Fails to mention potential risks or additional costs.
- Promotes products or procedures that have not been proven safe and effective.
- Neglects plans for weight maintenance following weight loss.

> TRY IT Review an advertisement for a popular weight-loss plan and explain why you think it might—or might not—be a fad diet.

CRITICAL THINKING QUESTIONS

A. What patterns are evident in fad weight-loss diets?

B. A fad diet website says it all: 30 ways to lose 5 pounds in a week. Millions of people have tried hundreds of crash diets in search of short-term fixes to their weight problems. It's amazing to think about what people are willing to do to avoid eating a well-balanced diet and exercising regularly—wire their jaws closed, swallow a parasite, drink nothing but salt water for a week. Why do you think consumers continue to pursue fad diets? How would you design a weight loss plan that would be appealing to most people *and* produce long-lasting results?

REFERENCES

1. L. Cusack and coauthors, Blood type diets lack supporting evidence: A systematic review, *American Journal of Clinical Nutrition* 98 (2013): 99–104.
2. R. Atallah and coauthors, Long-term effects of 4 popular diets on weight loss and cardiovascular risk factors: A systematic review of randomized controlled trials, *Circulation* 7 (2014): 815–827.
3. Weight loss market sheds some dollars in 2013, https://www.marketdataenterprises.com/wp-content/uploads/2014/01/Diet-Market-2014-Status-Report.pdf, February 4, 2014.
4. A. Astrup, A. Raben, and N. Geiker, The role of higher protein diets in weight control and obesity-related comorbidities, *International Journal of Obesity* 39 (2015): 721–726; D. H. Pesta and V. T. Samuel, A high-protein diet for reducing body fat: Mechanisms and possible caveats, *Nutrition and Metabolism* 11 (2014): 53.
5. P. Hernández-Alonso, High dietary protein intake is associated with an increased body weight and total death risk, *Clinical Nutrition* 35 (2016): 496–506.
6. B. C. Johnston and coauthors, Comparison of weight loss among named diet programs in overweight and obese adults, *Journal of the American Medical Association* 312 (2014): 923–933; M. L. Gow and coauthors, Impact of dietary macronutrient distribution on BMI and cardiometabolic outcomes in overweight and obese children and adolescents: A systematic review, *Nutrition Reviews* 72 (2014): 453–470.
7. Gut check: A reference guide for media on spotting false weight loss claims, https://www.ftc.gov/tips-advice/business-center/guidance/gut-check-reference-guide-media-spotting-false-weight-loss, January 2014.

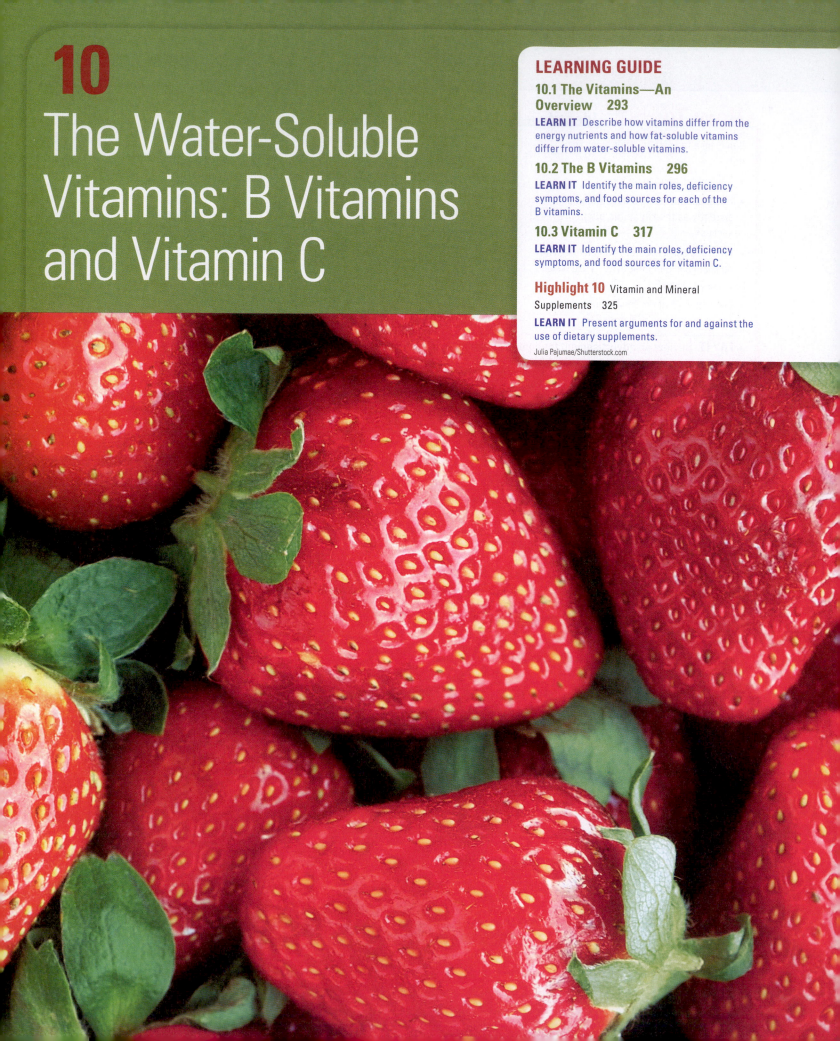

10 The Water-Soluble Vitamins: B Vitamins and Vitamin C

LEARNING GUIDE

Julia Pajumae/Shutterstock.com

Nutrition in Your Life

If you were playing a word game and your partner said "vitamins," how would you respond? If "pills" and "supplements" immediately come to mind, you may be missing the main message of the vitamin story—that hundreds of foods deliver more than a dozen vitamins that participate in thousands of activities throughout your body. Quite simply, foods supply vitamins to support all that you are and all that you do—and supplements of any one of them, or even a combination of them, can't compete with foods in keeping you healthy. As you read this chapter, consider whether the foods you are eating are meeting your water-soluble vitamin needs.

Earlier chapters focused on the energy-yielding nutrients—carbohydrates, fats, and proteins. This chapter begins with an overview of the **vitamins** and then examines each of the water-soluble vitamins; the next chapter features the fat-soluble vitamins. Researchers first recognized in the early 1900s that foods contain substances that are "vital to life." Since then, the world of vitamins has opened up dramatically.

Vitamins are powerful, as their *absence* attests. Vitamin A deficiency can cause blindness; a lack of the B vitamin niacin can cause dementia; and without vitamin D, bones fail to grow. The *presence* of vitamins also attests to their power. The B vitamin folate helps to prevent birth defects, and vitamin K helps blood to clot. Every year, people spend billions of dollars on supplements, hoping to cure their ailments (see Highlight 10). Vitamins do support good health, but they do not cure all ills nor do supplements provide all of the many disease-preventing benefits of vitamin-rich foods (as Highlight 11 explains).

10.1 The Vitamins—An Overview

LEARN IT Describe how vitamins differ from the energy nutrients and how fat-soluble vitamins differ from water-soluble vitamins.

The vitamins are a diverse group of essential nutrients that regulate most body processes involved in supporting growth and maintaining life. Notably, the vitamins differ from carbohydrates, fats, and proteins in the following ways:

- *Structure.* Vitamins are individual units; they are not linked together (as are molecules of glucose or amino acids). Appendix C presents the chemical structure for each of the vitamins.
- *Function.* Vitamins do not yield energy when metabolized; many of them do, however, assist the enzymes that participate in the release of energy from carbohydrates, fats, and proteins.
- *Food contents.* Like carbohydrates, fats, and proteins, vitamins are readily available from foods, but the amounts of vitamins people ingest from foods and the amounts they require daily are measured in *micrograms* (μg) or *milligrams* (mg), rather than grams (g).* For this reason, the vitamins are sometimes described as *micronutrients.*

Although small in size, the vitamins accomplish giant tasks. Obtaining enough, but not too much, of each vitamin is critical because both deficiencies and toxicities can be harmful.

As Chapter 1 described, the Dietary Reference Intakes (DRI) define the amounts of each vitamin that best support health. Research studies help to determine a vitamin's *requirement*—how much is needed to maintain adequacy. With this information, an Estimated Average Requirement (EAR) is calculated to estimate the

*For perspective, a dollar bill weighs about 1 g; 1 g = 1000 mg, and 1 mg = 1000 μg. Appendix H explains how to convert a measurement from one unit of measure to another.

vitamins: organic, essential nutrients required in small amounts by the body for health. Vitamins regulate body processes that support growth and maintain life.

- **vita** = life
- **amine** = containing nitrogen (the first vitamins discovered contained nitrogen)

average amount that appears sufficient for half of the population. Once an EAR is established, a *recommendation* can be made that will meet the needs of about 98 percent of the population—the Recommended Dietary Allowance (RDA). If there is insufficient evidence to determine an EAR (which is needed to set an RDA), a recommendation based on the average amount of a nutrient that a group of healthy people consumes—an Adequate Intake (AI)—may be used instead of an RDA. The Tolerable Upper Intake Level (UL) sets the highest amount that appears safe for regular consumption. (See Chapter 1 for more details on the DRI.)

Solubility As you may recall, carbohydrates and proteins are hydrophilic and lipids are hydrophobic. The vitamins divide along the same lines—the hydrophilic, water-soluble ones are the B vitamins (thiamin, riboflavin, niacin, biotin, pantothenic acid, vitamin B_6, folate, and vitamin B_{12}) and vitamin C; the hydrophobic, fat-soluble ones are vitamins A, D, E, and K. As each vitamin was discovered, it was given a name and sometimes a letter and number as well. Many of the vitamins have multiple names, which has led to some confusion. The summary tables throughout this chapter and the next provide both the standard and the common alternative names.

Solubility is apparent in the food sources of the different vitamins, and it affects their absorption, transport, storage, and excretion by the body. The water-soluble vitamins are found in the watery compartments of foods; the fat-soluble vitamins usually occur together in the fats and oils of foods. On being absorbed, the water-soluble vitamins move directly into the blood. Like fats, the fat-soluble vitamins must first enter the lymph, then the blood. Once in the blood, many of the water-soluble vitamins travel freely, whereas many of the fat-soluble vitamins require transport proteins. Upon reaching the cells, water-soluble vitamins freely circulate in the water-filled compartments whereas fat-soluble vitamins are held in fatty tissues and the liver until needed. The kidneys, monitoring the blood that flows through them, detect and remove small excesses of water-soluble vitamins; large excesses, however, may overwhelm the system, creating adverse effects. Fat-soluble vitamins tend to remain in fat-storage sites in the body rather than being excreted, and so are more likely to reach toxic levels when consumed in excess.

Because the body stores fat-soluble vitamins, they can be eaten in large amounts once in a while and still meet the body's needs over time. Water-soluble vitamins are retained in the body for varying lengths of time. The water-soluble vitamins must be eaten more regularly than the fat-soluble vitamins, although a single day's omission from the diet does not create a deficiency.

Bioavailability Some water-soluble vitamins are synthesized by GI tract bacteria and absorbed by the large intestine, but not in quantities great enough to meet the body's needs; foods must supply these essential nutrients. The amount available from foods depends not only on the quantity provided by a food but also on the vitamin's **bioavailability**—the amount absorbed and used by the body. The quantity of vitamins in a food can be determined relatively easily. Researchers analyze foods to determine the vitamin contents and publish the results in tables such as the USDA Food Composition Database (https://ndb.nal.usda.gov/). Determining the bioavailability of a vitamin is a more complex task because it depends on many factors, including:

- Efficiency of digestion and time of transit through the GI tract
- Previous nutrient intake and nutrition status
- Method of food preparation (raw, cooked, or processed)
- Source of the nutrient (synthetic, fortified, or naturally occurring)
- Other foods consumed at the same time

Chapters 10 through 13 describe factors that inhibit or enhance the absorption of individual vitamins and minerals. Experts consider these factors when estimating recommended intakes.

Precursors Some vitamins are available from foods in inactive forms known as **precursors**. Once inside the body, the precursor is converted to an active form

bioavailability: the rate at and the extent to which a nutrient is absorbed and used.

precursors: substances that precede others; with regard to vitamins, compounds that can be converted into active vitamins; also known as *provitamins.*

TABLE 10-1 Minimizing Nutrient Losses

- To slow the degradation of vitamins, refrigerate (most) fruits and vegetables.
- To minimize the oxidation of vitamins, store fruits and vegetables that have been cut in airtight wrappers, and store juices that have been opened in closed containers (and refrigerate them).
- To prevent vitamin losses during washing, rinse fruits and vegetables before cutting (not after).
- To minimize vitamin losses during cooking, use a microwave oven or steam vegetables in a small amount of water. Add vegetables after water has come to a boil. Use the cooking water in mixed dishes such as casseroles and soups. Avoid high temperatures and long cooking times.

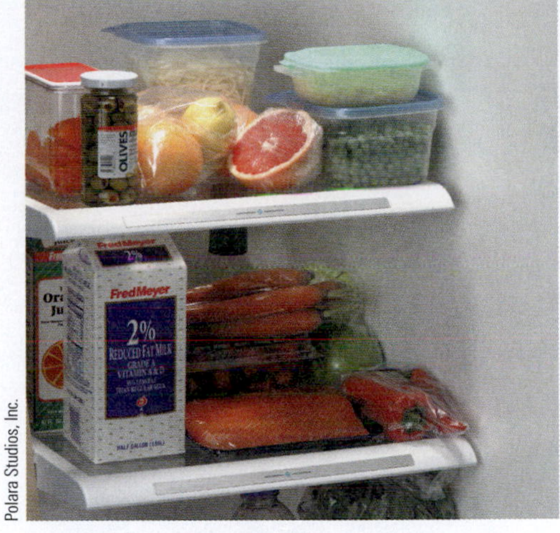
OLIVES
Fred Meyer
2%
REDUCED FAT MILK

> **PHOTO 10-1** To minimize vitamin losses, wrap cut fruits and vegetables or store them in airtight containers.

of the vitamin. For example, beta-carotene, a red-orange pigment found in fruits and vegetables, is a precursor to vitamin A. Thus, in measuring a person's vitamin intake, it is important to count both the amount of the active vitamin and the potential amount available from its precursors. The discussions and summary tables throughout this chapter and the next indicate which vitamins have precursors.

Organic Nature Fresh foods naturally contain vitamins, but because these vitamins are organic, they can be readily destroyed during processing. Therefore, processed foods should be used sparingly, and fresh foods should be handled with care during storage and in cooking (see Photo 10-1). Prolonged heating may destroy much of the thiamin in food. Because riboflavin can be destroyed by the ultraviolet rays of the sun or by fluorescent light, foods stored in transparent glass containers are most likely to lose riboflavin. Oxygen destroys vitamin C, so losses occur when foods are cut, processed, and stored; these losses may be enough to reduce its activity in the body. Table 10-1 summarizes ways to minimize nutrient losses in the kitchen, and Chapter 19 provides more details.

Toxicity Knowledge about some of the amazing roles of vitamins has prompted many people to take vitamin supplements, assuming that "more is better." Just as an inadequate intake can cause harm, so can an excessive intake. Even some of the water-soluble vitamins have adverse effects when taken in large doses.

That a vitamin can be both essential and harmful may seem surprising, but the same is true of most nutrients. The effects of every substance depend on its dose, and this is one reason consumers should not self-prescribe supplements. Figure 10-1 shows three possible relationships between dose levels and effects. The third diagram in Figure 10-1 represents the situation with nutrients—more is better up to a point, but beyond that point, still more can be harmful.

The DRI include Tolerable Upper Intake Levels (UL) to address the possibility of adverse effects from high doses of nutrients. The UL defines the highest amount

> **FIGURE 10-1 Dose Levels and Effects**

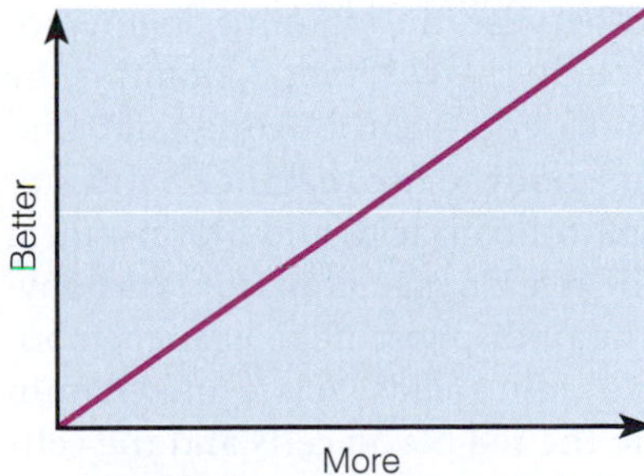
Better
More

As you progress in the direction of more, the effect gets better and better, with no end in sight (real life is seldom, if ever, like this).

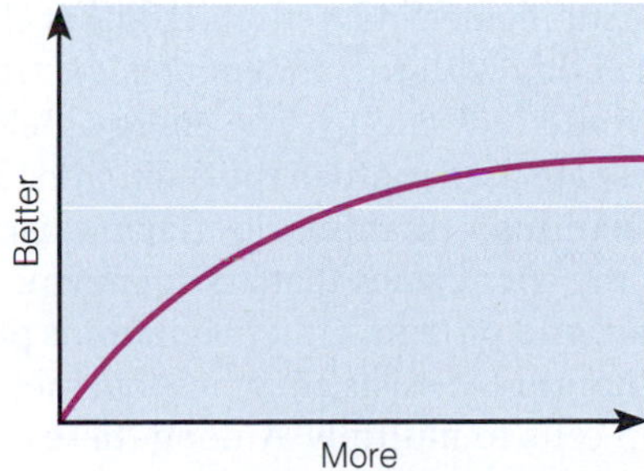
Better
More

As you progress in the direction of more, the effect reaches a maximum and then a plateau, becoming no better with higher doses.

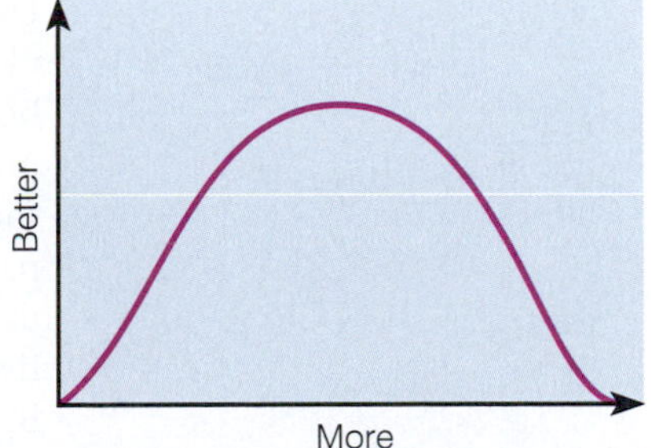
Better
More

As you progress in the direction of more, the effect reaches an optimum at some intermediate dose and then declines, showing that more is better up to a point and then harmful. That too much can be as harmful as too little is true for most nutrients.

TABLE 10-2 Water-Soluble and Fat-Soluble Vitamins Compared

	Water-Soluble Vitamins: B Vitamins and Vitamin C	Fat-Soluble Vitamins: Vitamins A, D, E, and K
Absorption	Directly into the blood	First into the lymph, then the blood
Transport	Travel freely	Many require transport proteins
Storage	Circulate freely in water-filled parts of the body	Stored in the cells associated with fat
Excretion	Kidneys detect and remove excess in urine	Less readily excreted; tend to remain in fat-storage sites
Toxicity	Possible to reach toxic levels when consumed from supplements	Likely to reach toxic levels when consumed from supplements
Requirements	Needed in frequent doses (perhaps 1 to 3 days)	Needed in periodic doses (perhaps weeks or even months)

NOTE: Exceptions occur, but these differences between the water-soluble and fat-solule vitamins are valid generalizations.

of a nutrient that is likely not to cause harm for most healthy people when consumed daily. The risk of harm increases as intakes rise above the UL. Of the nutrients discussed in this chapter, niacin, vitamin B_6, folate, choline, and vitamin C have UL, and these values are presented in their respective summary tables. Data are lacking to establish UL for the remaining B vitamins, but this does not mean that excessively high intakes would be without risk. (The insert pages present UL for the vitamins and minerals.)

REVIEW IT Describe how vitamins differ from the energy nutrients and how fat-soluble vitamins differ from water-soluble vitamins.

The vitamins are essential nutrients needed in tiny amounts in the diet both to prevent deficiency diseases and to support optimal health. The water-soluble vitamins are the B vitamins and vitamin C; the fat-soluble vitamins are vitamins A, D, E, and K. Table 10-2 summarizes the differences between the water-soluble and fat-soluble vitamins.

The following discussion of B vitamins begins with a brief description of each of them, then offers a look at the ways they work together. Thus, a preview of the individual vitamins is followed by a discussion of their interactions.

10.2 The B Vitamins

LEARN IT Identify the main roles, deficiency symptoms, and food sources for each of the B vitamins.

Despite supplement advertisements that claim otherwise, the vitamins do not provide the body with fuel for energy. It is true, though, that without B vitamins the body would lack energy. The energy-yielding nutrients—carbohydrate, fat, and protein—are used for fuel; the B vitamins help the body to use that fuel. Several of the B vitamins—thiamin, riboflavin, niacin, pantothenic acid, and biotin—form part of the **coenzymes** that assist enzymes in the release of energy from carbohydrate, fat, and protein. Other B vitamins play other indispensable roles in metabolism. Vitamin B_6 assists enzymes that metabolize amino acids. Folate and vitamin B_{12} help cells to multiply. Among these cells are the red blood cells and the cells lining the GI tract—cells that deliver energy to all the others.

The vitamin portion of a coenzyme allows a chemical reaction to occur; the remaining portion of the coenzyme binds to the enzyme. Without its coenzyme, an enzyme cannot function. Thus symptoms of B vitamin deficiencies directly reflect the disturbances of metabolism caused by a lack of coenzymes. Figure 10-2 illustrates coenzyme action.

coenzymes: complex organic molecules that work with enzymes to facilitate the enzymes' activity. Many coenzymes have B vitamins as part of their structures.

FIGURE 10-2 Coenzyme Action

Some vitamins form part of the coenzymes that enable enzymes either to synthesize compounds (as illustrated by the lower enzymes in this figure) or to dismantle compounds (as illustrated by the upper enzymes).

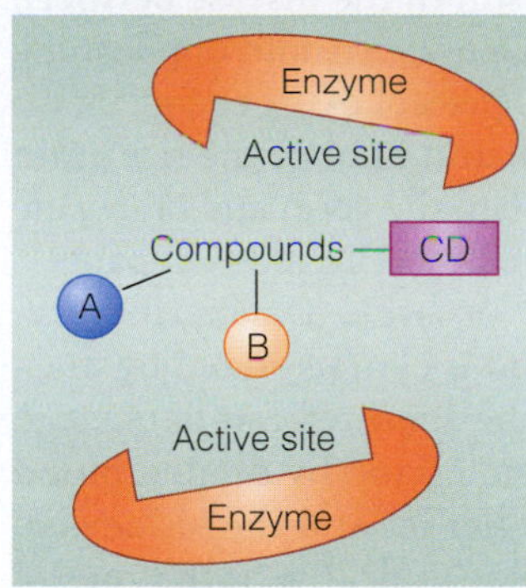

Enzyme
Active site
Compounds
CD
A
B
Active site
Enzyme

Without coenzymes, compounds A, B, and CD don't respond to their enzymes.

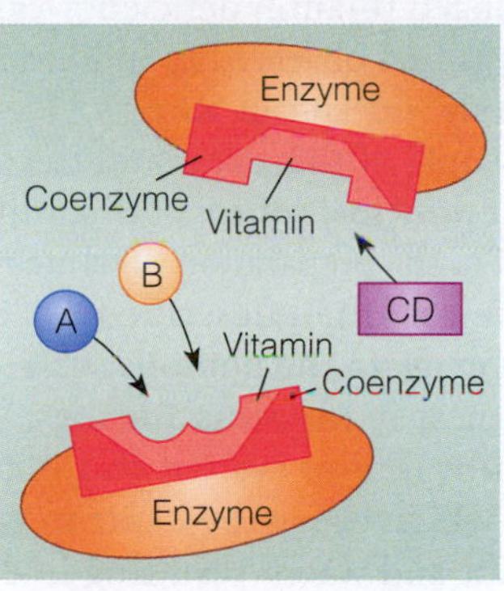

Enzyme
Coenzyme
Vitamin
B
CD
A
Vitamin
Coenzyme
Enzyme

With the coenzymes in place, compounds are attracted to their sites on the enzymes . . .

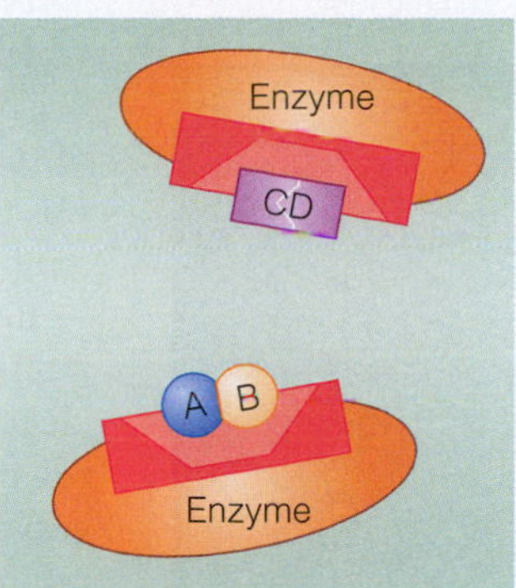

Enzyme
CD
A
B
Enzyme

. . . and the reactions proceed instantaneously. The coenzymes often donate or accept electrons, atoms, or groups of atoms.

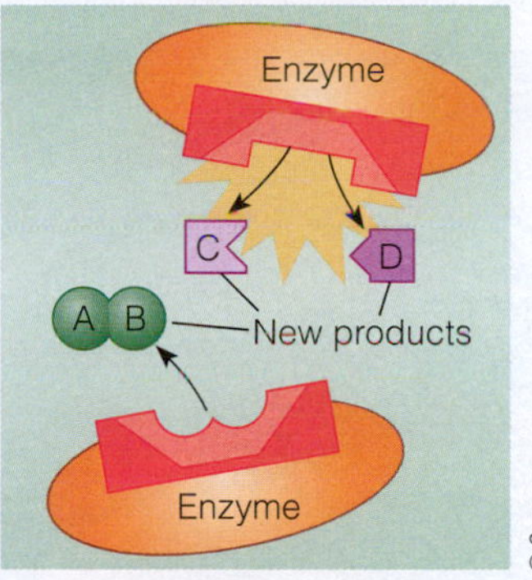

Enzyme
C
D
A
B
New products
Enzyme

The reactions are completed with either the formation of a new product, AB, or the breaking apart of a compound into two new products, C and D, and the release of energy.

The following sections describe the roles of individual B vitamins and note many coenzymes and metabolic pathways. Keep in mind that a later discussion assembles these pieces of information into a whole picture. The following sections also present the recommendations, deficiency and toxicity symptoms, and food sources for each vitamin. For thiamin, riboflavin, niacin, vitamin B_6, folate, vitamin B_{12}, and vitamin C, sufficient data were available to establish an RDA; for biotin, pantothenic acid, and choline, an Adequate Intake (AI) was set; only niacin, vitamin B_6, folate, choline, and vitamin C have UL. These values appear in the summary tables and figures that follow and on the pages of the insert.

Thiamin

Thiamin is the vitamin part of the coenzyme TPP (thiamin pyrophosphate) that assists in energy metabolism. The TPP coenzyme participates in the conversion of pyruvate to acetyl CoA (as Chapter 7 described). Recall how important this step is in allowing carbohydrate metabolism to proceed through the TCA cycle, thus producing much more ATP than during glycolysis alone. The reaction removes 1 carbon from the 3-carbon pyruvate to make the 2-carbon acetyl CoA and carbon dioxide (CO_2). In a similar step in the TCA cycle, TPP helps convert a 5-carbon compound to a 4-carbon compound. Besides playing these pivotal roles in energy metabolism, thiamin occupies a special site on the membranes of nerve cells. Consequently, nerve activity and muscle activity in response to nerves depend heavily on thiamin.

Thiamin Recommendations The thiamin RDA is based primarily on its role in enzyme activity. Generally, thiamin needs will be met if a person eats enough food to meet energy needs—if that energy comes from nutritious foods. The average thiamin intake in the United States meets or exceeds recommendations.

Thiamin Deficiency and Toxicity People who fail to eat enough food to meet energy needs risk nutrient deficiencies, including thiamin deficiency. Inadequate thiamin intakes have been reported among the nation's malnourished and homeless people. Similarly, people who derive most of their energy from empty-kcalorie foods and beverages risk thiamin deficiency. Alcohol provides a good example of how empty kcalories can lead to thiamin deficiency. Alcohol contributes energy but provides few, if any, nutrients and often displaces food. In addition, alcohol impairs thiamin absorption and enhances thiamin excretion in the

thiamin (THIGH-ah-min): a B vitamin. The coenzyme form is *TPP* (*thiamin pyrophosphate*).

> FIGURE 10-3 Thiamin-Deficiency Symptom—The Edema of Beriberi

Physical examination confirms that this person has wet beriberi. Notice how the impression of the physician's thumb remains on the foot.

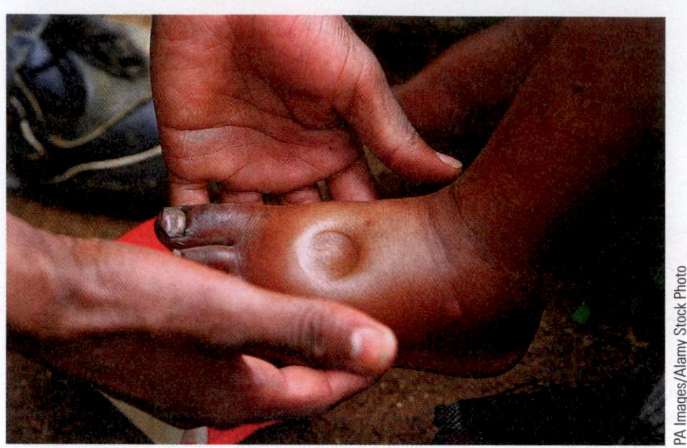

PA Images/Alamy Stock Photo

urine, doubling the risk of deficiency. An estimated four out of five alcoholics are thiamin deficient, which damages the brain's structure and impairs its function.*

Prolonged thiamin deficiency can result in the disease **beriberi,** which was first observed in Indonesia when the custom of polishing rice became widespread. Rice provided 80 percent of the energy intake of the people of that area, and the germ and bran of the rice grain was their principal source of thiamin. When the germ and bran were removed in the preparation of white rice, beriberi became rampant.

Beriberi is often described as "dry" or "wet." Dry beriberi reflects damage to the nervous system and is characterized by muscle weakness in the arms and legs. Wet beriberi reflects damage to the cardiovascular system and is characterized by dilated blood vessels, which cause the heart to work harder and the kidneys to retain salt and water, resulting in edema. Typically, both types of beriberi appear together, with one set of symptoms predominating. Figure 10-3 presents the edema of beriberi. No adverse effects have been associated with excesses of thiamin, and no UL has been determined.

Thiamin Food Sources Before examining Figure 10-4, you may want to read How To 10-1, which describes the content in this and similar figures found in this chapter and the next three chapters. When you look at Figure 10-4, notice that thiamin occurs in small quantities in many nutritious foods. The long red bar near the bottom of the graph shows that meats in the pork family are exceptionally rich in thiamin (see Photo 10-2). Yellow bars confirm that grains—whole grains or enriched—are a reliable source of thiamin.

beriberi: the thiamin-deficiency disease characterized by muscle weakness, edema, or both.

- **beri** = weakness
- **beriberi** = "I can't, I can't"

*Severe thiamin deficiency in alcohol abusers is called the *Wernicke-Korsakoff* (VER-nee-key KORE-sah-kof) *syndrome.* Symptoms include disorientation, loss of short-term memory, jerky eye movements, and staggering gait.

> How To 10-1 Evaluate Foods for Their Nutrient Contributions

Figure 10-4 is the first of a series of figures in this and the next three chapters that present the vitamins and minerals in foods. Each figure presents the same 24 foods, which were selected to ensure a variety of choices representative of each of the food groups as suggested by the USDA Food Patterns. For example, a bread, a cereal, and a pasta were chosen from the grain group. The suggestion to include a variety of vegetables was also considered: dark green vegetables (broccoli); orange and red vegetables (carrots); starchy vegetables (potatoes); legumes (pinto beans); and other vegetables (tomato juice). The selection of fruits followed suggestions to use whole fruits (bananas); citrus fruits (oranges); melons (watermelon); and berries (strawberries). Items were selected from the milk group and protein foods in a similar way. In addition to the 24 foods that appear in all of the figures, three different foods were selected for each of the nutrients to add variety and often reflect excellent, and sometimes unusual, sources.

Notice that the figures list the food, the serving size, and the food energy (kcalories) on the left. The amount of the nutrient per serving is presented in the graph on the right along with the RDA (or AI) for adults, so you can see how many servings would be needed to meet recommendations.

The colored bars show at a glance which food groups best provide a nutrient: yellow for grains; green for vegetables; purple for fruits; white for milk and milk products; brown for legumes; and red for protein foods. Because the USDA Food Patterns include legumes with both the protein foods group and the vegetable group and because legumes are especially rich in many vitamins and minerals, they have been given their own color to highlight their nutrient contributions.

Notice how the bar graphs shift in the various figures. Careful study of all of the figures taken together will confirm that variety is the key to nutrient adequacy.

Another way to evaluate foods for their nutrient contributions is to consider their nutrient density (their thiamin *per 100 kcalories*, for example). Quite often, vegetables rank higher on a nutrient-per-kcalorie list than they do on a nutrient-per-serving list (see pp. 36–37 to review how to evaluate foods based on nutrient density). The left column in the figure highlights about five foods that offer the best nutrient density. Notice how many of them are vegetables.

Realistically, people cannot eat for single nutrients. Fortunately, most foods deliver more than one nutrient, allowing people to combine foods into nourishing meals.

> TRY IT Calculate which food provides more riboflavin per 1-ounce serving—a pork chop (3 oz, 291 kcal, 0.25 mg riboflavin) or cheddar cheese (1½ oz, 165 kcal, 0.11 mg riboflavin). Which food is more nutrient dense with respect to riboflavin?

> **FIGURE 10-4** **Thiamin in Selected Foods**

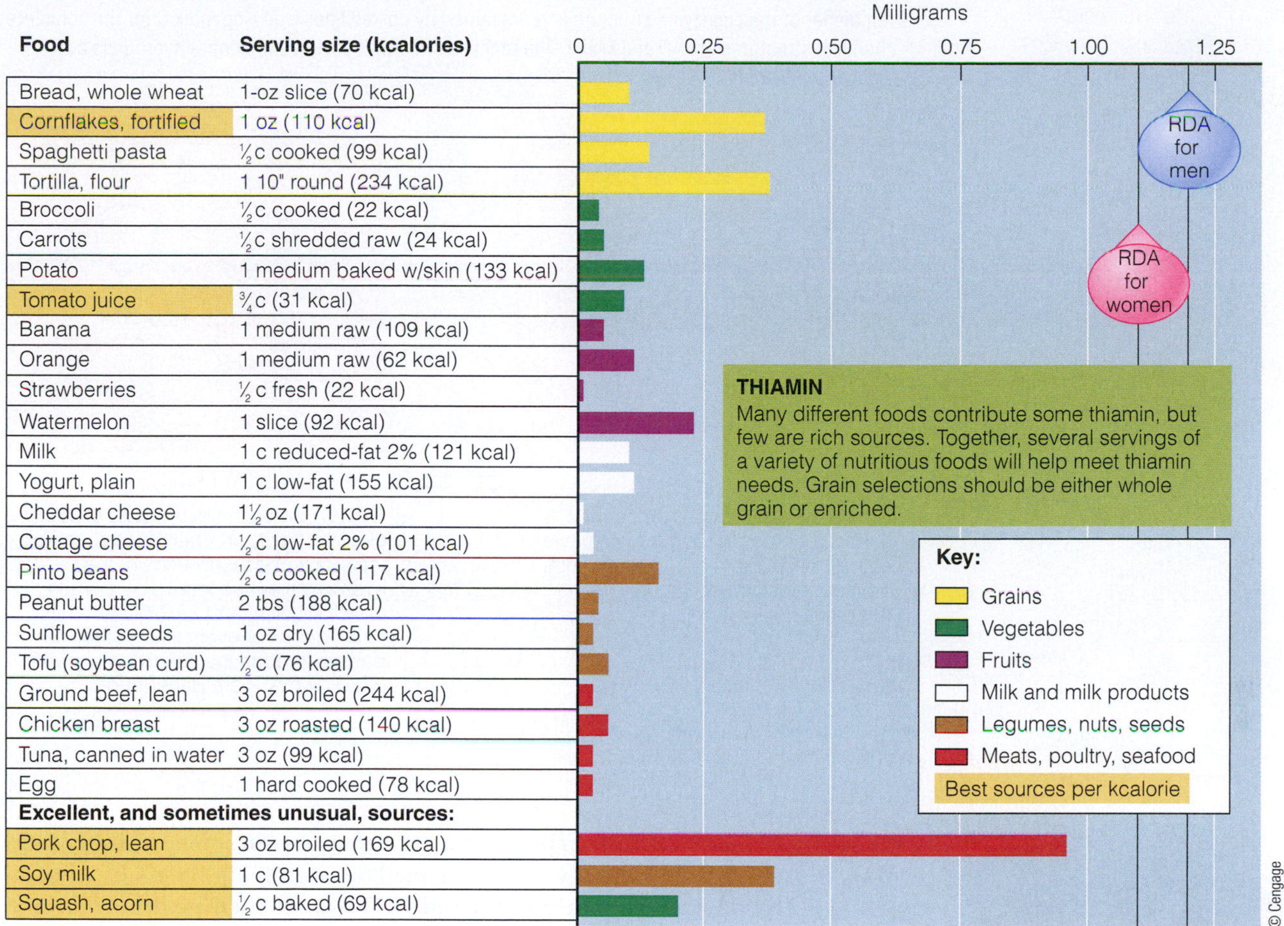

Food	Serving size (kcalories)
Bread, whole wheat	1-oz slice (70 kcal)
Cornflakes, fortified	1 oz (110 kcal)
Spaghetti pasta	½ c cooked (99 kcal)
Tortilla, flour	1 10" round (234 kcal)
Broccoli	½ c cooked (22 kcal)
Carrots	½ c shredded raw (24 kcal)
Potato	1 medium baked w/skin (133 kcal)
Tomato juice	¾ c (31 kcal)
Banana	1 medium raw (109 kcal)
Orange	1 medium raw (62 kcal)
Strawberries	½ c fresh (22 kcal)
Watermelon	1 slice (92 kcal)
Milk	1 c reduced-fat 2% (121 kcal)
Yogurt, plain	1 c low-fat (155 kcal)
Cheddar cheese	1½ oz (171 kcal)
Cottage cheese	½ c low-fat 2% (101 kcal)
Pinto beans	½ c cooked (117 kcal)
Peanut butter	2 tbs (188 kcal)
Sunflower seeds	1 oz dry (165 kcal)
Tofu (soybean curd)	½ c (76 kcal)
Ground beef, lean	3 oz broiled (244 kcal)
Chicken breast	3 oz roasted (140 kcal)
Tuna, canned in water	3 oz (99 kcal)
Egg	1 hard cooked (78 kcal)
Excellent, and sometimes unusual, sources:	
Pork chop, lean	3 oz broiled (169 kcal)
Soy milk	1 c (81 kcal)
Squash, acorn	½ c baked (69 kcal)

Milligrams
0
0.25
0.50
0.75
1.00
1.25
RDA for men
RDA for women
THIAMIN
Many different foods contribute some thiamin, but few are rich sources. Together, several servings of a variety of nutritious foods will help meet thiamin needs. Grain selections should be either whole grain or enriched.
Key:
Grains
Vegetables
Fruits
Milk and milk products
Legumes, nuts, seeds
Meats, poultry, seafood
Best sources per kcalorie

As mentioned earlier, prolonged cooking can destroy thiamin. Also, like other water-soluble vitamins, thiamin leaches into water when foods are boiled or blanched. Cooking methods that require little or no water such as steaming and microwave heating conserve thiamin and other water-soluble vitamins. The accompanying table provides a summary of thiamin.

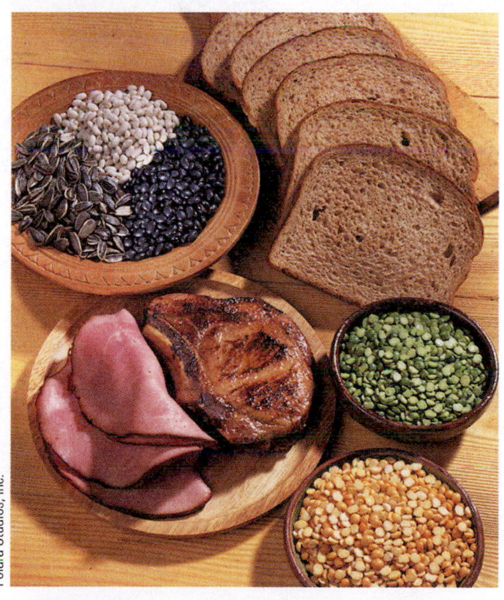

> **PHOTO 10-2** Pork is the richest source of thiamin, but enriched or whole-grain products typically make the greatest contribution to a day's intake because of the quantities eaten. Legumes such as split peas are also valuable sources of thiamin.

REVIEW IT Thiamin

Other Names
Vitamin B_1

RDA
Men: 1.2 mg/day
Women: 1.1 mg/day

Chief Functions in the Body
Part of coenzyme TPP (thiamin pyrophosphate) used in energy metabolism

Significant Sources
Whole-grain, fortified, or enriched grain products; moderate amounts in all nutritious food; pork
Easily destroyed by heat

Deficiency Disease
Beriberi (wet, with edema; dry, with muscle wasting)

Deficiency Symptoms[a]
Enlarged heart, cardiac failure; muscular weakness; apathy, poor short-term memory, confusion, irritability; anorexia, weight loss

Toxicity Symptoms
None reported

[a]Severe thiamin deficiency is often related to heavy alcohol consumption with limited food consumption (Wernicke-Korsakoff syndrome).

> **FIGURE 10-5 Riboflavin Coenzyme, Accepting and Donating Hydrogens**

This figure shows the chemical structure of the riboflavin portion of the coenzyme only; the remainder of the coenzyme structure is represented by dotted lines (see Appendix C for the complete chemical structures of FAD and FMN). The reactive sites that accept and donate hydrogens are highlighted in white.

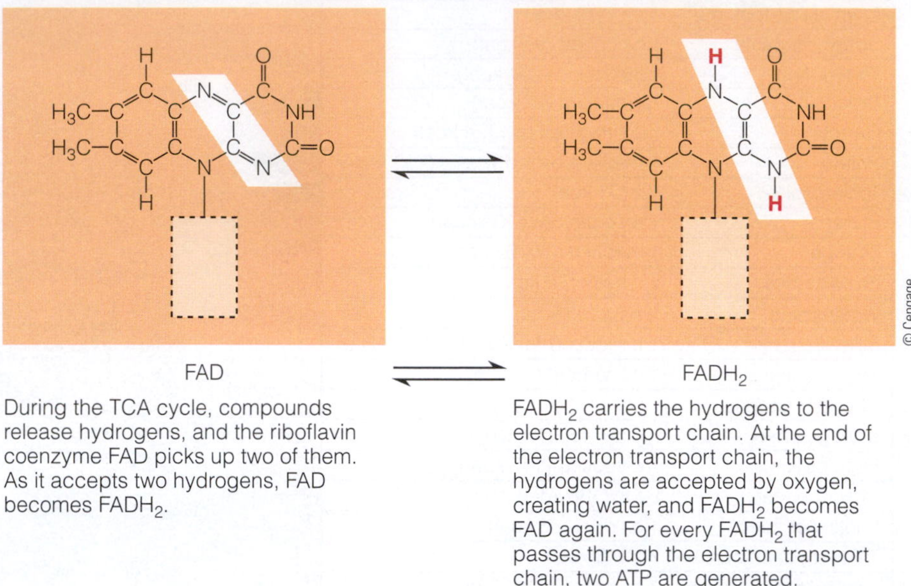

FAD
FADH2
© Cengage

During the TCA cycle, compounds release hydrogens, and the riboflavin coenzyme FAD picks up two of them. As it accepts two hydrogens, FAD becomes $FADH_2$.

$FADH_2$ carries the hydrogens to the electron transport chain. At the end of the electron transport chain, the hydrogens are accepted by oxygen, creating water, and $FADH_2$ becomes FAD again. For every $FADH_2$ that passes through the electron transport chain, two ATP are generated.

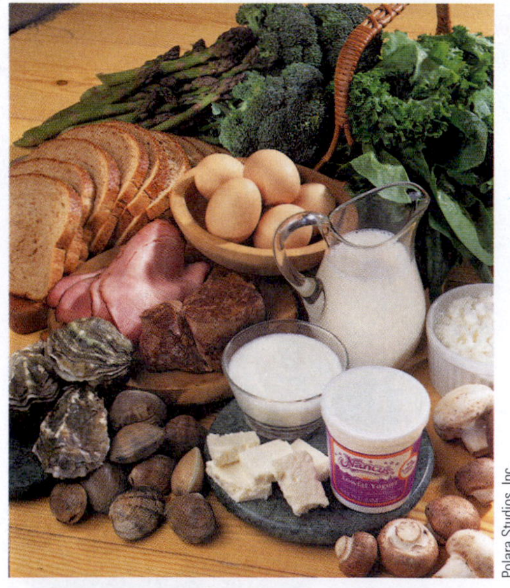

> **PHOTO 10-3** All of these foods are rich in riboflavin, but milk and milk products provide much of the riboflavin in the diets of most people.

Polara Studios, Inc.

riboflavin (RYE-boh-flay-vin): a B vitamin. The coenzyme forms are *FMN (flavin mononucleotide)* and *FAD (flavin adenine dinucleotide)*.

Riboflavin

Like thiamin, **riboflavin** serves as a coenzyme in many reactions, most notably in energy metabolism. The coenzyme forms of riboflavin are FMN (flavin mononucleotide) and FAD (flavin adenine dinucleotide); both can accept and then donate two hydrogens (see Figure 10-5). During energy metabolism, FAD picks up two hydrogens (with their electrons) from the TCA cycle and delivers them to the electron transport chain (as Chapter 7 described).

Riboflavin Recommendations Like thiamin's RDA, riboflavin's RDA is based primarily on its role in enzyme activity. Most people in the United States meet or exceed riboflavin recommendations.

Riboflavin Deficiency and Toxicity Lack of riboflavin causes inflammation of the membranes of the mouth, skin, eyes, and GI tract. Excesses of riboflavin appear to cause no harm, and no UL has been established.

Riboflavin Food Sources The greatest contributions of riboflavin come from milk and milk products (see Photo 10-3 and Figure 10-6). Whole-grain or enriched grains are also valuable sources because of the quantities people typically consume. When riboflavin sources are ranked by nutrient density (per kcalorie), many dark green, leafy vegetables (such as broccoli, turnip greens, asparagus, and spinach) appear high on the list. Vegans and others who don't use milk must rely on ample servings of dark greens and enriched grains for riboflavin. Nutritional yeast is another good source.

Ultraviolet light destroys riboflavin. For this reason, milk is sold in cardboard or opaque plastic containers, instead of clear glass bottles. In contrast, riboflavin is stable to heat, so cooking does not destroy it. The accompanying table provides a summary of riboflavin.

FIGURE 10-6 Riboflavin in Selected Foods

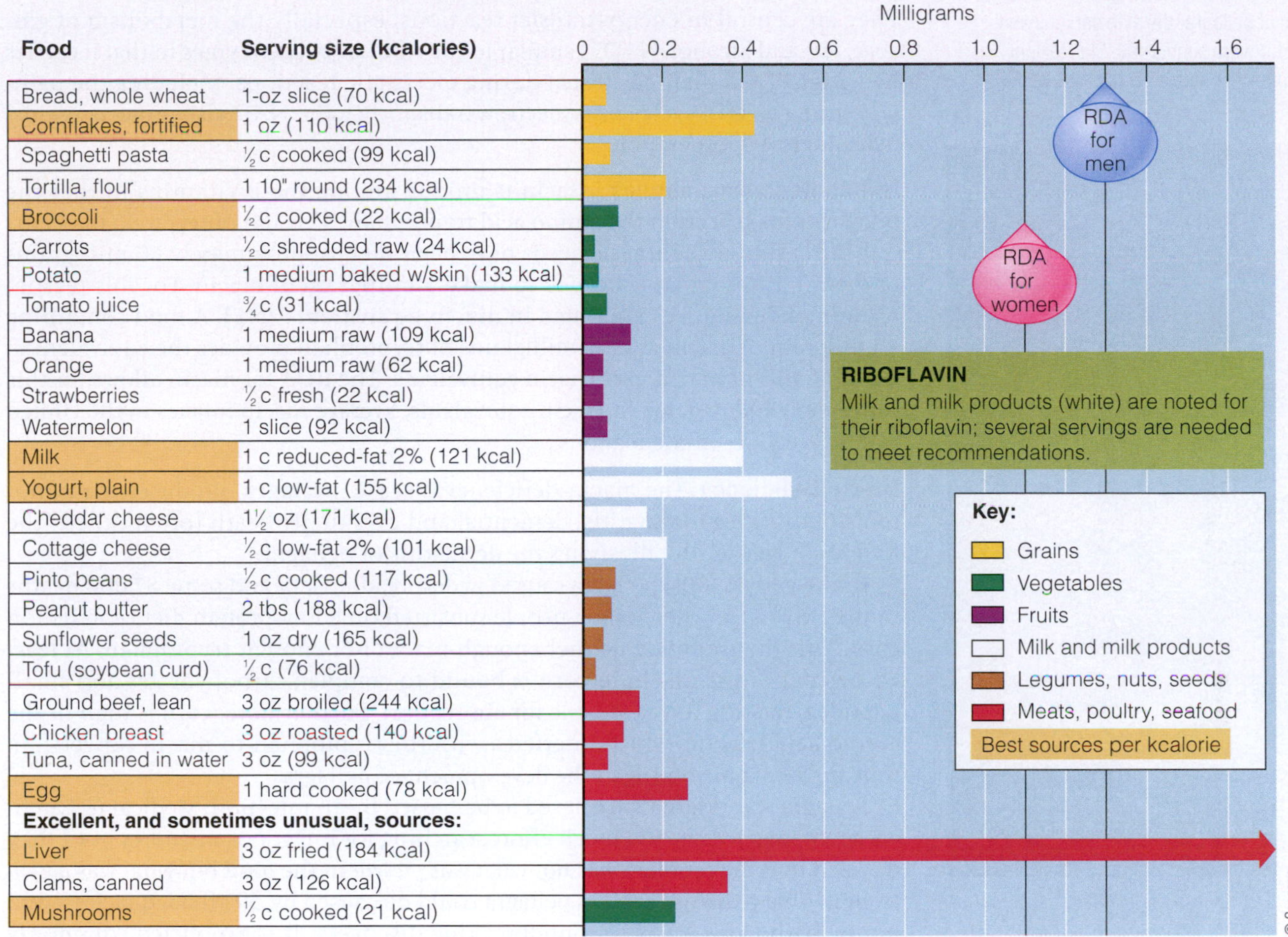

Milligrams
Food
Serving size (kcalories)
0
0.2
0.4
0.6
0.8
1.0
1.2
1.4
1.6
Bread, whole wheat
1-oz slice (70 kcal)
Cornflakes, fortified
1 oz (110 kcal)
Spaghetti pasta
½ c cooked (99 kcal)
Tortilla, flour
1 10" round (234 kcal)
Broccoli
½ c cooked (22 kcal)
Carrots
½ c shredded raw (24 kcal)
Potato
1 medium baked w/skin (133 kcal)
Tomato juice
¾ c (31 kcal)
Banana
1 medium raw (109 kcal)
Orange
1 medium raw (62 kcal)
Strawberries
½ c fresh (22 kcal)
Watermelon
1 slice (92 kcal)
Milk
1 c reduced-fat 2% (121 kcal)
Yogurt, plain
1 c low-fat (155 kcal)
Cheddar cheese
1½ oz (171 kcal)
Cottage cheese
½ c low-fat 2% (101 kcal)
Pinto beans
½ c cooked (117 kcal)
Peanut butter
2 tbs (188 kcal)
Sunflower seeds
1 oz dry (165 kcal)
Tofu (soybean curd)
½ c (76 kcal)
Ground beef, lean
3 oz broiled (244 kcal)
Chicken breast
3 oz roasted (140 kcal)
Tuna, canned in water
3 oz (99 kcal)
Egg
1 hard cooked (78 kcal)
Excellent, and sometimes unusual, sources:
Liver
3 oz fried (184 kcal)
Clams, canned
3 oz (126 kcal)
Mushrooms
½ c cooked (21 kcal)
RDA for men
RDA for women
RIBOFLAVIN
Milk and milk products (white) are noted for their riboflavin; several servings are needed to meet recommendations.
Key:
Grains
Vegetables
Fruits
Milk and milk products
Legumes, nuts, seeds
Meats, poultry, seafood
Best sources per kcalorie

REVIEW IT Riboflavin

Other Names

Vitamin B_2

RDA

Men: 1.3 mg/day

Women: 1.1 mg/day

Chief Functions in the Body

Part of coenzymes FMN (flavin mononucleotide) and FAD (flavin adenine dinucleotide) used in energy metabolism

Significant Sources

Milk products (yogurt, cheese); whole-grain, fortified, or enriched grain products; liver

Easily destroyed by ultraviolet light and irradiation

Deficiency Disease

Ariboflavinosis (ay-RYE-boh-FLAY-vin-oh-sis)

Deficiency Symptoms

Sore throat; cracks and redness at corners of mouth (cheilosis); painful, smooth, purplish red tongue (glossitis); inflammation characterized by skin lesions covered with greasy scales

Toxicity Symptoms

None reported

Niacin

Niacin refers to two chemical structures: nicotinic acid and nicotinamide (also known as niacinamide). The body can easily convert nicotinic acid to nicotinamide, which is the major form of niacin in the blood.

niacin (NIGH-a-sin): a B vitamin. The coenzyme forms are *NAD* (*nicotinamide adenine dinucleotide*) and *NADP* (*the phosphate form of NAD*). Niacin can be eaten preformed or made in the body from its precursor, tryptophan, an essential amino acid.

> **FIGURE 10-7 Niacin-Deficiency Symptom—The Dermatitis of Pellagra**

In the dermatitis of pellagra, the skin darkens and flakes away as if it were sunburned. Skin lesions typically develop only on those parts of the body exposed to the sun.

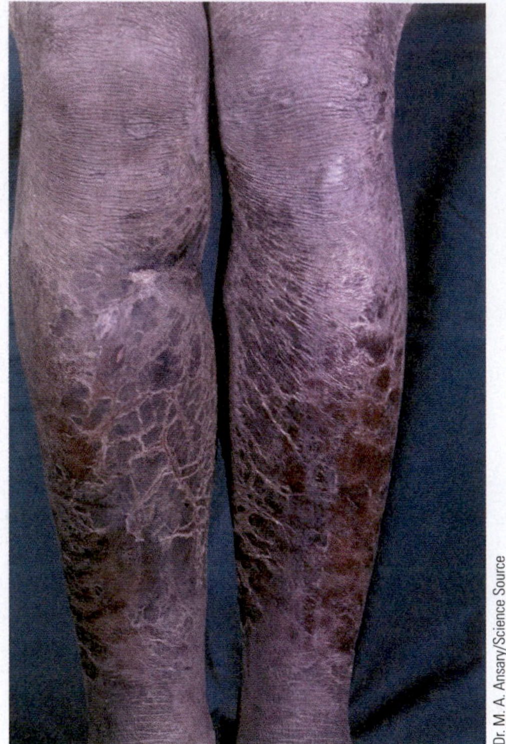

Dr. M. A. Ansary/Science Source

The two coenzyme forms of niacin, NAD (nicotinamide adenine dinucleotide) and NADP (the phosphate form), participate in numerous metabolic reactions. They are central in energy-transfer reactions, especially the metabolism of glucose, fat, and alcohol. NAD is similar to the riboflavin coenzymes in that it carries hydrogens (and their electrons) during metabolic reactions, including the pathway from the TCA cycle to the electron transport chain. NAD also protects against neurological degeneration.

Niacin Recommendations Niacin is unique among the B vitamins in that the body can make it from the amino acid tryptophan. This use of tryptophan occurs only after protein synthesis needs have been met. Approximately 60 milligrams of dietary tryptophan is needed to make 1 milligram of niacin. For this reason, recommended intakes are stated in **niacin equivalents (NE)**. A food containing 1 milligram of niacin and 60 milligrams of tryptophan provides the equivalent of 2 milligrams of niacin, or 2 niacin equivalents. The RDA for niacin allows for this conversion and is stated in niacin equivalents; average niacin intakes in the United States exceed recommendations.

Niacin Deficiency The niacin-deficiency disease, **pellagra**, produces the symptoms of diarrhea, dermatitis, dementia, and eventually death (often called "the four Ds"). Figure 10-7 illustrates the dermatitis of pellagra.

In the early 1900s, pellagra caused widespread misery and some 87,000 deaths in the US South, where many people subsisted on a low-protein diet centered on corn. This diet supplied neither enough niacin nor enough tryptophan. At least 70 percent of the niacin in corn is bound to complex carbohydrates and small peptides, making it unavailable for absorption. Furthermore, corn is high in the amino acid leucine, which interferes with the tryptophan-to-niacin conversion, thus further contributing to the development of pellagra.

Pellagra was originally believed to be caused by an infection. Medical researchers spent many years and much effort searching for infectious microbes until they realized that the problem was not what was *present* in the food but what was *absent* from it. That a disease such as pellagra could be caused by diet inadequacies—and not by pathogens—was a groundbreaking discovery. It contradicted commonly held medical opinions that diseases were caused only by infectious agents. By carefully following the scientific method (as Chapter 1 described), researchers advanced the science of nutrition dramatically.

Niacin Toxicity When a normal dose of a nutrient (levels commonly found in foods) provides a normal blood concentration, the nutrient is having a *physiological* effect. When a large dose (levels commonly available only from supplements) overwhelms the body and raises blood concentrations to abnormally high levels, the nutrient is acting like a drug and having a *pharmacological* effect. Naturally occurring niacin from foods has a physiological effect that causes no harm. Large doses of nicotinic acid from supplements or drugs, however, produce pharmacological effects, most notably **"niacin flush."** Niacin flush occurs when nicotinic acid is taken in doses only three to four times the RDA. It dilates the capillaries and causes a tingling sensation that can be painful. The nicotinamide form does not produce this effect.

Large doses of nicotinic acid can effectively raise HDL cholesterol, but may not benefit patients with heart disease whose blood lipids are already being controlled with statin drugs.[1] Because of possible side effects (such as liver damage), the use of niacin as a drug must be closely monitored.[2]

Niacin Food Sources Tables of food composition typically list preformed niacin only, but as mentioned, niacin can also be made in the body from the amino acid tryptophan. Dietary tryptophan could meet about half the daily niacin requirement for most people, but the average diet easily supplies enough preformed niacin.

Figure 10-8 presents niacin in selected foods. Meat, poultry, fish, legumes, and enriched and whole grains contribute about half the niacin people consume (see Photo 10-4). Mushrooms, potatoes, and tomatoes are among the

niacin equivalents (NE): the amount of niacin present in food, including the niacin that can theoretically be made from its precursor, tryptophan, present in the food.

- 1 NE = 1 mg niacin or 60 mg tryptophan

pellagra (pell-AY-gra): the niacin-deficiency disease, characterized by diarrhea, dermatitis, dementia, and eventually death.

- **pellis** = skin
- **agra** = rough

niacin flush: a temporary burning, tingling, and itching sensation that occurs when a person takes a large dose of nicotinic acid; often accompanied by a headache and reddened face, arms, and chest.

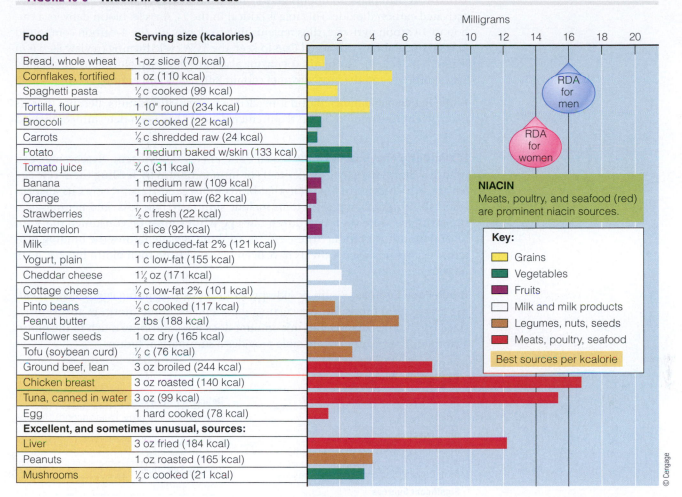

> **FIGURE 10-8 Niacin in Selected Foods**

Food	Serving size (kcalories)
Bread, whole wheat	1-oz slice (70 kcal)
Cornflakes, fortified	1 oz (110 kcal)
Spaghetti pasta	½ c cooked (99 kcal)
Tortilla, flour	1 10" round (234 kcal)
Broccoli	½ c cooked (22 kcal)
Carrots	½ c shredded raw (24 kcal)
Potato	1 medium baked w/skin (133 kcal)
Tomato juice	¾ c (31 kcal)
Banana	1 medium raw (109 kcal)
Orange	1 medium raw (62 kcal)
Strawberries	½ c fresh (22 kcal)
Watermelon	1 slice (92 kcal)
Milk	1 c reduced-fat 2% (121 kcal)
Yogurt, plain	1 c low-fat (155 kcal)
Cheddar cheese	1½ oz (171 kcal)
Cottage cheese	½ c low-fat 2% (101 kcal)
Pinto beans	½ c cooked (117 kcal)
Peanut butter	2 tbs (188 kcal)
Sunflower seeds	1 oz dry (165 kcal)
Tofu (soybean curd)	½ c (76 kcal)
Ground beef, lean	3 oz broiled (244 kcal)
Chicken breast	3 oz roasted (140 kcal)
Tuna, canned in water	3 oz (99 kcal)
Egg	1 hard cooked (78 kcal)
Excellent, and sometimes unusual, sources:	
Liver	3 oz fried (184 kcal)
Peanuts	1 oz roasted (165 kcal)
Mushrooms	½ c cooked (21 kcal)

Milligrams
0 2 4 6 8 10 12 14 16 18 20
RDA for men
RDA for women
NIACIN
Meats, poultry, and seafood (red) are prominent niacin sources.
Key:
Grains
Vegetables
Fruits
Milk and milk products
Legumes, nuts, seeds
Meats, poultry, seafood
Best sources per kcalorie

richest vegetable sources, and they can provide abundant niacin when eaten in generous amounts.

Niacin is less vulnerable to losses during food preparation and storage than other water-soluble vitamins. Being fairly heat resistant, niacin can withstand reasonable cooking times, but like other water-soluble vitamins, it will leach into cooking water. The accompanying table provides a summary of niacin.

REVIEW IT Niacin

Other Names

Nicotinic acid, nicotinamide, niacinamide, vitamin B_3; precursor is dietary tryptophan (an amino acid)

RDA

Men: 16 mg NE/day

Women: 14 mg NE/day

UL[a]

Adults: 35 mg/day

Chief Functions in the Body

Part of coenzymes NAD (nicotinamide adenine dinucleotide) and NADP (its phosphate form) used in energy metabolism

Significant Sources

Milk, eggs, meat, poultry, fish; whole-grain, fortified, and enriched grain products; nuts and all protein-containing foods

Deficiency Disease

Pellagra

Deficiency Symptoms

Diarrhea, abdominal pain, vomiting; inflamed, swollen, smooth, bright red tongue (glossitis); depression, apathy, fatigue, loss of memory, headache; bilateral symmetrical rash on areas exposed to sunlight

Toxicity Symptoms

Painful flush, hives, and rash ("niacin flush"); nausea and vomiting; liver damage; impaired glucose tolerance

[a]The UL applies to synthetic forms obtained from supplements, fortified foods, or a combination.

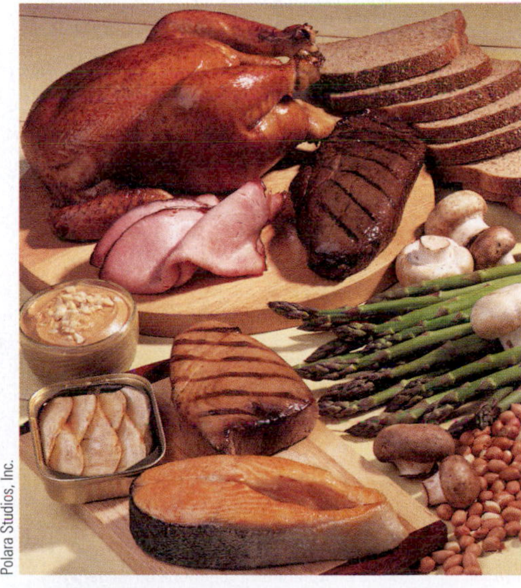

> **PHOTO 10-4** Protein-rich foods such as meat, fish, poultry, and peanut butter contribute much of the niacin in people's diets. Enriched breads and cereals and a few vegetables are also rich in niacin.

Biotin **Biotin** plays an important role in metabolism as a coenzyme that carries activated carbon dioxide. This role is critical in the TCA cycle: biotin delivers a carbon to 3-carbon pyruvate, thus replenishing oxaloacetate, the 4-carbon compound needed to combine with acetyl CoA to keep the TCA cycle turning (review Step 6 in Figure 7-15, p. 210). The biotin coenzyme also participates in gluconeogenesis, fatty acid synthesis, and the breakdown of certain fatty acids and amino acids.

Biotin Recommendations Biotin is needed in very small amounts. Because there is insufficient research on biotin requirements, an AI has been determined, instead of an RDA.

Biotin Deficiency and Toxicity Biotin deficiencies rarely occur. Researchers can induce a biotin deficiency in animals or human beings by feeding them raw egg whites, which contain a protein that binds biotin and thus prevents its absorption.* Biotin-deficiency symptoms include skin rash, hair loss, and neurological impairment. More than two dozen raw egg whites must be consumed daily for several months to produce these effects; cooking eggs denatures the binding protein. Because no adverse effects have been reported from high biotin intakes, a UL has not been set.

Biotin Food Sources Biotin is widespread in foods (including egg yolks), so eating a variety of foods protects against deficiencies. Some biotin is also synthesized by GI tract bacteria, but this amount does not contribute much to the biotin absorbed. The accompanying table provides a summary of biotin.

REVIEW IT Biotin

AI	Deficiency Symptoms
Adults: 30 µg/day	Depression, lethargy, hallucinations, numb or tingling sensation in the arms and legs; red, scaly rash around the eyes, nose, and mouth; hair loss
Chief Functions in the Body	**Toxicity Symptoms**
Part of a coenzyme used in energy metabolism, fat synthesis, amino acid metabolism, and glycogen synthesis	None reported
Significant Sources	
Widespread in foods; liver, egg yolks, soybeans, fish, whole grains; also produced by GI bacteria	

Pantothenic Acid **Pantothenic acid** is part of the chemical structure of coenzyme A—the same CoA that forms acetyl CoA, a key compound in several metabolic pathways featured in Chapter 7, including the TCA cycle. (Appendix C presents the chemical structures of these two molecules and shows that coenzyme A is made up in part of pantothenic acid.) As such, it is involved in more than 100 different steps in the synthesis of lipids, neurotransmitters, steroid hormones, and hemoglobin.

Pantothenic Acid Recommendations An AI for pantothenic acid has been set. It reflects the amount needed to replace daily losses.

Pantothenic Acid Deficiency and Toxicity Pantothenic acid deficiency is rare. Its symptoms involve a general failure of all the body's systems and include fatigue, GI distress, and neurological disturbances. The "burning feet" syndrome that affected prisoners of war in Asia during World War II is thought to have been caused by pantothenic acid deficiency. No toxic effects have been reported, and no UL has been established.

Pantothenic Acid Food Sources Pantothenic acid is widespread in foods, and typical diets seem to provide adequate intakes. Beef, poultry, whole grains, potatoes,

biotin (BY-oh-tin): a B vitamin that functions as a coenzyme in metabolism.

pantothenic (PAN-toe-THEN-ick) **acid:** a B vitamin. The principal active form is part of coenzyme A, called "CoA" throughout Chapter 7.

- **pantos** = everywhere

*The protein *avidin* (AV-eh-din) in egg whites binds biotin.

tomatoes, and broccoli are particularly good sources. Losses of pantothenic acid during food production can be substantial because it is readily destroyed by the freezing, canning, and refining processes. The accompanying table provides a summary of pantothenic acid.

REVIEW IT Pantothenic Acid

AI
Adults: 5 mg/day
Chief Functions in the Body
Part of coenzyme A, used in energy metabolism
Significant Sources
Widespread in foods; chicken, beef, potatoes, oats, tomatoes, liver, egg yolk, broccoli, whole grains
Easily destroyed by food processing
Deficiency Symptoms
Vomiting, nausea, stomach cramps; insomnia, fatigue, depression, irritability, restlessness, apathy; hypoglycemia, increased sensitivity to insulin; numbness, muscle cramps, inability to walk
Toxicity Symptoms
None reported

Vitamin B_6

Vitamin B_6 occurs in three forms—pyridoxal, pyridoxine, and pyridoxamine. All three can be converted to the coenzyme PLP (pyridoxal phosphate), which is active in more than 100 reactions, including carbohydrate, fatty acid, and amino acid metabolism. By using PLP to transfer amino groups (NH_2) from an amino acid to a keto acid, the body can make nonessential amino acids (review Figure 6-11, p. 181). The ability to add and remove amino groups makes PLP valuable in protein and urea metabolism as well. The conversions of the amino acid tryptophan to niacin or to the neurotransmitter serotonin also depend on PLP. In addition, PLP participates in the synthesis of heme (the nonprotein portion of hemoglobin), nucleic acids (such as DNA and RNA), and lecithin (a phospholipid).

Vitamin B_6 Recommendations The RDA for vitamin B_6 is based on the amounts needed to maintain adequate levels of its coenzymes. Unlike other water-soluble vitamins, vitamin B_6 is stored extensively in muscle tissue. Research does not support claims, however, that large doses of vitamin B_6 enhance muscle strength or physical endurance.

Vitamin B_6 Deficiency Without adequate vitamin B_6, synthesis of key neurotransmitters diminishes, and abnormal compounds produced during tryptophan metabolism accumulate in the brain. Early symptoms of vitamin B_6 deficiency include depression and confusion; advanced symptoms include abnormal brain wave patterns and convulsions.

Alcohol contributes to the destruction and loss of vitamin B_6 from the body. As Highlight 7 described, when the body breaks down alcohol, it produces acetaldehyde. If allowed to accumulate, acetaldehyde dislodges the PLP coenzyme from its enzymes; once loose, PLP breaks down and is excreted.

Vitamin B_6 Toxicity The first major report of vitamin B_6 toxicity appeared in the early 1980s. Until that time, most researchers and dietitians believed that, like the other water-soluble vitamins, vitamin B_6 could not reach toxic concentrations in the body. The report described neurological damage in people who had been taking more than 2 *grams* of vitamin B_6 daily (20 times the current UL of 100 *milligrams* per day) for 2 months or more.

Vitamin B_6 Food Sources As you can see from the colors in Figure 10-9 (p. 306), meats, fish, and poultry (red bars), potatoes and a few other vegetables (green bars), and fruits (purple bars) offer vitamin B_6 (see Photo 10-5). As is true of most of the other vitamins, fruits and vegetables rank considerably higher when foods are judged by nutrient density (vitamin B_6 per kcalorie). Several servings of vitamin B_6–rich foods are needed to meet recommended intakes.

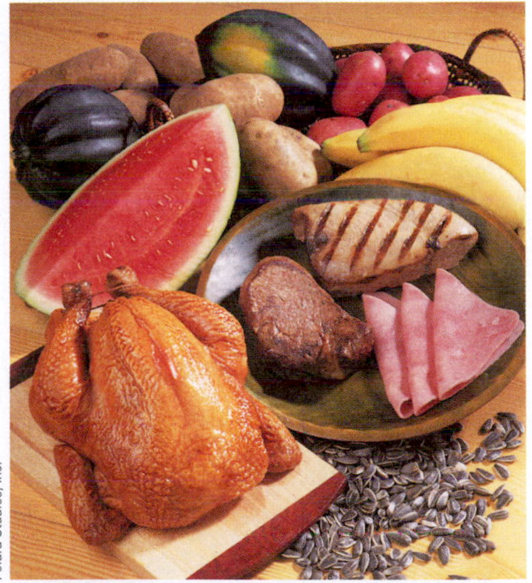

> **PHOTO 10-5** Most protein-rich foods such as meat, fish, and poultry provide ample vitamin B_6; some vegetables and fruits are good sources too.

vitamin B_6: a family of compounds—pyridoxal, pyridoxine, and pyridoxamine. The primary active coenzyme form is *PLP* (*pyridoxal phosphate*).

> **FIGURE 10-9 Vitamin B_6 in Selected Foods**

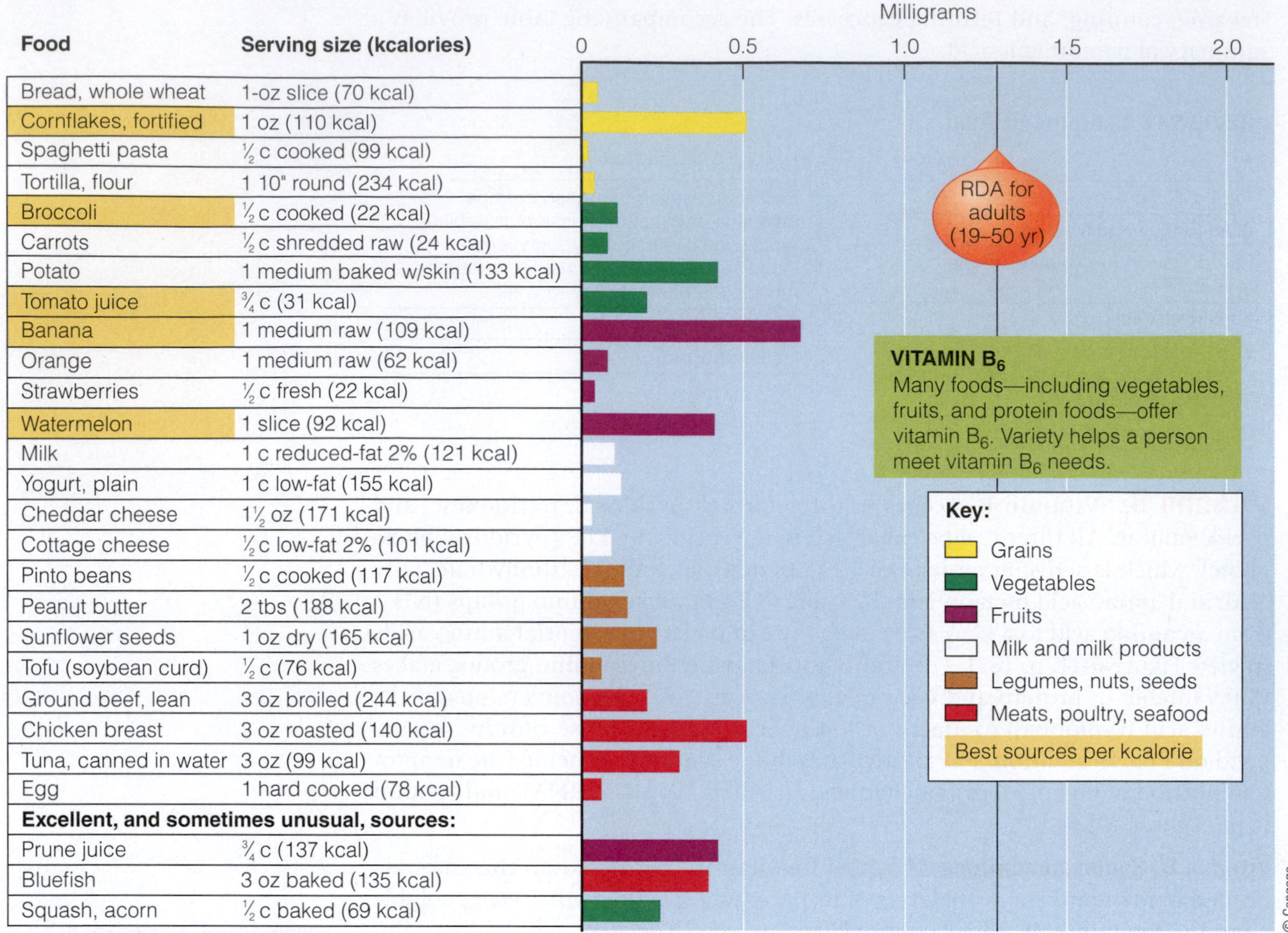

Milligrams
0 0.5 1.0 1.5 2.0
Food | Serving size (kcalories)
Bread, whole wheat | 1-oz slice (70 kcal)
Cornflakes, fortified | 1 oz (110 kcal)
Spaghetti pasta | ½ c cooked (99 kcal)
Tortilla, flour | 1 10" round (234 kcal)
Broccoli | ½ c cooked (22 kcal)
Carrots | ½ c shredded raw (24 kcal)
Potato | 1 medium baked w/skin (133 kcal)
Tomato juice | ¾ c (31 kcal)
Banana | 1 medium raw (109 kcal)
Orange | 1 medium raw (62 kcal)
Strawberries | ½ c fresh (22 kcal)
Watermelon | 1 slice (92 kcal)
Milk | 1 c reduced-fat 2% (121 kcal)
Yogurt, plain | 1 c low-fat (155 kcal)
Cheddar cheese | 1½ oz (171 kcal)
Cottage cheese | ½ c low-fat 2% (101 kcal)
Pinto beans | ½ c cooked (117 kcal)
Peanut butter | 2 tbs (188 kcal)
Sunflower seeds | 1 oz dry (165 kcal)
Tofu (soybean curd) | ½ c (76 kcal)
Ground beef, lean | 3 oz broiled (244 kcal)
Chicken breast | 3 oz roasted (140 kcal)
Tuna, canned in water | 3 oz (99 kcal)
Egg | 1 hard cooked (78 kcal)
Excellent, and sometimes unusual, sources:
Prune juice | ¾ c (137 kcal)
Bluefish | 3 oz baked (135 kcal)
Squash, acorn | ½ c baked (69 kcal)
RDA for adults (19–50 yr)
VITAMIN B6
Many foods—including vegetables, fruits, and protein foods—offer vitamin B6. Variety helps a person meet vitamin B6 needs.
Key:
Grains
Vegetables
Fruits
Milk and milk products
Legumes, nuts, seeds
Meats, poultry, seafood
Best sources per kcalorie

Foods lose vitamin B_6 when heated. Information is limited, but vitamin B_6 bioavailability from plant-derived foods seems to be lower than from animal-derived foods. The accompanying table provides a summary of vitamin B_6.

REVIEW IT Vitamin B_6

Other Names	Significant Sources
Pyridoxine, pyridoxal, pyridoxamine	Meats, fish, poultry, potatoes and other starchy vegetables, legumes, noncitrus fruits, fortified cereals, liver, soy products
RDA	Easily destroyed by heat
Adults (19–50 yr): 1.3 mg/day	**Deficiency Symptoms**
UL	Scaly dermatitis; microcytic anemia; depression, confusion, convulsions
Adults: 100 mg/day	**Toxicity Symptoms**
Chief Functions in the Body	Depression, fatigue, irritability, headaches, nerve damage causing numbness and muscle weakness leading to an inability to walk and convulsions; skin lesions
Part of coenzymes PLP (pyridoxal phosphate) and PMP (pyridoxamine phosphate) used in amino acid and fatty acid metabolism; helps to convert tryptophan to niacin and to serotonin; helps to make red blood cells	

folate (FOLE-ate): a B vitamin; also known as folic acid, folacin, or pteroylglutamic (tare-o-EEL-glue-TAM-ick) acid (PGA). The coenzyme forms are *DHF (dihydrofolate)* and *THF (tetrahydrofolate)*.

Folate

Folate, also known as folacin or folic acid, has a chemical name that would fit a flying dinosaur: pteroylglutamic acid (PGA for short). Its primary coenzyme form, THF (tetrahydrofolate), serves as part of an enzyme complex that transfers 1-carbon compounds that arise during metabolism. This action

> **FIGURE 10-10 Forms of Folate**

Chemically known as pteroylglutamic acid, folate consists of a ring structure (called a pteroyl) and one to six molecules of glutamate (an amino acid). (See Appendix C for the complete chemical structure.)

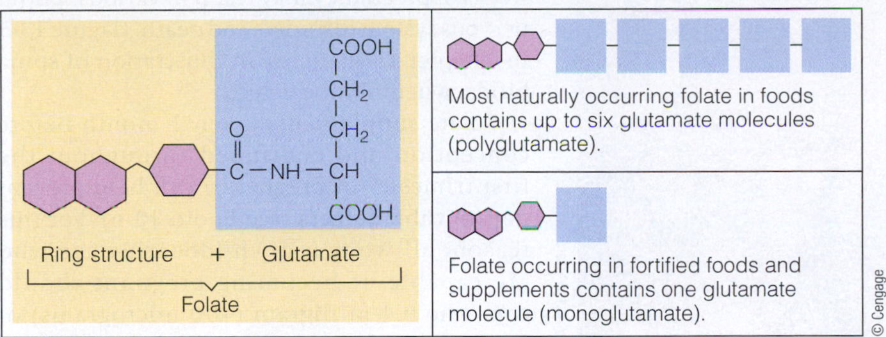
COOH
CH2
CH2
O
C—NH—CH
COOH
Ring structure + Glutamate
Folate
Most naturally occurring folate in foods contains up to six glutamate molecules (polyglutamate).
Folate occurring in fortified foods and supplements contains one glutamate molecule (monoglutamate).
© Cengage

converts vitamin B_{12} to one of its coenzyme forms, synthesizes the DNA required for all rapidly growing cells, and regenerates the amino acid methionine from homocysteine.

Figure 10-10 illustrates two forms of folate. It explains that folate in fortified foods and supplements is in its monoglutamate form (containing only one glutamate), whereas naturally occurring folate in foods contains up to six glutamates (known as a polyglutamate). During digestion, enzymes on the intestinal cell walls hydrolyze the polyglutamate to monoglutamate and several single glutamates. The monoglutamate is then attached to a methyl group (CH_3), which inactivates folate for storage in the liver and other body cells. To activate folate, the methyl group must be removed by an enzyme that requires the help of vitamin B_{12}. Without that help, folate remains trapped in its methyl form, unavailable to support DNA synthesis and cell growth. Figure 10-11 summarizes folate's absorption, activation, and relationship with vitamin B_{12}.

The liver incorporates excess folate into bile that is then sent to the gallbladder and GI tract. Thus folate travels in the same enterohepatic circulation as bile (review Figure 5-14, p. 141).

This complicated system for handling folate is vulnerable to GI tract injuries. Because folate is actively secreted back into the GI tract with bile, it can be reabsorbed repeatedly. If the GI tract cells are damaged, then folate is lost. Such is the case in alcohol abuse; folate deficiency rapidly develops and, ironically, further damages the GI tract. Remember, folate is active in cell multiplication—and the cells lining the GI tract are among the most rapidly replaced cells in the body. When unable to make new cells, the GI tract deteriorates and not only loses folate, but fails to absorb other nutrients as well.

> **FIGURE 10-11 Folate's Absorption and Activation**

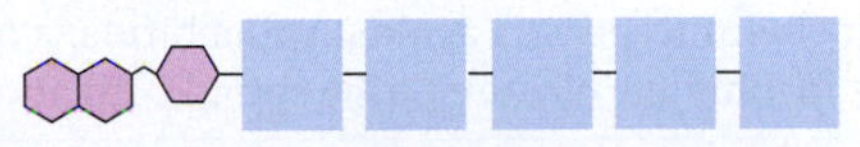
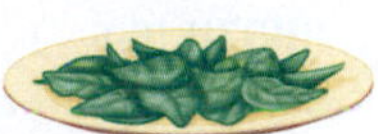

Spinach

In foods, folate naturally occurs as polyglutamate. (Folate occurs as monoglutamate in fortified foods and supplements.)

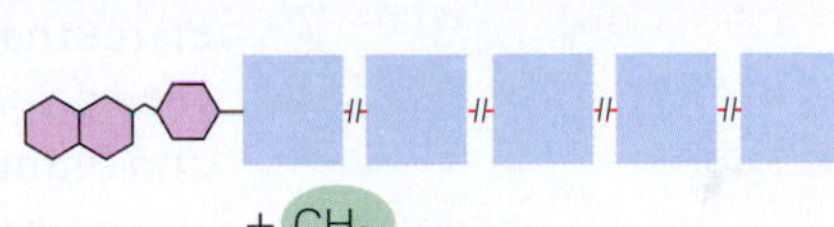
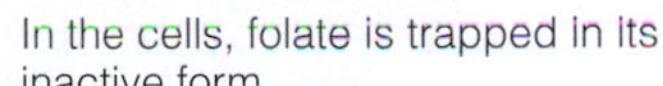
+ CH3
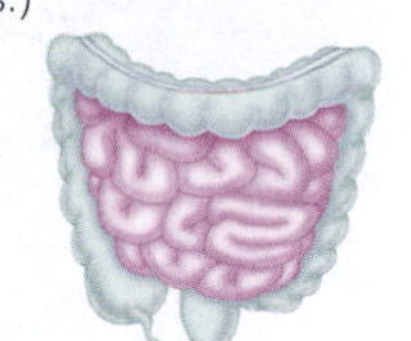

Intestine

In the intestine, digestion breaks glutamates off . . . and adds a methyl group. Folate is absorbed and delivered to cells.

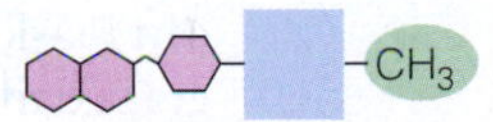
CH3
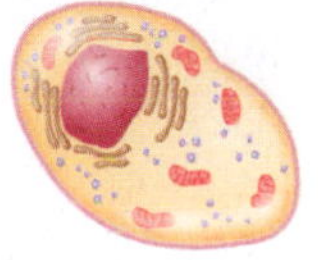

Cell

In the cells, folate is trapped in its inactive form.

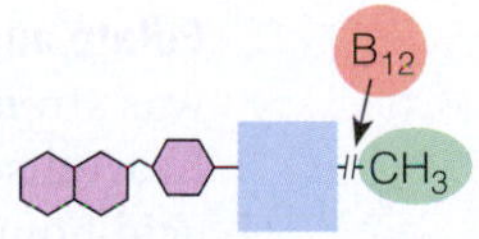
B12
CH3

To activate folate, vitamin B_{12} removes and keeps the methyl group, which activates vitamin B_{12}.

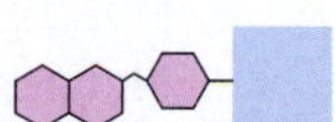
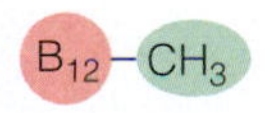
B12—CH3
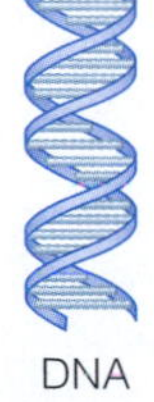

DNA

Both the folate coenzyme and the vitamin B_{12} coenzyme are now active and available for DNA synthesis.

© Cengage

Folate Recommendations The bioavailability of folate differs depending on the source, and these differences must be considered when establishing folate recommendations. The DRI committee gives naturally occurring folate from foods (polyglutamates) full credit. Synthetic folate from fortified foods and supplements (monoglutamates) is given extra credit because, on average, it is 1.7 times more available than naturally occurring food folate. Thus a person consuming 100 micrograms of folate from foods and 100 micrograms from a supplement (multiplied by 1.7) receives 270 **dietary folate equivalents (DFE)**. The need for folate rises considerably during pregnancy and whenever cells are multiplying, so the recommendations for pregnant women are considerably higher than for other adults.

dietary folate equivalents (DFE): the amount of folate available to the body from naturally occurring sources, fortified foods, and supplements, accounting for differences in the bioavailability from each source.

- DFE = μg food folate + (1.7 × μg synthetic folate)

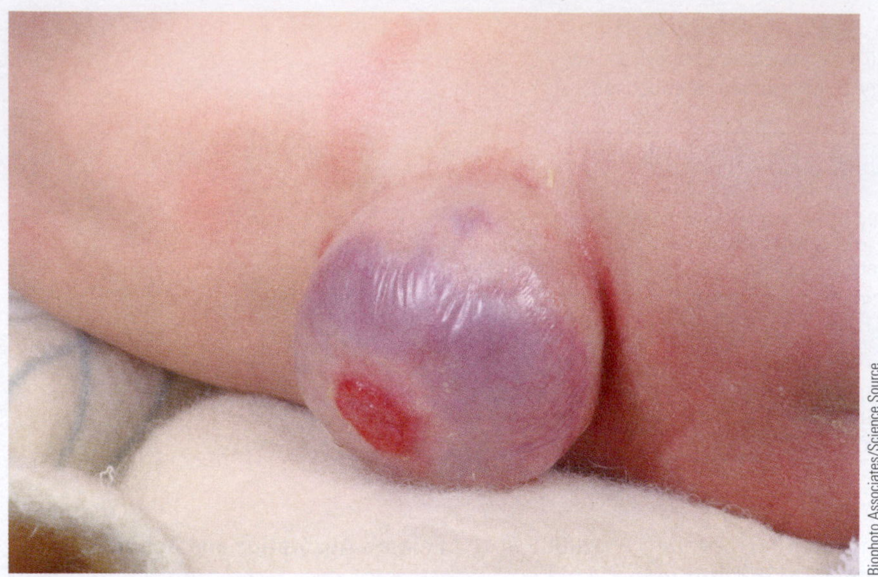
Biophoto Associates/Science Source

> **PHOTO 10-6** Folate helps to protect against spina bifida, a neural tube defect characterized by the incomplete closure of the spinal cord and its bony encasement.

Folate and Neural Tube Defects The brain and spinal cord develop from the **neural tube**, and defects in its orderly formation during the early weeks of pregnancy may result in various central nervous system disorders and death. (Figure 15-5 in Chapter 15 includes an illustration of spina bifida, a neural tube defect.)

Folate supplements taken 1 month before conception and continued throughout the first trimester of pregnancy can help prevent **neural tube defects** (see Photo 10-6). For this reason, all women of childbearing age who are capable of becoming pregnant should consume 0.4 milligram (400 micrograms) of folate daily—easily accomplished by eating folate-rich foods, folate-fortified foods, or a multivitamin supplement daily. Because half of the pregnancies each year are unplanned and because neural tube defects occur early in development before most women realize they are pregnant, the Food and Drug Administration (FDA) has mandated that grain products be fortified to deliver folate to the US population.* Labels on fortified products may claim that "adequate intake of folate has been shown to reduce the risk of neural tube defects." Fortification has improved folate status in women of childbearing age and dramatically lowered the prevalence rate of neural tube defects.

Some research suggests that folate taken before and during pregnancy may also prevent congenital heart disease; birth defects, such as cleft lip and cleft palate; and neurodevelopmental disorders, such as autism.[3] Such findings strengthen recommendations for women to pay attention to their folate needs.

Folate fortification raises safety concerns as well. Because high intakes of folate can mask a vitamin B_{12} deficiency, folate consumption should not exceed 1 milligram daily without close medical supervision. The risks and benefits of folate fortification continue to be a topic of current debate, especially given that 5 percent of the US population exceed the UL for folate.

Folate and Heart Disease The FDA's decision to fortify grain products with folate was strengthened by research suggesting a role for folate in protecting against heart disease. One of folate's key roles in the body is to break down the amino acid homocysteine. Without folate, homocysteine accumulates, which seems to enhance formation of blood clots and atherosclerotic lesions. Fortified foods and folate supplements raise blood folate and reduce blood homocysteine, but may not reduce the risk of heart attacks, strokes, or death from cardiovascular causes.

Folate and Cancer Because the synthesis of DNA and the transfer of methyl groups depend on folate, its relationships with cancer are complex, depending on the type of cancer and the timing of folate supplementation. Some research suggests that sufficient folate may protect against the initiation of cancer, whereas other studies report that high intakes may enhance progression once cancer has begun. In general, foods containing folate probably reduce the risk of pancreatic cancer. Limited evidence suggests that folate may also reduce the risk of esophageal and colorectal cancer.[4]

Folate Deficiency Folate deficiency impairs cell division and protein synthesis—processes critical to growing tissues. In a folate deficiency, the replacement of red

neural tube: the embryonic tissue that forms the brain and spinal cord.

neural tube defects: malformations of the brain, spinal cord, or both during embryonic development that often result in lifelong disability or death. The two main types of neural tube defects are *spina bifida* (literally "split spine") and *anencephaly* ("no brain").

*Bread products, flour, corn grits, cornmeal, farina, rice, macaroni, and noodles must be fortified with 140 micrograms of folate per 100 grams of grain. For perspective, 100 grams is roughly 3 slices of bread; 1 cup of flour; ½ cup of corn grits, cornmeal, farina, or rice; or ¾ cup of macaroni or noodles.

> **FIGURE 10-12 Normal Blood Cells and Blood Cells in Macrocytic Anemia Compared**

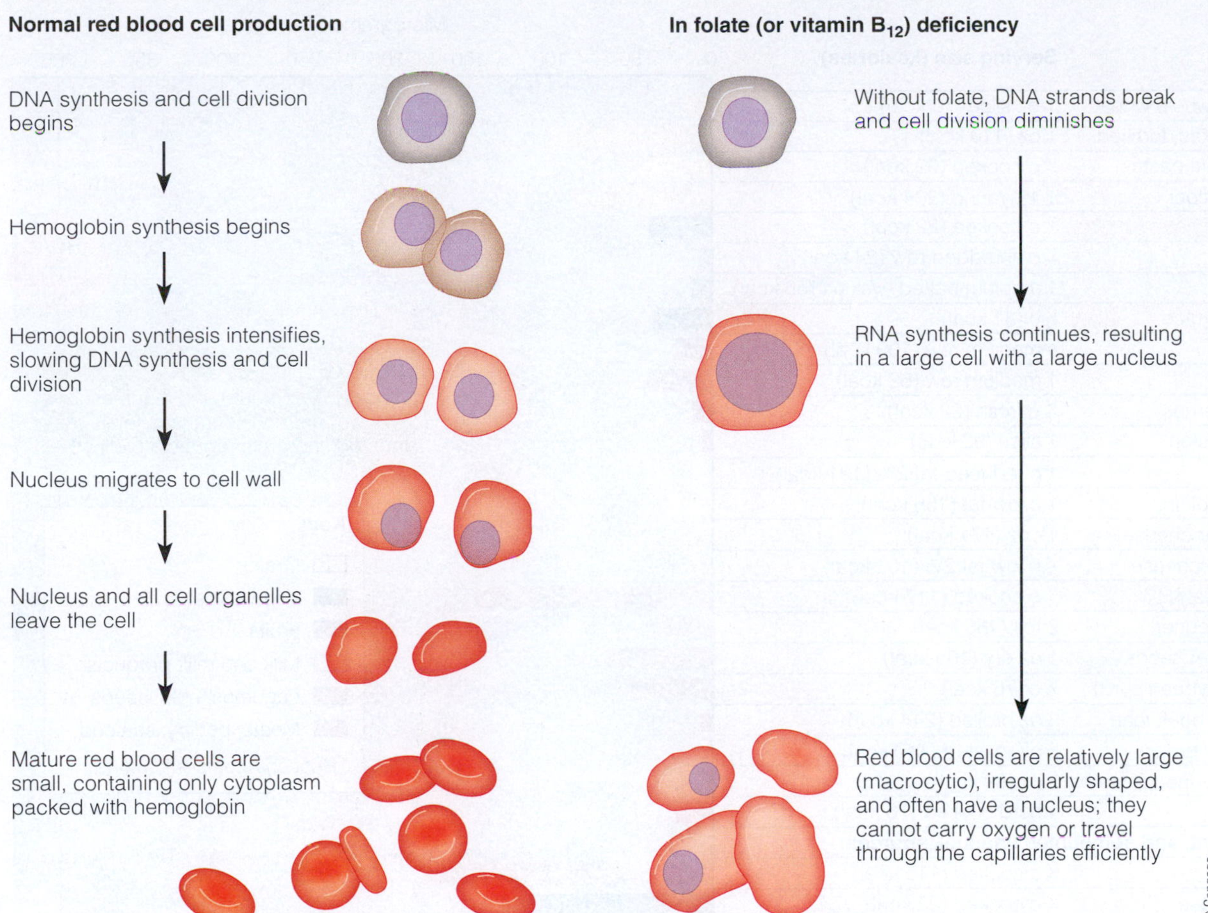

Normal red blood cell production
DNA synthesis and cell division begins
Hemoglobin synthesis begins
Hemoglobin synthesis intensifies, slowing DNA synthesis and cell division
Nucleus migrates to cell wall
Nucleus and all cell organelles leave the cell
Mature red blood cells are small, containing only cytoplasm packed with hemoglobin
In folate (or vitamin B_{12}) deficiency
Without folate, DNA strands break and cell division diminishes
RNA synthesis continues, resulting in a large cell with a large nucleus
Red blood cells are relatively large (macrocytic), irregularly shaped, and often have a nucleus; they cannot carry oxygen or travel through the capillaries efficiently

blood cells and GI tract cells falters. Not surprisingly, then, two of the first symptoms of a folate deficiency are **anemia** and GI tract deterioration.

The anemia of folate deficiency is known as *macrocytic* or *megaloblastic anemia* and is characterized by large, immature red blood cells (see Figure 10-12). Without folate, DNA damage interferes with the synthesis of the red blood cells as they attempt to divide and mature. The result is fewer, but larger, red blood cells that cannot carry oxygen or travel through the capillaries as efficiently as normal red blood cells. Since the implementation of folate fortification in the United States, the prevalence of macrocytic anemia has decreased dramatically.[5]

Of all the vitamins, folate appears to be most vulnerable to interactions with drugs, which can lead to a secondary deficiency.[6] Some medications, notably anticancer drugs, have a chemical structure similar to folate's structure and can displace the vitamin from enzymes and interfere with normal metabolism. (Highlight 17 discusses nutrient-drug interactions, and Figure H17-1 illustrates the similarities between the vitamin folate and the anticancer drug methotrexate.)

Aspirin and antacids also interfere with the body's folate status: aspirin inhibits the action of folate-requiring enzymes, and antacids limit the absorption of folate. Healthy adults who use these drugs to relieve an occasional headache or upset stomach need not be concerned, but people who rely heavily on aspirin or antacids should be aware of the nutrition consequences.

Folate Toxicity A UL has been established for folate from fortified foods or supplements (see the insert). Commonly consumed amounts of folate from both natural sources and fortified foods appear to cause no harm. The small percentage of adults who also take high-dose folate supplements, however, can reach levels

anemia (ah-NEE-me-ah): literally, "too little blood;" any condition in which there is reduced delivery of oxygen to the tissues. Anemia is not a disease itself but can be a consequence of many different disease conditions, including some nutrient deficiencies.

- **an** = without
- **emia** = blood

> FIGURE 10-13 Folate in Selected Foods

Food	Serving size (kcalories)
Bread, whole wheat	1-oz slice (70 kcal)
Cornflakes, fortified	1 oz (110 kcal)
Spaghetti pasta	½ c cooked (99 kcal)
Tortilla, flour	1 10" round (234 kcal)
Broccoli	½ c cooked (22 kcal)
Carrots	½ c shredded raw (24 kcal)
Potato	1 medium baked w/skin (133 kcal)
Tomato juice	½ c (31 kcal)
Banana	1 medium raw (109 kcal)
Orange	1 medium raw (62 kcal)
Strawberries	½ c fresh (22 kcal)
Watermelon	1 slice (92 kcal)
Milk	1 c reduced-fat 2% (121 kcal)
Yogurt, plain	1 c low-fat (155 kcal)
Cheddar cheese	1½ oz (171 kcal)
Cottage cheese	½ c low-fat 2% (101 kcal)
Pinto beans	½ c cooked (117 kcal)
Peanut butter	2 tbs (188 kcal)
Sunflower seeds	1 oz dry (165 kcal)
Tofu (soybean curd)	½ c (76 kcal)
Ground beef, lean	3 oz broiled (244 kcal)
Chicken breast	3 oz roasted (140 kcal)
Tuna, canned in water	3 oz (99 kcal)
Egg	1 hard cooked (78 kcal)
Excellent, and sometimes unusual, sources:	
Lentils	½ c cooked (115 kcal)
Asparagus	½ c cooked (22 kcal)
Orange juice	¾ c fresh (84 kcal)

Micrograms
0
50
100
150
200
250
300
350
400
RDA for adults
FOLATE
Vegetables (green) and legumes (brown) are rich sources of folate, as are fortified grain products (yellow).
Key:
Grains
Vegetables
Fruits
Milk and milk products
Legumes, nuts, seeds
Meats, poultry, seafood
Best sources per kcalorie

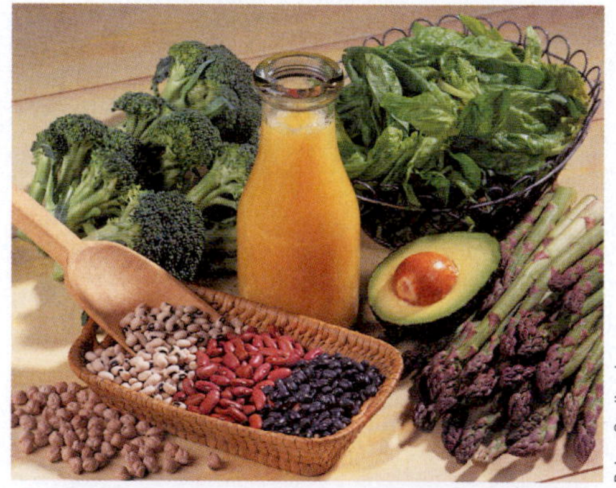

> PHOTO 10-7 Dark green and leafy vegetables (such as spinach and broccoli), legumes (such as black beans, kidney beans, and black-eyed peas), liver, and some fruits (notably citrus fruits and juices) are naturally rich in folate.

that are high enough to obscure a vitamin B_{12} deficiency and delay diagnosis of neurological damage.

Folate Food Sources Figure 10-13 shows that folate is especially abundant in legumes, fruits, and vegetables (see Photo 10-7). The vitamin's name suggests the word *foliage,* and indeed, dark green, leafy vegetables are outstanding sources. With fortification, grain products also contribute folate. The small red and white bars in Figure 10-13 indicate that meats and milk products are poor folate sources. Heat and oxidation during cooking and storage can destroy as much as half of the folate in foods. The table below provides a summary of folate.

REVIEW IT Folate

Other Names

Folic acid, folacin, pteroylglutamic acid (PGA)

RDA

Adults: 400 µg/day

UL[a]

Adults: 1000 µg/day

Chief Functions in the Body

Part of coenzymes THF (tetrahydrofolate) and DHF (dihydrofolate) used in DNA synthesis and therefore important in new cell formation

Significant Sources

Fortified grains, leafy green vegetables, legumes, seeds, liver

Easily destroyed by heat and oxygen

Deficiency Symptoms

Anemia (macrocytic); smooth, red tongue (glossitis); mental confusion, weakness, fatigue, irritability, headache; shortness of breath; elevated homocysteine

Toxicity Symptoms

Masks vitamin B_{12}–deficiency symptoms

[a]The UL applies to synthetic forms obtained from supplements, fortified foods, or a combination.

Vitamin B_{12} **Vitamin B_{12}** and folate are closely related: each depends on the other for activation. Recall that vitamin B_{12} removes a methyl group to activate the folate coenzyme. When folate gives up its methyl group, the vitamin B_{12} coenzyme becomes activated (review Figure 10-11, p. 307).

The regeneration of the amino acid methionine and the synthesis of DNA and RNA depend on both folate and vitamin B_{12}.* In addition, vitamin B_{12} maintains the sheath that surrounds and protects nerve fibers and promotes their normal growth. Bone cell activity and metabolism also depend on vitamin B_{12}.

The digestion and absorption of vitamin B_{12} depends on several steps. In the stomach, hydrochloric acid and the digestive enzyme pepsin release vitamin B_{12} from the proteins to which it is attached in foods. Then as vitamin B_{12} passes from the stomach to the small intestine, it binds with a stomach secretion called **intrinsic factor**. Bound together, intrinsic factor and vitamin B_{12} travel to the end of the small intestine, where receptors recognize the complex. Importantly, the receptors do not recognize vitamin B_{12} without intrinsic factor. The vitamin is gradually absorbed into the bloodstream as the intrinsic factor is degraded. Transport of vitamin B_{12} in the blood depends on specific binding proteins.

Like folate, vitamin B_{12} enters the enterohepatic circulation—continuously being secreted into bile and delivered to the intestine, where it is reabsorbed. Because most vitamin B_{12} is reabsorbed, healthy people rarely develop a deficiency even when their intake is minimal.

Vitamin B_{12} Recommendations The RDA for adults is only 2.4 micrograms of vitamin B_{12} a day—just over two-millionths of a gram. (For perspective, a single grain of sugar weighs several hundred micrograms.) As tiny as this amount appears to the human eye, it contains billions of molecules of vitamin B_{12}, enough to provide coenzymes for all the enzymes that need its help.

Vitamin B_{12} Deficiency and Toxicity Most vitamin B_{12} deficiencies reflect inadequate absorption, not poor intake. Inadequate absorption typically occurs for one of two reasons: a lack of hydrochloric acid or a lack of intrinsic factor. Without hydrochloric acid, the vitamin is not released from the dietary proteins and so is not available for binding with the intrinsic factor. Without the intrinsic factor, the vitamin cannot be absorbed.

Vitamin B_{12} deficiency is common among adults who use heartburn medications to suppress gastric acid production.[7] Deficiency is also common among the elderly.[8] Many older adults develop **atrophic gastritis**, a condition that damages the cells of the stomach. Atrophic gastritis may also develop in response to iron deficiency or infection with *Helicobacter pylori*, the bacterium implicated in ulcer formation. Without healthy stomach cells, production of hydrochloric acid and intrinsic factor diminishes. Even with an adequate intake from foods, vitamin B_{12} status suffers. The vitamin B_{12} deficiency caused by atrophic gastritis and a lack of intrinsic factor is known as **pernicious anemia**.

Some people inherit a defective gene for the intrinsic factor. In such cases, or when the stomach has been injured and cannot produce enough of the intrinsic factor, vitamin B_{12} must be given by injection to bypass the need for intestinal absorption. Alternatively, the vitamin may be delivered by nasal spray; absorption is rapid, high, and well tolerated.

Because vitamin B_{12} is found primarily in foods derived from animals, vegetarians, and especially vegans, are especially likely to develop a vitamin B_{12} deficiency.[9] It may take several years for people who stop eating animal-derived foods to develop deficiency symptoms because the body recycles much of its vitamin B_{12}, reabsorbing it over and over again and conserving its supply. When deficiency does occur, and vitamin B_{12} is no longer available, the consequences are dramatic. Neurological

---

*In the body, methionine serves as a methyl (CH_3) donor. In doing so, methionine can be converted to other amino acids. Some of these amino acids can regenerate methionine, but methionine is still considered an essential amino acid that is needed in the diet.

vitamin B_{12}: a B vitamin characterized by the presence of cobalt (see Figure 13-2). The active forms of coenzyme B_{12} are *methylcobalamin* and *deoxyadenosylcobalamin*.

intrinsic factor: a glycoprotein (a protein with short polysaccharide chains attached) secreted by the stomach cells that binds with vitamin B_{12} in the small intestine to aid in the absorption of vitamin B_{12}.

- **intrinsic** = on the inside

atrophic (a-TRO-fik) **gastritis** (gas-TRY-tis): chronic inflammation of the stomach accompanied by a diminished size and functioning of the mucous membranes and glands. This condition is also characterized by inadequate hydrochloric acid and intrinsic factor—two substances needed for vitamin B_{12} absorption.

- **atrophy** = wasting
- **gastro** = stomach
- **itis** = inflammation

pernicious (per-NISH-us) **anemia:** a macrocytic anemia that reflects a vitamin B_{12} deficiency caused by lack of intrinsic factor and characterized by abnormally large and immature red blood cells. Other symptoms include muscle weakness and irreversible neurological damage.

- **pernicious** = destructive

degeneration, a sign of vitamin B_{12} deficiency, appears rapidly in infants born to mothers with unsupplemented vegan diets.

Because vitamin B_{12} is required to convert folate to its active form, one of the most obvious vitamin B_{12}–deficiency symptoms is the anemia commonly seen in folate deficiency. This anemia is characterized by large, immature red blood cells, which indicate slow DNA synthesis and an inability to divide (review Figure 10-12, p. 309). When folate is trapped in its inactive form (methyl folate) because of vitamin B_{12} deficiency or is unavailable because of folate deficiency itself, DNA synthesis slows.

First to be affected in a vitamin B_{12} or folate deficiency are the rapidly growing blood cells. Either vitamin B_{12} or folate will clear up the anemia, but if folate is given when vitamin B_{12} is needed, the result is disastrous: devastating neurological symptoms. Remember that vitamin B_{12}, but not folate, maintains the sheath that surrounds and protects nerve fibers and promotes their normal growth. Folate "cures" the *blood* symptoms of a vitamin B_{12} deficiency, but cannot stop the *nerve* symptoms from progressing. By doing so, folate "masks" a vitamin B_{12} deficiency.

Even marginal vitamin B_{12} deficiency impairs memory and cognition.[10] Advanced neurological symptoms include a creeping paralysis that begins at the extremities and works inward and up the spine. Early detection and correction are necessary to prevent permanent nerve damage and paralysis. With sufficient folate in the diet, the neurological symptoms of vitamin B_{12} deficiency can develop without evidence of anemia and the cognitive decline is especially rapid. Such interactions between folate and vitamin B_{12} highlight some of the safety issues surrounding the use of supplements and the fortification of foods.[11] No adverse effects have been reported for excess vitamin B_{12}, and no UL has been set.

Vitamin B_{12} Food Sources Vitamin B_{12} is unique among the vitamins in being found almost exclusively in foods derived from animals. Its bioavailability is greatest from milk and fish. Anyone who eats reasonable amounts of animal-derived foods is most likely to have an adequate intake, including vegetarians who use milk products or eggs. Vegans, who restrict all foods derived from animals, need a reliable source, such as vitamin B_{12}–fortified soy milk or vitamin B_{12} supplements. Yeast grown on a vitamin B_{12}–enriched medium and mixed with that medium provides some vitamin B_{12}, but yeast itself does not contain active vitamin B_{12}. Similarly, neither fermented soy products such as miso (a soybean paste) nor sea algae such as spirulina provide active vitamin B_{12}. Extensive research shows that the amounts listed on the labels of these plant products are inaccurate and misleading because the vitamin B_{12} is in an inactive, unavailable form.

REVIEW IT Vitamin B_{12}

Other Names
Cobalamin (and related forms)

RDA
Adults: 2.4 µg/day

Chief Functions in the Body
Part of coenzymes methylcobalamin and deoxyadenosylcobalamin used in new cell synthesis; helps to maintain nerve cells; reforms folate coenzyme; helps to break down some fatty acids and amino acids

Significant Sources
Foods of animal origin (meat, fish, poultry, shellfish, milk, cheese, eggs), fortified cereals

Easily destroyed by microwave cooking

Deficiency Disease
Pernicious anemia[a]

Deficiency Symptoms
Anemia (macrocytic); fatigue, degeneration of peripheral nerves progressing to paralysis; sore tongue, loss of appetite, constipation

Toxicity Symptoms
None reported

[a]The name *pernicious anemia* refers to the vitamin B_{12} deficiency caused by atrophic gastritis and a lack of intrinsic factor, but not to that caused by inadequate dietary intake.

Choline Although not defined as a vitamin, choline is an essential nutrient that is commonly grouped with the B vitamins. The body uses choline to make the neurotransmitter acetylcholine and the phospholipid lecithin. During pregnancy, choline supports the neurological development of the fetus, and during adulthood, choline may improve cognition.[12]

Choline Recommendations The body can make choline from the amino acid methionine, but synthesis alone is insufficient to fully meet the body's needs; dietary choline is also needed. For this reason, the DRI Committee established an AI for choline.

Choline Deficiency and Toxicity Average choline intakes fall below the AI, but the impact of deficiencies are not fully understood. The UL for choline is based on its life-threatening effect in lowering blood pressure.

Choline Food Sources Choline is found in a variety of common foods such as milk, eggs, and peanuts and as part of lecithin, a food additive commonly used as an emulsifying agent (review Figure 5-8, p. 136). The accompanying table provides a summary of choline.

REVIEW IT Choline

AI	Deficiency Symptoms
Men: 550 mg/day	Liver damage
Women: 425 mg/day	**Toxicity Symptoms**
UL	Body odor, sweating, salivation, reduced growth rate, low blood pressure, liver damage
Adults: 3500 mg/day	**Significant Sources**
Chief Functions in the Body	Milk, liver, eggs, peanuts
Needed for the synthesis of the neurotransmitter acetylcholine and the phospholipid lecithin	

Nonvitamins

Some substances have been mistaken for vitamins, but they are not essential nutrients. Among them are the compounds **inositol** and **carnitine**, which can be made by the body. Inositol is a part of cell membrane structures, and carnitine transports long-chain fatty acids from the cytosol to the mitochondria for oxidation. Other nonvitamins include PABA (para-aminobenzoic acid, a component of folate's chemical structure), the bioflavonoids (vitamin P or hesperidin), pyrroloquinoline quinone (methoxatin), orotic acid, lipoic acid, and ubiquinone (coenzyme Q_{10}). Other names erroneously associated with vitamins are "vitamin O" (oxygenated saltwater), "vitamin B_5" (another name for pantothenic acid), "vitamin B_{15}" (also called "pangamic acid," a hoax), and "vitamin B_{17}" (laetrile, an alleged "cancer cure" and not a vitamin or a cure by any stretch of the imagination—in fact, laetrile is a potentially dangerous substance).

Interactions among the B Vitamins

This chapter has described some of the impressive ways that vitamins work individually, as if their many actions in the body could easily be disentangled. In fact, it is often difficult to tell which vitamin is truly responsible for a given effect because the nutrients are interdependent; the presence or absence of one affects another's absorption, metabolism, and excretion. You have already seen this interdependence with folate and vitamin B_{12}.

Riboflavin and vitamin B_6 provide another example. One of the riboflavin coenzymes, FMN, assists the enzyme that converts vitamin B_6 to its coenzyme form PLP. Consequently, a severe riboflavin deficiency can impair vitamin B_6 activity. Thus a deficiency of one nutrient may alter the action of another. Furthermore, a deficiency of one nutrient may create a deficiency of another. For example, both riboflavin and vitamin B_6 (as well as iron) are required for the conversion of

inositol (in-OSS-ih-tall): a nonessential nutrient that can be made in the body from glucose. Inositol is a part of cell membrane structures.

carnitine (CAR-neh-teen): a nonessential, nonprotein amino acid made in the body from lysine that helps transport fatty acids across the mitochondrial membrane.

tryptophan to niacin. Consequently, an inadequate intake of either riboflavin or vitamin B_6 can diminish the body's niacin supply. These interdependent relationships are evident in many of the roles B vitamins play in the body.

B Vitamin Roles Figure 10-14 summarizes the metabolic pathways introduced in Chapter 7 and conveys an *impression* of the many ways B vitamins assist in metabolic pathways. Metabolism is the body's work, and the B vitamin coenzymes are indispensable to every step. In scanning the pathways of metabolism

> **FIGURE 10-14 Metabolic Pathways Involving B Vitamins**

These metabolic pathways are introduced in Chapter 7 and are presented here to highlight the many coenzymes that facilitate the reactions. These coenzymes depend on the following vitamins:

- NAD and NADP: niacin
- TPP: thiamin
- CoA: pantothenic acid
- B_{12}: vitamin B_{12}
- FMN and FAD: riboflavin
- THF: folate
- PLP: vitamin B_6
- Biotin

Pathways leading toward acetyl CoA and the TCA cycle are catabolic, and those leading toward amino acids, glycogen, and fat are anabolic. For further details, see Appendix C.

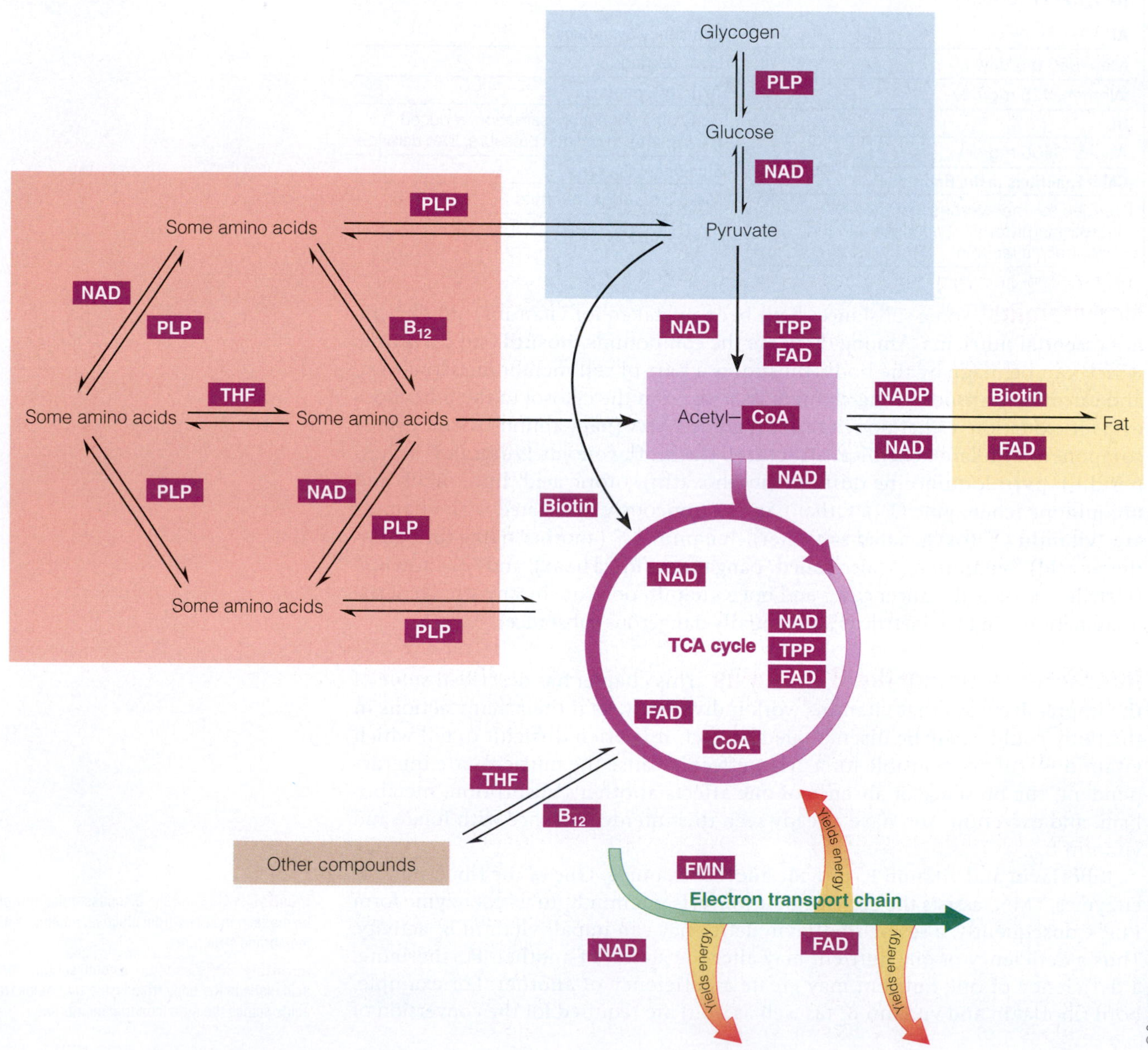

Glycogen
PLP
Glucose
NAD
Pyruvate
PLP
Some amino acids
NAD
PLP
B_{12}
THF
Some amino acids
Some amino acids
PLP
NAD
PLP
Some amino acids
PLP
NAD
TPP
FAD
Acetyl–CoA
NADP
Biotin
Fat
NAD
FAD
NAD
Biotin
NAD
NAD
TCA cycle
TPP
FAD
FAD
CoA
THF
B_{12}
Other compounds
FMN
Electron transport chain
Yields energy
NAD
FAD
Yields energy
Yields energy

depicted in the figure, note the many abbreviations for the coenzymes that keep the processes going.

Look at the now-familiar pathway of glucose breakdown. To break down glucose to pyruvate, the cells must have certain enzymes. For the enzymes to work, they must have the niacin coenzyme NAD. Cells can make NAD, but only if they have enough niacin (or enough of the amino acid tryptophan to make niacin).

The next step is the breakdown of pyruvate to acetyl CoA. The enzymes involved in this step require both NAD and the thiamin and riboflavin coenzymes TPP and FAD, respectively. The cells can manufacture the enzymes they need from the vitamins, if the vitamins are in the diet.

Another coenzyme needed for this step is CoA. Predictably, the cells can make CoA except for an essential part that must be obtained in the diet—pantothenic acid. Another coenzyme requiring biotin serves the enzyme complex involved in converting pyruvate to oxaloacetate, the compound that combines with acetyl CoA to start the TCA cycle.

These and other coenzymes participate throughout all the metabolic pathways. Vitamin B_6 is an indispensable part of PLP—a coenzyme required for many amino acid conversions, for a crucial step in the making of the iron-containing portion of hemoglobin for red blood cells, and for many other reactions. Folate becomes THF—the coenzyme required for the synthesis of new genetic material and therefore new cells. The vitamin B_{12} coenzyme, in turn, regenerates THF to its active form; thus vitamin B_{12} is also necessary for the formation of new cells.

Thus each of the B vitamin coenzymes is involved, directly or indirectly, in energy metabolism. Some facilitate the energy-releasing reactions themselves; others help build new cells to deliver the oxygen and nutrients that allow the energy reactions to occur.

B Vitamin Deficiencies Now suppose the body's cells lack one of these B vitamins—niacin, for example. Without niacin, the cells cannot make NAD. Without NAD, the enzymes involved in every step of the glucose-to-energy pathway cannot function. Then, because all the body's activities require energy, literally everything begins to grind to a halt. This is no exaggeration. The deadly disease pellagra, caused by niacin deficiency, produces the "devastating four Ds": dermatitis, which reflects a failure of the skin; dementia, a failure of the nervous system; diarrhea, a failure of digestion and absorption; and eventually, as would be the case for any severe nutrient deficiency, death. These symptoms are the obvious ones, but a niacin deficiency affects all other organs, too, because all are dependent on the energy pathways.

All the vitamins are as essential as niacin. With any B vitamin deficiency, many body systems become deranged, and similar symptoms may appear. A lack of any of them can have disastrous and far-reaching effects.

Deficiencies of single B vitamins seldom show up in isolation, however. After all, people do not eat nutrients singly; they eat foods, which contain mixtures of nutrients. For this reason, B vitamin deficiencies often coexist, and most typically occur among the elderly, vegetarians, and those with alcoholism, heart failure, and recent bariatric surgery.[13] Only in two cases described earlier—beriberi and pellagra—have dietary deficiencies associated with single B vitamins been observed on a large scale in human populations. Even in these cases, several vitamins were lacking even though one vitamin stood out above the rest. When foods containing the vitamin known to be needed were provided, the other vitamins that were in short supply came as part of the package.

Major deficiency diseases of epidemic proportions such as pellagra and beriberi are no longer seen in the United States, but lesser deficiencies of nutrients, including the B vitamins, sometimes occur in people whose food choices are poor because of poverty, ignorance, illness, or poor health habits like alcohol abuse. (Review Highlight 7 to fully appreciate how alcohol induces vitamin deficiencies and interferes with energy metabolism.) Remember from Chapter 1 that

FIGURE 10-15 B Vitamin–Deficiency Symptoms—The Smooth Tongue of Glossitis and the Skin Lesions of Cheilosis

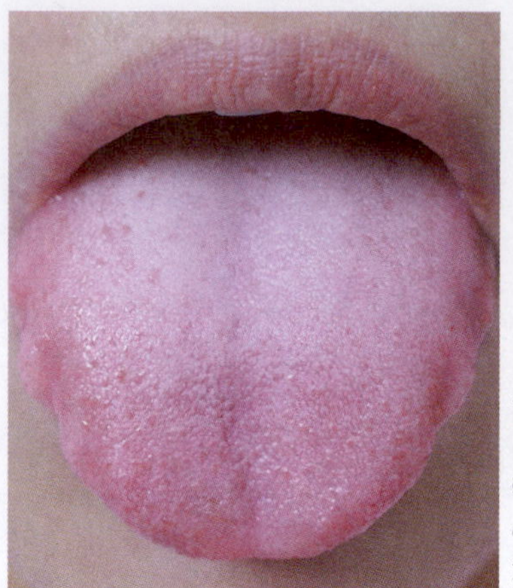

Shining Stars/Shutterstock.com

A healthy tongue has a rough and somewhat bumpy surface.

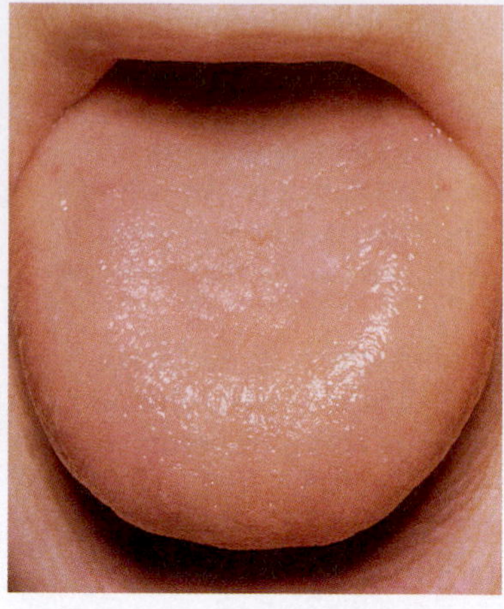

SPL/Science Source

In a B vitamin deficiency, the tongue becomes smooth and swollen due to atrophy of the tissue (glossitis).

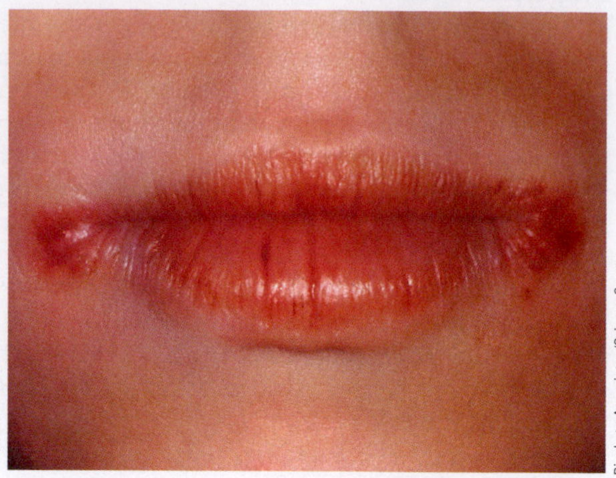

Biophoto Associates/Science Source

In a B vitamin deficiency, the corners of the mouth become irritated and inflamed (cheilosis).

deficiencies can arise not only from deficient intakes (primary causes), but also for other (secondary) reasons.

In identifying nutrient deficiencies, it is important to realize that a particular sign or symptom may not always have the same cause. The skin and the tongue (shown in Figure 10-15) appear to be especially sensitive to B vitamin deficiencies, but focusing on these body parts gives them undue emphasis. Both the skin and the tongue are readily visible in a physical examination.* The physician sees and reports the deficiency's outward signs, but the full impact of a vitamin deficiency occurs inside the cells of the body. If the skin develops a rash or lesions, other tissues beneath it may be degenerating too. Similarly, the mouth and tongue are the visible part of the digestive system; if they are abnormal, most likely the rest of the GI tract is as well.

Keep in mind that the cause of a sign or symptom is not always apparent. The summary tables in this chapter show that deficiencies of riboflavin, niacin, biotin, and vitamin B_6 can all cause skin rashes. So can a deficiency of protein, linoleic acid, or vitamin A. Because skin is on the outside and easy to see, it is a useful indicator of "things going wrong inside cells." By itself, a skin condition says nothing about its possible cause.

The same is true of anemia. Anemia is often caused by iron deficiency, but it can also be caused by a folate or vitamin B_{12} deficiency; by digestive tract failure to absorb any of these nutrients; or by such nonnutritional causes as infections, parasites, cancer, or loss of blood. No single nutrient will always cure a given symptom.

A person who feels chronically tired may be tempted to self-diagnose iron-deficiency anemia and self-prescribe an iron supplement. But this will relieve tiredness only if the cause is indeed iron-deficiency anemia. If the cause is a folate deficiency, taking iron will only prolong the fatigue. A person who is better informed may decide to take a multivitamin supplement with iron, covering the possibility of a vitamin deficiency. But the symptom may have a nonnutritional cause. If the cause of the tiredness is actually hidden blood loss due to cancer, the postponement of a diagnosis may be life-threatening. When fatigue is caused by a lack of sleep, of course, no nutrient or combination of nutrients can replace a good night's rest. A person who is chronically tired should see a physician rather than self-prescribe. If the condition is nutrition-related, a registered dietitian nutritionist should be consulted as well.

*The two common signs of B vitamin deficiencies are *glossitis* (gloss-EYE-tis), an inflammation of the tongue, and *cheilosis* (kye-LOH-sis or kee-LOH-sis), a condition of reddened lips with cracks at the corners of the mouth.

B Vitamin Toxicities Toxicities of the B vitamins from foods alone are unknown, but they can occur when people overuse dietary supplements. With supplements, the quantities can quickly overwhelm the cells. Consider that one small capsule can easily deliver 2 milligrams of vitamin B_6, but it would take more than 3000 bananas, 6600 cups of rice, or 3600 chicken breasts to supply an equivalent amount. When the cells become oversaturated with a vitamin, they must work to eliminate the excess. The cells dispatch water-soluble vitamins to the urine for excretion, but sometimes they cannot keep pace with the onslaught. Homeostasis becomes disturbed and symptoms of toxicity develop.

B Vitamin Food Sources Significantly, deficiency diseases, such as beriberi and pellagra, were resolved by providing foods. Dietary supplements advertise that vitamins are indispensable to life, but human beings obtained their nourishment from foods for centuries before supplements existed. If the diet lacks a vitamin, the first solution is to adjust food intake to obtain that vitamin.

The bar graphs of selected foods in this chapter, taken together, sing the praises of a balanced diet. The grains deliver thiamin, riboflavin, niacin, and folate. The fruit and vegetable groups excel in folate. Protein foods serve thiamin, niacin, vitamin B_6, and vitamin B_{12} well. The milk group stands out for riboflavin and vitamin B_{12}. A diet that offers a variety of foods from each group, prepared with reasonable care, serves up ample B vitamins.

REVIEW IT Identify the main roles, deficiency symptoms, and food sources for each of the B vitamins.

The B vitamins serve as coenzymes that facilitate the work of every cell. They are active in carbohydrate, fat, and protein metabolism and in the making of DNA and thus new cells. Historically famous B vitamin-deficiency diseases are beriberi (thiamin), pellagra (niacin), and pernicious anemia (vitamin B_{12}). Pellagra can be prevented by an adequate protein intake because the amino acid tryptophan can be converted to niacin in the body. A high intake of folate can mask the blood symptoms of a vitamin B_{12} deficiency, but it will not prevent the associated nerve damage. Vitamin B_6 participates in amino acid metabolism and can be harmful in excess. Biotin and pantothenic acid serve important roles in energy metabolism and are common in a variety of foods. Many substances that people claim as B vitamins are not. Fortunately, a variety of foods from each of the food groups provides an adequate supply of all of the B vitamins.

10.3 Vitamin C

LEARN IT Identify the main roles, deficiency symptoms, and food sources for vitamin C.

For many centuries, any man who joined the crew of a seagoing ship knew he had at best a 50–50 chance of returning alive—not because he might be slain by pirates or die in a storm, but because he might contract **scurvy**. As many as two-thirds of a ship's crew could die of scurvy during a long voyage. Only men on short voyages, especially around the Mediterranean Sea, were free of scurvy. No one knew the reason: that on long ocean voyages, the ship's cook used up the fresh fruits and vegetables early and then served only cereals and meats until the return to port.

In the mid-1700s, James Lind, a British physician serving in the navy, devised an experiment to find a cure for scurvy. He divided 12 sailors with scurvy into 6 pairs. Each pair received a different supplemental ration: cider, vinegar, sulfuric acid, seawater, oranges and lemons, or a strong laxative. Those receiving the citrus fruits quickly recovered, but sadly, it was almost 50 years before the British navy required all vessels to provide every sailor with lemon or lime juice daily. The tradition of providing British sailors with citrus juice daily to prevent scurvy gave them the nickname "limeys."

The antiscurvy "something" in citrus and other foods was dubbed the **antiscorbutic factor**. Centuries later, the factor was isolated and found to be a 6-carbon compound similar to glucose; it was named **ascorbic acid**.

scurvy: the vitamin C–deficiency disease.

antiscorbutic (AN-tee-skor-BUE-tik) **factor:** the original name for vitamin C.

- **anti** = against
- **scorbutic** = causing scurvy

ascorbic acid: one of the two active forms of vitamin C (see Figure 10-16). Many people refer to vitamin C by this name.

- **a** = without
- **scorbic** = having scurvy

> **FIGURE 10-16 Active Forms of Vitamin C**

The two hydrogens highlighted in yellow give vitamin C its acidity and its ability to act as an antioxidant.

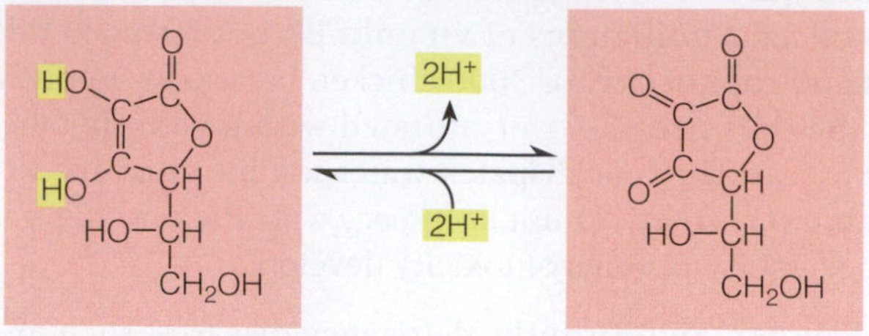

HO
HO
HO—CH
CH_2OH
$2H^+$
$2H^+$
HO—CH
CH_2OH
© Cengage

Ascorbic acid protects against oxidative damage by donating its two hydrogens with their electrons to free radicals (molecules with unpaired electrons). In doing so, ascorbic acid becomes dehydroascorbic acid.

Dehydroascorbic acid can readily accept hydrogens to become ascorbic acid. The reversibility of this reaction is key to vitamin C's role as an antioxidant.

Vitamin C Roles Vitamin C parts company with the B vitamins in its mode of action. In some settings, vitamin C serves as a **cofactor** helping specific enzymes perform their jobs, but in others, it acts as an antioxidant participating in more general ways.

As an Antioxidant Vitamin C loses electrons easily, a characteristic that allows it to perform as an antioxidant. In the body, **antioxidants** defend against free radicals. Free radicals are discussed fully in Highlight 11, but for now, a simple definition will suffice. A **free radical** is a molecule with one or more unpaired electrons, which makes it unstable and highly reactive. Antioxidants can neutralize free radicals by donating an electron or two. In doing so, antioxidants protect other substances from free radical damage. Figure 10-16 illustrates how vitamin C can give up electrons and then accept them again to become reactivated. This recycling of vitamin C is key to limiting losses and maintaining a reserve of antioxidants in the body. Other key antioxidant nutrients include vitamin E, beta-carotene, and selenium.

Vitamin C is like a bodyguard for water-soluble substances; it stands ready to sacrifice its own life to save theirs. In the cells and body fluids, vitamin C protects tissues from the **oxidative stress** of free radicals and thus may play an important role in preventing diseases. In the small intestine, vitamin C enhances iron absorption by protecting iron from oxidation. (Chapter 13 provides more details about the relationship between vitamin C and iron.)

As a Cofactor in Collagen Formation Vitamin C helps to form the fibrous structural protein of connective tissues known as **collagen**. Collagen serves as the matrix on which bones and teeth are formed. When a person is wounded, collagen glues the separated tissues together, forming scars. Cells are held together largely by collagen; this is especially important in the walls of the blood vessels, which must withstand the pressure of blood surging with each beat of the heart.

Chapter 6 described how the body makes proteins by stringing together chains of amino acids. During the synthesis of collagen, each time a proline or lysine is added to the growing protein chain, an enzyme hydroxylates it (adds an OH group), making the amino acid hydroxyproline or hydroxylysine, respectively. These two special amino acids facilitate the binding together of collagen fibers to make strong, ropelike structures. The conversion of proline to hydroxyproline requires both vitamin C and iron. Iron works as a cofactor in the reaction, and vitamin C protects iron from oxidation, thereby allowing iron to perform its job. Without vitamin C and iron, the hydroxylation step does not occur.

As a Cofactor in Other Reactions Vitamin C also serves as a cofactor in the synthesis of several other compounds. As in collagen formation, vitamin C helps in the hydroxylation of carnitine, a compound that transports fatty acids, especially

cofactor: a small, inorganic or organic substance that facilitates the action of an enzyme.

antioxidants: in the body, substances that significantly decrease the adverse effects of free radicals on normal physiological functions.

free radical: an unstable molecule with one or more unpaired electrons.

oxidative stress: a condition in which the production of oxidants and free radicals exceeds the body's ability to handle them and prevent damage.

collagen: the structural protein from which connective tissues such as scars, tendons, ligaments, and the foundations of bones and teeth are made.

long-chain fatty acids, across the inner membrane of mitochondria in cells. It also participates in the conversions of the amino acids tryptophan and tyrosine to the neurotransmitters serotonin and norepinephrine, respectively. Vitamin C also assists in the making of hormones, including thyroxine, which regulates the metabolic rate; when metabolism speeds up in times of extreme physical stress, the body's use of vitamin C increases.

In Stress Among the stresses known to increase vitamin C needs are infections; burns; extremely high or low temperatures; intakes of toxic heavy metals such as lead, mercury, and cadmium; the chronic use of certain medications, including aspirin, barbiturates, and oral contraceptives; and cigarette smoking. During stress, the adrenal glands—which contain more vitamin C than any other organ in the body—release vitamin C and hormones into the blood.*

When immune system cells are called into action, they use a great deal of oxygen and produce free radicals. In this case, free radicals are helpful. They act as ammunition in an "oxidative burst" that demolishes the offending viruses and bacteria and destroys the damaged cells. Vitamin C steps in as an antioxidant to control this oxidative activity.

In the Prevention and Treatment of the Common Cold Vitamin C has been a popular option for the prevention and treatment of the common cold for decades, but research supporting such claims has been conflicting and controversial. Some studies find no relationship between vitamin C and the occurrence of the common cold, whereas others report modest benefits—fewer colds, fewer days, and shorter duration of severe symptoms, especially for those exposed to physical and environmental stresses. A review of the research on the treatment and prevention of the common cold reveals a slight reduction in the duration and severity of the common cold in favor of those taking vitamin C supplements.[14] The question for consumers to consider is, "Is it enough to warrant routine daily supplementation?"

Discoveries about how vitamin C works in the body provide possible links between the vitamin and the common cold. Anyone who has ever had a cold knows the discomfort of a runny or stuffed-up nose. Nasal congestion develops in response to elevated blood **histamine**, and people commonly take antihistamines for relief. Like an antihistamine, vitamin C comes to the rescue and deactivates histamine.

In Disease Prevention Whether vitamin C may help in preventing or treating cancer, heart disease, cataract, and other diseases is still being studied, and findings are presented in Highlight 11's discussion on antioxidants. Conducting research in the United States can be difficult, however, because diets typically contribute enough vitamin C to provide optimal health benefits.

Vitamin C Recommendations

How much vitamin C does a person need? As is true of all the vitamins, recommendations are set generously above the minimum requirement to prevent deficiency disease and well below the toxicity level (see Figure 10-17).

The requirement—the amount needed to prevent the overt symptoms of scurvy—is only 10 milligrams daily. Consuming 10 milligrams a day does not saturate all the body tissues, however; higher intakes will increase the body's total vitamin C. At about 100 milligrams per day, 95 percent of the population reaches tissue saturation. (For perspective, 1 cup of orange juice provides more than 100 milligrams of vitamin C.) Recommendations are slightly lower, based on the amounts needed to provide antioxidant protection. At about 200 milligrams, absorption reaches a maximum, and there is little, if any, increase in blood concentrations at higher doses. Excess vitamin C is readily excreted.

*High amounts of vitamin C are also found in the pituitary glands; medium amounts in the liver, spleen, heart, kidneys, lungs, pancreas, and white blood cells; and small amounts in the muscles and red blood cells.

FIGURE 10-17 Vitamin C Intake (mg/day)

Recommendations for vitamin C are set generously above the minimum requirement and well below the toxicity level.

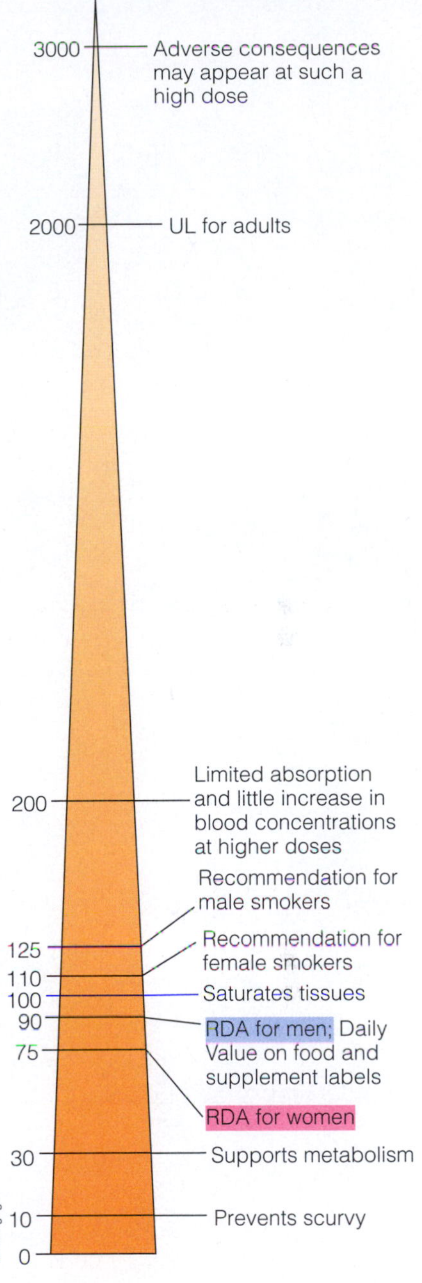

3000
Adverse consequences may appear at such a high dose
2000
UL for adults
200
Limited absorption and little increase in blood concentrations at higher doses
Recommendation for male smokers
125
Recommendation for female smokers
110
100
Saturates tissues
90
RDA for men; Daily Value on food and supplement labels
75
RDA for women
30
Supports metabolism
10
Prevents scurvy
0
© Cengage

histamine (HISS-tah-mean or HISS-tah-men): a substance produced by cells of the immune system as part of a local immune reaction to an antigen.

> **FIGURE 10-18 Vitamin C–Deficiency Symptoms—Scorbutic Gums and Pinpoint Hemorrhages**

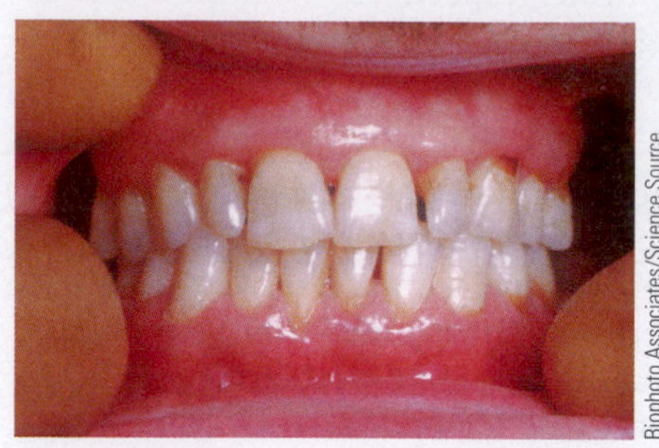
Biophoto Associates/Science Source

Scorbutic gums. Unlike other lesions of the mouth, scurvy presents a symmetrical appearance without infection.

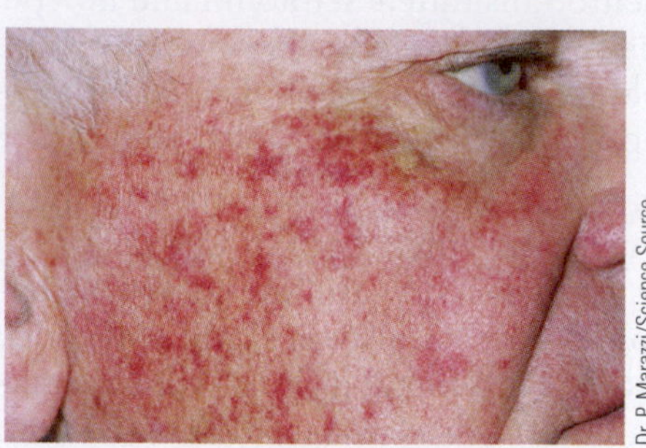
Dr. P. Marazzi/Science Source

Pinpoint hemorrhages. Small red spots appear in the skin, indicating spontaneous bleeding internally.

As mentioned earlier, cigarette smoking increases the need for vitamin C. Cigarette smoke contains oxidants, which greedily deplete this potent antioxidant. Exposure to cigarette smoke, especially when accompanied by low dietary intakes of vitamin C, depletes the body's vitamin C in both active and passive smokers. People who chew tobacco also have low levels of vitamin C. Because people who smoke cigarettes regularly suffer significant oxidative stress, their requirement for vitamin C is increased an additional 35 milligrams; nonsmokers regularly exposed to cigarette smoke should also be sure to meet their RDA for vitamin C. Smokers are among those most likely to suffer vitamin C deficiency.

Vitamin C Deficiency

Early signs of nutrient deficiencies can be difficult to recognize. Two of the most notable signs of a vitamin C deficiency reflect its role in maintaining the integrity of blood vessels. The gums bleed easily around the teeth, and capillaries under the skin break spontaneously, producing pinpoint hemorrhages (see Figure 10-18).

When vitamin C concentrations fall to about a fifth of optimal levels (this may take more than a month on a diet lacking vitamin C), scurvy symptoms begin to appear. Inadequate collagen synthesis causes further hemorrhaging. Muscles, including the heart muscle, degenerate. The skin becomes rough, brown, scaly, and dry. Wounds fail to heal because scar tissue will not form. Bone rebuilding falters; the ends of the long bones become softened, malformed, and painful, and fractures develop. The teeth become loose as the cartilage around them weakens. Anemia and infections are common. There are also characteristic psychological signs, including hysteria and depression. Sudden death is likely, caused by massive internal bleeding.

Once diagnosed, scurvy is readily resolved by increasing vitamin C intake. Moderate doses of 100 milligrams per day are sufficient, curing the scurvy within about 5 days. Such an intake is easily achieved by including vitamin C–rich foods in the diet.

Vitamin C Toxicity

The availability of vitamin C supplements and the publication of books recommending vitamin C to prevent colds and cancer have led many people to take large doses of vitamin C. Not surprisingly, side effects of vitamin C supplementation such as gastrointestinal distress and diarrhea have been reported. The UL for vitamin C was established based on these symptoms.

Several instances of interference with medical regimens are also known. Large amounts of vitamin C excreted in the urine obscure the results of tests used to detect glucose or ketones in the diagnosis of diabetes. In some instances, excess vitamin C gives a **false positive** result; in others, a **false negative**. People taking anticlotting medications may unwittingly counteract the effect if they also take

false positive: a test result indicating that a condition is present (positive) when in fact it is not present (therefore false).

false negative: a test result indicating that a condition is not present (negative) when in fact it is present (therefore false).

massive doses of vitamin C. Those with kidney disease, a tendency toward gout, or a genetic abnormality that alters vitamin C's breakdown to its excretion products are prone to forming kidney stones if they take large doses of vitamin C.*

Vitamin C supplements may adversely affect people with iron overload. As Chapter 13 explains, vitamin C enhances iron absorption and releases iron from body stores; too much free iron causes the kind of cellular damage typical of free radicals. These adverse consequences illustrate how vitamin C can act as a *pro*oxidant when quantities exceed the body's needs.

Vitamin C Food Sources Fruits and vegetables can easily provide a generous amount of vitamin C. A cup of orange juice at breakfast, a salad for lunch, and a stalk of broccoli and a potato for dinner alone provide more than 300 milligrams. (For perspective, review Figure 10-17, p. 319.) Clearly, a person making such food choices does not need vitamin C supplements.

Figure 10-19 shows the amounts of vitamin C in various common foods. The overwhelming abundance of purple and green bars reveals not only that the citrus fruits are justly famous for being rich in vitamin C, but that other fruits and vegetables are also in the same league (see Photos 10-8 and 10-9). A half cup of broccoli, bell

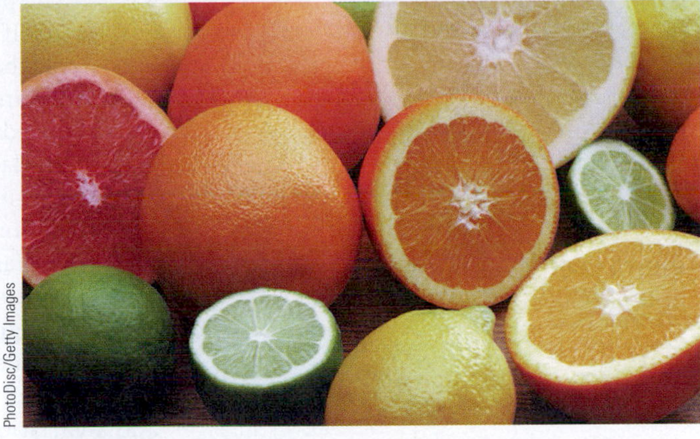
PhotoDisc/Getty Images

> PHOTO 10-8 When dietitians say "vitamin C," people think "citrus fruits."

> FIGURE 10-19 Vitamin C in Selected Foods

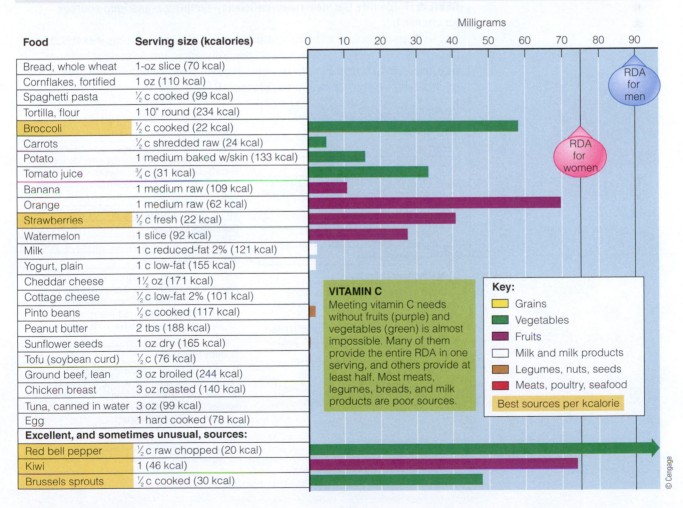

Food	Serving size (kcalories)
Bread, whole wheat	1-oz slice (70 kcal)
Cornflakes, fortified	1 oz (110 kcal)
Spaghetti pasta	½ c cooked (99 kcal)
Tortilla, flour	1 10" round (234 kcal)
Broccoli	½ c cooked (22 kcal)
Carrots	½ c shredded raw (24 kcal)
Potato	1 medium baked w/skin (133 kcal)
Tomato juice	¾ c (31 kcal)
Banana	1 medium raw (109 kcal)
Orange	1 medium raw (62 kcal)
Strawberries	½ c fresh (22 kcal)
Watermelon	1 slice (92 kcal)
Milk	1 c reduced-fat 2% (121 kcal)
Yogurt, plain	1 c low-fat (155 kcal)
Cheddar cheese	1½ oz (171 kcal)
Cottage cheese	½ c low-fat 2% (101 kcal)
Pinto beans	½ c cooked (117 kcal)
Peanut butter	2 tbs (188 kcal)
Sunflower seeds	1 oz dry (165 kcal)
Tofu (soybean curd)	½ c (76 kcal)
Ground beef, lean	3 oz broiled (244 kcal)
Chicken breast	3 oz roasted (140 kcal)
Tuna, canned in water	3 oz (99 kcal)
Egg	1 hard cooked (78 kcal)
Excellent, and sometimes unusual, sources:	
Red bell pepper	½ c raw chopped (20 kcal)
Kiwi	1 (46 kcal)
Brussels sprouts	½ c cooked (30 kcal)

Milligrams
0 10 20 30 40 50 60 70 80 90
RDA for men
RDA for women
VITAMIN C
Meeting vitamin C needs without fruits (purple) and vegetables (green) is almost impossible. Many of them provide the entire RDA in one serving, and others provide at least half. Most meats, legumes, breads, and milk products are poor sources.
Key:
Grains
Vegetables
Fruits
Milk and milk products
Legumes, nuts, seeds
Meats, poultry, seafood
Best sources per kcalorie

*Vitamin C is inactivated and degraded by several routes, and sometimes oxalate, which can form kidney stones, is produced along the way. People may also develop oxalate crystals in their kidneys regardless of vitamin C status.

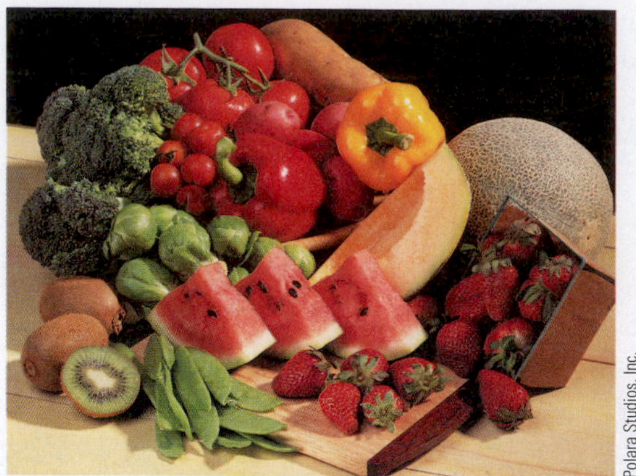

Polara Studios, Inc.

> **PHOTO 10-9** These fruits and vegetables are rich sources of vitamin C.

pepper, or strawberries provides more than 50 milligrams of the vitamin (and an array of other nutrients). Because vitamin C is vulnerable to heat, raw fruits and vegetables usually have a higher nutrient density than their cooked counterparts. Similarly, because vitamin C is readily destroyed by oxygen, foods and juices should be stored properly and consumed within a week of opening.

The potato is an important source of vitamin C, not because one potato by itself meets the daily need, but because potatoes are such a common staple that they make significant contributions. In fact, scurvy was unknown in Ireland until the potato blight of the mid-1840s, when some 2 million people died of malnutrition and infection.

The lack of yellow, white, brown, and red bars in Figure 10-19 confirms that grains, milk and milk products (except breast milk), and most protein foods are notoriously poor sources of vitamin C. Organ meats (liver, kidneys, and others) and raw meats contain some vitamin C, but most people don't eat large quantities of these foods. Raw meats and fish contribute enough vitamin C to be significant sources in parts of Alaska, Canada, and Japan, but elsewhere fruits and vegetables are necessary to supply sufficient vitamin C.

Because of vitamin C's antioxidant property, food manufacturers sometimes add a variation of vitamin C to some beverages and most cured meats, such as luncheon meats, to prevent oxidation and spoilage. This compound safely preserves these foods, but it does not have vitamin C activity in the body. Simply put, "Ham and bacon cannot replace fruits and vegetables."

REVIEW IT Identify the main roles, deficiency symptoms, and food sources for vitamin C.

Vitamin C acts primarily as an antioxidant and a cofactor. Recommendations are set well above the amount needed to prevent the deficiency disease scurvy. A variety of fruits and vegetables—most notably citrus fruits—provide generous amounts of vitamin C. The accompanying table provides a summary of vitamin C.

Vitamin C

Other Names

Ascorbic acid

RDA

Men: 90 mg/day

Women: 75 mg/day

Smokers: RDA + 35 mg/day

UL

Adults: 2000 mg/day

Chief Functions in the Body

Collagen synthesis (strengthens blood vessel walls, forms scar tissue, provides matrix for bone growth), antioxidant, thyroxine synthesis, amino acid metabolism, strengthens resistance to infection, helps in absorption of iron

Significant Sources

Citrus fruits, cabbage-type vegetables (such as brussels sprouts and cauliflower), dark green vegetables (such as bell peppers and broccoli), cantaloupe, strawberries, lettuce, tomatoes, potatoes, papayas, mangoes

Easily destroyed by heat and oxygen

Deficiency Disease

Scurvy

Deficiency Symptoms

Anemia (microcytic), atherosclerotic plaques, pinpoint hemorrhages; bone fragility, joint pain; poor wound healing, frequent infections; bleeding gums, loosened teeth; muscle degeneration, pain, hysteria, depression; rough skin, blotchy bruises

Toxicity Symptoms

Nausea, abdominal cramps, diarrhea; headache, fatigue, insomnia; hot flashes; rashes; interference with medical tests, aggravation of gout symptoms, urinary tract problems, kidney stones[a]

[a]People with kidney disease, a tendency toward gout, or a genetic abnormality that alters the breakdown of vitamin C are prone to forming kidney stones. Vitamin C is inactivated and degraded by several routes, sometimes producing oxalate, which can form stones in the kidneys.

Vita means life. After this discourse on the vitamins, who could dispute that they deserve their name? Their regulation of metabolic processes makes them vital to the normal growth, development, and maintenance of the body. The accompanying table condenses the information provided in this chapter for a quick review. The remarkable roles of the vitamins continue in the next chapter.

REVIEW IT The Water-Soluble Vitamins

Vitamin and Chief Functions	Deficiency Symptoms	Toxicity Symptoms	Food Sources
Thiamin Part of coenzyme TPP in energy metabolism	Beriberi (edema or muscle wasting), anorexia, weight loss, neurological disturbances, muscular weakness, heart enlargement and failure	None reported	Enriched, fortified, or whole-grain products; pork
Riboflavin Part of coenzymes FAD and FMN in energy metabolism	Inflammation of the mouth, skin, and eyelids	None reported	Milk products; enriched, fortified, or whole-grain products; liver
Niacin Part of coenzymes NAD and NADP in energy metabolism	Pellagra (diarrhea, dermatitis, and dementia)	Niacin flush, liver damage, impaired glucose tolerance	Protein-rich foods
Biotin Part of coenzyme in energy metabolism	Skin rash, hair loss, neurological disturbances	None reported	Widespread in foods; GI bacteria synthesis
Pantothenic acid Part of coenzyme A in energy metabolism	Digestive and neurological disturbances	None reported	Widespread in foods
Vitamin B_6 Part of coenzymes used in amino acid and fatty acid metabolism	Scaly dermatitis, depression, confusion, convulsions, anemia	Nerve degeneration, skin lesions	Protein-rich foods
Folate Activates vitamin B_{12}; helps synthesize DNA for new cell growth	Anemia, glossitis, neurological disturbances, elevated homocysteine	Masks vitamin B_{12} deficiency	Legumes, vegetables, fortified grain products
Vitamin B_{12} Activates folate; helps synthesize DNA for new cell growth; protects nerve cells	Anemia; nerve damage and paralysis	None reported	Foods derived from animals
Vitamin C Synthesis of collagen, carnitine, hormones, neurotransmitters; antioxidant	Scurvy (bleeding gums, pinpoint hemorrhages, abnormal bone growth, and joint pain)	Diarrhea, GI distress	Fruits and vegetables

What's Online

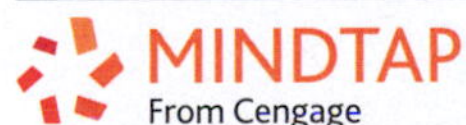
MINDTAP
From Cengage

Visit **www.cengagebrain.com** to access MindTap, a complete digital course that includes Diet & Wellness Plus, interactive quizzes, videos, and more.

REFERENCES

1. P. Mani and A. Rohatgi, Niacin therapy, HDL cholesterol, and cardiovascular disease: Is the HDL hypothesis defunct? *Current Atherosclerosis Reports* 17 (2015): 43.
2. U. Julius, Niacin as antidyslipidemic drug, *Canadian Journal of Physiology and Pharmacology* 93 (2015): 1043–1054.
3. S. Liu and coauthors, Effect of folic acid food fortification in Canada on congenital heart disease subtypes, *Circulation* 134 (2016): 647–655; R. Molina-Solana and coauthors, Current concepts on the effect of environmental factors on cleft lip and palate, *International Journal of Oral and Maxillofacial Surgery* 42 (2013): 177–184.
4. Q. Xiao and coauthors, Intakes of folate, methionine, vitamin B6, and vitamin B12 with risk of esophageal and gastric cancer in a large cohort study, *British Journal of Cancer* 110 (2014): 1328–1333.

5. O. A. Odewole and coauthors, Near-elimination of folate-deficiency anemia by mandatory folic acid fortification in older US adults: Reasons for Geographic and Racial Differences in Stroke study 2003–2007, *American Journal of Clinical Nutrition* 98 (2013): 1042–1047.
6. C. S. Hesdorffer and D. L. Longo, Drug-induced megaloblastic anemia, *New England Journal of Medicine* 373 (2015): 1649–1658.
7. J. R. Lam and coauthors, Proton pump inhibitor and histamine 2 receptor antagonist use and vitamin B12 deficiency, *Journal of the American Medical Association* 310 (2013): 2435–2442.
8. K. J. Pfisterer and coauthors, Vitamin B12 status in older adults living in Ontario long-term care homes: Prevalence and incidence of deficiency with supplementation a protective factor, *Applied Physiology, Nutrition, and Metabolism* 41 (2016): 219–222.
9. R. Pawlak, S. E. Lester, and T. Babatunde, The prevalence of cobalamin deficiency among vegetarians assessed by serum vitamin B12: A review of literature, *European Journal of Clinical Nutrition* 68 (2014): 541–548.
10. T. Köbe and coauthors, Vitamin B-12 concentration, memory performance, and hippocampal structure in patients with mild cognitive impairment, *American Journal of Clinical Nutrition* 103 (2016): 1045–1054.
11. A. L. Boyles and coauthors, Safe use of high intakes of folic acid: Research challenges and paths forward, *Nutrition Reviews* 74 (2016): 469–474; J. H. Choi and coauthors, Contemporary issues surrounding folic acid fortification initiatives, *Preventive Nutrition and Food Science* 19 (2014): 247–260.
12. E. T. M. Leermakers and coauthors, Effects of choline on health across the life course: A systematic review, *Nutrition Reviews* 73 (2016): 500–522; X. Jiang, A. A. West, and M. A. Caudill, Maternal choline supplementation: A nutritional approach for improving offspring health? *Trends in Endocrinology and Metabolism* 25 (2014): 263–273.
13. G. P. Sechi and coauthors, Advances in clinical determinants and neurological manifestations of B vitamin deficiency in adults, *Nutrition Reviews* 74 (2016): 281–300.
14. H. Hemilä and E. Chalker, Vitamin C for preventing and treating the common cold, *Cochrane Database of Systematic Reviews* (2013): CD000980.

 LEARN IT Present arguments for and against the use of dietary supplements.

Vitamin and Mineral Supplements

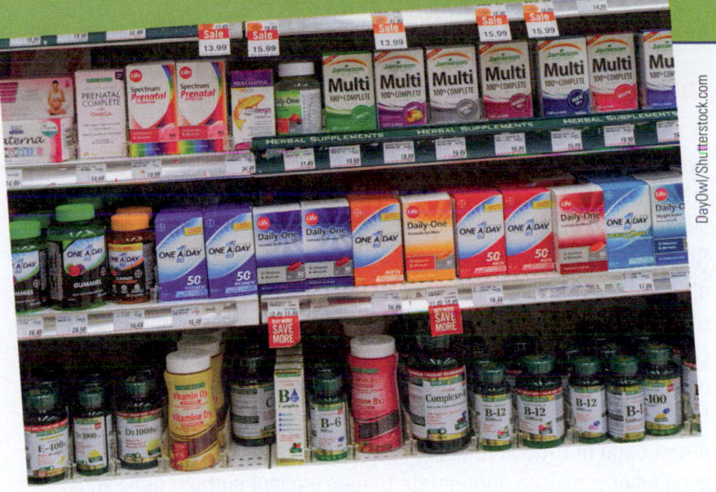
DayOwl/Shutterstock.com

More than half of the adults in the United States take a **dietary supplement** regularly, spending $37 billion each year. (Glossary H10-1 defines dietary supplements and related terms.) Most people take supplements as a part of their efforts to live a healthy life.[1] Yet most vitamin and mineral supplements do not prevent chronic disease or delay death.[2] This highlight focuses on vitamin and mineral supplements. (Amino acid and protein supplements are discussed in Chapter 6; weight loss products, in Chapter 9; ergogenic aids for athletes, in Highlight 14; and herbal supplements in Highlight 18.)

An estimated 30 percent of US adults take multivitamin-mineral supplements regularly.[3] Others take large doses of single nutrients, most commonly, vitamin D and calcium. In many cases, taking supplements is a costly but harmless practice; sometimes, it is both costly and harmful to health. Every year, more than 7000 emergency department visits in the United States are attributed to adverse effects of vitamin and/or mineral supplements; an additional 16,000 visits are attributed to other herbal and nutritional products.[4]

For the most part, people self-prescribe supplements, taking them on the advice of friends, advertisements, websites, or books that may or may not be reliable. Sometimes, they take supplements on the recommendation of a physician. When such advice follows a valid nutrition assessment, supplementation may be warranted, but even then the preferred course of action is to improve food choices and eating habits.[5] Without an assessment, the advice to take supplements may be inappropriate. A registered dietitian nutritionist can help with the decision.

This highlight asks several questions related to vitamin-mineral supplements. What are the arguments *for* taking supplements? What are the arguments *against* taking them? Finally, if people do take supplements, how can they choose the appropriate ones?

Arguments for Supplements

Vitamin-mineral supplements may be appropriate in some circumstances. In some cases, they can prevent or correct deficiencies; in others, they can reduce the risk of certain diseases. Consumers should discuss supplement use with their health-care providers, who can help monitor for adverse effects or nutrient-drug interactions.

Correct Overt Deficiencies

In the United States, adults rarely suffer nutrient deficiency diseases such as scurvy, pellagra, and beriberi, but nutrient deficiencies do still occur. To correct an overt deficiency disease, a physician may prescribe therapeutic doses two to ten times the RDA (or AI) of a nutrient. At such high doses, the supplement is having a pharmacological effect and acting as a drug.

Support Increased Nutrient Needs

As Chapters 15 through 17 explain, nutrient needs increase during certain stages of life, making it difficult to meet some of those needs without supplementation. For example, women who lose a lot of blood and therefore a lot of iron during menstruation each month may need an iron supplement. Women of childbearing age need folate supplements to reduce the risks of neural tube defects. Similarly, pregnant women and women who are breastfeeding their infants have exceptionally high nutrient needs and so usually need special supplements. Newborns routinely receive a single dose of vitamin K at birth to prevent abnormal bleeding. Infants may need other supplements as well, depending on whether they are breastfed or receiving formula, and on whether the water they drink contains fluoride.

GLOSSARY H10-1

dietary supplement: any pill, capsule, tablet, liquid, or powder that contains vitamins, minerals, herbs, or amino acids intended to increase dietary intake of these substances.

FDA (Food and Drug Administration): a part of the Department of Health and Human Services' Public Health Service that is responsible for ensuring the safety and wholesomeness of all dietary supplements and food processed and sold in interstate commerce except meat, poultry, and eggs (which are under the jurisdiction of the USDA); inspecting food plants and imported foods; and setting standards for food composition and product labeling.

high potency: 100% or more of the Daily Value for the nutrient in a single supplement and for at least two-thirds of the nutrients in a multinutrient supplement.

nanoceuticals: substances with extremely small particles that have been manufactured by nanotechnology.

nanotechnology: a manufacturing technology that manipulates atoms to change the structure of matter.

Improve Nutrition Status

In contrast to the classical deficiencies, which present a multitude of symptoms and are relatively easy to recognize, subclinical deficiencies are subtle and easy to overlook—and they are also more likely to occur. Without fortification or supplementation, many adults in the United States fall short of recommended intakes for several vitamins and minerals. People who do not eat enough food to deliver the needed amounts of nutrients, such as habitual dieters and the elderly, risk developing subclinical deficiencies. Similarly, vegetarians and vegans who restrict their use of entire food groups without appropriate substitutions may fail to fully meet their nutrient needs. If there is no way for these people to eat enough nutritious foods to meet their needs, then vitamin-mineral supplements may be appropriate to help prevent nutrient deficiencies.

Improve the Body's Defenses

Health-care professionals may provide special supplementation to people being treated for addictions to alcohol or other drugs and to people with prolonged illnesses, extensive injuries, or other severe stresses such as surgery. Illnesses and their treatments that interfere with appetite, eating, or nutrient absorption impair nutrition status. For example, the stomach condition atrophic gastritis often creates a vitamin B_{12} deficiency. In addition, nutrient needs may be heightened by diseases or medications. In all these cases, supplements are appropriate.

Reduce Disease Risks

Few people consume the optimal amounts of all the vitamins and minerals by diet alone. Inadequate intakes have been linked to chronic diseases such as heart disease, some cancers, and osteoporosis. For this reason, some physicians recommend that all adults take vitamin-mineral supplements. Such regular supplementation would provide an optimum intake to enhance metabolic harmony and prevent disease at relatively little cost. Others recognize the lack of conclusive evidence and the potential harm of supplementation and advise against such a recommendation. A statement from the National Institutes of Health acknowledges that evidence is insufficient to recommend either for or against the use of supplements to prevent chronic diseases.

Highlight 11 reviews the relationships between supplement use and disease prevention. It describes some of the accumulating evidence suggesting that intakes of certain nutrients at levels much higher than can be attained from foods alone may be beneficial in reducing some disease risks. It also presents research confirming the associated risks. Clearly, consumers must be cautious in taking supplements to prevent disease.

Who Needs Supplements?

In summary, the following list acknowledges that in these specific conditions, these people may need to take supplements:

- People with specific nutrient deficiencies may need specific nutrient supplements.
- People whose energy intakes are particularly low (fewer than 1600 kcalories per day) may need multivitamin-mineral supplements.
- Vegetarians who eat all-plant diets (vegans) and older adults with atrophic gastritis may need vitamin B_{12}.
- People who have lactose intolerance or milk allergies or who otherwise do not consume enough milk products to forestall extensive bone loss may need calcium and vitamin D.
- People in certain stages of the life cycle who have increased nutrient requirements may need specific nutrient supplements. For example, infants may need vitamin D, iron, and fluoride; women of childbearing age and pregnant women may need folate and iron; and the elderly may need vitamin B_{12} and vitamin D.
- People who have inadequate intakes of milk or milk products, limited sun exposure, or heavily pigmented skin may need vitamin D.
- People who have diseases, infections, or injuries or who have undergone surgery that interferes with the intake, absorption, metabolism, or excretion of nutrients may need specific nutrient supplements.
- People taking medications that interfere with the body's use of specific nutrients may need specific nutrient supplements.

Except for people in these circumstances, most adults can get all the nutrients they need by eating a variety of nutrient-dense foods. Even athletes can meet their nutrient needs without the help of supplements, as Chapter 14 explains.

Arguments against Supplements

Foods rarely cause nutrient imbalances or toxicities, but supplements can. The higher the dose, the greater the risk of harm. People's tolerances for high doses of nutrients vary, just as their risks of deficiencies do. Amounts that some can tolerate may be harmful for others, and no one knows who falls where along the spectrum. It is difficult to determine just how much of a nutrient is enough—or too much. The Tolerable Upper Intake Levels (UL) of the DRI answer the question "How much is too much?" by defining the highest amount that appears safe for most healthy people. Table H10-1 presents UL and Daily Values for selected vitamins and minerals.

Who Should Not Take Supplements?

The following list recognizes that in certain circumstances, these people may need to avoid specific supplements:

- Men and postmenopausal women should not take iron supplements given that excess iron is harmful and generally more likely than inadequacies.
- Smokers should not take beta-carotene supplements given that high doses have been associated with increased lung cancer and mortality.
- Postmenopausal women should not take vitamin A supplements given that excess retinol has been associated with increased risk of hip fractures and reduced bone density.
- Surgery patients should not take vitamin E supplements during the week before surgery because vitamin E acts as a blood thinner.

TABLE H10-1 Vitamin and Mineral Intakes for Adults

Nutrient	Tolerable Upper Intake Levels[a]	Daily Values
Vitamins		
Vitamin A	3000 µg[b]	900 µg
Vitamin D (as cholecalciferol)	100 µg	20 µg
Vitamin E (as alpha-tocopherol)	1000 mg[b]	15 mg
Vitamin K	—[c]	120 µg
Thiamin	—[c]	1.2 mg
Riboflavin	—[c]	1.3 mg
Niacin (as niacinamide)	35 mg[b]	16 mg
Vitamin B_6 (as pyridoxine)	100 mg	1.7 mg
Folate	1000 µg[b]	400 µg
Vitamin B_{12} (as cyanocobalamin)	—[c]	2.4 µg
Pantothenic acid	—[c]	5 mg
Biotin	—[c]	30 µg
Vitamin C (as ascorbic acid)	2000 mg	90 mg
Choline	3500 mg	550 mg
Minerals		
Chloride	3600 mg	2300 mg
Potasssium	—[c]	4700 mg
Calcium	2500 mg	1300 mg
Phosphorus	4000 mg	1250 mg
Magnesium	350 mg[b]	420 mg
Iron	45 mg	18 mg
Zinc	40 mg	11 mg
Iodine	1100 µg	150 µg
Selenium	400 µg	55 µg
Fluoride	10 mg	—
Copper	10 mg	0.9 mg
Manganese	11 mg	2.3 mg
Chromium	—[c]	35 µg
Molybdenum	2000 µg	45 µg

[a]Unless otherwise noted, Upper Levels represent total intakes from food, water, and supplements.
[b]Upper Levels for vitamin A are for preformed vitamin A only; for vitamin E, niacin, and folate, the UL represent intakes from supplements, fortified foods, or both; for magnesium, the UL represent intakes from supplements only and do not include intakes from food and water.
[c]These nutrients have been evaluated by the DRI Committee for Tolerable Upper Intake Levels, but none were established because of insufficient data. No adverse effects have been reported with intakes of these nutrients at levels typical of supplements, but caution is still advised, given the potential for harm that accompanies excessive intakes.

Toxicity

Supplement users may have excessive intakes of certain nutrients. The extent and severity of supplement toxicity remain unclear. Only a few alert health-care professionals can recognize toxicity, even when it is acute. When it is chronic, with the effects developing subtly and progressing slowly, it often goes unrecognized and unreported.[6] In view of the potential hazards, some authorities believe supplements should bear warning labels, advising consumers that large doses may be toxic.

At a minimum, manufacturers should be held to the same standards required of the drug industry, which may help to prevent toxicities. Consider that more than 200 people reported symptoms of diarrhea, fatigue, hair loss, and joint pain when the selenium supplements they had taken delivered up to 2.5 times the selenium concentration listed on the label.[7]

Toxic overdoses of vitamins and minerals in children are more readily recognized and, unfortunately, fairly common. Fruit-flavored, chewable vitamins shaped like cartoon characters entice young children to eat them like candy in amounts that can cause poisoning. Iron supplements (30 milligrams of iron or more per tablet) are especially toxic and have caused fatalities among children. Even mild overdoses cause GI distress, nausea, and black diarrhea, which reflects gastric bleeding. Severe overdoses result in bloody diarrhea, shock, liver damage, coma, and death.

Life-Threatening Misinformation

Another problem arises when people who are ill come to believe that high doses of vitamins or minerals can be therapeutic. Not only can high doses be toxic, but the person may also take them instead of seeking medical help. Furthermore, there are no guarantees that the supplements will be effective. Taking vitamin supplements instead of medication may sound appealing, but they do not protect against the progression of heart disease or cancers. In some cases, supplements may even be harmful. For example, supplements of vitamin E increase the risk of prostate cancer among healthy men.[8]

Marketing materials for supplements often make health statements that are required to be "truthful and not misleading," but they often fall far short of both. Highlight 18 revisits this topic and includes a discussion of herbal preparations and other alternative therapies.

Unknown Needs

Another argument against the use of supplements is that there are no standards and no one knows exactly how to formulate the "ideal" supplement. What nutrients should be included? Which, if any, of the phytochemicals should be included? How much of each? On whose needs should the choices be based? Surveys have repeatedly shown little relationship between the supplements people take and the nutrients they actually need.

False Sense of Security

Another argument against supplement use is that it may lull people into a false sense of security. A person might eat irresponsibly, thinking, "My supplement will ensure my needs are met." Or, experiencing a warning symptom of a disease, a person might postpone seeking a diagnosis, thinking, "I probably just need a supplement to make this go away." Such self-diagnosis is potentially dangerous.

Other Invalid Reasons

Other invalid reasons people might use for taking supplements include:

- The belief that the food supply or soil contains inadequate nutrients
- The belief that supplements can provide energy

- The belief that supplements can enhance athletic performance or build lean body tissues without physical work or faster than exercise alone (see Highlight 14)
- The belief that supplements will help a person cope with stress
- The belief that supplements can prevent, treat, or cure conditions ranging from the common cold to cancer

Ironically, people with health problems are more likely to take supplements than other people, yet today's health problems are more likely to be due to overnutrition and poor lifestyle choices than to nutrient deficiencies. The truth—that most people would benefit from improving their eating and activity patterns—is harder to swallow than a supplement pill.

Bioavailability and Antagonistic Actions

In general, the body absorbs nutrients best from foods in which the nutrients are diluted and dispersed among other substances that may facilitate their absorption. Taken in pure, concentrated form, nutrients are likely to interfere with one another's absorption or with the absorption of nutrients in foods eaten at the same time. Documentation of these effects is particularly extensive for minerals: zinc hinders copper and calcium absorption, iron hinders zinc absorption, calcium hinders magnesium and iron absorption, and magnesium hinders the absorption of calcium and iron. Similarly, binding agents in supplements limit mineral absorption.

Although minerals provide the most-familiar and best-documented examples, interference among vitamins is now being seen as supplement use increases. The vitamin A precursor beta-carotene, long thought to be nontoxic, interferes with vitamin E metabolism when taken over the long term as a dietary supplement. Vitamin E, on the other hand, antagonizes vitamin K activity and so should not be used by people being treated for blood-clotting disorders. Consumers who want the benefits of optimal absorption of nutrients should eat foods selected for nutrient density and variety.

Whenever the diet is inadequate, the person should first attempt to improve it so as to obtain the needed nutrients from foods. If that is truly impossible, then the person needs a multivitamin-mineral supplement that supplies between 50 and 150 percent of the Daily Value for each of the nutrients. These amounts reflect the ranges commonly found in foods and therefore are compatible with the body's normal handling of nutrients (its physiological tolerance). The next section provides some pointers to assist in the selection of an appropriate supplement.

Selection of Supplements

Whenever a physician or registered dietitian nutritionist recommends a supplement, follow the directions carefully. When selecting a supplement yourself, look for a single, balanced vitamin-mineral supplement. Supplements with a USP verification logo have been tested by the US Pharmacopeia (USP) to ensure that the supplement:

- Contains the declared ingredients and amounts listed on the label
- Does not contain harmful levels of contaminants
- Will disintegrate and release ingredients in the body
- Was made under safe and sanitary conditions

If you decide to take a vitamin-mineral supplement, ignore the eye-catching art and meaningless claims. Pay attention to the form the supplements are in, the list of ingredients, and the price. Here's where the truth lies, and from it you can make a rational decision based on facts. You have two basic questions to answer.

Form

The first question: What form do you want—chewable, liquid, or pills? If you'd rather drink your supplements than chew them, fine. If you choose a chewable form, though, be aware that chewable vitamin C can dissolve tooth enamel. If you choose pills, look for statements about the disintegration time. The USP suggests that supplements should completely disintegrate within 30 to 45 minutes. Obviously, supplements that don't dissolve have little chance of entering the bloodstream, so look for a brand that claims to meet USP disintegration standards.

Contents

The second question: What vitamins and minerals do you need? Generally, an appropriate supplement provides vitamins and minerals in amounts that do not exceed recommended intakes. Avoid supplements that, in a daily dose, provide more than the UL for *any* nutrient. Avoid preparations with more than 10 milligrams of iron per dose, except as prescribed by a physician. Iron is hard to get rid of once it's in the body, and an excess of iron can cause problems, just as a deficiency can (see Chapter 13).

Misleading Claims

Manufacturers of *organic* or natural vitamins boast that their pills are purified from real foods rather than synthesized in a laboratory. These supplements are no more effective than others and often cost more. The word *synthetic* may sound like "fake," but to synthesize just means to put together. Think back on the course of human evolution; it is not natural to take any kind of pill. In reality, the finest, most natural vitamin "supplements" available are whole grains, vegetables, fruits, meat, fish, poultry, eggs, legumes, nuts, and milk and milk products.

Avoid products that make **"high potency"** claims. More is not better (review Figure 10-1, p. 295). Remember that foods are also providing these nutrients. Nutrients can build up and cause unexpected problems. For example, a man who takes vitamins and begins to lose his hair may think his hair loss means he needs more vitamins, when in fact it may be the early sign of a vitamin A overdose. (Of course, it may be completely unrelated to nutrition as well.)

Be aware that fake vitamins and preparations that contain items not needed in human nutrition, such as carnitine and inositol, reflect a marketing strategy aimed at your pocket, not at your health. The manufacturer wants you to believe that its pills contain the latest "new" nutrient that other brands omit, but in reality, these substances are not known to be needed by human beings.

Realize that the claim that supplements "relieve stress" is another marketing ploy. If you give even passing thought to what people mean by "stress," you'll realize manufacturers could never design a supplement to meet everyone's needs. Is it stressful to take an exam? Well, yes. Is it stressful to survive a major car wreck with third-degree burns and multiple bone fractures? Definitely, yes. The body's responses to these stresses are different. The body does use vitamins and minerals in mounting a stress response, but a body fed a well-balanced diet can meet the needs of most minor stresses. For the major ones, medical intervention is needed. In any case, taking a dietary supplement won't make life any less stressful.

Other marketing tricks to sidestep are "green" pills that contain dehydrated, crushed parsley, alfalfa, and other fruit and vegetable extracts. The nutrients and phytochemicals advertised can be obtained from a serving of vegetables more easily and for less money. Such pills may also provide enzymes, but enzymes are inactivated in the stomach during protein digestion.

Recognize the latest nutrition buzzwords. Manufacturers were marketing "antioxidant" supplements before the print had time to dry on the first scientific reports of antioxidant vitamins' action in the body. Remember, too, that high doses can alter a nutrient's action in the body. An antioxidant in physiological quantities may be beneficial, but in pharmacological quantities, it may act as a prooxidant and cause harm. Highlight 11 explores antioxidants and supplement use in more detail.

Similarly, manufacturers began making dietary supplements using **nanotechnology** before the FDA had created guidelines defining their use in consumer products. These **nanoceuticals** promise enhanced nutrient absorption and activity. Such claims may sound good, but again, more does not always mean better.

Finally, be aware that advertising on the Internet is cheap and not closely regulated. Promotional e-mails can be sent to millions of people in an instant. Internet messages can easily cite references and provide links to other sites, implying an endorsement when in fact none has been given. Be cautious when examining unsolicited information and search for a balanced perspective.

Cost

When shopping for supplements, remember that local or store brands may be just as good as nationally advertised brands. If they are less expensive, it may be because the price does not have to cover the cost of national advertising.

Regulation of Supplements

Dietary supplements are regulated by the **FDA (Food and Drug Administration)** as foods. Details of supplement regulation are defined in the Dietary Supplement Health and Education Act of 1994, which was intended to enable consumers to make informed choices about dietary supplements. The act subjects supplements to the same general labeling requirements that apply to foods. Specifically:

- Nutrition labeling for dietary supplements is required.
- Labels may make nutrient claims (as "high" or "low") according to specific criteria (for example, "an excellent source of vitamin C").
- Labels may claim that the lack of a nutrient can cause a deficiency disease, but if they do, they must also include the prevalence of that deficiency disease in the United States.
- Labels may make health claims that are supported by significant scientific agreement and are not brand specific (for example, "folate protects against neural tube defects").
- Labels may claim to diagnose, treat, cure, or relieve common complaints such as menstrual cramps or memory loss, but may *not* make claims about specific diseases (except as noted previously).
- Labels may make structure-function claims about the role a nutrient plays in the body, how the nutrient performs its function, and how consuming the nutrient is associated with general well-being (see Photo H10-1). The manufacturer is responsible for ensuring that the claims are truthful and not misleading. Claims must be accompanied by an FDA disclaimer statement: "This statement has not been evaluated by the FDA. This product is not intended to diagnose, treat, cure, or prevent any disease."

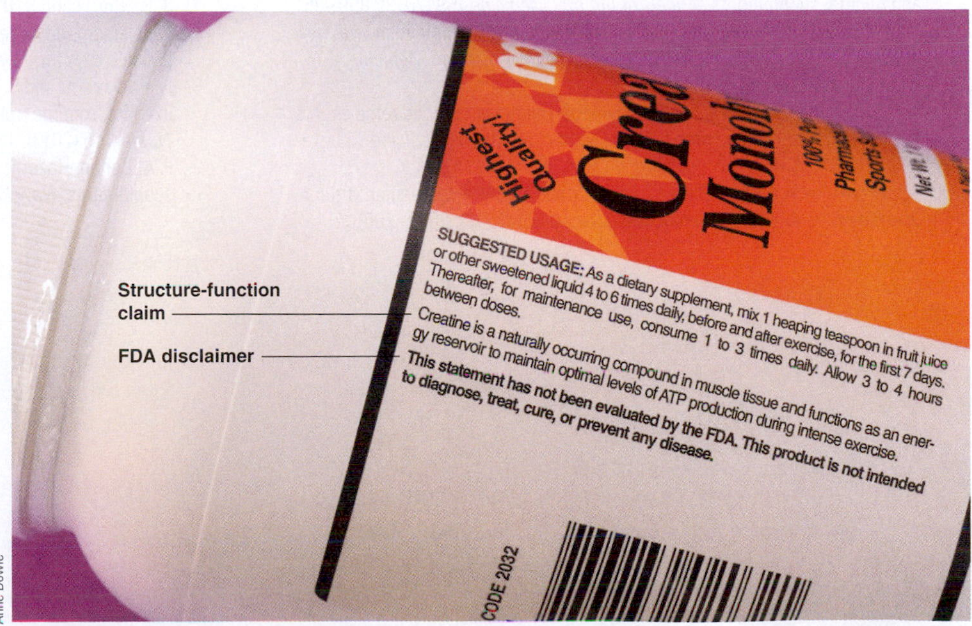
Highest Quality!
Crea
Monoh
SUGGESTED USAGE: As a dietary supplement, mix 1 heaping teaspoon in fruit juice or other sweetened liquid 4 to 6 times daily, before and after exercise, for the first 7 days. Thereafter, for maintenance use, consume 1 to 3 times daily. Allow 3 to 4 hours between doses.
Creatine is a naturally occuring compound in muscle tissue and functions as an energy reservoir to maintain optimal levels of ATP production during intense exercise.
This statement has not been evaluated by the FDA. This product is not intended to diagnose, treat, cure, or prevent any disease.
CODE 2032
Structure-function claim
FDA disclaimer
Anne Dowie

> **PHOTO H10-1** Structure-function claims do not need FDA authorization, but they must be accompanied by a disclaimer.

The multibillion-dollar-a-year supplement industry spends much money and effort influencing these regulations. The net effect of the Dietary Supplement Health and Education Act was a deregulation of the supplement industry. Unlike food additives or drugs, supplements do not need to be proved safe and effective, nor do they need the FDA's approval before being marketed. Furthermore, there are no standards for potency or dosage and no requirements for providing warnings of potential side effects. The FDA can only require good manufacturing practices: that dietary supplements be produced and packaged in a quality manner, do not contain contaminants or impurities, and are accurately labeled to reflect the actual contents.

Should a problem arise, the burden falls to the FDA to prove that the supplement poses a "significant or unreasonable risk of illness or injury." Only then would it be removed from the market. When asked, most Americans express support for greater regulation of dietary supplements. Health professionals agree.[9] To learn more about dietary supplements currently on the US market as well as those that have been recalled, consumers can visit the National Institutes of Health website (www.dsld.nlm.nih.gov/dsld/index.jsp).

If all the nutrients we need can come from food, why not just eat food? Foods have so much more to offer than supplements do. Nutrients in foods come in an infinite variety of combinations with a multitude of different carriers and absorption enhancers. They come with water, fiber, and an array of beneficial phytochemicals. Foods stimulate the GI tract to keep it healthy. They provide energy, and as long as you need energy each day, why not have nutritious foods deliver it? Foods offer pleasure, satiety, and opportunities for socializing while eating. Quite simply, foods meet human health needs far better than dietary supplements. For further proof, read Highlight 11.

CRITICAL THINKING QUESTIONS

A. What are the arguments for and against the use of dietary supplements?

B. According to the Health and Education Act of 1994, dietary supplements with familiar ingredients may be marketed without any evidence of effectiveness or safety. Supplements with new ingredients are supposed to provide the FDA with evidence of safety, but this part of the law is rarely enforced. Both the industry and the FDA acknowledge that most supplements are currently on the market without any assessment of safety. What is your position on this situation and what changes to the law, if any, would you propose to support your position?

REFERENCES

1. Dickenson and D. MacKay, Health habits and other characteristics of supplement users: A review, *Nutrition Journal* 13 (2014): 14.
2. E. Guallar and coauthors, Enough is enough: Stop wasting money on vitamin and mineral supplements, *Annals of Internal Medicine* 159 (2013): 850–851.
3. E. D. Kantor, C. D. Rehm, and M. Du, Trends in dietary supplement use among US adults from 1999-2012, *Journal of the American Medical Association* 316 (2016): 1464–1474.
4. A. I. Geller and coauthors, Emergency department visits for adverse events related to dietary supplements, *New England Journal of Medicine* 373 (2015): 1531–1540.
5. Position of the American Dietetic Association: Nutrient supplementation, *Journal of the American Dietetic Association* 109 (2009): 2073–2085.
6. M. Cellini and coauthors, Dietary supplements: Physician knowledge and adverse event reporting, *Medicine and Science in Sports and Exercise* 45 (2013): 23–28.
7. J. S. Morris and S. B. Crane, Selenium toxicity from a misformulated dietary supplement, adverse health effects, and the temporal response in the nail biologic monitor, *Nutrients* 5 (2013): 1024–1057.
8. H. L. Nicastro and B. K. Dunn, Selenium and prostate cancer prevention: Insights from the Selenium and Vitamin E Cancer Prevention Trial (SELECT), *Nutrients* 5 (2013): 1122–1148.
9. P. A. Cohen, Hazards of hindsight—Monitoring the safety of nutritional supplements, *New England Journal of Medicine* 370 (2014): 1277–1280.

11 The Fat-Soluble Vitamins: A, D, E, and K

LEARNING GUIDE

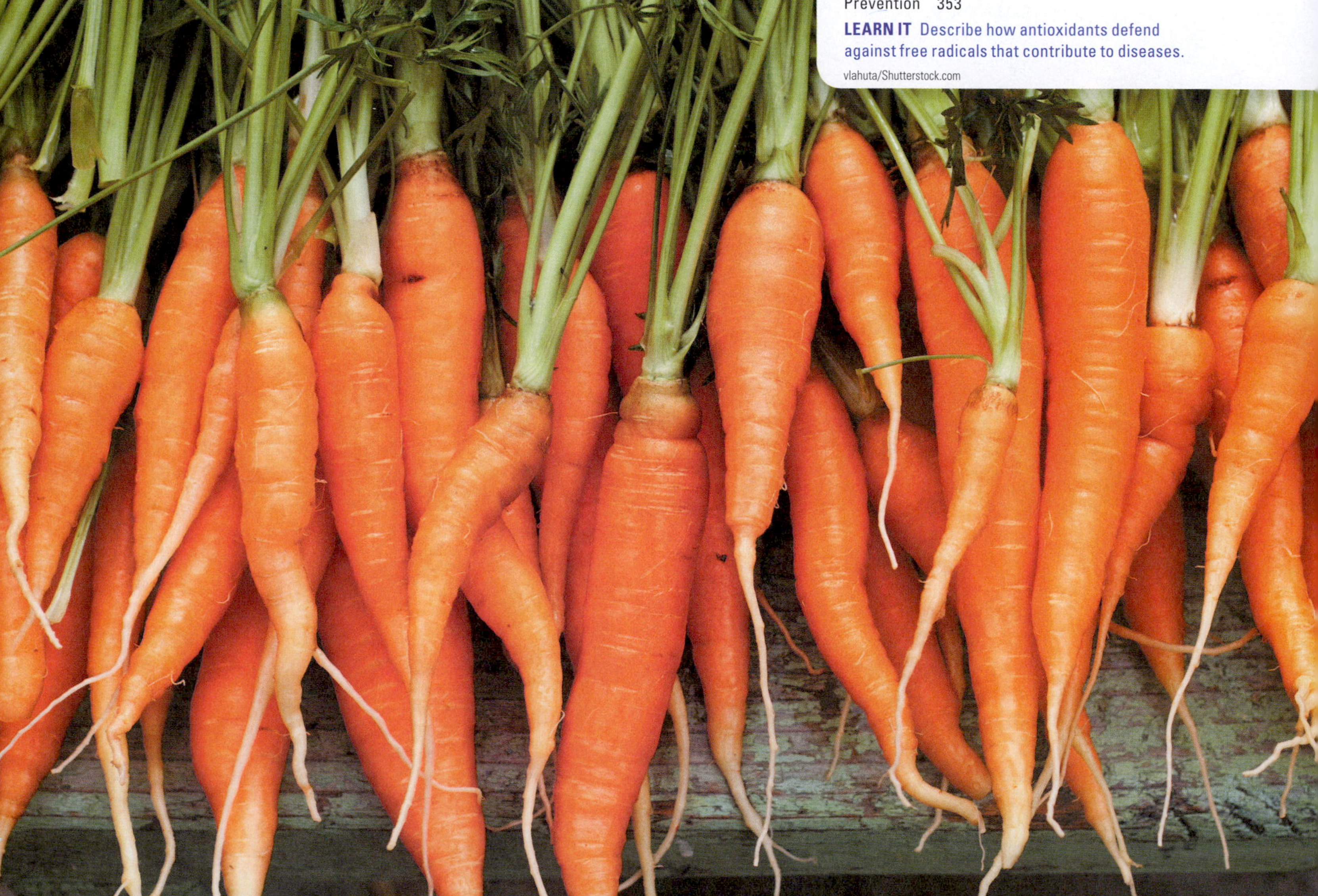

vlahuta/Shutterstock.com

Nutrition in Your Life

Realizing that vitamin A from vegetables participates in vision, a mom encourages her children to "eat your carrots" because "they're good for your eyes." A dad takes his children outside to "enjoy the fresh air and sunshine" because they need the vitamin D that is made with the help of the sun. A physician recommends that a patient use vitamin E to slow the progression of heart disease. Another physician gives a newborn a dose of vitamin K to protect against life-threatening blood loss. These common daily occurrences highlight some of the heroic work of the fat-soluble vitamins. As you read this chapter, consider whether the foods you are eating are meeting your fat-soluble vitamin needs.

The fat-soluble vitamins A, D, E, and K differ from the water-soluble vitamins in several significant ways (review Table 10-2, p. 296). Being insoluble in the watery fluids of the GI tract, the fat-soluble vitamins require bile for their digestion and absorption. Upon absorption, fat-soluble vitamins travel through the lymphatic system within chylomicrons before entering the bloodstream, where many of them require protein carriers for transport. The fat-soluble vitamins participate in numerous activities throughout the body, but excesses are stored primarily in the liver and adipose tissue. The body maintains blood concentrations by retrieving these vitamins from storage as needed; thus people can eat less than their daily need for days, weeks, or even months or years without ill effects. They need only ensure that, over time, *average* daily intakes approximate recommendations. By the same token, because fat-soluble vitamins are not readily excreted, the risk of toxicity is greater than it is for the water-soluble vitamins.

11.1 Vitamin A and Beta-Carotene

LEARN IT Identify the main roles, deficiency symptoms, and food sources for vitamin A.

Vitamin A was the first fat-soluble vitamin to be recognized. More than a century later, vitamin A and its precursor, **beta-carotene,** continue to intrigue researchers with their diverse roles and profound effects on health.

Three different forms of vitamin A are active in the body: **retinol, retinal,** and **retinoic acid.** Collectively known as **retinoids,** these compounds are commonly found in foods derived from animals. Foods derived from plants provide **carotenoids,** some of which can be converted to vitamin A.* The most studied of the carotenoids with **vitamin A activity** is beta-carotene, which can be split to form retinol in the intestine and liver. Figure 11-1 (p. 334) illustrates the structural similarities and differences of these vitamin A compounds and the cleavage of beta-carotene.

The cells can convert retinol and retinal to the other active forms of vitamin A as needed. The conversion of retinol to retinal is reversible, but the further conversion of retinal to retinoic acid is irreversible (see Figure 11-2, p. 334). This irreversibility is significant because each form of vitamin A performs a specific function that the others cannot.

Several proteins participate in the digestion and absorption of vitamin A. After absorption via the lymph system, vitamin A eventually arrives at the liver, where it is stored. There, a special transport protein, **retinol-binding protein (RBP),** picks up vitamin A from the liver and carries it in the blood. Cells that use vitamin A have special protein receptors for it, and its action within each cell may differ depending on the receptor. For example, retinoic acid can *stimulate* cell growth in the skin and *inhibit* cell growth in tumors.

*Carotenoids with vitamin A activity include alpha-carotene, beta-carotene, and beta-cryptoxanthin; carotenoids with no vitamin A activity include the phytochemicals lycopene, lutein, and zeaxanthin.

vitamin A: all naturally occurring compounds with the biological activity of *retinol*, the alcohol form of vitamin A.

beta-carotene (BAY-tah KARE-oh-teen): one of the carotenoids; an orange pigment and vitamin A precursor found in plants.

retinol (RET-ih-nol): the alcohol form of vitamin A.

retinal (RET-ih-nal): the aldehyde form of vitamin A.

retinoic (RET-ih-NO-ick) **acid:** the acid form of vitamin A.

retinoids (RET-ih-noyds): chemically related compounds with biological activity similar to that of retinol; metabolites of retinol.

carotenoids (kah-ROT-eh-noyds): pigments commonly found in plants and animals, some of which have vitamin A activity. The carotenoid with the greatest vitamin A activity is beta-carotene.

vitamin A activity: a term referring to both the active forms of vitamin A and the precursor forms in foods without distinguishing between them.

retinol-binding protein (RBP): the specific protein responsible for transporting retinol.

> **FIGURE 11-1 Forms of Vitamin A**

In this diagram, corners represent carbon atoms, as in all previous diagrams in this book. A further simplification here is that methyl groups (CH_3) are understood to be at the ends of the lines extending from corners. (See Appendix C for complete structures.)

Retinol, the alcohol form

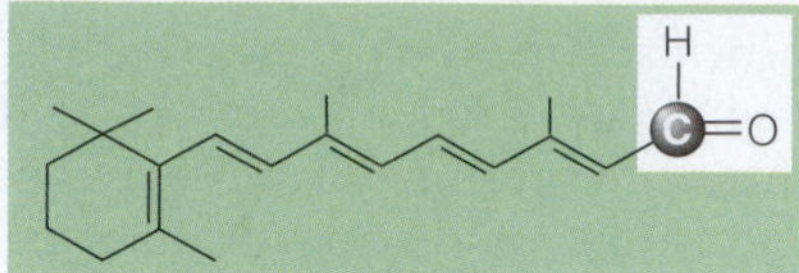
H
C
O

Retinal, the aldehyde form

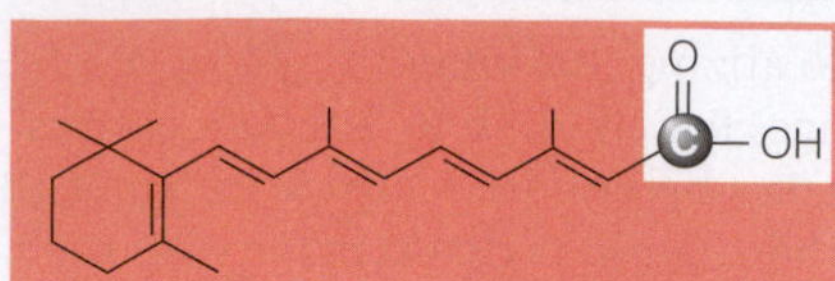
O
C
OH

Retinoic acid, the acid form

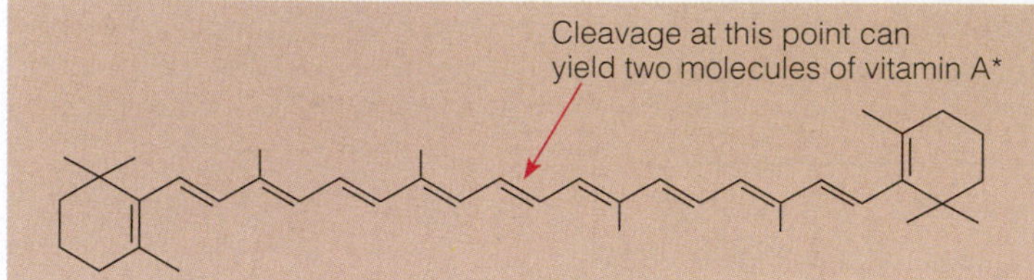
Cleavage at this point can yield two molecules of vitamin A*

Beta-carotene, a precursor

*Sometimes cleavage occurs at other points as well, so that one molecule of beta-carotene may yield only one molecule of vitamin A. Furthermore, not all beta-carotene is converted to vitamin A, and absorption of beta-carotene is not as efficient as that of vitamin A. For these reasons, 12 μg of beta-carotene is equivalent to 1 μg of vitamin A. Conversion of other carotenoids to vitamin A is even less efficient.

> **FIGURE 11-2 Conversion of Vitamin A Compounds**

Notice that the conversion from retinol to retinal is reversible, whereas the pathway from retinal to retinoic acid is not.

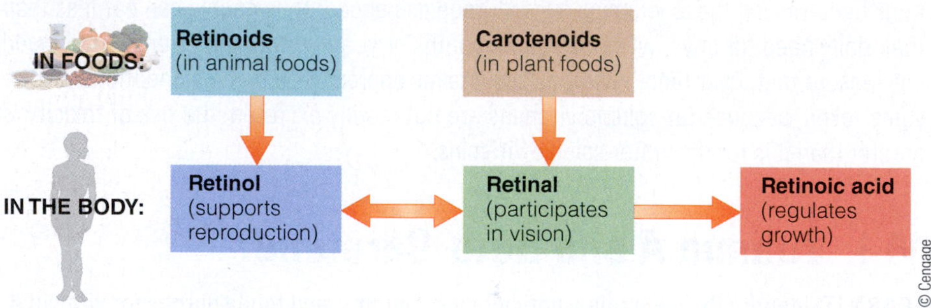
IN FOODS:
Retinoids (in animal foods)
Carotenoids (in plant foods)
IN THE BODY:
Retinol (supports reproduction)
Retinal (participates in vision)
Retinoic acid (regulates growth)

Roles in the Body

Vitamin A is a versatile vitamin, known to regulate the expression of several hundred genes. Its major roles include:

- Promoting vision
- Participating in protein synthesis and cell differentiation, thereby maintaining the health of epithelial tissues and skin
- Supporting reproduction and regulating growth

As mentioned, each form of vitamin A performs specific tasks. Retinol supports reproduction and is the major transport and storage form of the vitamin. Retinal is active in vision and is also an intermediate in the conversion of retinol to retinoic acid (review Figure 11-2). Retinoic acid acts like a hormone, regulating cell differentiation, growth, and embryonic development. Animals raised on retinoic acid as their only source of vitamin A can grow normally, but they become blind because retinoic acid cannot be converted to retinal (review Figure 11-2).

Vitamin A in Vision

Vitamin A plays two indispensable roles in the eye: it helps maintain a crystal-clear outer window, the **cornea,** and it participates in the conversion of light energy into nerve impulses at the **retina** (see Figure 11-3 for details). Some of the photosensitive cells of the retina contain **pigment** molecules called **rhodopsin.** Each rhodopsin molecule is composed of a protein called **opsin** bonded to a molecule of retinal, which plays a central role in vision. When light passes through the cornea of the eye and strikes the retina, rhodopsin responds. As it does, opsin is released and retinal shifts from a *cis* to a *trans* configuration,

cornea (KOR-nee-uh): the transparent membrane covering the outside of the eye.

retina (RET-in-uh): the innermost membrane of the eye, composed of several layers, including one that contains the rods and cones.

pigment: a molecule capable of absorbing certain wavelengths of light so that it reflects only those that we perceive as a certain color.

rhodopsin (ro-DOP-sin): a light-sensitive pigment of the retina that contains the retinal form of vitamin A and the protein opsin.

- **rhod** = red (pigment)
- **opsin** = visual protein

opsin (OP-sin): the protein portion of visual pigment molecules.

> FIGURE 11-3 Vitamin A's Role in Vision

More than 100 million photosensitive cells reside in the retina, and each contains about 30 million molecules of vitamin A–containing visual pigments. The rods contain the rhodopsin pigment and respond to faint light; the cones contain the iodopsin pigment and function in color vision.

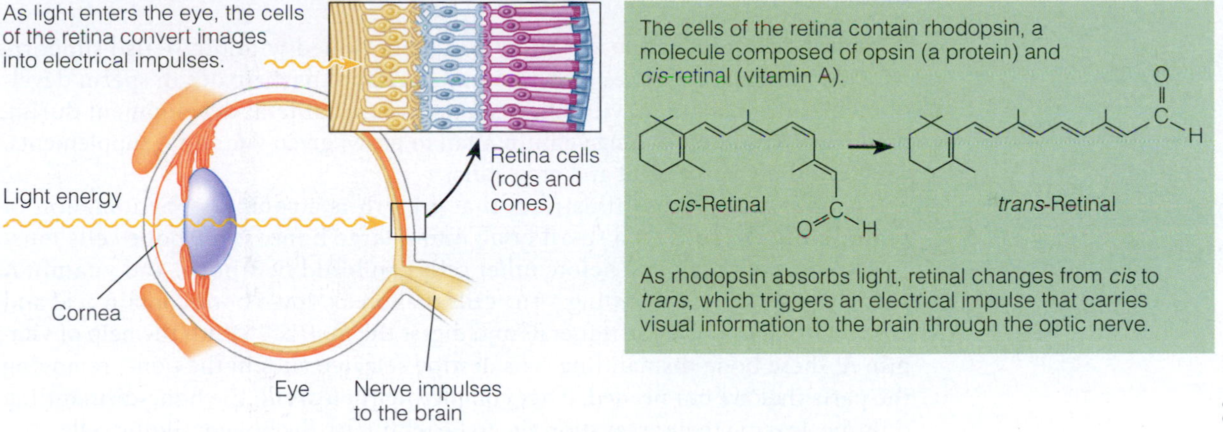
As light enters the eye, the cells of the retina convert images into electrical impulses.
Retina cells (rods and cones)
Light energy
Cornea
Eye
Nerve impulses to the brain
The cells of the retina contain rhodopsin, a molecule composed of opsin (a protein) and cis-retinal (vitamin A).
cis-Retinal
trans-Retinal
As rhodopsin absorbs light, retinal changes from cis to trans, which triggers an electrical impulse that carries visual information to the brain through the optic nerve.
© Cengage

just as fatty acids do during hydrogenation (see p. 135). These changes generate an electrical impulse that conveys the message to the brain. Much of the retinal is then converted back to its active *cis* form and combined with the opsin protein to regenerate rhodopsin. Some retinal, however, may be oxidized to retinoic acid, a biochemical dead end for the visual process. Visual activity leads to repeated small losses of retinal, necessitating its constant replenishment either directly from foods or indirectly from retinol stores.

Vitamin A in Protein Synthesis and Cell Differentiation Despite its important role in vision, only one-thousandth of the body's vitamin A is in the retina. Much more is in the cells lining the body's surfaces. There, the vitamin participates in protein synthesis and **cell differentiation,** a process by which each type of cell develops to perform a specific function.

All body surfaces, both inside and out, are covered by layers of cells known as **epithelial cells.** The **epithelial tissue** on the outside of the body is, of course, the skin—and vitamin A and beta-carotene help protect against skin damage from sunlight. The epithelial tissues that line the inside of the body are the **mucous membranes:** the linings of the mouth, stomach, and intestines; the linings of the lungs and the passages leading to them; the linings of the urinary bladder and urethra; the linings of the uterus and vagina; and the linings of the eyelids and sinus passageways. Within the body, the mucous membranes line an area larger than a tennis court, and vitamin A helps to maintain their integrity (see Figure 11-4).

> FIGURE 11-4 Mucous Membrane Integrity

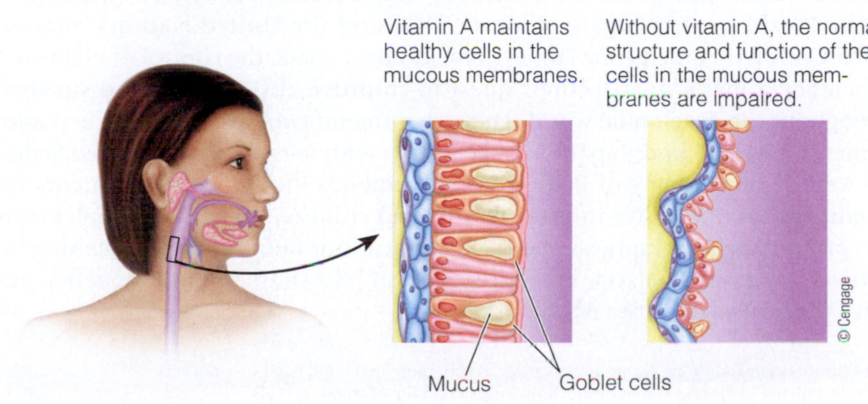
Vitamin A maintains healthy cells in the mucous membranes.
Without vitamin A, the normal structure and function of the cells in the mucous membranes are impaired.
Mucus
Goblet cells
© Cengage

cell differentiation (DIF-er-EN-she-AY-shun): the process by which immature cells develop specific functions different from those of the original that are characteristic of their mature cell type.

epithelial (ep-i-THEE-lee-ul) **cells:** cells on the surface of the skin and mucous membranes.

epithelial tissue: the layer of the body that serves as a selective barrier between the body's interior and the environment. Examples are the cornea of the eyes, the skin, the respiratory lining of the lungs, and the lining of the digestive tract.

mucous (MYOO-kus) **membranes:** the membranes, composed of mucus-secreting cells, that line the surfaces of body tissues.

Vitamin A promotes differentiation of epithelial cells and goblet cells, one-celled glands that synthesize and secrete mucus. Mucus coats and protects the epithelial cells from invasive microorganisms and other potentially damaging substances, such as gastric juices.

Vitamin A in Reproduction and Growth As mentioned, vitamin A also supports reproduction and regulates growth. In men, retinol participates in sperm development, and in women, vitamin A supports normal fetal development during pregnancy. Children lacking vitamin A fail to grow; given vitamin A supplements, these children gain weight and grow taller.

The growth of bones illustrates that growth is a complex phenomenon of **remodeling**. To convert a small bone into a large bone, some bone cells must "undo" parts of the bone before other cells can build new bone, and vitamin A participates in the dismantling.* The cells that break down bone contain acid and enzymes that dissolve the minerals and digest the matrix.** With the help of vitamin A, these bone-dismantling cells destroy selected sites in the bone, removing the parts that are not needed. After completing their work, the bone-dismantling cells die, leaving their excavation site to be rebuilt by the bone-building cells.

Beta-Carotene as a Precursor and an Antioxidant Beta-carotene plays two primary roles in the body. First, it serves as a vitamin A precursor, as Figure 11-1 (p. 334) illustrates. Second, some beta-carotene acts as an antioxidant capable of protecting the body against disease, as Highlight 11 explains.

Vitamin A Deficiency

Vitamin A status depends mostly on the adequacy of vitamin A stores, 90 percent of which are in the liver. Vitamin A status also depends on a person's protein status because retinol-binding protein serves as the vitamin's transport carrier inside the body.

If a person were to stop eating vitamin A–containing foods, deficiency symptoms would not begin to appear until after stores were depleted—1 to 2 years for a healthy adult but much sooner for a growing child. Then the consequences would be profound and severe. Vitamin A deficiency is uncommon in the United States, but it is a major nutrition problem in many developing countries, responsible for a million or more unnecessary deaths and cases of blindness each year. Many countries around the world nourish their people with biofortified corn, rice, and cassava to protect against vitamin A deficiencies; Highlight 19 describes the controversies surrounding genetic modification and biofortification of our foods.[1] Routine vitamin A supplementation and food fortification saves the sight and lives of an estimated half a million children every year.[2]

Infectious Diseases Vitamin A supports immune function and inhibits replication of the measles virus. In developing countries around the world, measles is a devastating infectious disease, killing 367 children each day.[3] The severity of the illness often correlates with the degree of vitamin A deficiency; deaths are usually due to related infections such as pneumonia and severe diarrhea. Providing vitamin A to children diagnosed with measles reduces the risk of dying by half.

The World Health Organization (WHO) and the United Nations International Children's Emergency Fund (UNICEF) have made the control of vitamin A deficiency a major goal in their quest to improve child health and survival throughout the developing world. They recommend two doses of vitamin A supplements, given 24 hours apart, for all children with measles. In the United States, the American Academy of Pediatrics recommends vitamin A supplements for certain groups of measles-infected infants and children. Vitamin A supplements also protect against blindness and the complications of other life-threatening infections, including malaria, lung diseases, and HIV (human immunodeficiency virus, the virus that causes AIDS).

---

*The cells that dismantle bone during growth are *osteoclasts;* those that build bone are *osteoblasts.*

**The degradative enzymes are contained within *lysosomes* (LYE-so-zomes).

remodeling: the dismantling and re-formation of a structure.

Night Blindness **Night blindness** is one of the first detectable signs of vitamin A deficiency and permits early diagnosis. In night blindness, the person loses the ability to recover promptly from the temporary blinding that follows a flash of bright light at night or to see after dark. In many parts of the world, after the sun goes down, vitamin A–deficient people become night-blind. They often cling to others or sit still, afraid that they may trip and fall or lose their way if they try to walk alone. Treatment with vitamin A rapidly corrects night blindness.

Blindness (Xerophthalmia) Beyond night blindness is total blindness—failure to see at all. Night blindness is caused by a lack of vitamin A at the back of the eye, the retina; total blindness is caused by a lack of vitamin A at the front of the eye, the cornea. Severe vitamin A deficiency is the leading cause of preventable blindness in the world, causing as many as half a million children to lose their sight each year; an estimated half of them die within a year of losing their sight.[4]

Blindness due to vitamin A deficiency, known as **xerophthalmia,** develops in stages. At first, the cornea becomes dry and hard because of inadequate mucus production—a condition known as **xerosis.** Then xerosis quickly progresses to **keratomalacia,** the softening of the cornea that leads to irreversible blindness. For this reason, prompt correction of vitamin A deficiency is essential to preserving eyesight.

Keratinization Elsewhere in the body, vitamin A deficiency affects other surfaces. On the body's outer surface, the epithelial cells of the skin change shape and begin to secrete the protein **keratin**—the same hard, inflexible protein commonly found in hair and nails. As Figure 11-5 shows, the skin becomes dry, rough, and scaly as lumps of keratin accumulate (**keratinization**). Without vitamin A, the goblet cells in the GI tract diminish in number and activity, limiting their secretion of mucus. With less mucus, normal digestion and absorption of nutrients falter, and this, in turn, worsens malnutrition by limiting the absorption of whatever nutrients the diet may deliver. Similar changes in the cells of other epithelial tissues weaken defenses, making infections of the respiratory tract, the GI tract, the urinary tract, the vagina, and inner ear likely.

Vitamin A Toxicity

Just as a deficiency of vitamin A affects all body systems, so does a toxicity. Symptoms of toxicity begin to develop when all the binding proteins are loaded, and vitamin A is free to damage cells. Such effects are unlikely when a person depends on a balanced diet for nutrients, but toxicity is a real possibility when concentrated amounts of **preformed vitamin A** in foods derived from animals, fortified foods, or supplements are consumed. Children are most vulnerable to toxicity because they need less vitamin A and are more sensitive to overdoses. An Upper Level (UL) of 3000 micrograms has been set for adults and applies only to the preformed vitamin. Multivitamin supplements typically provide 1200 to 1500 micrograms—much more vitamin A than most people need. (For perspective, the RDA for vitamin A is 700 micrograms for women and 900 micrograms for men.)

Beta-carotene, which is found in a wide variety of fruits and vegetables, is not converted efficiently enough in the body to cause vitamin A toxicity; instead, it is stored in the fat just under the skin. Although overconsumption of beta-carotene from foods may turn the skin yellow, this is not harmful (see Figure 11-6). In contrast, overconsumption of beta-carotene from supplements may be quite harmful. In excess, this antioxidant may act as a prooxidant (as Highlight 11 explains). Adverse effects of beta-carotene supplements are most evident in people who drink alcohol and smoke cigarettes.

Bone Defects Excessive intakes of preformed vitamin A may weaken the bones and contribute to fractures and osteoporosis.[5] Vitamin A suppresses bone-building activity, stimulates bone-dismantling activity, and interferes with vitamin D's ability to maintain normal blood calcium.

> **FIGURE 11-5 Vitamin A–Deficiency Symptom—The Rough Skin of Keratinization**

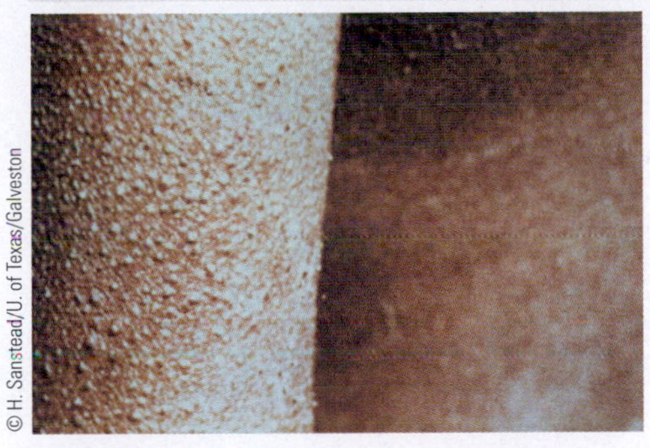

© H. Sanstead/U. of Texas/Galveston

In vitamin A deficiency, the epithelial cells secrete the protein keratin in a process known as *keratinization.* (Keratinization doesn't occur in the GI tract, but mucus-producing cells dwindle and mucus production declines.) The extreme of this condition is *hyperkeratinization* or *hyperkeratosis.* When keratin accumulates around hair follicles, the condition is known as *follicular hyperkeratosis.*

> **FIGURE 11-6 Symptom of Beta-Carotene Excess—Discoloration of the Skin**

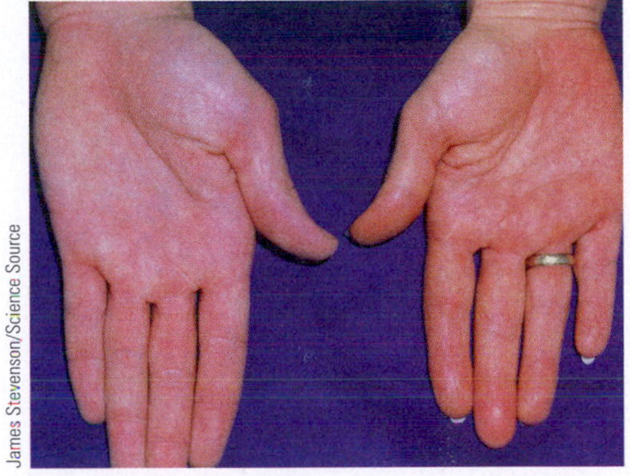

James Stevenson/Science Source

The hand on the right shows the skin yellowing that occurs when blood levels of beta-carotene rise in response to a diet that features carrots, pumpkins, and orange juice. (The hand on the left belongs to someone else and is shown here for comparison.)

night blindness: slow recovery of vision after flashes of bright light at night or an inability to see in dim light; an early symptom of vitamin A deficiency.

xerophthalmia (zer-off-THAL-mee-uh): progressive blindness caused by inadequate mucus production due to severe vitamin A deficiency.

- **xero** = dry
- **ophthalm** = eye

xerosis (zee-ROW-sis): abnormal drying of the skin and mucous membranes; a sign of vitamin A deficiency.

keratomalacia (KARE-ah-toe-ma-LAY-shuh): softening of the cornea that leads to irreversible blindness; a sign of severe vitamin A deficiency.

keratin (KARE-uh-tin): a water-insoluble protein; the normal protein of hair and nails.

keratinization: accumulation of keratin in a tissue; a sign of vitamin A deficiency.

preformed vitamin A: dietary vitamin A in its active form.

Birth Defects Excessive vitamin A during pregnancy leads to abnormal cell death in the spinal cord, which increases the risk of birth defects such as spina bifida and cleft palate.[6] In such cases, vitamin A is considered a **teratogen.** High intakes (daily supplemental intakes of vitamin A equivalent to roughly four times the RDA for women) before the seventh week of pregnancy appear to be the most damaging. For this reason, vitamin A is not given as a supplement in the first trimester of pregnancy without specific evidence of deficiency, which is rare.

Not for Acne Adolescents need to know that massive doses of vitamin A have no beneficial effect on **acne.** The prescription medicine Accutane is made from vitamin A but is chemically different.* Taken orally, Accutane is effective against the deep lesions of cystic acne. It is highly toxic, however, especially during growth, and has caused birth defects in infants when women have taken it during pregnancy. For this reason, women taking Accutane must agree to pregnancy testing and to using two forms of contraception from at least 1 month before taking the drug through at least 1 month after discontinuing its use. Should they become pregnant, they need to stop taking Accutane immediately and notify their physician.

Another vitamin A relative, Retin-A, fights acne, the wrinkles of aging, and other skin disorders.** Applied topically, this ointment smooths and softens skin; it also lightens skin that has become darkly pigmented after inflammation. During treatment, the skin becomes red and tender and peels.

Vitamin A Recommendations

Because the body can derive vitamin A from both retinoids and carotenoids, its content in foods and its recommendations are expressed as **retinol activity equivalents (RAE).** One microgram of retinol counts as 1 RAE, as does 12 micrograms of dietary beta-carotene.*** This difference recognizes that beta-carotene's absorption and conversion are significantly less efficient than those of the retinoids. Food and supplement labels sometimes report vitamin A contents using International Units (IU), a measure of vitamin activity used before direct chemical analysis was possible. The glossary on the insert provides factors that can be used to convert IU to a weight measurement.

Vitamin A in Foods

The richest sources of the retinoids are foods derived from animals—liver, fish liver oils, milk and milk products, butter, and eggs. Because vitamin A is fat soluble, it is lost when milk is skimmed. To compensate, reduced-fat, low-fat, and fat-free milks are fortified so as to provide the amount found in whole milk. Margarine is usually fortified to provide the same amount of vitamin A as butter.

Plants contain no retinoids, but many vegetables and some fruits contain vitamin A precursors—the carotenoids. Only a few carotenoids have vitamin A activity; the carotenoid with the greatest vitamin A activity is beta-carotene. Beta-carotene is a rich, deep yellow, almost orange, compound. The beta-carotene in dark green, leafy vegetables is abundant, but masked by large amounts of the green pigment **chlorophyll.** Attractive meals that include colorful fruits and vegetables rich in beta-carotene are likely to provide vitamin A (see Photo 11-1).

The Colors of Vitamin A Foods Dark leafy greens (like broccoli and spinach—not celery or cabbage) and rich yellow or deep orange vegetables and fruits (such as cantaloupe, carrots, and sweet potatoes—not corn or bananas) help people meet their vitamin A needs (see Figure 11-7). A diet including several servings of such carotene-rich sources helps ensure a sufficient intake.

Bright color is not always a sign of vitamin A activity, however. Beets and corn, for example, derive their colors from the red and yellow **xanthophylls,**

*The generic name for Accutane is *isotretinoin.*

**The generic name for Retin-A is *tretinoin topical.*

***For beta-carotene from supplements, 2 micrograms equal 1 microgram RAE and for other vitamin A precursor carotenoids, 24 micrograms equal 1 microgram RAE.

teratogen (ter-AT-oh-jen): a substance that causes abnormal fetal development and birth defects.

acne: a chronic inflammation of the skin's follicles and oil-producing glands, which leads to an accumulation of oils inside the ducts that surround hairs; usually associated with the maturation of young adults.

retinol activity equivalents (RAE): a measure of vitamin A activity; the amount of retinol that the body will derive from a food containing preformed retinol or its precursor, beta-carotene.

chlorophyll (KLO-row-fil): the green pigment of plants, which absorbs light and transfers the energy to other molecules, thereby initiating photosynthesis.

xanthophylls (ZAN-tho-fills): pigments found in plants responsible for the color changes seen in autumn leaves.

which have no vitamin A activity. As for white plant foods such as potatoes, cauliflower, pasta, and rice, they also offer little or no vitamin A. Similarly, fast foods often lack vitamin A. Anyone who dines frequently on hamburgers, french fries, and colas is wise to emphasize colorful vegetables and fruits at other meals.

Vitamin A–Rich Liver People sometimes wonder if eating liver too frequently can cause vitamin A toxicity. Liver is a rich source because vitamin A is stored in the livers of animals, just as in humans.* Arctic explorers who have eaten large quantities of polar bear liver have become ill with symptoms suggesting vitamin A toxicity. Liver offers many nutrients, and eating it periodically may improve a person's nutrition status, but caution is warranted not to eat too much too often, especially for pregnant women. With 1 ounce of beef liver providing more than three times the RDA for vitamin A, intakes can increase quickly.

Golden Rice and Biofortified Foods As mentioned earlier, vitamin A deficiency is a major problem in developing countries, impairing growth, causing blindness, and suppressing the immune system. In these developing regions of the world, fruits and vegetables are a scarcity, and rice, which contains no beta-carotene or vitamin A, is the staple food. Through biotechnology, scientists have been able to genetically modify rice (and other staple foods) to be a significant source

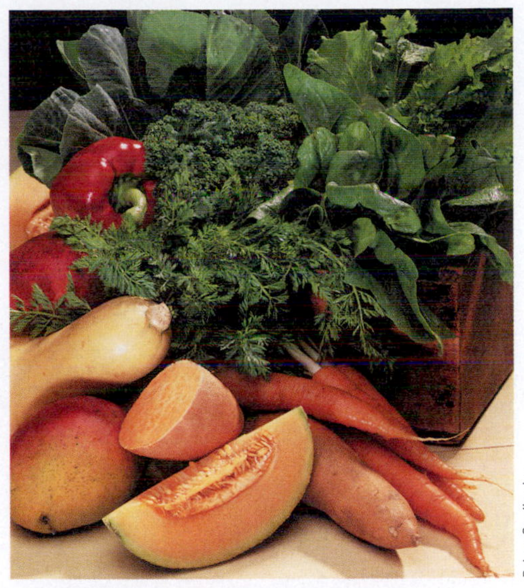

Polara Studios Inc.

> **PHOTO 11-1** The carotenoids in foods bring colors to meals; the retinoids in our eyes allow us to see them.

> **FIGURE 11-7 Vitamin A in Selected Foods**

Food	Serving size (kcalories)
Bread, whole wheat	1-oz slice (70 kcal)
Cornflakes, fortified	1 oz (110 kcal)
Spaghetti pasta	½ c cooked (99 kcal)
Tortilla, flour	1 10" round (234 kcal)
Broccoli	½ c cooked (22 kcal)
Carrots	½ c shredded raw (24 kcal)
Potato	1 medium baked w/skin (133 kcal)
Tomato juice	¾ c (31 kcal)
Banana	1 medium raw (109 kcal)
Orange	1 medium raw (62 kcal)
Strawberries	½ c fresh (22 kcal)
Watermelon	1 slice (92 kcal)
Milk, fortified	1 c reduced-fat 2% (121 kcal)
Yogurt, plain	1 c low-fat (155 kcal)
Cheddar cheese	1½ oz (171 kcal)
Cottage cheese	½ c low-fat 2% (101 kcal)
Pinto beans	½ c cooked (117 kcal)
Peanut butter	2 tbs (188 kcal)
Sunflower seeds	1 oz dry (165 kcal)
Tofu (soybean curd)	½ c (76 kcal)
Ground beef, lean	3 oz broiled (244 kcal)
Chicken breast	3 oz roasted (140 kcal)
Tuna, canned in water	3 oz (99 kcal)
Egg	1 hard cooked (78 kcal)
Excellent, and sometimes unusual, sources:	
Beef liver	3 oz fried (184 kcal)
Sweet potatoes	½ c cooked (116 kcal)
Mango	1 (135 kcal)

Micrograms RAE
0
100
200
300
400
500
600
700
800
900
1000
RDA for women
RDA for men
VITAMIN A
Dark green and deep orange vegetables (green) and fruits (purple) and fortified foods such as milk contribute vitamin A. Some foods are rich enough in vitamin A to provide the RDA and more in a single serving.
Key:
Grains
Vegetables
Fruits
Milk and milk products
Legumes, nuts, seeds
Meats, poultry, seafood
Best sources per kcalorie

*The liver is not the only organ that stores vitamin A. The kidneys, adrenal glands, and other organs do, too, but the liver stores the most and is the most commonly eaten organ meat.

of beta-carotene. Commonly called *golden rice* because of its yellowish tinge, this rice offers a promising solution to world malnutrition, but it also raises questions about potential risks to the environment. More details are provided in Highlight 19's review of food biotechnology and Chapter 20's presentation of world hunger and possible solutions.

REVIEW IT Identify the main roles, deficiency symptoms, and food sources for vitamin A.

Vitamin A is found in the body in three forms: retinol, retinal, and retinoic acid. Together, they are essential to vision, healthy epithelial tissues, and growth. Vitamin A deficiency is a major health problem worldwide, leading to infections, blindness, and keratinization. Toxicity can also cause problems and is most often associated with supplement abuse. Animal-derived foods such as liver and whole or fortified milk provide retinoids, whereas brightly colored plant-derived foods such as spinach, carrots, and pumpkins provide beta-carotene and other carotenoids. In addition to serving as a precursor for vitamin A, beta-carotene acts as an antioxidant in the body. The accompanying table provides a summary of vitamin A.

Vitamin A

Other Names	Chief Functions in the Body
Retinol, retinal, retinoic acid; precursors are carotenoids such as beta-carotene	Vision; maintenance of cornea, epithelial cells, mucous membranes, skin; bone and tooth growth; reproduction; immunity
RDA	**Significant Sources**
Men: 900 µg RAE/day Women: 700 µg RAE/day	Retinol: fortified milk, cheese, cream, butter, fortified margarine, eggs, liver
UL	
Adults: 3000 µg/day (preformed vitamin A)	Beta-carotene: spinach and other dark green, leafy vegetables, broccoli, deep orange fruits (apricots, cantaloupe) and vegetables (squash, carrots, sweet potatoes, pumpkin)
Deficiency Disease	**Toxicity Disease**
Hypovitaminosis A	Hypervitaminosis A[a]
Deficiency Symptoms	**Chronic Toxicity Symptoms**
Night blindness, corneal drying (xerosis), triangular gray spots on eye (Bitot's spots), softening of the cornea (keratomalacia), and corneal degeneration and blindness (xerophthalmia); impaired immunity (infectious diseases); plugging of hair follicles with keratin, forming white lumps (hyperkeratosis)	Increased activity of osteoclasts[b] causing reduced bone density; liver abnormalities; birth defects **Acute Toxicity Symptoms** Blurred vision, nausea, vomiting, vertigo; increase of pressure inside skull, mimicking brain tumor; headaches; muscle incoordination

[a]A related condition, *hypercarotenemia,* is caused by the accumulation of too much of the vitamin A precursor beta-carotene in the blood, which turns the skin noticeably yellow. Hypercarotenemia is not, strictly speaking, a toxicity symptom.
[b]*Osteoclasts* are the cells that destroy bone during its growth. Those that build bone are *osteoblasts.*

11.2 Vitamin D

LEARN IT Identify the main roles, deficiency symptoms, and sources for vitamin D.

Vitamin D differs from the other nutrients in that the body can synthesize it, with the help of sunlight, from a precursor that the body makes from cholesterol. Therefore, vitamin D is not an essential nutrient; given enough time in the sun, people need no vitamin D from foods.

Also known as **calciferol,** vitamin D comes in two major forms.[7] **Vitamin D_2** derives primarily from plant foods in the diet. **Vitamin D_3** derives from animal

calciferol (kal-SIF-er-ol): vitamin D.

vitamin D_2: vitamin D derived from plant foods in the diet; also called *ergocalciferol* (ER-go-kal-SIF-er-ol).

vitamin D_3: vitamin D derived from animal foods in the diet or made in the skin from 7-dehydrocholesterol, a precursor of cholesterol, with the help of sunlight; also called *cholecalciferol* (KO-lee-kal-SIF-er-ol) or *calciol.* After hydroxylation in the liver, calciol becomes *calcidiol* and after hydroxylation in the kidneys, calcidiol becomes *calcitriol.*

> FIGURE 11-8 Vitamin D Synthesis and Activation

The final activation step in the kidneys is tightly regulated by hormones. (Appendix C presents the chemical structures for these various forms of vitamin D and related compounds.)

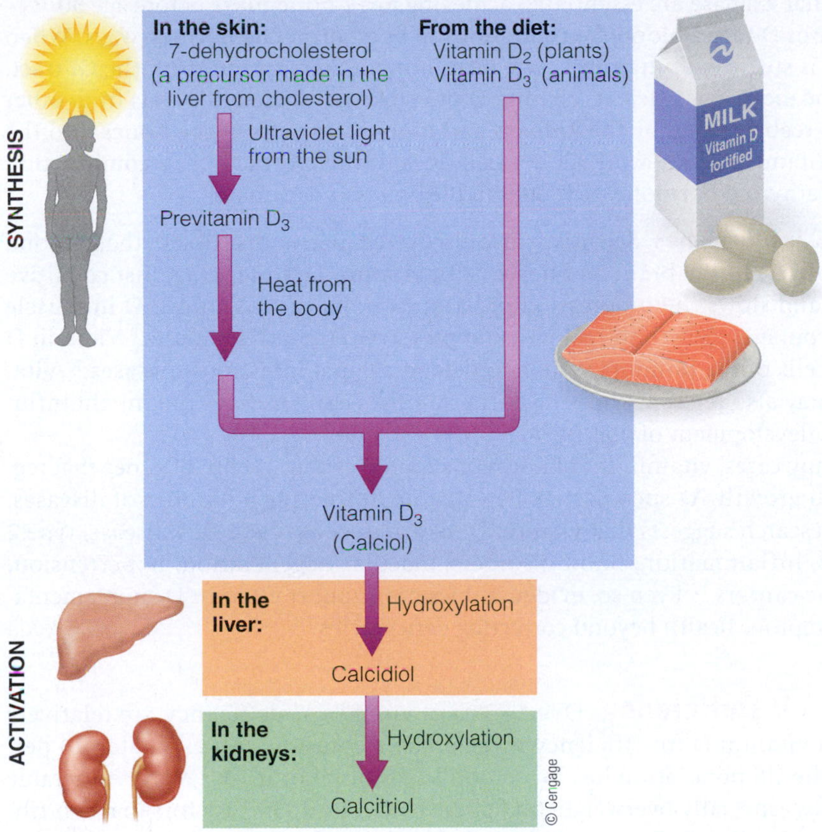
SYNTHESIS
In the skin:
7-dehydrocholesterol
(a precursor made in the liver from cholesterol)
Ultraviolet light from the sun
Previtamin D_3
Heat from the body
From the diet:
Vitamin D_2 (plants)
Vitamin D_3 (animals)
MILK
Vitamin D fortified
Vitamin D_3
(Calciol)
ACTIVATION
In the liver:
Hydroxylation
Calcidiol
In the kidneys:
Hydroxylation
Calcitriol
© Cengage

foods in the diet and from synthesis in the skin. These two forms of vitamin D are similar and both must be activated before they can fully function.

Figure 11-8 diagrams the pathway for making and activating vitamin D in the body. To make vitamin D, ultraviolet rays from the sun hit a precursor in the skin and convert it to previtamin D_3, which is converted to vitamin D_3 with the help of the body's heat. To activate vitamin D—whether made in the body or consumed from the diet—two hydroxylation reactions must occur. First, the liver adds an OH group, and then the kidneys add another OH group to produce the active vitamin. As you might expect, diseases affecting either the liver or the kidneys can interfere with the activation of vitamin D and produce symptoms of deficiency.

Roles in the Body Though called a vitamin, the active form of vitamin D is actually a hormone—a compound manufactured by one part of the body that travels through the blood and triggers a response from another part of the body. Like vitamin A, vitamin D has a binding protein that carries it to the target organs—most notably, the intestines, the kidneys, and the bones. All respond to vitamin D by making the minerals needed for bone growth and maintenance available.

Vitamin D in Bone Growth Vitamin D is a member of a large and cooperative bone-making and maintenance team composed of nutrients and other compounds, including vitamins A and K; the hormones parathyroid hormone and calcitonin; the protein collagen; and the minerals calcium, phosphorus, magnesium, and fluoride. Vitamin D's specific role in bone health is to assist in the absorption of calcium and phosphorus, thus helping to maintain blood concentrations of these minerals. The bones grow denser and stronger as they absorb and deposit these minerals. Details of calcium balance and mineral deposition appear in Chapter 12, but here's a sneak preview: adequate nutrition and regular exercise are essential to achieving **peak bone mass** before age 30.

Vitamin D raises blood concentrations of bone minerals in three ways. When the diet is sufficient, vitamin D enhances mineral absorption from the GI tract. When the diet is insufficient, vitamin D provides the needed minerals from other sources: reabsorption by the kidneys and mobilization from the bones into the blood. Vitamin D may work alone, as it does in the GI tract, or in combination with parathyroid hormone, as it does in the bones and kidneys.

Vitamin D in Other Roles Scientists have discovered many other tissues that respond to vitamin D. In the brain and nerve cells, vitamin D protects against cognitive decline and slows the progression of Parkinson disease.[8] Vitamin D in muscle cells encourages growth in children and preserves strength in adults.[9] Vitamin D signals cells of the immune system to defend against infectious diseases.[10] Vitamin D may also regulate the cells of the adipose tissue in ways that might influence the development of obesity.[11]

In many cases, vitamin D enhances or suppresses the activity of genes that regulate cell growth. As such, it may be valuable in treating a number of diseases. Recent research suggests that vitamin D may protect against heart disease, type 2 diabetes, inflammation, brain disorders, macular degeneration, hypertension, and some cancers.[12] Even so, evidence does not support vitamin D supplementation to improve health beyond correcting deficiencies.[13]

Vitamin D Deficiency

Overt signs of vitamin D deficiency are relatively rare, but vitamin D insufficiency is remarkably common. An estimated 16 percent of the US population has low blood levels of vitamin D.[14] Most vulnerable are blacks, especially overweight and obese black children.[15] Factors that contribute to vitamin D deficiency include dark skin, breastfeeding without supplementation, lack of sunlight, and not using fortified milk. In vitamin D deficiency, production of **calbindin**, a protein that binds calcium in the intestinal cells, slows. Thus, even when calcium in the diet is adequate, it passes through the GI tract unabsorbed, leaving the bones undersupplied. Consequently, a vitamin D deficiency creates a calcium deficiency and increases the risks of several chronic diseases and osteoporosis. Vitamin D–deficient adolescents do not reach their peak bone mass.

Rickets Worldwide, the prevalence of the vitamin D–deficiency disease **rickets** is extremely high, affecting more than half of the children in some countries. In the United States, rickets is not common, but when it occurs, black children and adolescents—especially females and overweight teens—are the ones most likely to be affected. To prevent rickets, the American Academy of Pediatrics recommends a supplement for all infants, children, and adolescents who do not receive enough vitamin D.

In rickets, the bones fail to calcify normally, causing growth impairments and skeletal abnormalities. The bones become so weak that they bend when they have to support the body's weight (see Figure 11-9). A child with rickets who is old enough to walk characteristically develops bowed legs, often the most obvious sign of the disease. Another sign is the beaded ribs that result from the poorly formed attachments of the bones to the cartilage.*

Osteomalacia In adults, the poor mineralization of bone results in the painful bone disease **osteomalacia.** The bones become increasingly soft, flexible, brittle, and deformed.

*Because the poorly formed rib attachments resemble rosary beads, this symptom is commonly known as *rachitic* (ra-KIT-ik) *rosary* ("the rosary of rickets").

peak bone mass: the highest attainable bone density for an individual, developed during the first three decades of life.

calbindin: a calcium-binding transport protein that requires vitamin D for its synthesis.

rickets: the vitamin D–deficiency disease in children characterized by inadequate mineralization of bone (manifested in bowed legs or knock-knees, outward-bowed chest, and "beads" on ribs). A rare type of rickets, not caused by vitamin D deficiency, is known as *vitamin D–refractory rickets.*

osteomalacia (OS-tee-oh-ma-LAY-shuh): a bone disease characterized by softening of the bones. Symptoms include bending of the spine and bowing of the legs. The disease occurs most often in adult women.

- **osteo** = bone
- **malacia** = softening

> **FIGURE 11-9 Vitamin D–Deficiency Symptoms—Bowed Legs and Beaded Ribs of Rickets**

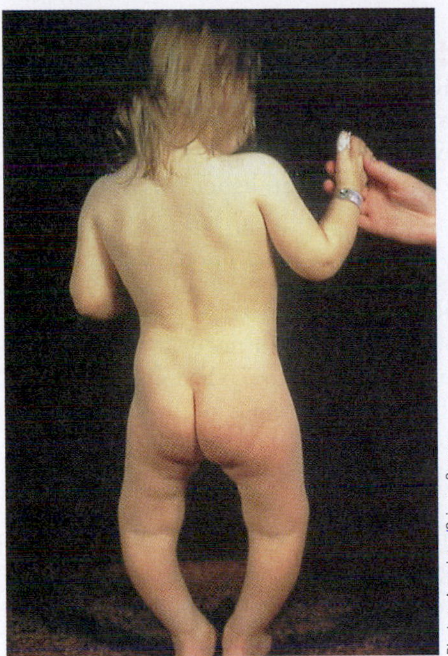

Biophoto Associates/Science Source

Bowed legs. In rickets, the poorly formed long bones of the legs bend outward as weight-bearing activities such as walking begin.

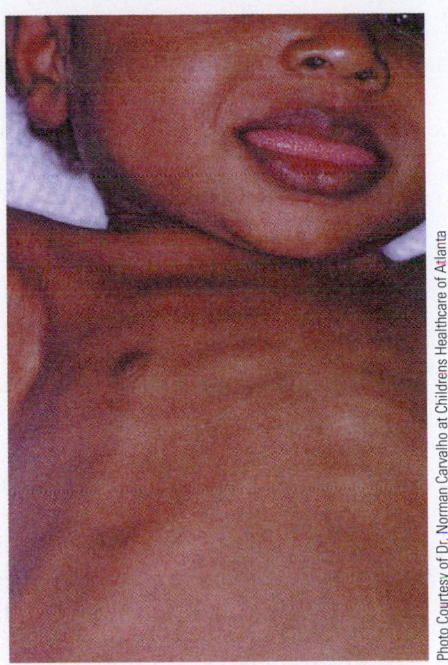

Photo Courtesy of Dr. Norman Carvalho at Childrens Healthcare of Atlanta

Beaded ribs. In rickets, a series of "beads" develop where the cartilages and bones attach.

Osteoporosis Any failure to synthesize adequate vitamin D or obtain enough from foods sets the stage for a loss of calcium from the bones, which can result in fractures. Highlight 12 describes the many factors that lead to osteoporosis, a condition of reduced bone density.

The Elderly Vitamin D deficiency is especially likely in older adults for several reasons. For one, the skin, liver, and kidneys lose their capacity to make and activate vitamin D with advancing age. For another, older adults typically drink little or no milk—the main dietary source of vitamin D. And finally, older adults typically spend much of the day indoors, and when they do venture outside, many of them cautiously wear protective clothing or apply sunscreen to all sun-exposed areas of their skin. Dark-skinned adults living in northern regions are particularly vulnerable. All of these factors increase the likelihood of vitamin D deficiency and its consequences: bone losses, osteoporotic fractures, and muscle weakness. Vitamin D supplementation helps raise blood levels, reduce bone loss, improve muscle performance, and lower the risks of falls and fractures in elderly persons.

Vitamin D Toxicity

Vitamin D clearly illustrates how nutrients in optimal amounts support health, but both inadequacies and excesses create harm. Vitamin D is among the most likely of the vitamins to have toxic effects when consumed in excessive amounts. The amounts of vitamin D made by the skin and found in foods are well within the safe limits set by the UL, but supplements containing the vitamin in concentrated form should be kept out of the reach of children and used cautiously by adults.[16]

Excess vitamin D raises the concentration of blood calcium.[17]* Excess blood calcium tends to precipitate in the soft tissue, forming stones, especially in the

*High blood calcium is known as *hypercalcemia* and may develop from a variety of disorders, including vitamin D toxicity. It does *not* develop from too much calcium in the diet.

kidneys, where calcium is concentrated in an effort to excrete it. Calcification may also harden the blood vessels and is especially dangerous in the major arteries of the brain, heart, and lungs, where it can cause death.

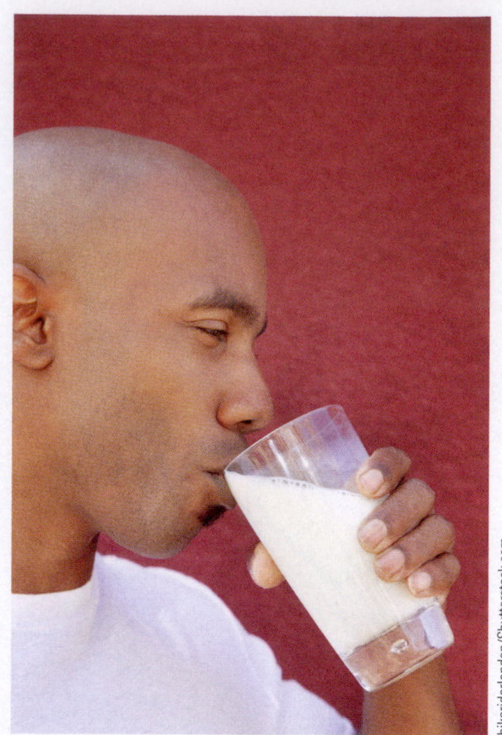

bikeriderlondon/Shutterstock.com

> **PHOTO 11-2** A cold glass of milk refreshes as it replenishes vitamin D and other bone-building nutrients.

Vitamin D Recommendations and Sources

Only a few foods contain vitamin D naturally. Fortunately, the body can make vitamin D with the help of a little sunshine. In setting dietary recommendations, however, the DRI Committee assumed that no vitamin D was available from skin synthesis. Some research suggests that the vitamin D RDA is insufficient, especially for African Americans.[18]

Vitamin D in Foods The *Dietary Guidelines* advise consumers to drink vitamin D–fortified milk (see Photo 11-2). The fortification of milk and other foods with vitamin D is the best guarantee that people will meet their needs.[19]* Consumers using alternatives such as soy milk or almond milk need to read labels carefully to ensure they are getting vitamin D–fortified products. Despite vitamin D fortification, the average intake in the United States falls short of recommendations. Egg yolks and oily fish such as salmon, mackerel, and sardines are the best natural sources of vitamin D.

Meeting vitamin D needs is difficult without adequate sunshine, fortification, or supplementation. Importantly, feeding infants and young children nonfortified "health beverages" instead of milk or infant formula can create severe nutrient deficiencies, including rickets.

Vitamin D from the Sun Most of the world's population relies on natural exposure to sunlight to maintain adequate vitamin D nutrition. The sun imposes no risk of vitamin D toxicity; prolonged exposure to sunlight degrades the vitamin D precursor in the skin, preventing its conversion to the active vitamin.

Prolonged exposure to sunlight can, however, prematurely wrinkle the skin and cause skin cancer. Sunscreens help reduce these risks, but sunscreens with a sun protection factor (SPF) of 8 and higher can also reduce vitamin D synthesis. Still, even with an SPF 15 to 30 sunscreen, sufficient vitamin D synthesis can be obtained in 10 to 20 minutes of sun exposure. Alternatively, a person could apply sunscreen after enough time has elapsed to provide sufficient vitamin D synthesis. For most people, exposing hands, face, and arms on a clear summer day for 5 to 10 minutes two or three times a week should be sufficient to maintain vitamin D nutrition (see Photo 11-3). Avoiding sun exposure completely may be harmful to health.[20]

The pigments of dark skin provide some protection from the sun's damage, but they also reduce vitamin D synthesis. Dark-skinned people require more sunlight exposure than light-skinned people—perhaps as much as 4 to 6 times longer. Latitude, season, and time of day also have dramatic effects on vitamin D synthesis and status (see Figure 11-10). Heavy cloud cover, smoke, or smog block the ultraviolet (UV) rays of the sun that promote vitamin D synthesis. People who stay in the shade and wear long-sleeved clothing are twice as likely to develop vitamin D deficiency as those who rarely do so. Vitamin D deficiency is especially prevalent in the winter and in the Arctic and Antarctic regions of the world. To ensure an adequate vitamin D status, supplements may be needed. The body's vitamin D supplies from summer synthesis alone are insufficient to meet winter needs.

Depending on the radiation used, the UV rays from tanning lamps and tanning beds may also stimulate vitamin D synthesis. The potential hazards of skin damage, however, may outweigh any possible benefits.** The Food and Drug

*Vitamin D fortification of milk in the United States is 10 micrograms per quart.

**The best wavelengths for vitamin D synthesis are UV-B rays between 290 and 310 nanometers. Some tanning parlors advertise "UV-A rays only, for a tan without the burn," but UV-A rays can damage the skin.

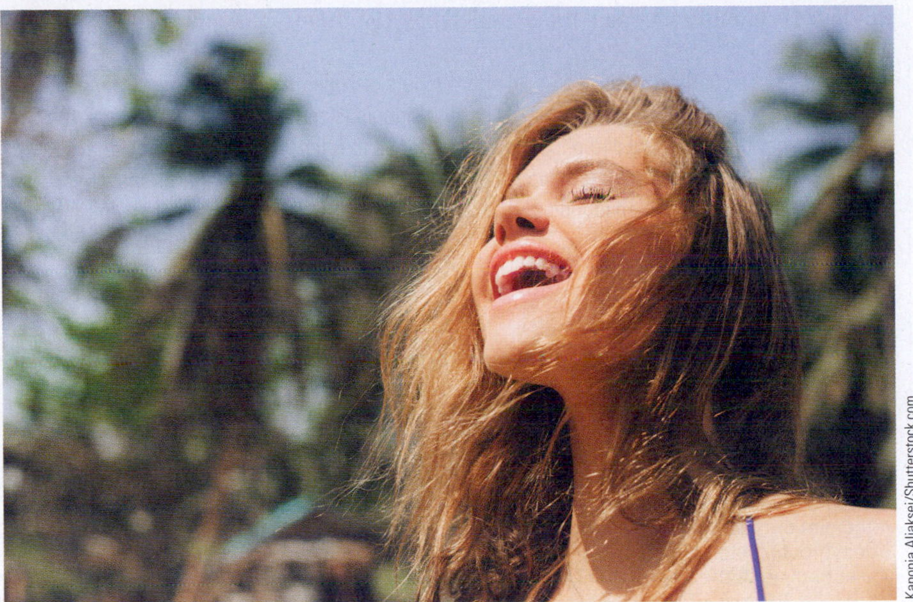
Kaponia Aliaksei/Shutterstock.com

> **PHOTO 11-3** The body can make vitamin D with a little help from sunshine.

Administration (FDA) warns that if the lamps are not properly filtered, people using tanning booths risk burns, damage to the eyes and blood vessels, and skin cancer.

Vitamin D from Supplements As mentioned, some people may benefit from taking vitamin D supplements. Vitamin D can be found in multivitamin-mineral supplements as well as a high-dose single supplement. As a single supplement, vitamin D_3 is less expensive, more commonly available, and more effective than vitamin D_2.[21]

> **FIGURE 11-10 Vitamin D Synthesis and Latitude**

Above 40° north latitude (and below 40° south latitude in the southern hemisphere), vitamin D synthesis essentially ceases for the 4 months of winter. Synthesis increases as spring approaches, peaks in summer, and declines again in the fall. People living in regions of extreme northern (or extreme southern) latitudes may miss as much as 6 months of vitamin D production every year.

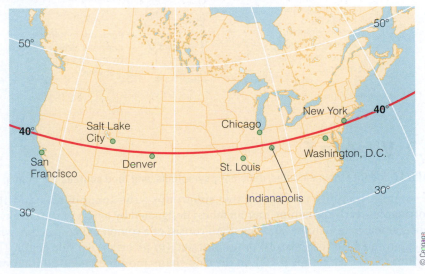
50°
50°
40°
40°
Salt Lake City
Chicago
New York
San Francisco
Denver
St. Louis
Washington, D.C.
Indianapolis
30°
30°
© Cengage

REVIEW IT Identify the main roles, deficiency symptoms, and sources for vitamin D.

Vitamin D can be synthesized in the body with the help of sunlight or obtained from some foods, most notably fortified milk. Vitamin D sends signals to three primary target sites: the GI tract to absorb more calcium and phosphorus, the bones to release more, and the kidneys to retain more. These actions maintain blood calcium concentrations and support bone density. A deficiency causes rickets in childhood and osteomalacia in later life. The accompanying table provides a summary of vitamin D.

Vitamin D

Other Names

calciferol (vitamin D)

ergocalciferol (vitamin D_2): vitamin D derived from plant foods in the diet and made from the yeast and plant sterol ergosterol.

cholecalciferol (vitamin D_3 or **calciol):** vitamin D from animal-derived foods in the diet or made in the skin from 7-dehydrocholesterol, a precursor of cholesterol, with the help of sunlight.

calcidiol (25-hydroxyvitamin D): vitamin D found in the blood that is made from the hydroxylation of calciol in the liver.

calcitriol (1,25-dihydroxyvitamin D): vitamin D that is made from the hydroxylation of calcidiol in the kidneys; the biologically active hormone, sometimes called *active vitamin D.*

RDA

Adults: 15 µg/day or 600 IU/day (19–70 yr)
20 µg/day or 800 IU/day (>70 yr)

UL

Adults: 100 µg/day or 4000 IU/day

Chief Functions in the Body

Mineralization of bones (raises blood calcium and phosphorus by increasing absorption from digestive tract, withdrawing calcium from bones, stimulating retention by kidneys)

Significant Sources

Synthesized in the body with the help of sunlight; fortified milk, margarine, butter, juices, cereals, and chocolate mixes; veal, beef, egg yolks, liver, fatty fish (herring, salmon, sardines) and their oils

Deficiency Diseases

Rickets, osteomalacia

Deficiency Symptoms

Rickets in children:

Inadequate calcification, resulting in misshapen bones (bowing of legs); enlargement of ends of long bones (knees, wrists); deformities of ribs (bowed, with beads or knobs); delayed closing of fontanel, resulting in rapid enlargement of head (see figure below); lax muscles resulting in protrusion of abdomen; muscle spasms

Osteomalacia or osteoporosis in adults:

Loss of calcium, resulting in soft, flexible, brittle, and deformed bones; progressive weakness; pain in pelvis, lower back, and legs

Toxicity Disease

Hypervitaminosis D

Toxicity Symptoms

Elevated blood calcium; calcification of soft tissues (blood vessels, kidneys, heart, lungs, tissues around joints)

Fontanel
A fontanel is an open space in the top of a baby's skull before the bones have grown together. In rickets, closing of the fontanel is delayed.

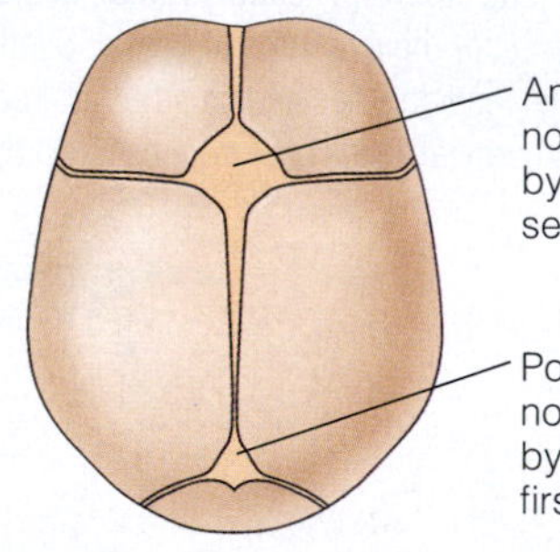
Anterior fontanel normally closes by the end of the second year.
Posterior fontanel normally closes by the end of the first year.

11.3 Vitamin E

LEARN IT Identify the main roles, deficiency symptoms, and food sources for vitamin E.

The vitamin E family consists of two subgroups—the **tocopherols** and the **tocotrienols**—each containing four members designated by letters of the Greek alphabet (alpha, beta, gamma, and delta). All consist of a complex ring structure with a long saturated (in tocopherols) or unsaturated (in tocotrienols) side chain. The positions of methyl groups (CH_3) on the side chain and their chemical rotations

tocopherols (tuh-KOFF-uh-rawls): members of the vitamin E family having the chemical structure of a complex ring structure with a long saturated side chain. (See Appendix C for chemical structures.)

tocotrienols (TOE-koh-try-EE-nawls): members of the vitamin E family having the chemical structure of a complex ring structure with a long unsaturated side chain. (See Appendix C for chemical structures.)

distinguish the four members within each subgroup. (Appendix C provides the chemical structures.)

Of all the members of the vitamin E family, only **alpha-tocopherol** is maintained in the body and can meet the body's needs for the vitamin. The others are not converted to alpha-tocopherol in the body, nor are they recognized by its transport protein. For these reasons, the RDA is based only on alpha-tocopherol. Most vitamin E research has focused on alpha-tocopherol, but recent studies suggest that the other tocopherols and tocotrienols have unique antioxidant and anti-inflammatory roles that better protect against chronic diseases such as cancer.[22] In addition to preventing cancer, tocotrienols may also protect against osteoporosis, diabetes, heart disease, and neurological disorders.

Vitamin E as an Antioxidant Vitamin E is a fat-soluble antioxidant and one of the body's primary defenders against the adverse effects of free radicals. Its main action is to stop the chain reaction of free radicals from producing more free radicals (see Highlight 11). In doing so, vitamin E protects the vulnerable components of the cells and their membranes from destruction. Most notably, vitamin E prevents the oxidation of the polyunsaturated fatty acids, but it protects other lipids and related compounds (for example, vitamin A) as well.

Accumulating evidence suggests that vitamin E may reduce the risk of heart disease by protecting low-density lipoproteins (LDL) against oxidation and reducing inflammation.[23] The oxidation of LDL and associated inflammation have been implicated as key factors in the development of heart disease. Highlight 11 explains how vitamin E and other antioxidants might protect against chronic diseases, such as heart disease and cancer, and explores whether foods or supplements might be most helpful—or harmful.

Vitamin E Deficiency A primary deficiency of vitamin E (from poor dietary intake) is rare; deficiency is usually associated with diseases of fat malabsorption such as cystic fibrosis. Without vitamin E, the red blood cells break and spill their contents as the polyunsaturated fatty acids in their membranes become oxidized. This classic sign of vitamin E deficiency, known as **erythrocyte hemolysis,** is seen in premature infants born before the transfer of vitamin E from the mother to the infant that takes place in the last weeks of pregnancy. Vitamin E treatment corrects **hemolytic anemia.**

Prolonged vitamin E deficiency, as can occur with some genetic disorders, also causes neuromuscular dysfunction.[24] Common symptoms include loss of muscle coordination and reflexes and impaired vision and speech. Vitamin E treatment helps to correct these neurological symptoms of vitamin E deficiency.

Vitamin E Toxicity Vitamin E supplement use has risen in recent years as its protective actions against chronic diseases have been recognized, although research shows no benefits of supplementation in healthy people.[25] Fortunately, the liver carefully regulates vitamin E concentrations. Toxicity is rare, and vitamin E appears safe across a broad range of intakes. The UL for vitamin E (1000 milligrams) is more than 65 times greater than the recommended intake for adults (15 milligrams). Extremely high doses of vitamin E may interfere with the blood-clotting action of vitamin K and enhance the effects of drugs used to oppose blood clotting, causing hemorrhage.

Vitamin E Recommendations The RDA for vitamin E is based on the alpha-tocopherol form only. As mentioned earlier, the other tocopherols and

alpha-tocopherol: the active vitamin E compound.

erythrocyte (eh-RITH-ro-cite) **hemolysis** (he-MOLL-uh-sis): the breaking open of red blood cells (erythrocytes); a symptom of vitamin E–deficiency disease in human beings.

- **erythro** = red
- **cyte** = cell
- **hemo** = blood
- **lysis** = breaking

hemolytic (HE-moh-LIT-ick) **anemia:** the condition of having too few red blood cells as a result of erythrocyte hemolysis.

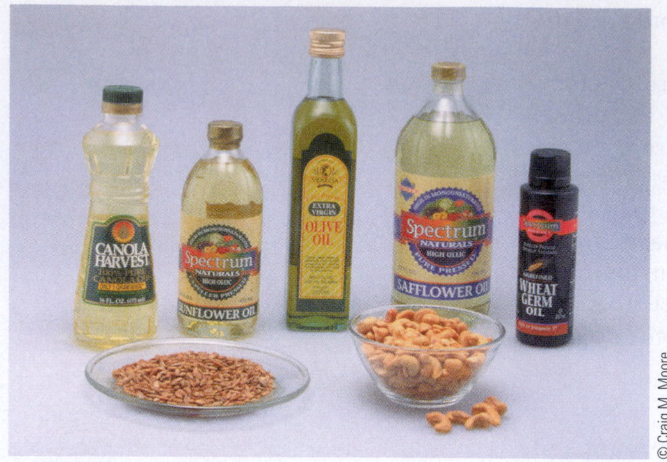
CANOLA HARVEST
Spectrum
OLIVE OIL
Spectrum
SAFFLOWER OIL
WHEAT GERM OIL
© Craig M. Moore

> **PHOTO 11-4** Fat-soluble vitamin E is found predominantly in vegetable oils, seeds, and nuts.

tocotrienols cannot be converted to alpha-tocopherol, nor do they perform the same metabolic roles in the body. A person who consumes large quantities of polyunsaturated fatty acids needs more vitamin E. Fortunately, vitamin E and polyunsaturated fatty acids tend to occur together in the same foods.

Vitamin E in Foods Vitamin E is widespread in foods. Much of the vitamin E in the diet comes from vegetable oils and products made from them, such as margarine and salad dressings (see Photo 11-4). Wheat germ oil is especially rich in vitamin E.

Because vitamin E is readily destroyed by heat and oxidation, fresh foods are preferable sources. Most processed and convenience foods do not contribute enough vitamin E to ensure an adequate intake.

REVIEW IT Identify the main roles, deficiency symptoms, and food sources for vitamin E.

Vitamin E acts as an antioxidant, defending lipids and other components of the cells against oxidative damage. Deficiencies are rare, but they do occur in premature infants, the primary symptom being erythrocyte hemolysis. Vitamin E is found predominantly in vegetable oils and appears to be one of the least toxic of the fat-soluble vitamins. The accompanying table provides a summary of vitamin E.

Vitamin E

Other Names	**Significant Sources**
Alpha-tocopherol	Polyunsaturated plant oils (margarine, salad dressings), dark green, leafy vegetables (spinach, turnip greens, collard greens, broccoli), wheat germ, whole grains, liver, egg yolks, nuts, seeds, fatty meats
RDA	Easily destroyed by heat and oxygen
Adults: 15 mg/day	**Deficiency Symptoms**
UL	Red blood cell breakage (erythrocyte hemolysis), nerve damage
Adults: 1000 mg/day	**Toxicity Symptoms**
Chief Functions in the Body	Augments the effects of anticlotting medication
Antioxidant (stabilization of cell membranes, regulation of oxidation reactions, protection of polyunsaturated fatty acids [PUFA] and vitamin A)	

11.4 Vitamin K

LEARN IT Identify the main roles, deficiency symptoms, and sources for vitamin K.

Vitamin K appropriately gets its name from the Danish word *koagulation* ("coagulation" or "clotting"). Its primary action is blood clotting, in which its presence can make the difference between life and death. Blood has a remarkable ability to remain liquid, but it can clot within seconds when the integrity of that system is disturbed.

Roles in the Body More than a dozen different proteins and the mineral calcium are involved in making a blood clot. Vitamin K is essential for the activation of several of these proteins, among them prothrombin, made by the liver as a precursor of the protein thrombin (see Figure 11-11). When any of the blood-clotting factors is lacking, **hemorrhagic disease** results. If an artery or vein is cut or broken, bleeding goes unchecked. Of course, this is not to say that hemorrhaging is always caused by vitamin K deficiency. Another cause is the genetic disorder **hemophilia,** which is neither caused nor cured by vitamin K.

hemorrhagic (hem-oh-RAJ-ik) **disease:** a disease characterized by excessive bleeding.

hemophilia (HE-moh-FEEL-ee-ah): a hereditary disease in which the blood is unable to clot because it lacks the ability to synthesize certain clotting factors.

> **FIGURE 11-11 Blood-Clotting Process**

Vitamin K is essential for the synthesis of prothrombin and several other clotting factors. Blood clots are formed by a cascade of reactions, with each step creating a compound that activates the next step.

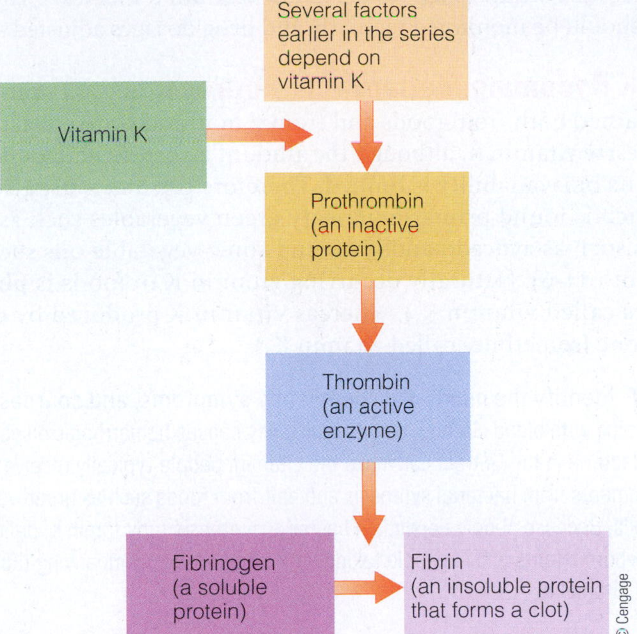

Several factors earlier in the series depend on vitamin K
Vitamin K
Prothrombin (an inactive protein)
Thrombin (an active enzyme)
Fibrinogen (a soluble protein)
Fibrin (an insoluble protein that forms a clot)
© Cengage

Vitamin K also participates in the metabolism of bone proteins, most notably **osteocalcin.** Without vitamin K, osteocalcin cannot bind to the minerals that normally form bones, resulting in low bone density.* An adequate intake of vitamin K helps decrease bone turnover and protect against fractures. The effectiveness of vitamin K supplements on bone health is inconclusive.[26]

Vitamin K is historically known for its role in blood clotting, and more recently for its participation in bone building, but additional roles continue to be discovered. Recent research suggests that vitamin K may be associated with a reduced risk of heart disease, some cancers, and all-cause mortality.[27]

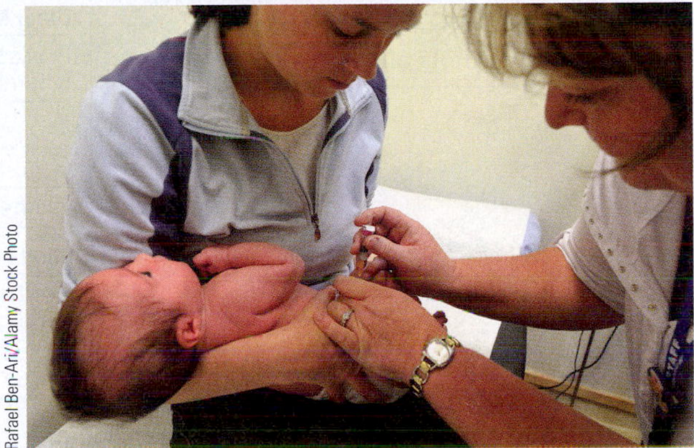
Rafael Ben-Ari/Alamy Stock Photo

> **PHOTO 11-5** Soon after birth, newborn infants receive a dose of vitamin K to prevent hemorrhagic disease.

Vitamin K Deficiency

Chapter 1 explains that a *primary deficiency* develops in response to an inadequate dietary intake whereas a *secondary deficiency* occurs for other reasons. A primary deficiency of vitamin K is rare, but a secondary deficiency may occur in two circumstances. First, whenever fat absorption falters, as occurs when bile production fails, vitamin K absorption diminishes. Second, some drugs disrupt vitamin K's synthesis and action in the body: antibiotics kill the vitamin K–producing bacteria in the intestine, and anticoagulant drugs interfere with vitamin K metabolism and activity. Excessive bleeding due to a vitamin K deficiency can be fatal.

Newborn infants present a unique case of vitamin K nutrition because they are born with a **sterile** intestinal tract, and the vitamin K–producing bacteria take weeks to establish themselves. Furthermore, vitamin K is minimally transported across the placenta and its concentration in breast milk is low. At the same time, plasma prothrombin concentrations are low, which reduces the likelihood of fatal blood clotting during the stress of birth. To prevent hemorrhagic disease in the newborn, a single dose of vitamin K is given at birth by intramuscular injection (see Photo 11-5).[28] Concerns that vitamin K given at birth raises the risks of childhood cancer are unfounded.

Vitamin K Toxicity

Toxicity is not common, and no adverse effects have been reported with high intakes of vitamin K. Therefore, a UL has not been established.

*Vitamin K is a cofactor for a carboxylase enzyme. When vitamin K is inadequate, osteocalcin is undercarboxylated and therefore less effective in binding calcium.

osteocalcin (os-teo-KAL-sen): a calcium-binding protein in bones, essential for normal mineralization.

sterile: free of microorganisms, such as bacteria.

High doses of vitamin K can, however, reduce the effectiveness of anticoagulant drugs used to prevent blood clotting. People taking these drugs should try to eat the same amount of vitamin K-rich foods daily; unfortunately, many avoid eating green vegetables instead, which results in low vitamin K intakes.[29] Their blood clotting times should be monitored regularly and drug dosages adjusted accordingly.

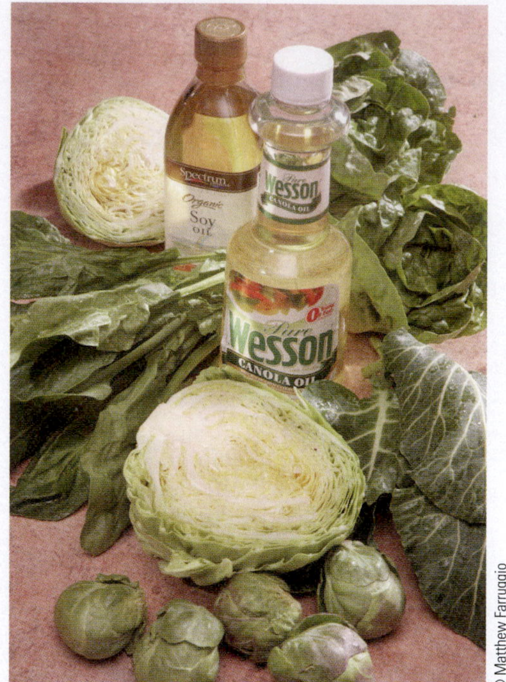

Spectrum
Organic
Soy
Oil
Wesson
CANOLA OIL
Wesson
CANOLA OIL

© Matthew Farruggio

> **PHOTO 11-6** Notable food sources of vitamin K include green vegetables such as collards, spinach, bib lettuce, brussels sprouts, and cabbage and vegetable oils such as soybean oil and canola oil.

Vitamin K Recommendations and Sources Like vitamin D, vitamin K can be obtained both from foods and from a nonfood source. Bacteria in the GI tract synthesize vitamin K, although the amount is insufficient to meet the body's needs and its bioavailability is limited. Therefore the diet must also supply vitamin K, which is found primarily in leafy green vegetables such as spinach and kale, fruits such as avocado and kiwi, and some vegetable oils such as soybean oil (see Photo 11-6). Naturally occurring vitamin K in foods is **phylloquinone** (sometimes called vitamin K_1), whereas vitamin K produced by GI bacteria is **menaquinone** (sometimes called vitamin K_2).

REVIEW IT Identify the main roles, deficiency symptoms, and sources for vitamin K.
Vitamin K helps with blood clotting, and its deficiency causes hemorrhagic disease (uncontrolled bleeding). Bacteria in the GI tract can make the vitamin; people typically receive about half of their requirements from bacterial synthesis and half from foods such as green vegetables and vegetable oils. Because people depend on bacterial synthesis for vitamin K, deficiency is most likely in newborn infants and in people taking antibiotics. The accompanying table provides a summary of vitamin K.

Vitamin K

Other Names
Phylloquinone (vitamin K_1), menaquinone (vitamin K_2), menadione (in supplements)

AI
Men: 120 μg/day
Women: 90 μg/day

Chief Functions in the Body
Synthesis of blood-clotting proteins and bone proteins

Significant Sources
Bacterial synthesis in the digestive tract (although not enough to fully meet needs); liver; dark green, leafy vegetables, cabbage-type vegetables; milk

Deficiency Symptoms
Hemorrhaging

Toxicity Symptoms
None known

The four fat-soluble vitamins play many specific roles in the growth and maintenance of the body. Their presence affects the health and function of the eyes, skin, GI tract, lungs, bones, teeth, nervous system, and blood; their deficiencies become apparent in these same areas. Toxicities of the fat-soluble vitamins are possible, especially when people use supplements, because the body stores excesses.

As with the water-soluble vitamins, the function of one fat-soluble vitamin often depends on the presence of another. Recall that vitamin E protects vitamin A from oxidation. In vitamin E deficiency, vitamin A absorption and storage are impaired. Three of the four fat-soluble vitamins—A, D, and K—play important roles in bone growth and remodeling. As mentioned, vitamin K helps synthesize a specific bone protein, and vitamin D regulates that synthesis. Vitamin A, in turn, may control which bone-building genes respond to vitamin D. Vitamin E and vitamin K share some metabolic pathways, which can create problems, especially in blood clotting.

Fat-soluble vitamins also interact with minerals. Vitamin D and calcium cooperate in bone formation, and zinc is required for the synthesis of vitamin A's transport protein, retinol-binding protein. Zinc also assists the enzyme that regenerates retinal from retinol in the eye. Vitamin A deficiency and iron deficiency often occur together and each seems to interfere with the other's metabolism.

The roles of the fat-soluble vitamins differ from those of the water-soluble vitamins, and they appear in different foods—yet they are just as essential to life. The need for them underlines the importance of eating a wide variety of nourishing foods daily. The accompanying table provides a summary of the fat-soluble vitamins.

phylloquinone (fill-oh-KWYN-own): the plant form of vitamin K; also called *vitamin* K_1.

menaquinone (men-ah-KWYN-own): the bacteria-produced form of vitamin K; also called *vitamin* K_2.

REVIEW IT The Fat-Soluble Vitamins

Vitamin and Chief Functions	Deficiency Symptoms	Toxicity Symptoms	Significant Sources
Vitamin A			
Vision; maintenance of cornea, epithelial cells, mucous membranes, skin; bone and tooth growth; reproduction; immunity	Infectious diseases, night blindness, blindness (xerophthalmia), keratinization	Reduced bone mineral density, liver abnormalities, birth defects	Retinol: milk and milk products Beta-carotene: dark green, leafy and deep yellow/orange vegetables
Vitamin D			
Mineralization of bones (raises blood calcium and phosphorus by increasing absorption from digestive tract, withdrawing calcium from bones, stimulating retention by kidneys)	Rickets, osteomalacia	Calcium imbalance (calcification of soft tissues and formation of stones)	Synthesized in the body with the help of sunshine; fortified milk
Vitamin E			
Antioxidant (stabilization of cell membranes, regulation of oxidation reactions, protection of polyunsaturated fatty acids [PUFA] and vitamin A)	Erythrocyte hemolysis, nerve damage	Hemorrhagic effects	Vegetable oils
Vitamin K			
Synthesis of blood-clotting proteins and bone proteins	Hemorrhage	None known	Synthesized in the body by GI bacteria; dark green, leafy vegetables

What's Online

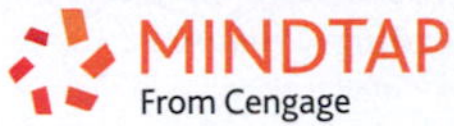
MINDTAP
From Cengage

Visit **www.cengagebrain.com** to access MindTap, a complete digital course that includes Diet & Wellness Plus, interactive quizzes, videos, and more.

REFERENCES

1. F. F. DeMoura and coauthors, Biofortified β-carotene rice improves vitamin A intake and reduces the prevalence of inadequacy among women and young children in a simulated analysis in Bangladesh, Indonesia, and the Philippines, *American Journal of Clinical Nutrition* 104 (2016): 769–775; A. C. Palmer and coauthors, Provitamin A-biofortified maize increases serum β-carotene, but not retinol, in marginally nourished children: A cluster-randomized trial in rural Zambia, *American Journal of Clinical Nutrition* 104 (2016): 181–190; E. F. Talsma and coauthors, Biofortified yellow cassava and vitamin A status of Kenyan children: A randomized controlled trial, *American Journal of Clinical Nutrition* 103 (2016): 258–267.
2. A. Sommer, Preventing blindness and saving lives: The centenary of vitamin A, *JAMA Ophthalmology* 132 (2014): 115–117.
3. World Health Organization, Measles fact sheet, January 2017, www.who.int/mediacentre/factsheets/fs286/en.
4. World Health Organization, Micronutrient deficiencies, January 2017, www.who.int/nutrition/topics/vad/en.
5. S. A. Tanumihardjo, Vitamin A and bone health: The balancing act, *Journal of Clinical Densitometry* 16 (2013): 414–419.
6. J. Okano, J. Udagawa, and K. Shiota, Roles of retinoic acid signaling in normal and abnormal development of the palate and tongue, *Congenital Anomalies* 54 (2014): 69–76.
7. G. Jones, Extrarenal vitamin D activation and interactions between vitamin D_2, vitamin D_3, and vitamin D analogs, *Annual Review of Nutrition* 33 (2013): 23–44.
8. L. Wang and coauthors, Vitamin D from different sources is inversely associated with Parkinson disease, *Movement Disorders* 30 (2015): 560–566; X. Cui and coauthors, Low vitamin D concentration exacerbates adult brain dysfunction, *American Journal of Clinical Nutrition* 97 (2013): 907–908.
9. A. S. Grimaldi and coauthors, 25(OH) Vitamin D is associated with greater muscle strength in healthy men and women, *Medicine and Science in Sports and Exercise* 45 (2013): 157–162.
10. C. Kroner-Jde, A. Sommer, and M. Fabri, Vitamin D every day to keep the infection away? *Nutrients* 7 (2015): 4170–4188.
11. L. K. Pourshahidi, Vitamin D and obesity: Current perspectives and future directions, *Proceedings of the Nutrition Society* 74 (2015): 115–124.
12. M. Song and coauthors, Plasma 25-hydroxyvitamin D and colorectal cancer risk according to tumour immunity status, *Gut* 65 (2016): 296–304; S. L. McDonnell and coauthors, Serum 25-hydroxyviatmin D concentrations ≥40 ng/ml are associated with >65% lower cancer risk: Pooled analysis of randomized trial and prospective cohort study, *PLoS One* 11 (2016): e0152441; J. P. Reis and coauthors, Race, vitamin D-binding protein gene polymorphisms, 25-hydroxyvitamin D, and incident diabetes: The Atherosclerosis Risk in Communities (ARIC) Study, *American Journal of Clinical Nutrition* 101 (2015): 1232–1240; L. Ke and coauthors, Vitamin D status and hypertension: A review, *Integrated Blood Pressure Control* 8 (2015): 13–35; A. E. Millen and coauthors, Association between vitamin D status and age-related macular degeneration by genetic risk, *JAMA Ophthalmology* 133 (2015): 1171–1179; I. Mozos and O. Marginean, Links between vitamin D deficiency and cardiovascular diseases, *BioMed Research International* 2015 (2015): 109275; C. Mathieu, Vitamin D and diabetes: Where do we stand? *Diabetes Research and Clinical Practice* 108 (2015): 201–209; P. Autier and coauthors, Vitamin D status and ill health: A systematic review, *Lancet Diabetes and Endocrinology* 2 (2014): 76–89; K. S. Vimaleswaran and coauthors, Association of vitamin D status with arterial blood pressure and hypertension risk: A mendelian randomisation study, *Lancet Diabetes and Endocrinology* 2 (2014): 719–729; N. J. Groves, J. J. McGrath, and T. H. J. Burne, Vitamin D as a

neurosteroid affecting the developing and adult brain, *Annual Review of Nutrition* 34 (2014): 117–141.

13. L. A. Beveridge and coauthors, Effect of vitamin D supplementation on blood pressure: A systematic review and meta-analysis incorporating individual patient data, *JAMA Internal Medicine* 175 (2015): 745–754; M. R. Hoffman, P. A. Senior, and D. R. Mager, Vitamin D supplementation and health-related quality of life: A systematic review of the literature, *Journal of the Academy of Nutrition and Dietetics* 115 (2015): 406–418; K. Amrein and coauthors, Effect of high-dose vitamin D_3 on hospital length of stay in critically ill patients with vitamin D deficiency: The VITdAL-ICU Randomized Clinical Trial, *Journal of the American Medical Association* 312 (2014): 1520–1530; J. R. Rees and coauthors, Vitamin D_3 supplementation and upper respiratory tract infections in a randomized, controlled trial, *Clinical Infectious Diseases* 57 (2013): 1384–1392.
14. R. L. Schleicher and coauthors, The vitamin D status of the US population from 1988 to 2010 using standardized serum concentrations of 25-hydroxyvitamin D shows recent modest increases, *American Journal of Clinical Nutrition* 104 (2016): 454–461.
15. L. E. Au and coauthors, Associations of vitamin D intake with 25-hydroxyvitamin D in overweight and racially/ethnically diverse US children, *Journal of the Academy of Nutrition and Dietetics* 113 (2013): 1511–1516.
16. J. C. Gallagher, L. M. Smith, and V. Yalamanchili, Incidence of hypercalciuria and hypercalcemia during vitamin D and calcium supplementation in older women, *Menopause* 21 (2014): 1173–1180.
17. Z. Malihi and coauthors, Hypercalcemia, hypercalciuria, and kidney stones in long-term studies of vitamin D supplementation: A systematic review and meta-analysis, *American Journal of Clinical Nutrition* 104 (2016): 1039–1051; J. R. Genzen, Hypercalcemic crisis due to vitamin D toxicity, *Lab Medicine* 45 (2014): 147–150.
18. K. D. Cashman, The vitamin D RDA for African American adults: Higher than that for white persons? *American Journal of Clinical Nutrition* 99 (2014): 427–428; K. Ng and coauthors, dose response to vitamin D supplementation in African Americans: Results of a 4-arm, randomized placebo-controlled trial, *American Journal of Clinical Nutrition* 99 (2014): 587–598.
19. K. H. Madsern and coauthors, Randomized controlled trial of the effects of vitamin D-fortified milk and bread on serum 25-hydroxyvitamin D concentrations in families in Denmark during winter: The VitmaD study, *American Journal of Clinical Nutrition* 98 (2013): 374–382.
20. P. G. Lindqvist, Avoidance of sun exposure is a risk factor for all-cause mortality: Results from the Melanoma in Southern Sweden cohort, *Journal of Internal Medicine* 276 (2014): 77–86.
21. U. Lehmann and coauthors, Bioavailability of vitamin D2 and D3 in healthy volunteers, a randomised placebo-controlled trial, *Journal of Clinical Endocrinology and Metabolism* 98 (2013): 4339–4345.
22. Q. Jiang, Natural forms of vitamin E: Metabolism, antioxidant, and anti-inflammatory activities and their role in disease prevention and therapy, *Free Radical Biology and Medicine* 72 (2014): 76–90.
23. P. Y. Zhang, X. Xu, and X. C. Li, Cardiovascular diseases: Oxidative damage and antioxidant protection, *European Review for Medical and Pharmacological Sciences* 18 (2014): 3091–3096.
24. R. F. Pfeiffer, Neurologic manifestations of malabsorption syndromes, *Handbook of Clinical Neurology* 120 (2014): 621–632; D. Bromley, P. C. Anderson, and V. Daggett, Structural consequences of mutations to the a-tocopherol transfer protein associated with the neurodegenerative disease ataxia with vitamin E deficiency, *Biochemistry* 52 (2013): 4264–4273.
25. A. J. Curtis and coauthors, Vitamin E supplementation and mortality in healthy people: A meta-analysis of randomised controlled trials, *Cardiovascular Drugs and Therapy* 28 (2014): 563–573.
26. M. S. Hamidi, O. Gajic-Velijanoski, and A. M. Cheung, Vitamin K and bone health, *Journal of Clinical Densitometry* 16 (2013): 409–413.
27. M. Juanola-Falgarona and coauthors, Dietary intake of vitamin K is inversely associated with mortality risk, *Journal of Nutrition* 144 (2014): 743–750.
28. M. Witt and coauthors, Prophylactic dosing of vitamin K to prevent bleeding, *Pediatrics* 137 (2016): e20154222; M. Weddle and coauthors, Are pediatricians complicit in vitamin K deficiency bleeding? *Pediatrics* 136 (2015): 753–757.
29. C. Leblanc and coauthors, Avoidance of vitamin K-rich foods is common among warfarin users and translates into lower usual vitamin K intakes, *Journal of the Academy of Nutrition and Dietetics* 116 (2016): 1000–1007.

 LEARN IT Describe how antioxidants defend against free radicals that contribute to diseases.

Antioxidant Nutrients in Disease Prevention

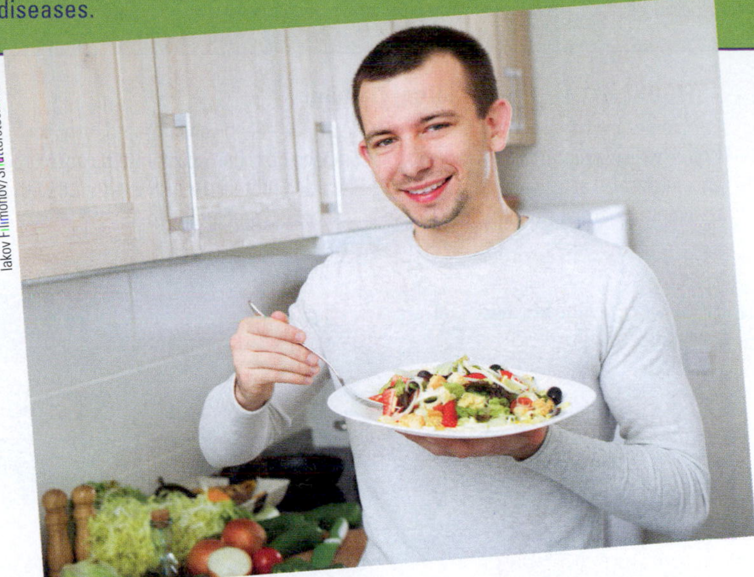
Iakov Filimonov/Shutterstock.com

Count on supplement manufacturers to exploit the day's hot topics in nutrition. The moment bits of research news surface, new supplements appear—and terms such as *antioxidants* and *lycopene* become household words. Friendly faces in TV commercials try to persuade us that these supplements hold magic in the fight against aging and disease. New supplements hit the market and sales soar.

In the meantime, scientists and medical experts around the world continue their work to clarify and confirm the roles of antioxidants in preventing chronic diseases. This highlight summarizes some of the accumulating evidence. It also revisits the advantages of foods over supplements. But first it is important to introduce the troublemaker—an unstable molecule known as a **free radical.** (Glossary H11-1 defines free radical and related terms.)

Free Radicals and Disease

Chapter 7 describes how the body's cells use oxygen in metabolic reactions. In the process, oxygen reacts with body compounds and produces highly unstable molecules known as free radicals. In addition to normal body processes, environmental factors such as ultraviolet radiation, air pollution, and tobacco smoke generate free radicals.

A free radical is a molecule with one or more unpaired electrons.* An electron without a partner is unstable and highly reactive. To regain its stability, the free radical quickly finds a stable but vulnerable compound from which to steal an electron.

With the loss of an electron, the formerly stable molecule becomes a free radical itself and steals an electron from another nearby molecule. Thus an electron-snatching chain reaction is under way with free radicals producing more free radicals. **Antioxidants** neutralize free radicals by donating one of their own electrons, thus ending the chain reaction. When they lose electrons, antioxidants do not become free radicals because they are stable in either form. (Review Figure 10-16, p. 318, to see how ascorbic acid can give up two hydrogens with their electrons and become dehydroascorbic acid.)

Free radicals attack. Occasionally, these free-radical attacks are helpful. For example, cells of the immune system use free radicals as ammunition in an "oxidative burst" that demolishes disease-causing viruses and bacteria. Most often, however, free-radical attacks cause widespread damage. They commonly damage the polyunsaturated fatty acids in lipoproteins and in cell membranes, disrupting the transport of substances into and out of cells. Free radicals also alter DNA, RNA, and proteins, creating excesses and deficiencies of specific proteins, impairing cell functions, and eliciting an inflammatory response. All of these actions contribute to cell damage, disease progression, and aging (see Figure H11-1, p. 354).

The body's natural defenses and repair systems try to control the destruction caused by free radicals, but these systems are not 100 percent effective. In fact, they become less effective with age, and the unrepaired damage accumulates. To some extent, dietary antioxidants defend the body against **oxidative stress,** but if antioxidants are unavailable or if free-radical production becomes excessive, health problems may develop. Oxygen-derived free radicals may cause diseases, not only by indiscriminately destroying the valuable components of cells, but also by serving as signals for specific activities within the cells. Studies suggest that oxidative stress may be a causative factor and antioxidants may be a protective factor in cognitive performance and the aging process as well as in the development of diseases such as cancer, arthritis, cataracts, diabetes, hypertension, and heart disease.[1]

*Many free radicals exist, but oxygen-derived free radicals are most common in the human body. Examples of oxygen-derived free radicals include superoxide radical (O_2^{-}), hydroxyl radical (OH·), and nitric oxide (NO·). (The dots in the symbols represent the unpaired electrons.) Technically, hydrogen peroxide (H_2O_2) and singlet oxygen are not free radicals because they contain paired electrons, but the unstable conformation of their electrons makes radical-producing reactions likely. Scientists sometimes use the term *reactive oxygen species (ROS)* to describe all of these compounds.

GLOSSARY H11-1

antioxidants: in the body, substances that significantly decrease the adverse effects of free radicals on normal physiological functions.

free radical: an unstable molecule with one or more unpaired electrons.

(See Appendix B for a review of basic chemistry concepts.)

oxidants (OKS-ih-dants): compounds (such as oxygen itself) that oxidize other compounds. Compounds that prevent oxidation are called *antioxidants,* whereas those that promote it are called *prooxidants.*

- **anti** = against
- **pro** = for

oxidative stress: a condition in which the production of oxidants and free radicals exceeds the body's ability to handle them and prevent damage.

phytochemicals: nonnutrient compounds found in plants. Some phytochemicals have biological activity in the body.

prooxidants: substances that significantly induce oxidative stress.

> **FIGURE H11-1 Free-Radical Damage**

Free radicals are highly reactive. They might attack the polyunsaturated fatty acids in a cell membrane, which generates lipid radicals that damage cells and accelerate disease progression. Free radicals might also attack and damage DNA, RNA, and proteins, which interferes with the body's ability to maintain normal cell function, causing disease and premature aging.

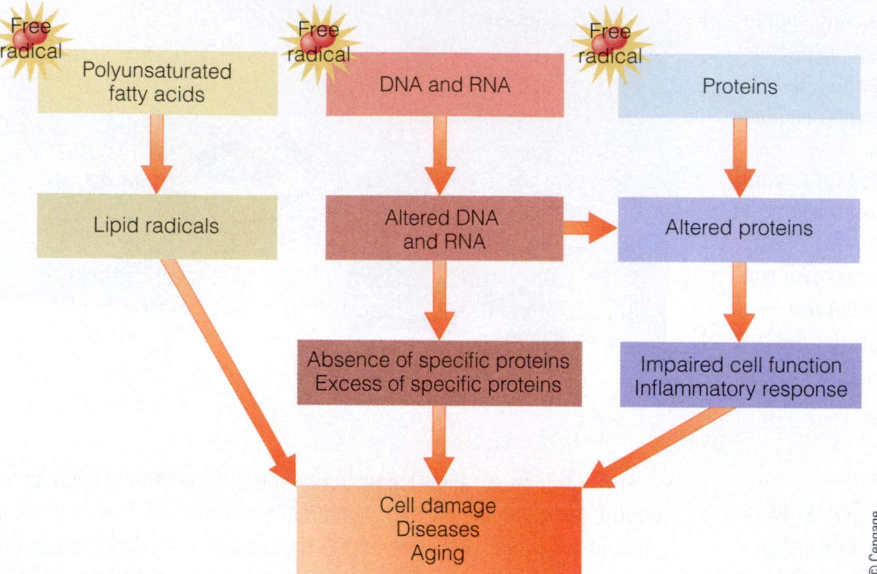
Free radical
Polyunsaturated fatty acids
Free radical
DNA and RNA
Free radical
Proteins
Lipid radicals
Altered DNA and RNA
Altered proteins
Absence of specific proteins
Excess of specific proteins
Impaired cell function
Inflammatory response
Cell damage
Diseases
Aging
© Cengage

Defending against Free Radicals

The body maintains a couple lines of defense against free-radical damage. A system of enzymes disarms the most harmful **oxidants.*** The action of these enzymes depends on the minerals selenium, copper, manganese, and zinc. If the diet fails to provide adequate supplies of these minerals, this line of defense weakens. The body also uses the antioxidant vitamins—vitamin E, beta-carotene, and vitamin C. Vitamin E defends the body's lipids (cell membranes, nervous tissues, and lipoproteins, for example) by efficiently stopping the free-radical chain reaction. Beta-carotene also acts as an antioxidant in lipid membranes. Vitamin C protects other tissues, such as the skin and fluid of the blood, against free-radical attacks. Vitamin C seems especially adept at neutralizing free radicals from polluted air and cigarette smoke; it also restores oxidized vitamin E to its active state.

Dietary antioxidants also include some of the **phytochemicals** (as Highlight 13 describes). Together, nutrients and phytochemicals with antioxidant activity minimize damage and prevent disease in the following ways:

- Limiting free-radical formation
- Destroying free radicals or their precursors
- Stimulating antioxidant enzyme activity
- Repairing oxidative damage
- Stimulating repair enzyme activity
- Supporting a healthy immune system

*These enzymes include *glutathione peroxidase, thioredoxin reductase, superoxide dismutase,* and *catalase.*

These actions play key roles in defending the body against chronic diseases such as cancer and heart disease.

Defending against Cancer

Cancers arise when cellular DNA is damaged—sometimes by free-radical attacks. Antioxidants may reduce cancer risks by protecting DNA from this damage. Many researchers have reported low rates of cancer in people whose diets include abundant vegetables and fruits, rich in antioxidants.

Foods rich in vitamin C seem to protect against certain types of cancers, especially those of the head and neck.[2] Such a correlation may reflect the benefits of a diet rich in fruits and vegetables; evidence that vitamin C supplements reduce the risk of cancer is lacking.

Researchers hypothesize that vitamin E might inhibit cancer formation by attacking free radicals that damage DNA. Analysis of several studies finds an inverse association between vitamin E and prostate cancer.[3] Evidence that vitamin E supplements help guard against cancer, however, is lacking. In fact, research has found no lower—and possibly a higher—risk of some cancers in people taking high doses of vitamin E (and other antioxidant) supplements.[4]

Several studies report a cancer-preventing benefit of vegetables and fruits rich in beta-carotene and the other carotenoids as well. Carotenoids may protect against oxidative damage to DNA. Some research suggests that high blood concentrations of beta-carotene and the other carotenoids are associated with lower rates of some cancers.[5] Studies do not, however, find a reduction in cancer risk with beta-carotene supplementation. Benefits most likely reflect a healthy diet abundant in fruits and vegetables. In fact, a major review of several large research studies concluded that none produced evidence to justify the use of antioxidant supplements for cancer prevention. Furthermore, recommendations caution *against* the use of beta-carotene or vitamin E supplements for the prevention of cancer or heart disease.[6]

Defending against Heart Disease

Decades of research have contributed to our understanding of how oxidative stress contributes to atherosclerosis and how antioxidants might protect against heart disease, yet questions remain.[7] High blood cholesterol carried in LDL (low-density lipoproteins) is a major risk factor for cardiovascular disease, but how do LDL exert their damage? One scenario is that free radicals within the arterial walls oxidize LDL, changing their structure and function. The oxidized LDL then accelerate the formation of artery-clogging plaques. These free radicals also oxidize the polyunsaturated fatty acids of the cell membranes, sparking additional changes in the arterial walls, which impede the flow of blood. Susceptibility to such oxidative damage within the arterial walls is heightened by a diet high in saturated fat and by cigarette smoke. In contrast, diets that include plenty of fruits and vegetables, especially when saturated fat is low, strengthen antioxidant defenses against LDL oxidation. Similarly, supplements of antioxidant vitamins may protect against arterial stiffness.[8]

Antioxidants, especially vitamin E, may protect against hypertension and cardiovascular disease. Epidemiological studies suggest that people who eat foods rich in vitamin E have relatively few atherosclerotic plaques and low rates of death from heart disease. Among its many protective roles, vitamin E defends against LDL oxidation, inflammation, arterial injuries, and blood clotting. Whether vitamin E supplements slow the progression of heart disease is less clear.

Some studies suggest that vitamin C protects against LDL oxidation, raises HDL, lowers total cholesterol, and improves blood pressure. Vitamin C may also minimize inflammation and the free-radical action within the arterial wall. The association of a lower risk of heart disease and all-cause mortality with a diet rich in fruits and vegetables may, in part, be attributed to high concentrations of vitamin C.[9] Like vitamin E, the role of vitamin C supplements in reducing the risk of heart disease remains uncertain. One study reports improvements with supplements of vitamin C and vitamin E when taken individually, but not when taken together—illustrating, once again, that the relationships between nutrients and diseases are complex and that attention to dietary patterns may be more effective than supplement use.[10]

Foods, Supplements, or Both?

In the process of scavenging and quenching free radicals, antioxidants themselves become oxidized. To some extent, they can be regenerated, but losses still occur and free radicals attack continuously. To maintain defenses, a person must replenish dietary antioxidants regularly. But should antioxidants be replenished from foods or from supplements?

Foods—especially fruits and vegetables—offer not only antioxidants, but also an array of other valuable vitamins and minerals as well (see Photo H11-1). Importantly, deficiencies of these nutrients can damage DNA as readily as free radicals can. Eating fruits and vegetables in abundance protects against both deficiencies and diseases—and may protect against inflammation and DNA damage. Three dietary strategies seem most effective in preventing heart disease:

- Use unsaturated fats instead of saturated or *trans* fats (see Highlight 5).
- Select foods rich in omega-3 fatty acids (see Chapter 5).
- Consume a diet high in fruits, vegetables, nuts, and whole grains and low in refined grain products.

Such a diet combined with physical activity, weight control, and not smoking serves as the best prescription for health. Note that taking supplements is not among these disease-prevention recommendations.

Diets that deliver sufficient quantities of antioxidant vitamins may protect against cancer and heart disease—but only a small fraction of the US population consumes recommended amounts. Some research suggests a protective effect from as little as a daily glass of orange juice or carrot juice (rich sources of vitamin C and beta-carotene, respectively). Other intervention studies, however, have used levels of nutrients that far exceed current recommendations and can be achieved only by taking supplements. In making their recommendations for the antioxidant nutrients, the DRI Committee considered these studies and determined they do not support taking supplements over eating a healthy diet.

Clearly, fruits and vegetables containing antioxidant nutrients and phytochemicals have been associated with a diminished risk of many chronic diseases, but supplements have not always proved beneficial. In fact, the benefits are often more apparent when the vitamins come from foods rather than from supplements. In other words, the antioxidant actions of fruits and vegetables are greater than their nutrients alone can explain. Without data to confirm the benefits of supplements, we cannot accept the potential risks. And the risks are real.

Consider the findings from a meta-analysis of the relationships between supplements of vitamin A, vitamin E, beta-carotene, or combinations and total mortality. Researchers concluded that supplements provided no benefits and actually *increased* mortality.[11] Beta-carotene *increases* the risk of lung cancer and overall mortality in smokers.[12] One study on cancer prevention was prematurely terminated when researchers noted a trend toward developing diabetes in subjects receiving selenium and a slight increased risk of prostate cancer in those receiving vitamin E; another study concluded that vitamin E supplements increase the risk of some strokes, but reduce the risk of others, making its indiscriminate use unwise.

Even if research clearly proves that a particular nutrient is the ultimate protective ingredient in foods, supplements would not be the answer because their contents are limited. Vitamin E supplements, for

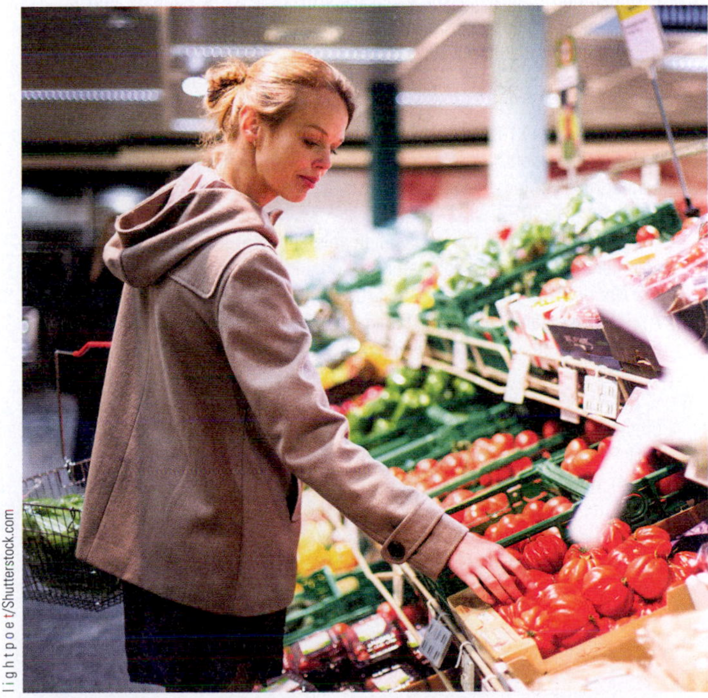

lightpoet/Shutterstock.com

> **PHOTO H11-1** Many disease-fighting products are available now at your local produce counter.

example, usually contain alpha-tocopherol, but foods provide an assortment of tocopherols and tocotrienols among other nutrients, many of which provide valuable protection against free-radical damage. In addition to a full array of nutrients, foods provide phytochemicals that also fight against many diseases. Supplements shortchange users. Furthermore, supplements should be used only as an adjunct to other measures such as smoking cessation, weight control, physical activity, and medication as needed.

Clearly, much more research is needed to define optimal and harmful levels of intake. This much we know: antioxidants behave differently under various conditions. At physiological levels typical of a healthy diet, they act as antioxidants, but at pharmacological doses typical of supplements, they may act as **prooxidants,** stimulating the production of free radicals and altering metabolism in a way that may promote disease. Until the optimum intake of antioxidant nutrients can be determined, the risks of supplement use remain unclear. A review of the relationships between antioxidants and chronic diseases—sorted by foods or supplements—would reveal a decrease in risk attributed to foods 9 out of 10 times. Any increase in risk is always from supplement use, and often in smokers. Clearly, the best way to add antioxidants to the diet is to eat generous servings of fruits and vegetables daily.

It should be clear by now that we cannot know the identity and action of every chemical in every food. Even if we did, why create a supplement to replicate a food? Why not eat foods and enjoy the pleasure, nourishment, and health benefits they provide? The potential for antioxidant activity is widespread among plants.[13] Among the fruits, pomegranates, berries, and citrus rank high in antioxidants; top antioxidant vegetables include kale, spinach, and brussels sprouts; millet and oats contain the most antioxidants among the grains; pinto beans and soybeans are outstanding legumes; and walnuts outshine the other nuts. But don't try to single out one particular food for its "magical" nutrient, antioxidant, or phytochemical. Instead, eat a wide variety of fruits, vegetables, grains, legumes, and nuts every day—and get *all* the benefits these foods have to offer.

CRITICAL THINKING QUESTIONS

A. What are the arguments for obtaining antioxidants from foods, supplements, or both?

B. The American Heart Association and other health organizations have concluded that consumers should get their antioxidants from foods rather than supplements. They add that taking supplements may even be harmful. Supplement manufacturers claim that such statements are unfair and that their natural botanical extracts provide numerous health benefits. In fact, some suggest that beneficial effects can only be achieved by taking high-dose supplements. Given that there are currently no DRI defining the kinds of antioxidants or the daily quantities needed, how might you ensure a healthy intake of antioxidants? If you decide to take an antioxidant supplement, how might you research the product to determine its safety and effectiveness?

REFERENCES

1. P. Ghezzi and coauthors, The oxidative stress theory of disease: Levels of evidence and epistemological aspects, *British Journal of Clinical Pharmacology* (2016): doi:10.1111/bph.13544.
2. L. deMunter and coauthors, Vitamin and carotenoid intake and risk of head-neck cancer subtypes in the Netherlands Cohort Study, *American Journal of Clinical Nutrition* 102 (2015): 420–432.
3. T. J. Key and coauthors, Carotenoids, retinol, tocopherols, and prostate cancer risk: Pooled analysis of 15 studies, *American Journal of Clinical Nutrition* 102 (2015): 1142–1157.
4. A. R. Kristal and coauthors, Baseline selenium status and effects of selenium and vitamin E supplementation on prostate cancer risk, *Journal of the National Cancer Institute* 106 (2014): djt456.
5. A. H. Eliassen and coauthors, Plasma carotenoids and risk of breast cancer over 20 y of follow-up, *American Journal of Clinical Nutrition* 101 (2015): 1197–205.
6. V. A. Moyer, Vitamin, mineral, and multivitamin supplements for the primary prevention of cardiovascular disease and cancer: U.S. Preventive Services Task Force Recommendation Statement, *Annals of Internal Medicine* 160 (2014): 558–564.
7. H. N. Siti, Y. Kamisah, and J. Kamsiah, The role of oxidative stress, antioxidants and vascular inflammation in cardiovascular disease: A review, *Vascular Pharmacology* 71 (2015): 40–56.
8. A. W. Ashor and coauthors, Antioxidant vitamin supplementation reduces arterial stiffness in adults: A systematic review and meta-analysis of randomized controlled trials, *Journal of Nutrition* 144 (2014): 1594–1602.
9. C. J. Kobylecki and coauthors, Genetically high plasma vitamin C, intake of fruit and vegetables, and risk of ischemic heart disease and all-cause mortality: A Mendelian randomization study, *American Journal of Clinical Nutrition* 101 (2015): 1135–1143.
10. A. W. Ashor and coauthors, Effect of vitamin C and vitamin E supplementation on endothelial function: A systematic review and meta-analysis of randomised controlled trials, *British Journal of Nutrition* 113 (2015): 1182–1194; Y. Wang, O. K. Chun, and W. O. Song, Plasma and dietary antioxidant status as cardiovascular disease risk factors: A review of human studies, *Nutrients* 5 (2013): 2969–3004.
11. G. Bjelakovic, D. Nikolova, and C. Gluud, Antioxidant supplements to prevent mortality, *Journal of the American Medical Association* 310 (2013): 1178–1179.
12. A. M. Mondul and coauthors, Metabolomic profile of response to supplementation with b-carotene in the Alpha-Tocopherol, Beta-Carotene Cancer Prevention Study, *American Journal of Clinical Nutrition* 98 (2013): 488–493.
13. D. M. Kasote and coauthors, Significance of antioxidant potential of plants and its relevance to therapeutic applications, *International Journal of Biological Sciences* 11 (2015): 982–991.

12 Water and the Major Minerals

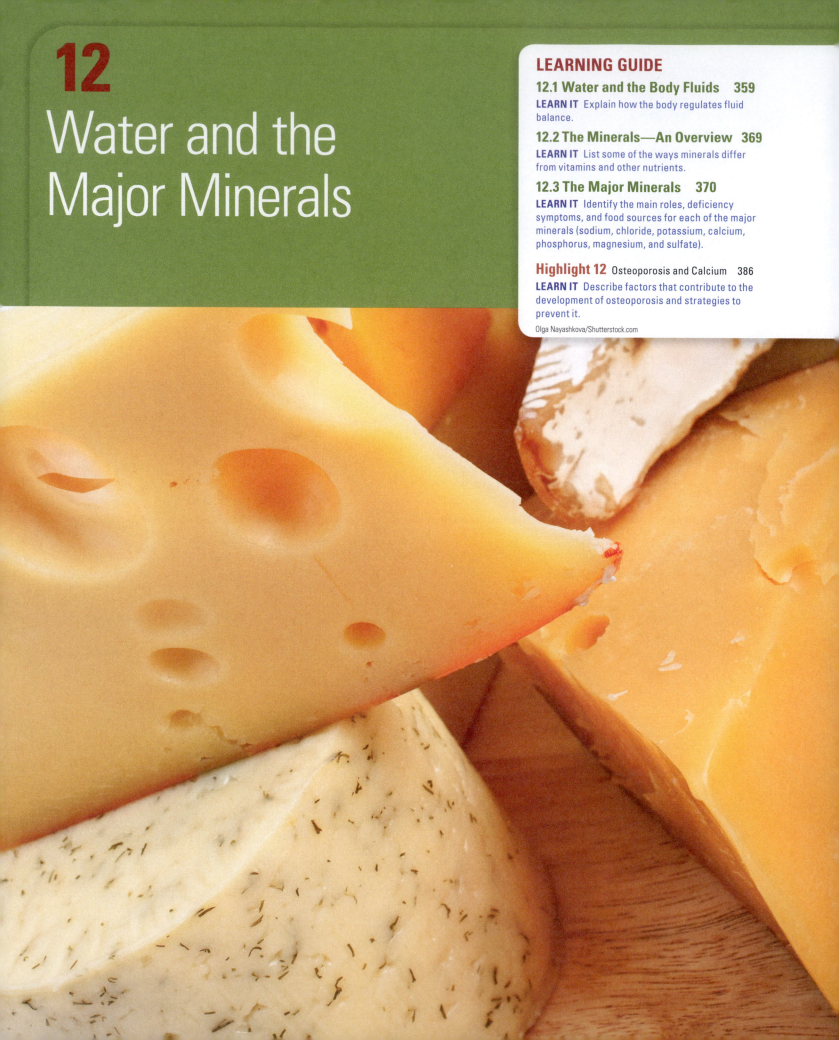

LEARNING GUIDE

Olga Nayashkova/Shutterstock.com

Nutrition in Your Life

What's your beverage of choice? If you said water, then congratulate yourself for recognizing its importance in maintaining your body's fluid balance. If you answered milk, then pat yourself on the back for taking good care of your bones. Without water, you would realize within days how vital it is to your survival. The consequences of a lack of milk (or other calcium-rich foods) are also dramatic, but may not become apparent for decades. Water, calcium, and all the other major minerals support fluid balance and bone health. Before getting too comfortable reading this chapter, pour yourself a glass of water or milk. Your body will thank you. As you read this chapter, consider whether the foods you are eating are meeting your water and major mineral needs.

Water is an essential nutrient, more important to life than any of the others (see Photo 12-1). The body needs more water each day than any other nutrient. Furthermore, you can survive only a few days without water, whereas a deficiency of the other nutrients may take weeks, months, or even years to develop.

This chapter begins with a look at water and the body's fluids. The body maintains an appropriate balance and distribution of fluids with the help of another class of nutrients—the minerals. In addition to introducing the minerals that help regulate body fluids, this chapter describes many of the other important functions minerals perform in the body. Chapter 19 revisits water as a beverage and addresses consumer concerns about its safety; Chapter 20 looks at water usage in agriculture and food production and examines the impending water shortages we face.

12.1 Water and the Body Fluids

LEARN IT Explain how the body regulates fluid balance.

Water constitutes about 60 percent of an adult's body weight and a higher percentage of a child's (see Figure 1-1, p. 7). Because water makes up about 75 percent of the weight of lean tissue and less than 25 percent of the weight of fat, a person's body composition influences how much of the body's weight is water. The proportion of water is generally smaller in females, obese people, and the elderly because of their smaller proportion of lean tissue.

In the body, water is the fluid in which all life processes occur. The water in the body fluids:

- Carries nutrients and waste products throughout the body
- Maintains the structure of large molecules such as proteins and glycogen
- Participates in metabolic reactions
- Serves as the solvent for minerals, vitamins, amino acids, glucose, and many other small molecules so that they can participate in metabolic activities
- Acts as a lubricant and cushion around joints and inside the eyes, the spinal cord, and, in pregnancy, the amniotic sac surrounding the fetus in the womb
- Aids in the regulation of normal body temperature, as the evaporation of sweat from the skin removes excess heat from the body
- Maintains blood volume

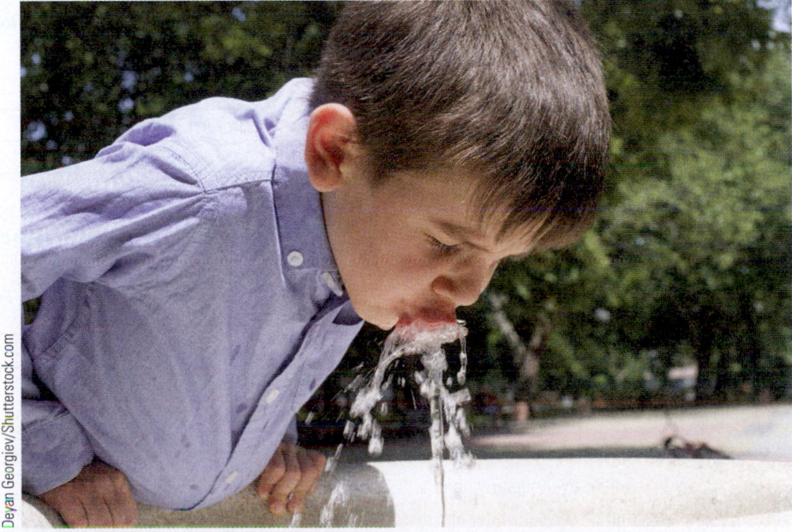

Deyan Georgiev/Shutterstock.com

> **PHOTO 12-1** Water is the most indispensable nutrient.

> **FIGURE 12-1 One Cell and Its Associated Fluids**

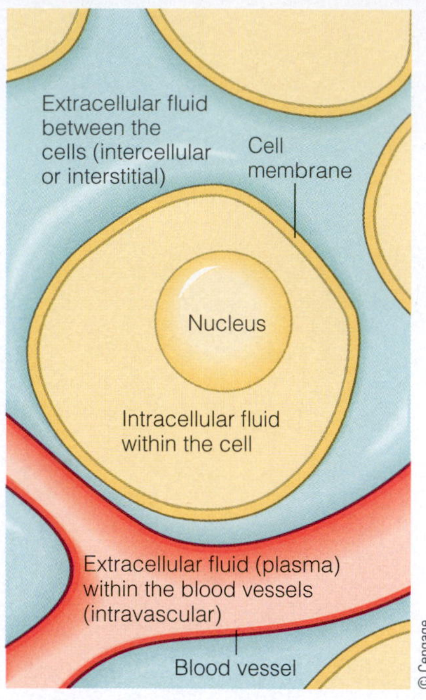
Extracellular fluid between the cells (intercellular or interstitial)
Cell membrane
Nucleus
Intracellular fluid within the cell
Extracellular fluid (plasma) within the blood vessels (intravascular)
Blood vessel
© Cengage

These activities take place in fluids that are carefully distributed in various compartments throughout the body.

Distribution and Movement of Body Fluids

Every cell contains fluid of the exact composition that is best for that cell. Fluid inside cells is called **intracellular fluid**, whereas fluid outside cells is called **extracellular fluid**. The extracellular fluid that surrounds each cell is called **interstitial fluid**, whereas the extracellular fluid in the blood vessels is called **intravascular fluid**. Figure 12-1 illustrates a cell and its associated fluids. The compositions of intercellular and extracellular fluids differ from one another. They continuously lose and replace their components, yet the composition in each compartment remains remarkably constant under normal conditions. Maintaining a balance of about two-thirds of the body fluids inside the cells and one-third outside is vital to the life of the cells. If too much water were to enter the cells, they might rupture; if too much water were to leave, they would collapse.

Electrolytes

When a mineral **salt** such as sodium chloride (NaCl) dissolves in water, it separates **(dissociates)** into **ions**—positively and negatively charged particles (Na^+ and Cl^-). The positive ions are **cations**; the negative ones are **anions**. (To remember the difference between cations and anions, think of the "t" in cations as a "plus" sign and the "n" in anions as a "negative.") Unlike pure water, which conducts electricity poorly, ions dissolved in water carry electrical current. For this reason, salts that dissociate into ions are called **electrolytes**, and fluids that contain them are **electrolyte solutions**.

In all electrolyte solutions, anion and cation concentrations are balanced (the number of negative and positive charges are equal). If a fluid contains 1000 negative charges, it must also contain 1000 positive charges. If an anion enters the fluid, a cation must accompany it or another anion must leave so that electrical neutrality will be maintained. For example, whenever sodium (Na^+) ions leave a cell, potassium (K^+) ions enter. In fact, it's a good bet that whenever Na^+ and K^+ ions are moving, they are going in opposite directions.

Table 12-1 shows that, indeed, the positive and negative charges inside and outside cells are perfectly balanced, even though the numbers of each kind of

TABLE 12-1 Important Body Electrolytes

Electrolytes	Intracellular (inside cells) Concentration (mEq/L)	Extracellular (outside cells) Concentration (mEq/L)
Cations (positively charged ions)		
Sodium (Na^+)	10	142
Potassium (K^+)	150	5
Calcium (Ca^{++})	2	5
Magnesium (Mg^{++})	40	3
	202	155
Anions (negatively charged ions)		
Chloride (Cl^-)	2	103
Bicarbonate (HCO_3^-)	10	27
Phosphate ($HPO_4^=$)	103	2
Sulfate ($SO_4^=$)	20	1
Organic acids (lactate, pyruvate)	10	6
Proteins	57	16
	202	155

© Cengage

NOTE: The numbers of positive and negative charges in a given fluid are the same. For example, in extracellular fluid, the cations and anions both equal 155 milliequivalents per liter (mEq/L). Of the cations, sodium ions make up 142 mEq/L; and potassium, calcium, and magnesium ions make up the remainder. Of the anions, chloride ions number 103 mEq/L; bicarbonate ions number 27; and the rest are provided by phosphate ions, sulfate ions, organic acids, and protein.

intracellular fluid: fluid inside the cells, usually high in potassium and phosphate. Intracellular fluid accounts for approximately two-thirds of the body's water.
- **intra** = within

extracellular fluid: fluid outside the cells. Extracellular fluid includes two main components—the interstitial fluid between cells and the intravascular fluid inside blood vessels. Extracellular fluid accounts for approximately one-third of the body's water.
- **extra** = outside

interstitial (IN-ter-STISH-al) **fluid:** fluid between the cells (intercellular), usually high in sodium and chloride. Interstitial fluid is a large component of extracellular fluid.
- **inter** = in the midst, between

intravascular fluid: fluid within blood vessels.
- **intra** = within

salt: a compound composed of a positive ion other than H^+ and a negative ion other than OH^-. An example is sodium chloride (Na^+Cl^-).
- **Na** = sodium
- **Cl** = chloride

dissociates (dis-SO-see-aites): physically separates.

ions (EYE-uns): atoms or molecules that have gained or lost electrons and therefore have electrical charges. Examples include the positively charged sodium ion (Na^+) and the negatively charged chloride ion (Cl^-). For a closer look at ions, see Appendix B.

cations (CAT-eye-uns): positively charged ions.

anions (AN-eye-uns): negatively charged ions.

electrolytes: salts that dissolve in water and dissociate into charged particles called ions.

electrolyte solutions: solutions that can conduct electricity.

ion differ over a wide range. Inside the cells, the positive charges total 202 and the negative charges balance these perfectly. Outside the cells, the amounts and proportions of the ions differ from those inside, but again the positive and negative charges balance. Scientists count these charges in **milliequivalents per liter (mEq/L)**.

As Figure 12-2 shows, some electrolytes are concentrated primarily outside the cells (notably, sodium, chloride, and calcium), whereas others are concentrated predominantly inside the cells (notably, potassium, magnesium, phosphate, and sulfate). Cell membranes are *selectively permeable*, meaning that they allow the passage of some molecules, but not others.

> **FIGURE 12-2 A Cell and Its Electrolytes**

All of these electrolytes are found both inside and outside the cells, but each can be found mostly on one side or the other of the cell membrane.

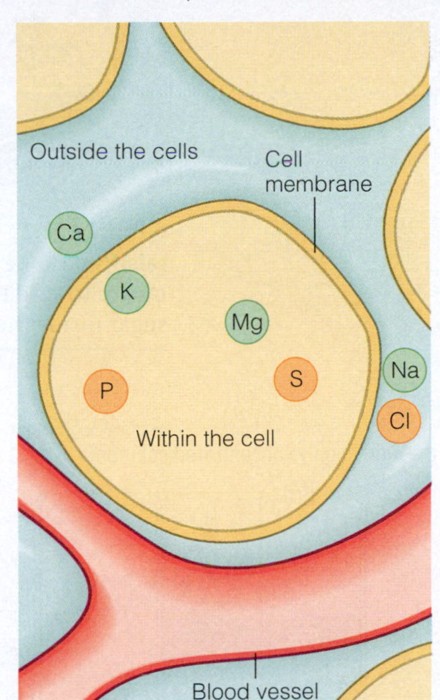
Outside the cells
Cell membrane
Ca
K
Mg
P
S
Na
Cl
Within the cell
Blood vessel

Chemical symbols:
Ca = calcium
Cl = chloride
K = potassium
Mg = magnesium
Na = sodium
P = phosphorus
S = sulfate

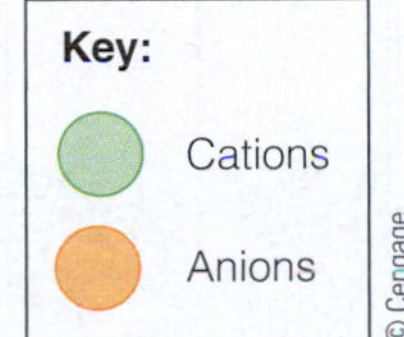
Key:
Cations
Anions

© Cengage

Electrolytes Attract Water Whenever electrolytes move across the membrane, water follows because electrolytes attract water. Each water molecule has a net charge of zero, but the oxygen side of the molecule has a slightly negative charge, and the hydrogen molecules have a slightly positive charge. Figure 12-3 shows the result in an electrolyte solution: both positive and negative ions attract clusters of water molecules around them. This attraction allows salts to dissolve in water and enables the body to move fluids into appropriate compartments.

Solutes Attract Water The concentration of a solution reflects the amount of a **solute** relative to its fluid. Consider saltwater, for example. One cup of water with one teaspoon salt dissolved in it has the same concentration as one-half cup water with one-half teaspoon salt dissolved in it; the proportions of salt to water are the same in the two solutions and they would taste the same with respect to their saltiness. Adding more water would dilute the solution, making it less concentrated; it wouldn't taste as salty. Adding more salt would make the solution more concentrated; it would taste saltier.

Solutes attract water. The movement of water across a membrane toward the more concentrated solutes is called **osmosis**. The amount of pressure needed to prevent the movement of water across a membrane is called the **osmotic pressure**. Figure 12-4 (p. 362) illustrates osmosis, and Photos 12-2 and 12-3 (p. 362) provide familiar examples.

> **FIGURE 12-3 Water Dissolves Salts and Follows Electrolytes**

The structural arrangement of the two hydrogen atoms and one oxygen atom enables water to dissolve salts. Water's role as a solvent is one of its most valuable characteristics.

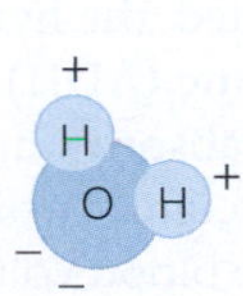
+
H
O
H
+
–
–

The negatively charged electrons that bond the hydrogens to the oxygen spend most of their time near the oxygen atom. As a result, the oxygen is slightly negative, and the hydrogens are slightly positive (see Appendix B).

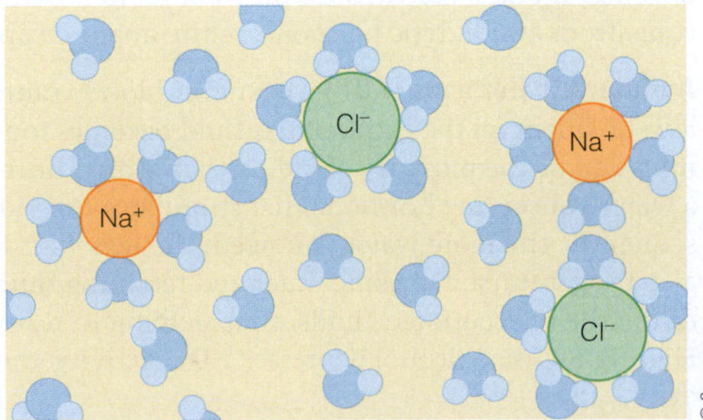
Cl⁻
Na⁺
Na⁺
Cl⁻

© Cengage

In an electrolyte solution, water molecules are attracted to both anions and cations. Notice that the negative oxygen atoms of the water molecules are drawn to the sodium cation (Na^+), whereas the positive hydrogen atoms of the water molecules are drawn to the chloride ions (Cl^-).

milliequivalents per liter (mEq/L): the concentration of electrolytes in a volume of solution. Milliequivalents reveal characteristics about the solution that are not evident when the concentration is expressed in terms of weight.

solutes (SOLL-yutes): the substances that are dissolved in a solution. The number of molecules in a given volume of fluid is the *solute concentration*.

osmosis: the movement of water across a membrane *toward* the side where the solutes are more concentrated.

osmotic pressure: the amount of pressure needed to prevent the movement of water across a membrane.

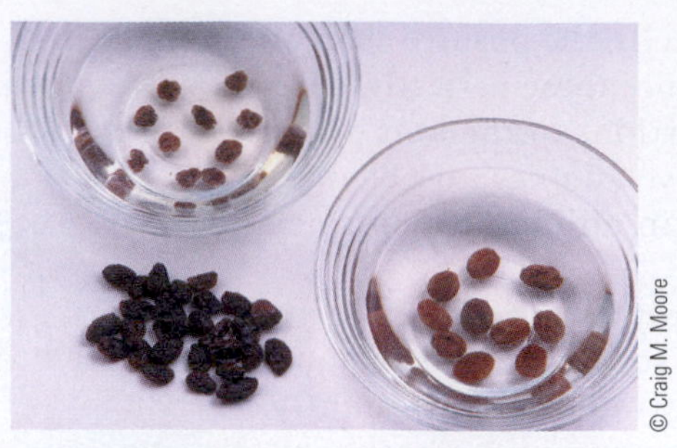

© Craig M. Moore

> **PHOTO 12-2** When immersed in water, raisins become plump because water moves toward the higher concentration of sugar inside the raisins.

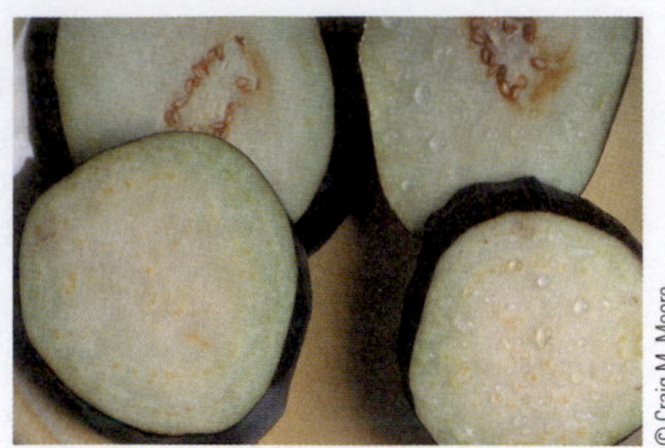

© Craig M. Moore

> **PHOTO 12-3** When sprinkled with salt, eggplant and other vegetables "sweat" because water moves toward the higher concentration of salt outside the vegetable.

> **FIGURE 12-4 Osmosis**

Water flows in the direction of the more highly concentrated solution.

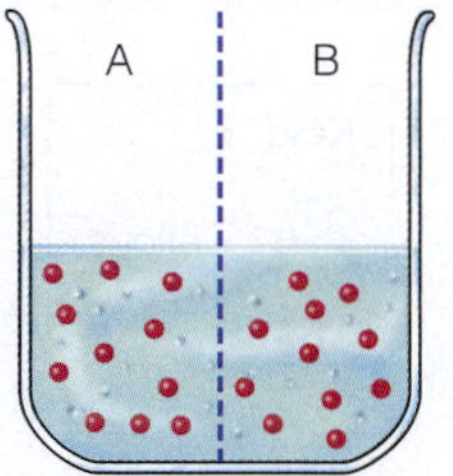

A
B

1 With equal numbers of solute particles on both sides of the semipermeable membrane, the concentrations are equal, and the tendency of water to move in either direction is about the same.

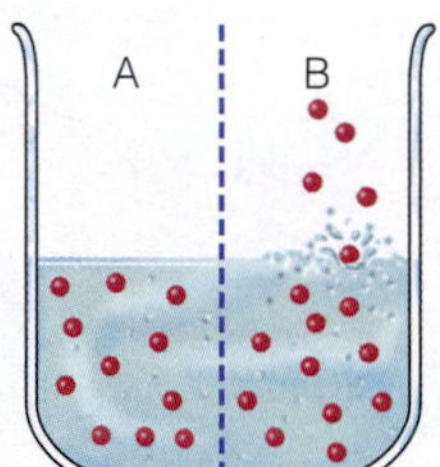

A
B

2 Now additional solute is added to side B. Solute cannot flow across the divider (in the case of a cell, its membrane).

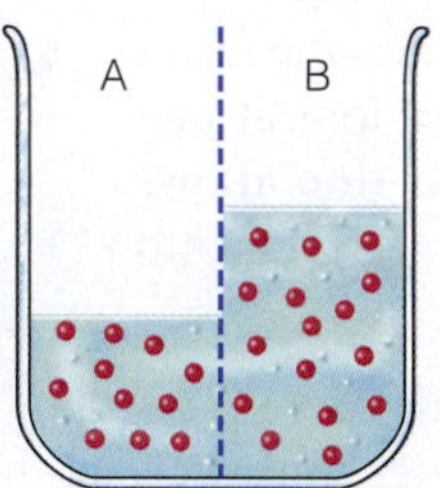

A
B

3 Water can flow both ways across the divider, but has a greater tendency to move from side A to side B, where there is a greater concentration of solute. The volume of water becomes greater on side B, and the concentrations on side A and B become equal.

© Cengage

Proteins Attract Water Chapter 6 described how proteins attract water and help regulate fluid movement. It explains that when proteins leak out of the blood vessels into the spaces between the cells, fluids follow and cause the swelling of edema. In addition, transport proteins in the cell membranes regulate the passage of positive ions and other substances from one side of the membrane to the other. Negative ions follow positive ions, and water flows toward the more concentrated solution.

An example of a protein that regulates the flow of fluids and ions in and out of cells is the sodium-potassium pump. The pump actively exchanges sodium for potassium across the cell membrane, using ATP as an energy source. Figure 6-10 (p. 179) illustrates this action.

Regulation of Fluid Balance

Fluids maintain the blood volume, which in turn influences blood pressure. The kidneys are central to the regulation of blood volume and blood pressure. All day, every day, the kidneys reabsorb needed substances and water and excrete wastes with some water in the urine (see Figure 12-5). The kidneys meticulously adjust the volume and the concentration of the urine to accommodate changes in the body, including variations in the day's food and beverage intakes. Instructions on whether to retain or release substances or water come from antidiuretic hormone, renin, angiotensin, and aldosterone.

Antidiuretic Hormone (ADH) Whenever blood volume or blood pressure falls too low, or whenever the extracellular fluid becomes too concentrated, the **hypothalamus** signals the pituitary gland to release **antidiuretic hormone (ADH)**. ADH is a water-conserving hormone that stimulates the kidneys to reabsorb water. Consequently, the more water you need, the less your kidneys excrete. These events also trigger thirst. Drinking water and retaining fluids raise the blood volume and dilute the concentrated fluids, thus helping to restore homeostasis. (Recall from Highlight 7 that alcohol depresses ADH activity, thus promoting fluid losses and dehydration.)

Renin Cells in the kidneys respond to low blood pressure by releasing an enzyme called **renin**. Through a complex series of events, renin causes the kidneys to reabsorb sodium. Sodium reabsorption, in turn, is always accompanied by water retention, which helps to raise blood volume and blood pressure.

hypothalamus (high-po-THAL-ah-mus): a brain center that controls activities such as maintenance of water balance, regulation of body temperature, and control of appetite.

antidiuretic hormone (ADH): a water-conserving hormone produced by the pituitary gland in response to dehydration (or a high sodium concentration in the blood) that stimulates the kidneys to reabsorb more water and therefore to excrete less. In addition to its antidiuretic effect, ADH elevates blood pressure and so is also called *vasopressin* (VAS-oh-PRES-in).

- **vaso** = vessel
- **press** = pressure

renin (REN-in): an enzyme from the kidneys that hydrolyzes the protein angiotensinogen to angiotensin I, which results in the kidneys reabsorbing sodium.

> **FIGURE 12-5 A Nephron, One of the Kidney's Many Functioning Units**

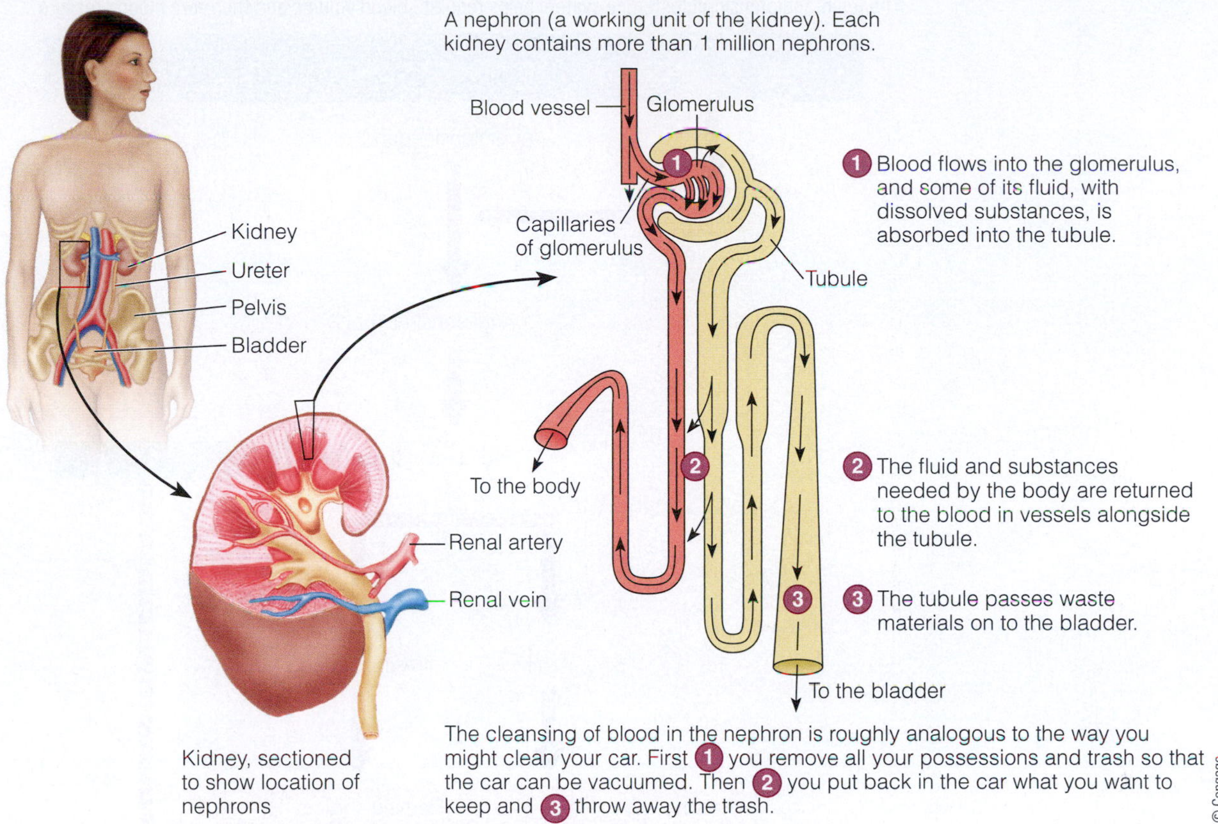

A nephron (a working unit of the kidney). Each kidney contains more than 1 million nephrons.
Blood vessel
Glomerulus
Capillaries of glomerulus
Tubule
Kidney
Ureter
Pelvis
Bladder
To the body
Renal artery
Renal vein
To the bladder
1 Blood flows into the glomerulus, and some of its fluid, with dissolved substances, is absorbed into the tubule.
2 The fluid and substances needed by the body are returned to the blood in vessels alongside the tubule.
3 The tubule passes waste materials on to the bladder.
Kidney, sectioned to show location of nephrons
The cleansing of blood in the nephron is roughly analogous to the way you might clean your car. First 1 you remove all your possessions and trash so that the car can be vacuumed. Then 2 you put back in the car what you want to keep and 3 throw away the trash.
© Cengage

Angiotensin In addition to its role in sodium retention, renin hydrolyzes **angiotensinogen** (a protein from the liver) to **angiotensin I**. Angiotensin I is inactive until another enzyme converts it to its active form—**angiotensin II**. Angiotensin II is a powerful **vasoconstrictor** that narrows the diameters of blood vessels, thereby raising the blood pressure.

Aldosterone In addition to acting as a vasoconstrictor, angiotensin II stimulates the release of the hormone **aldosterone** from the **adrenal glands**. Aldosterone signals the kidneys to excrete potassium and to retain more sodium, and therefore water, because when sodium moves, water follows. Again, the effect is that when more water is needed, less is excreted.

All of these actions are presented in Figure 12-6 (p. 364) and help explain why high-sodium diets aggravate conditions such as hypertension and edema. Too much sodium causes water retention and an accompanying rise in blood pressure, swelling in the interstitial spaces, or both. Chapter 18 discusses hypertension in detail.

Fluid and Electrolyte Imbalance

Normally, the body defends itself successfully against fluid and electrolyte imbalances. With minor imbalances, people can replace the fluids and minerals lost in sweat or in a temporary bout of diarrhea, for example, by drinking plain cool water and eating regular foods. Certain situations and some medications, however, may overwhelm the body's ability to compensate. Severe, prolonged vomiting and diarrhea as well as heavy sweating, burns, and traumatic wounds may incur such great fluid and electrolyte losses as to precipitate a medical emergency.

Appropriate medical intervention depends on the circumstances surrounding the loss of fluids and their solutes. If fluid is lost by vomiting or diarrhea, sodium is lost indiscriminately. If the adrenal glands oversecrete aldosterone, as may occur when

angiotensinogen: a precursor protein that is hydrolyzed to angiotensin I by renin.

angiotensin I (AN-gee-oh-TEN-sin): an inactive precursor that is converted by an enzyme to yield active angiotensin II.

angiotensin II: a hormone involved in blood pressure regulation.

vasoconstrictor (VAS-oh-kon-STRIK-tor): a substance that constricts or narrows the blood vessels.

aldosterone (al-DOS-ter-own): a hormone secreted by the adrenal glands that regulates blood pressure by increasing the reabsorption of sodium by the kidneys. Aldosterone also regulates chloride and potassium concentrations.

adrenal glands: glands adjacent to, and just above, each kidney.

> **FIGURE 12-6 How the Body Regulates Blood Volume and Blood Pressure**

The renin-angiotensin-aldosterone system helps regulate blood volume and therefore blood pressure.

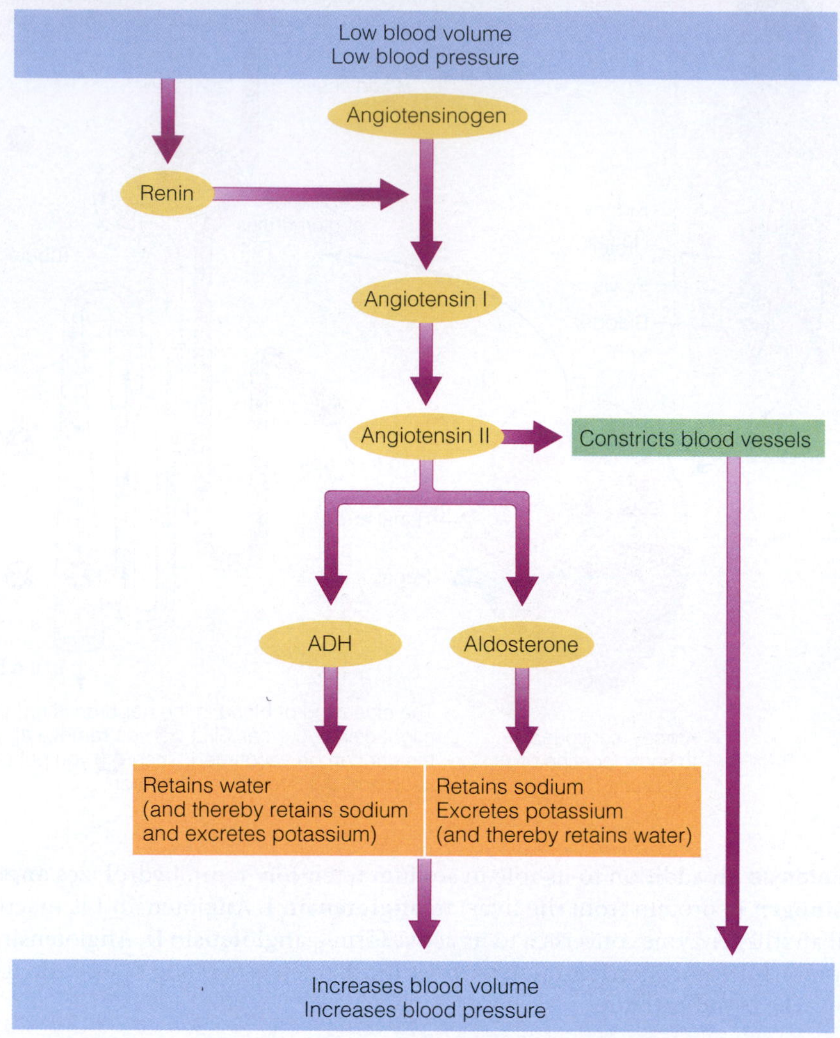

Low blood volume
Low blood pressure
Angiotensinogen
Renin
Angiotensin I
Angiotensin II
Constricts blood vessels
ADH
Aldosterone
Retains water (and thereby retains sodium and excretes potassium)
Retains sodium Excretes potassium (and thereby retains water)
Increases blood volume
Increases blood pressure
© Cengage

a tumor develops, the kidneys may excrete too much potassium. A person with uncontrolled diabetes may lose glucose (a solute not normally excreted) and large amounts of fluid with it. Each situation results in dehydration, but drinking water alone will not restore balance. Medical intervention is required to restore balance.

In some cases, restoring balance demands rapid replacement of fluids and electrolytes—for example, when diarrhea threatens the life of a malnourished child. Caregivers around the world have learned to use **oral rehydration therapy (ORT)**—a simple solution of sugar, salt, and water, taken by mouth—to treat dehydration caused by severe diarrhea. These lifesaving formulas do not require hospitalization and can be prepared from ingredients available locally. Caregivers need only learn to measure ingredients carefully and use sanitary water. Once rehydrated, a person can begin eating foods. (Chapter 14 presents a discussion of sport drinks.)

Acid–Base Balance

The body uses its ions not only to help maintain fluid and electrolyte balance, but also to regulate the acidity (pH) of its fluids. The pH scale introduced in Chapter 3 is repeated here in Figure 12-7 with the normal and abnormal pH ranges of the blood added. As you can see, the body must maintain the pH within a narrow range to avoid life-threatening consequences. Slight deviations in either direction can denature proteins, rendering them useless—for example, enzymes couldn't catalyze reactions and hemoglobin couldn't carry oxygen.

oral rehydration therapy (ORT): the administration of a simple solution of sugar, salt, and water, taken by mouth, to treat dehydration caused by diarrhea. A simple ORT recipe (cool before giving):

- ½ L boiling water
- A small handful of sugar (4 tsp)
- 3 pinches of salt (½ tsp)

> FIGURE 12-7 The pH Scale

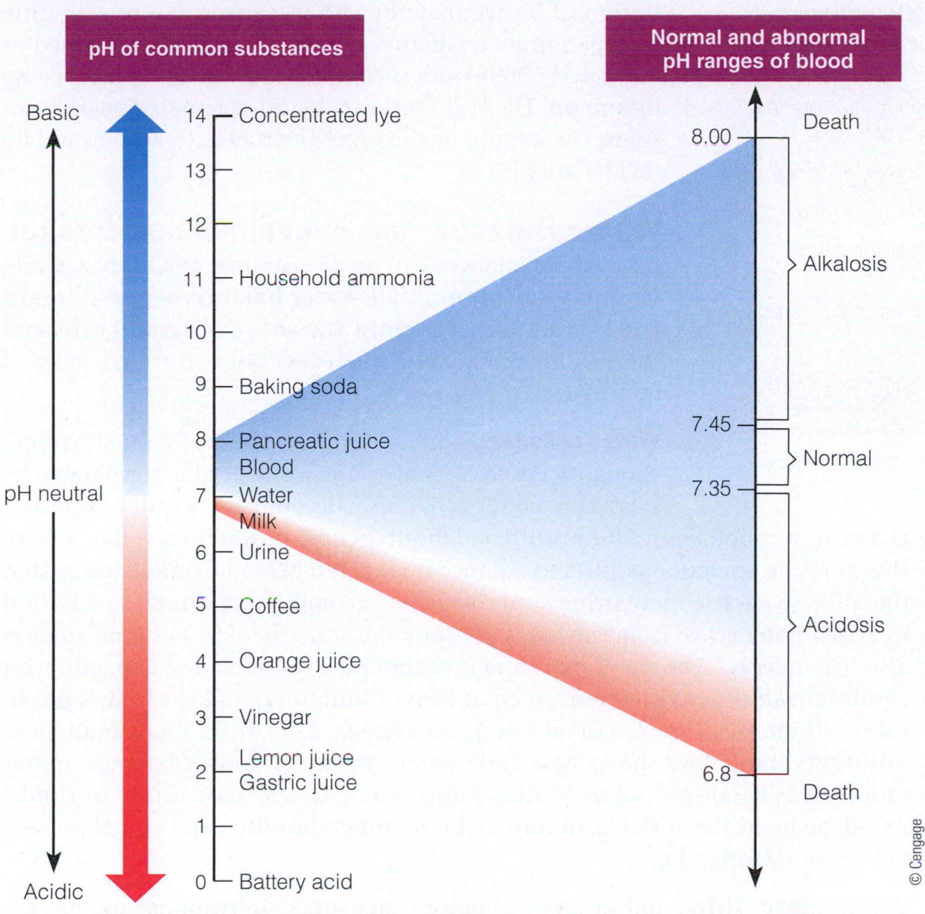

pH of common substances
Normal and abnormal pH ranges of blood
Basic
pH neutral
Acidic
14 Concentrated lye
13
12
11 Household ammonia
10
9 Baking soda
8 Pancreatic juice
Blood
7 Water
Milk
6 Urine
5 Coffee
4 Orange juice
3 Vinegar
2 Lemon juice
Gastric juice
1
0 Battery acid
8.00
7.45
7.35
6.8
Death
Alkalosis
Normal
Acidosis
Death
© Cengage

NOTE: Each step is 10 times as concentrated in base (1⁄10 as much acid, or H^+) as the one below it.

The acidity of the body's fluids is determined by the concentration of hydrogen ions (H^+).* A high concentration of hydrogen ions is acidic. Normal energy metabolism generates hydrogen ions, as well as many other acids, that must be neutralized. Three systems defend the body against fluctuations in pH—buffers in the blood, respiration in the lungs, and excretion in the kidneys.

Regulation by the Buffers **Bicarbonate** (a base) and **carbonic acid** (an acid) in the body fluids, as well as some proteins, protect the body against changes in acidity by acting as **buffers**—substances that can neutralize acids or bases. Carbon dioxide, which is formed all the time during energy metabolism, dissolves in water to form carbonic acid in the blood. Carbonic acid, in turn, dissociates to form hydrogen ions and bicarbonate ions. The appropriate balance between carbonic acid and bicarbonate is essential to maintaining optimal blood pH. Figure 12-8 (p. 366) presents the chemical reactions of this buffer system, which is primarily under the control of the lungs and kidneys.

Respiration in the Lungs The lungs control the concentration of carbonic acid by raising or lowering the respiration rate, depending on whether the pH needs to be increased or decreased. If too much carbonic acid builds up, the respiration rate speeds up; this hyperventilation increases the amount of carbon dioxide exhaled, thereby lowering the carbonic acid concentration and restoring homeostasis. Conversely, if bicarbonate builds up, the respiration rate slows; carbon dioxide is retained and forms more carbonic acid. Again, homeostasis is restored.

*The lower the pH, the higher the H^+ ion concentration and the stronger the acid. A pH above 7 is alkaline, or base—a solution in which OH^- ions predominate.

bicarbonate: an alkaline compound with the formula HCO_3 that is produced in all cell fluids from the dissociation of carbonic acid to help maintain the body's acid–base balance. Bicarbonate is also secreted from the pancreas as part of the pancreatic juice.

carbonic acid: a compound with the formula H_2CO_3 that results from the combination of carbon dioxide (CO_2) and water (H_2O); of particular importance in maintaining the body's acid–base balance.

buffers: compounds that keep a solution's pH constant when acids or bases are added.

FIGURE 12-8 Bicarbonate–Carbonic Acid Buffer System

The reversible reactions of the bicarbonate–carbonic acid buffer system help to regulate the body's pH and maintain homeostasis. Recall from Chapter 7 that carbon dioxide and water are formed during energy metabolism.

Carbon dioxide (CO_2) is a volatile gas that quickly dissolves in water (H_2O), forming carbonic acid (H_2CO_3), which lowers the body's pH:

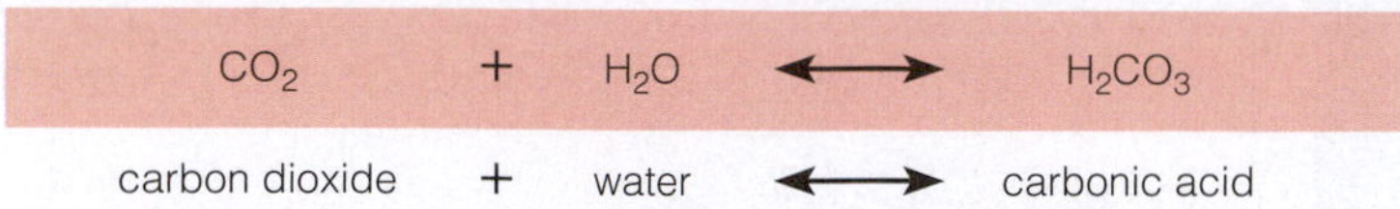
CO_2 + H_2O ⟷ H_2CO_3
carbon dioxide + water ⟷ carbonic acid

Carbonic acid readily dissociates to a hydrogen ion (H^+) and a bicarbonate ion (HCO_3^-), which raises the body's pH:

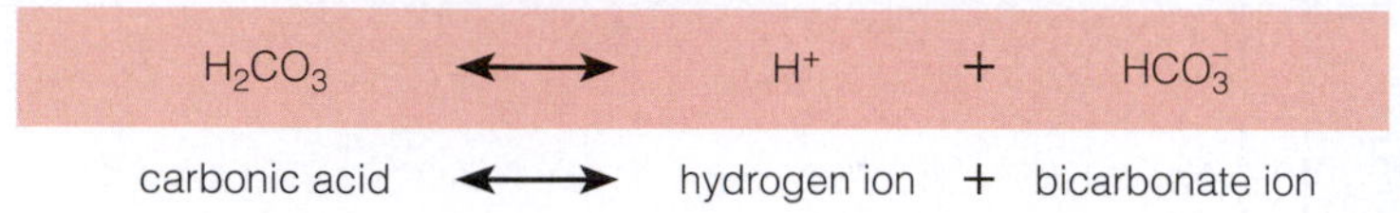
H_2CO_3 ⟷ H^+ + HCO_3^-
carbonic acid ⟷ hydrogen ion + bicarbonate ion

Excretion in the Kidneys The kidneys control the concentration of bicarbonate by either reabsorbing or excreting it, depending on whether the pH needs to be increased or decreased. Their work is complex, but the net effect is easy to sum up. The *body's* total acid burden remains nearly constant; the acidity of the *urine* fluctuates to accommodate that balance.

Water Balance and Recommended Intakes

Because imbalances can be devastating, the body actively maintains an appropriate **water balance** between intake and output. Consequently, the entire system of cells and their fluids remains in a delicate, but controlled, state of homeostasis.

Water Losses At the very least, the body must excrete enough water to carry away the waste products generated by a day's metabolic activities. This **obligatory water excretion** is a minimum of about 500 milliliters (about 2 cups) of water each day. Above this amount, excretion adjusts to balance intake. If a person drinks more water, the kidneys excrete more urine, and the urine becomes more dilute. In addition to urine, water is lost from the lungs as vapor and from the skin as sweat; some is also lost in feces.* The amount of fluid lost from each source varies, depending on conditions in the environment (such as heat or humidity) and the body's physical condition (such as exercise or fever). On average, daily losses total about 2500 milliliters. Table 12-2 shows how daily water losses and intakes balance; maintaining this balance requires healthy kidneys and an adequate intake of fluids. An adequate intake of fluids, in turn, helps maintain healthy kidneys and prevent kidney stone formation.

Water Intake **Thirst** and satiety influence water intake in response to changes sensed by the mouth, hypothalamus, and nerves. When water intake is inadequate, the blood becomes concentrated (having lost water but not the solutes within it), the mouth becomes dry, and the hypothalamus initiates drinking behavior. When water intake is excessive, the stomach expands, and stretch receptors send signals to stop drinking. Similar signals are sent from receptors in the heart as blood volume increases.

When too much water is lost from the body and not replaced, **dehydration** develops. A first sign of dehydration is thirst, the signal that the body has lost some fluid. If a person is unable to obtain water or, as in many elderly people, fails to perceive the thirst message, the symptoms of dehydration may progress rapidly from thirst to weakness, exhaustion, and delirium—and end in death if not corrected (see Table 12-3). Notice that an early sign of dehydration is fatigue; keep that in mind when considering caffeinated beverages for an afternoon "pick-me-up" and choose water instead. Dehydration develops with either inadequate water

TABLE 12-2 Water Balance

Water Sources	Amount (mL)	Water Losses	Amount (mL)
Beverages	550 to 1500	Kidneys (urine)	500 to 1400
Foods	700 to 1000	Skin (sweat)	450 to 900
Metabolism	200 to 300	Lungs (breath)	350
		GI tract (feces)	150
Total	1450 to 2800	Total	1450 to 2800

NOTE: For perspective, 100 milliliters is a little less than ½ cup and 1000 milliliters is a little more than 1 quart (1 mL = 0.03 oz).

*Water lost from the lungs and skin accounts for almost half of the daily losses even when a person is not visibly perspiring; these losses are commonly referred to as *insensible water losses*.

water balance: the balance between water intake and output (losses).

obligatory (ah-BLIG-ah-TORE-ee) **water excretion:** the minimum amount of water the body has to excrete each day to dispose of its wastes—about 500 milliliters (about 2 cups, or 1 pint).

thirst: a conscious desire to drink.

dehydration: the condition in which body water output exceeds water input. Symptoms include thirst, dry skin and mucous membranes, rapid heartbeat, low blood pressure, and weakness.

TABLE 12-3 Signs of Dehydration

Body Weight Lost (%)	Symptoms
1–2	Thirst, fatigue, weakness, vague discomfort, loss of appetite
3–4	Impaired physical performance, dry mouth, reduction in urine, flushed skin, impatience, apathy
5–6	Difficulty concentrating, headache, irritability, sleepiness, impaired temperature regulation, increased respiratory rate
7–10	Dizziness, spastic muscles, loss of balance, delirium, exhaustion, collapse

NOTE: The onset and severity of symptoms at various percentages of body weight lost depend on the activity, fitness level, degree of acclimation, temperature, and humidity. If not corrected, dehydration can lead to death.

intake or excessive water losses. Figure 12-9 illustrates how the color of urine may indicate possible dehydration. (Chapter 14 revisits dehydration and the fluid needs of athletes.)

Water intoxication, on the other hand, is rare but can occur with excessive water intake and kidney disorders that reduce urine production. The symptoms may include confusion, convulsions, and even death in extreme cases. Excessive water ingestion (10 to 20 liters) within a few hours dilutes the sodium concentration of the blood and contributes to a dangerous condition known as **hyponatremia**. For this reason, guidelines suggest limiting fluid intake during times of heavy sweating to between 1 and 1.5 liters per hour. (Chapter 14 revisits the possibility of hyponatremia in endurance athletes.)

Water Sources The obvious dietary source of water is water itself, which provides about one-third of the total water intake in the United States. In addition, other beverages and nearly all foods also contain water. Most fruits and vegetables contain up to 90 percent water, and many meats and cheeses contain at least 50 percent. See Table 12-4 for selected foods. Also, **metabolic water** is generated as an end product during condensation reactions and the oxidation of energy-yielding nutrients. Recall from Chapter 7 that when the energy-yielding nutrients break down, their carbon and hydrogen molecules combine with oxygen to yield carbon dioxide (CO_2) and water (H_2O). As Table 12-2 shows, the water derived daily from these three sources—beverages, foods, and metabolism—averages about 2500 milliliters (roughly 2.5 quarts, or 10.5 cups).

Water Recommendations Because water needs vary depending on diet, activity, environmental temperature, and humidity, a general water requirement is difficult to establish. Recommendations are sometimes expressed in proportion to the amount of energy expended under average environmental conditions; for adults, for example, 1.0 to 1.5 milliliters per kcalorie expended (roughly one-half cup per 100 kcalories). The recommended water intake for a person who expends 2000 kcalories a day, then, is 2 to 3 liters of water (about 8 to 12 cups). This recommendation is in line with the Adequate Intake (AI) for *total* water set by the DRI Committee. Total water includes not only drinking water, but water in other beverages and in foods as well. On average, most adults in the United States consume about the AI for total water; older adults tend to consume less.[1] Because a wide range of water intakes will prevent dehydration and its harmful consequences, the AI is based on average intakes. People who are physically active or who live in hot environments may need more (see Photo 12-4, p. 368).

Which beverages are best? Any beverage can readily meet the body's fluid needs, but those with few or no kcalories do so without contributing to weight gain. Given that obesity is a major health problem and that beverages currently represent more than 20 percent of the total energy intake in the United States, water is the best choice for most people. Other choices include tea, coffee, nonfat and low-fat milk and soymilk, artificially sweetened beverages, fruit and vegetable juices, sports drinks, and lastly, sweetened nutrient-poor beverages.

> FIGURE 12-9 The Color of Urine in Relation to Hydration

The color of urine gives a hint to a person's hydration status, but cannot be used for diagnosis. In addition to dehydration, the color of urine may indicate the presence of food dyes; blood; bladder, liver, or kidney disease; and medications.

Color	Hydration
Transparent	Possible over-hydration
Pale straw	Normal, well hydrated
Transparent yellow	Normal
Dark yellow	Normal, possible mild dehydration
Deep amber or honey	Normal, possible moderate dehydration
Orange	Possible severe dehydration

TABLE 12-4 Percentage of Water in Selected Foods

100%	Water
90–99%	Fat-free milk, strawberries, watermelon, lettuce, cabbage, celery, spinach, broccoli
80–89%	Fruit juice, yogurt, apples, grapes, oranges, carrots
70–79%	Shrimp, bananas, corn, potatoes, avocados, cottage cheese, ricotta cheese
60–69%	Pasta, legumes, salmon, ice cream, chicken breast
50–59%	Ground beef, hot dogs, feta cheese
40–49%	Pizza
30–39%	Cheddar cheese, bagels, bread
20–29%	Pepperoni sausage, cake, biscuits
10–19%	Butter, margarine, raisins
1–9%	Crackers, cereals, pretzels, taco shells, peanut butter, nuts
0%	Oils, sugars

water intoxication: the rare condition in which body water contents are too high in all body fluid compartments.

hyponatremia (HIGH-po-na-TREE-me-ah): a decreased concentration of sodium in the blood.

metabolic water: water generated during metabolism.

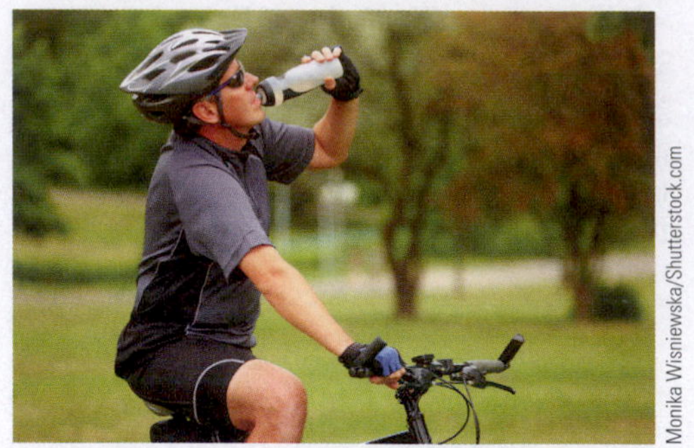

> **PHOTO 12-4** Physically active people must remember to replace their body fluids.

Monika Wisniewska/Shutterstock.com

Because caffeine acts as a diuretic, people who drink caffeinated beverages may lose slightly more fluid than when drinking water, but the losses are relatively insignificant. The DRI Committee considered such findings in their recommendations for water intake and concluded that caffeinated beverages contribute to the daily total water intake similar to that contributed by noncaffeinated beverages. In other words, it doesn't seem to matter whether people rely on caffeine-containing beverages or other beverages to meet their fluid needs.

As Highlight 7 (p. 219) explained, alcohol acts as a diuretic and can impair a person's health. To limit the risks associated with alcoholic beverages, consumers should keep intake moderate and drink plenty of water as well.

Health Effects of Water Water supports good health. Physical and mental performances depend on it, as does the optimal functioning of the GI tract, kidneys, heart, and other body systems. The kind of water a person drinks may also make a difference to health. Water is usually either hard or soft. **Hard water** has high concentrations of calcium and magnesium; the principal mineral of **soft water** is sodium or potassium. (See Glossary 12-1 for other common terms used to describe water.) In practical terms, soft water makes more bubbles with less soap; hard water leaves a ring on the tub, a crust of rocklike crystals in the teakettle, and a gray residue in the laundry.

Soft water may seem more desirable around the house, and some homeowners purchase water softeners that replace magnesium and calcium with sodium. In the body, however, soft water with sodium may aggravate hypertension and heart disease. In contrast, the minerals in hard water may benefit these conditions. Soft water also more easily dissolves certain contaminant minerals, such as cadmium and lead, from old plumbing pipes. As Chapter 13 explains, these contaminant minerals harm the body by displacing the nutrient minerals from their normal sites of action.

Many people select **bottled water**, believing it to be safer than tap water and therefore worth its substantial cost. Chapter 19 offers a discussion of bottled water safety and regulations.

REVIEW IT Explain how the body regulates fluid balance.

Water makes up about 60 percent of the adult body's weight. It assists with the transport of nutrients and waste products throughout the body, participates in chemical reactions, acts as a solvent, serves as a shock absorber, and regulates body temperature. To maintain water balance, intake from liquids, foods, and metabolism must equal losses from the kidneys, skin, lungs, and GI tract. Whenever the body experiences low blood volume, low blood pressure, or highly concentrated body fluids, the actions of ADH, renin, angiotensin, and aldosterone restore homeostasis. Electrolytes (charged minerals) in the fluids help distribute the fluids inside and outside the cells, thus ensuring the appropriate water balance and acid–base balance to support all life processes. Excessive losses of fluids and electrolytes upset these balances, and the kidneys play a key role in restoring homeostasis.

hard water: water with a high calcium and magnesium content.

soft water: water with a high sodium or potassium content.

bottled water: drinking water sold in bottles.

GLOSSARY 12-1
WATER TERMS

artesian water: water drawn from a well that taps a confined aquifer in which the water is under pressure.

carbonated water: water that contains carbon dioxide gas, either naturally occurring or added, that causes bubbles to form in it; also called *bubbling* or *sparkling water.* The FDA defines seltzer, soda, and tonic waters as soft drinks; they are not regulated as water.

distilled water: water that has been vaporized and recondensed, leaving it free of dissolved minerals.

filtered water: water treated by filtration, usually through *activated carbon filters* that reduce the lead in tap water, or by *reverse osmosis* units that force pressurized water across a membrane, removing lead, arsenic, and some microorganisms from tap water.

mineral water: water from a spring or well that naturally contains at least 250 parts per million (ppm) of minerals. Minerals give water a distinctive flavor. Many mineral waters are high in sodium.

natural water: water obtained from a spring or well that is certified to be safe and sanitary. The mineral content may not be changed, but the water may be treated in other ways such as with ozone or by filtration.

public water: water from a municipal or county water system that has been treated and disinfected.

purified water: water that has been treated by distillation or other physical or chemical processes that remove dissolved solids. Because purified water contains no minerals or contaminants, it is useful for medical and research purposes.

spring water: water originating from an underground spring or well. It may be bubbly (carbonated), or "flat" or "still," meaning not carbonated. Brand names such as "Spring Pure" do not necessarily mean that the water comes from a spring.

well water: water drawn from groundwater by tapping into an aquifer.

12.2 The Minerals—An Overview

LEARN IT List some of the ways minerals differ from vitamins and other nutrients.

Figure 12-10 shows the amounts of the **major minerals** found in the body and, for comparison, some of the **trace minerals.** The distinction between the major and trace minerals does not mean that one group is more important than the other—all minerals are vital. The major minerals are so named because they are present, and needed, in larger amounts in the body. They are shown at the top of the figure and are discussed in this chapter. The trace minerals, shown at the bottom of the figure, are discussed in Chapter 13. A few generalizations pertain to all of the minerals and distinguish them from the vitamins. Especially notable is their chemical nature.

> **FIGURE 12-10 Minerals in a 60-kilogram (132-pound) Human Body**

Not only are the major minerals needed by the body in larger amounts, but they are also present in the body in larger amounts than the trace minerals.

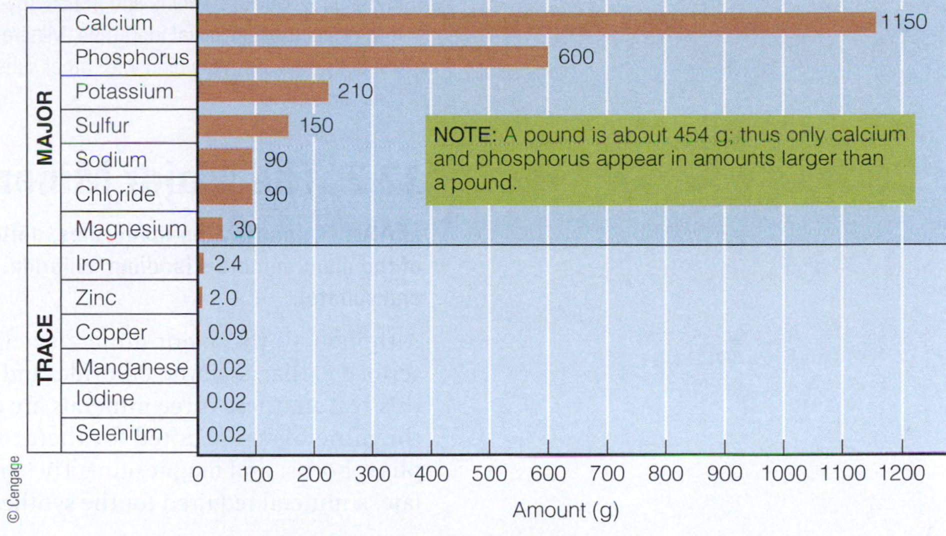

MAJOR
Calcium 1150
Phosphorus 600
Potassium 210
Sulfur 150
Sodium 90
Chloride 90
Magnesium 30
TRACE
Iron 2.4
Zinc 2.0
Copper 0.09
Manganese 0.02
Iodine 0.02
Selenium 0.02
NOTE: A pound is about 454 g; thus only calcium and phosphorus appear in amounts larger than a pound.
0 100 200 300 400 500 600 700 800 900 1000 1100 1200
Amount (g)

Inorganic Elements Unlike the organic vitamins, which are easily destroyed, minerals are inorganic elements that always retain their chemical identity. Once minerals enter the body, they remain there until excreted; they cannot be changed into anything else. Iron, for example, may temporarily combine with other charged elements in salts, but it is always iron. Neither can minerals be destroyed by heat, air, acid, or mixing. Consequently, little care is needed to preserve minerals during food preparation. In fact, the ash that remains when a food is burned contains all the minerals that were in the food originally. Minerals can be lost from food only when they leach into cooking water that is then poured down the drain.

The Body's Handling of Minerals The minerals also differ from the vitamins in the amounts the body can absorb and in the extent to which they must be specially handled. Some minerals, such as potassium, are easily absorbed into the blood, transported freely, and readily excreted by the kidneys, much like the water-soluble vitamins. Other minerals, such as calcium, are more like fat-soluble vitamins in that they must have carriers to be absorbed and transported. And, like some of the fat-soluble vitamins, minerals consumed in excess can be toxic.

Variable Bioavailability The **bioavailability** of minerals varies. Some foods contain **binders** that combine chemically with minerals, preventing their absorption and carrying them out of the body with other wastes. Examples of binders include phytates, which are found primarily in legumes, seeds, nuts, and grains, and oxalates, which are present in rhubarb, beet greens, sweet potatoes, and spinach, among other vegetables. These foods contain more minerals than the body actually receives for use.

Nutrient Interactions Chapter 10 described how the presence or absence of one vitamin can affect another's absorption, metabolism, and excretion. The same is true of the minerals. The interactions between sodium and calcium, for example, cause both to be excreted when sodium intakes are high. Phosphorus binds with magnesium in the GI tract, so magnesium absorption is limited when phosphorus intakes are high. These are just two examples of the interactions involving minerals featured in this chapter. Discussions in both this chapter and the next point out additional problems that arise from such interactions. Notice how often they reflect an excess of one mineral creating an inadequacy of another and how supplements—not foods—are most often to blame.

major minerals: essential mineral nutrients the human body requires in relatively large amounts (greater than 100 milligrams per day); sometimes called *macrominerals.*

trace minerals: essential mineral nutrients the human body requires in relatively small amounts (less than 100 milligrams per day); sometimes called *microminerals.*

bioavailability: the rate at and the extent to which a nutrient is absorbed and used.

binders: chemical compounds in foods that combine with nutrients (especially minerals) to form complexes the body cannot absorb. Examples include *phytates* (FYE-tates) and *oxalates* (OCK-sa-lates).

REVIEW IT List some of the ways minerals differ from vitamins and other nutrients.

Compared with the trace minerals, major minerals are found, and needed, in larger quantities in the body. Unlike vitamins and the energy-yielding nutrients, minerals are inorganic elements that retain their chemical identities. Minerals usually receive special handling and regulation in the body, and they may bind with other substances or interact with other minerals, thus limiting their absorption.

12.3 The Major Minerals

LEARN IT Identify the main roles, deficiency symptoms, and food sources for each of the major minerals (sodium, chloride, potassium, calcium, phosphorus, magnesium, and sulfate).

Although all the major minerals help maintain the body's fluid balance as described earlier, sodium, chloride, and potassium are most noted for that role. For this reason, these three minerals are discussed first here. Later sections describe the minerals most noted for their roles in bone growth and health—calcium, phosphorus, and magnesium. The chapter closes with a brief discussion on sulfate, a mineral required for the synthesis of several sulfur-containing compounds.

Sodium

People have held salt (sodium chloride) in high regard throughout recorded history. We describe someone we admire as "the salt of the earth" and people who are not productive as "not worth their salt." The word *salary* comes from the Latin word for salt, a valued commodity.

Cultures vary in their use of salt, but most people find its taste innately appealing. Salt brings its own tangy taste and enhances other flavors, most likely by suppressing the bitter flavors. You can taste this effect for yourself: tonic water with its bitter quinine tastes sweeter with a little salt added.

Sodium Roles in the Body **Sodium** is the principal cation of the extracellular fluid and the primary regulator of its volume.[2] Sodium also helps maintain acid–base balance and is essential to nerve impulse transmission and muscle contraction.*

Sodium is readily absorbed by the intestinal tract and travels freely in the blood until it reaches the kidneys, which filter all the sodium out of the blood. Then, with great precision, the kidneys return to the blood the exact amount of sodium the body needs. Normally, the amount excreted is approximately equal to the amount ingested on a given day. When blood sodium rises, as when a person eats salted foods, thirst signals the person to drink until the appropriate sodium-to-water concentration is restored. Then the kidneys excrete both the excess water and the excess sodium together. Both too much and too little sodium in the diet can be harmful. The key to good health, then, is finding the balance that meets the relatively small need for this essential nutrient but does not exceed the amount that leads to hypertension and heart disease.[3]

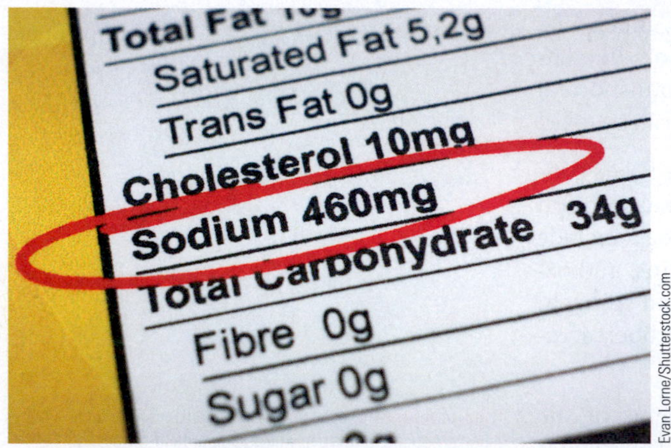
Total Fat
Saturated Fat 5,2g
Trans Fat 0g
Cholesterol 10mg
Sodium 460mg
Total Carbohydrate 34g
Fibre 0g
Sugar 0g

Evan Lorne/Shutterstock.com

> **PHOTO 12-5** Food labels indicate the sodium content of foods, making it easier for consumers to select products with less sodium.

Sodium Recommendations Diets rarely lack sodium, and even when intakes are low, the body adapts by reducing sodium losses in urine and sweat, thus making deficiencies unlikely. Sodium recommendations are set low enough to protect against high blood pressure, but high enough to allow an adequate intake of other nutrients with a typical diet. Because high sodium intakes correlate with high blood pressure, the Upper Level (UL) for adults is set at 2300 milligrams per day, as is the Daily Value used on food labels (see Photo 12-5). An estimated 90 percent of the US population exceeds the recommended intake for sodium.[4]

sodium: the principal cation in the extracellular fluids of the body; critical to the maintenance of fluid balance, nerve impulse transmissions, and muscle contractions.

*One of the ways the kidneys regulate acid–base balance is by excreting hydrogen ions (H^+) in exchange for sodium ions (Na^+).

Sodium and Hypertension Most sodium is consumed as salt (sodium chloride), and a high salt intake correlates strongly with high blood pressure and heart disease. A salt-restricted diet lowers blood pressure and improves heart disease risk in healthy people as well as in those with hypertension.[5] For this reason, the *Dietary Guidelines for Americans* advise limiting daily *salt* intake to about 1 teaspoon (the equivalent of about 2.3 grams or 2300 milligrams of *sodium*).[6] For adults with prehypertension and hypertension, a reduction to 1500 milligrams of sodium per day is of even greater benefit. Most people will benefit from a sodium intake within this range (1500 to 2300 milligrams).[7] Limited evidence suggests lower sodium intakes may be associated with health problems for some groups of people.[8]

Because sodium is so prevalent in the food supply, consumers need to use multiple strategies to lower their intake.[9] How To 12-1 offers several tips for cutting salt (and therefore sodium) intake.

Given the current US food supply and typical eating habits, creating a nutritionally balanced diet that meets sodium recommendations can be a challenge. One eating pattern, known as the DASH (Dietary Approaches to Stop Hypertension) Eating Plan, is especially effective in lowering blood pressure. Like other USDA Food Patterns, the DASH Eating Plan reflects the *Dietary Guidelines* and allows people to stay within their energy allowance, meet nutrient needs, and lower disease risk. The DASH approach emphasizes potassium-rich fruits, vegetables, and low-fat milk products; includes whole grains, nuts, poultry, and fish; and calls for reduced intakes of sodium, red and processed meats, sweets, and sugar-containing beverages. Chapter 18 offers a complete discussion of hypertension and the dietary recommendations for its prevention and treatment.

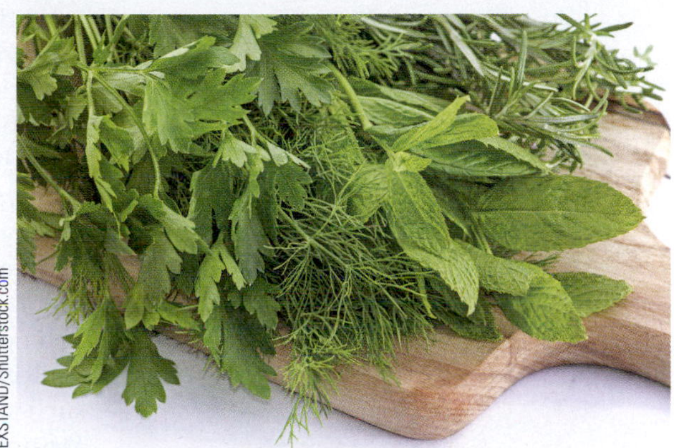
ALEXSTAND/Shutterstock.com

> **PHOTO 12-6** Fresh herbs add flavor to a recipe without adding salt.

> How To 12-1 Cut Salt (and Sodium) Intake

Salt (sodium chloride) is about 40% sodium and 60% chloride.

- 1 g salt contributes about 400 mg sodium and 600 mg chloride
- 6 g salt = 1 tsp
- 1 tsp salt contributes about 2300 mg sodium and 3700 mg chloride

Most people eat more salt (and therefore sodium) than they need. Some people can lower their blood pressure by avoiding highly salted foods and removing the salt shaker from the table. Foods eaten without salt may seem less tasty at first, but with repetition, people can learn to enjoy the natural flavors of many unsalted foods. Strategies to cut salt intake include:

- Read labels with an eye open for sodium. (See Glossary 2-1, p. 59, for terms used to describe the sodium contents of foods on labels.)
- Select products with less sodium and buy low-salt or salt-free products when available.
- Select fresh or frozen vegetables. If buying canned vegetables, drain and rinse in water to remove some of the sodium or select those labeled low-sodium or no-salt-added.
- Select fresh or frozen meat, fish, and poultry instead of processed items or select products labeled low-sodium or no-salt-added.
- Cook foods from scratch at home more often; limit sauces, mixes, and instant products.
- Cook with little or no added salt.
- Prepare foods with sodium-free herbs and spices such as basil, bay leaves, curry, garlic, ginger, mint, oregano, pepper, rosemary, and thyme; lemon juice; vinegar; or wine (see Photo 12-6).
- Add little or no salt at the table; taste foods before adding salt.

Use these foods sparingly:

- Foods prepared in brine, such as pickles, olives, and sauerkraut
- Salty or smoked meats, such as bologna, corned or chipped beef, bacon, frankfurters, ham, lunchmeats, salt pork, sausage, and smoked tongue
- Salty or smoked fish, such as anchovies, caviar, salted and dried cod, herring, sardines, and smoked salmon
- Snack items such as potato chips, pretzels, salted popcorn, salted nuts, and crackers
- Condiments such as bouillon cubes; seasoned salts; MSG; soy, teriyaki, Worcestershire, and barbeque sauces; prepared horseradish, ketchup, and mustard
- Cheeses, especially processed types
- Canned and instant soups
- Packaged instant or flavored rice, pasta, and cereal mixes

> **TRY IT** Compare the sodium contents of 1 ounce of the following foods: a plain bagel, potato chips, and animal crackers.

Sodium and Bone Loss (Osteoporosis) A high salt intake is also associated with increased calcium excretion, but its influence on bone loss is less clear. In addition, potassium may prevent the calcium excretion caused by a high-salt diet. For these reasons, dietary advice to prevent bone loss parallels that suggested for hypertension—a DASH eating pattern that is low in sodium and abundant in potassium-rich fruits and vegetables and calcium-rich low-fat milk.

Sodium in Foods In general, processed foods have the most sodium, whereas unprocessed foods such as fresh fruits and vegetables have the least. In fact, most of the sodium in people's diets comes from salt added to foods during food processing and preparation; only a small proportion comes from salt added during cooking and at the table or from the natural content in foods. Among foods with the highest sodium density (milligrams of sodium per kcalorie) are mixed foods such as sandwiches, pizza, tacos, and soups. Because sodium intake tends to increase as kcalories increase, making food choices based on low sodium density is a practical and effective way to meet sodium recommendations.[10]

To help consumers limit their intake, public health organizations and policymakers worldwide have called for manufacturers and restaurants to reduce sodium in the food supply. Quite simply, removing salt from processed foods is a more effective option than educating consumers.[11] Unfortunately, several studies report that these voluntary reductions in sodium by the food industry are slow and not particularly meaningful.[12]

Because processed foods may contain sodium without chloride, as in additives such as sodium bicarbonate or sodium saccharin, they do not always taste salty. Most people are surprised to learn that 1 ounce of some cereals contains more sodium than 1 ounce of salted peanuts—and that ½ cup of instant chocolate pudding contains still more. The peanuts taste saltier because the salt is all on the surface, where the tongue's taste receptors immediately pick it up.

Figure 12-11 shows that processed foods not only contain more sodium than their less-processed counterparts but also have less potassium. Low potassium

> **FIGURE 12-11 What Processing Does to the Sodium and Potassium Contents of Foods**

People who eat foods high in salt often happen to be eating fewer potassium-containing foods at the same time. Notice how potassium is lost and sodium is gained as foods become more processed, causing the potassium-to-sodium ratio to fall dramatically. Even when potassium isn't lost, the addition of sodium still lowers the potassium-to-sodium ratio. Selecting fresh, unprocessed foods lowers blood pressure in two ways, then—by lowering sodium intakes and by raising potassium intakes.

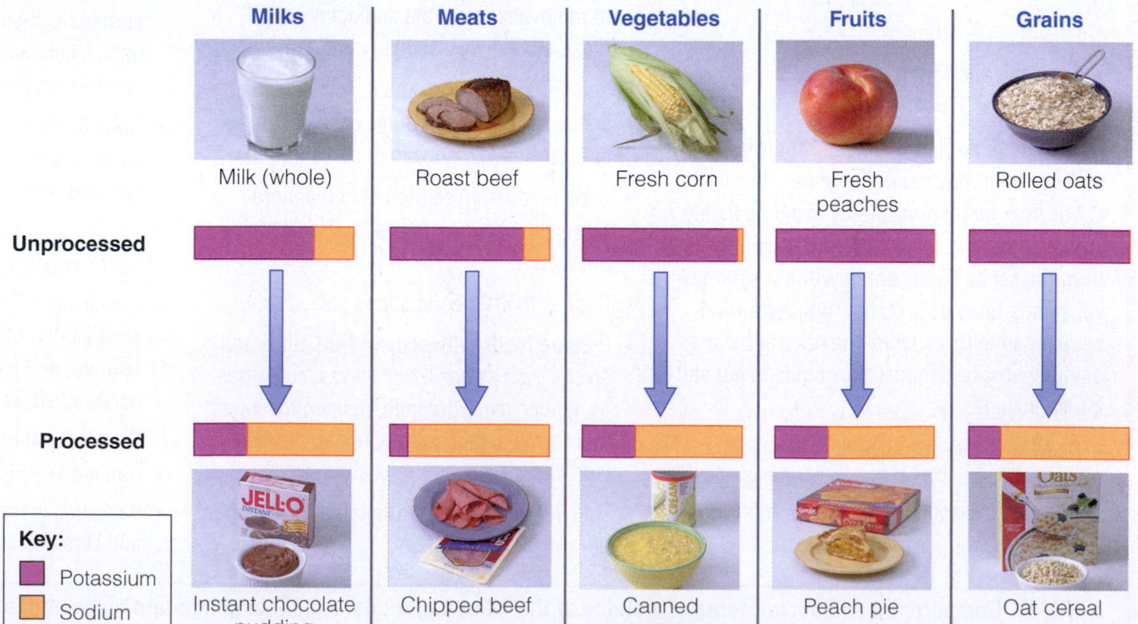

Milks
Meats
Vegetables
Fruits
Grains
Milk (whole)
Roast beef
Fresh corn
Fresh peaches
Rolled oats
Unprocessed
Processed
JELL-O
Instant chocolate pudding
Chipped beef
Canned cream corn
Peach pie
Oat cereal
Key:
Potassium
Sodium

Matthew Farruggio

may be as significant as high sodium when it comes to blood pressure regulation, so processed foods have (at least) two strikes against them.

Sodium Deficiency Sodium deficiency does not develop from an inadequate diet. The body only needs a little and typical diets provide more than enough. Blood sodium may drop with vomiting, diarrhea, or heavy sweating, and in these cases, both sodium and water must be replenished. Under normal conditions of sweating due to physical activity, salt losses can easily be replaced later in the day with ordinary foods. Salt tablets are not recommended because too much salt, especially if taken with too little water, can induce dehydration. During intense activities, such as ultra-endurance events, athletes can lose so much sodium and drink so much water that they develop hyponatremia—the dangerous condition of having too little sodium in the blood. Symptoms of hyponatremia include headache, confusion, stupor, seizures, and coma. Importantly, hyponatremia is caused by excessive sodium losses, not from inadequate sodium intake. (Chapter 14 offers details about hyponatremia and guidelines for ultra-endurance athletes.)

Sodium Toxicity and Excessive Intakes The immediate symptoms of acute sodium toxicity are edema and high blood pressure. Prolonged excessive sodium intake contributes to hypertension, as explained earlier. In addition, a high-sodium intake damages the blood vessels, kidneys, brain, and heart, thus increasing the risk of death from heart disease as well as from other causes.[13]

REVIEW IT Sodium is the main cation outside cells and one of the primary electrolytes responsible for maintaining fluid balance. Dietary deficiency is unlikely, and excesses raise blood pressure. For this reason, health professionals advise a diet moderate in salt and sodium. The accompanying table provides a summary of sodium.

Sodium

AI	
Adults:	1500 mg/day (19–50 yr)
	1300 mg/day (51–70 yr)
	1200 mg/day (>70 yr)

UL
Adults: 2300 mg/day

Chief Functions in the Body
Maintains normal fluid and electrolyte balance; assists in nerve impulse transmission and muscle contraction

Deficiency Symptoms
Not from inadequate intakes Hyponatremia from excessive losses

Toxicity Symptoms
Edema, acute hypertension

Significant Sources
Table salt, soy sauce; moderate amounts in meats, milks, breads, and vegetables; large amounts in processed foods

Chloride

The element *chlorine* (Cl_2) is a poisonous gas. When chlorine reacts with sodium or hydrogen, however, it forms the negative chloride ion (Cl^-). *Chloride,* an essential nutrient, is required in the diet.

Chloride Roles in the Body **Chloride** is the major anion of the extracellular fluids (outside the cells), where it occurs mostly in association with sodium. Chloride moves passively across membranes through channels and so also associates with potassium inside cells. Like sodium and potassium, chloride maintains fluid and electrolyte balance.

In the stomach, the chloride ion is part of hydrochloric acid, which maintains the strong acidity of gastric juice. One of the most serious consequences of vomiting is the loss of this acid from the stomach, which upsets the acid–base balance. Such imbalances are commonly seen in bulimia nervosa, as described in Highlight 8.

Chloride Recommendations and Intakes Chloride is abundant in foods (especially processed foods) as part of sodium chloride and other salts. Chloride recommendations are slightly higher than, but still equivalent to, those of

chloride (KLO-ride): the major anion in the extracellular fluids of the body. Chloride is the ionic form of chlorine, Cl^-. See Appendix B for a description of the chlorine-to-chloride conversion.

sodium. In other words, ¾ teaspoon of salt will deliver some sodium, more chloride, and still meet the AI for both.

Chloride Deficiency and Toxicity Diets rarely lack chloride. Like sodium losses, chloride losses may occur in conditions such as heavy sweating, chronic diarrhea, and vomiting. The only known cause of elevated blood chloride concentrations is dehydration due to water deficiency. In both cases, consuming ordinary foods and beverages can restore chloride balance.

REVIEW IT Chloride is the major anion outside cells, and it associates closely with sodium. In addition to its role in fluid balance, chloride is part of the stomach's hydrochloric acid. The accompanying table provides a summary of chloride.

Chloride

AI	Deficiency Symptoms
Adults: 2300 mg/day (19–50 yr) 2000 mg/day (51–70 yr) 1800 mg/day (>70 yr)	Do not occur under normal circumstances
UL	**Toxicity Symptoms**
Adults: 3600 mg/day	Vomiting
Chief Functions in the Body	**Significant Sources**
Maintains normal fluid and electrolyte balance; part of hydrochloric acid found in the stomach, necessary for proper digestion	Table salt, soy sauce; moderate amounts in meats, milks, eggs; large amounts in processed foods

Potassium

Like sodium, **potassium** is a positively charged ion. In contrast to sodium, potassium is the body's principal intracellular cation, *inside* the body cells.

Potassium Roles in the Body Potassium plays a major role in maintaining fluid and electrolyte balance and cell integrity. During nerve transmissions and muscle contractions, potassium and sodium briefly trade places across the cell membrane. The cell then quickly pumps them back into place. Controlling potassium distribution is a high priority for the body because it affects many aspects of homeostasis, including a steady heartbeat.

Potassium Recommendations and Intakes Potassium is abundant in all living cells. Because cells remain intact unless foods are processed, the richest sources of potassium are *fresh* foods—as Figure 12-12 shows. In contrast, most processed foods such as canned vegetables, ready-to-eat cereals, and luncheon meats contain less potassium—and more sodium (recall Figure 12-11, p. 372). To meet the AI for potassium, most people need to increase their intake of fruits and vegetables (see Photo 12-7).

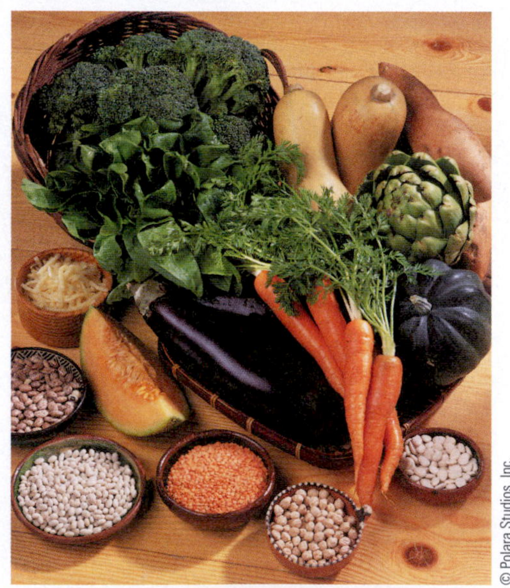

© Polara Studios, Inc.

> **PHOTO 12-7** Fresh foods, especially fruits and vegetables, provide potassium in abundance.

potassium: the principal cation within the body's cells; critical to the maintenance of fluid balance, nerve impulse transmissions, and muscle contractions.

Potassium and Hypertension Diets low in potassium, especially when combined with high sodium intakes, raise blood pressure and increase the risk of death from heart disease.[14] In contrast, high potassium intakes reduce the risks of hypertension, heart disease, stroke, and related deaths.[15] Unfortunately, most US adults consume too much sodium and too little potassium. Recall that the DASH eating pattern used to lower blood pressure emphasizes potassium-rich foods such as fruits and vegetables.

Potassium Deficiency Potassium deficiency is characterized by an increase in blood pressure, kidney stones, and bone turnover. As deficiency progresses, symptoms include irregular heartbeat, muscle weakness, and glucose intolerance.

Potassium Toxicity Potassium toxicity does not result from overeating foods high in potassium; therefore a UL has not been set. It can result from overconsumption of potassium salts or supplements (including some "energy fitness shakes") and

FIGURE 12-12 Potassium in Selected Foods

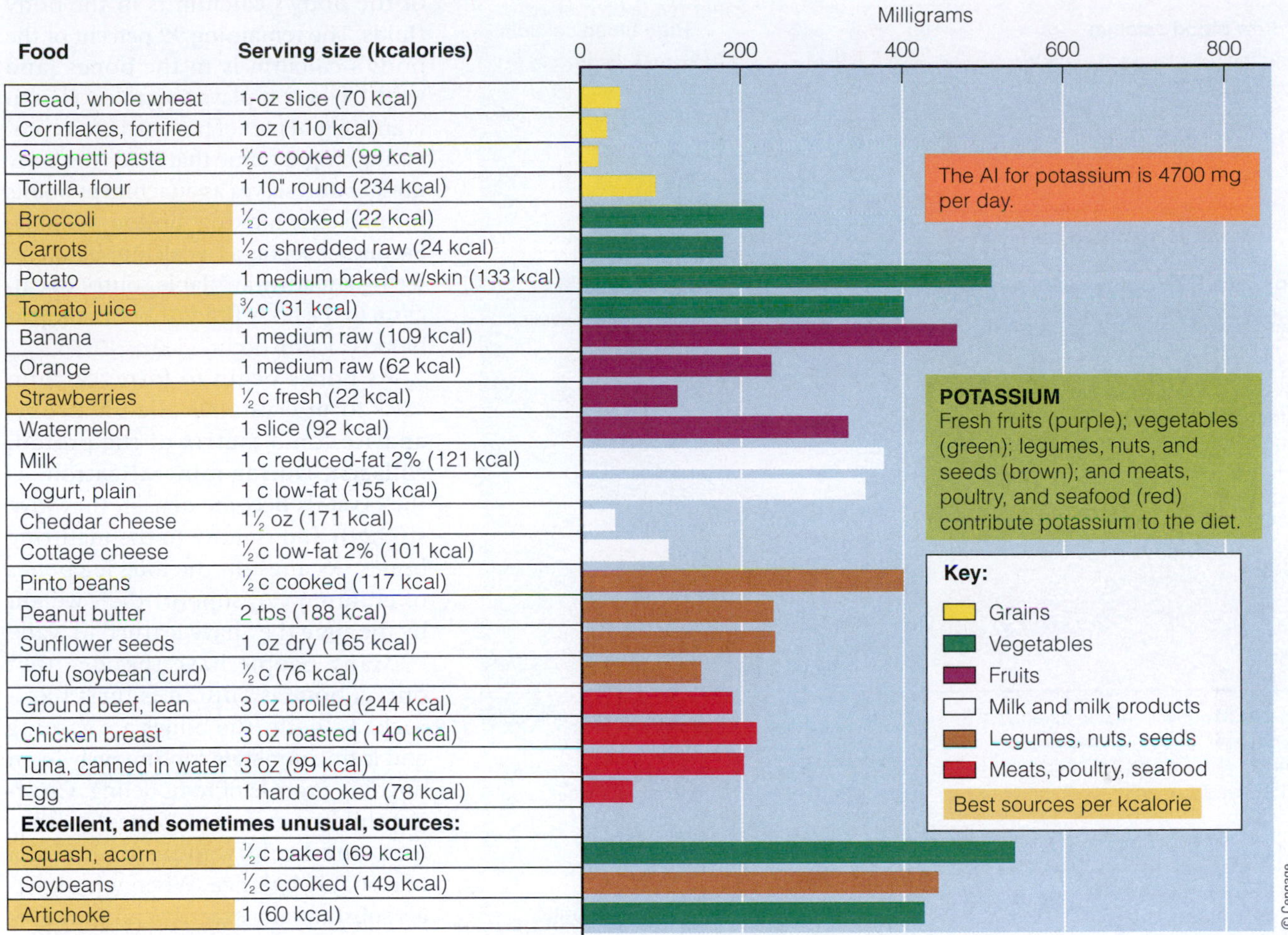
Milligrams
Food
Serving size (kcalories)
0
200
400
600
800
Bread, whole wheat 1-oz slice (70 kcal)
Cornflakes, fortified 1 oz (110 kcal)
Spaghetti pasta ½ c cooked (99 kcal)
Tortilla, flour 1 10" round (234 kcal)
Broccoli ½ c cooked (22 kcal)
Carrots ½ c shredded raw (24 kcal)
Potato 1 medium baked w/skin (133 kcal)
Tomato juice ¾ c (31 kcal)
Banana 1 medium raw (109 kcal)
Orange 1 medium raw (62 kcal)
Strawberries ½ c fresh (22 kcal)
Watermelon 1 slice (92 kcal)
Milk 1 c reduced-fat 2% (121 kcal)
Yogurt, plain 1 c low-fat (155 kcal)
Cheddar cheese 1½ oz (171 kcal)
Cottage cheese ½ c low-fat 2% (101 kcal)
Pinto beans ½ c cooked (117 kcal)
Peanut butter 2 tbs (188 kcal)
Sunflower seeds 1 oz dry (165 kcal)
Tofu (soybean curd) ½ c (76 kcal)
Ground beef, lean 3 oz broiled (244 kcal)
Chicken breast 3 oz roasted (140 kcal)
Tuna, canned in water 3 oz (99 kcal)
Egg 1 hard cooked (78 kcal)
Excellent, and sometimes unusual, sources:
Squash, acorn ½ c baked (69 kcal)
Soybeans ½ c cooked (149 kcal)
Artichoke 1 (60 kcal)
The AI for potassium is 4700 mg per day.
POTASSIUM
Fresh fruits (purple); vegetables (green); legumes, nuts, and seeds (brown); and meats, poultry, and seafood (red) contribute potassium to the diet.
Key:
Grains
Vegetables
Fruits
Milk and milk products
Legumes, nuts, seeds
Meats, poultry, seafood
Best sources per kcalorie
© Cengage

from certain diseases or treatments. Given more potassium than the body needs, the kidneys accelerate excretion. If potassium is injected directly into a vein, however, it can stop the heart.

REVIEW IT Potassium, like sodium and chloride, is an electrolyte that plays an important role in maintaining fluid balance. Potassium is the primary cation inside cells; fresh foods, notably fruits and vegetables, are its best sources. The accompanying table provides a summary of potassium.

Potassium

AI

Adults: 4700 mg/day

Chief Functions in the Body

Maintains normal fluid and electrolyte balance; facilitates many reactions; supports cell integrity; assists in nerve impulse transmission and muscle contractions

Deficiency Symptoms[a]

Irregular heatbeat, muscular weakness, glucose intolerance

Toxicity Symptoms

Muscular weakness; vomiting; if given into a vein, can stop the heart

Significant Sources

All whole foods: meats, milks, fruits, vegetables, grains, legumes

[a]Deficiency accompanies dehydration.

Calcium

Calcium is the most abundant mineral in the body. It receives much emphasis in this chapter and in the highlight that follows because an adequate intake helps grow a healthy skeleton in early life and minimize bone loss in later life.

calcium: the most abundant mineral in the body; found primarily in the body's bones and teeth.

> **FIGURE 12-13 Calcium Balance**

Low blood calcium			**High blood calcium**
Signals the parathyroid glands to secrete parathyroid hormone into the blood		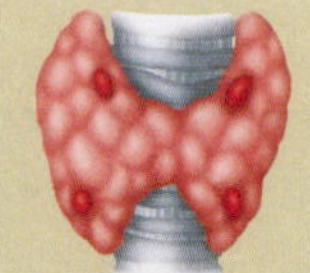 Thyroid gland with parathyroid glands embedded	Signals the thyroid gland to secrete calcitonin
Vitamin D	**Parathyroid hormone**		**Calcitonin**
	Stimulates the activation of vitamin D		Inhibits the activation of vitamin D
Stimulates calcium reabsorption from the kidneys into the blood	Stimulates calcium reabsorption from the kidneys into the blood	Kidneys	Prevents calcium reabsorption in the kidneys
Enhances calcium absorption in the intestines		Intestines	Limits calcium absorption in the intestines
Stimulates osteoclast cells to break down bone, releasing calcium into the blood	Stimulates osteoclast cells to break down bone, releasing calcium into the blood	Bones	Inhibits osteoclast cells from breaking down bone, preventing the release of calcium
End results			**End results**
Raised blood calcium	Raised blood calcium		Lower blood calcium
	Parathyroid hormone secretion inhibited		Calcitonin secretion inhibited

NOTE: Calcitonin plays a major role in defending infants and young children against the dangers of rising blood calcium that can occur when regular feedings of milk deliver large quantities of calcium to a small body. In contrast, calcitonin plays a relatively minor role in adults because their absorption of calcium is less efficient and their bodies are larger, making elevated blood calcium unlikely.

Calcium Roles in the Body Only 1 percent of the body's calcium is in the body fluids. The remaining 99 percent of the body's calcium is in the bones (and teeth), where it plays two roles. First, it is an integral part of bone structure, providing a rigid frame that holds the body upright and serves as attachment points for muscles, making motion possible. Second, it serves as a calcium bank, offering a readily available source of calcium to the body fluids should a drop in blood calcium occur.

As bones begin to form, calcium salts form crystals, called **hydroxyapatite**, on a matrix of the protein collagen. During **mineralization**, as the crystals become denser, they give strength and rigidity to the maturing bones. As a result, the long leg bones of children can support their weight by the time they have learned to walk.

Many people have the idea that once a bone is built, it is inert like a rock. Actually, the bones are gaining and losing minerals continuously in an ongoing process of remodeling. Growing children gain more bone than they lose, and healthy adults maintain a reasonable balance. When withdrawals substantially exceed deposits, problems such as osteoporosis develop (as described in Highlight 12).

The formation of teeth follows a pattern similar to that of bones. The turnover of minerals in teeth is not as rapid as in bone, however; fluoride hardens and stabilizes the crystals of teeth, opposing the withdrawal of minerals from them.

Although only 1 percent of the body's calcium circulates in the extracellular and intracellular fluids, its presence there is vital to life. Calcium in the extracellular fluids helps maintain normal blood pressure and participates in blood clotting.

The calcium in intracellular fluids binds to proteins within the cells and activates them. For example, when the protein **calmodulin** binds with calcium, it activates the enzymes involved in breaking down glycogen, which releases energy for muscle contractions. Many such proteins participate in the regulation of muscle contractions, the transmission of nerve impulses, the secretion of hormones, and the activation of some enzyme reactions.

Calcium Balance Calcium homeostasis involves a system of hormones and vitamin D. Whenever blood calcium falls too low or rises too high, three body systems respond: the intestines, bones, and kidneys. Figure 12-13 illustrates how vitamin D and two hormones—**parathyroid hormone** and **calcitonin**—return blood calcium to normal.

The calcium in bones provides a nearly inexhaustible bank of calcium for the blood. The blood borrows and returns calcium as needed so that even with an

hydroxyapatite (high-drox-ee-APP-ah-tite): crystals made of calcium and phosphorus.

mineralization: the process in which calcium, phosphorus, and other minerals crystallize on the collagen matrix of a growing bone, hardening the bone.

calmodulin (cal-MOD-you-lin): a calcium-binding protein that regulates such cell activities as muscle contractions.

parathyroid hormone: a hormone from the parathyroid glands that regulates blood calcium by raising it when levels fall too low; also known as *parathormone* (PAIR-ah-THOR-moan).

calcitonin (KAL-seh-TOE-nin): a hormone secreted by the thyroid gland that regulates blood calcium by lowering it when levels rise too high.

inadequate diet, *blood* calcium remains normal—even as *bone* calcium diminishes (see Figure 12-14). Blood calcium changes only in response to abnormal regulatory control, not to diet. A person can have an inadequate calcium intake for years and have no noticeable symptoms. Only later in life does it become apparent that bone integrity has been compromised.

Blood calcium above normal results in **calcium rigor**: the muscles contract and cannot relax. Similarly, blood calcium below normal causes **calcium tetany**—also characterized by uncontrolled muscle contraction. These conditions do *not* reflect a *dietary* excess or lack of calcium; they are caused by a lack of vitamin D or by abnormal secretion of the regulatory hormones. A chronic *dietary* deficiency of calcium, or a chronic deficiency due to poor absorption over the years, depletes the bones. Again: the *bones*, not the blood, are robbed by a calcium deficiency.

Calcium Absorption Because many factors affect calcium absorption, the most effective way to ensure adequacy is to increase calcium intake. On average, adults absorb about 30 percent of the calcium they ingest. The stomach's acidity helps keep calcium soluble, and vitamin D helps make the **calcium-binding protein** needed for absorption. This relationship explains why calcium-rich milk is a good choice for vitamin D fortification.

Whenever calcium is needed, the body increases its calcium absorption. The result is obvious in the case of a newborn infant, whose calcium absorption is 55 to 60 percent. Similarly, a pregnant woman doubles her absorption of calcium. Growing children and teens absorb up to 50 percent of the calcium they consume. Then, when bone growth slows or stops, absorption falls to the adult level of about 30 percent. In addition, absorption becomes more efficient during times of inadequate intakes.

Many of the conditions that enhance calcium absorption limit its absorption when they are absent. For example, sufficient vitamin D supports absorption, and a deficiency impairs it. In addition, fiber in general, and the binders phytate and oxalate in particular, interfere with calcium absorption, but their effects are relatively minor in typical US diets. Vegetables with oxalates and whole grains with phytates are nutritious foods, of course, but they are not useful calcium sources.

Calcium Recommendations Calcium is unlike most other nutrients in that hormones maintain its *blood* concentration regardless of dietary intake. As Figure 12-14 shows, when calcium intake is high, the *bones* benefit; when intake is low, the *bones* suffer. Calcium recommendations are therefore based on the amount needed to retain the most calcium in bones. By retaining the most calcium possible, the bones can develop to their fullest potential in size and density—their **peak bone mass**—within genetic limits.

Calcium recommendations have been set high enough to accommodate a 30 percent absorption rate. Because obtaining enough calcium during growth helps ensure that the skeleton will be strong and dense, the recommendation for adolescents to the age of 18 years is 1300 milligrams daily. Between the ages of 19 and 50, recommendations are lowered to 1000 milligrams a day; for women older than 50 and all adults older than 70, recommendations are raised again to 1200 milligrams a day to minimize the bone loss that tends to occur later in life. Almost half of the people in the United States have calcium intakes below current recommendations.[16] Those meeting recommendations for calcium are likely to be using calcium supplements. High intakes of calcium from supplements may have adverse effects such as kidney stone formation. For this reason, a UL has been established.

A high-protein diet increases urinary calcium losses, but does not seem to impair bone health. In fact, protein may even improve calcium absorption and bone strength. The DRI Committee considered these nutrient interactions in

> FIGURE 12-14 Maintaining Blood Calcium from the Diet and from the Bones

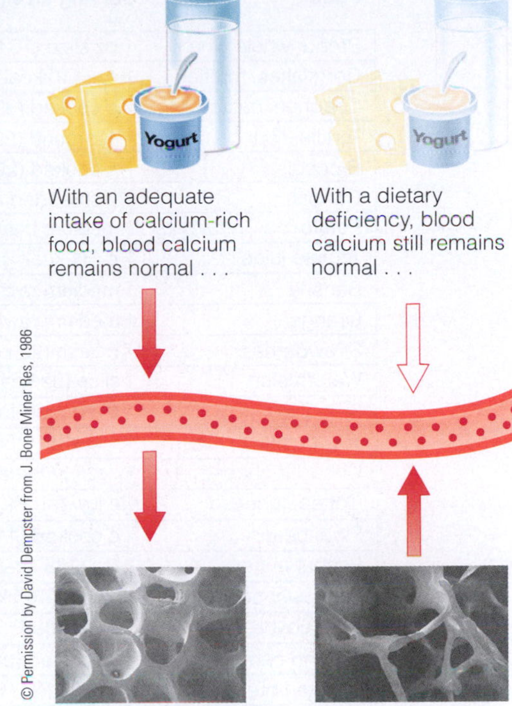
Yogurt
Yogurt
With an adequate intake of calcium-rich food, blood calcium remains normal . . .
With a dietary deficiency, blood calcium still remains normal . . .
. . . and bones deposit calcium. The result is strong, dense bones.
. . . because bones give up calcium to the blood. The result is weak, osteoporotic bones.

calcium rigor: hardness or stiffness of the muscles caused by high blood calcium concentrations.

calcium tetany (TET-ah-nee): intermittent spasm of the extremities due to nervous and muscular excitability caused by low blood calcium concentrations.

calcium-binding protein: a protein in the intestinal cells, made with the help of vitamin D, that facilitates calcium absorption.

peak bone mass: the highest attainable bone density for an individual, developed during the first three decades of life.

> FIGURE 12-15 Calcium in Selected Foods

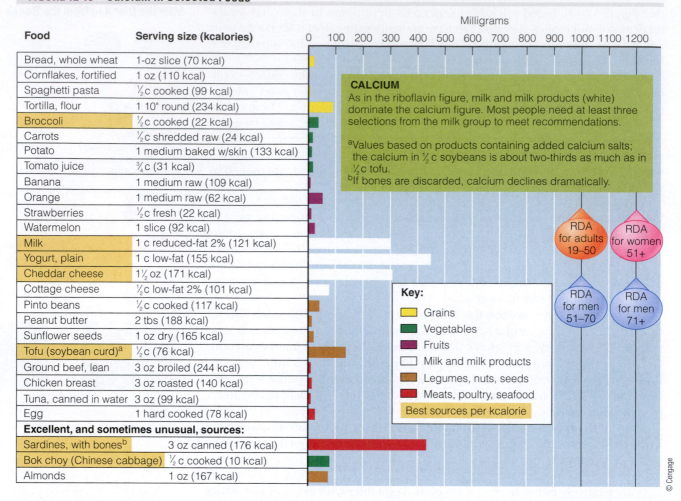

Food	Serving size (kcalories)
Bread, whole wheat	1-oz slice (70 kcal)
Cornflakes, fortified	1 oz (110 kcal)
Spaghetti pasta	½c cooked (99 kcal)
Tortilla, flour	1 10" round (234 kcal)
Broccoli	½c cooked (22 kcal)
Carrots	½c shredded raw (24 kcal)
Potato	1 medium baked w/skin (133 kcal)
Tomato juice	¾c (31 kcal)
Banana	1 medium raw (109 kcal)
Orange	1 medium raw (62 kcal)
Strawberries	½c fresh (22 kcal)
Watermelon	1 slice (92 kcal)
Milk	1 c reduced-fat 2% (121 kcal)
Yogurt, plain	1 c low-fat (155 kcal)
Cheddar cheese	1½ oz (171 kcal)
Cottage cheese	½c low-fat 2% (101 kcal)
Pinto beans	½c cooked (117 kcal)
Peanut butter	2 tbs (188 kcal)
Sunflower seeds	1 oz dry (165 kcal)
Tofu (soybean curd)[a]	½c (76 kcal)
Ground beef, lean	3 oz broiled (244 kcal)
Chicken breast	3 oz roasted (140 kcal)
Tuna, canned in water	3 oz (99 kcal)
Egg	1 hard cooked (78 kcal)
Excellent, and sometimes unusual, sources:	
Sardines, with bones[b]	3 oz canned (176 kcal)
Bok choy (Chinese cabbage)	½c cooked (10 kcal)
Almonds	1 oz (167 kcal)

Milligrams: 0, 100, 200, 300, 400, 500, 600, 700, 800, 900, 1000, 1100, 1200

RDA for adults 19–50; RDA for women 51+; RDA for men 51–70; RDA for men 71+

CALCIUM
As in the riboflavin figure, milk and milk products (white) dominate the calcium figure. Most people need at least three selections from the milk group to meet recommendations.

[a]Values based on products containing added calcium salts; the calcium in ½c soybeans is about two-thirds as much as in ½c tofu.
[b]If bones are discarded, calcium declines dramatically.

Key:
- Grains
- Vegetables
- Fruits
- Milk and milk products
- Legumes, nuts, seeds
- Meats, poultry, seafood
- Best sources per kcalorie

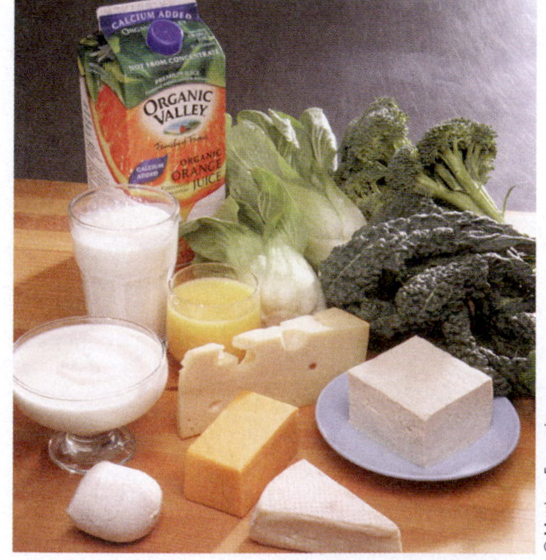
ORGANIC VALLEY
ORANGE JUICE

> **PHOTO 12-8** Milk and milk products are well known for their calcium, but calcium-set tofu, bok choy, kale, calcium-fortified orange juice, and broccoli are also rich in calcium.

establishing the RDA for calcium and did not adjust dietary recommendations based on this information.

Calcium Food Sources Figure 12-15 and Photo 12-8 show that calcium is found most abundantly in one food group—milk and milk products. The person who doesn't like to drink milk may prefer to eat cheese or yogurt. Alternatively, milk and milk products can be concealed in foods. Powdered fat-free milk can be added to casseroles, soups, and other recipes during preparation. This simple step is an excellent way to obtain not only extra calcium, but more protein, vitamins, and minerals as well.

Many people, for a variety of reasons, cannot or do not drink milk. Some cultures do not use milk in their cuisines; some vegetarians exclude milk as well as meat; and some people are allergic to milk protein or are lactose intolerant. Others simply do not enjoy the taste of milk. It is possible for people who do not drink milk to obtain adequate calcium, but only if they carefully select other calcium-rich foods. Some brands of tofu, corn tortillas, some nuts (such as almonds), and some seeds (such as sesame seeds) can supply calcium for the person who doesn't use milk products. A slice of most breads contains only about 5 to 10 percent of the calcium found in milk, but it can be a major source for people who eat many slices because the calcium is well absorbed. Oysters are also a rich source of calcium, as are small fish eaten with their bones, such as canned sardines.

Among the vegetables, mustard and turnip greens, bok choy, kale, parsley, watercress, and broccoli are good sources of available calcium. So are some seaweeds such as the nori popular in Japanese cooking. Some dark green, leafy vegetables—notably spinach and Swiss chard—appear to be calcium-rich but actually provide little, if any, calcium because they contain binders that limit absorption. It would take 8 cups of spinach—containing six times as much calcium as 1 cup of milk—to deliver the equivalent in *absorbable* calcium.

With the exception of foods, such as spinach, that contain calcium binders, the calcium content of foods is usually more important than bioavailability. Consequently, recognizing that people eat a variety of foods containing calcium, the DRI Committee did not adjust for calcium bioavailability when setting recommendations. Figure 12-16 ranks selected foods according to their calcium bioavailability.

Some mineral waters provide as much as 500 milligrams of calcium per liter, offering a convenient way to meet both calcium and water needs. Similarly, calcium-fortified orange juice and other fruit and vegetable juices allow a person to obtain both calcium and vitamins easily. Other examples of calcium-fortified foods include high-calcium milk (milk with extra calcium added) and calcium-fortified cereals. Fortified juices and foods help consumers increase calcium intakes, but depending on the calcium sources, the bioavailability may be significantly less than quantities listed on food labels. Highlight 12 discusses calcium supplements.

A generalization that has been gaining strength throughout this book is supported by the information given here about calcium. A balanced diet that supplies a variety of foods is the best plan to ensure adequacy for all essential nutrients. All food groups should be included, and none should be overemphasized. In our culture, calcium intake is usually inadequate wherever milk is lacking in the diet. By contrast, iron is usually lacking whenever milk is overemphasized, as Chapter 13 explains.

Calcium Deficiency A low calcium intake during the growing years limits the bones' ability to reach their peak bone mass. Most people achieve a peak bone mass by their late 20s, and dense bones best protect against age-related bone loss and fractures (see Figure 12-17). All adults lose bone as they grow older, beginning between the ages of 30 and 40. When bone losses reach the point of causing fractures under common, everyday stresses, the condition is known as **osteoporosis.** Osteoporosis and **osteopenia** affect an estimated 54 million people in the United States, mostly older women.[17]

Unlike many diseases that make themselves known through symptoms such as pain, shortness of breath, skin lesions, tiredness, and the like, osteoporosis is silent. The body sends no signals saying bones are losing their calcium and, as a result, their integrity. Blood samples offer no clues because blood calcium remains normal regardless of bone content, and measures of bone density are

> FIGURE 12-16 Bioavailability of Calcium from Selected Foods

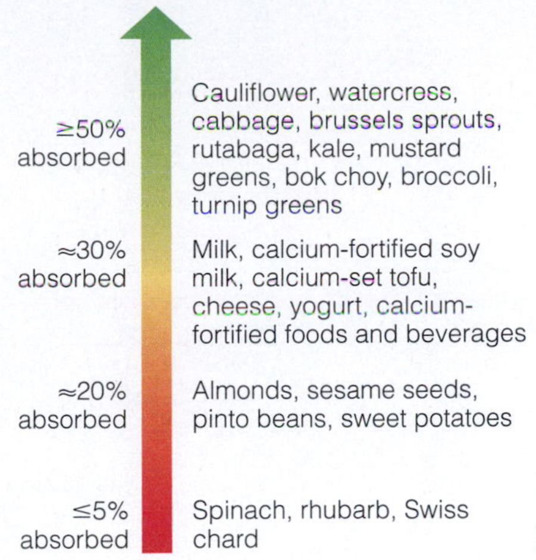
≥50% absorbed
Cauliflower, watercress, cabbage, brussels sprouts, rutabaga, kale, mustard greens, bok choy, broccoli, turnip greens
≈30% absorbed
Milk, calcium-fortified soy milk, calcium-set tofu, cheese, yogurt, calcium-fortified foods and beverages
≈20% absorbed
Almonds, sesame seeds, pinto beans, sweet potatoes
≤5% absorbed
Spinach, rhubarb, Swiss chard
© Cengage

> FIGURE 12-17 Phases of Bone Development throughout Life

The active growth phase occurs from birth to approximately age 20. The phase of peak bone mass development occurs between the ages of 12 and 30. The final phase, when bone resorption exceeds formation, begins between the ages of 30 and 40 and continues through the remainder of life.

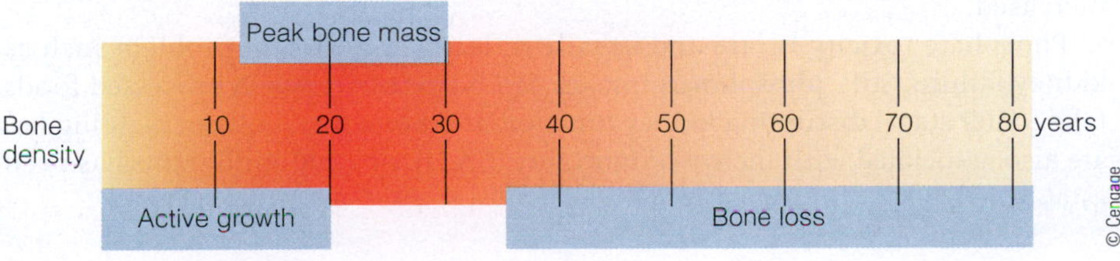
Peak bone mass
Bone density
10
20
30
40
50
60
70
80 years
Active growth
Bone loss
© Cengage

osteoporosis (OS-tee-oh-pore-OH-sis): a disease in which the bones become porous and fragile due to a loss of minerals; also called *adult bone loss.*

- **osteo** = bone
- **porosis** = porous

osteopenia (OS-tee-oh-PEE-nee-ah): a bone condition in which bone loss is significant, but not as severe as in osteoporosis.

not routinely taken until later in life. Highlight 12 suggests strategies to protect against bone loss, of which eating calcium-rich foods is only one.

REVIEW IT Most of the body's calcium is in the bones, where it provides a rigid structure and a reservoir of calcium for the blood. Blood calcium participates in muscle contraction, blood clotting, and nerve impulses, and it is closely regulated by a system of hormones and vitamin D. Calcium is found predominantly in milk and milk products. Even when calcium intake is inadequate, blood calcium remains normal, but at the expense of bone loss, which can lead to osteoporosis. The accompanying table provides a summary of calcium.

Calcium

RDA	Deficiency Symptoms
Adults: 1000 mg/day (adults, 19–50 yr) 1000 mg/day (men, 51–70 yr) 1200 mg/day (men, ≥71 yr) 1200 mg/day (women, ≥51 yr)	Stunted growth in children; bone loss (osteoporosis) in adults
UL	**Toxicity Symptoms**
Adults: 2500 mg/day (adults, 19–50 yr) 2000 mg/day (adults, ≥51 yr)	Constipation; increased risk of urinary stone formation and kidney dysfunction; interference with absorption of other minerals
Chief Functions in the Body	**Significant Sources**
Mineralization of bones and teeth; also involved in muscle contraction and relaxation, nerve functioning, blood clotting, blood pressure	Milk and milk products, small fish (with bones), calcium-set tofu (bean curd), greens (bok choy, broccoli, chard, kale), legumes

Phosphorus

Phosphorus is the second most abundant mineral in the body. About 85 percent of it is found combined with calcium in the hydroxyapatite crystals of bones and teeth.

Phosphorus Roles in the Body

Phosphorus is found not only in bones and teeth, but also in all body cells as part of a major buffer system. Phosphorus is also part of DNA and RNA and is therefore necessary for all growth.

Phosphorus assists in energy metabolism. The high-energy compound ATP uses three phosphate groups to do its work. Many enzymes and the B vitamins become active only when a phosphate group is attached.

Phospholipids provide stability to the lipoprotein vehicles that help transport lipids in the blood. Phospholipids are also the major structural components of cell membranes, where they control the transport of nutrients into and out of the cells. Some proteins, such as the casein in milk, contain phosphorus as part of their structures (phosphoproteins).

Phosphorus Recommendations and Intakes

Because phosphorus is commonly found in almost all foods, dietary deficiencies are unlikely. As Figure 12-18 shows, foods rich in proteins—such as meat, poultry, fish, milk, and cheese—are the best sources of phosphorus. Many processed foods and soft drinks contain phosphate-based additives, and phosphorus intakes in the United States have increased as consumption of processed foods and beverages has increased.

Phosphate toxicity is rare and usually reflects a significant problem such as kidney failure. Still, phosphorus intakes can be excessive when processed foods take center stage, disrupting kidney function and bone metabolism; high intakes are also associated with increased mortality.[18] A UL of 4000 milligrams has been established.

phosphorus: a major mineral found mostly in the body's bones and teeth.

> **FIGURE 12-18** Phosphorus in Selected Foods

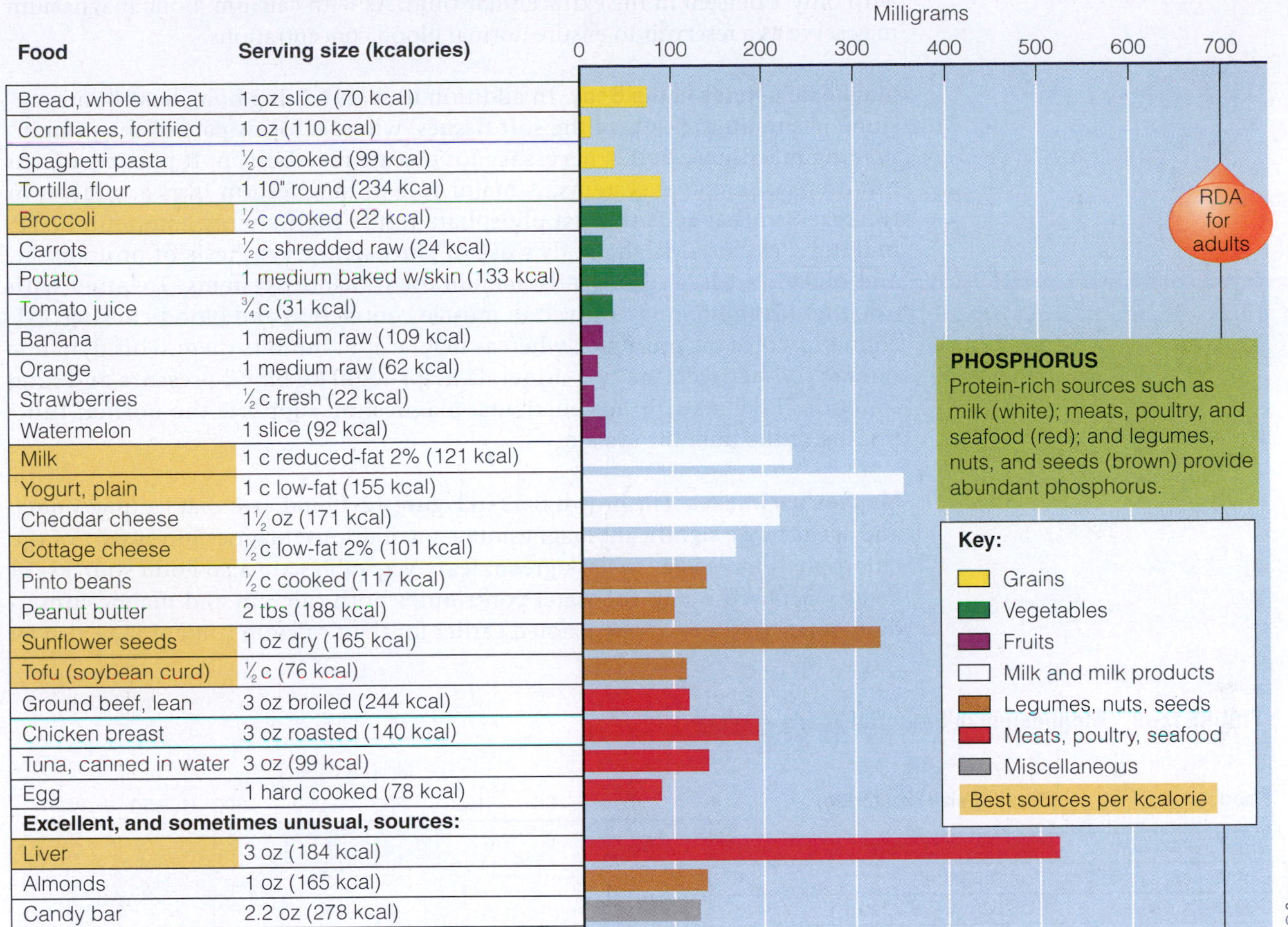

Milligrams
Food
Serving size (kcalories)
0
100
200
300
400
500
600
700
Bread, whole wheat
1-oz slice (70 kcal)
Cornflakes, fortified
1 oz (110 kcal)
Spaghetti pasta
½ c cooked (99 kcal)
Tortilla, flour
1 10" round (234 kcal)
Broccoli
½ c cooked (22 kcal)
Carrots
½ c shredded raw (24 kcal)
Potato
1 medium baked w/skin (133 kcal)
Tomato juice
¾ c (31 kcal)
Banana
1 medium raw (109 kcal)
Orange
1 medium raw (62 kcal)
Strawberries
½ c fresh (22 kcal)
Watermelon
1 slice (92 kcal)
Milk
1 c reduced-fat 2% (121 kcal)
Yogurt, plain
1 c low-fat (155 kcal)
Cheddar cheese
1½ oz (171 kcal)
Cottage cheese
½ c low-fat 2% (101 kcal)
Pinto beans
½ c cooked (117 kcal)
Peanut butter
2 tbs (188 kcal)
Sunflower seeds
1 oz dry (165 kcal)
Tofu (soybean curd)
½ c (76 kcal)
Ground beef, lean
3 oz broiled (244 kcal)
Chicken breast
3 oz roasted (140 kcal)
Tuna, canned in water
3 oz (99 kcal)
Egg
1 hard cooked (78 kcal)
Excellent, and sometimes unusual, sources:
Liver
3 oz (184 kcal)
Almonds
1 oz (165 kcal)
Candy bar
2.2 oz (278 kcal)
RDA for adults
PHOSPHORUS
Protein-rich sources such as milk (white); meats, poultry, and seafood (red); and legumes, nuts, and seeds (brown) provide abundant phosphorus.
Key:
Grains
Vegetables
Fruits
Milk and milk products
Legumes, nuts, seeds
Meats, poultry, seafood
Miscellaneous
Best sources per kcalorie

REVIEW IT Phosphorus accompanies calcium both in the crystals of bone and in many foods such as milk. Phosphorus is also important in energy metabolism as part of ATP, in lipid structures as part of phospholipids, and in genetic materials as part of DNA and RNA. The accompanying table provides a summary of phosphorus.

Phosphorus

RDA	Deficiency Symptoms
Adults: 700 mg/day	Muscular weakness, bone pain[a]
UL	**Toxicity Symptoms**
Adults (19–70 yr): 4000 mg/day	Calcification of nonskeletal tissues, particularly the kidneys
Chief Functions in the Body	**Significant Sources**
Mineralization of bones and teeth; part of every cell; important in genetic material, part of phospholipids, used in energy transfer and in buffer systems that maintain acid-base balance	Foods derived from animals (meat, fish, poultry, eggs, milk)

[a]Dietary deficiency rarely occurs, but some drugs can bind with phosphorus, making it unavailable and resulting in bone loss that is characterized by weakness and pain.

Magnesium

Only about 1 ounce of **magnesium** is present in the body of a 132-pound person (review Figure 12-10, p. 369). More than half of the body's

magnesium: a cation within the body's cells, active in many enzyme systems.

magnesium is in the bones. Much of the rest is in the muscles and soft tissues, with only 1 percent in the extracellular fluid. As with calcium, bone magnesium may serve as a reservoir to ensure normal blood concentrations.

Magnesium Roles in the Body In addition to maintaining bone health, magnesium acts in all the cells of the soft tissues, where it forms part of the protein-making machinery and is necessary for energy metabolism. It participates in hundreds of enzyme systems. A major role of magnesium is as a catalyst in the reaction that adds the last phosphate to the high-energy compound ATP, making it essential to the body's use of glucose; the synthesis of protein, fat, and nucleic acids; and the cells' membrane transport systems. Together with calcium, magnesium is involved in muscle contraction and blood clotting: calcium promotes the processes, whereas magnesium inhibits them. This dynamic interaction between the two minerals helps regulate blood pressure and lung function. Like many other nutrients, magnesium supports the normal functioning of the immune system.

Magnesium Intakes The brown bars in Figure 12-19 indicate that legumes, nuts, and seeds make significant magnesium contributions. Magnesium is part of the chlorophyll molecule, so dark green, leafy vegetables are also good sources. In areas with hard water, the water contributes both calcium and magnesium to daily intakes. Mineral waters noted earlier for their calcium content may also be

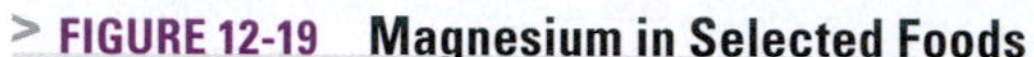

> FIGURE 12-19 Magnesium in Selected Foods

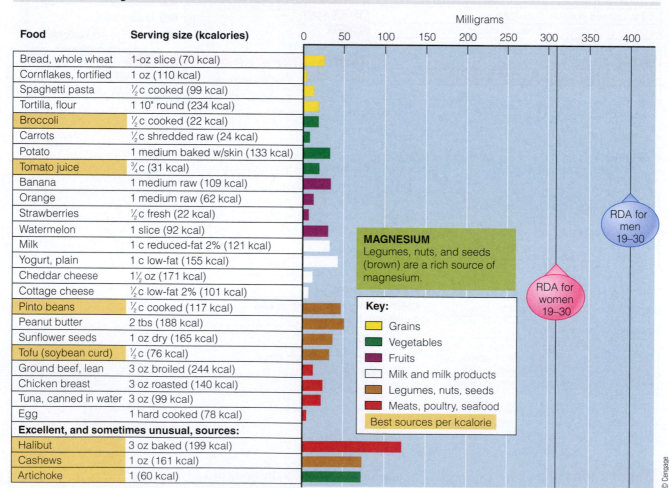

Food	Serving size (kcalories)
Bread, whole wheat	1-oz slice (70 kcal)
Cornflakes, fortified	1 oz (110 kcal)
Spaghetti pasta	½ c cooked (99 kcal)
Tortilla, flour	1 10" round (234 kcal)
Broccoli	½ c cooked (22 kcal)
Carrots	½ c shredded raw (24 kcal)
Potato	1 medium baked w/skin (133 kcal)
Tomato juice	¾ c (31 kcal)
Banana	1 medium raw (109 kcal)
Orange	1 medium raw (62 kcal)
Strawberries	½ c fresh (22 kcal)
Watermelon	1 slice (92 kcal)
Milk	1 c reduced-fat 2% (121 kcal)
Yogurt, plain	1 c low-fat (155 kcal)
Cheddar cheese	1½ oz (171 kcal)
Cottage cheese	½ c low-fat 2% (101 kcal)
Pinto beans	½ c cooked (117 kcal)
Peanut butter	2 tbs (188 kcal)
Sunflower seeds	1 oz dry (165 kcal)
Tofu (soybean curd)	½ c (76 kcal)
Ground beef, lean	3 oz broiled (244 kcal)
Chicken breast	3 oz roasted (140 kcal)
Tuna, canned in water	3 oz (99 kcal)
Egg	1 hard cooked (78 kcal)
Excellent, and sometimes unusual, sources:	
Halibut	3 oz baked (199 kcal)
Cashews	1 oz (161 kcal)
Artichoke	1 (60 kcal)

Milligrams
0 50 100 150 200 250 300 350 400
MAGNESIUM
Legumes, nuts, and seeds (brown) are a rich source of magnesium.
Key:
Grains
Vegetables
Fruits
Milk and milk products
Legumes, nuts, seeds
Meats, poultry, seafood
Best sources per kcalorie
RDA for women 19–30
RDA for men 19–30

magnesium-rich and can be important sources of this mineral for those who drink them. Bioavailability of magnesium from mineral water is about 50 percent, but it improves when the water is consumed with a meal.

Magnesium Deficiency Average magnesium intakes typically fall below recommendations, which may exacerbate inflammation and contribute to chronic diseases such as heart disease, stroke, hypertension, diabetes, and cancer.[19] A severe magnesium deficiency causes a tetany similar to the calcium tetany described earlier. Magnesium deficiencies also impair central nervous system activity and may be responsible for the hallucinations experienced during alcohol withdrawal.

Magnesium and Hypertension Magnesium is critical to heart function and seems to protect against hypertension and support heart health.[20] Interestingly, people living in areas of the country with hard water, which contains high concentrations of calcium and magnesium, tend to have low rates of heart disease. With magnesium deficiency, the walls of the arteries and capillaries tend to constrict—a possible explanation for the hypertensive effect.

Magnesium Toxicity Magnesium toxicity is rare, but it can be fatal. The UL for magnesium applies only to nonfood sources such as supplements or magnesium salts.

REVIEW IT Like calcium and phosphorus, magnesium supports bone mineralization. Magnesium is also involved in numerous enzyme systems and in heart function. It is found abundantly in legumes and dark green, leafy vegetables and, in some areas, in water. The accompanying table offers a summary of magnesium.

Magnesium

RDA	Deficiency Symptoms
Men (19–30 yr): 400 mg/day Women (19–30 yr): 310 mg/day	Weakness; confusion; if extreme, convulsions, bizarre muscle movements (especially of eye and face muscles), hallucinations, and difficulty in swallowing; in children, growth failure[a]
UL	**Toxicity Symptoms**
Adults: 350 mg nonfood magnesium/day	From nonfood sources only; diarrhea, alkalosis, dehydration
Chief Functions in the Body	**Significant Sources**
Bone mineralization, building of protein, enzyme action, normal muscle contraction, nerve impulse transmission, maintenance of teeth, and functioning of immune system	Nuts, legumes, whole grains, dark green vegetables, seafood, chocolate, cocoa

[a]A still more severe deficiency causes tetany, an extreme, prolonged contraction of the muscles similar to that caused by low blood calcium.

Sulfate

Sulfate is the oxidized form of the mineral **sulfur,** as it exists in foods and water. The body's need for sulfate is easily met by a variety of foods and beverages. In addition, the body receives sulfate from the amino acids methionine and cysteine, which are found in dietary proteins. These sulfur-containing amino acids help determine the contour of protein molecules. The sulfur-containing side chains in cysteine molecules can link to each other via disulfide bridges, which stabilize the protein structure. (See the drawing of insulin with its disulfide bridges in Figure 6-4, p. 171.) Skin, hair, and nails contain some of the body's more rigid proteins, which have a high sulfur content.

Because the body's sulfate needs are easily met with normal protein intakes, there is no recommended intake for sulfate. Deficiencies do not occur when diets contain protein. Only when people lack protein to the point of severe deficiency will they lack the sulfur-containing amino acids.

sulfate: a salt produced from the oxidation of sulfur.

sulfur: a mineral present in the body as part of some proteins.

REVIEW IT Identify the main roles, deficiency symptoms, and food sources for each of the major minerals (sodium, chloride, potassium, calcium, phosphorus, magnesium, and sulfate).

Like the other nutrients, minerals' actions are coordinated to get the body's work done. The major minerals, especially sodium, chloride, and potassium, influence the body's fluid balance; whenever an anion moves, a cation moves—always maintaining homeostasis. Sodium, chloride, potassium, calcium, and magnesium are key members of the team of nutrients that direct nerve impulse transmission and muscle contraction. They are also the primary nutrients involved in regulating blood pressure. Phosphorus and magnesium participate in many reactions involving glucose, fatty acids, amino acids, and the vitamins. Calcium, phosphorus, and magnesium combine to form the structure of the bones and teeth. Each major mineral also plays other specific roles in the body. The accompanying table provides a summary of the major minerals.

REVIEW IT The Major Minerals

Chief Functions	Deficiency Symptoms	Toxicity Symptoms	Significant Sources
Sodium			
Maintains normal fluid and electrolyte balance; assists in nerve impulse transmission and muscle contraction	Muscle cramps, mental apathy, loss of appetite	Edema, acute hypertension	Table salt, soy sauce; moderate amounts in meats, milks, breads, and vegetables; large amounts in processed foods
Chloride			
Maintains normal fluid and electrolyte balance; part of hydrochloric acid found in the stomach, necessary for proper digestion	Do not occur under normal circumstances	Vomiting	Table salt, soy sauce; moderate amounts in meats, milks, eggs; large amounts in processed foods
Potassium			
Maintains normal fluid and electrolyte balance; facilitates many reactions; supports cell integrity; assists in nerve impulse transmission and muscle contractions	Irregular heartbeat, muscular weakness, glucose intolerance	Muscular weakness; vomiting; if injected into a vein, can stop the heart	All whole foods; meats, milks, fruits, vegetables, grains, legumes
Calcium			
Mineralization of bones and teeth; also involved in muscle contraction and relaxation, nerve functioning, blood clotting, and blood pressure	Stunted growth in children; bone loss (osteoporosis) in adults	Constipation; increased risk of urinary stone formation and kidney dysfunction; interference with absorption of other minerals	Milk and milk products, small fish (with bones), tofu, greens (bok choy, broccoli, chard), legumes
Phosphorus			
Mineralization of bones and teeth; part of every cell; important in genetic material, part of phospholipids, used in energy transfer and in buffer systems that maintain acid–base balance	Muscular weakness, bone pain[a]	Calcification of nonskeletal tissues, particularly the kidneys	All animal tissues (meat, fish, poultry, eggs, milk)
Magnesium			
Bone mineralization, building of protein, enzyme action, normal muscle contraction, nerve impulse transmission, maintenance of teeth, and functioning of immune system	Weakness; confusion; if extreme, convulsions, bizarre muscle movements (especially of eye and face muscles), hallucinations, and difficulty in swallowing; in children, growth failure[b]	From nonfood sources only; diarrhea, alkalosis, dehydration	Nuts, legumes, whole grains, dark green vegetables, seafood, chocolate, cocoa
Sulfate			
As part of proteins, stabilizes their shape by forming disulfide bridges; part of the vitamins biotin and thiamin and the hormone insulin	None known; protein deficiency would occur first	Toxicity would occur only if sulfur-containing amino acids were eaten in excess; this (in animals) suppresses growth	All protein-containing foods (meats, fish, poultry, eggs, milk, legumes, nuts)

[a]Dietary deficiency rarely occurs, but some drugs can bind with phosphorus, making it unavailable and resulting in bone loss that is characterized by weakness and pain.
[b]A still more severe deficiency causes tetany, an extreme, prolonged contraction of the muscles similar to that caused by low blood calcium.

With all of the tasks these minerals perform, they are of great importance to life. Consuming enough of each of them every day is easy, given a variety of foods from each of the food groups. Whole-grain breads supply magnesium; fruits, vegetables, and legumes provide magnesium and potassium too; milk products offer calcium and phosphorus; meats, poultry, and seafood offer phosphorus and sulfate as well; all foods provide sodium and chloride, with excesses being more problematic than inadequacies. The message is quite simple and has been repeated throughout this text: for an adequate intake of all the nutrients, including the major minerals, choose a variety of foods from each of the five food groups. And drink plenty of water.

What's Online

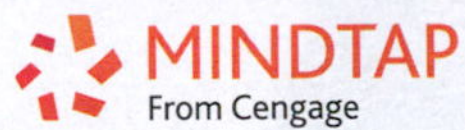
MINDTAP
From Cengage

Visit **www.cengagebrain.com** to access MindTap, a complete digital course that includes Diet & Wellness Plus, interactive quizzes, videos, and more.

REFERENCES

1. Daily water intake among US men and women, 2009-2012, NCHS Data Brief No. 242, April 2016.
2. R. H. Sterns, Disorders of plasma sodium: Causes, consequences, and correction, *New England Journal of Medicine* 372 (2015): 55–65.
3. T. A. Kotchen, A. W. Cowley, and E. D. Frohlich, Salt in health and disease: A delicate balance, *New England Journal of Medicine* 368 (2013): 1229–1237.
4. Prevalence of excess sodium intake in the United States: NHANES, 2009–2012, *Morbidity and Mortality Weekly Report* 64 (2016): 1393–1397.
5. F. J. He, J. Li, and G. A. Macgregor, Effect of longer-term modest salt reduction on blood pressure, *Cochrane Database of Systematic Reviews* 4 (2013): CD004937; Salt restriction, *Journal of the American Medical Association* 311 (2014): 2229.
6. US Department of Health and Human Services and US Department of Agriculture, *2015-2020 Dietary Guidelines for Americans*, 8th ed. (2015), www.health.gov/dietaryguidelines/2015/guidelines.
7. J. Merino and coauthors, Is complying with the recommendations of sodium intake beneficial for health in individuals at high cardiovascular risk? Findings from the PREDIMED Study, *American Journal of Clinical Nutrition* 101 (2015): 440–448; N. R. Cook, L. J. Appel, and P. K. Whelton, Lower levels of sodium intake and reduced cardiovascular risk, *Circulation* 129 (2014): 981–989.
8. B. M. Davy, T. M. Halliday, and K. P. Davy, Sodium intake and blood pressure: New controversies, new labels . . . new guidelines? *Journal of the Academy of Nutrition and Dietetics* 115 (2015): 200–203; S. Oparil, Low sodium intake: Cardiovascular health benefit or risk? *New England Journal of Medicine* 371 (2014): 677–679; M. O'Donnell and coauthors, Urinary sodium and potassium excretion, mortality, and cardiovascular events, *New England Journal of Medicine* 371 (2014): 612–623.
9. C. A. M. Anderson and coauthors, Effects of a behavioral intervention that emphasizes spices and herbs on adherence to recommended sodium intake: Results of the SPICE randomized clinical trial, *American Journal of Clinical Nutrition* 102 (2015): 671–679.
10. P. M Guenther, J. M. G. Lyon, and L. J. Appel, Modeling dietary patterns to assess sodium recommendations for nutrient adequacy, *American Journal of Clinical Nutrition* 97 (2013): 842–847.
11. M. A. H. Hendriksen and coauthors, Potential effect of salt reduction in processed foods on health, *American Journal of Clinical Nutrition* 99 (2014): 446–453.
12. A. Rudelt, S. French, and L. Harnack, Fourteen-year trends in sodium content of menu offerings at eight leading fast-food restaurants in the USA, *Public Health Nutrition* 17 (2014): 1682–1688; H. W. Wu and R. Sturm, Changes in the energy and sodium content of main entrées in US chain restaurants from 2010 to 2011, *Journal of the Academy of Nutrition and Dietetics* 114 (2014): 209–219; M. F. Jacobson, S. Havas, and R. McCarter, Changes in sodium levels in processed and restaurant foods, 2005-2011, *JAMA Internal Medicine* 173 (2013): 1285–1291.
13. N. R. Cook, L. J. Appel, and P. K. Whelton, Sodium intake and all-cause mortality over 20 years in the trials of hypertension prevention, *Journal of the American College of Cardiology* 68 (2016): 1609–1617; W. B. Farquhar and coauthors, Dietary sodium and health: More than just blood pressure, *Journal of the American College of Cardiology* 65 (2015): 1042–105; D. Mozaffarian and coauthors, Global sodium consumption and death from cardiovascular causes, *New England Journal of Medicine* 371 (2014): 624–634; K. J. Aaron and P. W. Sanders, Role of dietary salt and potassium intake in cardiovascular health and disease: A review of the evidence, *Mayo Clinical Proceedings* 88 (2013): 987–995.
14. Z. Zhang and coauthors, Association between usual sodium and potassium intake and blood pressure and hypertension among U.S. adults: NHANES 2005-2010, *PLoS One* 8 (2013): e75289.
15. A. Seth and coauthors, Potassium intake and risk of stroke in women with hypertension and nonhypertension in the Women's Health Initiative, *Stroke* 45 (2014): 2874–2880; K. J. Aaron and P. W. Sanders, Role of dietary salt and potassium intake in cardiovascular health and disease: A review of the evidence, *Mayo Clinic Proceedings* 88 (2013): 987–995; N. J. Aburto and coauthors, Effect of increased potassium intake on cardiovascular risk factors and disease: Systematic review and meta-analyses, *British Medical Journal* 346 (2013): f1387.
16. M. K. Hoy and J. D. Goldman, Calcium intake of the U. S. population: *What We Eat in America*, NHANES 2009-2010, September 2014.
17. National Osteoporosis Foundation, www.nof.org, January 2017.
18. A. R. Chang and coauthors, High dietary phosphorus intake is associated with all-cause mortality: Results from NHANES III, *American Journal of Clinical Nutrition* 99 (2014): 320–327; E. Takeda and coauthors, Increasing dietary phosphorus intake from food additives: Potential for negative impact on bone health, *Advances in Nutrition* 5 (2014): 92–97; M. S. Calvo and K. L. Tucker, Is phosphorus intake that exceeds dietary requirements a risk factor in bone health? *Annals of the New York Academy of Sciences* 1301 (2013): 29–35.
19. M. M. Joosten and coauthors, Urinary and plasma magnesium and risk of ischemic heart disease, *American Journal of Clinical Nutrition* 97 (2013): 1299–1306; L. C. Del Gobbo and coauthors, Circulating and dietary magnesium and risk of cardiovascular disease: A systematic review and meta-analysis of prospective studies, *American Journal of Clinical Nutrition* 98 (2013): 160–173.
20. X. Zhang and coauthors, Effects of magnesium supplementation on blood pressure: A meta-analysis of randomized double-blind placebo-controlled trials, *Hypertension* 68 (2016): 324–333; P. J. Joris and coauthors, Long-term magnesium supplementation improves arterial stiffness in overweight and obese adults: Results of a randomized, double-blind placebo-controlled intervention trial, *American Journal of Clinical Nutrition* 103 (2016): 1260–1266.

HIGHLIGHT > 12

LEARN IT Describe factors that contribute to the development of osteoporosis and strategies to prevent it.

Osteoporosis and Calcium

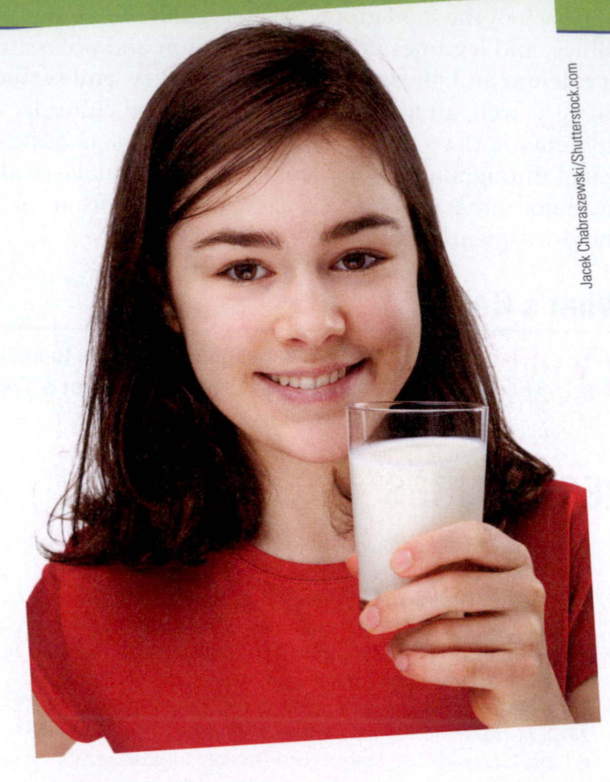

Jacek Chabraszewski/Shutterstock.com

Osteoporosis becomes apparent during the later years, but it develops much earlier—and without warning. Few people are aware that their bones are being robbed of their strength. The problem often first becomes evident when someone's hip suddenly gives way. People say, "She fell and broke her hip," but in fact the hip may have been so fragile that it broke *before* she fell. Even bumping into a table may be enough to shatter a porous bone into fragments so numerous and scattered that they cannot be reassembled. Removing them and replacing them with an artificial joint requires major surgery. An estimated 300,000 people in the United States are hospitalized each year because of hip fractures related to osteoporosis. About one in five die of complications within a year; one in three will never walk or live independently again.[1] Their quality of life slips downward.[2]

This highlight examines low bone density and osteoporosis, one of the most prevalent diseases of aging, affecting more than 53 million people in the United States—most of them women older than 50.[3] It reviews the many factors that contribute to the 2 million fractures in the bones of the hips, vertebrae, wrists, arms, and ankles each year. And it presents strategies to reduce the risks, paying special attention to the role of dietary calcium.

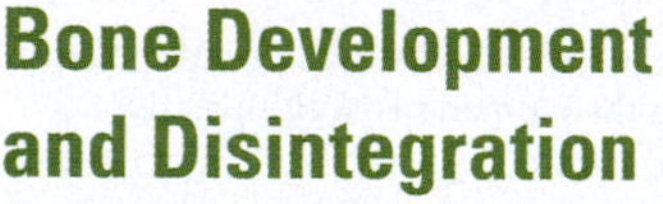

Bone Development and Disintegration

Bone has two compartments: the outer, hard shell of **cortical bone** and the inner, lacy matrix of **trabecular bone**. (Glossary H12-1 defines these and other related terms.) Both types of bone can lose minerals, but in different ways and at different rates. The first photograph in Figure H12-1 shows a human leg bone sliced lengthwise, exposing the lacy, calcium-containing crystals of trabecular bone. These crystals give up calcium to the blood when the diet runs short, and they take up calcium again when the supply is plentiful (review Figure 12-14, p. 377). For people who have eaten calcium-rich foods throughout the bone-forming years of their youth, these deposits make bones dense and provide a rich reservoir of calcium.

A close look at the first photograph in Figure H12-1 reveals that protecting the trabecular bone is a dense, ivorylike exterior shell—the cortical bone. Cortical bone composes the shafts of the long bones, and a thin cortical shell caps the ends of the bones too. Both compartments confer strength on bone: cortical bone provides the sturdy outer wall, and trabecular bone provides support along the lines of stress.

The two types of bone handle calcium in different ways. Supplied with blood vessels and metabolically active, trabecular bone is sensitive to hormones that govern day-to-day deposits and withdrawals of calcium. It readily gives up minerals whenever blood calcium needs replenishing. Losses of trabecular bone start becoming significant for men and women in their 30s, although losses can occur whenever calcium withdrawals exceed deposits. Cortical bone also gives up calcium, but slowly and at a steady pace. Cortical bone losses typically begin at about age 40 and continue slowly but surely thereafter.

As bone loss continues, **bone density** declines, and osteoporosis becomes apparent (see Figure H12-1). Bones become so

GLOSSARY H12-1

antacids: medications used to relieve indigestion by neutralizing acid in the stomach.

bone density: a measure of bone strength. When minerals fill the bone matrix (making it dense), they give it strength.

bone meal or **powdered bone:** crushed or ground bone preparations intended to supply calcium to the diet. Calcium from bone is not well absorbed and is often contaminated with toxic minerals such as arsenic, mercury, lead, and cadmium.

cortical bone: the very dense bone tissue that forms the outer shell surrounding trabecular bone and comprises the shaft of a long bone.

dolomite: a compound of minerals (calcium magnesium carbonate) found in limestone and marble. Dolomite is powdered and is sold as a calcium-magnesium supplement. However, it may be contaminated with toxic minerals, is not well absorbed, and interferes with absorption of other essential minerals.

osteoporosis (OS-tee-oh-pore-OH-sis)**:** a disease in which the bones become porous and fragile due to loss of minerals; also called *adult bone loss*.

oyster shell: a product made from the powdered shells of oysters that is sold as a calcium supplement, but it is not well absorbed by the digestive system.

trabecular (tra-BECK-you-lar) **bone:** the lacy inner structure of calcium crystals that supports the bone's structure and provides a calcium storage bank.

> **FIGURE H12-1 Healthy and Osteoporotic Trabecular Bones**

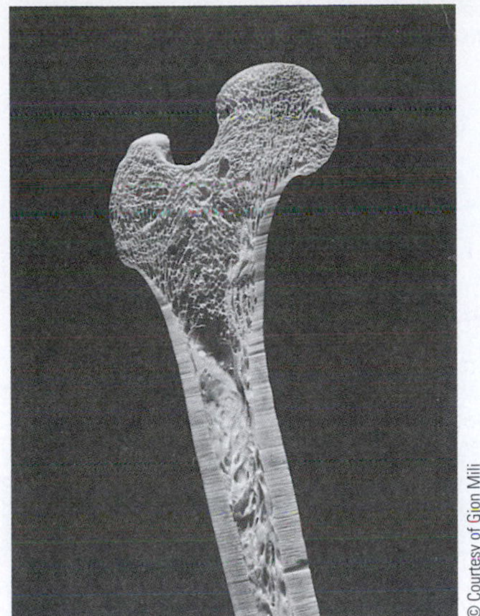

© Courtesy of Gjon Mili

Trabecular bone is the lacy network of calcium-containing crystals that fills the interior. Cortical bone is the dense, ivorylike bone that forms the exterior shell.

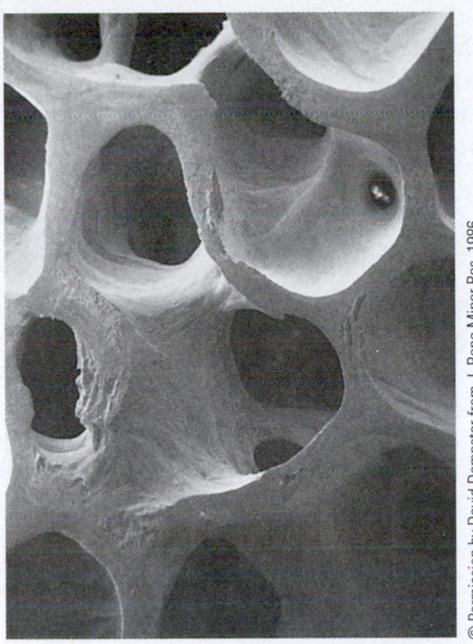

© Permission by David Dempster from J. Bone Miner Res, 1986

Electron micrograph of healthy trabecular bone.

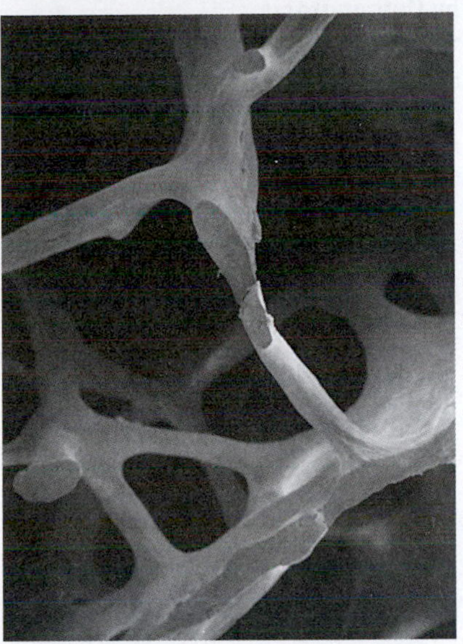

© Permission by David Dempster from J. Bone Miner Res, 1986

Electron micrograph of trabecular bone affected by osteoporosis.

fragile that even the body's own weight can overburden the spine—vertebrae may suddenly disintegrate and crush down, painfully pinching major nerves. Or the vertebrae may compress into wedge shapes, forming what is often called a "dowager's hump," the posture many older people assume as they "grow shorter." Figure H12-2 (p. 388) shows the effect of compressed spinal bone on a woman's height and posture. Because both the cortical shell and the trabecular interior weaken, breaks most often occur in the hip, as mentioned in the opening paragraph.

Physicians can determine bone loss and diagnose osteoporosis by measuring bone density using dual-energy X-ray absorptiometry (DEXA) scanning (see Photo H12-1). They also consider risk factors for osteoporosis, including age, personal and family history of fractures, and physical inactivity. Table H12-1 (p. 388) summarizes the major risk factors for osteoporosis. The more risk factors that apply to a person, the greater the chances of bone loss. Notice that several risk factors that are influential in the development of osteoporosis—such as age, gender, and genetics—cannot be changed. Other risk factors—such as diet, physical activity, body weight, smoking, and alcohol use—are personal behaviors that can be changed. By eating a calcium-rich, well-balanced diet; being physically active; abstaining from smoking; and drinking alcohol in moderation (if at all), people can defend themselves against osteoporosis. These decisions are particularly important for those with other risk factors that cannot be changed.

Whether a person develops osteoporosis seems to depend on the interactions of several factors, including nutrition. The strongest predictor of bone density is age.

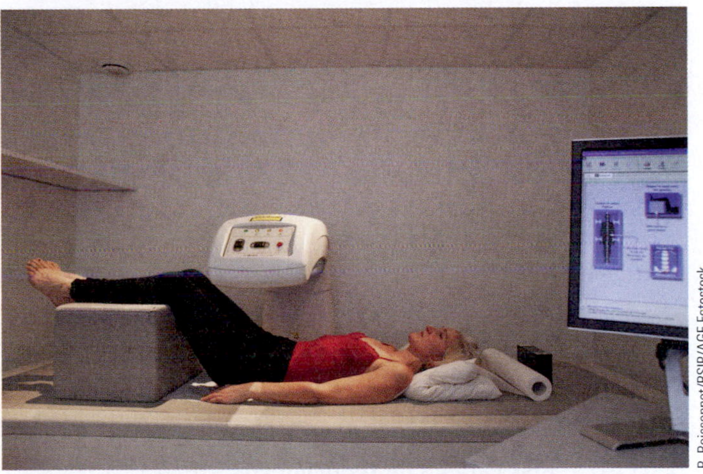

B. Boissonnet/BSIP/AGE Fotostock

> **PHOTO H12-1** Using a DEXA (dual-energy X-ray absorpiometry) test to measure bone mineral density identifies osteoporosis, determines risks for fractures, and tracks responses to treatment.

Age and Bone Calcium

Two major stages of life are critical in the development of osteoporosis. The first is the bone-acquiring stage of childhood and adolescence. The second is the bone-losing decades of late adulthood, especially in women after menopause. The bones gain strength and density all through the growing years and into young adulthood. As people age, the cells that build bone gradually become less active, but those that

> **FIGURE H12-2 Loss of Height in a Woman Caused by Osteoporosis**

The woman on the left is about 50 years old. On the right, she is 80 years old. Her legs have not grown shorter. Instead, her back has lost length due to collapse of her spinal bones (vertebrae). Collapsed vertebrae cannot protect the spinal nerves from pressure that causes excruciating pain.

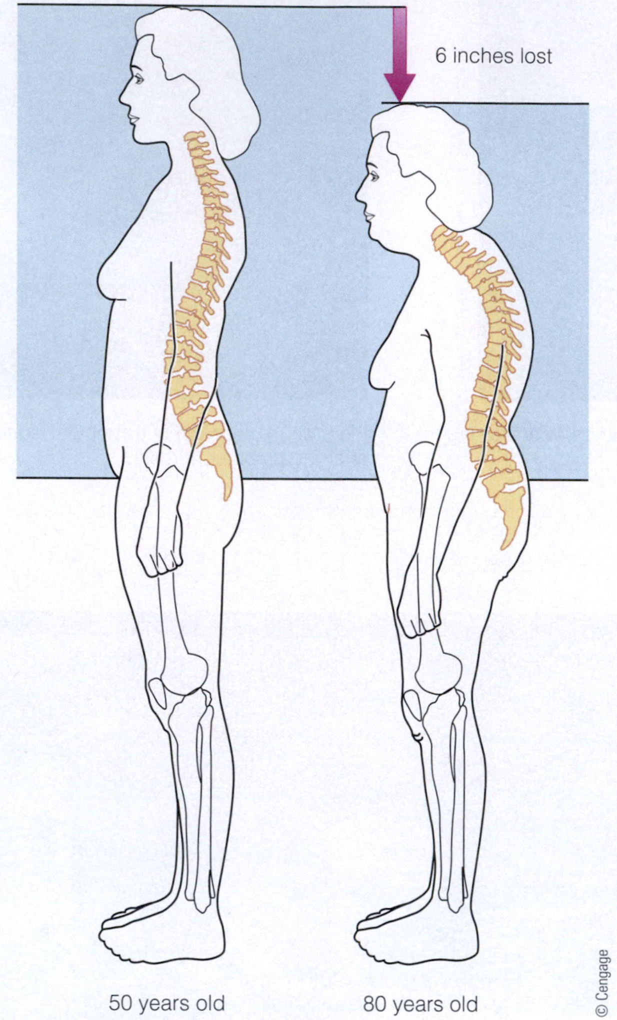
6 inches lost
50 years old
80 years old
© Cengage

TABLE H12-1 Risk Factors for Osteoporosis

Nonmodifiable	Modifiable
• Female gender • Older age (>50 yr) • Small frame • Caucasian, Asian, or Hispanic/Latino • Family history of osteoporosis or fractures • Personal history of fractures • Estrogen deficiency in women (amenorrhea or menopause, especially early or surgically induced); testosterone deficiency in men	• Sedentary lifestyle • Diet inadequate in calcium and vitamin D • Diet excessive in protein, sodium, caffeine • Cigarette smoking • Alcohol abuse • Low body weight • Certain medications, such as glucocorticoids, aluminum-containing antacids, and antiseizure drugs

> **FIGURE H12-3 Bone Losses over Time Compared**

Peak bone mass is achieved by age 30. Women gradually lose bone mass until menopause, when losses accelerate dramatically and then gradually taper off.

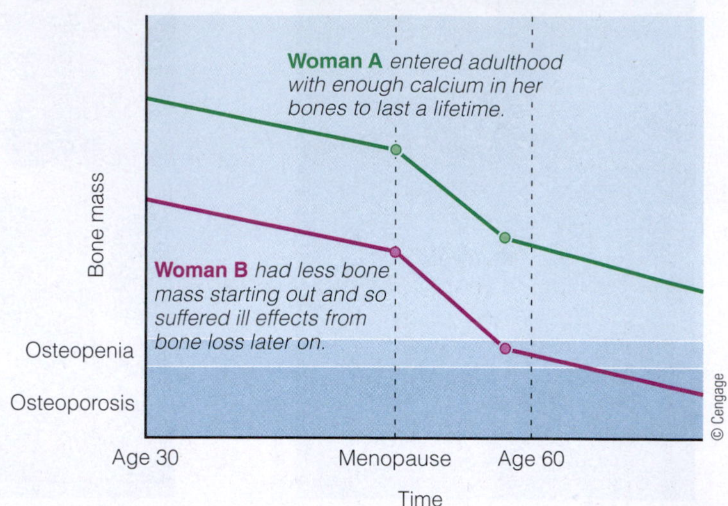
Woman A entered adulthood with enough calcium in her bones to last a lifetime.
Woman B had less bone mass starting out and so suffered ill effects from bone loss later on.
Bone mass
Osteopenia
Osteoporosis
Age 30
Menopause
Age 60
Time
© Cengage

dismantle bone continue working. The result is that bone loss exceeds bone formation. Some bone loss is inevitable, but losses can be curtailed by maximizing bone mass.

Maximizing Bone Mass

To maximize bone mass, the diet must deliver an adequate supply of calcium during the first three decades of life. Children and teens who consume milk products and get enough calcium have denser bones than those with inadequate intakes.[4] With little or no calcium from the diet, the body must depend on bone to supply calcium to the blood—bone mass diminishes, and bones lose their density, integrity, and strength. When people reach the bone-losing years of middle age, those who formed dense bones during their youth have the advantage. They simply have more bone starting out and can lose more before suffering ill effects. Figure H12-3 demonstrates this effect.

Minimizing Bone Loss

Not only does dietary calcium build strong bones in youth, but it remains important in protecting against losses in the later years. Unfortunately, calcium intakes of older adults are typically low, and calcium absorption declines after menopause. The kidneys do not activate vitamin D as well as they did earlier (recall that vitamin D enhances calcium absorption). Also, sunlight is needed to form vitamin D, and many older people spend little or no time outdoors in the sunshine. For these reasons, and because intakes of vitamin D are typically low anyway, blood levels of vitamin D decline.

Some of the hormones that influence bone and calcium metabolism—parathyroid hormone, calcitonin, estrogen, and testosterone—also change with age and accelerate bone loss. Together, these age-related factors contribute to bone loss: inefficient bone remodeling, reduced calcium intakes, impaired calcium absorption, poor vitamin D status, and hormonal changes that favor bone mineral withdrawal.

Gender and Hormones

After age, gender is the next strongest predictor of osteoporosis. The sex hormones play a major role in regulating the rate of bone turnover. In general, men have greater bone density than women at maturity, and women have greater losses than men in later life. Consequently, men develop bone problems about 10 years later than women, and women account for two out of three cases of osteoporosis.

Menopause imperils women's bones. Bone dwindles rapidly when the hormone estrogen diminishes and menstruation ceases. The lack of estrogen contributes to the release of cytokines that produce inflammation and accelerate bone loss. Women may lose up to 20 percent of their bone mass during the 6 to 8 years following menopause. Eventually, losses taper off so that women again lose bone at the same rate as men their age. Losses of bone minerals continue throughout the remainder of a woman's lifetime, but not at the free-fall pace of the menopause years (review Figure H12-3).

Rapid bone losses also occur when *young* women's ovaries fail to produce enough estrogen, causing menstruation to cease. In some cases, diseased ovaries are to blame and must be removed; in others, the ovaries fail to produce sufficient estrogen because the women suffer from anorexia nervosa and have unreasonably restricted their body weight (see Highlight 8, p. 252). The amenorrhea and low body weights explain much of the bone loss seen in these young women, even years after diagnosis and treatment.

Estrogen therapy may help some women prevent further bone loss and reduce the incidence of fractures. Because estrogen therapy may increase the risks for breast cancer, women must carefully weigh any potential benefits against the possible dangers. Several drug therapies have been developed to inhibit bone loss and enhance bone formation. A combination of drugs or of hormone replacement and a drug may be most beneficial.

Some women who choose not to use estrogen therapy turn to soy as an alternative treatment. Interestingly, the phytochemicals commonly found in soy mimic the actions of estrogen in the body. Research results have been mixed and controversial, but overall seem to indicate a lack of benefit for soy and its phytochemicals in helping to prevent the rapid bone losses of the menopause years.[5] As is true of all dietary supplements and herbal products, there may be risks associated with their use; in the case of soy, research suggests relative safety with modest benefit.[6] Because the risks and benefits vary depending on each person's medical history, women should discuss soy options with their physicians.

As in women, sex hormones appear to play a key role in men's bone loss as well. Other common causes of osteoporosis in men include excessive use of corticosteroids and alcohol.[7]

Genetics

The role of genetics in osteoporosis is strong, although still unclear.[8] Most likely, genes influence both the peak bone mass achieved during growth and the bone loss incurred during the later years. The extent to which a given genetic potential is realized, however, depends on many outside factors. Diet and physical activity, for example, can maximize peak bone density during growth, whereas alcohol and tobacco abuse can accelerate bone losses later in life. Importantly, these factors are within a person's control.

Physical Activity and Body Weight

Physical activity may be the single most important factor supporting bone growth during adolescence. Active adolescents have stronger bones in adulthood.[9] Muscle strength and bone strength go together. When muscles work, they pull on the bones, stimulating them to grow denser. The hormones that promote new muscle growth also support bone growth. As a result, active bones are denser and stronger than sedentary bones.

Both the muscle contraction and the gravitational pull of the body's weight create a load that benefits bone metabolism. As Photo H12-2 shows, to keep bones healthy, a person should engage in weight training or weight-bearing endurance activities (such as tennis and jogging or sprint cycling) regularly.[10] Regular physical activity combined with an adequate calcium intake helps maximize bone density in children and adolescents.[11] Adults can also maximize and maintain bone density with a regular program of weight training. Even past menopause, when most women are losing bone, weight training improves bone density.

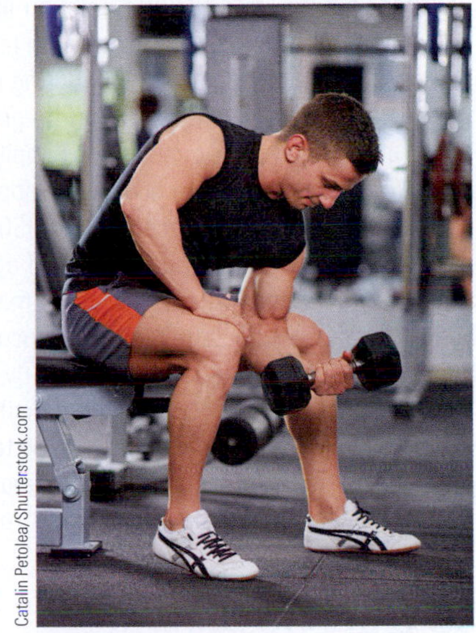
Catalin Petolea/Shutterstock.com

> **PHOTO H12-2** Strength training helps build strong bones.

Heavier body weights and weight gains place a similar stress on the bones and promote their density. In contrast, weight losses reduce bone density and increase the risk of fractures—in part because energy restriction diminishes calcium absorption and compromises calcium balance. As mentioned in Highlight 8, the relative energy deficiency that results from a combination of restricted energy intake and extreme daily exercise reliably predicts bone loss.

Smoking and Alcohol

Add bone damage to the list of ill consequences associated with smoking. The bones of smokers are less dense than those of nonsmokers—even after controlling for differences in age, body weight, and physical activity habits. Fortunately, the damaging effects can be reversed with smoking cessation. Blood indicators of beneficial bone activity are apparent 6 weeks after a person stops smoking. In time, bone density is similar for former smokers and nonsmokers.

People who abuse alcohol often suffer from osteoporosis and experience more bone breaks than others. Several factors appear to be involved. Alcohol enhances fluid excretion, leading to excessive calcium losses in the urine; upsets the hormonal balance required for healthy bones; slows bone formation, leading to lower bone density; stimulates bone breakdown; and increases the risk of falling.

Dietary Calcium

For older adults, an adequate calcium intake alone cannot protect against bone fractures.[12] Bone strength later in life depends primarily on how well the bones were built during childhood and adolescence. Adequate calcium nutrition during the growing years is essential to achieving optimal peak bone mass. Simply put, growing children who do not get enough calcium do not develop strong bones. For this reason, the DRI Committee recommends 1300 milligrams of calcium per day for everyone 9 through 18 years of age. Unfortunately, few girls meet the recommendations for calcium during these bone-forming years. (Boys generally obtain intakes close to those recommended because they eat more food.) Consequently, most girls start their adult years with less-than-optimal bone density. As adults, women rarely meet their recommended intakes of 1000 to 1200 milligrams from food. Some authorities suggest 1500 milligrams of calcium for postmenopausal women who are not receiving estrogen.

Other Nutrients

Much research has focused on calcium, but other nutrients support bone health too. Adequate protein protects bones and reduces the likelihood of hip fractures. As mentioned earlier, vitamin D is needed to maintain calcium metabolism and optimal bone health. Vitamin K regulates bone and cartilage mineralization and decreases bone turnover.[13] Vitamin C may slow bone losses. The minerals magnesium and potassium also help maintain bone mineral density. Vitamin A is needed in the bone-remodeling process, but too much vitamin A may be associated with osteoporosis. Carotenoids may inhibit bone loss. Omega-3 fatty acids may help preserve bone integrity.[14] Additional research points to the bone benefits not of a specific nutrient, but of a diet rich in fruits, vegetables, and whole grains. In contrast, diets containing too much salt are associated with bone losses. Similarly, diets containing too many sodas or commercially baked snack and fried foods are associated with low bone mineral density. Clearly, a well-balanced diet that depends on all the food groups to supply a full array of nutrients is central to bone health.

A Perspective on Calcium Supplements

Bone health depends, in part, on calcium. People who do not consume milk products or other calcium-rich foods in amounts that provide even half the recommendation should consider consulting a registered dietitian nutritionist who can assess the diet and suggest food choices to correct any inadequacies. Calcium from foods may support bone health better than calcium from supplements. For those who are unable to consume enough calcium-rich foods, however, taking calcium supplements—especially in combination with vitamin D—may help enhance bone density and protect against bone loss and fractures.[15] Because some research suggests that calcium from supplements may increase the risk of heart attacks and strokes, women should consult their physicians when making this decision.[16]

Selecting a calcium supplement requires a little investigative work to sort through the many options. Before examining calcium supplements, recognize that multivitamin-mineral pills contain little or no calcium. The label may list a few milligrams of calcium, but remember that the recommended intake is a gram (1000 milligrams) or more for adults.

Calcium supplements are typically sold as compounds of calcium carbonate (common in **antacids** and fortified chocolate candies), citrate, gluconate, lactate, malate, or phosphate. These supplements often include magnesium, vitamin D, or both. In addition, some calcium supplements are made from **bone meal, oyster shell**, or **dolomite** (limestone). Many calcium supplements, especially those derived from these natural products, contain lead—which impairs health in numerous ways, as Chapter 13 points out. Fortunately, calcium interferes with the absorption and action of lead in the body.

The first question to ask is how much calcium the supplement provides. Most calcium supplements provide between 250 and 1000 milligrams of calcium. To be safe, total calcium intake from both foods and supplements should not exceed the UL. Read the label to find out how much a dose supplies. Unless the label states otherwise, supplements of calcium carbonate are 40 percent calcium; those of calcium citrate are 21 percent; lactate, 13 percent; and gluconate, 9 percent. Select a low-dose supplement and take it several times a day rather than taking a large-dose supplement all at once. Taking calcium supplements in doses of 500 milligrams or less improves absorption. Small doses also help ease the GI distress (constipation, intestinal bloating, and excessive gas) that sometimes accompanies calcium supplement use.

The next question to ask is how well the body absorbs and uses the calcium from various supplements. Most healthy people absorb calcium equally well from milk and any of these supplements: calcium carbonate, citrate, or phosphate. More important than supplement solubility is tablet disintegration. When manufacturers compress large quantities of calcium into small pills, the stomach acid has difficulty penetrating the pill. To test a supplement's ability to dissolve, drop it into a 6-ounce cup of vinegar, and stir occasionally. A high-quality formulation will dissolve within a half-hour.

Finally, people who choose supplements must take them regularly. Furthermore, consideration should be given to the best time to take the supplements. To circumvent adverse nutrient interactions, take calcium supplements between, not with, meals. (Importantly, do not take calcium supplements with iron supplements or iron-rich meals; calcium inhibits iron absorption.) To enhance calcium absorption, take supplements with meals. If such contradictory advice drives you crazy, reconsider the benefits of food sources of calcium. Most experts agree that foods are the best source of most nutrients.

Some Closing Thoughts

Unfortunately, many of the strongest risk factors for osteoporosis are beyond a person's control: age, gender, and genetics. But several strategies are effective for prevention.[17] First, ensure an optimal peak bone mass during childhood and adolescence by eating a balanced diet rich in calcium and vitamin D and by engaging in regular physical activity. Then, maintain that bone mass in early adulthood by continuing those healthy diet and activity habits, abstaining from cigarette smoking and using alcohol moderately, if at all. Finally, minimize bone loss in later life by maintaining an adequate nutrition and exercise regimen, and, especially for older women, consult a physician about bone density tests, calcium supplements, or drug therapies that may be effective both in preventing bone loss and in restoring lost bone. The reward is the best possible chance of preserving bone health throughout life.

CRITICAL THINKING QUESTIONS

A. What behaviors would be most helpful in preventing osteoporosis?

B. Osteoporosis typically develops in old age, yet the time to optimize bone density is during childhood and adolescence—decades away from the realities of hip fractures and spinal collapses. What plan of action might you develop to encourage teens to adopt strategies that will enhance bone development? Be sure to address potential obstacles and reluctances typical of that age.

REFERENCES

1. Centers for Disease Control and Prevention (CDC), www.cdc.gov /HomeandRecreationalSafety/Falls/adulthipfx.html, September 20, 2016.
2. D. M. Black and C. J. Rosen, Postmenopausal osteoporosis, *New England Journal of Medicine* 374 (2016): 254–62.
3. N. C. Wright and coauthors, The recent prevalence of osteoporosis and low bone mass in the United States based on bone mineral density at the femoral neck or lumbar spine, *Journal of Bone and Mineral Research* 29 (2014): 2520–2526.
4. D. K. Dror and L. H. Allen, Dairy product intake in children and adolescents in developed countries: Trends, nutritional contribution, and a review of association with health outcomes, *Nutrition Reviews* 72 (2013): 68–81.
5. V. S. Lagari and S. Levis, Phytoestrogens in the prevention of postmenopausal bone loss, *Journal of Clinical Densitometry* 16 (2013): 445–449.
6. D. L. Alekel and coauthors, Soy isoflavones for reducing bone loss study: Effects of a 3-year trial on hormones, adverse events, and endometrial thickness in postmenopausal women, *Menopause* 22 (2015): 185–197; J. W. Pawlowski and coauthors, Impact of equol-producing capacity and soy-isoflavone profiles of supplements on bone calcium, retention in postmenopausal women: A randomized crossover trial, *American Journal of Clinical Nutrition* 102 (2015): 695–703; E. Poluzzi and coauthors, Phytoestrogens in postmenopause: The state of the art from a chemical pharmacological and regulatory perspective, *Current Medicinal Chemistry* 21 (2014): 417–436.
7. T. Wilson and coauthors, The clinical epidemiology of male osteoporosis: A review of the recent literature, *Clinical Epidemiology* 7 (2015): 65–76.
8. G. R. Clark and E. L. Duncan, The genetics of osteoporosis, *British Medical Bulletin* 113 (2015): 73–81; N. Alonso and S. H. Ralston, Unveiling the mysteries of the genetics of osteoporosis, *Journal of Endocrinological Investigation* 37 (2014): 925–934.
9. S. A. Jackowski and coauthors, Adolescent physical activity and bone strength at the proximal femur in adulthood, *Medicine and Science in Sports and Exercise* 46 (2014): 736–744.
10. E. A. Marques and coauthors, Response of bone mineral density, inflammatory cytokines, and biochemical bone markers to a 32-week combined loading exercise programme in older men and women, *Archives of Gerontology and Geriatrics* 57 (2013): 226–233.
11. C. Julián-Almárcegui and coauthors, Combined effects of interaction between physical activity and nutrition on bone health in children and adolescents: A systematic review, *Nutrition Reviews* 73 (2015): 127–139.
12. M. J. Bolland and coauthors, Calcium intake and risk of fracture: Systematic review, *British Medical Journal* 351 (2015): h4580; V. Tai and coauthors, Calcium intake and bone mineral density: Systematic review and meta-analysis, *British Medical Journal* 351 (2015): h4183.
13. M. S. Hamidi and A. M. Cheung, Vitamin K and musculoskeletal health in postmenopausal women, *Molecular Nutrition and Food Research* 58 (2014): 1647–1657.
14. T. S. Orchard and coauthors, The association of red blood cell n-3 and n-6 fatty acids with bone mineral density and hip fracture risk in the women's health initiative, *Journal of Bone and Mineral Research* 28 (2013): 505–515.
15. R. L. Prentice and coauthors, Health risks and benefits from calcium and vitamin D supplementation Women's Health Initiative clinical trial and cohort study, *Osteoporosis International* 24 (2013): 567–580.
16. J. J. B. Anderson and coauthors, Calcium intake from diet and supplements and the risk of coronary artery calcification and its progression among older adults: 10-year follow-up of the Multi-Ethnic Study of Atherosclerosis (MESA), *Journal of the American Heart Association* 5 (2016): e003815; C. S. Shin and K. M. Kim, The risks and benefits of calcium supplementation, *Endocrinology and Metabolism* 30 (2015): 27–34; D. Challoumas and coauthors, Effects of combined vitamin D-calcium supplements on the cardiovascular system: Should we be cautious? *Atherosclerosis* 238 (2015): 388–398; M. J. Bolland, A. Grey, and I. R. Reid, Calcium supplements and cardiovascular risk: 5 years on, *Therapeutic Advances in Drug Safety* 4 (2013): 199–210.
17. P. J. Mitchell and coauthors, Life-course approach to nutrition, *Osteoporosis International* 26 (2015): 2723–2742.

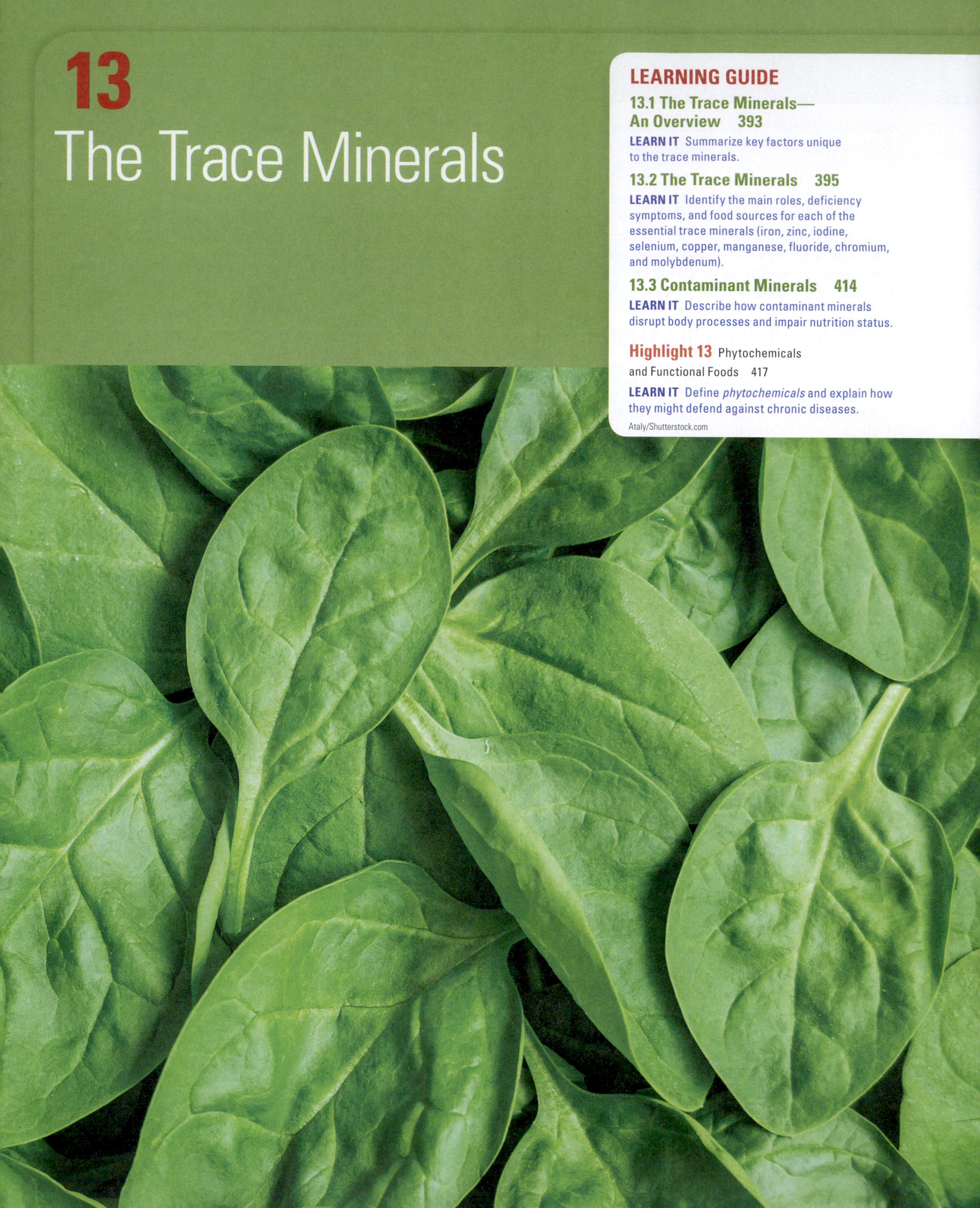

13 The Trace Minerals

LEARNING GUIDE

Ataly/Shutterstock.com

Nutrition in Your Life

Trace—barely a perceptible amount. But the trace minerals tackle big jobs. Your blood can't carry oxygen without iron, and insulin can't deliver glucose without chromium. Teeth become decayed without fluoride, and thyroid glands develop goiter without iodine. Together, the trace minerals keep you healthy and strong. Where can you get these amazing minerals? A variety of foods, especially those from the protein foods group, sprinkled with a little iodized salt and complemented by a glass of fluoridated water will do the trick. It's remarkable what your body can do with only a few milligrams—or even micrograms—of the trace minerals. As you read this chapter, consider whether the foods you are eating are meeting your trace mineral needs.

This chapter features the essential **trace minerals**—iron, zinc, iodine, selenium, copper, manganese, fluoride, chromium, and molybdenum. Figure 12-10 in Chapter 12 (p. 369) showed the tiny quantities of trace minerals in the human body. The trace minerals are so named because they are present, and needed, in relatively small amounts in the body. All together, they would hardly fill a teaspoon. Yet they are no less important than the major minerals or any of the other nutrients. Each of the trace minerals performs a vital role. A deficiency of any of them may be fatal, and excesses are equally deadly. Remarkably, a well-balanced diet supplies enough of these minerals to maintain health.

This chapter also mentions other trace minerals—such as arsenic, boron, nickel, bromine, and vanadium—that are not considered nutrients. These minerals may have beneficial roles in the body, but research on them is insufficient to determine essentiality. Also mentioned in this chapter are contaminant minerals that disrupt body processes and impair nutrition status. The highlight that follows examines phytochemicals—compounds that also are not essential nutrients, but that have biological activity in the body. Again, a well-balanced diet—especially one abundant in fruits and vegetables—supplies a full array of phytochemicals to support good health.

13.1 The Trace Minerals—An Overview

LEARN IT Summarize key factors unique to the trace minerals.

The body requires the trace minerals in small amounts. They participate in diverse tasks all over the body, each having special duties that only it can perform.

Food Sources The trace mineral contents of foods depend on soil and water composition and on how foods are processed. Furthermore, many factors in the diet and within the body affect the minerals' **bioavailability.** Still, outstanding food sources for each of the trace minerals, just like those for the other nutrients, include a wide variety of foods.

Deficiencies Assessing trace mineral status is challenging. Severe deficiencies of the better-known minerals are relatively easy to recognize. Deficiencies of the others may be harder to diagnose, and for all minerals, mild deficiencies are easy to overlook. Because the minerals are active in many body systems—digestive, cardiovascular, circulatory, muscular, skeletal, and nervous—deficiencies can have wide-reaching effects and can affect people of all ages. The most common result of a deficiency in children is failure to grow and thrive.

Toxicities Most of the trace minerals are toxic at intakes only two and a half to eleven times above current recommendations (see Figure 13-1, p. 394). Thus it is important not to habitually exceed the Upper Level (UL) of recommended

trace minerals: essential mineral nutrients the human body requires in relatively small amounts (less than 100 milligrams per day); sometimes called *microminerals.*

bioavailability: the rate at and the extent to which a nutrient is absorbed and used.

> **FIGURE 13-1 RDA (or AI) and UL Compared for Selected Trace Minerals**

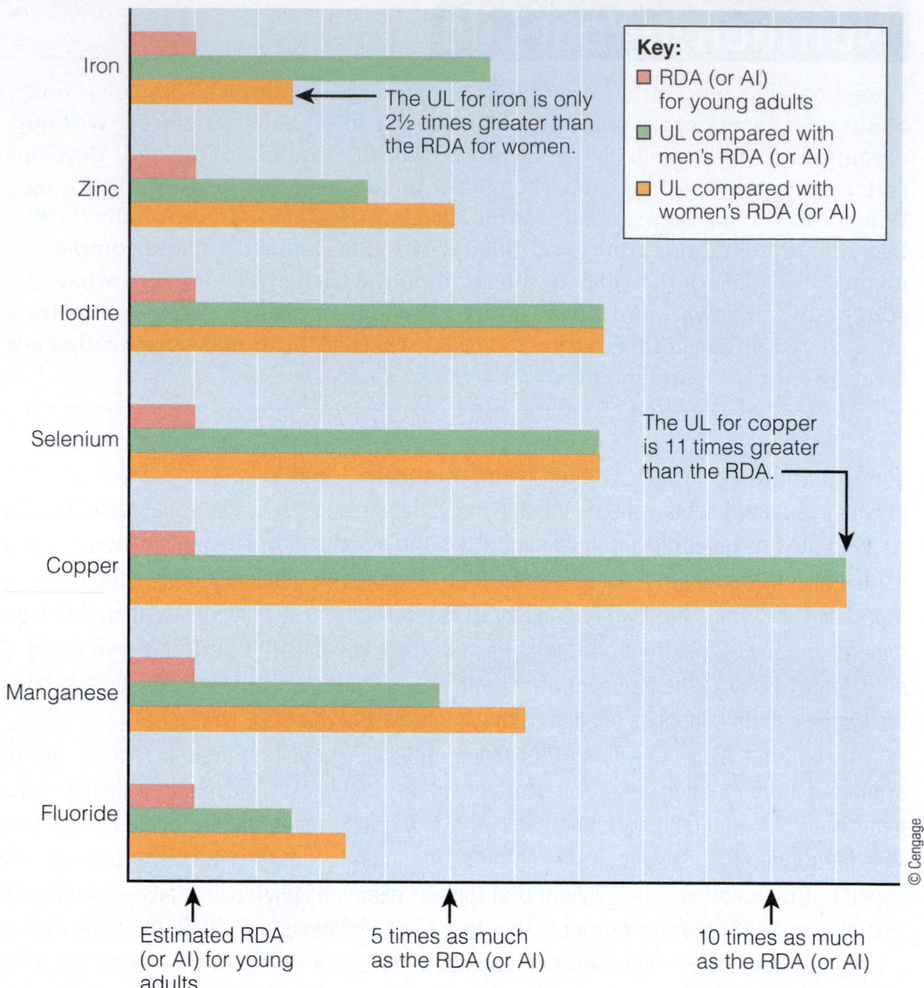
Iron
Zinc
Iodine
Selenium
Copper
Manganese
Fluoride
The UL for iron is only 2½ times greater than the RDA for women.
Key:
RDA (or AI) for young adults
UL compared with men's RDA (or AI)
UL compared with women's RDA (or AI)
The UL for copper is 11 times greater than the RDA.
Estimated RDA (or AI) for young adults
5 times as much as the RDA (or AI)
10 times as much as the RDA (or AI)
© Cengage

intakes (see inside front pages). Many dietary supplements contain trace minerals, making it easy for users to exceed their needs. Highlight 10 discussed supplement use and some of the regulations included in the Dietary Supplement Health and Education Act. As that discussion notes, consumers have demanded the freedom to choose their own doses of nutrients. By law, the Food and Drug Administration (FDA) has no authority to limit the amounts of trace minerals in supplements. Individuals who take supplements must therefore be aware of the possible dangers and select supplements that do not exceed 100 percent of the Daily Value by much. It is easier and safer to meet nutrient needs by selecting a variety of foods than by combining an assortment of supplements.

Interactions Interactions among the trace minerals are common and often well coordinated to meet the body's needs. For example, several of the trace minerals support insulin's work, influencing its synthesis, storage, release, and action.

At other times, interactions lead to nutrient imbalances. An excess of one may cause a deficiency of another. (A slight manganese overload, for example, may aggravate an iron deficiency.) A deficiency of one may interfere with the work of another. (A selenium deficiency halts the activation of the iodine-containing thyroid hormones.) A deficiency of a trace mineral may even open the way for a contaminant mineral to cause a toxic reaction. (Iron deficiency, for example, makes the body more vulnerable to lead poisoning.) These examples of nutrient interactions highlight one of the many reasons why people should use supplements conservatively, if at all: supplementation can easily create imbalances.

A good food source of one nutrient may be a poor food source of another, and factors that enhance the action of some trace minerals may interfere with others. Meats, for example, are a good source of iron but a poor source of calcium; vitamin C enhances the absorption of iron but hinders that of copper.

Nonessential Trace Minerals The essential trace minerals featured in this chapter have been well studied; researchers understand the primary roles in the body and the consequences of deficiencies and toxicities. Enough information is available to determine DRI. In contrast, research to determine whether other trace minerals are essential is challenging because quantities in the body are so small and also because human deficiencies are unknown. Identifying their functions in the body can be particularly problematic. Much of the available knowledge comes from research using animals.

Research is currently insufficient to determine the DRI for nickel, bromine, vanadium, cobalt, and boron, even though they may play beneficial roles in the human body. Nickel may serve as a cofactor for certain enzymes. Bromine is involved in the formation of collagen, which gives tissues their structure.[1] Vanadium is necessary for growth and bone development and for normal reproduction. Cobalt is a key mineral in the large vitamin B_{12} molecule (see Figure 13-2). Boron may play a key role in bone health, brain activities, and immune response.

In the future, we may discover that these and other trace minerals are essential to growth and health. Even arsenic—famous as a poison used by murderers and known to be a carcinogen—may turn out to be essential for human beings in tiny quantities. It has already proved useful in the treatment of some types of leukemia.[2] Research on all the trace minerals is active, suggesting that we have much more to learn about them.

REVIEW IT Summarize key factors unique to the trace minerals.

Although the body uses only tiny amounts of the trace minerals, they are vital to health. Because so little is required, the trace minerals can be toxic at levels not far above estimated requirements—a consideration for supplement users. Like the other nutrients, the trace minerals are best obtained by eating a variety of foods.

> **FIGURE 13-2 Cobalt in Vitamin B_{12}**

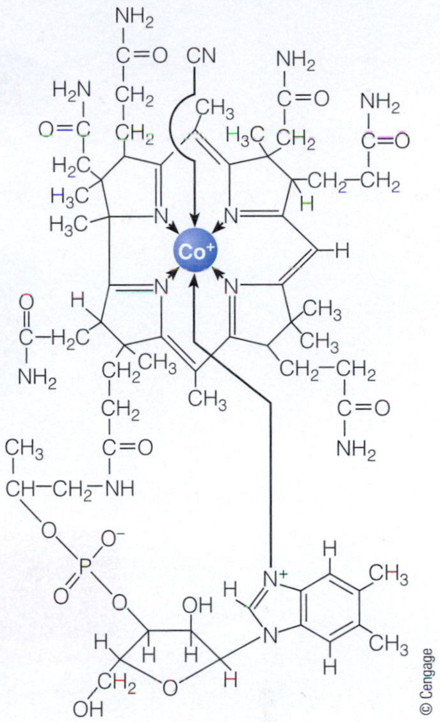

NH2
C=O
CN
NH2
H2N
CH2
CH3
C=O
NH2
O=C
CH2
H3C
CH2
C=O
H2C
CH2–CH2
H
H3C
H3C
N
N
Co+
H
N
N
O
H
CH3
C–H2C
CH3
NH2
CH2
CH3
CH2–CH2
CH3
CH2
C=O
CH3
C=O
NH2
CH–CH2–NH
O
O–
P
H
N+
CH3
O
O
H
OH
N
H
H
H
CH3
H
H
CH2
O
OH
© Cengage

The intricate vitamin B_{12} molecule contains one atom of the mineral cobalt. The alternative name for vitamin B_{12}, cobalamin, reflects the presence of cobalt in its structure.

13.2 The Trace Minerals

LEARN IT Identify the main roles, deficiency symptoms, and food sources for each of the essential trace minerals (iron, zinc, iodine, selenium, copper, manganese, fluoride, chromium, and molybdenum).

Iron

Iron is an essential nutrient, vital to many of the cells' activities, but it poses a problem for millions of people. Some people simply don't eat enough iron-containing foods to support their health optimally, whereas others absorb so much iron that it threatens their health. Iron exemplifies the principle that both too little and too much of a nutrient in the body can be harmful. In its efforts to protect against both deficiency and toxicity, the body has several ways to regulate iron transport and maintain iron balance.[3]

Iron Roles in the Body Iron has the ability to switch back and forth between two ionic states. In the reduced state, iron has lost two electrons and therefore has a net positive charge of two; it is known as *ferrous iron* (Fe^{++}). In the oxidized state, iron has lost a third electron, has a net positive charge of three, and is known as *ferric iron* (Fe^{+++}). Ferrous iron can be oxidized to ferric iron, and ferric iron can be reduced to ferrous iron. By doing so, iron can serve as a **cofactor** to enzymes involved in the numerous oxidation-reduction reactions that commonly occur in all cells. Enzymes involved in making amino acids, collagen, hormones, and neurotransmitters all require iron. (For details about ions, oxidation, and reduction, see Appendix B.)

iron: an essential trace mineral that is needed for the transport of oxygen and the metabolism of energy nutrients.

cofactor: a small, inorganic or organic substance that facilitates the action of an enzyme.

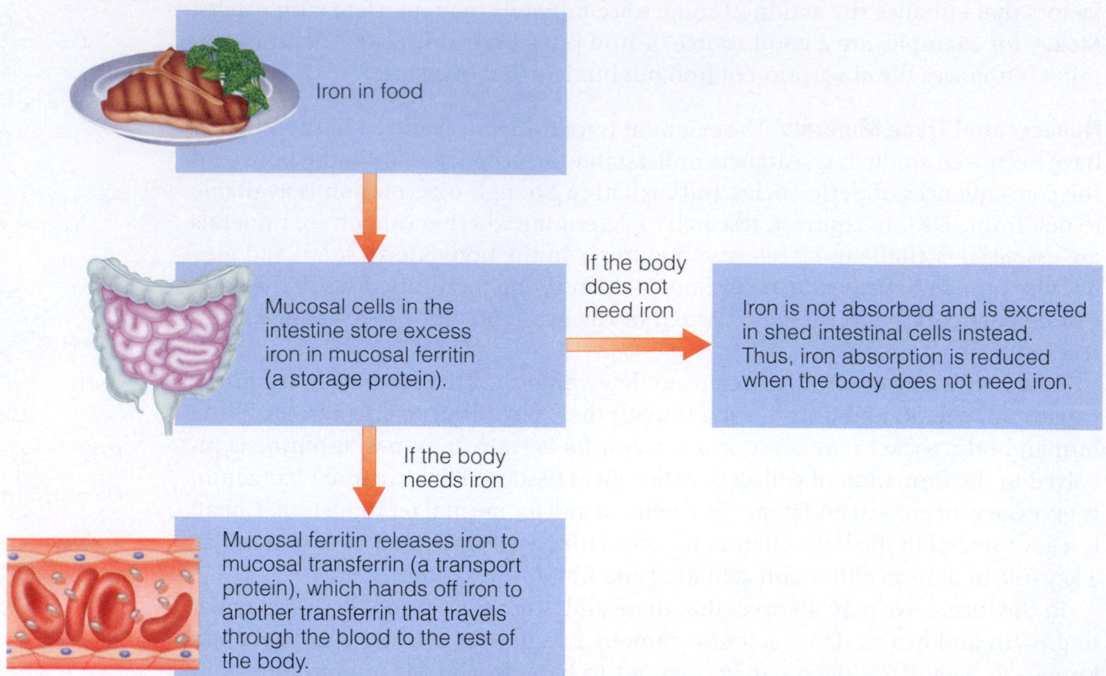
Iron in food
Mucosal cells in the intestine store excess iron in mucosal ferritin (a storage protein).
If the body does not need iron
Iron is not absorbed and is excreted in shed intestinal cells instead. Thus, iron absorption is reduced when the body does not need iron.
If the body needs iron
Mucosal ferritin releases iron to mucosal transferrin (a transport protein), which hands off iron to another transferrin that travels through the blood to the rest of the body.
© Cengage

> FIGURE 13-3 Iron Absorption

Iron forms a part of the electron carriers that participate in the electron transport chain (discussed in Chapter 7).* These carriers transfer hydrogens and electrons to oxygen, forming water, and in the process, make ATP for the cells' energy use.

Most of the body's iron is found in two proteins: **hemoglobin** in the red blood cells and **myoglobin** in the muscle cells. In both, iron helps accept, carry, and then release oxygen.

Iron Absorption The body conserves iron. Because it is difficult to excrete iron once it is in the body, balance is maintained primarily through absorption. More iron is absorbed when stores are empty and less is absorbed when stores are full.Special proteins help the body absorb iron from food (see Figure 13-3). The iron-storage protein **ferritin** captures iron from food and stores it in the cells of the small intestine. When the body needs iron, ferritin releases some iron to an iron transport protein called **transferrin.** If the body does not need iron, it is carried out when the intestinal cells are shed and excreted in the feces; intestinal cells are replaced about every 3 to 5 days. By holding iron temporarily, these cells control iron absorption by either delivering iron when it is needed or disposing of it when stores are full.

Iron absorption depends in part on its dietary source. Iron occurs in two forms in foods: as **heme iron,** which is found only in foods derived from the flesh of animals, such as meats, poultry, and fish and as **nonheme iron,** which is found in both plant-derived and animal-derived foods (see Figure 13-4). On average, heme iron represents about 10 percent of the iron a person consumes in a day. Even though heme iron accounts for only a small proportion of the intake, it is so well absorbed that it contributes significant iron. About 25 percent of heme iron and 17 percent of nonheme iron is absorbed, depending on dietary factors and the body's iron stores. In iron deficiency, absorption increases. In iron overload, absorption declines.

Heme iron has a high bioavailability and is not influenced by dietary factors. In contrast, several dietary factors influence nonheme iron absorption (see Table 13-1).[4] Meat, fish, and poultry contain not only the well-absorbed heme iron, but also a peptide (sometimes called the **MFP factor**) that promotes

*The iron-containing electron carriers of the electron transport chain are known as *cytochromes.* See Appendix C for details on the electron transport chain.

TABLE 13-1 Factors That Influence Nonheme Iron Absorption

Enhancing Factors	Inhibiting Factors
• MFP factor • Vitamin C (ascorbic acid) • Acids (citric and lactic) • Sugars (fructose)	• Phytates (legumes, grains, nuts, seeds) • Vegetable proteins (soybeans, legumes, nuts) • Calcium (milk) • Tannic acid (and other polyphenols in tea and coffee)

© Cengage

hemoglobin (HE-moh-GLO-bin): the globular protein of the red blood cells that transports oxygen from the lungs to tissues throughout the body; hemoglobin accounts for 80 percent of the body's iron.

myoglobin: the oxygen-holding protein of the muscle cells.
- **myo** = muscle

ferritin (FAIR-ih-tin): the iron storage protein.

transferrin (trans-FAIR-in): the iron transport protein.

heme (HEEM) **iron:** the iron in foods that is bound to the hemoglobin and myoglobin proteins; found only in meat, fish, and poultry.

nonheme iron: the iron in foods that is not bound to proteins; found in both plant-derived and animal-derived foods.

MFP factor: a peptide released during the digestion of meat, fish, and poultry that enhances nonheme iron absorption.

> **FIGURE 13-4 Heme and Nonheme Iron in Foods**

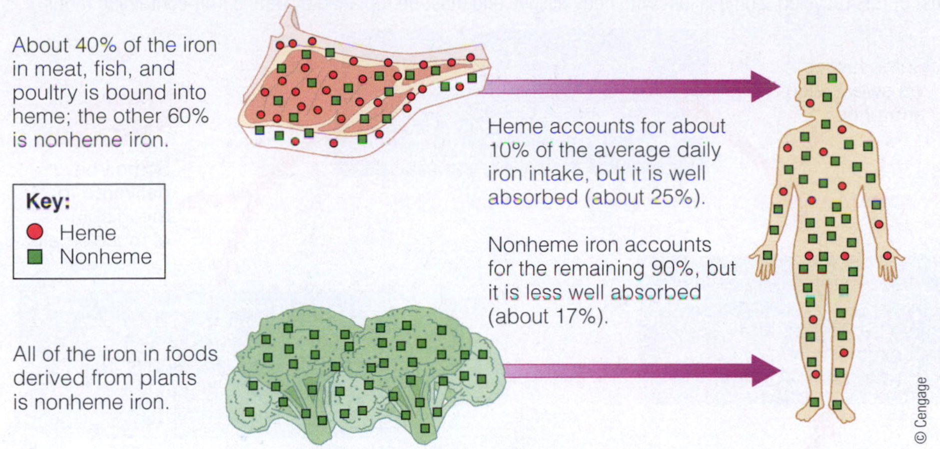
About 40% of the iron in meat, fish, and poultry is bound into heme; the other 60% is nonheme iron.
Key:
Heme
Nonheme
Heme accounts for about 10% of the average daily iron intake, but it is well absorbed (about 25%).
Nonheme iron accounts for the remaining 90%, but it is less well absorbed (about 17%).
All of the iron in foods derived from plants is nonheme iron.
© Cengage

the absorption of nonheme iron from other foods eaten at the same meal. Vitamin C (ascorbic acid) also enhances nonheme iron absorption from foods eaten at the same meal by capturing the iron and keeping it in the reduced ferrous form, ready for absorption. Some acids (such as citric acid) and sugars (such as fructose) also enhance nonheme iron absorption. Overall, about 18 percent of dietary iron is absorbed from mixed diets and only about 10 percent from vegetarian diets. As you might expect, vegetarian diets do not have the benefit of easy-to-absorb heme iron or the help of the MFP factor in enhancing absorption.

Some dietary factors bind with nonheme iron, inhibiting absorption. These factors include the phytates in legumes, whole grains, and rice; the vegetable proteins in soybeans, other legumes, and nuts; the calcium in milk; and the polyphenols (such as tannic acid) in tea, coffee, grain products, oregano, and red wine.

The many dietary enhancers, inhibitors, and their combined effects make it difficult to estimate iron absorption. Most of these factors exert a strong influence individually, but not when combined with the others in a meal. Furthermore, the impact of the combined effects diminishes when a diet is evaluated over several days. When multiple meals are analyzed together, three factors appear to be most relevant: MFP factor and vitamin C as enhancers (see Photo 13-1) and phytates as inhibitors.

In addition to dietary influences, iron absorption also depends on an individual's health, stage in the life cycle, and iron status. Absorption can be as low as 2 percent in a person with GI disease or as high as 35 percent in a rapidly growing, healthy child. The body adapts to absorb more iron when a person's iron stores fall short or when the need increases for any reason (such as pregnancy). The body makes more ferritin to absorb more iron from the small intestine and more transferrin to carry more iron around the body. Similarly, when iron stores are sufficient, the body adapts to absorb less iron.

Iron Transport and Storage The blood transport protein transferrin delivers iron to the bone marrow and other tissues. The bone marrow uses large quantities of iron to make new red blood cells, whereas other tissues use less. Surplus iron is stored in the protein ferritin, primarily in the liver; other storage locations include the bone marrow and spleen. When dietary iron has been plentiful, ferritin is constantly and rapidly made and broken down, providing an ever-ready supply of iron. When iron concentrations become abnormally high, the liver converts some ferritin into another storage protein called **hemosiderin.** Hemosiderin releases iron more slowly than ferritin does. Storing excess iron in hemosiderin protects the body against the damage that free iron can cause. Free iron acts as a free radical, attacking cell lipids, DNA, and protein. (See Highlight 11, p. 353, for more information on free radicals and the damage they can cause.)

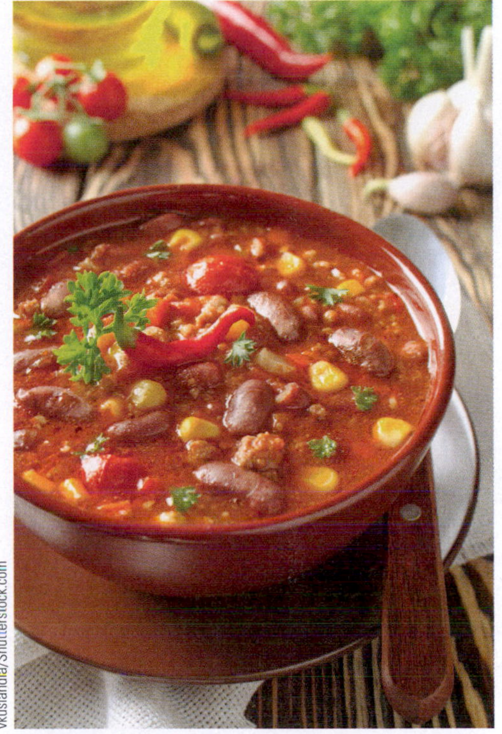
vkuslandia/Shutterstock.com

> **PHOTO 13-1** This chili dinner provides several sources of iron and factors that may enhance its absorption: heme and nonheme iron and the MFP factor from meat, nonheme iron from legumes, and vitamin C from tomatoes.

hemosiderin (heem-oh-SID-er-in): an iron-storage protein primarily made in times of iron overload.

> **FIGURE 13-5 Iron Recycled in the Body**

Once iron enters the body, most of it is recycled. Some is lost with body tissues and must be replaced by eating iron-containing foods.

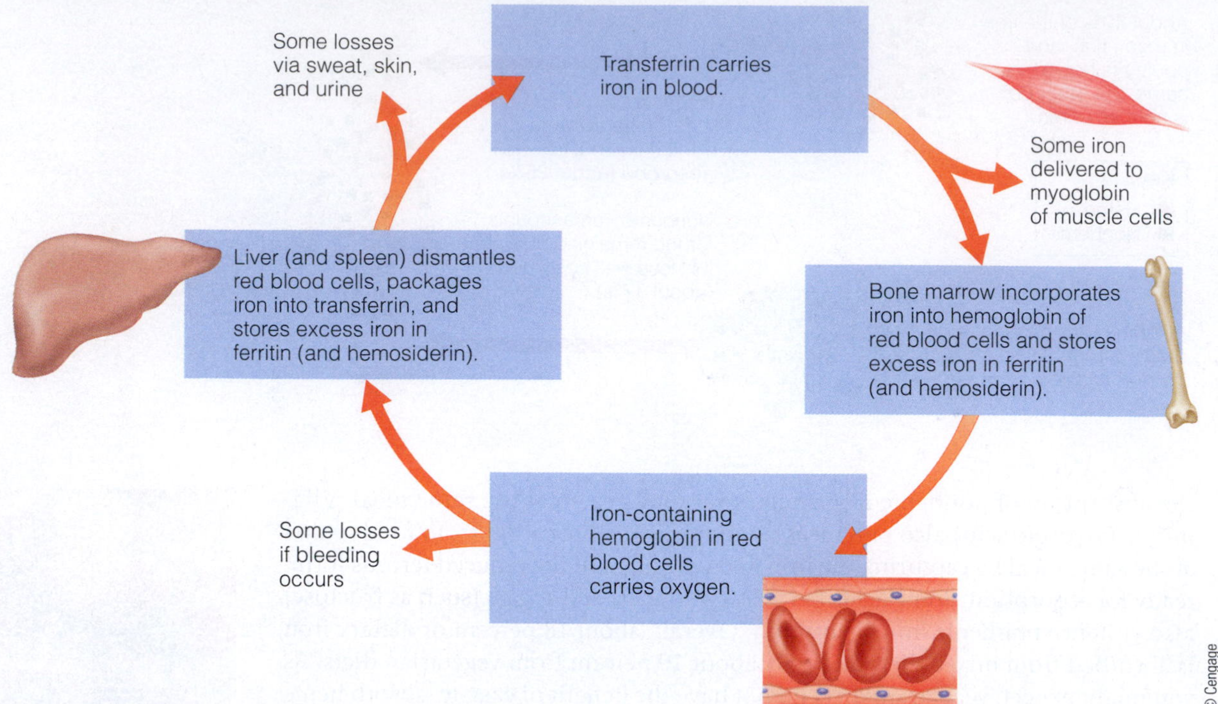

Some losses via sweat, skin, and urine
Transferrin carries iron in blood.
Some iron delivered to myoglobin of muscle cells
Liver (and spleen) dismantles red blood cells, packages iron into transferrin, and stores excess iron in ferritin (and hemosiderin).
Bone marrow incorporates iron into hemoglobin of red blood cells and stores excess iron in ferritin (and hemosiderin).
Some losses if bleeding occurs
Iron-containing hemoglobin in red blood cells carries oxygen.
© Cengage

The average red blood cell lives about 4 months; then the spleen and liver cells remove it from the blood, take it apart, and prepare the degradation products for excretion or recycling. The iron is salvaged: the liver attaches it to transferrin, which transports it back to the bone marrow to be reused in making new red blood cells. Thus, although red blood cells live for only about 4 months, the iron recycles through each new generation of cells (see Figure 13-5). The body loses some iron daily via the GI tract and, if bleeding occurs, in blood. Only tiny amounts of iron are lost in urine, sweat, and shed skin. Iron excretion differs for men and women. On average, men and women lose about 1.0 milligram of iron per day, with women losing additional iron in menses; menstrual losses vary considerably, but over a month, they average about 0.5 milligram per day.

Maintaining iron balance depends on the careful regulation of iron absorption, transport, storage, recycling, and losses. Central to the regulation of iron balance is the hormone **hepcidin.** Produced by the liver, hepcidin helps maintain blood iron within the normal range by limiting absorption from the small intestine and controlling release from the liver, spleen, and bone marrow. Hepcidin production increases in iron overload and decreases in iron deficiency.

Iron Deficiency Worldwide, **iron deficiency** is the most common nutrient deficiency, with **iron-deficiency anemia** affecting an estimated 30 percent of the population, more than 2 billion people—mostly preschool children and pregnant women.[5] In the United States, iron deficiency is less prevalent, but it still affects about 10 percent of the population—primarily toddlers, adolescent girls, and women of childbearing age. Iron deficiency is also relatively common among those who are overweight and obese. The association between iron deficiency and obesity has yet to be explained, but researchers are currently examining the relationships between the inflammation, hepcidin, and reduced iron absorption.[6] Preventing and correcting iron deficiency are high priorities.

Some stages of life demand more iron but provide less, making deficiency likely. Women in their reproductive years are especially prone to iron deficiency because

hepcidin: a hormone produced by the liver that regulates iron balance.

iron deficiency: the state of having depleted iron stores.

iron-deficiency anemia: severe depletion of iron stores that results in low hemoglobin and small, pale red blood cells. Iron-deficiency anemia is a *microcytic* (my-cro-SIT-ic) *hypochromic* (high-po-KROME-ic) *anemia.*

- **micro** = small
- **cytic** = cell
- **hypo** = too little
- **chrom** = color

of repeated blood losses during menstruation. Pregnancy demands additional iron to support the added blood volume, growth of the fetus, and blood loss during childbirth. Infants and young children receive little iron from their high-milk diets, yet need extra iron to support their rapid growth and brain development.* Iron deficiency among toddlers in the United States is common. The rapid growth of adolescence, especially for males, and the menstrual losses of females also demand extra iron that a typical teen diet may not provide. An adequate iron intake is especially important during these stages of life.

Bleeding from any site incurs iron losses.** As mentioned, menstrual losses can be considerable as they tap women's iron stores regularly. In some cases, such as an active ulcer, the bleeding may not be obvious, but even small chronic blood losses significantly deplete iron reserves. In developing countries, blood loss is often brought on by malaria and parasitic infections of the GI tract. People who donate blood regularly also incur losses and may benefit from iron supplements.[7]

Assessment of Iron Deficiency Iron deficiency develops in stages. This section provides a brief overview of how to detect these stages, and Appendix E provides more details. In the first stage of iron deficiency, iron stores diminish. Measures of serum ferritin (in the blood) reflect iron stores and are most valuable in assessing iron status at this earliest stage. Unfortunately, serum ferritin increases with infections, which interferes with an accurate diagnosis and estimates of prevalence.

The second stage of iron deficiency is characterized by a decrease in transport iron: the iron-carrying protein transferrin *increases* (an adaptation that enhances iron absorption). Together, measurements of serum ferritin and transferrin can determine the severity of the deficiency—the more transferrin and the less serum ferritin, the more advanced the deficiency is. Transferrin saturation—the percentage of transferrin that is saturated with iron—decreases as iron stores decline.

The third stage of iron deficiency occurs when the lack of iron limits hemoglobin production. Now the hemoglobin precursor, **erythrocyte protoporphyrin,** begins to accumulate as hemoglobin and **hematocrit** values decline. Hemoglobin and hematocrit tests are easy, quick, and inexpensive, so they are the tests most commonly used in evaluating iron status. Their usefulness in detecting iron deficiency is limited, however, because they are late indicators. Furthermore, other nutrient deficiencies and medical conditions can influence their values.

Iron Deficiency and Anemia Notice that iron deficiency and iron-deficiency anemia are not the same: people may be iron deficient without being anemic. The term *iron deficiency* refers to depleted iron stores; the term *iron-deficiency anemia* refers to the severe depletion of iron stores that results in a low hemoglobin concentration.[8] In iron-deficiency anemia, hemoglobin synthesis decreases, resulting in red blood cells that are pale (hypochromic) and small (microcytic), as shown in Figure 13-6 (p. 400). Without adequate iron, these cells can't carry enough oxygen from the lungs to the tissues. Energy metabolism in the cells falters. The result is fatigue, weakness, headaches, apathy, pallor, and poor resistance to cold temperatures. Because hemoglobin is the bright red pigment of the blood, the skin of a fair person who is anemic may become noticeably pale. In a dark-skinned person, the tongue and eye lining, normally pink, are very pale.

The fatigue that accompanies iron-deficiency anemia differs from the tiredness a person experiences from a simple lack of sleep. People with anemia feel fatigue only when they exert themselves. Consequently, their work productivity, voluntary activities, and athletic performance decline.[9] Iron supplementation can relieve the fatigue and improve the body's response to physical activity. (The iron needs of physically active people and the special iron deficiency known as *sports anemia* are discussed in Chapter 14.)

*The condition of developing iron-deficiency anemia because iron-poor milk displaces iron-rich foods in the diet is sometimes called *milk anemia*.

**The iron content of blood is about 0.5 milligram/100 milliliters of blood. A person donating a pint of blood (approximately 500 milliliters) loses about 2.5 milligrams of iron.

erythrocyte protoporphyrin (PRO-toe-PORE-fe-rin): a precursor to hemoglobin.

hematocrit (hee-MAT-oh-krit): the percentage of total blood volume that consists of red blood cells.

> FIGURE 13-6 Normal Blood Cells and Blood Cells in Iron-Deficiency Anemia Compared

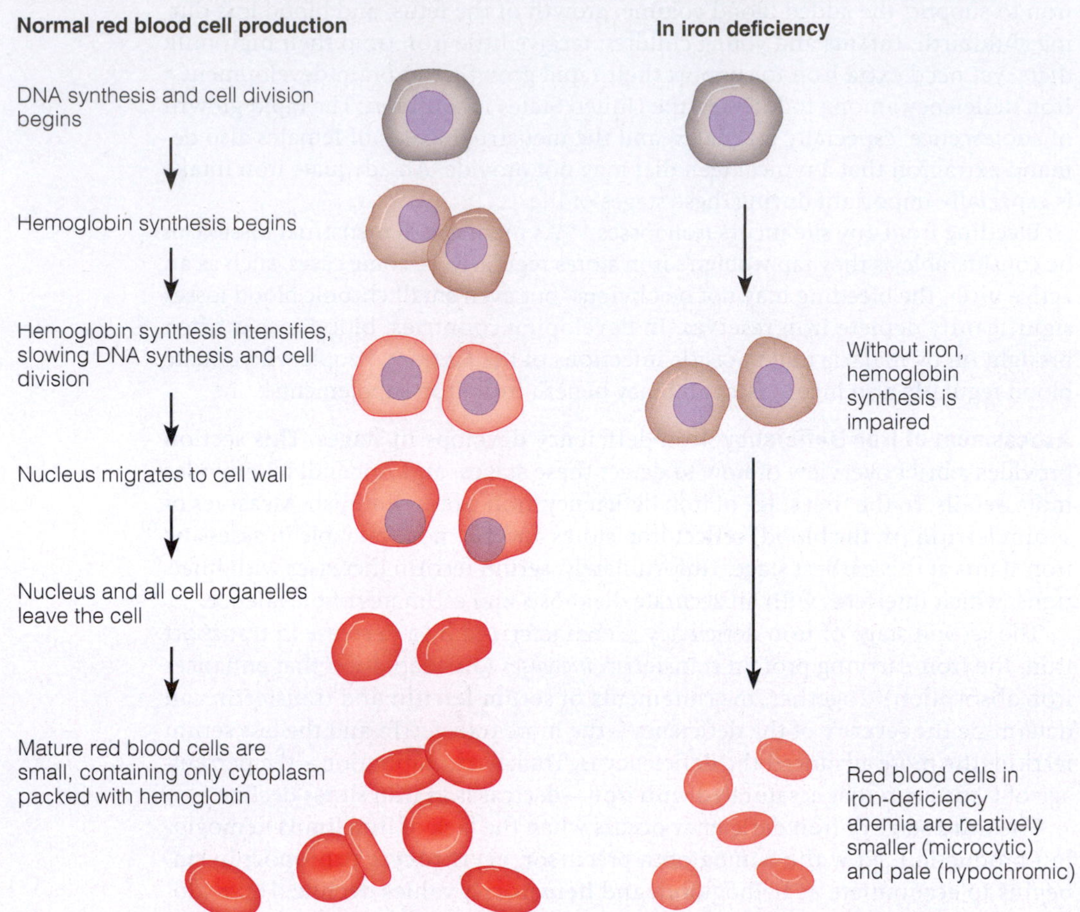
Normal red blood cell production
In iron deficiency
DNA synthesis and cell division begins
Hemoglobin synthesis begins
Hemoglobin synthesis intensifies, slowing DNA synthesis and cell division
Without iron, hemoglobin synthesis is impaired
Nucleus migrates to cell wall
Nucleus and all cell organelles leave the cell
Mature red blood cells are small, containing only cytoplasm packed with hemoglobin
Red blood cells in iron-deficiency anemia are relatively smaller (microcytic) and pale (hypochromic)
© Cengage

Iron Deficiency and Behavior Long before the red blood cells are affected and anemia is diagnosed, a developing iron deficiency affects behavior. Even at slightly lowered iron levels, energy metabolism is impaired and neurotransmitter synthesis is altered, reducing physical work capacity and mental productivity. Without the physical energy and mental alertness to work, plan, think, play, sing, or learn, people simply do less. They have no obvious deficiency symptoms; they just appear unmotivated and apathetic.

Many of the symptoms associated with iron deficiency are easily mistaken for behavioral or motivational problems. A restless child who fails to pay attention in class might be thought contrary. An apathetic homemaker who has let housework pile up might be thought lazy. No responsible dietitian would ever claim that all behavioral problems are caused by nutrient deficiencies, but poor nutrition is always a possible contributor to problems like these. When investigating a behavioral problem, check the adequacy of the diet and seek a routine physical examination before undertaking more expensive, and possibly more harmful, treatment options. If iron deficiency is the problem, then treatment with an iron-rich diet and iron supplements may improve mood, cognitive skills, and physical performance. The effects of iron deficiency on children's behavior are discussed further in Chapter 16.

Iron Deficiency and Pica A curious behavior seen in some iron-deficient people, especially in women and children of low-income groups, is **pica**—the craving and consumption of ice, chalk, starch, and other nonfood substances. These substances contain no iron and cannot remedy a deficiency; in fact, these substances may actually inhibit iron absorption, which may explain the iron deficiency that accompanies pica.[10]

pica (PIE-ka): a craving for and consumption of nonfood substances. Pica is known as *geophagia* (gee-oh-FAY-gee-uh) when referring to eating clay, baby powder, chalk, ash, ceramics, paper, paint chips, or charcoal; *pagophagia* (pag-oh-FAY-gee-uh) when referring to eating large quantities of ice; and *amylophagia* (AM-ee-low-FAY-gee-ah) when referring to eating uncooked starch (flour, laundry starch, or raw rice).

Iron Overload As mentioned earlier, because too much iron can be toxic, its levels in the body are closely regulated and absorption normally decreases when iron stores are full. Even a diet that includes fortified foods usually poses no risk for most people, but some individuals are vulnerable to excess iron. Once considered rare, **iron overload** has emerged as an important disorder of iron metabolism and regulation.

The most likely cause of iron overload is a disorder known as **hemochromatosis**, which is caused by a genetic failure to prevent unneeded iron in the diet from being absorbed.[11] People who use alcohol excessively are particularly vulnerable because alcohol damages the small intestine, further impairing its defenses against absorbing excess iron. Just as insulin supports normal glucose homeostasis and its absence or ineffectiveness causes diabetes, the hormone hepcidin supports iron homeostasis and its deficiency or (rarely) resistance causes hemochromatosis. Other causes of iron overload include repeated blood transfusions (which bypass the intestinal defense), massive doses of supplementary iron (which overwhelm the intestinal defense), and other rare metabolic disorders.

Some of the signs and symptoms of iron overload are similar to those of iron deficiency: apathy, lethargy, and fatigue. Therefore, taking iron supplements before assessing iron status is clearly unwise; hemoglobin tests alone would fail to make the distinction because excess iron accumulates in storage. Iron overload assessment tests measure transferrin saturation and serum ferritin.

Iron overload is characterized by a toxic accumulation of iron in the liver, heart, joints, and other tissues. Excess iron in these tissues causes free-radical damage. Infections are likely because viruses and bacteria thrive on iron-rich blood. Untreated iron overload can lead to cirrhosis, liver cancer, heart failure, and arthritis.[12] In addition to selecting a low-iron diet and limiting absorption-enhancing factors, treatment involves **phlebotomy**, which removes blood from the body, and chelation therapy, which uses a **chelate** to form a complex with iron and promote its excretion. Research targeting the activity of hepcidin is active and promising.[13]

Iron overload is much more common in men than in women and is twice as prevalent among men as iron deficiency. The widespread fortification of foods with iron makes it difficult for people with hemochromatosis to follow a low-iron diet, and greater dangers lie in the indiscriminate use of iron and vitamin C supplements. Vitamin C not only enhances iron absorption, but also releases iron from ferritin, allowing free iron to wreak the damage typical of free radicals. Thus vitamin C acts as a *pro*oxidant when taken in high doses. (See Highlight 11 for a discussion of free radicals and their effects on chronic diseases.)

Iron and Chronic Diseases Some research suggests a link between heart disease and heme iron.[14] Limited evidence suggests an association between iron and some cancers.[15] Excess iron might contribute to these chronic diseases by increasing oxidative stress.[16] One of the benefits of a high-fiber diet may be that the accompanying phytates bind iron, making it less available for such reactions.

Iron Poisoning Large doses of iron supplements cause GI distress, including constipation, nausea, vomiting, and diarrhea. These effects may not be as serious as other consequences of iron toxicity, but they are consistent enough to establish a UL of 45 milligrams per day for adults.

Ingestion of iron-containing supplements is a common cause of accidental poisoning in young children. Symptoms of toxicity include nausea, vomiting, diarrhea, a rapid heartbeat, a weak pulse, dizziness, shock, and confusion. As few as five iron tablets containing as little as 200 milligrams of iron have caused death in young children. The exact cause of death is uncertain, but excessive free-radical damage is thought to play a role in heart failure and respiratory distress. Autopsy reports reveal iron deposits and cell death in the stomach, small intestine, liver, and blood vessels (which can cause internal bleeding). As with medicines and other potentially toxic substances, keep iron-containing tablets out of the reach of children. If you suspect iron poisoning, call the nearest poison control center or a physician immediately.

iron overload: toxicity from excess iron.

hemochromatosis (HE-moh-KRO-ma-toe-sis): a genetically determined failure to prevent absorption of unneeded dietary iron that is characterized by iron overload and tissue damage.

phlebotomy: the withdrawal of blood from the body.

chelate (KEY-late): a substance that can grasp the positive ions of a mineral.

- **chele** = claw

Iron Recommendations The usual diet in the United States provides about 6 to 7 milligrams of iron for every 1000 kcalories. The recommended daily intake for men is 8 milligrams, and because most men eat more than 2000 kcalories a day, they can meet their iron needs with little effort. Women in their reproductive years, however, need 18 milligrams a day.

Because women have higher iron needs and lower energy needs, they sometimes have trouble obtaining enough iron. On average, women receive only 12 to 13 milligrams of iron per day, which is not enough iron for women until after menopause. To meet their iron needs from foods, premenopausal women need to select iron-rich foods at every meal.

Vegetarians need 1.8 times as much iron to make up for the low bioavailability typical of their diets. Good vegetarian sources of iron include soy foods (such as soybeans and tofu), legumes (such as lentils and kidney beans), nuts (such as cashews and almonds), seeds (such as pumpkin seeds and sunflower seeds), cereals (such as cream of wheat and oatmeal), dried fruit (such as apricots and raisins), vegetables (such as mushrooms and potatoes), and blackstrap molasses.

Iron Food Sources To obtain enough iron, people must first select iron-rich foods—both naturally occurring and enriched or fortified—and then take advantage of factors that maximize iron absorption. This discussion begins by identifying iron-rich foods and then reviews the factors affecting absorption. Figure 13-7 shows the amounts of iron in selected foods. Meats, fish, and poultry

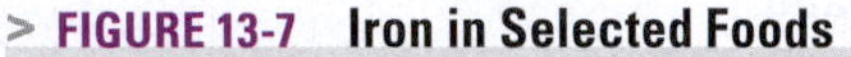

> FIGURE 13-7 **Iron in Selected Foods**

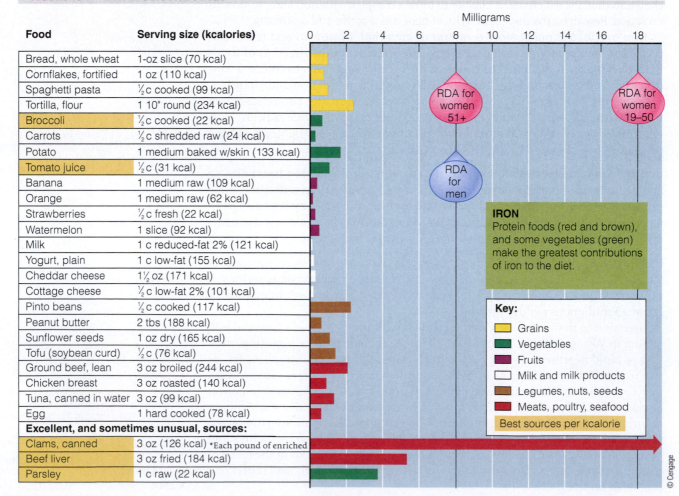

Food	Serving size (kcalories)
Bread, whole wheat	1-oz slice (70 kcal)
Cornflakes, fortified	1 oz (110 kcal)
Spaghetti pasta	½ c cooked (99 kcal)
Tortilla, flour	1 10" round (234 kcal)
Broccoli	½ c cooked (22 kcal)
Carrots	½ c shredded raw (24 kcal)
Potato	1 medium baked w/skin (133 kcal)
Tomato juice	½ c (31 kcal)
Banana	1 medium raw (109 kcal)
Orange	1 medium raw (62 kcal)
Strawberries	½ c fresh (22 kcal)
Watermelon	1 slice (92 kcal)
Milk	1 c reduced-fat 2% (121 kcal)
Yogurt, plain	1 c low-fat (155 kcal)
Cheddar cheese	1½ oz (171 kcal)
Cottage cheese	½ c low-fat 2% (101 kcal)
Pinto beans	½ c cooked (117 kcal)
Peanut butter	2 tbs (188 kcal)
Sunflower seeds	1 oz dry (165 kcal)
Tofu (soybean curd)	½ c (76 kcal)
Ground beef, lean	3 oz broiled (244 kcal)
Chicken breast	3 oz roasted (140 kcal)
Tuna, canned in water	3 oz (99 kcal)
Egg	1 hard cooked (78 kcal)
Excellent, and sometimes unusual, sources:	
Clams, canned	3 oz (126 kcal) *Each pound of enriched
Beef liver	3 oz fried (184 kcal)
Parsley	1 c raw (22 kcal)

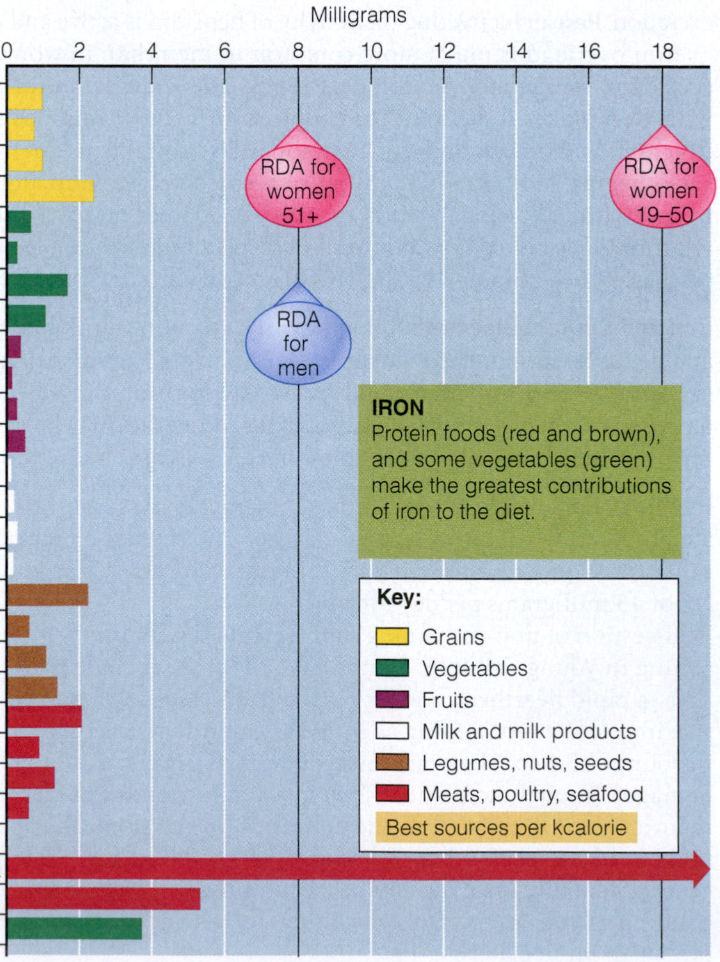

Milligrams
0
2
4
6
8
10
12
14
16
18
RDA for women 51+
RDA for women 19–50
RDA for men
IRON
Protein foods (red and brown), and some vegetables (green) make the greatest contributions of iron to the diet.
Key:
Grains
Vegetables
Fruits
Milk and milk products
Legumes, nuts, seeds
Meats, poultry, seafood
Best sources per kcalorie

contribute the most iron per serving; other protein-rich foods such as legumes and eggs are also good sources. Although an indispensable part of the diet, foods in the milk group are notoriously poor in iron. Grain products vary, with whole-grain, enriched, and fortified breads and cereals contributing significantly to iron intakes. Finally, dark greens (such as broccoli) and dried fruits (such as raisins) contribute some iron.

The FDA does not mandate iron enrichment, but most states require manufacturers to enrich flour and grain products with iron (see Photo 13-2).* One serving of enriched bread or cereal provides only a little iron, but because people eat many servings of these foods, the contribution can be significant. Iron fortification of grain products effectively reduces the prevalence of iron deficiency.[17] Iron added to foods is nonheme iron, which is not absorbed as well as heme iron, but when eaten with absorption-enhancing foods, enrichment iron can increase iron stores and reduce iron deficiency. In cases of iron overload, enrichment may exacerbate the problem.

Craig M. Moore

> **PHOTO 13-2** When the label on a grain product says "enriched," it means iron and several B vitamins have been added to meet FDA standards.

In general, the bioavailability of iron is high in meats, fish, and poultry, intermediate in grains and legumes, and low in most vegetables, especially those containing oxalates, such as spinach. As mentioned earlier, the amount of iron ultimately absorbed from a meal depends on the combined effects of several enhancing and inhibiting factors. For maximum absorption of nonheme iron, eat meat for the MFP factor and fruits or vegetables for vitamin C. The iron of baked beans, for example, will be enhanced by the MFP factor in a piece of pork served with them. The iron of bread will be enhanced by the vitamin C in a slice of tomato on a sandwich.

Iron Contamination In addition to the iron from foods, **contamination iron** from nonfood sources of inorganic iron salts can contribute to the day's intakes. Foods cooked in iron cookware take up iron salts. The more acidic the food and the longer it is cooked in iron cookware, the higher the iron content. The iron content of eggs can triple in the time it takes to scramble them in an iron pan. Admittedly, the absorption of this iron may be poor (perhaps only 1 to 2 percent), but every little bit helps a person who is trying to increase iron intake (see Photo 13-3).

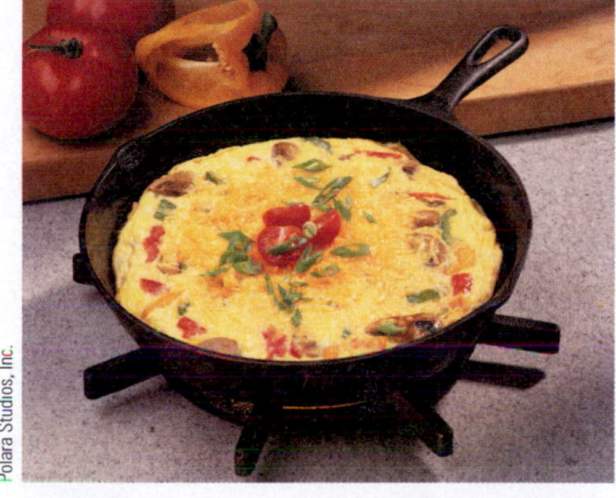

Polara Studios, Inc.

> **PHOTO 13-3** An old-fashioned iron skillet adds iron to foods. Increase in iron content (mg) for selected foods (3 oz) after cooking in iron skillet:

Beef stew	0.66→3.40
Chili	0.96→6.27
Cornbread	0.67→0.86
Hamburger	1.49→2.29
Pancake	0.63→1.31
Rice	0.67→1.97
Scrambled egg	1.49→4.76
Spaghetti sauce	0.61→5.77

Iron Supplementation People who are iron deficient may need supplements as well as an iron-rich, absorption-enhancing diet. Many physicians routinely recommend iron supplements to pregnant women, infants, and young children. Iron from supplements is less well absorbed than that from food, so the doses must be high. The absorption of iron taken as ferrous sulfate is better than that from other iron supplements. Absorption also improves when supplements are taken between meals, at bedtime on an empty stomach, and with liquids (other than milk, tea, or coffee, which inhibit absorption). Taking iron supplements in a single dose instead of several doses per day is equally effective and may improve a person's willingness to take it regularly.

There is no benefit to taking iron supplements with orange juice because vitamin C does not enhance absorption from supplements as it does from foods. Vitamin C enhances iron absorption by converting insoluble ferric iron in foods to the more soluble ferrous iron, and supplemental iron is already in the ferrous form. Constipation is a common side effect of iron supplementation; drinking plenty of water helps relieve this problem. The best strategy to ensure compliance is to individualize the dose, formulation, and schedule. Most importantly, iron supplements should be taken only when prescribed by a physician who has assessed an iron deficiency.

contamination iron: iron found in foods as the result of contamination by inorganic iron salts from iron cookware, iron-containing soils, and the like.

*Each pound of enriched flour contains at least 20 milligrams of iron.

REVIEW IT

Most of the body's iron is in hemoglobin and myoglobin, where it carries oxygen for use in energy metabolism; some iron is also required for enzymes involved in a variety of reactions. Special proteins assist with iron absorption, transport, and storage—all helping to maintain an appropriate balance—because both too little and too much iron can be damaging. Iron deficiency is most common among infants and young children, teenagers, women of childbearing age, and pregnant women. Symptoms include fatigue and anemia. Iron overload is most common in men. Heme iron, which is found only in meat, fish, and poultry, is better absorbed than nonheme iron, which occurs in most foods. Nonheme iron absorption is improved by eating iron-containing foods with foods containing the MFP factor and vitamin C; absorption is limited by phytates and oxalates. The accompanying table provides a summary of iron.

Iron

RDA

Men: 8 mg/day

Women: 18 mg/day (19–50 yr)
8 mg/day (51+)

UL

Adults: 45 mg/day

Chief Functions in the Body

Part of the protein hemoglobin, which carries oxygen in the blood; part of the protein myoglobin in muscles, which makes oxygen available for muscle contraction; necessary for the utilization of energy as part of the cells' metabolic machinery

Significant Sources

Red meats, fish, poultry, shellfish, eggs, legumes, dried fruits

Deficiency Symptoms

Anemia: weakness, fatigue, headaches; impaired work performance and cognitive function; impaired immunity; pale skin, nail beds, mucous membranes, and palm creases; concave nails; inability to regulate body temperature; pica

Toxicity Symptoms

GI distress

Iron overload: infections, fatigue, joint pain, skin pigmentation, organ damage

Zinc

Zinc is an essential trace element required for numerous metabolic reactions. Virtually all cells contain zinc, but the highest concentrations are found in muscle and bone.

Zinc Roles in the Body Zinc supports the work of thousands of proteins in the body, such as the **metalloenzymes,** which participate in a variety of metabolic processes, and **transcription factors,** which regulate gene expression.[18] In addition, zinc stabilizes cell membranes and DNA, helping to strengthen antioxidant defenses against free-radical attacks. Zinc also assists in immune function and in growth and development.[19] Zinc participates in the synthesis, storage, and release of the hormone insulin in the pancreas, although it does not appear to play a direct role in insulin's action. Zinc interacts with platelets in blood clotting, affects thyroid hormone function, and influences behavior and learning performance. It is needed to produce the active form of vitamin A (retinal) in visual pigments and the retinol-binding protein that transports vitamin A. It is essential to normal taste perception, wound healing, sperm production, and fetal development. A zinc deficiency impairs all these and other functions, underlining the vast importance of zinc in supporting the body's proteins.

Zinc Absorption The body's handling of zinc resembles that of iron in some ways and differs in others. A key difference is the circular passage of zinc from the small intestine to the body and back again.

The rate of zinc absorption varies from about 15 to 40 percent, depending on the amount of zinc consumed—as zinc intake increases, the rate of absorption decreases, and as zinc intake decreases, the rate of absorption increases. Like iron, dietary factors such as phytates influence absorption, limiting its bioavailability.

Upon absorption into an intestinal cell, zinc has two options. Zinc may participate in the metabolic functions of the intestinal cell itself, or it may be retained within the intestinal cells by **metallothionein** until the body needs zinc. Metallothionein plays a key role in storing and distributing zinc throughout the body.

zinc: an essential trace mineral that is part of many enzymes and a constituent of insulin.

metalloenzymes (meh-TAL-oh-EN-zimes): enzymes that contain one or more minerals as part of their structures.

transcription factors: proteins that bind to specific sites in DNA and alter gene expression.

metallothionein (meh-TAL-oh-THIGH-oh-neen): a sulfur-rich protein that avidly binds with and transports metals such as zinc.

- **metallo** = containing a metal
- **thio** = containing sulfur
- **ein** = a protein

> **FIGURE 13-8 Enteropancreatic Circulation of Zinc**

Some zinc from food is absorbed by the small intestine and sent to the pancreas to be incorporated into digestive enzymes that return to the small intestine. This cycle is called the *enteropancreatic circulation* of zinc.

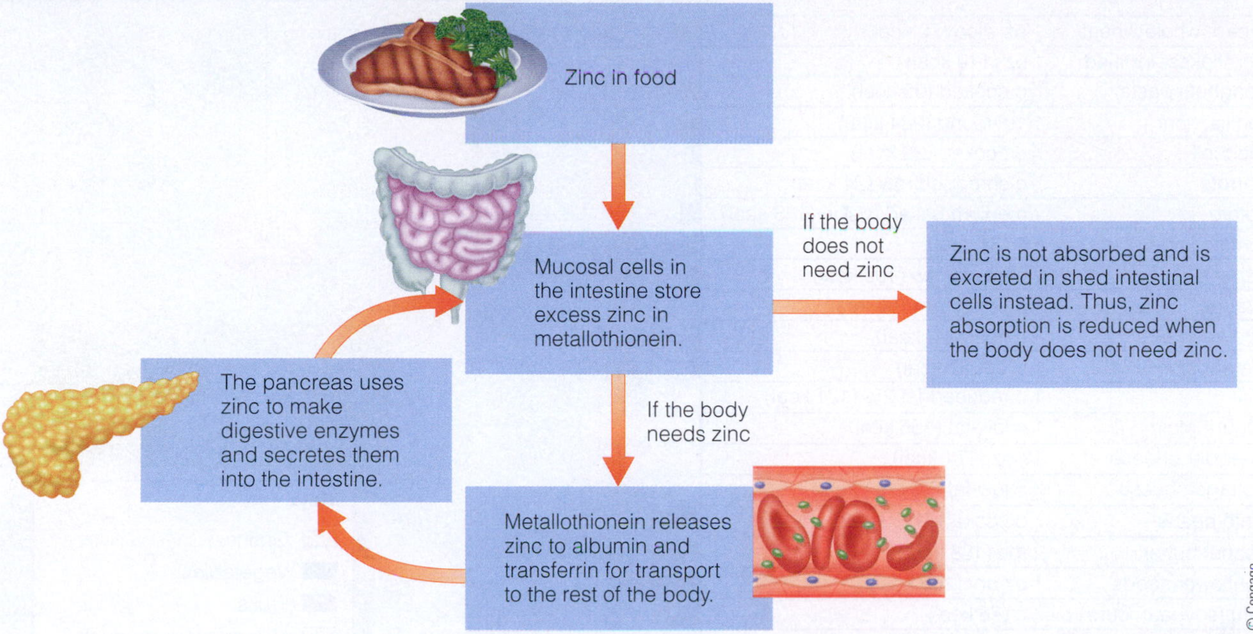

Zinc in food
Mucosal cells in the intestine store excess zinc in metallothionein.
If the body does not need zinc
Zinc is not absorbed and is excreted in shed intestinal cells instead. Thus, zinc absorption is reduced when the body does not need zinc.
If the body needs zinc
Metallothionein releases zinc to albumin and transferrin for transport to the rest of the body.
The pancreas uses zinc to make digestive enzymes and secretes them into the intestine.
© Cengage

Zinc Transport After being absorbed, some zinc eventually reaches the pancreas, where it is incorporated into many of the digestive enzymes that the pancreas releases into the small intestine at mealtimes. The small intestine thus receives two doses of zinc with each meal—one from foods and the other from the zinc-rich pancreatic juices. The recycling of zinc in the body from the pancreas to the small intestine and back to the pancreas is referred to as the **enteropancreatic circulation** of zinc. Each time zinc circulates through the small intestine, it may be excreted in shed intestinal cells or reabsorbed into the body (see Figure 13-8). The body loses zinc primarily in feces. Smaller losses occur in urine, shed skin, hair, sweat, menstrual fluids, and semen.

Numerous proteins participate in zinc transport. Zinc's main transport vehicle in the blood is the protein albumin. Some zinc also binds to transferrin—the same transferrin that carries iron in the blood.

Zinc Deficiency Zinc deficiency is not widespread in developed countries, but an estimated 17 percent of the world's population has inadequate zinc intakes.[20] Human zinc deficiency was first reported in the 1960s in children and adolescent boys in Egypt, Iran, and Turkey. Children have especially high zinc needs because they are growing rapidly and synthesizing many zinc-containing proteins, and Middle Eastern diets are traditionally low in the richest zinc source—meats. Furthermore, the staple foods in these diets are legumes, unleavened breads, and other whole-grain foods—all high in fiber and phytates, which inhibit zinc absorption.*

Figure 13-9 shows stunted growth and mentions the immature sexual development characteristic of zinc deficiency. In addition, zinc deficiency hinders digestion and absorption, causing diarrhea, which worsens malnutrition not only for zinc, but for other nutrients as well. It also impairs the immune response, making infections likely—among them, pneumonia and GI tract infections, which worsen malnutrition, including zinc malnutrition (a classic downward spiral of events).[21] Chronic zinc deficiency damages the central nervous system and brain and may lead to poor motor development and cognitive

*Unleavened bread contains no yeast, which normally breaks down phytates during fermentation.

> **FIGURE 13-9 Zinc-Deficiency Symptom—Stunted Growth**

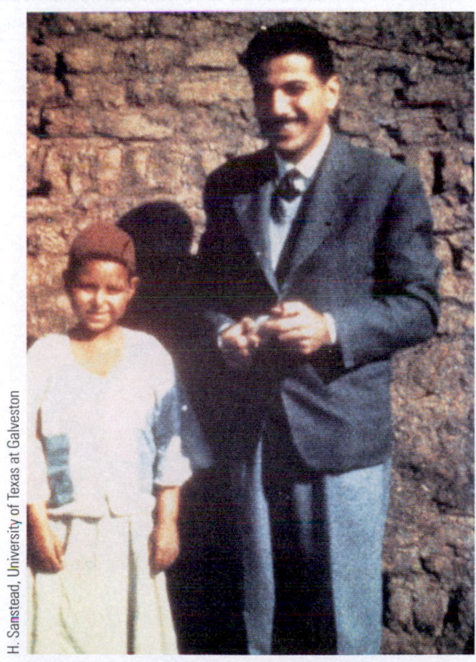

H. Sanstead, University of Texas at Galveston

The Egyptian man on the right is an adult of average height. The Egyptian boy on the left is 17 years old but is only 4 feet tall, like a 7-year-old in the United States. His genitalia are like those of a 6-year-old.

enteropancreatic (EN-ter-oh-PAN-kree-AT-ik) circulation: the circulatory route from the pancreas to the small intestine and back to the pancreas.

> **FIGURE 13-10 Zinc in Selected Foods**

Food	Serving size (kcalories)
Bread, whole wheat	1-oz slice (70 kcal)
Cornflakes, fortified	1 oz (110 kcal)
Spaghetti pasta	½ c cooked (99 kcal)
Tortilla, flour	1 10" round (234 kcal)
Broccoli	½ c cooked (22 kcal)
Carrots	½ c shredded raw (24 kcal)
Potato	1 medium baked w/skin (133 kcal)
Tomato juice	¾ c (31 kcal)
Banana	1 medium raw (109 kcal)
Orange	1 medium raw (62 kcal)
Strawberries	½ c fresh (22 kcal)
Watermelon	1 slice (92 kcal)
Milk	1 c reduced-fat 2% (121 kcal)
Yogurt, plain	1 c low-fat (155 kcal)
Cheddar cheese	1½ oz (171 kcal)
Cottage cheese	½ c low-fat 2% (101 kcal)
Pinto beans	½ c cooked (117 kcal)
Peanut butter	2 tbs (188 kcal)
Sunflower seeds	1 oz dry (165 kcal)
Tofu (soybean curd)	½ c (76 kcal)
Ground beef, lean	3 oz broiled (244 kcal)
Chicken breast	3 oz roasted (140 kcal)
Tuna, canned in water	3 oz (99 kcal)
Egg	1 hard cooked (78 kcal)
Excellent, and sometimes unusual, sources:	
Oysters	3 oz cooked (139 kcal)
Sirloin steak, lean	3 oz broiled (172 kcal)
Crab	3 oz cooked (94 kcal)

Milligrams
0
2
4
6
8
10
12
RDA for men
RDA for women
ZINC
Meat, seafood, and poultry (red) are concentrated sources of zinc. Milk (white) and legumes, nuts, and seeds (brown) contain some zinc.
Key:
Grains
Vegetables
Fruits
Milk and milk products
Legumes, nuts, seeds
Meats, poultry, seafood
Best sources per kcalorie

performance. Because zinc deficiency directly impairs vitamin A metabolism, vitamin A–deficiency symptoms often appear. Zinc deficiency also disturbs thyroid function and the metabolic rate. It alters taste, causes loss of appetite, and slows wound healing—in fact, its symptoms are so pervasive that generalized malnutrition and sickness are more likely to be the diagnosis than simple zinc deficiency.

Zinc Toxicity High doses (more than 50 milligrams) of zinc may cause vomiting, diarrhea, headaches, exhaustion, and other symptoms. The UL for adults was set at 40 milligrams based on zinc's interference in copper metabolism—an effect that, in animals, leads to degeneration of the heart muscle.

Zinc Recommendations and Sources Figure 13-10 shows zinc amounts in selected foods per serving. Zinc is highest in protein-rich foods such as shellfish (especially oysters), meats, poultry, milk, and cheese (see Photo 13-4). Plant-based diets tend to be low in zinc, although legumes and whole-grain products are good sources of zinc if eaten in large quantities.[22] In typical US diets, the phytate content of grains is not high enough to impair zinc absorption. Vegetables vary in zinc content depending on the soil in which they are grown. Average zinc intakes in the United States are slightly higher than recommendations.

Zinc Supplementation In developed countries, most people obtain enough zinc from the diet without resorting to supplements. In developing countries, zinc supplementation plays a major role in effectively reducing the incidence of disease and death associated with diarrhea and pneumonia.[23]

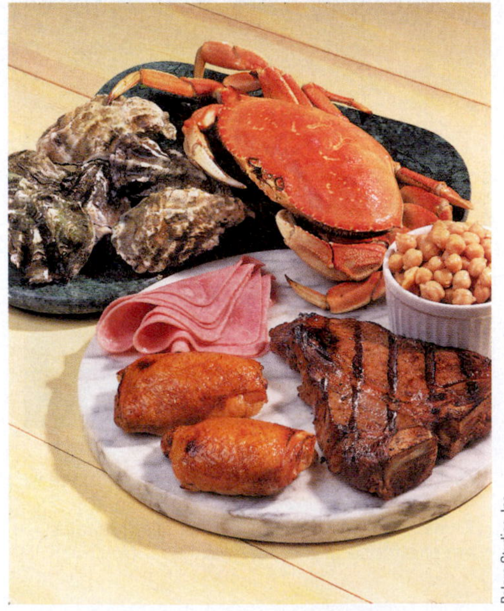

> **PHOTO 13-4** Zinc is highest in protein-rich foods such as oysters, beef, poultry, legumes, and nuts.

Zinc lozenges may shorten the duration, but not the severity, of common cold symptoms.[24] Lozenges of zinc acetate or zinc gluconate are most effective, whereas other zinc compounds, including those with flavor enhancers, are much less effective. In addition to the appropriate zinc formulation, effectiveness depends on relatively high doses (75 milligrams) taken within 24 hours of the onset of symptoms and continued daily throughout the duration of the cold. Common side effects of zinc lozenges include nausea and bad taste reactions.

REVIEW IT

Zinc-requiring enzymes participate in a multitude of reactions affecting growth, vitamin A activity, and pancreatic digestive enzyme synthesis, among others. After a meal, both dietary zinc and zinc-rich pancreatic secretions (via enteropancreatic circulation) are absorbed. Absorption is regulated by a special binding protein (metallothionein) in the small intestine. Protein-rich foods derived from animals are the best sources of bioavailable zinc. Fiber and phytates in cereals bind zinc, limiting absorption. Stunted growth and sexual immaturity are hallmark symptoms of zinc deficiency. The accompanying table provides a summary of zinc.

Zinc

RDA	Significant Sources
Men: 11 mg/day Women: 8 mg/day	Protein-containing foods: red meats, shellfish, whole grains; some fortified cereals
UL	**Deficiency Symptoms[a]**
Adults: 40 mg/day	Stunted growth, delayed sexual maturation, impaired immune function, hair loss, eye and skin lesions, loss of appetite
Chief Functions in the Body	**Toxicity Symptoms**
Part of many enzymes; associated with the hormone insulin; involved in making genetic material and proteins, immune reactions, transport of vitamin A, taste perception, wound healing, the making of sperm, and the normal development of the fetus	Loss of appetite, impaired immunity, low HDL, copper and iron deficiencies

[a]A rare inherited disease of zinc malabsorption, *acrodermatitis* (AK-roh-der-ma-TIE-tis) *enteropathica* (EN-ter-oh-PATH-ick-ah), causes additional and more severe symptoms.

Iodine

Traces of **iodine** are indispensable to life. It commonly occurs as the anion iodide or as part of an iodate salt.

Iodine Roles in the Body Iodine is an integral part of the thyroid hormones that regulate body temperature, metabolic rate, reproduction, growth, blood cell production, nerve and muscle function, and more.* By controlling the rate at which the cells use oxygen, these hormones influence the amount of energy expended during basal metabolism.

Iodine Deficiency The hypothalamus regulates thyroid hormone production by controlling the release of the pituitary's thyroid-stimulating hormone (TSH).** With iodine deficiency, thyroid hormone production diminishes, and the body responds by secreting more TSH in a futile attempt to accelerate iodine uptake by the thyroid gland. If a deficiency persists, the cells of the thyroid gland enlarge to trap as much iodine as possible. Sometimes the gland enlarges until it makes a visible lump in the neck, a **goiter** (shown in Figure 13-11).

Almost all cases of goiter are caused by iodine deficiency. A relatively small percent of the world's population have goiter because they regularly eat excessive amounts of foods that contain phytochemicals that interfere with iodine uptake

*The thyroid gland releases tetraiodothyronine (T_4), commonly known as *thyroxine* (thigh-ROCKS-in), to its target tissues. Upon reaching the cells, T_4 loses one iodine, becoming triiodothyronine (T_3), which is the active form of the hormone.
**Thyroid-stimulating hormone is also called *thyrotropin*.

> **FIGURE 13-11 Iodine-Deficiency Symptom—The Enlarged Thyroid of Goiter**

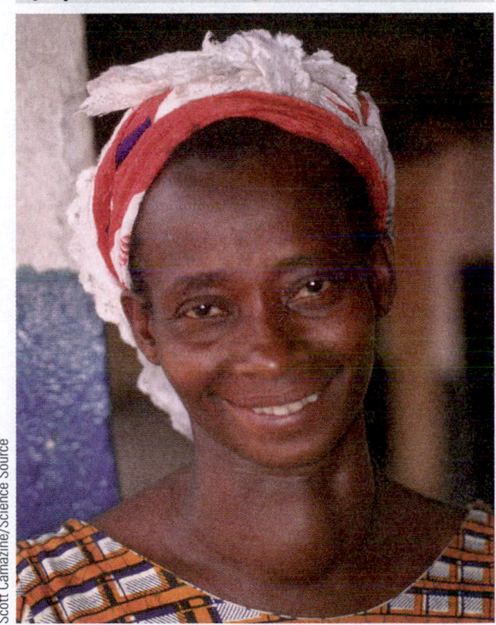

Scott Camazine/Science Source

In iodine deficiency, the thyroid gland enlarges—a condition known as simple goiter. Iodine toxicity also enlarges the thyroid gland, creating a similar-looking goiter.

iodine: an essential trace mineral that is needed for the synthesis of thyroid hormones; the anion (I^-) form of iodine is *iodide.*

goiter (GOY-ter): an enlargement of the thyroid gland due to an iodine deficiency, malfunction of the gland, or overconsumption of a goitrogen. Goiter caused by iodine deficiency is sometimes called *simple goiter.*

by the thyroid and thus limit its hormone production. These phytochemicals act as **goitrogens**, and their effect is not counteracted by dietary iodine. Goitrogen-containing foods include vegetables such as collards, brussels sprouts, and kale. The goitrogens present in plants remind us that even natural components of foods can cause harm when eaten in excess.

Goiter may be the earliest and most obvious sign of iodine deficiency, but the most tragic and prevalent damage occurs in the brain.[25] Iodine deficiency is the most common cause of *preventable* mental impairment and brain damage in the world. Nearly one-third of the world's school-age children have iodine deficiency. Children with even a mild iodine deficiency typically have goiters and perform poorly in school.[26] With sustained treatment, however, mental performance in the classroom as well as thyroid function improves.

A severe iodine deficiency during pregnancy causes the extreme and irreversible mental impairment and stunted physical growth known as **cretinism.**[27]* The near eradication of cretinism in the United States and other developed countries is a great triumph, but cretinism still affects approximately 2 million children worldwide every year.[28] A worldwide effort to provide iodized salt to people living in iodine-deficient areas has been dramatically successful. An estimated 70 percent of all households in developing countries have access to iodized salt.[29] Because iron deficiency is common among people with iodine deficiency and because iron deficiency reduces the effectiveness of iodized salt, dual fortification with both iron and iodine may be most beneficial.

Iodine Toxicity Excessive intakes of iodine can interfere with thyroid function and enlarge the gland, just as deficiency can. During pregnancy, exposure to excessive iodine from foods, prenatal supplements, or medications is especially damaging to the developing infant. An infant exposed to toxic amounts of iodine during gestation may develop a goiter so severe as to block the airways and cause suffocation. The UL is 1100 micrograms per day for an adult—several times higher than average or recommended intakes (review Figure 13-1, p. 394). For perspective, most foods provide 3 to 75 micrograms of iodine per serving.

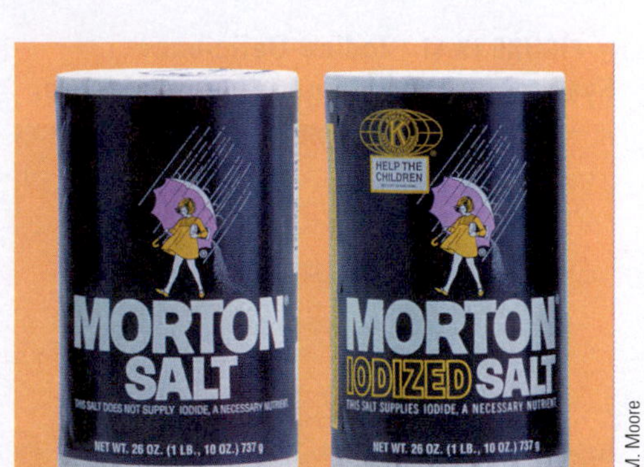
MORTON
SALT
MORTON
IODIZED SALT
HELP THE CHILDREN
NET WT. 26 OZ. (1 LB., 10 OZ.) 737 g
NET WT. 26 OZ. (1 LB., 10 OZ.) 737 g

Craig M. Moore

> **PHOTO 13-5** Only "iodized salt" has had iodine added. Labels on salt that do not provide added iodine must state "This salt does not supply iodide, a necessary nutrient."

Iodine Recommendations and Sources The ocean is the world's major source of iodine. In coastal areas, kelp, seafood, water, and even iodine-containing sea mist are dependable iodine sources. Further inland, the amount of iodine in foods is variable and generally reflects the amount present in the soil in which plants are grown or on which animals graze. Landmasses that were once under the ocean have soils rich in iodine; those in flood-prone areas where water leaches iodine from the soil are poor in iodine. In the United States, the iodization of salt provides about 60 micrograms of iodine per gram of salt (see Photo 13-5). This tiny amount eliminated the widespread misery caused by iodine deficiency during the 1930s, but iodized salt is not available in many parts of the world. Some countries add iodine to bread, fish paste, or drinking water instead.

Although the average consumption of iodine in the United States exceeds recommendations, it falls below toxic levels. Some of the excess iodine in the US diet stems from fast foods, which use iodized salt liberally. Some iodine comes from bakery products and from milk. The baking industry uses iodates (iodine salts) as dough conditioners, and most dairies feed cows iodine-containing medications and use iodine to disinfect milking equipment. Processed foods in the United States use regular salt, not iodized salt.

The recommended intake of iodine for adults is a minuscule amount that is easily met by consuming seafood, vegetables grown in iodine-rich soil, and iodized salt. Just one-half teaspoon of iodized salt provides the RDA for iodine. In the United States, labels indicate whether salt is iodized.

goitrogens (GOY-troh-jenz): substances that enlarge the thyroid gland and cause *toxic goiter*. Goitrogens occur naturally in such foods as cabbage, kale, brussels sprouts, cauliflower, broccoli, and kohlrabi.

cretinism (CREE-tin-ism): a congenital disease characterized by limited mental and physical development and commonly caused by maternal iodine deficiency during pregnancy.

*The underactivity of the thyroid gland is known as *hypothyroidism* and may be caused by iodine deficiency or any number of other causes. Without treatment, an infant with *congenital hypothyroidism* will develop *cretinism*.

REVIEW IT

Iodine is an essential component of the thyroid hormones. An iodine deficiency can lead to simple goiter (enlargement of the thyroid gland) and can impair fetal development, causing cretinism. Iodization of salt has largely eliminated iodine deficiency in the United States. The accompanying table provides a summary of iodine.

Iodine

RDA	Deficiency Disease
Adults: 150 μg/day	Simple goiter, cretinism
UL	**Deficiency Symptoms**
1100 μg/day	Underactive thyroid gland, goiter, limited mental and physical development in infants (cretinism)
Chief Functions in the Body	**Toxicity Symptoms**
A component of two thyroid hormones that help regulate growth, development, and metabolic rate	Underactive thyroid gland, elevated TSH, goiter
Significant Sources	
Iodized salt, seafood, bread, dairy products, plants grown in iodine-rich soil and animals fed those plants	

Selenium

The essential mineral **selenium** shares some of the chemical characteristics of the mineral sulfur. This similarity allows selenium to substitute for sulfur in the amino acids methionine, cysteine, and cystine.

Selenium Roles in the Body Selenium is one of the body's antioxidant nutrients, working primarily as a part of proteins—most notably, the glutathione peroxidase enzymes. Glutathione peroxidase and vitamin E work in tandem. Glutathione peroxidase prevents free-radical formation, thus blocking the chain reaction before it begins; if free radicals do form and a chain reaction starts, vitamin E stops it. (Highlight 11 described free-radical formation, chain reactions, and antioxidant action.) Other selenium-containing enzymes selectively activate or inactivate the thyroid hormones.

Selenium Deficiency Selenium deficiency is associated with **Keshan disease**—a heart disease that was prevalent in regions of China where the soil and foods lack selenium. Although a virus also contributes to the development of Keshan disease, selenium deficiency is a factor and adequate selenium prevents it.[30]

Selenium and Cancer Whereas low levels of selenium may increase the risk of some cancers, the antioxidant action of higher levels may protect against some cancers.[31] Selenium supplements, however, have not proved effective in preventing cancer and may in fact damage DNA and cause harm.

Selenium Recommendations and Sources Selenium is found in the soil, and therefore in the crops grown for consumption. People living in regions with selenium-poor soil may still get enough selenium, partly because they eat vegetables and grains transported from other regions and partly because they eat meats, milk, and eggs, which are reliable sources of selenium. Eating as few as two Brazil nuts a day effectively improves selenium status. Average intakes in the United States exceed the RDA, which is based on the amount needed to maximize glutathione peroxidase activity.

Selenium Toxicity The body carefully regulates selenium metabolism and transport to help ensure a healthy balance.[32] Because high doses of selenium are toxic, a UL has been set. Selenium toxicity causes loss and brittleness of hair and nails, garlic breath odor, and nervous system abnormalities.

selenium (se-LEEN-ee-um): an essential trace mineral that is part of an antioxidant enzyme.

Keshan (KESH-an or ka-SHAWN) **disease:** the heart disease associated with selenium deficiency; named for one of the provinces of China where it was first studied. Keshan disease is characterized by heart enlargement and insufficiency; fibrous tissue replaces the muscle tissue that normally composes the middle layer of the walls of the heart.

REVIEW IT

Selenium is an antioxidant nutrient that works closely with the glutathione peroxidase enzyme and vitamin E. Selenium is found in association with protein in foods. Deficiencies are associated with a heart abnormality known as Keshan disease. The accompanying table provides a summary of selenium.

Selenium

RDA

Adults: 55 μg/day

UL

Adults: 400 μg/day

Chief Functions in the Body

Defends against oxidation; regulates thyroid hormone

Significant Sources

Seafood, meat, whole grains, fruits, and vegetables (depending on soil content)

Deficiency Symptoms

Predisposition to heart disease characterized by cardiac tissue becoming fibrous (Keshan disease)

Toxicity Symptoms

Loss and brittleness of hair and nails; skin rash, fatigue, irritability, and nervous system disorders; garlic breath odor

Copper

The body contains about 100 milligrams of **copper** in a variety of cells and tissues. Copper balance and transport depend on a system of proteins.

Copper Roles in the Body

Copper serves as a constituent of several enzymes. The copper-containing enzymes have diverse metabolic roles with one common characteristic: all involve reactions that consume oxygen or oxygen radicals. For example, copper-containing enzymes catalyze the oxidation of ferrous iron to ferric iron, which allows iron to bind to transferrin. Copper's role in iron metabolism makes it a key factor in hemoglobin synthesis. Copper- and zinc-containing enzymes participate in the body's natural defenses against the oxidative damage of free radicals. Still other copper enzymes help to manufacture collagen, inactivate histamine, and degrade serotonin. Copper, like iron, is needed in many of the reactions involved in energy metabolism.[33]

Copper Deficiency and Toxicity

Typical US diets provide adequate amounts of copper, and deficiency is rare. In animals, copper deficiency raises blood cholesterol and damages blood vessels, raising questions about whether low dietary copper might contribute to cardiovascular disease in humans.

Some genetic disorders create a copper toxicity, but excessive intakes from foods are unlikely. Excessive intakes from supplements may cause liver damage, and therefore a UL has been set.

Two rare genetic disorders affect copper status in opposite directions. In **Menkes disease,** the intestinal cells absorb copper, but cannot release it into circulation, causing a life-threatening deficiency. Treatment involves giving copper intravenously. In **Wilson's disease,** copper accumulates in the liver and brain, creating a life-threatening toxicity. Wilson's disease can be controlled by reducing copper intake, using chelating agents such as penicillamine, and taking zinc supplements, which interfere with copper absorption.

Copper Recommendations and Sources

The richest food sources of copper are legumes, whole grains, nuts, shellfish, and seeds. More than half of the copper from foods is absorbed, and the major route of elimination appears to be bile. Water may also provide copper, depending on the type of plumbing pipe and the hardness of the water.

REVIEW IT

Copper is a component of several enzymes, all of which are involved in some way with oxygen or oxidation. Some act as antioxidants; others are essential to iron metabolism. Legumes,

copper: an essential trace mineral that is part of many enzymes.

Menkes disease: a genetic disorder of copper transport that creates a copper deficiency and results in mental impairment, poor muscle tone, seizures, brittle kinky hair, and failure to thrive.

Wilson's disease: a genetic disorder of copper metabolism that creates a copper toxicity and results in neurologic symptoms such as tremors, impaired speech, inappropriate behaviors, and personality changes.

whole grains, and shellfish are good sources of copper. The accompanying table provides a summary of copper.

Copper

RDA	Significant Sources
Adults: 900 µg/day	Seafood, nuts, whole grains, seeds, legumes
UL	**Deficiency Symptoms**
Adults: 10,000 µg/day (10 mg/day)	Anemia, bone abnormalities
Chief Functions in the Body	**Toxicity Symptoms**
Necessary for the absorption and use of iron in the formation of hemoglobin; part of several enzymes	Liver damage

Manganese

Manganese The human body contains a mere 20 milligrams of **manganese**. Most of it can be found in the bones and metabolically active organs such as the liver, kidneys, and pancreas.

Manganese Roles in the Body Manganese acts as a cofactor for many enzymes that facilitate the metabolism of carbohydrate, lipids, and amino acids. In addition, manganese-containing metalloenzymes assist in bone formation and the conversion of pyruvate to a TCA cycle compound. Its essential role in maintaining healthy nerves has sparked a flurry of activity in Parkinson's disease and Huntington's disease research.[34]

Manganese Deficiency and Toxicity Manganese requirements are low, and many plant foods contain significant amounts of this trace mineral, so deficiencies are rare. As is true of other trace minerals, however, dietary factors such as phytates inhibit its absorption. In addition, high intakes of iron and calcium limit manganese absorption, so people who use supplements of those minerals regularly may impair their manganese status.

Manganese toxicity is more likely to occur from a contaminated environment than from an excessive dietary intake. Miners who inhale large quantities of manganese dust on the job over prolonged periods show symptoms of a brain disease, along with abnormalities in appearance and behavior. A UL has been established based on intakes from food, water, and supplements.

Manganese Recommendations and Sources Grain products make the greatest contribution of manganese to the diet. With insufficient information to establish an RDA, an AI was set based on average intakes.

REVIEW IT

Manganese-dependent enzymes are involved in bone formation and various metabolic processes. Because manganese is widespread in plant foods, deficiencies are rare, although regular use of calcium and iron supplements may limit manganese absorption. The accompanying table provides a summary of manganese.

Manganese

AI	Significant Sources
Men: 2.3 mg/day	Nuts, whole grains, leafy vegetables, tea
Women: 1.8 mg/day	**Deficiency Symptoms**
UL	Rare
Adults: 11 mg/day	**Toxicity Symptoms**
Chief Functions in the Body	Nervous system disorders
Cofactor for several enzymes; bone formation	

manganese: an essential trace mineral that acts as a cofactor for many enzymes.

> FIGURE 13-12 US Population Receiving Fluoridated Water

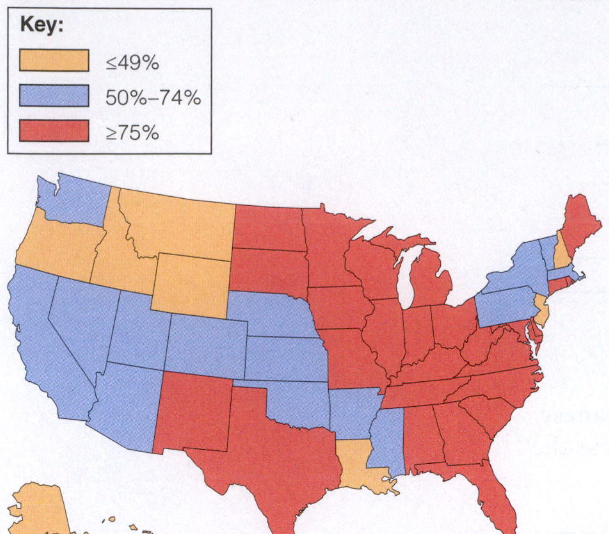
Key:
≤49%
50%–74%
≥75%
© Cengage

> FIGURE 13-13 Fluoride-Toxicity Symptom—The Mottled Teeth of Fluorosis

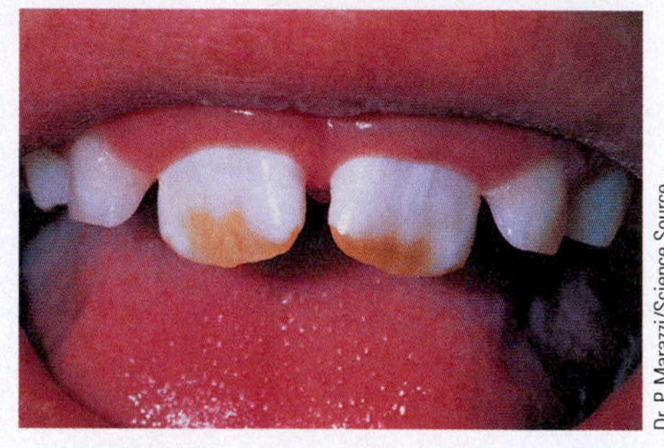
Dr. P. Marazzi/Science Source

Fluoride

Fluoride is present in virtually all soils, water supplies, plants, and animals. The body contains only a trace of fluoride, but with this amount, the crystalline deposits in teeth are larger and more perfectly formed.

Fluoride Roles in the Body As Chapter 12 explained, during the mineralization of bones and teeth, calcium and phosphorus form crystals called hydroxyapatite. Fluoride can replace the hydroxyl (OH) portions of the hydroxyapatite crystal, forming **fluorapatite,** which makes the teeth stronger and more resistant to decay.

Dental caries ranks as the nation's most widespread public health problem: an estimated 95 percent of the population have decayed, missing, or filled teeth. These dental problems can quickly lead to a multitude of nutrition problems by interfering with a person's ability to chew and eat a wide variety of foods. Where fluoride is lacking, dental decay is common.

Drinking water is usually the best source of fluoride, and 75 percent of the US population served by community water systems receives fluoridated water (see Figure 13-12).[35] Fluoridation of drinking water (to raise the concentration to 0.7 milligram per liter of water) protects against dental caries and supports oral health.[36] By fluoridating the drinking water, a community offers its residents, particularly the children, a safe, economical, practical, and effective way to defend against dental caries. Most bottled waters lack fluoride.

Fluoride Toxicity Too much fluoride can damage the teeth, causing **fluorosis.** For this reason, a UL has been established. In mild cases, the teeth develop small white flecks; in severe cases, the enamel becomes pitted and permanently stained (as shown in Figure 13-13). Fluorosis occurs only during tooth development and cannot be reversed, making its prevention during the first 3 years of life a high priority. To limit fluoride ingestion, take care not to swallow fluoride-containing dental products such as toothpaste and mouthwash and use fluoride supplements only as prescribed by a physician.

Fluoride Recommendations and Sources As mentioned earlier, much of the US population has access to water with an optimal fluoride concentration, which typically delivers about 1 milligram per person per day. Fish and most teas contain appreciable amounts of natural fluoride.

REVIEW IT

Fluoride makes teeth stronger and more resistant to decay. Fluoridation of public water supplies can significantly reduce the incidence of dental caries, but excess fluoride during tooth development can cause fluorosis—discolored and pitted tooth enamel. The accompanying table provides a summary of fluoride.

Fluoride

AI	Significant Sources
Men: 4 mg/day Women: 3 mg/day	Drinking water (if fluoride containing or fluoridated), tea, seafood
UL	**Deficiency Symptoms**
Adults: 10 mg/day	Susceptibility to tooth decay
Chief Functions in the Body	**Toxicity Symptoms**
Strengthens teeth; helps to make teeth resistant to decay	Fluorosis (pitting and discoloration of teeth)

fluoride: an essential trace mineral that makes teeth stronger and more resistant to decay.

fluorapatite (floor-APP-uh-tite): the stabilized form of tooth crystal, in which fluoride has replaced the hydroxyl groups of hydroxyapatite.

fluorosis (floor-OH-sis): discoloration and pitting of tooth enamel caused by excess fluoride during tooth development.

Chromium

Chromium is an essential mineral that participates in carbohydrate and lipid metabolism. Like iron, chromium assumes different charges. For chromium, the Cr^{+++} ion is the most stable and most commonly found in foods.

Chromium Roles in the Body Chromium helps maintain glucose homeostasis by enhancing the activity of the hormone insulin.* When chromium is lacking, a diabetes-like condition may develop, with elevated blood glucose and impaired glucose tolerance, insulin response, and glucagon response. Research suggests that chromium supplements provide little or no benefit to people with type 2 diabetes.[37]

Chromium Recommendations and Sources Chromium is present in a variety of foods. The best sources are unrefined foods, particularly liver, brewer's yeast, and whole grains. The more refined foods people eat, the less chromium they ingest.

REVIEW IT

Chromium enhances insulin's action. A deficiency can impair glucose homeostasis. Chromium is widely available in unrefined foods including brewer's yeast, whole grains, and liver. The accompanying table provides a summary of chromium.

Chromium

AI	Significant Sources
Men: 35 µg/day Women: 25 µg/day	Meats (especially liver), whole grains, brewer's yeast
Chief Functions in the Body	**Deficiency Symptoms**
Enhances insulin action and may improve glucose tolerance	Diabetes-like condition
	Toxicity Symptoms
	None reported

Molybdenum

Molybdenum acts as a working part of several metalloenzymes. Dietary deficiencies of molybdenum are unknown because the amounts needed are so small—as little as 0.1 part per million parts of body tissue. Legumes, breads and other grain products, leafy green vegetables, milk, and liver are molybdenum-rich foods. Average daily intakes fall within the suggested range of intakes.

Molybdenum toxicity in people is rare. It has been reported in animal studies, and a UL has been established. Characteristics of molybdenum toxicity include kidney damage and reproductive abnormalities.

REVIEW IT

Molybdenum is found in a variety of foods and participates in several metabolic reactions. The accompanying table provides a summary of molybdenum.

Molybdenum

RDA	Significant Sources
Adult: 45 µg/day	Legumes, cereals, nuts
UL	**Deficiency Symptoms**
Adults: 2 mg/day	Unknown
Chief Functions in the Body	**Toxicity Symptoms**
Cofactor for several enzymes	None reported; reproductive effects in animals

*Small organic compounds that enhance insulin's actions are called *glucose tolerance factors (GTF)*. Some glucose tolerance factors contain chromium.

chromium (KRO-mee-um): an essential trace mineral that enhances the activity of insulin.

molybdenum (mo-LIB-duh-num): an essential trace mineral that acts as a cofactor for many enzymes.

13.3 Contaminant Minerals

LEARN IT Describe how contaminant minerals disrupt body processes and impair nutrition status.

Chapter 12 and this chapter explain the many ways minerals serve the body—maintaining fluid and electrolyte balance, providing structural support to the bones, transporting oxygen, and assisting enzymes. In contrast to the essential minerals that the body requires, contaminant minerals impair the body's growth, work capacity, and general health. Contaminant minerals include the **heavy metals** lead, mercury, and cadmium, which enter the food supply by way of soil, water, and air pollution. This section focuses on lead poisoning because it is a serious environmental threat to young children and because reducing blood lead levels in children is a goal of the Healthy People initiative. Much of the information on lead applies to the other contaminant minerals as well—they all disrupt body processes and impair nutrition status similarly.

Like other minerals, lead is indestructible; the body cannot change its chemistry. Chemically similar to nutrient minerals such as iron, calcium, and zinc (cations with two positive charges), lead displaces them from some of the metabolic sites they normally occupy so they are then unable to perform their roles. For example, lead competes with iron in heme, but it cannot carry oxygen. Similarly, lead competes with calcium in the brain, but it cannot signal messages from nerve cells. Excess lead in the blood also deranges the structure of red blood cell membranes, making them leaky and fragile. Lead interacts with white blood cells, too, impairing their ability to fight infection, and it binds to antibodies, thwarting their effort to resist disease.

Children with iron deficiency are particularly vulnerable to lead toxicity. Chapter 16 examines the damaging effects of iron deficiency and lead toxicity on a child's growth and development. Chapter 19 includes mercury in its discussion of environmental contamination of foods.

REVIEW IT Describe how contaminant minerals disrupt body processes and impair nutrition status.

Lead typifies the ways all heavy metals behave in the body: they interfere with nutrients that are trying to do their jobs. The "good guy" nutrients are shoved aside by the "bad guy" contaminants. Then, when the contaminants cannot perform the roles of the nutrients, health diminishes. To safeguard our health, we must defend ourselves against contamination by eating nutrient-rich foods and preserving a clean environment.

This chapter completes the introductory lessons on the nutrients. Each nutrient from the amino acids to zinc has been described rather thoroughly—its chemistry, roles in the body, sources in the diet, symptoms of deficiency and toxicity, and influences on health and disease. Such a detailed examination is informative, but it can also be misleading. It is important to step back from the detailed study of the individual nutrients to look at them as a whole. After all, people eat foods, not nutrients, and most foods deliver dozens of nutrients. Furthermore, nutrients work cooperatively with one another in the body; their actions are most often *inter*actions. This chapter alone mentioned how iron depends on vitamin C to keep it in its active form and copper to incorporate it into hemoglobin, how zinc is needed to activate and transport vitamin A, and how both iodine and selenium are needed for the synthesis of thyroid hormones. The table on p. 415 provides a summary of the trace minerals for your review. Highlight 13 explores the benefits of phytochemicals.

heavy metals: mineral ions such as mercury and lead, so called because they are of relatively high atomic weight. Many heavy metals are poisonous.

REVIEW IT The Trace Minerals

Mineral and Chief Functions	Deficiency Symptoms	Toxicity Symptoms[a]	Significant Sources
Iron			
Part of the protein hemoglobin, which carries oxygen in the blood; part of the protein myoglobin in muscles, which makes oxygen available for muscle contraction; necessary for energy metabolism	Anemia: weakness, fatigue, headaches; impaired work performance; impaired immunity; pale skin, nail beds, mucous membranes, and palm creases; concave nails; inability to regulate body temperature; pica	GI distress; iron overload: infections, fatigue, joint pain, skin pigmentation, organ damage	Red meats, fish, poultry, shellfish, eggs, legumes, dried fruits
Zinc			
Part of insulin and many enzymes; involved in making genetic material and proteins, immune reactions, transport of vitamin A, taste perception, wound healing, the making of sperm, and normal fetal development	Stunted growth, delayed sexual maturation, impaired immune function, hair loss, eye and skin lesions, loss of appetite	Loss of appetite, impaired immunity, low HDL, copper and iron deficiencies	Protein-containing foods: red meats, fish, shellfish, poultry, whole grains; fortified cereals
Iodine			
A component of the thyroid hormones that help to regulate growth, development, and metabolic rate	Underactive thyroid gland, goiter, limited mental and physical development (cretinism)	Underactive thyroid gland, elevated TSH, goiter	Iodized salt; seafood; plants grown in iodine-rich soil and animals fed those plants
Selenium			
Part of an enzyme that defends against oxidation; regulates thyroid hormone	Associated with Keshan disease	Nail and hair brittleness and loss; fatigue, irritability, and nervous system disorders, skin rash, garlic breath odor	Seafoods, organ meats; other meats, whole grains, fruits, and vegetables (depending on soil content)
Copper			
Helps form hemoglobin; part of several enzymes	Anemia, bone abnormalities	Liver damage	Seafood, nuts, legumes, whole grains, seeds
Manganese			
Cofactor for several enzymes; bone formation	Rare	Nervous symptom disorders	Nuts, whole grains, leafy vegetables, tea
Fluoride			
Maintains health of bones and teeth; confers decay resistance on teeth	Susceptibility to tooth decay	Fluorosis (pitting and discoloration) of teeth	Drinking water (if fluoridated), tea, seafood
Chromium			
Enhances insulin action, may improve glucose intolerance	Diabetes-like condition	None reported	Meats (liver), whole grains, brewer's yeast
Molybdenum			
Cofactor for several enzymes	Unknown	None reported	Legumes, cereals, nuts

[a]Acute toxicities of many minerals cause abdominal pain, nausea, vomiting, and diarrhea.

What's Online

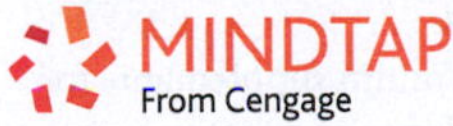
MINDTAP
From Cengage

Visit **www.cengagebrain.com** to access MindTap, a complete digital course that includes Diet & Wellness Plus, interactive quizzes, videos, and more.

REFERENCES

1. A. S. McCall and coauthors, Bromine is an essential trace element for assembly of collagen IV scaffolds in tissue development and architecture, *Cell* 157 (2014): 1380–1392.
2. A. Kritharis, T. P. Bradley, and D. R. Budman, The evolving use of arsenic in pharmacotherapy of malignant disease, *Annals of Hematology* 92 (2013): 719–730.
3. D. M. Frazer and G. J. Anderson, The regulation of iron transport, *Biofactors* 40 (2014): 206–214.
4. R. Collings and coauthors, The absorption of iron from whole diets: A systematic review, *American Journal of Clinical Nutrition* 98 (2013): 65–81.
5. World Health Organization, Micronutrients: Iron Deficiency Anaemia, www.who.int/nutrition/topics/ida/en, January 2017.
6. A. C. Cepeda-Lopez and coauthors, In overweight and obese women, dietary iron absorption is reduced and the enhancement of iron absorption by ascorbic acid is one-half that in normal-weight women, *American Journal of Clinical Nutrition* 102 (2015): 1389–1397; C. Becker and coauthors, Iron metabolism in obesity: How interaction between homeostatic mechanisms can interfere with their original purpose, *Journal of Trace Elements in Medicine and Biology* 30 (2015): 195–201.
7. J. E. Kiss and coauthors, Oral iron supplementation after blood donation: A randomized clinical trial, *Journal of the American Medical Association* 313 (2015): 575–583.
8. C. Camaschella, Iron-deficiency anemia, *New England Journal of Medicine* 372 (2015): 1832–1843.
9. P. Buratti and coauthors, Recent advances in iron metabolism: Relevance for health, exercise, and performance, *Medicine and Science in Sports and Exercise* 47 (2015): 1596–1604; J. P. McClung and L. E. Murray-Kolb, Iron nutrition and premenopausal women: Effects of poor iron status on physical and neuropsychological performance, *Annual Review of Nutrition* 33 (2013): 271–288.
10. R. A. Lumish and coauthors, Gestational iron deficiency is associated with pica behaviors in adolescents, *Journal of Nutrition* 144 (2014): 1533–1539.
11. L. B. VanWagner and R. M. Green, Elevated serum ferritin, *Journal of the American Medical Association* 312 (2014): 743–744.
12. P. C. Adams, Epidemiology and diagnostic testing for hemochromatosis and iron overload, *International Journal of Laboratory Hematology* 37 (2015): 25–30; E. Gammella and coauthors, Iron-induced damage in cardiomyopathy: Oxidative-dependent and independent mechanisms, *Oxidative Medicine and Cellular Longevity* 2015 (2015): 230182.
13. C. Camaschella, Treating iron overload, *New England Journal of Medicine* 368 (2013): 2325–2327.
14. J. Hunnicutt, K. He, and P. Xun, Dietary iron intake and body iron stores are associated with risk of coronary heart disease in a meta-analysis of prospective cohort studies, *Journal of Nutrition* 144 (2014): 359–366; W. Yang and coauthors, Is heme iron intake associated with risk of coronary heart disease? A meta-analysis of prospective studies, *European Journal of Nutrition* 53 (2014): 395–400.
15. H. Padmanabhn, M. J. Brookes, and T. Iqbal, Iron and colorectal cancer: Evidence from in vitro and animal studies, *Nutrition Reviews* 73 (2015): 308–317.
16. H. Aljwaid and coauthors, Non-transferrin-bound iron is associated with biomarkers of oxidative stress, inflammation and endothelial dysfunction in type 2 diabetes, *Journal of Diabetes and Its Complications* 29 (2015): 943–949.
17. H. Pachón and coauthors, Evidence of the effectiveness of flour fortification programs on iron status and anemia: A systematic review, *Nutrition Reviews* 73 (2015): 780–795.
18. A. S. Prasad, Discovery of human zinc deficiency: Its impact on human health and disease, *Advances in Nutrition* 4 (2013): 176–190.
19. N. W. Solomons, Update on zinc biology, *Annals of Nutrition and Metabolism* 62 (2013): 8–17.
20. R. L. Bailey, K. P. West, Jr., and R. E. Black, The epidemiology of global micronutrient deficiencies, *Annals of Nutrition and Metabolism* 66 (2015): 22–33.
21. H. Haase and L. Rink, Multiple impacts of zinc on immune function, *Metallomics* 6 (2014): 1175–1180.
22. M. Foster and coauthors, Effect of vegetarian diets on zinc status: A systematic review and meta-analysis of studies in humans, *Journal of the Science of Food and Agriculture* 93 (2013): 2362–2371.
23. M. E. Penny, Zinc supplementation in public health, *Annals of Nutrition and Metabolism* 62 (2013): 31–42.
24. R. R. Das and M. Singh, Oral zinc for the common cold, *Journal of the American Medical Association* 311 (2014): 1440–1441.
25. K. Redman and coauthors, Iodine deficiency and the brain: Effects and mechanisms, *Critical Reviews in Food Science and Nutrition* 56 (2016): 2695–2713; M. Puig-Domingo and L. Vila, The implications of iodine and its supplementation during pregnancy in fetal brain development, *Current Clinical Pharmacology* 8 (2013): 97–109.
26. J. H. Lazarus, The importance of iodine in public health, *Environmental Geochemistry and Health* 37 (2015): 605–618.
27. E. N. Pearce and coauthors, Consequences of iodine deficiency and excess in pregnant women: An overview of current knowns and unknowns, *American Journal of Clinical Nutrition* 104 (2016): 918S–923S.
28. S. Syed, Iodine and the "near" eradication of cretinism, *Pediatrics* 135 (2015): 594–596.
29. GAIN-UNICEF Universal Salt Iodization Partnership Program. Retrieved January 2014 from www.gainhealth.org/programs/USI.
30. J. Loscalzo, Keshan disease, selenium deficiency, and the selenoproteome, *New England Journal of Medicine* 370 (2014): 1756–1760.
31. C. Méplan, Selenium and chronic diseases: A nutritional genomics perspective, *Nutrients* 7 (2015): 3621–3651; M. Vinceti and coauthors, Selenium for preventing cancer, *Cochrane Database of Systematic Reviews* 30 (2014): CD005195; K. L. Penney and coauthors, Selenoprotein P genetic variants and mRNA expression, circulating selenium, and prostate cancer risk and survival, *Prostate* 73 (2013): 700–705.
32. R. F. Burk and K. E. Hill, Regulation of selenium metabolism and transport, *Annual Review of Nutrition* 35 (2015): 109–134.
33. S. Gulec and J. F. Collins, Molecular mediators governing iron-copper interactions, *Annual Review of Nutrition* 34 (2014): 95–116.
34. K. J. Horning and coauthors, Manganese is essential for neuronal health, *Annual Review of Nutrition* 35 (2015): 71–108.
35. Water Fluoridation Data and Statistics, www.cdc.gov/fluoridation/statistics/index.htm, updated September 7, 2016.
36. U.S. Public Health Service recommendation for fluoride concentration in drinking water for the prevention of dental caries, *Public Health Reports* 130 (2015): 318–331; Fluoride use in caries prevention in the primary care setting, *Pediatrics* 134 (2014): 626–633.
37. R. B. Costello, J. T. Dwyer, and R. L. Bailey, Chromium supplements for glycemic control in type 2 diabetes: Limited evidence of effectiveness, *Nutrition Reviews* 74 (2016): 455–468; C. H. Bailey, Improved meta-analytic methods show no effect of chromium supplements on fasting glucose, *Biological Trace Element Research* 157 (2014): 1–8.

HIGHLIGHT > 13

LEARN IT Define *phytochemicals* and explain how they might defend against chronic diseases.

Phytochemicals and Functional Foods

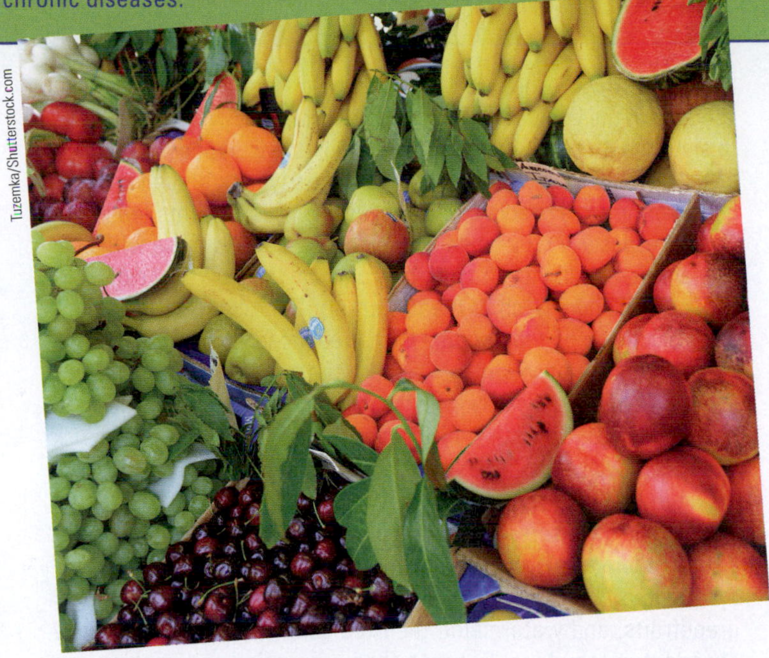
Tuzemka/Shutterstock.com

Chapter 13 completes the introductory lessons on the six classes of nutrients—carbohydrates, lipids, proteins, vitamins, minerals, and water. In addition to these nutrients, foods contain thousands of other compounds, including the **phytochemicals.** Chapter 1 introduced the phytochemicals as compounds found in plant-derived foods that have biological activity in the body. Research on phytochemicals is unfolding daily, adding to our knowledge of their roles in human health, but there are still many questions and only tentative answers. Just a few of the tens of thousands of phytochemicals have been researched at all, and only a sampling are mentioned in this highlight—enough to illustrate their wide variety of food sources and roles in supporting health.

The concept that foods provide health benefits beyond those of the nutrients emerged from numerous epidemiological studies showing the protective effects of plant-based diets on cancer and heart disease. People have been using foods to maintain health and prevent disease for years, but now these foods are sometimes called **functional foods**, suggesting these foods provide health benefits beyond their nutrient contributions. (Glossary H13-1 defines this and other terms.)

As Chapter 1 explained, functional foods include all foods (whole, fortified, enriched, or enhanced foods) that have a potentially beneficial effect on health.[1] Whole foods—as natural and familiar as oatmeal or tomatoes—are the simplest functional foods. In some cases, foods have been modified to provide health benefits, perhaps by lowering the *trans* fat contents. In other cases, manufacturers have fortified foods by adding nutrients or phytochemicals that provide health benefits. Examples of these functional foods include orange juice fortified with calcium to help build strong bones and margarine made with a plant sterol that lowers blood cholesterol.

Much of this text touts the benefits of nature's functional foods—whole grains rich in dietary fibers, oily fish rich in omega-3 fatty acids, and fresh fruits rich in phytochemicals, for example. This highlight begins with a look at foods, the phytochemicals they contain, and their roles in disease prevention. Then the discussion turns to examine the most controversial of functional foods—novel foods to which phytochemicals have been added to promote health. How these foods fit into a healthy diet is still unclear.

The Phytochemicals

In foods, phytochemicals impart tastes, aromas, colors, and other characteristics. They give hot peppers their burning sensation, garlic its pungent flavor, and tomatoes their red color. In the body, phytochemicals can have profound physiological effects—acting as antioxidants, mimicking hormones, stimulating enzymes, interfering with DNA replication, suppressing inflammation, destroying bacteria, and binding to cell walls. Any of these actions may prevent the development of chronic diseases, depending in part on how genetic factors interact with the phytochemicals. Phytochemicals might also have adverse effects when consumed in excess as a dietary supplement.

Defending against Cancer

A variety of phytochemicals from a variety of foods appear to protect against DNA damage and defend the body against cancer.[2] A few examples follow.

Soy may protect against breast and prostate cancers.[3] Soybeans—as well as **flaxseeds**—are a rich source of the **phytoestrogens.** Because the chemical structure of phytoestrogens is similar to the

GLOSSARY H13-1

carotenoids (kah-ROT-eh-noyds): pigments commonly found in plants and animals, some of which have vitamin A activity. The carotenoid with the greatest vitamin A activity is beta-carotene.

flavonoids (FLAY-von-oyds): yellow pigments in foods; phytochemicals that may exert physiological effects on the body.

flaxseeds: the small brown seeds of the flax plant; valued in nutrition as a source of fiber, lignans, and omega-3 fatty acids.

functional foods: foods that have a potentially beneficial effect on health when consumed as part of a varied diet on a regular basis at effective levels.

lignans: phytochemicals present in flaxseed that are converted to phytosterols by intestinal bacteria and are under study as possible anticancer agents.

lutein (LOO-teen): a plant pigment of yellow hue; a phytochemical believed to play roles in eye functioning and health.

lycopene (LYE-koh-peen): a pigment responsible for the red color of tomatoes and other red-hued vegetables; a phytochemical that may act as an antioxidant in the body.

phytochemicals: nonnutrient compounds found in plants. Some phytochemicals have biological activity in the body.

- **phyto** = plant

phytoestrogens: phytochemicals structurally similar to human estrogen that weakly mimic or modulate estrogen's action in the body. Phytoestrogens include the isoflavones *genistein, daidzein,* and *glycitein.*

plant sterols: phytochemicals that have structural similarities to cholesterol and lower blood cholesterol by interfering with cholesterol absorption. Plant sterols include *sterol esters* and *stanol esters.*

hormone estrogen, they can weakly mimic or modulate the effects of estrogen in the body. They also have antioxidant activity that appears to slow the growth of some cancers. Soy foods appear to be most effective when consumed in moderation early and throughout life.[4] Importantly, soy extracts and phytoestrogen supplements are ill-advised—especially for women with breast cancer and those with high risk factors—as phytoestrogens may promote the growth of estrogen-dependent tumors (such as breast cancer). The American Cancer Society recommends that women with breast cancer should consume only *moderate* amounts of soy as part of a healthy plant-based diet and should not intentionally ingest high levels of soy or supplements of phytoestrogens. Consistently high intakes of soy may increase the risk of stroke in women.[5]

Limited evidence suggests that tomatoes may offer protection against some cancers. Among the phytochemicals thought to be responsible for this effect is **lycopene,** one of the many **carotenoids.**[6] Lycopene is the pigment that gives apricots, guava, papaya, pink grapefruits, and watermelon their red color—and it is especially abundant in tomatoes. Because food processing and cooking can improve carotenoid absorption, cooked tomato products, such as spaghetti sauce, provide even more lycopene. Lycopene is a powerful antioxidant that seems to inhibit the growth of cancer cells. Importantly, the benefits of lycopene have been seen when people have eaten *foods* containing lycopene; lycopene supplements may interfere with cancer treatments.

Soybeans and tomatoes are only two of the many fruits and vegetables credited with providing anticancer activity. Strong and convincing evidence shows that the risk of many cancers, and perhaps of cancer in general, decreases when diets include an abundance of fruits and vegetables. To that end, current recommendations urge consumers to eat five to nine servings of fruits and vegetables a day.

Defending against Heart Disease

Diets based primarily on fruits and vegetables appear to support heart health better than those founded on highly refined foods—perhaps because of the abundance of nutrients, fiber, and phytochemicals such as the **flavonoids.**[7] Flavonoids, a large group of phytochemicals known for their health-promoting qualities, are found in whole grains, legumes, soy, vegetables, fruits, herbs, spices, teas, cocoa (chocolate), nuts, olive oil, and red wines. Flavonoids are powerful antioxidants that may help protect LDL cholesterol against oxidation, minimize inflammation, and reduce blood platelet stickiness, thereby slowing the progression of atherosclerosis and making blood clots less likely. Whereas an abundance of flavonoid-containing *foods* in the diet may lower the risks of chronic diseases, no claims can be made for flavonoids extracted from foods and sold as supplements. In fact, purified flavonoids may even be harmful.

In addition to flavonoids, fruits and vegetables are rich in carotenoids such as beta-carotene, lycopene, and **lutein.** Studies suggest that a diet rich in carotenoids may lower the risk of heart disease by decreasing inflammation and oxidative stress.[8]

The **plant sterols** of soy and the **lignans** of flaxseed may also protect against heart disease.[9] These cholesterol-like molecules are naturally found in all plants and inhibit cholesterol absorption in the body. As a result, blood cholesterol levels decline.[10] These phytochemicals also seem to protect against heart disease by reducing inflammation and lowering blood pressure.[11]

Defending against Other Diseases

Most research on phytochemicals has focused on cancer and heart disease, but phytochemicals defend against other diseases as well. The orange-yellow pigment curcumin, commonly found in curry powder, may help reverse insulin resistance, inflammation, and other symptoms associated with obesity. The carotenoids lutein and zeaxanthin may protect the eyes and skin from ultraviolet light damage.[12]

The Phytochemicals in Perspective

Foods are complex. They deliver thousands of phytochemicals in addition to dozens of nutrients. For this reason, researchers must be careful in giving credit for particular health benefits to any one compound. Diets rich in whole grains, legumes, vegetables, fruits, and nuts seem to protect against heart disease and cancer, but identifying *the* specific foods or components of foods that are responsible is difficult. Each food possesses a unique array of phytochemicals—citrus fruits provide monoterpenes; grapes, resveratrol; cocoa, flavonoids; and flaxseed, lignans, to name just a few. Broccoli may contain as many as 10,000 different phytochemicals—each with the potential to influence some action in the body. Beverages such as wine, spices such as oregano, and oils such as olive oil (especially virgin olive oil) contain many phytochemicals that may explain, in part, why people who eat a traditional Mediterranean diet have reduced risks of heart disease and cancer. Phytochemicals might also explain why the DASH diet is so effective in lowering blood pressure and blood lipids. Even identifying all of the phytochemicals and their effects doesn't answer all the questions because the actions of phytochemicals may be complementary or overlapping—which reinforces the principle of variety in diet planning. For an appreciation of the array of phytochemicals offered by a variety of foods, see Figure H13-1.

Functional Foods

Because foods naturally contain thousands of phytochemicals that are biologically active in the body, virtually all of them have some value in supporting health. In other words, even simple, whole foods, in reality, are functional foods. Ginger may quell nausea; blueberries may lower blood pressure; garlic may lower blood cholesterol; grapes may reduce inflammation; coffee may reduce the risk of prostate cancer; and black tea may protect against bone fractures, just to name a few examples.[13] Functional foods rich in phytochemicals are easy to find in the produce section of grocery stores. Just look for the colorful fruits and vegetables (see Table H13-1, p. 420). But food manufacturers continue to market and create functional foods as well.

Many processed foods become functional foods when they are fortified with nutrients or enhanced with phytochemicals or herbs

> **FIGURE H13-1** **An Array of Phytochemicals in a Variety of Foods and Beverages**

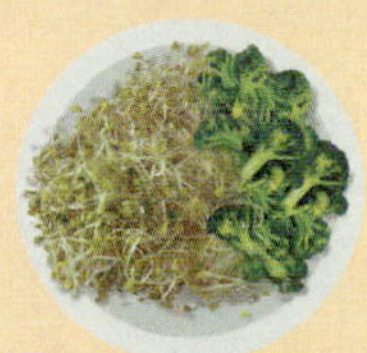

Broccoli and broccoli sprouts (and brussels sprouts, bok choy, cabbage, cauliflower, kale, collard greens, swiss chard, turnips, and watercress) contain an abundance of the cancer-fighting phytochemicals sulforaphane and indoles.

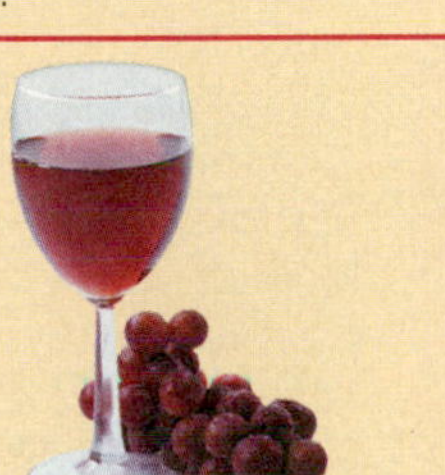

The phytochemical resveratrol found in grapes (and nuts) improves glucose control, inhibits cancer cell growth, and limits blood clot formation and inflammation.

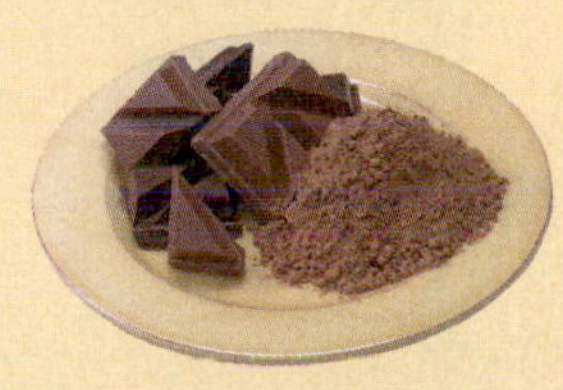

The flavonoids in cocoa and chocolate defend against oxidation and reduce the tendency of blood to clot.

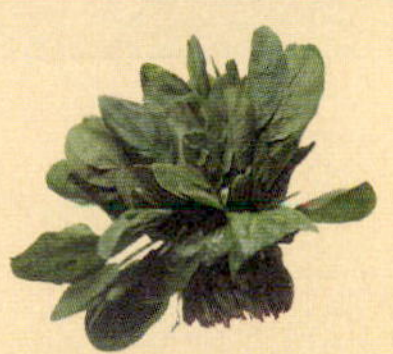

Spinach (and collard greens, corn, swiss chard, and winter squash) contains the carotenoids lutein and zeaxanthin, which help protect the eyes against macular degeneration.

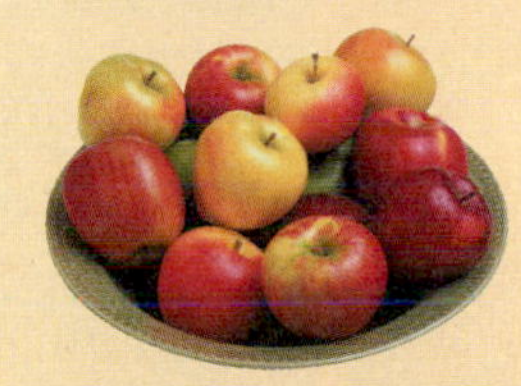

An apple a day—rich in phenolic acids—may protect against heart disease.

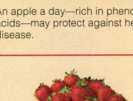

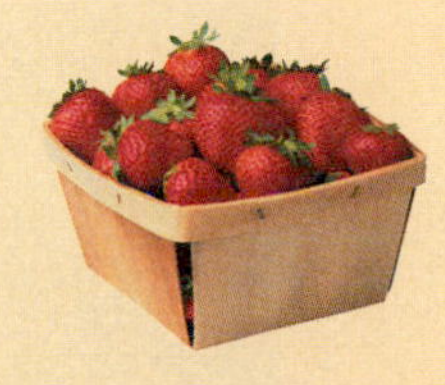

The ellagic acid of strawberries (and blackberries, blueberries, raspberries, and grapes) may inhibit certain types of cancer and decrease cholesterol levels.

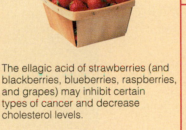

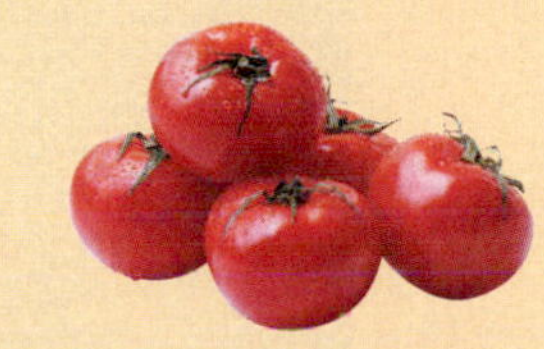

Tomatoes (and pink grapefruit, red peppers, and watermelons), with their abundant lycopene, may defend against cancer and heart disease by protecting DNA from oxidative damage.

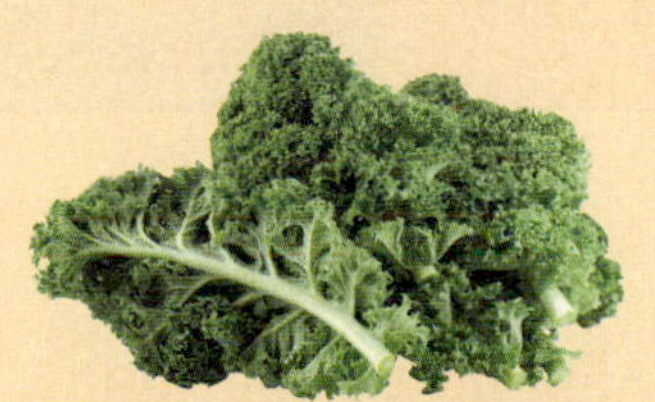

Quercetins—commonly found in kale (and onions, pears, and grapes)—reduce inflammation from allergies, inhibit tumor growth, and protect the lungs.

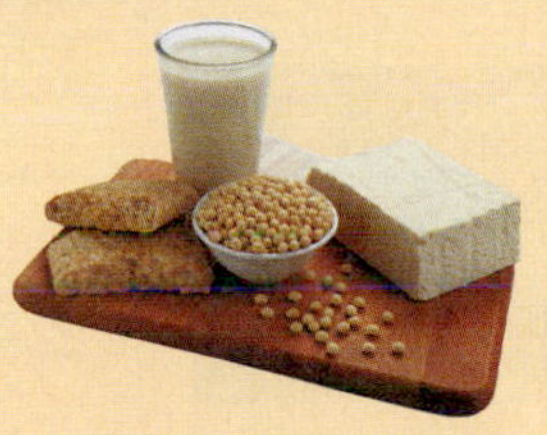

The phytoestrogens of soybeans seem to starve cancer cells and inhibit tumor growth; the plant sterols may lower blood cholesterol and protect cardiac arteries.

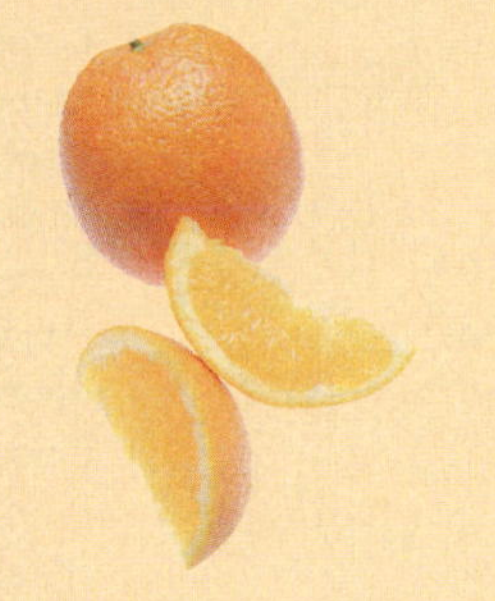

The monoterpenes of citrus fruits (and cherries) may protect the lungs.

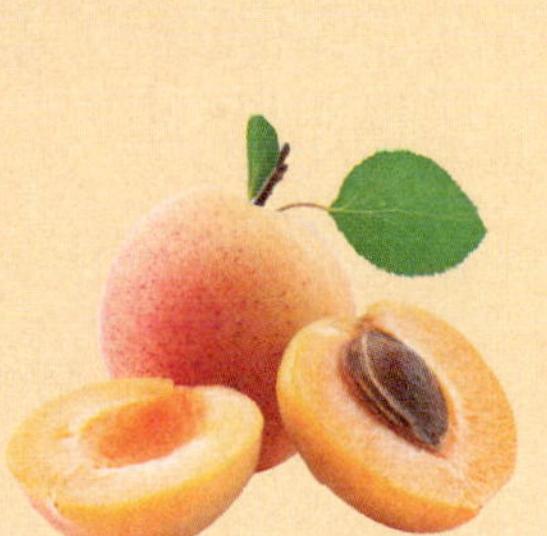

Colorful foods such as apricots (and cantaloupes, carrots, kale, kiwifruit, mangoes, papaya, pumpkins, spinach, sweet potatoes, and winter squash) contain beta-carotene, which may help slow aging, protect against some cancers, improve lung function, and reduce complications of diabetes.

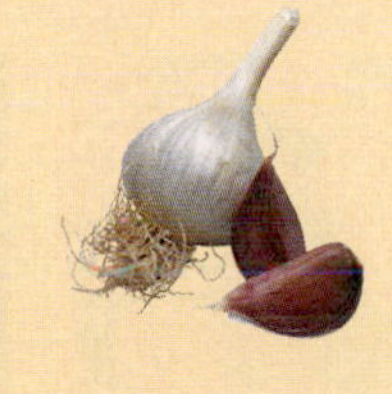

Garlic (and chives, leeks, onions, and scallions), with its abundant organosulfur compounds, may lower blood cholesterol and blood pressure and protect against stomach cancer.

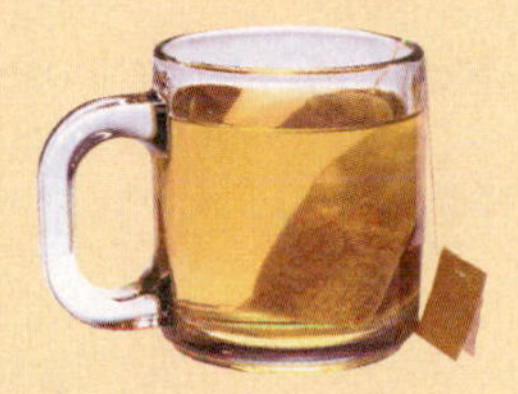

The flavonoids in black tea may protect against heart disease, whereas those in green tea may defend against cancer.

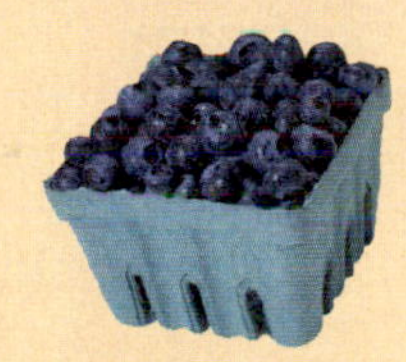

Blueberries (and cherries, plums, and strawberries), a rich source of anthocyanins, may protect against the effects of aging.

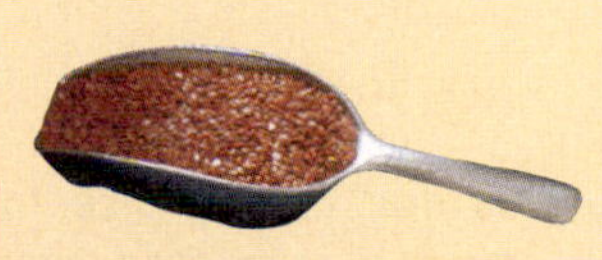

Flaxseed, the richest source of lignans, may prevent the spread of cancer.

HIGHLIGHT > 13

TABLE H13-1 The Colors of Foods Rich in Phytochemicals

Red	White-Brown	Orange-Yellow	Blue-Purple	Green
Anthocyanins Lycopene	Allicin Allyl sulfides	Beta-carotene Limonene	Anthocyanins Ellagic acid Phenolics	Beta-carotene Lutein Indoles
Beets Cherries Cranberries Pink grapefruit Pomegranates Radicchio Radishes Raspberries Red apples Red peppers Red potatoes Rhubarb Strawberries Tomatoes Watermelon	Bananas Brown pears Cauliflower Chives Dates Garlic Ginger Leeks Mushrooms Onions Parsnips Shallots Turnips	Apricots Cantaloupe Carrots Lemons Mangoes Nectarines Oranges Papayas Peaches Persimmons Pineapple Pumpkin Rutabagas Squash Sweet potatoes Tangerines Yellow peppers	Black currants Blackberries Blueberries Dried plums Eggplant Elderberries Plums Purple figs Purple peppers Raisins Purple cabbage Purple grapes	Artichokes Arugula Asparagus Avocados Broccoli Brussels sprouts Cabbage Celery Cucumbers Endive Green apples Green beans Green grapes Green onions Green pears Green peppers Honeydew melon Kiwifruit Leafy greens Limes Okra Peas Snow peas Spinach Sugar snap peas Watercress Zucchini

Africa Studio/Shutterstock.com; Elena Veselova/Shutterstock.com; Denizya/Shutterstock.com; J. R. Bale/Alamy Stock Photo; D. Hurst/Alamy Stock Photo

(calcium-fortified orange juice, for example). Less frequently, an entirely new food is created, as in the case of a meat substitute made of mycoprotein—a protein derived from a fungus.* This functional food not only provides dietary fiber, polyunsaturated fats, and high-quality protein, but it also lowers LDL cholesterol, raises HDL cholesterol, improves glucose response, and prolongs satiety after a meal. Such a novel functional food raises the question—is it a food or a drug?

*This mycoprotein product is marketed under the trade name Quorn (pronounced KWORN).

Foods as Pharmacy

Hippocrates is credited with saying, "Let food be thy medicine and medicine be thy food." This simple message, uttered thousands of years ago, recognizes how good food supports good health (see Photo H13-1).

Not too long ago, most of us could agree on what was a food and what was a drug. Today, functional foods blur the distinctions. They have characteristics similar to both foods and drugs, but do not fit neatly into either category. Consider margarine, for example.

Eating nonhydrogenated margarine sparingly instead of butter generously may lower blood cholesterol slightly over several months and

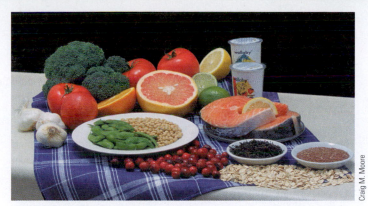

Craig M. Moore

> **PHOTO H13-1** Nature offers a variety of functional foods that provide us with many health benefits.

clearly falls into the food category. Taking a statin drug, on the other hand, lowers blood cholesterol significantly within weeks and clearly falls into the drug category. But margarine enhanced with a plant sterol that lowers blood cholesterol moderately is in a gray area between the two. The margarine looks and tastes like a food, but it acts like a drug.

The use of functional foods as drugs creates a whole new set of diet-planning challenges. Not only must foods provide an adequate intake of all the nutrients to support good health, but they must also deliver druglike ingredients to protect against disease. Like drugs used to treat chronic diseases, functional foods may need to be eaten several times a day for several months or even years to have a beneficial effect. Sporadic users may be disappointed in the results. Margarine enriched with plant sterols may reduce cholesterol by up to 15 percent, much more than regular margarine does, but not nearly as much as the more than 30 percent reduction seen with cholesterol-lowering drugs. For this reason, functional foods may be more useful for prevention and mild cases of disease than for intervention and more severe cases. In any case, because prescription medicines are so much more effective and because people respond to plant sterols so differently, consumers should always make treatment decisions in consultation with their health care providers.

Foods and drugs differ dramatically in cost as well. Functional foods such as fruits and vegetables incur no added costs, but foods that have been manufactured with added phytochemicals can be expensive, costing up to six times as much as their conventional counterparts—yet still below that of medicines.

Unanswered Questions

To achieve a desired health effect, which is the better choice: to eat a novel functional food created to affect a specific body function or to adjust the diet? Does it make more sense to use a margarine enhanced with a plant sterol that lowers blood cholesterol or simply to limit the amount of butter eaten?* Is it smarter to eat eggs enriched with omega-3 fatty acids or to restrict egg consumption? Might functional foods offer a sensible solution for improving our nation's health—if done correctly? Perhaps so, but the problem is that the food industry moves faster than either scientists or the Food and Drug Administration. Consumers were able to buy soup with St. John's wort that claimed to enhance mood and fruit juice with echinacea that was supposed to fight colds while scientists were still conducting their studies on these ingredients. Research to determine the safety and effectiveness of these substances is still in progress. Until this work is complete, consumers are on their own in finding answers to the following questions:

- *Does it work?* Research is generally lacking and findings are often inconclusive.
- *How much does it contain?* Food labels are not required to list the quantities of added phytochemicals. Even if they were, consumers have no standard for comparison and cannot deduce whether the amounts listed are a little or a lot. Most importantly, until research is complete, food manufacturers do not know what amounts (if any) are most effective—or most toxic.
- *Is it safe?* Functional foods can act like drugs. They contain ingredients that can alter body functions and cause allergies, drug interactions, and other side effects. Yet, unlike drug labels, food labels do not provide instructions for the dosage, frequency, or duration of treatment.
- *Is it healthy?* Adding phytochemicals to a food does not magically make it a healthy choice. A candy bar fortified with phytochemicals—or even a piece of chocolate rich in natural flavonoids—is still made mostly of sugar and fat.[14]

Critics suggest that the designation "functional foods" may be nothing more than a marketing tool (see Photo H13-2). After all, even the most experienced researchers cannot yet identify the perfect combination of nutrients and phytochemicals to support optimal health. Yet manufacturers are freely experimenting with various concoctions

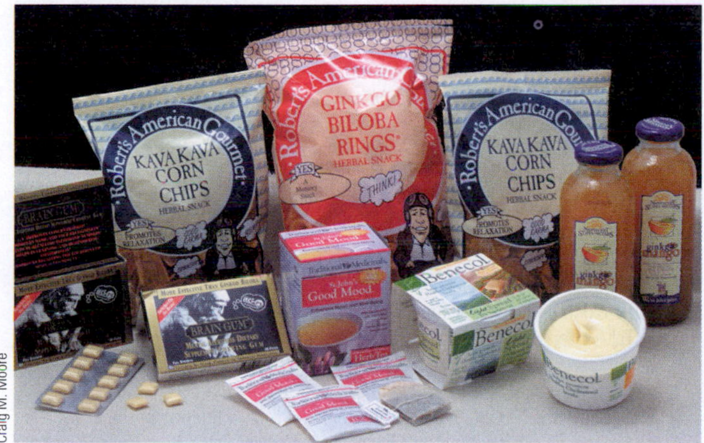
Robert's American Gourmet
KAVA KAVA CORN CHIPS
HERBAL SNACK
GINKGO BILOBA RINGS
Good Mood
Benecol

Craig M. Moore

> **PHOTO H13-2** Some functional foods currently on the market promise to "enhance mood," "promote relaxation and good karma," "increase alertness," and "improve memory," among other claims.

*Margarine products that lower blood cholesterol contain either sterol esters from vegetable oils, soybeans, and corn or stanol esters from wood pulp.

as if they possessed that knowledge. Is it okay for them to sprinkle phytochemicals on fried snack foods or caramel candies and label them "functional," thus implying health benefits?

Future Foods

Nature has elegantly designed foods to provide us with a complex array of dozens of nutrients and thousands of phytochemicals that may benefit health—most of which we have yet to identify or understand. Over the years, we have taken those foods, deconstructed them, and then reconstructed them in an effort to "improve" them. With new scientific understandings of how nutrients—and the myriad other compounds in foods—interact with genes, we may someday be able to design *specific* eating patterns to meet the *exact* health needs of *each* individual. Indeed, our knowledge of the human genome and of human nutrition may well merge to allow specific recommendations for individuals based on their predisposition to diet-related diseases.

If the present trend continues, someday physicians may be able to prescribe the perfect foods to enhance health, and farmers will be able to grow them. As Highlight 19 explains, scientists have already developed gene technology to alter the composition of food crops. They can grow rice enriched with vitamin A and tomatoes containing a hepatitis vaccine, for example. It seems quite likely that foods can be created to meet every possible human need. But then, in a sense, that was largely true 100 years ago when we relied on the bounty of nature.

CRITICAL THINKING QUESTIONS

A. Which is the better choice—to eat processed foods that have been enhanced with phytochemicals or to eat natural foods that are rich in phytochemicals?

B. Some research suggests that cranberries may help prevent urinary tract infections, but what about cranberry supplements? Limited research suggests that *foods* rich in phytoestrogens may benefit heart, bone, breast, and menopausal health, but *phytoestrogen supplements* or *phytoestrogen-enhanced functional foods* are not recommended, particularly for women at high risk of breast cancer. How can you determine whether a phytochemical and/or functional food offers a safe and sensible solution to improving your health?

REFERENCES

1. Position of the Academy of Nutrition and Dietetics: Functional foods, *Journal of the Academy of Nutrition and Dietetics* 113 (2013): 1096–1103.
2. M. González-Vallinas and coauthors, Dietary phytochemicals in cancer prevention and therapy: A complementary approach with promising perspectives, *Nutrition Reviews* 71 (2013): 585–599.
3. J. M. Pavese, S. N. Krishna, and R. C. Bergan, Genistein inhibits human prostate cancer cell detachment, invasion, and metastasis, *American Journal of Clinical Nutrition* 100 (2014): 431S–436S; X. O. Liu and coauthors, Association between dietary factors and breast cancer risk among Chinese females: Systematic review and meta-analysis, *Asian Pacific Journal of Cancer Prevention* 15 (2014): 1291–1298; M. Adjakly and coauthors, Genistein and daidzein: Different molecular effects on prostate cancer, *Anticancer Research* 33 (2013): 39–44.
4. M. Messina, Soy foods, isoflavones, and the health of postmenopausal women, *American Journal of Clinical Nutrition* 100 (2014): 423S–430S.
5. D. Yu and coauthors, Dietary isoflavones, urinary isoflavonoids, and risk of ischemic stroke in women, *American Journal of Clinical Nutrition* 102 (2015): 680–686.
6. J. Chen and coauthors, The effect of lycopene on the PI3K/Akt signalling pathway in prostate cancer, *Anticancer Agents in Medicinal Chemistry* 14 (2014): 800–805.
7. C. P. Bondonno and coauthors, Dietary flavonoids and nitrate: Effects on nitric oxide and vascular function, *Nutrition Reviews* 73 (2015): 216–235.
8. E. T. M. Leermakers and coauthors, The effects of lutein on cardiometabolic health across the life course: A systematic review and meta-analysis, *American Journal of Clinical Nutrition* 103 (2016): 481–494; L. Müller and coauthors, Lycopene and its antioxidant role in the prevention of cardiovascular diseases: A critical review, *Critical Reviews in Food Science and Nutrition* 56 (2016): 1868–1879; M. A. Gammone, G. Riccioni, and N. D'Orazio, Carotenoids: Potential allies of cardiovascular health? *Food and Nutrition Research* 59 (2015): 26762; M. M. Ciccone and coauthors, Dietary intake of carotenoids and their antioxidant and anti-inflammatory effects in cardiovascular care, *Mediators of Inflammation* 2013 (2013): 782137.
9. R. U. Almario and S. E. Karakas, Lignan content of the flaxseed influences its biological effects in healthy men and women, *Journal of the American College of Nutrition* 32 (2013): 194–199.
10. J. M. McKenney and coauthors, A softgel dietary supplement containing esterified plant sterols and stanols improves the blood lipid profile of adults with primary hypercholesterolemia: A randomized, double-blind, placebo-controlled replication study, *Journal of the Academy of Nutrition and Dietetics* 114 (2014): 244–249; M. A. Shaghaghi, S. S. Abumweis, and P. J. H. Jones, Cholesterol lowering efficacy of plant sterols/stanols provided in capsule and tablet formats: Results of a systematic review and meta-analysis, *Journal of the Academy of Nutrition and Dietetics* 113 (2013): 1494–1503.
11. D. Rodriguez-Leyva and coauthors, Potent antihypertensive action of dietary flaxseed in hypertensive patients, *Hypertension* 62 (2013): 1081–1089.
12. J. Mares, Lutein and zeaxanthin isomers in eye health and disease, *Annual Review of Nutrition* 36 (2016): 571–602; S. M. Abdel-Aal and coauthors, Dietary sources of lutein and zeaxanthin carotenoids and their role in eye health, *Nutrients* 5 (2013): 1169–1185.
13. G. Myers and coauthors, Tea and flavoid intake predict osteoporotic fracture risk in elderly Australian women: A prospective study, *American Journal of Clinical Nutrition* 102 (2015): 958–965; H. Liu and coauthors, Coffee consumption and prostate cancer risk: A meta-analysis of cohort studies, *Nutrition and Cancer* 67 (2015): 392–400; S. A. Johnson and coauthors, Daily blueberry consumption improves blood pressure and arterial stiffness in postmenopausal women with pre- and stage 1-hypertension: A randomized, double-blind, placebo-controlled clinical trial, *Journal of the Academy of Nutrition and Dietetics* 115 (2015): 369–377; K. Ried, C. Toben, and P. Fakler, Effect of garlic on serum lipids: An updated meta-analysis, *Nutrition Reviews* 71 (2013): 282–299; W. M. Marx and coauthors, Ginger (*Zingiber officinale*) and chemotherapy-induced nausea and vomiting: A systematic literature review, *Nutrition Reviews* 71 (2013): 245–254.
14. S. Ellam and G. Williamson, Cocoa and human health, *Annual Review of Nutrition* 33 (2013): 105–128.

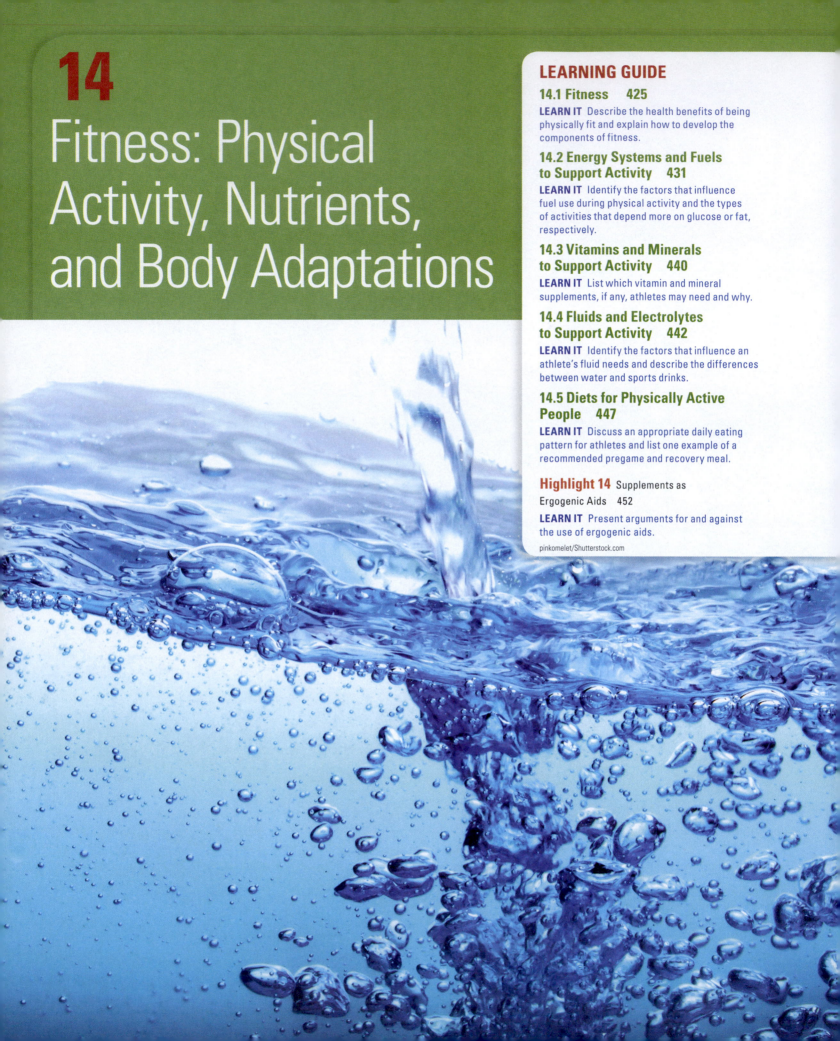

14

Fitness: Physical Activity, Nutrients, and Body Adaptations

LEARNING GUIDE

pinkomelet/Shutterstock.com

Nutrition in Your Life

Every day, you choose whether to be physically active or not, and your choices over time can influence how well you feel and how long you live. Today's world makes it easy to be inactive—too easy in fact—but the many health rewards of being physically active make it well worth the effort. You may even discover how much fun it is to be active, and with a little perseverance, you may become physically fit as well. The choice is yours. As you read this chapter, consider whether your physical activities meet current recommendations and whether your daily food, fluid, and nutrient intakes are appropriate to support those activities.

Are you physically fit? If so, your joints are flexible, your muscles are strong, and your body is lean with enough, but not too much, fat. You have the endurance to engage in daily physical activities with enough reserve energy to handle added challenges. Carrying heavy suitcases, opening a stuck window, or climbing four flights of stairs, which might strain an unfit person, is easy for you. What's more, you are prepared to meet mental and emotional challenges too. All these characteristics of **fitness** describe the same wonderful condition of a healthy body.

Or perhaps you are **sedentary**. Today's world fosters inactivity, and people who exert minimal physical effort become weak and unhealthy. In fact, a sedentary lifestyle contributes to the development of several chronic diseases.[1]

Regardless of your level of fitness, this chapter is written for you, whoever you are and whatever your goals—whether you want to improve your health, lose weight, hone your athletic skills, or simply adopt an active lifestyle. This chapter begins by discussing fitness and its benefits, and then explains how the body uses energy nutrients to fuel physical activity. Finally, it describes diets to support fitness.

14.1 Fitness

LEARN IT Describe the health benefits of being physically fit and explain how to develop the components of fitness.

Fitness depends on a certain minimum amount of **physical activity** or **exercise.** Both physical activity and exercise involve body movement, muscle contraction, and enhanced energy expenditure, but "exercise" is often used to describe structured, planned physical activity. This chapter focuses on how the active body uses energy nutrients—whether that body is pedaling a bike across campus or pedaling a stationary bike in a gym. Thus, for our purposes, the terms *physical activity* and *exercise* are used interchangeably.

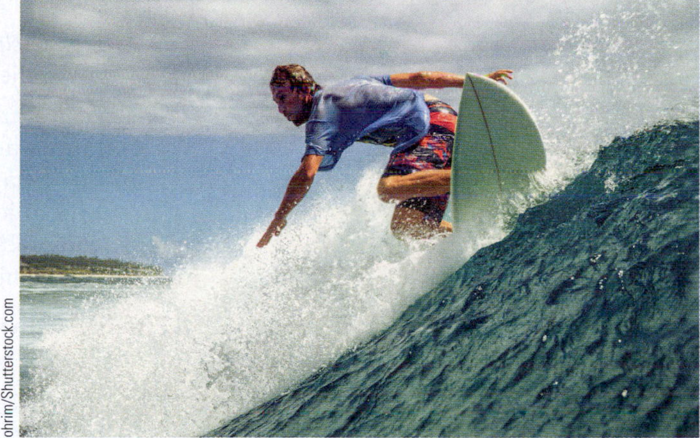

ohrim/Shutterstock.com

> **PHOTO 14-1** Physical activity, or lack of it, exerts a significant and pervasive influence on nutrition and health.

Benefits of Fitness The health benefits of increasing physical activities and reducing sedentary times cannot be overemphasized (see Photo 14-1). Extensive evidence confirms that regular physical activity promotes health and reduces the risk of developing a number of diseases.[2] Yet, despite an increasing awareness of the health benefits that physical activity confers, only about 20 percent of adults in the United States meet physical activity guidelines.[3] Like smoking and obesity, physical inactivity is linked to the major degenerative diseases—heart disease, cancer, stroke, diabetes, and hypertension—the primary killers of adults in developed countries.[4]

fitness: the characteristics that enable the body to perform physical activity; more broadly, the ability to meet routine physical demands with enough reserve energy to rise to a physical challenge; or the body's ability to withstand stress of all kinds.

sedentary: physically inactive (literally, "sitting down a lot").

physical activity: bodily movement produced by muscle contractions that substantially increase energy expenditure.

exercise: planned, structured, and repetitive body movements that promote or maintain physical fitness.

As a person becomes physically fit, the health of the entire body improves. In general, physically fit people enjoy:

- *Restful sleep.* Rest and sleep occur naturally after periods of physical activity.
- *Nutritional health.* Physical activity expends energy and thus allows people to eat more food. If they choose wisely, active people will consume more nutrients and be less likely to develop nutrient deficiencies.
- *Improved body composition.* A balanced program of physical activity limits body fat and increases or maintains lean tissue. Thus physically active people have relatively less body fat than sedentary people at the same body weight.[5]
- *Improved bone density.* Weight-bearing physical activity builds bone strength and protects against osteoporosis.[6]
- *Resistance to colds and other infectious diseases.* Fitness enhances immunity.[7]*
- *Low risks of some cancers.* Lifelong physical activity may help protect against colon cancer, breast cancer, and some other cancers.[8]
- *Strong circulation and lung function.* Physical activity that challenges the heart and lungs strengthens the circulatory system.
- *Low risk of cardiovascular disease.* Physical activity lowers blood pressure, slows resting pulse rate, and lowers blood cholesterol, thus reducing the risks of heart attacks and strokes.[9] Some research suggests that physical activity may reduce the risk of cardiovascular disease in another way as well—by reducing visceral fat stores.[10]
- *Low risk of type 2 diabetes.* Physical activity normalizes glucose tolerance.[11] Regular physical activity improves glucose control and reduces the risk of developing type 2 diabetes.
- *Reduced risk of gallbladder disease.* Regular physical activity reduces the risk of gallbladder disease—perhaps by facilitating weight control and lowering blood lipid levels.[12]
- *Low incidence and severity of anxiety and depression.* Physical activity may improve mood and enhance the quality of life by reducing depression and anxiety.[13]
- *Strong self-image.* The sense of achievement that comes from meeting physical challenges promotes self-confidence.
- *Long life and high quality of life in the later years.* In general, active people live longer, healthier lives than sedentary people do.[14] Even as little as 15 minutes a day of moderate-intensity activity can add years to a person's life.[15] In addition to extending longevity, physical activity supports independence and mobility in later life by reducing the risk of falls and minimizing the risk of injury should a fall occur.[16]

Physical Activity Benefits Revealed The health benefits of regular physical activity have long been known, but the mechanisms underlying such benefits have, until recently, been difficult to elucidate. As discussed above, regular physical activity may protect against major chronic diseases by positively influencing metabolic risk factors such as obesity, blood pressure, insulin resistance, inflammation, and blood lipids. Exactly how physical activity may exert such widespread improvements to health has recently begun to be revealed.

As discussed in Chapter 5, adipose tissue actively secretes proteins known as adipokines that help regulate energy balance and other body functions and in turn influence health. Similarly, researchers now know that during or immediately after physical activity, skeletal muscles release proteins known as **myokines**; over time, these myokines elicit systemic changes.[17] Myokines released by skeletal muscle during physical activity signal changes in skeletal

myokines: signaling proteins secreted by skeletal muscles.

*Moderate physical activity can stimulate immune function. Intense, vigorous, prolonged activity such as marathon running, however, may compromise immune function.

TABLE 14-1 Levels of Physical Activity Intensity Compared

Level of Intensity	Breathing and/or Heart Rate	Perceived Exertion (on a Scale of 0 to 10)	Talk Test	Energy Expenditure	Walking Pace
Light	Little to no increase	<5	Able to sing	<3.5 kcal/min	<3 mph
Moderate	Some increase	5 or 6	Able to have a conversation	3.5 to 7 kcal/min	3 to 4.5 mph
Vigorous	Large increase	7 or 8	Conversation is difficult or "broken"	>7 kcal/min	>4.5 mph

SOURCE: Centers for Disease Control and Prevention, www.cdc.gov/physicalactivity/everyone; updated March 30, 2011.

muscle as well as in adipose tissue and organs such as the liver. For example, one myokine is thought to reduce insulin sensitivity in both the liver and adipose tissue. The identification and function of skeletal muscle myokines requires much more research, but the limited evidence thus far provides promise for a greater understanding of the relationships between regular physical activity and adaptive changes that enhance health and prevent chronic diseases.

Physical Activity Guidelines What does a person have to do to reap the health rewards of physical activity? To gain substantial *health* benefits, most guidelines recommend a minimum amount of time performing **aerobic physical activity.** The minimum amount of time depends on whether the activity is **moderate-intensity physical activity** or **vigorous-intensity physical activity.** Table 14-1 compares intensity levels. Whether moderate or vigorous, a minimum length of 10 minutes of aerobic physical activity is recommended.[18] Of course, more time and greater intensity bring greater health benefits—maintaining a healthy body weight (BMI of 18.5 to 24.9) and further reducing the risk of chronic diseases.[19]

In addition to providing health benefits, physical activity helps develop and maintain *fitness*. Table 14-2 presents the American College of Sports Medicine

aerobic physical activity: activity in which the body's large muscles move in a rhythmic manner for a sustained period of time. Aerobic activity, also called *endurance activity*, improves cardiorespiratory fitness. Brisk walking, running, swimming, and bicycling are examples.

moderate-intensity physical activity: physical activity that requires some increase in breathing and/or heart rate and expends 3.5 to 7 kcalories per minute. Walking at a speed of 3 to 4.5 miles per hour (about 15 to 20 minutes to walk 1 mile) is an example.

vigorous-intensity physical activity: physical activity that requires a large increase in breathing and/or heart rate and expends more than 7 kcalories per minute. Walking at a very brisk pace (>4.5 miles per hour) or running at a pace of at least 5 miles per hour are examples.

TABLE 14-2 ACSM Guidelines for Physical Fitness

	Cardiorespiratory	Strength	Flexibility
	Steve Cole/PhotoDisc/Getty Images	David Hanover Photography	David Hanover Photography
Type of Activity	Aerobic activity that uses large-muscle groups and can be maintained continuously	Resistance activity that is performed at a controlled speed and through a full range of motion	Stretching activity that uses the major muscle groups
Frequency	5 to 7 days per week	2 to 3 nonconsecutive days per week	2 to 7 days per week
Intensity	Moderate (equivalent to walking at a pace of 3 to 4 miles per hour)[a]	Enough to enhance muscle strength and improve body composition	Enough to feel tightness or slight discomfort
Duration	At least 30 minutes per day	2 to 4 sets of 8 to 12 repetitions involving each major muscle group	2 to 4 repetitions of 15 to 30 seconds per muscle group
Examples	Running, cycling, dancing, swimming, inline skating, rowing, power walking, cross-country skiing, kickboxing, water aerobics, jumping rope; sports activities such as basketball, soccer, racquetball, tennis, volleyball	Pull-ups, push-ups, sit-ups, weightlifting, pilates	Yoga

[a]For those who prefer vigorous-intensity aerobic activity such as walking at a very brisk pace (>4.5 mph) or running (≥5 mph), a minimum of 20 minutes per day, 3 days per week is recommended.
SOURCE: American College of Sports Medicine position stand: Quantity and quality of exercise for developing and maintaining cardiorespiratory, musculoskeletal, and neuromotor fitness in apparently healthy adults—Guidance for prescribing exercise, *Medicine and Science in Sports and Exercise* 43 (2011): 1334–1359; W. L. Haskell and coauthors, Physical activity and public health: Updated recommendation for adults from the American College of Sports Medicine and the American Heart Association, *Medicine & Science in Sports & Exercise* 39 (2007): 1423–1434.

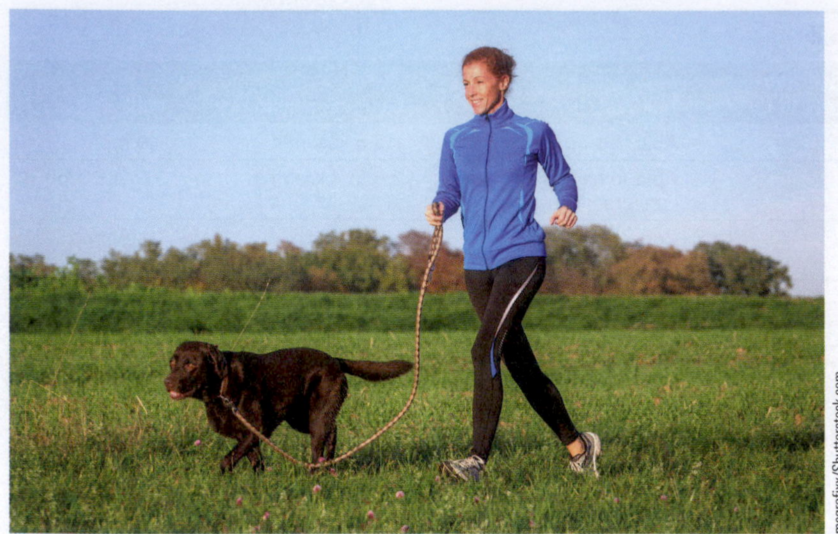

msgrafixx/Shutterstock.com

> **PHOTO 14-2** Choose an active lifestyle. Use the stairs; walk or bike to work, class, or shops; wash and wax the car; mow the grass; rake the leaves; shovel snow; walk the dog; play with children. Be active and have fun.

(ACSM) guidelines for physical activity.[20] Following these guidelines will help adults improve their cardiorespiratory endurance, body composition, strength, and flexibility. At this level of fitness, a person can reap still greater health benefits (substantially lower risk of premature death compared with those who are inactive, improved cardiorespiratory fitness, and improved body composition, for example).[21] Fitness and health both depend on maintaining an active lifestyle every day.

The bottom line is that any physical activity, even moderate activity, *beyond* activities of daily living, provides some health benefits, and these benefits follow a dose-response relationship (see Photo 14-2). In other words, some activity is better than none, and more activity is better still—up to a point. Pursued in excess, intense physical activity, especially when combined with poor eating habits, can undermine health, as Highlight 8, Eating Disorders, explains (pp. 252–254).

Developing Fitness

A person who practices a physical activity *adapts* by becoming better able to perform that activity after each session. People shape their bodies by what they choose to do (see Photo 14-3). Muscle cells and tissues respond to a physical activity **overload** by building, within genetic limits, the structures needed to perform it.[22]

Muscles are continually under renovation. Every day, particularly during the fasting periods between meals, a healthy body degrades a small portion of its muscle protein and then rebuilds new muscle with available amino acids during feeding periods.[23] This balance between protein degradation and synthesis maintains the body's muscle tissue. To *gain* muscle tissue, protein synthesis must be greater than degradation, a condition called **hypertrophy.** When protein degradation is greater than synthesis, the result is **atrophy.** Physical activity tips the balance toward muscle hypertrophy. The opposite is also true: unused muscles diminish in size and weaken over time, tipping the balance toward muscle atrophy.

The muscles adapt and build only the proteins they need to cope with the work performed.[24] Muscles engaged in activities that require strength develop more of the proteins needed for greater muscle mass; body builders have large, well-developed muscles. By comparison, those engaged in endurance activities develop more of the proteins needed to combat muscle fatigue; distance cyclists can pedal for many hours before fatigue sets in.

Strategies to Build Fitness and Prevent Injuries

A variety of physical activities produces the best overall fitness, and to this end, people need to work different muscle groups from day to day. This strategy provides a day or two of rest for different muscle groups, allowing time to replenish nutrients and to repair any minor damage incurred by the activity.

Other tips for building fitness and minimizing the risk of overuse injuries are:

- Be active all week, not just on the weekends.
- Use proper equipment and wear proper attire.
- Perform exercises using proper form.
- Include **warm-up** and **cool-down** activities in each session. Warming up helps prepare muscles, ligaments, and tendons for the upcoming activity and mobilizes fuels to support strength and endurance activities. Cooling down reduces muscle cramping and allows the heart rate to slow gradually.

overload: an extra physical demand placed on the body; an increase in the frequency, duration, or intensity of an activity. A principle of training that states for a body system to improve, it must be worked at frequencies, durations, or intensities that increase by increments.

hypertrophy (high-PER-tro-fee)**:** growing larger; with regard to muscles, an increase in size (and strength) in response to use.

atrophy (AT-ro-fee)**:** becoming smaller; with regard to muscles, a decrease in size (and strength) because of disuse, undernutrition, or wasting diseases.

warm-up: 5 to 10 minutes of light activity, such as easy jogging or cycling, prior to a workout to prepare the body for more vigorous activity.

cool-down: 5 to 10 minutes of light activity, such as walking or stretching, following a vigorous workout to gradually return the body's core to near-normal temperature.

- Train hard enough to challenge your strength or endurance a few times each week rather than every time you work out. Between challenges, do moderate workouts and include at least one day of rest each week.
- Pay attention to body signals. Symptoms such as abnormal heartbeat, dizziness, lightheadedness, cold sweat, confusion, or pain or pressure in the middle of the chest, teeth, jaw, neck, or arm demand immediate medical attention.
- Work out wisely. Do not start with activities so demanding that pain stops you within a day or two. Learn to enjoy small steps toward improvement. Fitness builds slowly.

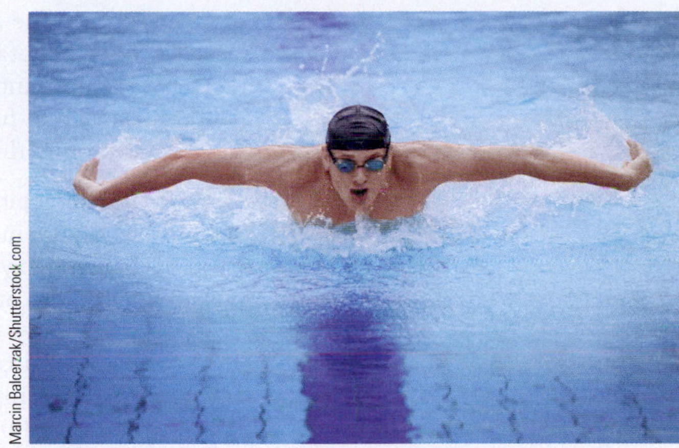

Marcin Balcerzak/Shutterstock.com

> **PHOTO 14-3** People's bodies are shaped by the activities they perform.

Cautions on Starting a Fitness Program Before beginning a fitness program, make sure it is safe for you to do so.[25] Most apparently healthy people can begin a moderate exercise program such as walking or increasing daily activities without a medical examination, but people with any of the following coronary risk factors may need medical advice:

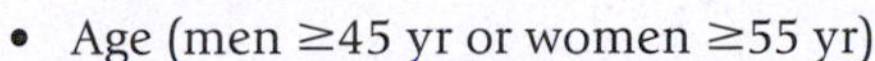

- Age (men ≥45 yr or women ≥55 yr)
- Family history of heart disease
- Cigarette smoking
- Hypertension
- Blood cholesterol ≥200 mg/dL, LDL ≥130 mg/dL or HDL ≤40 mg/dL, or taking lipid-lowering medication
- Prediabetes or diabetes (fasting plasma glucose ≥100 mg/dL)
- Sedentary lifestyle
- Obesity (BMI ≥30), or waist circumference >40 inches for men and >35 inches for women

The Components of Fitness

To be physically fit, a person must develop enough flexibility, muscle strength and endurance, and cardiorespiratory endurance to meet the everyday demands of life with some to spare, and achieve a healthy body composition. **Flexibility** allows the joints to move freely, reducing the risk of injury. **Cardiorespiratory endurance** supports the ongoing activity of the heart and lungs. **Muscle strength** and **muscle endurance** enable muscles to work harder and longer without fatigue. **Body composition** improves as physical activity supports lean body tissues and reduces excess body fat.

Although nutrition influences each component of fitness to some extent, its role in flexibility is not as apparent as for the others. For this reason, cardiorespiratory endurance and muscle strength and endurance are emphasized in the following sections. As the heart and lungs improve their capacity to sustain physical activity and the muscles become stronger and less readily fatigued, body composition improves: body fat decreases and lean body mass increases. (Chapter 8 discusses body composition and the health risks of too much body fat.)

Cardiorespiratory Endurance

The length of time a person can remain active with an elevated heart rate—that is, the ability of the heart, lungs, and blood to sustain a given demand—defines a person's cardiorespiratory endurance. Cardiorespiratory endurance training improves a person's ability to sustain vigorous activities such as running, brisk walking, or swimming. Such training enhances the capacity of the heart, lungs, and blood to deliver oxygen to, and remove waste from, the body's cells.[26] Cardiorespiratory endurance training, therefore, is *aerobic*, meaning oxygen requiring. As the cardiorespiratory system gradually adapts to the demands of aerobic activity, the body delivers oxygen more efficiently.

flexibility: the capacity of the joints to move through a full range of motion; the ability to bend and recover without injury.

cardiorespiratory endurance: the ability to perform large-muscle, dynamic exercise of moderate to high intensity for prolonged periods.

muscle strength: the ability of muscles to work against resistance.

muscle endurance: the ability of a muscle to contract repeatedly without becoming exhausted.

body composition: the proportions of muscle, bone, fat, and other tissues that make up a person's total body weight.

In fact, the accepted measure of a person's cardiorespiratory fitness is maximal oxygen uptake (VO_{2max}). The benefits of cardiorespiratory training are not just physical, though, because all of the body's cells, including the brain cells, require oxygen to function. When the cells receive more oxygen more readily, both the body and the mind benefit.

Cardiorespiratory Conditioning **Cardiorespiratory conditioning** occurs as aerobic workouts improve heart and lung function. **Cardiac output** increases, thus enhancing oxygen delivery. The heart becomes stronger, and each beat pumps more blood. Because the heart pumps more blood with each beat, fewer beats are necessary, and the resting heart rate slows down. The average resting pulse rate for adults is around 70 beats per minute, but people who achieve cardiorespiratory conditioning may have resting pulse rates of 50 or even lower. The muscles that work the lungs become stronger, too, so breathing becomes more efficient. Circulation through the arteries and veins improves. Blood moves easily, and blood pressure declines.[27] In short, cardiorespiratory conditioning:

- Increases cardiac output and oxygen delivery
- Increases blood volume per heart beat (stroke volume)
- Slows resting pulse rate
- Increases breathing efficiency
- Improves circulation
- Reduces blood pressure

Cardiorespiratory endurance reflects the health of the heart and circulatory system, on which all other body systems depend. To improve cardiorespiratory endurance, activities must be sustained for 20 minutes or longer and use most of the large-muscle groups of the body (legs, buttocks, and abdomen). The level of training must be intense enough to elevate heart rate.

A person's own perceived effort is usually a reliable indicator of the intensity of an activity. In general, workouts should be at an intensity that raises your heart rate but still leaves you able to talk comfortably. For those who are more competitive and want to work to their limits on some days, a treadmill test can reveal the maximum heart rate. Workouts are safe at up to 85 percent of that rate. Table 14-2 (p. 427) includes the ACSM guidelines for developing and maintaining cardiorespiratory fitness.

Muscle Conditioning One of the benefits of cardiorespiratory training is that fit muscles use oxygen efficiently, reducing the heart's workload. An added bonus is that muscles that use oxygen efficiently can burn fat longer—a plus for body composition and weight control.

Muscle Strength and Endurance

Resistance training has long been recognized as a means to build and maintain muscle mass, strength, power, and endurance. Additional benefits of resistance training, however, have also emerged. Progressive resistance training helps prevent and manage several chronic diseases, including cardiovascular disease, and enhances psychological well-being.[28] Resistance training can also help maximize and maintain bone mass.[29] Even in women past menopause (when most women are losing bone), resistance training can improve bone density, especially in combination with adequate dietary calcium and vitamin D intake.[30]

By promoting strong muscles in the back and abdomen, resistance training can improve posture and reduce the risk of back injury. Resistance training can also help prevent the decline in physical mobility that often accompanies aging.[31] Older adults, even those in their 80s, who participate in resistance training programs not only gain muscle strength but also improve their muscle endurance, which enables them to walk longer before exhaustion. Leg strength and walking endurance are powerful indicators of an older adult's physical abilities.

VO_{2max}: the maximum rate of oxygen consumption by an individual at sea level.

cardiorespiratory conditioning: improvements in heart and lung function and increased blood volume, brought about by aerobic training.

cardiac output: the volume of blood discharged by the heart each minute; determined by multiplying the stroke volume by the heart rate. The stroke volume is the amount of oxygenated blood the heart ejects toward the tissues at each beat. Cardiac output (volume/minute) = stroke volume (volume/beat) × heart rate (beats/minute)

resistance training: the use of free weights or weight machines to provide resistance for developing muscle strength, power, and endurance; also called *weight training*. A person's own body weight may also be used to provide resistance such as when a person does push-ups, pull-ups, or abdominal crunches.

Resistance training builds muscle strength, **muscle power**, and muscle endurance. To emphasize muscle strength, combine high resistance (heavy weight) with a low number of repetitions (8 to 12).[32] To emphasize muscle power, combine moderate resistance (light to medium weight) with high velocity (as fast as safely possible). To emphasize muscle endurance, combine less resistance (lighter weight) with more repetitions (15 to 20). Resistance training enhances performance in other sports too. Swimmers can develop a more efficient stroke and tennis players a more powerful serve when they train with weights, for example.

A Balanced Fitness Program The intensity and type of physical activities that are best for one person may not be good for another. A person who has been sedentary will initially perform at a dramatically different level of intensity than a fit person.

The type of physical activity that is best for you depends, too, on what you want to achieve and what you enjoy doing (see Photo 14-4). Some people love walking, whereas others prefer to dance or ride a bike. Those who want to be stronger and firmer, lift weights. Keep in mind that muscle is more metabolically active than body fat, so the more muscle you have, the more energy you'll expend.

In a balanced fitness program, aerobic activity improves cardiorespiratory fitness, stretching enhances flexibility, and resistance training develops muscle strength, muscle power, and muscle endurance. Table 14-3 provides an example of a balanced fitness program.

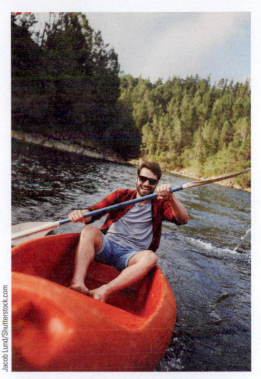

Jacob Lund/Shutterstock.com

> PHOTO 14-4 The key to regular physical activity is finding an activity you enjoy.

REVIEW IT Describe the health benefits of being physically fit and explain how to develop the components of fitness.

Physical activity brings good health and long life. To develop fitness—whose components are flexibility, cardiorespiratory endurance, muscle strength and endurance, and body composition—a person must condition the body, through training, to adapt to the activity performed.

TABLE 14-3 A Sample Balanced Fitness Program

Monday, Tuesday, Wednesday, Thursday, Friday:

- 5 minutes of warm-up activity
- 30–60 minutes of aerobic activity
- 10 minutes of cool-down activity and stretching

Tuesday, Thursday, Saturday:

- 5 minutes of warm-up activity
- 30 minutes of resistance training
- 10 minutes of cool-down activity and stretching

Saturday and/or Sunday:

- Sports, walking, hiking, biking, or swimming

14.2 Energy Systems and Fuels to Support Activity

LEARN IT Identify the factors that influence fuel use during physical activity and the types of activities that depend more on glucose or fat, respectively.

Nutrition and physical activity go hand in hand. Activity demands carbohydrate and fat as fuel, protein to build and maintain lean tissues, vitamins and minerals to support both energy metabolism and tissue building, and water to help distribute the fuels and to dissipate the resulting heat and wastes. This section describes how nutrition supports a person who decides to get up and go.

The Energy Systems of Physical Activity

As Chapter 7 described, the high-energy compound ATP provides the energy that powers all the activities of living cells. ATP is present in small amounts in all body tissues all the time, and it can deliver energy instantly. Muscle cells may need additional ATP to power their many activities. When an ATP molecule is split in the muscle cells, the energy released contracts muscles and generates heat. Thus, physical exertion uses ATP. Three major energy systems enable muscle cells to regenerate ATP during different types of physical activity:

- the phosphagen system (also called the creatine phosphate system)
- the lactic acid system (anaerobic glycolysis)
- the aerobic system (aerobic glycolysis, fatty acid oxidation, and TCA cycle)

All three energy systems function at all times, but depending on the intensity of the activity and the conditioning of the athlete, one system will predominate at any given time. The following sections describe each of these systems.

muscle power: the product of force generation (strength) and movement velocity (speed); the speed at which a given amount of exertion is completed.

The Phosphagen System Immediately after the onset of a demand, before muscle ATP pools dwindle, a muscle enzyme begins to break down another high-energy compound that is stored in the muscle, **creatine phosphate (CP).** CP is made from creatine, a compound commonly found in muscles, with a phosphate group attached. CP can split anaerobically (not requiring oxygen) to release phosphate, which can be used to replenish ATP. Supplies of CP in a muscle last for only about 10 seconds, producing enough quick energy, without oxygen, for a 100-meter dash.

When activity ceases and the muscles are resting, ATP gives up one of its phosphate groups to creatine. Thus, CP is produced during rest by reversing the process that occurs during muscular activity. (Highlight 14 includes creatine supplements in its discussion of substances commonly used in the pursuit of fitness.)

The Lactic Acid System After the first 10 seconds or so of intense activity, energy from the phosphagen system diminishes, so muscle cells call upon the lactic acid system to produce more ATP. As Chapter 7 described, the lactic acid system involves the anaerobic breakdown of glucose to pyruvate (and then of pyruvate to lactate). The primary source of glucose is muscle glycogen. This system can generate a small amount of ATP quickly for high-intensity activity lasting up to 3 minutes. A later section describes the consequences of lactate accumulation.

The Aerobic System To meet the more prolonged demands of sustained activity, the muscles rely on the aerobic system to provide ATP for muscle contraction (see Photo 14-5). As Chapter 7 described, carbohydrate, fat, and some amino acids are continuously oxidized to ensure an uninterrupted supply of ATP.

During rest, the body derives more than half of its ATP from the oxidation of fatty acids, most of the rest from the complete oxidation of glucose, and a small percentage from the oxidation of amino acids. During physical activity, the body adjusts its mixture of fuels. Muscles always use a mixture of fuels—never just one. How much of which fuel the muscles use during physical activity depends on an interplay among the fuels available from the diet, the intensity and duration of the activity, and the degree to which the body is conditioned to perform that activity. The next sections explain these relationships by examining each of the energy-yielding nutrients individually, but keep in mind that although one fuel may predominate at a given time, the other two will still be involved. Table 14-4 shows how fuel use changes according to the intensity and duration of the activity.

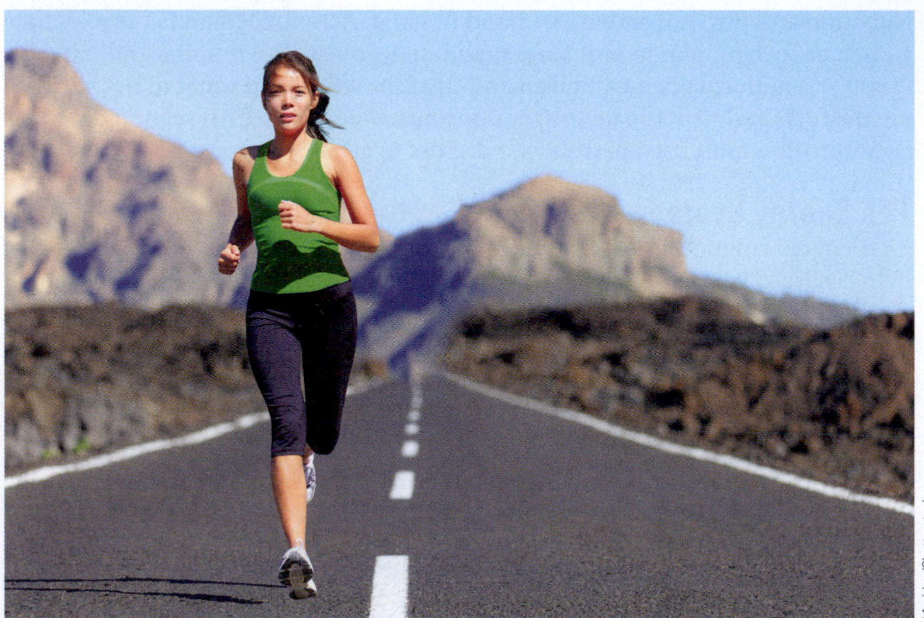
Maridav/Shutterstock.com

> **PHOTO 14-5** Sustained muscular efforts as in a long-distance run involve *aerobic* work.

creatine phosphate (CP): a high-energy compound in muscle cells that acts as a reservoir of energy that can maintain a steady supply of ATP. CP provides the energy for short bursts of activity; also called *phosphocreatine*.

- During rest: ATP + creatine → CP
- During activity: CP → ATP + creatine

TABLE 14-4 Primary Fuels Used for Activities of Different Intensities and Durations

Activity Intensity	Activity Duration	Energy System	Preferred Fuel Source	Oxygen Needed?	Activity Example
Extreme	5 to 10 sec	Phosphagen system	ATP-CP (immediate availability)	No	100-meter sprint, shot put, golf or baseball bat swing, tennis or volleyball serve
Very high	20 sec to 2 min	Lactic acid system	ATP from carbohydrate (anaerobic glycolysis)	No	400-meter run, 100-meter swim, gymnastic routine
High	2 min to 20 min	Aerobic system	ATP from carbohydrate (glycolysis and TCA cycle)	Yes	Cycling, swimming, running
Moderate	> 20 min	Aerobic system	ATP from fat (fatty acid-oxidation and TCA cycle)	Yes	Hiking

NOTE: All energy systems function at all times, but depending on the intensity of the activity and the conditioning of the athlete, one system will predominate at any given time.

Anaerobic versus Aerobic Oxygen—or its lack—is central to the energy systems just described. The phosphagen and lactic acid systems are anaerobic—meaning without oxygen. As its name suggests, the aerobic system uses oxygen. As you read the following pages, notice how the fuel mixture shifts depending on whether the activity is anaerobic or aerobic.

Anaerobic activities are associated with strength, agility, and split-second surges of power (see Photo 14-6). The jump of a slam dunk, the power of a tennis serve, and the heave of a bench press all involve anaerobic work. Such high-intensity, short-duration activities depend mostly on glucose as the chief energy fuel in the lactic acid system.

Endurance activities of low to moderate intensity and long duration depend more on fat to provide energy through the aerobic system. The ability to continue swimming to the shore, to keep on hiking to the top of the mountain, or to continue pedaling all the way home reflects aerobic capacity. As mentioned earlier, aerobic capacity is also crucial to maintaining a healthy heart and circulatory system. Because various physical activities use different energy systems and quantities of nutrients to various degrees, a person's food choices can greatly influence performance.

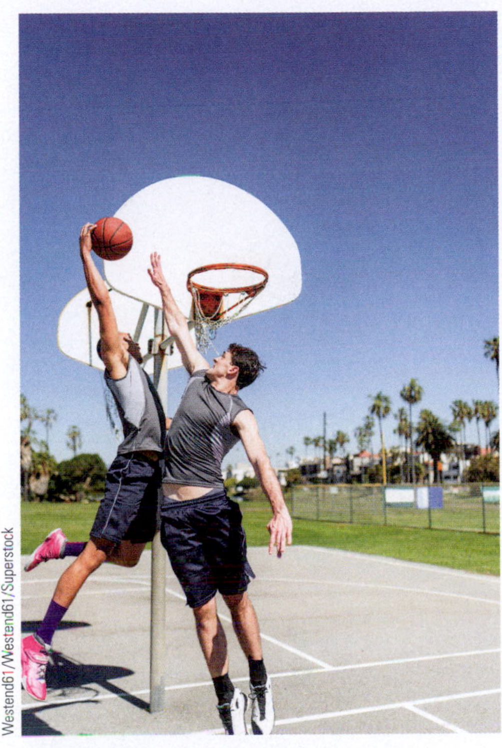

> **PHOTO 14-6** Split-second surges of power as in the jump of a basketball player involve *anaerobic* work.

Glucose Use during Physical Activity

Glucose, stored in the liver and muscles as glycogen, is vital to physical activity. During exertion, the liver breaks down its glycogen and releases glucose into the bloodstream. The muscles use this glucose as well as their own private glycogen stores to fuel their work. Glycogen stores can easily support everyday activities but are limited to less than 2000 kcalories of energy, enough for about 20 miles of running. The more athletes can fill muscle glycogen stores, the longer the glycogen will last during physical activity, which in turn influences performance. When glycogen is depleted, the muscles become fatigued.

Diet Affects Glycogen Storage and Use How much carbohydrate a person eats influences how much glycogen is stored. A classic study compared fuel use during activity among three groups of runners on different diets.[33] For several days before testing, one group consumed a normal mixed diet, a second group consumed a high-carbohydrate diet, and the third group consumed a no-carbohydrate diet (fat and protein diet). As Figure 14-1 (p. 434) shows, the high-carbohydrate diet allowed the runners to keep going longer before becoming exhausted. This study and many others that followed have confirmed that high-carbohydrate diets enhance endurance by ensuring ample glycogen stores. Thus, to fill glycogen stores, eat plenty of carbohydrate-rich foods.

Intensity of Activity Affects Glycogen Use How long glycogen stores will last depends not only on diet, but also on the intensity of the activity. Moderate activities such as jogging use glycogen slowly. The lungs and circulatory system have no trouble keeping up with the muscles' need for oxygen. The individual breathes

> **FIGURE 14-1 The Effect of Diet on Physical Endurance**

A high-carbohydrate diet can increase an athlete's endurance. In this study, the fat and protein diet provided 94 percent of kcalories from fat and 6 percent from protein; the normal mixed diet provided 55 percent of kcalories from carbohydrate; and the high-carbohydrate diet provided 83 percent of kcalories from carbohydrate.

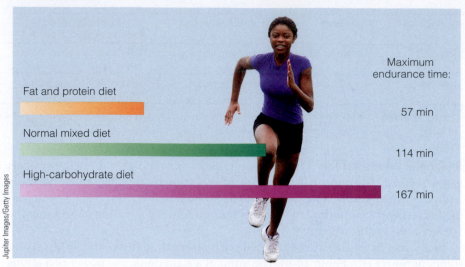

Maximum endurance time:
Fat and protein diet
57 min
Normal mixed diet
114 min
High-carbohydrate diet
167 min
Jupiter Images/Getty Images

easily, and the heart beats steadily—the activity is aerobic. The muscles derive their energy from both glucose and fatty acids. By depending partly on fatty acids, moderate aerobic activity conserves glycogen.

Intense activities—the kind that make it difficult "to catch your breath," such as a quarter-mile race—use glycogen quickly. In such activities, the muscles rely on the lactic acid system to break down glucose to pyruvate anaerobically, producing ATP quickly.

Lactate Lactate is the product of anaerobic glycolysis. When the rate of glycolysis exceeds the capacity of the mitochondria to accept hydrogens with their electrons for the electron transport chain, the accumulating pyruvate molecules are converted to lactate. At low intensities, lactate is readily cleared from the blood, but at higher intensities, lactate accumulates. When the rate of lactate production exceeds the rate of clearance, intense activity can be maintained for only 1 to 3 minutes (as in a 400- to 800-meter race or a boxing match). Lactate has long been blamed for muscle fatigue, but research disputes this idea. Working muscles may produce lactate and experience fatigue, but the lactate does not cause the fatigue.[34] In contrast, depletion of muscle glycogen by about 80 percent reliably produces fatigue.[35]

Lactate quickly leaves the muscles and travels in the blood to the liver. There, liver enzymes convert the lactate back into glucose. Glucose can then return to the muscles to fuel additional activity. This recycling process that regenerates glucose from lactate is known as the *Cori cycle,* and is shown in Figure 7-7 (p. 204).

Duration of Activity Affects Glycogen Use Glycogen use depends not only on the intensity of an activity, but also on its duration (see Photo 14-7). Initially, a person uses mostly glycogen for fuel. As the muscles devour their own glycogen, they become ravenous for more glucose. Glucagon signals the liver to empty out its glycogen stores to provide the muscles with more glucose.

A person who continues exercising moderately (mostly aerobically) begins to use less and less glucose and more and more fat for fuel (review Table 14-4, p. 433). Still, glucose use continues, and if the activity lasts long enough and is intense enough, blood glucose declines and muscle and liver glycogen stores become depleted. Physical activity can continue for a short time thereafter only because glucagon signals the liver to produce, from lactate and certain amino acids, the minimum amount of glucose needed to briefly forestall total depletion.

Gluconeogenesis could support an activity of low intensity, such as walking, but cannot support continued strenuous activity. After a couple of hours of strenuous activity, glucose stores are depleted. When depletion occurs, it brings nervous system function to a near halt, making continued exertion at the same intensity almost impossible. Marathon runners refer to this point of glucose exhaustion as "hitting the wall."

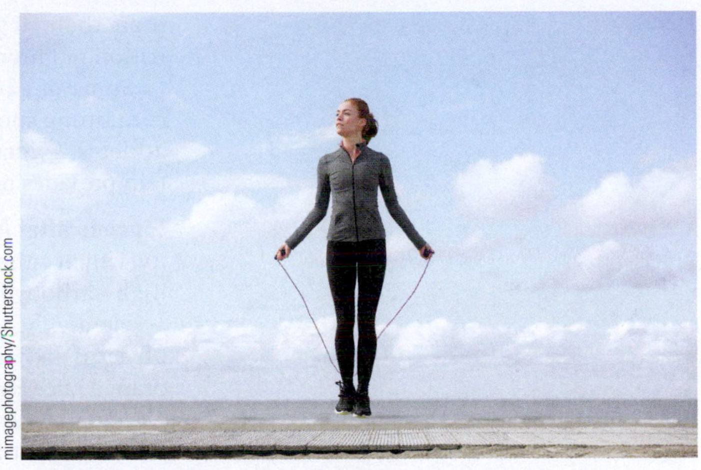
mimagephotography/Shutterstock.com

> **PHOTO 14-7** Moderate- to high-intensity aerobic exercises that can be sustained for only a short time (less than 20 minutes) use some fat, but more glucose for fuel.

Training Affects Glycogen Use Training, too, affects how much glycogen muscles will store. Muscle cells that repeatedly deplete their glycogen through hard work adapt to store greater amounts of glycogen to support that work. Conditioned muscles also rely less on glucose and more on fat for energy, so glycogen breakdown and glucose use occur more slowly in trained than in untrained individuals at a given activity intensity. A person who is attempting an activity for the first time uses much more glucose than an athlete who is trained to perform the same activity. Oxygen delivery to the muscles by the heart and lungs plays a role, too, but equally importantly, trained muscles are better equipped to use the oxygen because their cells contain more mitochondria, the structures within a cell that are responsible for producing ATP (review Figure 7-14, p. 209). Untrained muscles depend more heavily on anaerobic glucose breakdown, even when physical activity is just moderate.

Glucose before Activity Most of an athlete's glucose is provided by carbohydrate-rich meals consumed throughout the day. In addition, glucose consumed within a few hours before training or competition is thought to "top off" the athlete's glycogen stores, providing the greatest possible glucose supply to support sustained activity. The pregame meal to provide glucose can take many forms, as a later section describes.

Glucose during Activity Muscles can obtain the glucose they need not only from glycogen stores, but also from foods and beverages consumed during activity. Consuming carbohydrate is especially useful during exhausting endurance activities (lasting more than 1 hour) and during games such as soccer or hockey, which last for hours and demand repeated bursts of intense activity.[36]

Interestingly, during high-intensity activity lasting less than an hour, some research suggests that merely rinsing the mouth with a carbohydrate solution may be enough to improve performance.[37] In such instances, the benefit is not related to muscle glycogen availability as when athletes ingest carbohydrate during prolonged events. Rather, researchers speculate that there may be receptors in the mouth that sense potential carbohydrate availability and relay this message to areas of the brain involved with reward and motor control.[38]

Endurance athletes often run short of glucose by the end of competitive events. To ensure optimal carbohydrate intake, sports nutrition experts recommend 30 to 60 grams of carbohydrate per hour during prolonged events.[39] Carbohydrate-based sports drinks offer a convenient way to meet this recommendation and also help replace water and electrolyte losses, as a later section explains. Thus, to ensure optimal hydration and carbohydrate intake, endurance athletes are advised to drink one-half to one liter of a 4 to 8 percent carbohydrate-based sports drink per hour, in small, frequent doses during activity.[40] During the last stages of an endurance competition, when glycogen is running low, glucose consumed during the event can slowly make its way from the digestive tract to the muscles and augment the body's supply of glucose enough to forestall exhaustion. Athletes who participate in endurance events lasting longer than 3 hours may tolerate more than 60 grams of carbohydrate per hour, but such athletes have specific nutrition requirements beyond the scope of this chapter.

Some researchers have questioned whether adding protein to carbohydrate-containing sports beverages would offer a performance advantage to endurance athletes. Evidence so far suggests that when carbohydrate intake is optimal, protein provides no additional performance benefit.[41]

Glucose after Activity Muscles depleted of glycogen have greater insulin sensitivity, which enhances glucose uptake and promotes glycogen synthesis. Thus, eating high-carbohydrate foods *after* physical activity also enlarges glycogen stores. To accelerate the rate of glycogen storage, train normally; then, within 2 hours after physical activity, consume a high-carbohydrate meal or snack, such as a glass of orange juice and some graham crackers, toast, or cereal.[42] After 2 hours, the rate of glycogen storage declines by almost half. This strategy is particularly important to athletes who train hard more than once a day.

Chapter 4 introduced the glycemic response and discussed the possible health benefits of eating a *low*-glycemic diet. Such a diet may also benefit endurance performance. Some research indicates that foods with a low glycemic response enhance fatty acid availability and use during subsequent activity, thereby reducing reliance on the muscles' own lipid and glycogen stores.[43] More research is needed to confirm these findings.

Carbohydrate Recommendations for Athletes To postpone fatigue and maximize performance, athletes must maintain available glucose supplies for as long as they can. To do so, athletes need abundant carbohydrate each day. Recent research supports a range of carbohydrate intakes for athletes based on the athlete's total energy needs, training needs, and performance (see Table 14-5).

Fat Use during Physical Activity

Sports nutrition experts recommend that athletes consume 20 to 35 percent of their energy from fat to meet nutrient and energy needs—the same recommendation as for others.[44] Athletes who restrict fat below 20 percent of total energy intake may fail to consume adequate energy and nutrients. Recommendations to include vegetable oils, nuts, olives, fatty fish, and other sources of health-promoting fats in the diet apply to athletes as well as to everyone else.

Diets high in saturated fat carry risks of heart disease. Physical activity offers some protection against cardiovascular disease, but athletes may still suffer heart attacks and strokes. Limiting saturated fat intake to less than 10 percent of total energy intake is another way athletes can protect themselves from heart disease.

TABLE 14-5 Recommended Daily Carbohydrate Intakes for Athletes

These general research-based guidelines should be adjusted to an athlete's energy needs, training regimen, and performance.

Activity Intensity and Duration	Recommendations (g/kg/day)	Carbohydrate Intakes	
		Males	Females
Low-intensity	3–5	210–350 g (840–1400 kcal)	165–275 g (660–1100 kcal)
Moderate intensity, ≤1 hr/day	5–7	350–490 g (1400–1960 kcal)	275–385 g (1100–1540 kcal)
Moderate to high intensity, 1–3 hr/day	6–10	420–700 g (1680–2800 kcal)	330–550 g (1320–2200 kcal)
Moderate to high intensity, >4–5 hr/day	8–12	560–840 g (2240–3360 kcal)	440–660 g (1760–2640 kcal)

NOTE: Daily carbohydrate intakes are based on a 70-kilogram (154-pound) man and 55-kilogram (121-pound) woman.
SOURCE: Position of the Academy of Nutrition and Dietetics, Dietitians of Canada, and the American College of Sports Medicine: Nutrition and athletic performance, *Journal of the Academy of Nutrition and Dietetics* 116 (2016): 501–528.

In contrast to *dietary* fat, *body* fat stores are extremely important during physical activity, as long as the activity is not too intense. Unlike glycogen stores, the body's fat stores can usually provide more than 70,000 kcalories and fuel hours of activity without running out.

The fat used in physical activity is liberated as fatty acids from the internal fat stores and from the fat under the skin. Areas that have the most fat to spare donate the greatest amounts to the blood (although they may not be the areas that appear fattiest). Thus, "spot reducing" doesn't work because muscles do not "own" the fat that surrounds them. Fat cells release fatty acids into the blood, not into the underlying muscles. Then the blood gives to each muscle the amount of fat that it needs. Proof of this is found in a tennis player's arms—the skinfold measures of fat are the same in both arms, even though the muscles of one arm work much harder and may be larger than those of the other. A balanced fitness program that includes strength training will tighten muscles underneath the fat, improving the overall appearance. Keep in mind that some body fat is essential to good health. (Chapter 8 discussed the health risks of too little body fat.)

Duration of Activity Affects Fat Use Early in an activity, as the muscles draw on fatty acids, blood levels fall. If the activity continues for more than a few minutes, the hormone epinephrine signals the fat cells to begin breaking down their stored triglycerides and liberating fatty acids into the blood. As physical activity continues, the blood fatty acid concentration surpasses the normal resting concentration. Thereafter, sustained, moderate activity uses body fat stores as its major fuel (see Photo 14-8).

Intensity of Activity Affects Fat Use The intensity of physical activity also affects fat use. As the intensity of activity increases, fat makes less and less of a contribution to the fuel mixture. Remember that fat can be broken down for energy only by aerobic metabolism. For fat to fuel activity, then, oxygen must be abundantly available. If a person is breathing easily during activity, the muscles are getting all the oxygen they need and are able to use more fat in the fuel mixture.

Training Affects Fat Use Training—repeated aerobic activity—produces the adaptations that permit the body to draw more heavily on fat for fuel. Training stimulates the muscle cells to manufacture more and larger mitochondria, the "powerhouse" structures of the cells that produce ATP for energy. Another adaptation: the heart and lungs become stronger and better able to deliver oxygen to muscles at high activity intensities. Still another: hormones in the body of a trained person slow glucose release from the liver and speed up the use of fat instead. These adaptations reward not only trained athletes but all active people; a person who trains in aerobic activities such as distance running or cycling becomes well suited to the activity.

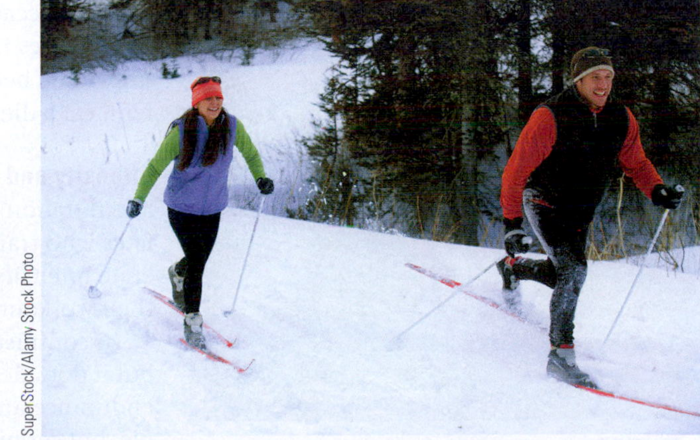

SuperStock/Alamy Stock Photo

> **PHOTO 14-8** Low- to moderate-intensity aerobic exercises that can be sustained for a long time (more than 20 minutes) use some glucose, but more fat, for fuel.

Protein Use during Physical Activity—and between Times

Table 14-4 (p. 433) summarizes the fuel uses discussed so far, but does not include the third energy-yielding nutrient, protein, because protein is not a major fuel for physical activity. Nevertheless, physically active people use protein just as other people do—to build muscle and other lean tissues and, to some extent, to fuel activity. The body does, however, handle protein differently during activity than during rest.

Protein Used in Muscle Building Synthesis of body proteins is suppressed during activity. In the hours of recovery following activity, though, protein synthesis accelerates beyond normal resting levels. As noted earlier, eating high-carbohydrate foods immediately after exercise accelerates muscle glycogen storage. Similarly, research shows that eating high-quality protein, either by itself or together with carbohydrate, enhances muscle protein synthesis.[45] With food intake, of course, insulin is secreted. Insulin not only stimulates muscle protein synthesis, but also greatly inhibits muscle protein breakdown. Remember that the body adapts and builds the molecules, cells, and tissues it needs for the next period of activity. Whenever the body remodels a part of itself, it tears down old structures to make way for new ones. Repeated activity, with just a slight overload, triggers the protein-dismantling and protein-synthesizing equipment of each muscle cell to make needed changes—that is, to adapt.

The physical work of each muscle cell acts as a signal to its DNA and RNA to begin producing the kinds of proteins that will best support that work. Take running, for example. In the first difficult sessions, the body is not yet equipped to perform aerobic work easily, but with each session, the cells' genetic material gets the message that an overhaul is needed. In the hours that follow the session, the genes send molecular messages to the protein-building equipment that tell it what old structures to break down and what new structures to build. Within the limits of its genetic potential, the body responds. Running (or any aerobic activity) stimulates synthesis of mitochondria to facilitate efficient aerobic metabolism. Over time, the body adapts and running becomes easier.

The body of a weightlifter responds to training as well, but the response differs from that of aerobic training. Weightlifting stimulates synthesis of muscle fiber protein to enhance muscle mass and strength—with little change in mitochondria. An athlete may add between ¼ ounce and 1 ounce (between 7 and 28 grams) of protein to muscle mass each day during active muscle-building phases of training.

Protein Used as Fuel Not only do athletes retain more protein in their muscles, but they also use more protein as fuel. Muscles speed up their use of amino acids for energy during physical activity, just as they speed up their use of fat and carbohydrate. Still, protein contributes only about 10 percent of the total fuel used, both during activity and during rest. The most active people of all—endurance athletes—use large amounts of all energy fuels, including protein, during performance, but they also eat more food and therefore usually consume enough protein.

Diet Affects Protein Use during Activity Diet influences how much protein is used during physical activity. People who consume diets adequate in energy and rich in *carbohydrate* use less protein than those who eat protein- and fat-rich diets. Recall that carbohydrates spare proteins from being broken down to make glucose when needed. Because physical activity requires glucose, a diet lacking in carbohydrate necessitates the conversion of amino acids to glucose. The same is true for a diet high in fat because fatty acids can never provide glucose. In short, to conserve protein, eat a diet adequate in energy and rich in carbohydrate.

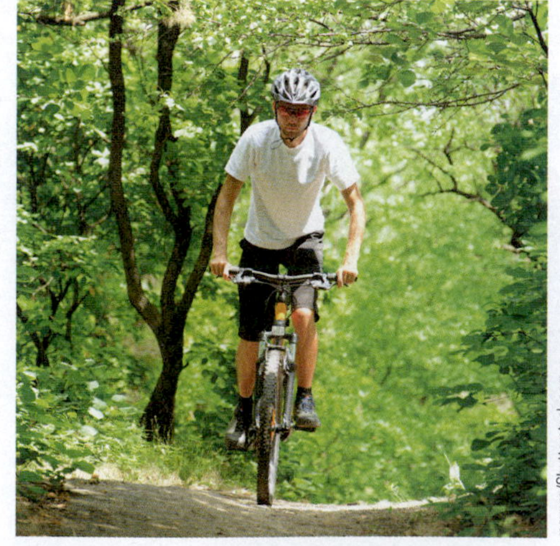

maxpro/Shutterstock.com

> PHOTO 14-9 Protein contributes more to the fuel mix when aerobic activity is at least moderately intense and lasts longer than an hour.

Intensity and Duration of Activity Affect Protein Use during Activity The intensity and duration of activity also modifies protein use (see Photo 14-9). Endurance athletes who train for more than an hour a day, engaging in aerobic activity of moderate intensity and long duration, may deplete their glycogen stores by the end of their workouts and become somewhat more dependent on body protein for energy.

In contrast, anaerobic strength training does not use more protein for energy, but it does demand more protein to build muscle. Thus, the protein needs of both endurance and strength athletes are slightly higher than those of sedentary people, but certainly not as high as the protein intakes many athletes consume.

Protein Recommendations for Active People As mentioned, all active people, and especially athletes in training, probably need more protein than sedentary people

TABLE 14-6 Recommended Daily Protein Intakes for Athletes

	Recommendations (g/kg/day)	Protein Intakes (g/day)	
		Males	Females
RDA for adults	0.8	56	44
Recommended intake for athletes	1.2–2.0	84–140	66–110
US average intake		99	68

NOTE: Daily protein intakes are based on a 70-kilogram (154-pound) man and 55-kilogram (121-pound) woman.
SOURCES: Position of the Academy of Nutrition and Dietetics, Dietitians of Canada, and the American College of Sports Medicine: Nutrition and athletic performance, *Journal of the Academy of Nutrition and Dietetics* 116 (2016): 501–528; US Department of Agriculture, Agricultural Research Service, 2014, Nutrient intakes from food and beverages: Mean amounts consumed per individual, by gender and age, *What We Eat in America*, NHANES, 2011–2012. http://www.ars.usda.gov/nea/bhnrc/fsrg; Committee on Dietary Reference Intakes, *Dietary Reference Intakes for Energy, Carbohydrate, Fiber, Fat, Fatty Acids, Cholesterol, Protein and Amino Acids* (Washington, D.C.: National Academies Press, 2005), pp. 660–661.

do. Endurance athletes, such as long-distance runners and cyclists, use more protein for fuel than strength or power athletes do, and they retain some, especially in the muscles used for their sport. Strength athletes, such as weightlifters, and power athletes, such as football players, use less protein for fuel, but they still use some and retain much more. Therefore, *all* athletes in training should attend to protein needs, but they should first meet their energy needs with adequate carbohydrate intakes. Without adequate carbohydrate intake, athletes will burn off as fuel the very protein they wish to retain in muscle.

How much protein, then, should an active person consume? The DRI Committee does not recommend greater than normal protein intakes for athletes, but other authorities do.[46] Recent research supports a range of protein intakes for athletes based on training experience, frequency and intensity of training sessions, and importantly, energy and carbohydrate availability (see Table 14-6).[47] Daily protein intake goals are best met by a meal plan that includes moderate amounts (20 to 30 grams) of high-quality protein in 4 to 5 small meals throughout the day, including within 2 hours following strenuous training sessions. Table 14-7 presents foods and beverages that provide 20 grams of high-quality protein. Even the highest protein recommendations can be met without protein supplements, or even excessive servings of meat. Chapter 6 reviewed the potential dangers of using protein and amino acid supplements (see pp. 187–188).

TABLE 14-7 Selected Foods and Beverages Providing 20 Grams of High-Quality Protein

The indicated portion of any of these foods provides approximately 20 grams of protein and varying amounts of energy as shown.

Food or Beverage	Amount	Energy (kcal)
Almonds	3 oz	500
Beef, cooked lean ground	3 oz	145
Cheese, cheddar	3 oz	345
Chicken, cooked skinless breast	3 oz	130
Eggs (white)	6 large	100
Eggs (whole)	3 large	270
Milk, low-fat	20 oz	255
Tofu	8 oz	185
Tuna, light canned in water	3 oz	70
Yogurt, Greek-style	8 oz	130

SOURCE: USDA National Nutrient Database for Standard Reference. Release 28. http://ndb.nal.usda.gov.

REVIEW IT Identify the factors that influence fuel use during physical activity and the types of activities that depend more on glucose or fat, respectively.

The mixture of fuels the muscles use during physical activity depends on diet, the intensity and duration of the activity, and training. During intense activity, the fuel mix contains mostly glucose, whereas during less intense, moderate activity, fat makes a greater contribution. With endurance training, muscle cells adapt to store more glycogen and to rely less on glucose and more on fat for energy. Athletes in training may need more protein than sedentary people do, but they typically eat more food as well and therefore obtain enough protein without taking supplements.

14.3 Vitamins and Minerals to Support Activity

LEARN IT List which vitamin and mineral supplements, if any, athletes may need and why.

Many of the vitamins and minerals assist in releasing energy from fuels and in transporting oxygen. This knowledge has led many people to believe, mistakenly, that vitamin and mineral *supplements* offer physically active people both health benefits and athletic advantages. (Review Highlight 10 for a discussion of vitamin and mineral supplements, and see Highlight 14, which explores supplements and other products people use in the hope of enhancing athletic performance.)

Dietary Supplements Nutrient supplements do not enhance the performance of well-nourished people. Deficiencies of vitamins and minerals, however, do impede performance. Regular, strenuous, physical activity increases the demand for energy, and athletes and active people tend to eat more food. If they select nutrient-dense foods to meet those increased energy needs, they will, in most cases, also meet their vitamin and mineral needs (see Photo 14-10). Remember, however, that nutrient recommendations are based on the needs of healthy people in different life stages and do not reflect the potentially greater needs that some athletes may incur.

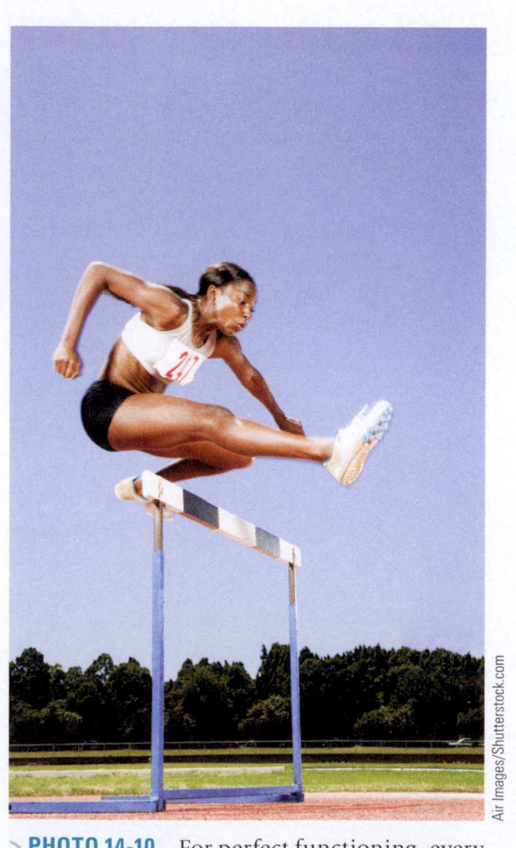

> **PHOTO 14-10** For perfect functioning, every nutrient is needed.

Air Images/Shutterstock.com

As Highlight 8 mentioned, some athletes who struggle to meet low body-weight requirements may eat so little food that they fail to obtain all the nutrients they need.[48] The practice of "making weight" is opposed by many health and fitness organizations, but for athletes who choose this course of action, a single daily multivitamin-mineral supplement that provides no more than the DRI recommendations for nutrients may be beneficial. In addition, some athletes simply do not eat enough food to maintain a healthy body weight during times of intense training or competition. For these athletes as well, a daily multivitamin-mineral supplement can be helpful.

Some athletes believe that taking vitamin or mineral supplements directly before competition will enhance performance. These beliefs are contrary to scientific reality. Most vitamins and minerals function as small parts of larger working units. After absorption into the blood, these nutrients travel to the cells for assembly with their appropriate other parts before they can do their work. This takes time—hours or days. Vitamins or minerals taken right before an event are useless for improving performance, even if the person is actually suffering deficiencies of them.

Nutrients of Concern In general, active people who eat well-balanced meals do not need vitamin or mineral supplements. Two nutrients, vitamin E and iron, do merit special mention here, however, each for a different reason. Vitamin E is discussed because so many athletes take vitamin E supplements. Iron is discussed because some athletes may be unaware that they need iron supplements.

Vitamin E During prolonged, high-intensity physical activity, the muscles' consumption of oxygen increases tenfold or more, which increases the production of free radicals in the body. As Highlight 11 explained, vitamin E is a potent antioxidant that vigorously defends cell membranes against the oxidative damage of free radicals.

Does vitamin E supplementation protect against exercise-induced oxidative stress? Some studies find that it does; others show no effect, and still others report enhanced oxidative stress.[49] Recent research may offer some insight into these inconsistencies. Although free radicals are usually damaging, during repeated episodes of endurance activities, they may actually be beneficial. Free radicals activate powerful antioxidant enzymes, which may enhance the athlete's tolerance to oxidative stresses. Researchers speculate that antioxidant supplements such as vitamin E interfere with this protective adaptation. This may explain why, in some studies, athletes taking vitamin E show signs of increased oxidative stress. Clearly, more research is needed on supplements, but in the meantime, active people can benefit by using vitamin E–rich vegetable oils and eating generous servings of antioxidant-rich fruits and vegetables regularly. Beta-carotene and vitamin C in fruits and vegetables, as well as many of the phytochemicals in these foods, are also potent antioxidants.

Iron Deficiency Physically active young women, especially those who engage in endurance activities such as distance running, are prone to iron deficiency.[50] Habitually low intakes of iron-rich foods, high iron losses through menstruation, and the high demands of muscles for the iron-containing electron carriers of the mitochondria and the muscle protein myoglobin can contribute to iron deficiency in physically active young women. In addition, endurance activities temporarily increase the release of hepcidin, which limits iron absorption (see Chapter 13).[51]

Adolescent female athletes who eat vegetarian diets may be particularly vulnerable to iron deficiency. As Chapter 13 explained, the bioavailability of iron is often poor in vegetarian diets. To protect against iron deficiency, vegetarian athletes need to select good dietary sources of iron (fortified cereals, legumes, nuts, and seeds) and include vitamin C–rich foods with each meal. So long as vegetarian athletes, like all athletes, consume enough nutrient-dense foods, they can perform as well as anyone.

Iron-Deficiency Anemia Iron-deficiency anemia impairs physical performance because iron is an essential component of hemoglobin. Without adequate iron, hemoglobin in red blood cells cannot deliver oxygen to the cells for energy metabolism. Without adequate oxygen, an active person cannot perform aerobic activities and tires easily. Iron deficiency without clinical signs of anemia may also impair physical performance.[52]

Sports Anemia Early in training, athletes may develop low blood hemoglobin for a while. This condition, sometimes called **sports anemia,** is not a true iron-deficiency condition. Strenuous aerobic activity promotes destruction of the more fragile, older red blood cells, and the resulting cleanup work reduces the blood's iron content temporarily. Strenuous activity also expands the blood's plasma volume, thereby reducing the red blood cell count per unit of blood. This low hematocrit looks like iron-deficiency anemia, but it is not the same. In sports anemia, the red blood cells do not diminish in size or number as in anemia, so the oxygen-carrying capacity is not hindered. Most researchers view sports anemia as an *adaptive,* temporary response to endurance training. Iron-deficiency anemia requires iron supplementation, but sports anemia does not.

Iron Recommendations for Athletes The best strategy for maintaining adequate iron nutrition depends on the individual. Menstruating women may border on iron deficiency even without the iron losses incurred by physical activity. Active teens of both genders have high iron needs because they are growing. Especially for women and teens, then, prescribed supplements may be needed to correct iron deficiencies. Physicians use the results of blood tests to determine whether such supplementation is needed. (Review Chapter 13 for many more details about iron, and see Appendix E for a description of the tests used in assessing anemia.)

sports anemia: a transient condition of low hemoglobin in the blood, associated with the early stages of sports training or other strenuous activity.

REVIEW IT List which vitamin and mineral supplements, if any, athletes may need and why.

With the possible exception of iron, well-nourished active people and athletes do not need nutrient supplements. Women and teens may need to pay special attention to their iron needs.

14.4 Fluids and Electrolytes to Support Activity

LEARN IT Identify the factors that influence an athlete's fluid needs and describe the differences between water and sports drinks.

The need for water far surpasses the need for any other nutrient. The body relies on watery fluids as the medium for all of its life-supporting activities, and if it loses too much water, its well-being will be compromised.

Obviously, the body loses water via sweat. Breathing uses water, too, exhaled as vapor. During physical activity, water losses from both sources are significant, and dehydration becomes a threat. Dehydration's first symptom is fatigue: a water loss of greater than 2 percent of body weight can reduce a person's capacity to do muscular work.[53] With a water loss of about 7 percent, a person is likely to collapse. For perspective, a water loss of 2 percent in a person weighing 150 pounds is equal to 3 pounds; a water loss of 7 percent is equal to 10.5 pounds.

Temperature Regulation As Chapter 7 discussed, working muscles produce heat as a by-product of energy metabolism. During intense activity, muscle heat production can be 15 to 20 times greater than at rest. The body cools itself by sweating. Each liter of sweat dissipates almost 600 kcalories of heat, preventing a rise in body temperature of almost 10 degrees on the Celsius scale.* The body routes its blood supply through the capillaries just under the skin, and the skin secretes sweat to evaporate and cool the skin and the underlying blood. The blood then flows back to cool the deeper body chambers.

Hyperthermia In hot, humid weather, sweat doesn't evaporate well because the surrounding air is already laden with water. In **hyperthermia,** body heat builds up and triggers maximum sweating, but without sweat evaporation, little cooling takes place. In such conditions, active people must take precautions to prevent **heat stroke.** To reduce the risk of heat stroke, drink enough fluid before and during the activity, rest in the shade when tired, and wear lightweight clothing that allows sweat to evaporate. (Hence the danger of rubber or heavy suits that supposedly promote weight loss during physical activity—they promote profuse sweating, prevent sweat evaporation, and invite heat stroke.) If you ever experience any of the symptoms of heat stroke listed in Table 14-8 stop your activity, ask for help,

TABLE 14-8 Symptoms of Heat Stroke and Hypothermia Compared

Heat Stroke	Hypothermia
• Clumsiness, stumbling	• Clumsiness, loss of coordination
• Confusion, dizziness, other mental changes, loss of consciousness	• Confusion, disorientation, other mental changes, loss of consciousness
• Flushed skin (skin may turn red as body temperature rises)	• Drowsiness
• Muscle cramping (early symptom)	• Shivering (early symptom)
• Nausea and vomiting	• Cessation of shivering (late symptom)
• Rapid breathing	• Slurred speech
• Rapid heart rate	• Slow breathing
• Sudden cessation of sweating (hot, dry, skin)	• Slow heart rate
• Throbbing headache	

SOURCE: Adapted from Centers for Disease Control and Prevention, www.cdc.gov.

hyperthermia: an above-normal body temperature.

heat stroke: a dangerous accumulation of body heat with accompanying loss of body fluid.

*10 degrees on the Celcius scale is about 18 degrees on the Fahrenheit scale.

and cool down as quickly as possible. Heat stroke can be fatal, people often die of it, and these symptoms demand attention.

Hypothermia In cold weather, **hypothermia,** or low body temperature, can be as serious as heat stroke is in hot weather. Inexperienced, slow runners participating in long races on cold or wet, chilly days are especially vulnerable to hypothermia. Slow runners who produce little heat can become too cold if clothing is inadequate. Early symptoms of hypothermia include feeling cold, shivering, apathy, and social withdrawal. As body temperature continues to fall, shivering may stop, and disorientation, slurred speech, and change in behavior or appearance set in (review Table 14-8). People with these symptoms soon become helpless to protect themselves from further body heat losses. Even in cold weather, however, the active body still sweats and still needs fluids. The fluids should be warm or at room temperature to help protect against hypothermia.

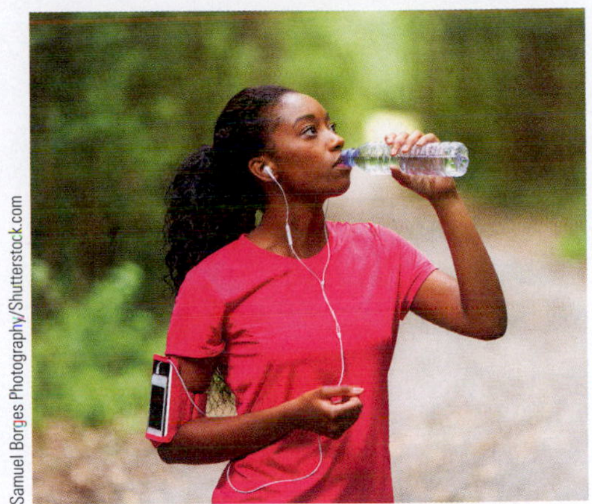

Samuel Borges Photography/Shutterstock.com

> **PHOTO 14-11** To prevent dehydration and the fatigue that accompanies it, drink liquids before, during, and after physical activity.

Fluid Replacement via Hydration Endurance athletes can easily lose 1.5 liters or more of fluid during *each hour* of activity. Table 14-9 presents a suggested schedule of hydration for physical activity. To prepare for fluid losses, a person must hydrate before activity; to replace fluid losses, the person must rehydrate during and after activity (see Photo 14-11). Even then, in hot weather, the GI tract may not be able to absorb enough water fast enough to keep up with sweat losses, and some degree of dehydration may be inevitable. Athletes who know their body's **hourly sweat rate** can strive to replace the total amount of fluid lost during activity to prevent dehydration.

Athletes who are preparing for competition are often advised to drink extra fluids in the *days* immediately before the event, especially if they are still training. The extra water is not stored in the body, but drinking extra water ensures maximum hydration at the start of the event. Full hydration is imperative for every athlete both in training and in competition. The athlete who arrives at an event even slightly dehydrated begins with a disadvantage.

What is the best fluid for an exercising body? For noncompetitive, everyday active people, plain, cool water is recommended, especially in warm weather, for two reasons: (1) water rapidly leaves the digestive tract to enter the tissues where it is needed, and (2) it cools the body from the inside out. For endurance athletes, carbohydrate-containing beverages may be appropriate. Fluid ingestion during the event has the dual purposes of replenishing water lost through sweating and providing a source of carbohydrate to supplement the body's limited glycogen stores. Many carbohydrate-containing sports drinks are marketed for active people; a later section compares them with water.

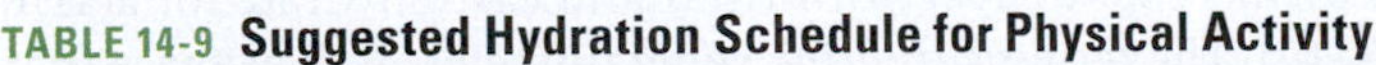

TABLE 14-9 Suggested Hydration Schedule for Physical Activity

Timing	Recommended Intakes (based on body weight)	Males	Females
≥4 hours before activity	1 oz/10 lb	16 oz	12 oz
2 hours before activity, if heavy sweating is expected	Add 0.6 oz/10 lb	+9 oz	+7 oz
Every 15 min during activity	Drink enough to minimize loss of body weight, but don't drink too much	8 oz	4 oz
After activity	≥2 cups for each pound of body weight lost[a]		

NOTE: Intakes are based on a 70-kilogram (154-pound) man and a 55-kilogram (121-pound) woman.

[a]Drinking 2 cups of fluid every 20 to 30 minutes after exercise until the total amount required is consumed is more effective for rehydration than drinking the needed amount all at once. Rapid fluid replacement after exercise stimulates urine production and results in less body water retention.

SOURCE: Position of the Academy of Nutrition and Dietetics, Dietitians of Canada, and the American College of Sports Medicine: Nutrition and athletic performance, *Journal of the Academy of Nutrition and Dietetics* 116 (2016): 501–528; C. A. Rosenbloom and E. J. Coleman, eds., *Sports Nutrition: A Practice Manual for Professionals* (Chicago: Academy of Nutrition and Dietetics, 2012), p. 115; American College of Sports Medicine, Position stand; Exercise and fluid replacement, *Medicine and Science in Sports and Exercise* 39 (2007): 377–390.

hypothermia: a below-normal body temperature.

hourly sweat rate: the amount of weight lost plus fluid consumed during exercise per hour. One pound equals roughly 2 cups (500 milliliters) of fluid.

Electrolyte Losses and Replacement When a person sweats, small amounts of electrolytes—the electrically charged minerals sodium, potassium, chloride, and magnesium—are lost from the body along with water. Losses are greatest in beginners; training improves electrolyte retention.

To replenish lost electrolytes, a person ordinarily needs only to eat a regular diet that meets energy and nutrient needs. In events lasting more than 1 hour, sports drinks may be needed to replace fluids and electrolytes. Salt tablets can worsen dehydration and impair performance; they increase potassium losses, irritate the stomach, and cause vomiting. Endurance athletes considering the use of salt tablets to replace sodium are advised to consult with a health care professional before doing so.

Hyponatremia When athletes compete in endurance sports lasting longer than 3 hours, replenishing electrolytes is crucial. If athletes sweat profusely over a long period of time and do not replace lost sodium, a dangerous condition known as **hyponatremia** may result. Research shows that some athletes who sweat profusely may also lose more sodium in their sweat than others—and are prone to debilitating heat cramps. These athletes lose twice as much sodium in sweat as athletes who don't cramp. Depending on individual variation, exercise intensity, and changes in ambient temperature and humidity, sweat rates for these athletes can exceed 2 liters per hour.

Hyponatremia also occurs when endurance athletes drink such large amounts of water over the course of a long event that they overhydrate, diluting the body's fluids to such an extent that the sodium concentration becomes extremely low. New recommendations advise athletes to use their thirst as a guide to avoid overhydration and hyponatremia.[54] During long competitions, when athletes lose sodium through heavy sweating *and* consume excessive amounts of liquids, especially water, hyponatremia becomes likely.

Some athletes may still be vulnerable to hyponatremia even when they consume sports drinks during an event. Sports drinks do contain sodium, but in some cases, too little to replace sweat losses. Still, sports drinks do offer more sodium than plain water.

To prevent hyponatremia, athletes need to replace sodium during prolonged events. Sports drinks, salty pretzels, and other sodium sources can provide sodium during long competitions. Some athletes may need beverages with higher sodium concentrations than commercial sports drinks. In the days before the event, especially an event in the heat, athletes should not restrict salt in their diets. The symptoms of hyponatremia are similar to, but not the same as, those of dehydration (see Table 14-10).

TABLE 14-10 Symptoms of Hyponatremia

- Bloating, puffiness from water retention (shoes tight, rings tight)
- Confusion
- Seizure
- Severe headache
- Vomiting

Sports Drinks

Hydration is critical to optimal performance. As stated earlier, water best meets the fluid needs of most people, yet manufacturers market many good-tasting sports drinks that deliver both fluid and carbohydrate for active people (see Photo 14-12). The term *sports drink* generally refers to beverages that contain carbohydrates and electrolytes in specific concentrations, and they are the focus of this discussion.

Many sports drinks compete for their share of the multi-billion-dollar market. What do sports drinks have to offer?

Fluid Sports drinks offer fluids to help offset the loss of fluids during physical activity, but plain water can do this too. Alternatively, diluted fruit juices or flavored water can be used if preferred to plain water.

Glucose Sports drinks offer simple sugars or **glucose polymers** that help maintain hydration and blood glucose and enhance performance as effectively as, or in some circumstances, even better than, water. Such measures are especially beneficial for strenuous endurance activities lasting longer than 1 hour, during intense activities, or during prolonged competitive games that demand repeated intermittent activity.[55] Sports drinks may also be used for events lasting less than 1 hour, although plain water is appropriate as well.

hyponatremia (HIGH-poe-na-TREE-mee-ah): a decreased concentration of sodium in the blood.

- **hypo** = below
- **natrium** = sodium (Na)
- **emia** = blood

glucose polymers: compounds that supply glucose, not as single molecules, but linked in chains somewhat like starch. The objective is to attract less water from the body into the digestive tract (osmotic attraction depends on the number, not the size, of particles).

> How To 14-1 Calculate the Carbohydrate Concentration of Sports Drinks

Sports drinks with a carbohydrate concentration of 6 to 8 percent best support athletes participating in events lasting 1 hour or longer. To calculate the carbohydrate concentration of a sports drink, divide the grams of carbohydrates per serving by the serving size (in milliliters) and multiply by 100.

Consider a sports drink that contains 22 grams of carbohydrates per serving and lists the serving size as 360 milliliters (12 ounces):

$$\frac{22 \text{ grams carbohydrate}}{360 \text{ milliliters}} = 0.06$$

$$0.06 \times 100 = 6\% \text{ carbohydrates}$$

> TRY IT Calculate the carbohydrate concentration of a sports drink that contains 20 grams of carbohydrate per serving (240 milliliters).

Fluid transport to the tissues from beverages containing up to 8 percent glucose is rapid. Most sports drinks contain about 7 percent carbohydrate (about half the sugar of ordinary soft drinks, or about 5 teaspoons in each 12 ounces). Less than 6 percent carbohydrate may not enhance performance, and more than 8 percent may cause abdominal cramps, nausea, and diarrhea. How To 14-1 describes how to calculate the carbohydrate concentration of sports drinks.

Although glucose can enhance endurance and performance in strenuous competitive events, for the moderate exerciser, it can be counterproductive if weight loss is the goal. Glucose is sugar, and like candy, it provides only empty kcalories—no vitamins or minerals. Most sports drinks provide between 50 and 100 kcalories per 8-ounce cup.

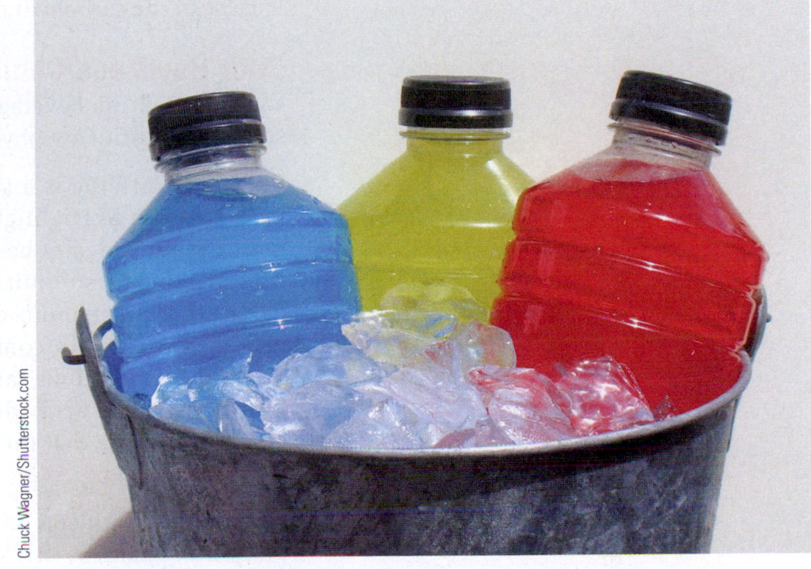

Chuck Wagner/Shutterstock.com

> **PHOTO 14-12** Water is the best fluid for most physically active people, but some consumers prefer the flavors of sports drinks.

Sodium and Other Electrolytes Sports drinks offer sodium and other electrolytes to help replace those lost during physical activity. Sodium in sports drinks also helps increase the rate of fluid absorption from the GI tract and maintain plasma volume during activity and recovery. Most physically active people do not need to replace the minerals lost in sweat immediately; a meal eaten within hours after competition replaces these minerals soon enough. Most sports drinks are relatively low in sodium, however, so those who choose to use these beverages run little risk of excessive intake.

Good Taste Manufacturers reason that if a drink tastes good, people will drink more, thereby ensuring adequate hydration. For athletes who prefer the flavors of sports drinks over water, it may be worth paying for good taste to replace lost fluids.

For athletes who exercise for 1 hour or more, sports drinks provide an advantage over water. Sports drinks may also be beneficial for athletes who:

- Exercise on an empty stomach
- Do not consume enough carbohydrate
- Want to load carbohydrates
- Want to gain weight
- Train at altitude or in extreme weather

- Had diarrhea (or vomiting) recently
- Do not drink adequate amounts of water

For most physically active people, though, water is the best fluid to replenish the body's lost fluids. The most important thing to do is drink when you feel thirsty.

Enhanced Water Another beverage often marketed to athletes and active people is **enhanced water.** Enhanced waters are lightly flavored waters with added sugars, vitamins, minerals, and in some cases, protein. Many enhanced waters are neither natural nor healthy, as marketing ads claim. In fact, most enhanced waters contain small amounts of only a few minerals, some of the B vitamins, and sometimes vitamin C or vitamin E. In the context of daily needs, the vitamins and minerals in these drinks do not add up to much. For example, it takes a quart of most of these beverages to provide only 10 percent of the RDA for iron or calcium. Quite simply, enhanced waters are not a substitute for eating nutrient-rich fruits and vegetables. Enhanced waters may not be harmful, but they can be expensive and most people do not need them. If the flavor of enhanced waters encourages greater fluid intake, then they may offer some advantage. Serious endurance athletes need the carbohydrate-electrolyte sports drinks discussed earlier.

Poor Beverage Choices: Caffeine and Alcohol

Athletes, like others, sometimes drink beverages that contain caffeine or alcohol. Each of these substances can influence physical performance.

Caffeine Caffeine is a stimulant, and athletes sometimes use it to enhance performance, as Highlight 14 explains. Carbonated soft drinks, with or without caffeine, may not be a wise choice for athletes: bubbles make a person feel full quickly and so limit fluid intake. Some of the increasingly popular energy drinks contain amounts of caffeine equivalent to a cup or more of coffee. When used in excess or in combination with stimulants or other unregulated substances, energy drinks can hinder performance and are potentially dangerous.[56] Another reason energy drinks should not be used for fluid replacement during athletic events is that the carbohydrate concentrations are too high for optimal fluid absorption.

Alcohol Some athletes mistakenly believe that they can replace fluids and load up on carbohydrates by drinking beer. Beer is not carbohydrate-rich. A 12-ounce beer provides 13 grams of carbohydrate—one-third the amount of carbohydrate in a glass of orange juice the same size. In addition to carbohydrate, beer also contains alcohol, of course. Energy from alcohol breakdown generates heat, but it does not fuel activity because alcohol is metabolized in the liver, not in the muscles.

Beer is not rich in vitamins or minerals. Beer contains traces of some B vitamins, but it cannot compete with food sources. As for minerals, beer contains a few minerals, but to replace the minerals lost in sweat, athletes need good sources such as fruit juices or sports drinks.

Alcohol's diuretic effect impairs the body's fluid balance, making dehydration likely. After physical activity, a person needs to replace fluids, not lose them by drinking beer. Alcohol also impairs the body's ability to regulate its temperature, increasing the likelihood of hypothermia or heat stroke.

It is difficult to overstate alcohol's detrimental effects on physical activity. Alcohol alters perceptions; slows reaction time; reduces strength, power, and endurance; and hinders accuracy, balance, eye-hand coordination, and coordination in general—all opposing optimal athletic performance. In addition, it deprives people of their judgment, thereby compromising safety in sports. Many sports-related fatalities and injuries involve alcohol or other drugs.

Clearly, alcohol impairs performance. For those who do drink, do not drink alcohol before exercising and drink plenty of water after exercising before drinking alcohol.

enhanced water: water that is fortified with ingredients such as vitamins, minerals, protein, oxygen, or herbs. Enhanced water is marketed as *vitamin water, sports water, oxygenated water,* and *protein water.*

REVIEW IT Identify the factors that influence an athlete's fluid needs and describe the differences between water and sports drinks.

Active people need to drink plenty of water; endurance athletes need to drink both water and carbohydrate-containing beverages, especially during training and competition. During events lasting longer than 3 hours, athletes need to pay special attention to replace sodium losses to prevent hyponatremia.

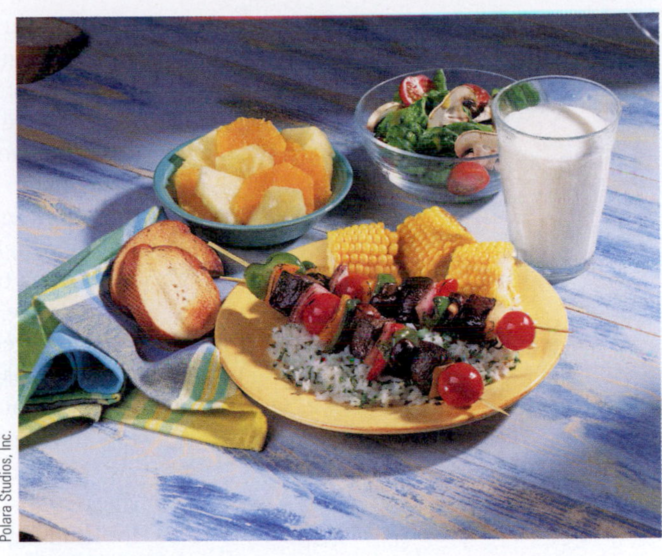

Polara Studios, Inc.

> **PHOTO 14-13** A variety of foods is the best source of nutrients for athletes.

14.5 Diets for Physically Active People

LEARN IT Discuss an appropriate daily eating pattern for athletes and list one example of a recommended pregame and recovery meal.

No one diet best supports physical performance. Active people who choose foods within the framework of the diet-planning principles presented in Chapter 2 can design many excellent diets.

Choosing a Diet to Support Fitness Above all, keep in mind that water is depleted more rapidly than any other nutrient. A diet to support fitness must provide water, energy, and all the other nutrients.[57]

Water Even casual exercisers must attend conscientiously to their fluid needs. A thirsty athlete should not wait to hydrate. As mentioned earlier, however, overhydration may lead to hyponatremia. Adequate hydration is crucial for every athlete, both in training and in competition. To find out how much water is needed to replenish activity losses, weigh yourself before and after the activity—the difference is almost all water. One pound equals roughly 2 cups (500 milliliters) of fluid.

Nutrient Density A healthful diet is based on nutrient-dense foods—foods that supply adequate vitamins and minerals for the energy they provide (see Photo 14-13). Active people need to eat both for nutrient adequacy and for energy—and energy needs can be extremely high. For example, during training, meals for some Olympic athletes provide as much as 10,000 kcalories a day. Still, a nutrient-rich diet remains central for adequacy's sake. Though vital, energy alone is not enough to support performance. Table 14-11 offers convenient, nutrient-dense snack ideas for athletes and active people.

Carbohydrate Full glycogen stores are critical to athletes and other highly active people. Guidelines to provide high carbohydrate availability for athletes are based on the athlete's weight and the characteristics of training sessions

TABLE 14-11 Nutrient-Dense Snacks for Athletes and Active People

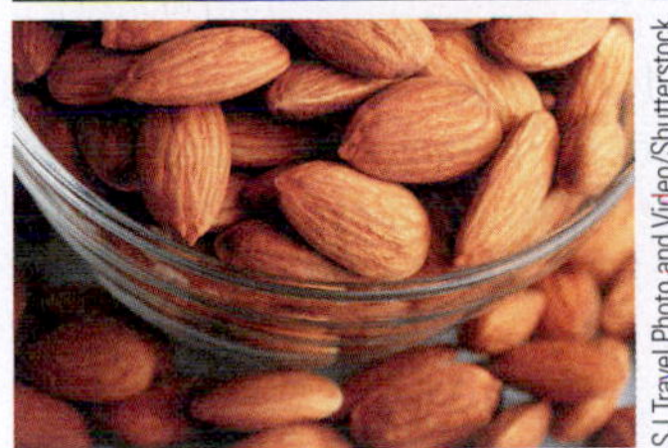

SJ Travel Photo and Video/Shutterstock

One ounce of almonds provides protein, fiber, calcium, vitamin E, and healthy unsaturated fats. Similar choices include other nuts or trail mix consisting of dried fruit, nuts, and seeds.

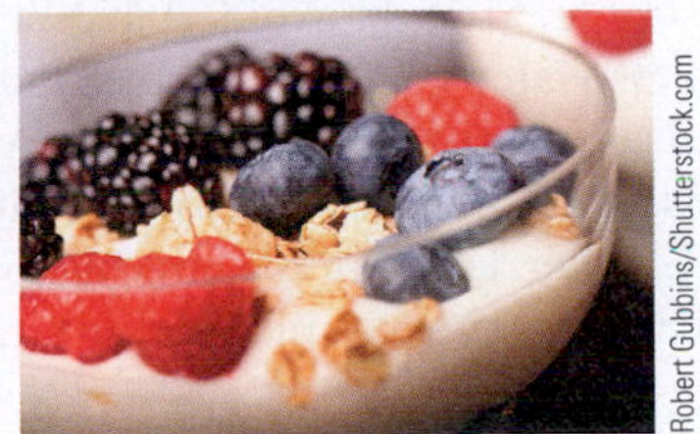

Robert Gubbins/Shutterstock.com

Low-fat Greek yogurt contains more protein per serving than regular yogurt, but a little less calcium. A small amount of fresh fruit adds fiber and vitamins. A similar choice is low-fat cheese paired with fresh fruit.

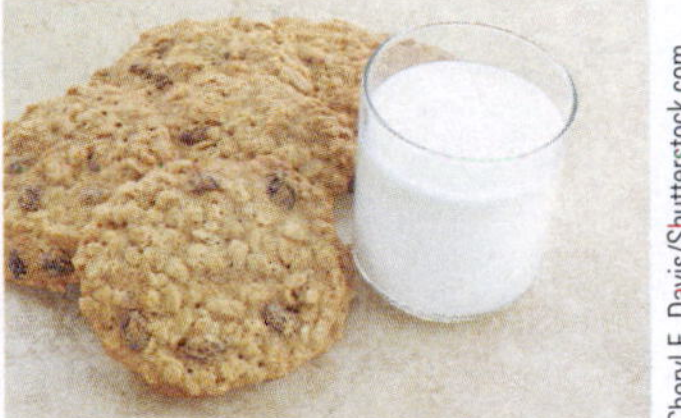

Cheryl E. Davis/Shutterstock.com

Low-fat milk or chocolate milk together with fig bars or oatmeal-raisin cookies offer protein and fiber. A similar choice is whole-grain cereal with low-fat milk.

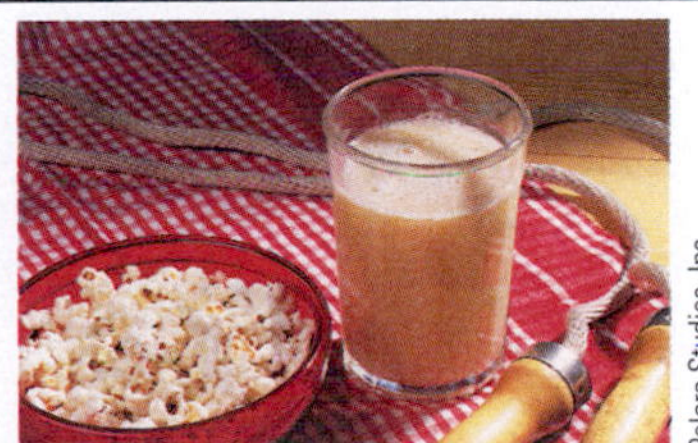

Polara Studios, Inc.

Popcorn offers fiber and a fruit smoothie quenches thirst and provides valuable vitamins. A similar choice is pretzels and fruit juice.

and competitions (review Table 14-5, p. 436). As discussed earlier, the timing of carbohydrate intake is also important for maximizing carbohydrate availability. On two occasions, the active person's regular high-carbohydrate, fiber-rich diet may require temporary adjustment. Both of these exceptions involve training for competition rather than for fitness in general. One special occasion is the pregame meal, when fiber-rich, bulky foods are best avoided. The pregame meal is discussed in a later section.

The other occasion is during intensive training, when energy needs may be so high as to outstrip the person's capacity to eat enough food to meet them. In this case, the athlete may want to rely on concentrated carbohydrate foods, such as dried fruits, sweet potatoes, and nectars, and even high-fat foods, such as avocados and nuts. Some athletes use commercial high-carbohydrate liquid supplements to obtain the carbohydrate and energy needed for intense training and top performance. These supplements do not *replace* regular food; they are meant to be used in *addition* to it. Unlike the sports drinks discussed earlier, these high-carbohydrate supplement beverages are too concentrated to be used for fluid replacement.

Protein In addition to carbohydrate and some fat (and the energy they provide), physically active people need protein. Meats and milk products are rich protein sources, but even highly active people must limit intakes of the fat-rich varieties of these foods to protect against heart disease. Lean protein-rich foods such as skinless poultry, fish and seafood, eggs, low-fat milk products, low-fat cheeses, legumes, and nuts boost protein intakes while keeping saturated fat intakes within bounds.

Meals before and after Competition

No single food improves speed, strength, or skill in competitive events, although some *kinds* of foods do support performance better than others, as already explained. Still, a competitor may eat a particular food before or after an event for psychological reasons. One eats a steak the night before wrestling. Another eats a spoonful of honey within 5 minutes before diving. So long as these practices remain harmless, they should be respected.

Pregame Meals Science indicates that the pregame meal or snack should include plenty of fluids and be light and easy to digest. It should provide between 300 and 800 kcalories, primarily from carbohydrate-rich foods that are familiar and well tolerated by the athlete. The meal should end 1 to 4 hours before competition to allow time for the stomach to empty before exertion. The larger the meal, the more time needed for digestion. Thus, a full meal providing plenty of carbohydrate may be eaten 3 or more hours before an event, a small meal (400 to 500 kcalories) may be eaten 2 to 3 hours before an event, and a small, high-carbohydrate snack may be appropriate 1 hour before an event.

Breads, potatoes, pasta, and fruit juices—that is, carbohydrate-rich foods low in fat and fiber—form the basis of the best pregame meal (see Figure 14-2 for some examples). Bulky, fiber-rich foods such as raw vegetables or high-bran cereals, although usually desirable, are best avoided just before competition. Fiber in the digestive tract attracts water and can cause stomach discomfort during performance. Liquid meals are easy to digest, and many such meals are commercially available. Alternatively, athletes can mix low-fat milk or fruit juices, frozen fruits, and flavorings in a blender. For example, mixing low-fat milk or apple juice with a frozen banana and cinnamon or vanilla makes a tasty, high-carbohydrate, liquid pregame meal.

Recovery Meals Athletes who perform intense practice sessions several times a day or compete for hours on consecutive days need to quickly replenish glycogen to be ready for the next activity. As mentioned earlier, eating high-carbohydrate foods *after* physical activity enhances glycogen storage, just as eating high-quality protein foods helps stimulate protein synthesis. Because people are usually

> **FIGURE 14-2 Examples of High-Carbohydrate Pregame Meals**

Pregame meals may be eaten 1 to 4 hours before the event and provide 300 to 800 kcalories, primarily from carbohydrate-rich foods.

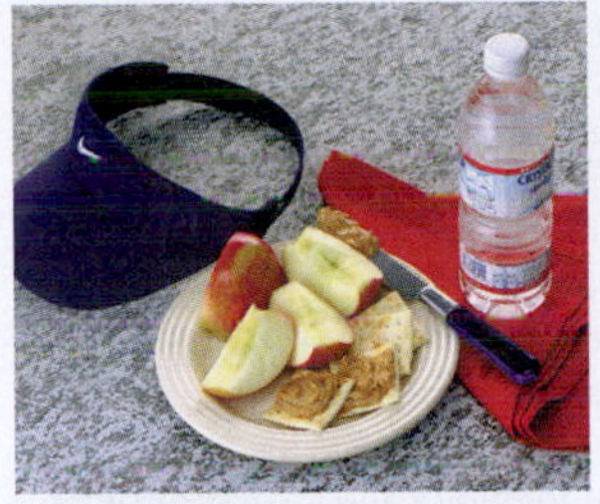

300-kcalorie meal
1 large apple
4 saltine crackers
1½ tbs reduced-fat peanut butter

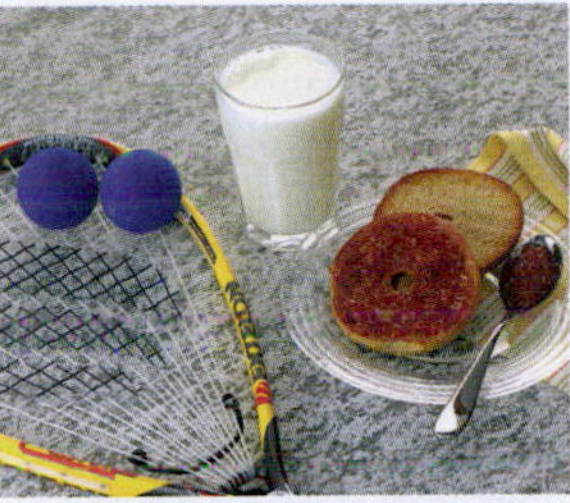

500-kcalorie meal
1 large whole-wheat bagel
2 tbs jelly
1½ c low-fat milk

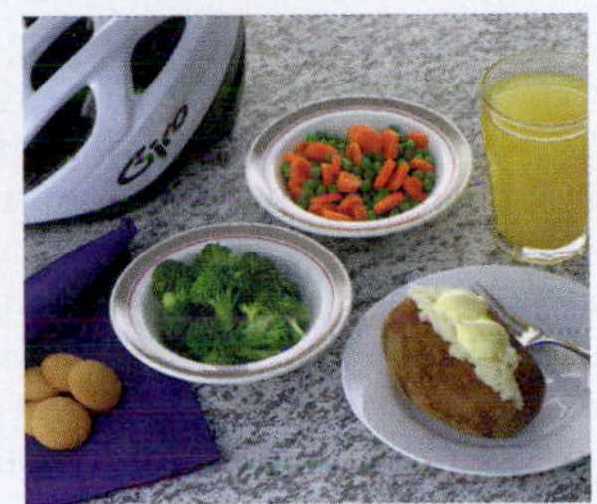

Matthew Farruggio

750-kcalorie meal
1 large baked potato
2 tsp margarine
1 c steamed broccoli
1 c mixed carrots and green peas
5 vanilla wafers
1½ c apple or pineapple juice

not hungry immediately following physical activity, a carbohydrate-containing beverage such as low-fat milk may be preferred. A two-cup serving of chocolate milk, taken within an hour or two following exercise has been shown to both maintain muscle glycogen stores and increase muscle protein synthesis.[58] If an active person does feel hungry after an event, then foods high in carbohydrate, moderate in protein, and low in fat and fiber are the ones to choose—similar to those recommended prior to competition.

REVIEW IT Discuss an appropriate daily eating pattern for athletes and list one example of a recommended pregame and recovery meal.

The person who wants to excel physically will apply accurate nutrition knowledge along with dedication to rigorous training. A diet that provides ample fluid and includes a variety of nutrient-dense foods in quantities to meet energy needs will enhance not only athletic performance, but overall health as well. Carbohydrate-rich foods that are light and easy to digest are recommended for both the pregame and recovery meal.

Training and genetics being equal, who will win a competition? The athlete who habitually consumes inadequate amounts of needed nutrients will lag behind the competitor who arrives at the event with a long history of full nutrient stores and well-met metabolic needs. Some athletes learn that nutrition can support physical performance and turn to pills and powders instead of foods. In case you need further convincing that a healthful diet surpasses such potions, the following highlight addresses this issue.

What's Online

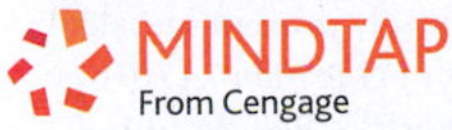

MINDTAP
From Cengage

Visit **www.cengagebrain.com** to access MindTap, a complete digital course that includes Diet & Wellness Plus, interactive quizzes, videos, and more.

REFERENCES

1. K. Lyden and coauthors, Discrete features of sedentary behavior impact cardiometabolic risk factors, *Medicine and Science in Sports and Exercise* 47 (2015): 1079–1086; C. E. Matthews and coauthors, Mortality benefits for replacing sitting time with different physical activities, *Medicine and Science in Sports and Exercise* 47 (2015): 1833–1840; S. Saurabh and coauthors, Effect of prolonged sitting and breaks in sitting time on endothelial function, *Medicine and Science in Sports and Exercise* 47 (2015): 843–849; B. A. Larsen and coauthors, Associations of physical activity and sedentary behavior with regional fat deposition, *Medicine and Science in Sports and Exercise* 46 (2015): 520–528.
2. U. Ekelund and coauthors, Does physical activity attenuate, or even eliminate, the detrimental association of sitting time with mortality? A

harmonised meta-analysis of data from more than 1 million men and women, *Lancet* 2016, doi:10.1016/S0140-6736(16)30370-1; D. Schmid and coauthors, Replacing sedentary time with physical activity in relation to mortality, *Medicine and Science in Sports and Exercise* 48 (2016): 1312–1319; C. Y. Wu and coauthors, The association of physical activity with all-cause, cardiovascular, and cancer mortality among older adults, *Preventive Medicine* 72 (2015): 23–29; U. Ekelund and coauthors, Physical activity and all-cause mortality across levels of overall and abdominal adiposity in European men and women: The European Prospective Investigation into Cancer and Nutrition Study (EPIC), *American Journal of Clinical Nutrition* 101 (2015): 613–621; H. Nakahara, S. Y. Ueda, and T. Miyamoto, Low-frequency severe-intensity interval training improves cardiorespiratory functions, *Medicine and Science in Sports and Exercise* 47 (2015): 789–798; P. T. Williams, Dose-response relationship between exercise and respiratory disease mortality, *Medicine and Science in Sports and Exercise* 46 (2014): 711–717; E. H. Bell and coauthors, Physical activity and cardiovascular disease in African Americans in Atherosclerosis Risk in Communities, *Medicine and Science in Sports and Exercise* 45 (2013): 901–907.

3. Centers for Disease Control and Prevention, *Facts about Physical Activity*, www.cdc.gov/physicalactivity/data/facts.htm; updated May 23, 2014.
4. P. Ladenvall and coauthors, Low aerobic capacity in middle-aged men associated with increased mortality rates during 45 years of follow-up, *European Journal of Preventive Cardiology*, 2016, doi:10.1177/2047487316655466; S. C. Moore and coauthors, Association of leisure-time physical activity with risk of 26 types of cancer in 1.44 million adults, *JAMA Internal Medicine*, May 16, 2016, doi:10.1001/jamainternmed.2016.1548; R. Cannioto and coauthors, Chronic recreational physical inactivity and epithelial ovarian cancer risk: Evidence from the ovarian cancer association consortium, *Cancer, Epidemiology, Biomarkers, and Prevention* 25 (2016): 1114–1124; Wu and coauthors, 2015; S. W. Farrell and coauthors, Is there a gradient of mortality risk among men with low cardiorespiratory fitness? *Medicine and Science in Sports and Exercise* 47 (2015): 1825–1832; C. H. Lin and coauthors, Moderate physical activity level as a protective factor against metabolic syndrome in middle-aged and older women, *Journal of Clinical Nursing* 24 (2015): 1234–1245.
5. Ekelund and coauthors, 2016; A. Philipsen and coauthors, Associations of objectively measured physical activity and abdominal fat distribution, *Medicine and Science in Sports and Exercise* 47 (2015): 983–989; D. L. Swift and coauthors, The role of exercise and physical activity in weight loss and maintenance, *Progress in Cardiovascular Diseases* 56 (2014): 441–447.
6. S. J. Warden and coauthors, Physical activity when young provides lifelong benefits to cortical bone size and strength in men, *Proceedings of the National Academy of Sciences of the United States of America* 111 (2014): 5337–5342; M. T. Korhonen and coauthors, Bone density, structure and strength, and their determinants in aging sprint athletes, *Medicine and Science in Sports and Exercise* 44 (2012): 2340–2349.
7. R. J. Simpson and coauthors, Exercise and the regulation of immune functions, *Progress in Molecular Biology and Translational Science* 135 (2015): 355–380.
8. Moore and coauthors, 2016; Cannioto and coauthors, 2016; C. Eheman and coauthors, Annual Report to the Nation on the status of cancer, 1975–2008, featuring cancers associated with excess weight and lack of sufficient physical activity, *Cancer* 118 (2012): 2338–2366.
9. Wu and coauthors, 2015; Nakahara, Ueda, and Miyamoto, 2015; M. E. G. Armstrong and coauthors, Frequent physical activity may not reduce vascular disease risk as much as moderate activity: Large prospective study of UK women, *Circulation* 131 (2015): 721–729; Bell and coauthors, 2013.
10. Philipsen and coauthors, 2015; V. Lévesque and coauthors, Targeting abdominal adiposity and cardiorespiratory fitness in the workplace, *Medicine and Science in Sports and Exercise* 47 (2015): 1342–1350; C. H. Lin and coauthors, Moderate physical activity level as a protective factor against metabolic syndrome in middle-aged and older women, *Journal of Clinical Nursing* 24 (2015): 1234–1245.
11. S. Fan and coauthors, Physical activity level and incident type 2 diabetes among Chinese adults, *Medicine and Science in Sports and Exercise* 47 (2015): 751–756; D. T. Lackland and J. H. Voeks, Metabolic syndrome and hypertension: Regular exercise as part of lifestyle management, *Current Hypertension Reports* 16 (2014): 492; C. P. Earnest and coauthors, Aerobic and strength training in concomitant metabolic syndrome and type 2 diabetes, *Medicine and Science in Sports and Exercise* 46 (2014): 1293–1301; C. K. Roberts, J. P. Little, and J. P. Thyfault, Modification of insulin sensitivity and glycemic control by activity and exercise, *Medicine and Science in Sports and Exercise* 45 (2013): 1868–1877.
12. D. Aune, M. Leitzmann, and L. J. Vatten, Physical activity and the risk of gallbladder disease: A systematic review and meta-analysis of cohort studies, *Journal of Physical Activity and Health*, 2016, doi:10.1123/jpah.2015-0456; R. J. Shephard, Physical activity and the biliary tract in health and disease, *Sports Medicine* 45 (2015): 1295–1309.
13. E. M. McMahon and coauthors, Physical activity in European adolescents and associations with anxiety, depression and well-being, *European Child and Adolescent Psychiatry*, 2016, doi:10.1007/s00787-016-0875-9; M. B. Powers, G. J. Asmundson, and J. A. J. Smits, Exercise for mood and anxiety disorders: The state-of-the-science, *Cognitive Behavior Therapy* 44 (2015): 237–239.
14. Ekelund and coauthors, 2016; Ladenvall and coauthors, 2016; L. M. León-Muñoz and coauthors, Continued sedentariness, change in sitting time and mortality in older adults, *Medicine and Science in Sports and Exercise* 45 (2013): 1501–1507.
15. H. Arem and coauthors, Leisure time physical activity and mortality: A detailed pooled analysis of the dose-response relationship, *JAMA Internal Medicine* 175 (2015): 959–967.
16. K. Uusi-Rasi and coauthors, Exercise and vitamin D in fall prevention among older women, *JAMA Internal Medicine* 175 (2015): 703–711; M. Pahor and coauthors, Effect of structured physical activity on prevention of major mobility disability in older adults, *Journal of the American Medical Association* 311 (2014): 2387–2396; L. Krist, F. Dimeo, and T. Keil, Can progressive resistance training twice a week improve mobility, muscle strength, and quality of life in very elderly nursing-home residents with impaired mobility? A pilot study, *Clinical Interventions in Aging* 8 (2013): 443–448.
17. M. Catoire and S. Kersten, The search for exercise factors in humans, *FASEB Journal* 29 (2015): 1615–1628.
18. American College of Sports Medicine position stand, Quantity and quality of exercise for developing and maintaining cardiorespiratory, musculoskeletal, and neuromotor fitness in apparently healthy adults: Guidance for prescribing exercise, *Medicine and Science in Sports and Exercise* 43 (2011): 1334–1359.
19. H. H. Kyu and coauthors, Physical activity and risk of breast cancer, colon, diabetes, ischemic heart disease, and ischemic stroke events: Systematic review and dose-response meta-analysis for the Global Burden of Disease Study, 2013, *BMJ* 354 (2016): i3857; Arem and coauthors, 2015; Wu and coauthors, 2015; F. L. Miller and coauthors, Exercise dose, exercise adherence, and associated health outcomes in the TIGER Study, *Medicine and Science in Sports and Exercise* 46 (2014): 69–75.
20. American College of Sports Medicine position stand, 2011.
21. C. A. Brawner and coauthors, Change in maximal exercise capacity is associated with survival in men and women, *Mayo Clinic Proceedings* 92 (2017): 383–390; Centers for Disease Control and Prevention, www.cdc.gov/physicalactivity/everyone/health; updated June 4, 2015.
22. C. Porter and coauthors, Resistance exercise training alters mitochondrial function human skeletal muscle, *Medicine and Science in Sports and Exercise* 47 (2015):1922–1931; P. J. Atherton and K. Smith, Muscle protein synthesis in response to nutrition and exercise, *Journal of Physiology* 590.5 (2012): 1049–1047.
23. W. K. Mitchell and coauthors, Human skeletal muscle protein metabolism responses to amino acid nutrition, *Advances in Nutrition* 7 (2016): 828S–838S; B. E. Phillips, D. S. Hill, and P. J. Atherton, Regulation of muscle protein synthesis in humans, *Current Opinion in Clinical Nutrition and Metabolic Care* 15 (2012): 58–63.
24. D. M. Camera, W. J. Smiles, and J. A. Hawley, Exercise-induced skeletal muscle signaling pathways and human athletic performance, *Free Radical Biology and Medicine*, 2016, doi:10.1016/j.freeradbiomed.2016.02.007; J. C. Drake, R. J. Wilson, and Z. Yan, Molecular mechanisms for mitochondrial adaptation to exercise training in skeletal muscle, *FASEB Journal* 30 (2016): 13–22.
25. American College of Sports Medicine, *ACSM's Guidelines for Exercise Testing and Prescription*, 9th ed. (Philadelphia, PA: Lippincott, Williams & Wilkins, 2013), pp. 19–38.

26. N. M. Johannsen and coauthors, Combined aerobic resistance training effects on glucose homeostasis, fitness, and other major health indices: A review of current guidelines, *Sports Medicine,* 2016, doi:10.1007/s40279-016-0548-3; G. Huang and coauthors, Dose-response relationship of cardiorespiratory fitness adaptation to controlled endurance training in sedentary older adults, *European Journal of Preventive Cardiology* 23 (2016): 518–529; Z. Milanovic, G. Sporis, and M. Weston, Effectiveness of high-intensity interval training (HIT) and continuous endurance training for VO2 max improvements: A systematic review and meta-analysis of controlled trials, *Sports Medicine* 45 (2015): 1469–1481.
27. X. Lin and coauthors, Leisure time physical activity and cardio-metabolic health: Results from the Brazilian Longitudinal Study of Adult Health (ELSA-Brasil), *Journal of the American Heart Association* 5 (2016): 6; D. M. Bhammar, S. S. Angadi, and G. A. Gaesser, Effects of fractionized and continuous exercise on 24-h ambulatory blood pressure, *Medicine and Science in Sports and Exercise* 44 (2012): 2270–2276; S. Liu and coauthors, Blood pressure responses to acute and chronic exercise are related in prehypertension, *Medicine and Science in Sports and Exercise* 44 (2012): 1644–1652.
28. Johannsen and coauthors, 2016; C. K. Roberts and coauthors, Strength fitness and body weight status on markers of cardiometabolic health, *Medicine and Science in Sports and Exercise* 47 (2015): 1211–1218; M. D. Ross and coauthors, Resistance exercise increases endothelial progenitor cells and angiogenic factors, *Medicine and Science in Sports and Exercise* 46 (2014): 16–23; American College of Sports Medicine position stand, 2011; American College of Sports Medicine position stand: Progression models in resistance training for healthy adults, *Medicine and Science in Sports and Exercise* 41 (2009): 687–708.
29. J. Xu and coauthors, Effects of exercise on bone status in female subjects, from young girls to postmenopausal women: An overview of systematic reviews and meta-analyses, *Sports Medicine* 46 (2016): 1165-1182; American College of Sports Medicine position stand, 2011.
30. V. P. Nicholson and coauthors, Low-load very high-repetition resistance training attenuates bone loss at the lumbar spine in active post-menopausal women, *Calcified Tissue International,* 2015, doi:10.1007/s00223-015-9976-6; E. A. Marques and coauthors, Response of bone mineral density, inflammatory cytokines, and biochemical bone markers to a 32-week combined loading exercise programme in older men and women, *Archives of Gerontology and Geriatrics* 57 (2013): 226–233.
31. B.J. Nicklas and coauthors, Effects of resistance training with and without caloric restriction on physical function and mobility in overweight and obese older adults: a randomized controlled trial, *American Journal of Clinical Nutrition* 101 (2015): 991–999; L. Krist, F. Dimeo, and T. Keil, Can progressive resistance training twice a week improve mobility, muscle strength, and quality of life in very elderly nursing-home residents with impaired mobility? A pilot study, *Clinical Interventions in Aging* 8 (2013): 443–448.
32. American College of Sports Medicine position stand, Progression models in resistance training for healthy adults, *Medicine and Science in Sports and Exercise* 41 (2009): 687–708.
33. J. Bergstrom and coauthors, Diet, muscle glycogen and physical performance, *Acta Physiologica Scandinavica* 71 (1967): 140–150.
34. J. F. Moxnes and Ø. Sandbakk, The kinetics of lactate production and removal during whole-body exercise, *Theoretical Biology and Medical Modeling* 9 (2012): 7.
35. K. D. Gejl and coauthors, Muscle glycogen content modifies SR Ca2+ release rate in elite endurance athletes, *Medicine and Science in Sports and Exercise* 46 (2014): 496–505; N. Ortenblad, H. Westerblad, and J. Nielsen, Muscle glycogen stores and fatigue, *Journal of Physiology* 591 (2013): 4405–4413.
36. Position of the Academy of Nutrition and Dietetics, Dietitians of Canada, and American College of Sports Medicine: Nutrition and athletic performance, *Journal of the Academy of Nutrition and Dietetics* 116 (2016): 501–528; N. M. Cermak, L. J. C. van Loon, The use of carbohydrates during exercise as an ergogenic aid, *Sports Medicine* 43 (2013): 1139–1155.
37. T. Stellingwerff and G. R. Cox, Systematic review: Carbohydrate supplementation on exercise performance or capacity of varying durations, *Applied Physiology, Nutrition, and Metabolism* 39 (2014): 998–1011; Cermak and van Loon, 2013; A. Jeukendrup, The new carbohydrate intake recommendations, *Nestle' Nutrition Workshop Series* 75 (2013): 63–71.
38. Stellingwerff and Cox, 2014.
39. Position of the Academy of Nutrition and Dietetics, Dietitians of Canada, and American College of Sports Medicine, 2016.
40. Stellingwerff and Cox, 2014.
41. T. M. McLellan, S. M. Pasiakos, and H. R. Lieberman, Effects of protein in combination with carbohydrate supplements on acute or repeat endurance exercise performance: A systematic review, *Sports Medicine* 44 (2014): 535–550; Cermak and van Loon, 2013.
42. Position of the Academy of Nutrition and Dietetics, Dietitians of Canada, and the American College of Sports Medicine, 2016.
43. M. J. Ormsbee, C. W. Bach, and D. A. Baur, Pre-exercise nutrition: The role of macronutrients, modified starches and supplements on metabolism and endurance performance, *Nutrients* 6 (2014): 1782–1808.
44. Position of the Academy of Nutrition and Dietetics, Dietitians of Canada, and the American College of Sports Medicine, 2016.
45. D. M. Camera and coauthors, Protein ingestion increases myofibrillar protein synthesis after concurrent exercise, *Medicine and Science in Sports and Exercise* 47 (2015): 82–91; C. Rosenbloom, Protein power, *Nutrition Today* 50 (2015): 72–77; O. C. Witard and coauthors, Myofibrillar muscle protein synthesis rates subsequent to a meal in response to increasing doses of whey protein at rest and after resistance exercise, *American Journal of Clinical Nutrition* 99 (2014): 86–95.
46. Position of the Academy of Nutrition and Dietetics, Dietitians of Canada, and the American College of Sports Medicine, 2016; S. M. Phillips, S. Chevalier, and H. J. Leidy, Protein "requirements" beyond the RDA: Implications for optimizing health, *Applied Physiology, Nutrition, and Metabolism* 41 (2016): 565–572.
47. Position of the Academy of Nutrition and Dietetics, Dietitians of Canada, and the American College of Sports Medicine, 2016; Phillips, Chevalier, and Leidy, 2016; Rosenbloom, 2015.
48. Position of the Academy of Nutrition and Dietetics, Dietitians of Canada, and the American College of Sports Medicine, 2016.
49. R. T. Makowski and coauthors, Dietary antioxidants as modifiers of physiologic adaptations to exercise, *Medicine and Science in Sports and Exercise* 47 (2015): 1857–1868.
50. G. Bruinvels and coauthors, The prevalence and impact of heavy menstrual bleeding (menorrhagia) in elite and non-elite athletes, *PLoS One* 11 (2016): e0149881; I. Alaunyte, V. Stojceska, and A. Plunkett, Iron and the female athlete: A review of dietary treatment methods for improving iron status and exercise performance, *Journal of the International Society of Sports Nutrition* 12 (2015): 38.
51. W.N. Kong, G. Gao, and Y.Z. Chang, Hepcidin and sports anemia, *Cell and Bioscience* 4 (2014): 19.
52. R. J. Burden and coauthors, Is iron treatment beneficial in iron-deficient but non-anaemic (IDNA) endurance athletes? A systematic review and meta-analysis, *British Journal of Sports Medicine* 49 (2015): 1389–1397; D. M. Dellavalle and J. D. Haas, Iron supplementation improves energetic efficiency in iron-depleted female rowers, *Medicine and Science in Sports and Exercise* 46 (2014): 1204–1215.
53. Position of the Academy of Nutrition and Dietetics, Dietitians of Canada, and the American College of Sports Medicine, 2016; American College of Sports Medicine, *ACSM's Guidelines for Exercise Testing and Prescription,* 9th ed. (Philadelphia, PA: Lippincott, Williams & Wilkins, 2013), pp. 216–222.
54. T. Hew-Butler and coauthors, Statement of Third International Exercise-Associated Hyponatremia Consensus Development Conference, Carlsbad, California, 2015, *Clinical Journal of Sport Medicine* 25 (2015): 303–320; M. D. Hoffman and K. J. Stuempfle, Sodium supplementation and exercise-associated hyponatremia during prolonged exercise, *Medicine and Science in Sports and Exercise* 47 (2015): 1781–1787.
55. Position of the Academy of Nutrition and Dietetics, Dietitians of Canada, and the American College of Sports Medicine, 2016.
56. C. Rosenbloom, Energy drinks, caffeine, and athletes, *Nutrition Today* 49 (2014): 49–54.
57. S. A. Herring and coauthors, Selected issues for nutrition and the athlete: A team physician consensus statement, *Medicine and Science in Sports and Exercise* 45 (2013): 2378–2386.
58. W. R. Lunn and coauthors, Chocolate milk and endurance exercise recovery: Protein balance, glycogen, and performance, *Medicine and Science in Sports and Exercise* 44 (2012): 682–691.

LEARN IT Present arguments for and against the use of ergogenic aids.

Supplements as Ergogenic Aids

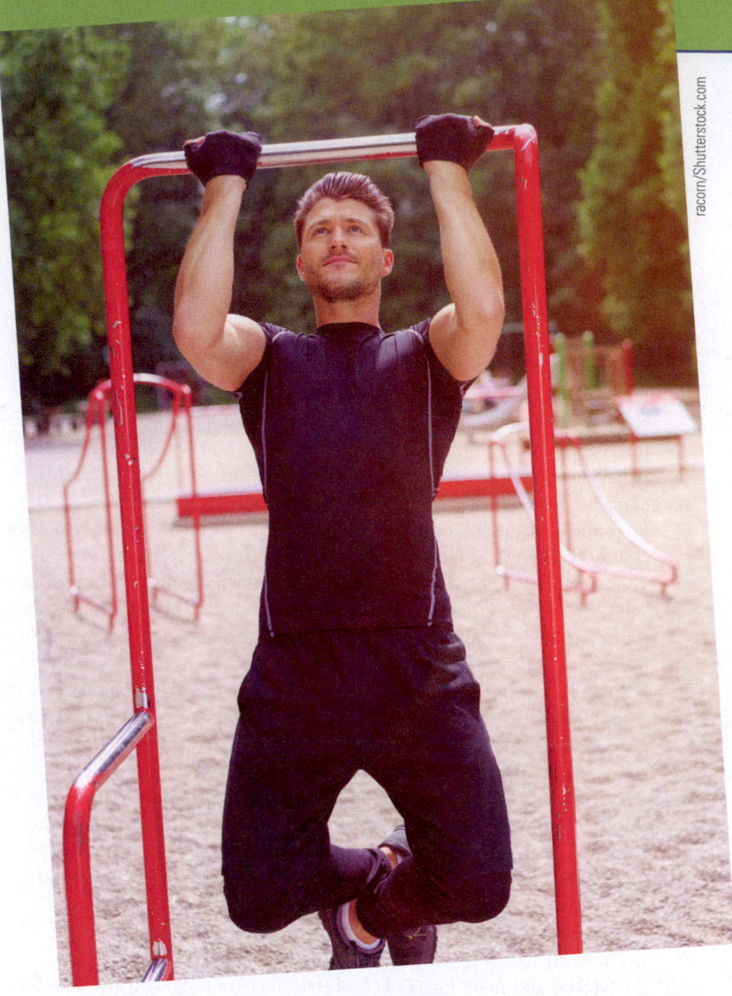
racorn/Shutterstock.com

Athletes gravitate to promises that they can enhance their performance by taking pills, powders, or potions. Unfortunately, they often hear such promises from their coaches and peers, who advise them to use dietary supplements, take drugs, or follow procedures that claim to deliver results with little effort. When such performance-enhancing aids are harmless, they are only a waste of money; when they impair performance or harm health, they waste athletic potential and cost lives. This highlight looks at scientific evidence for and against dietary supplements and other preparations available to athletes.

Many substances or treatments claim to be *ergogenic*, meaning work enhancing. In connection with athletic performance, **ergogenic aids** are substances or treatments that purportedly improve athletic performance above and beyond what is possible through training. For practical purposes, most ergogenic aids can be categorized as follows:

- Those that perform as claimed
- Those that may perform as claimed but for which there is insufficient evidence at this time
- Those that do not perform as claimed
- Those that are dangerous, banned, or illegal, and therefore should not be used

Glossary H14-1 defines several of the commonly used ergogenic aids discussed in this highlight.

For the vast majority of ergogenic aids, research findings do not support the claims made.[1] Athletes who hear that a product is ergogenic should ask who is making the claim and who will profit from the sale. Chapter 6 included a discussion on protein powders and amino acid supplements (pp. 187–188).

Athletes who supplement their diets with products promoted to improve athletic performance should be aware that some supplements are contaminated with illegal substances such as steroids or stimulants that are not listed on the label.[2] Supplements contaminated with illegal substances pose health risks to those who use them as well as the risk of positive drug testing for athletes subject to such tests.

GLOSSARY H14-1

anabolic steroids: drugs related to the male sex hormone, testosterone, that stimulate the development of lean body mass.

- **anabolic** = promoting growth
- **sterols** = compounds chemically related to cholesterol

androstenedione: *See DHEA.*

beta-alanine: a nonessential amino acid that is the rate-limiting precursor for the synthesis of the dipeptide carnosine. Carnosine acts primarily as a buffer in skeletal muscle. Beta-alanine supplements raise carnosine concentrations, which enhance the muscles' buffering capacity.

beta-hydroxymethylbutyrate (HMB): a metabolite of the amino acid leucine promoted to increase muscle mass and strength.

caffeine: a natural stimulant found in many common foods and beverages, including coffee, tea, and chocolate; may enhance endurance by stimulating fatty acid release. High doses cause headaches, trembling, rapid heart rate, and other undesirable side effects.

carnitine: a nonessential nonprotein amino acid made in the body from lysine that helps transport fatty acids across the mitochondrial membrane. As a supplement, carnitine supposedly "burns" fat and spares glycogen during endurance events, but in reality it does neither.

convenient dietary supplements: liquid meal replacers, energy drinks, energy bars, and energy gels that athletes and active people use to replenish energy and nutrients when time is limited.

creatine (KREE-ah-tin)**:** a nitrogen-containing compound that combines with phosphate to form the high-energy compound creatine phosphate (or phosphocreatine) in muscles.

DHEA (dehydroepiandrosterone) and **androstenedione:** hormones made in the adrenal glands that serve as precursors to the male sex hormone, testosterone; falsely promoted as burning fat, building muscle, and slowing aging.

dietary nitrate: an inorganic compound composed of nitrogen and oxygen found in water and foods such as spinach, beets, celery, radishes, and lettuce. Dietary nitrate supplementation may reduce the oxygen cost of exercise, thereby improving exercise performance and tolerance.

ergogenic (ER-go-JEN-ick) **aids:** substances or techniques used in an attempt to enhance physical performance.

- **ergo** = work
- **genic** = gives rise to

hGH (human growth hormone): a hormone produced by the brain's pituitary gland that regulates normal growth and development; also called *somatotropin.*

sodium bicarbonate (baking soda): a white crystalline powder that is used to buffer acid that accumulates in the muscles and blood during high-intensity exercise.

Dietary Supplements that Perform as Claimed

Among the extensive array of dietary supplements and other ergogenic aids that athletes use, a few seem to live up to the claims made for them, based on research so far. Convenient dietary supplements, caffeine, creatine, sodium bicarbonate, beta-alanine, and dietary nitrate are the examples discussed here.

Convenient Dietary Supplements

Ready-to-drink supplements such as liquid meal replacers and energy drinks, energy bars, and energy gels are **convenient dietary supplements** for athletes and active people, especially when time is limited. Many such products appeal to athletes by claiming to provide "complete" nutrition. These supplements usually taste good and provide extra carbohydrate and food energy, but they fall short of providing "complete" nutrition. They can be useful as a pregame meal or a between-meal snack, but they should not replace regular meals.

Liquid meal replacers may help a nervous athlete who cannot tolerate solid food on the day of an event. A liquid meal 2 to 3 hours before competition can supply some of the fluid and carbohydrate needed in a pregame meal, but a shake of fat-free milk or juice (such as apple or papaya) and frozen fat-free yogurt or frozen fruit (such as strawberries or bananas) can do the same thing less expensively.

Caffeine

Some research supports the use of **caffeine** to enhance endurance and, to some extent, to enhance short-term, high-intensity exercise performance.[3] Many athletes consume caffeine in coffee, tea, energy drinks, energy shots, gels, gums, and other products to provide an energy boost during sports. In fact, caffeinated energy drinks and low-volume, concentrated energy shots are widely marketed to college students and athletes by way of sport sponsorships, generating billions of dollars in sales each year.[4]

Caffeine is a stimulant that elicits a number of physiological and psychological effects in the body. Caffeine may enhance alertness and concentration, and reduce the perception of fatigue.[5]

The possible benefits of caffeine use must be weighed against its adverse effects—stomach upset, nervousness, irritability, headaches, and diarrhea. Caffeine-containing beverages should be used in moderation, if at all, and *in addition* to other fluids, not as a substitute for them.

Caffeine is a *restricted* substance by the National Collegiate Athletic Association, which allows urine concentrations of 15 milligrams per liter or less (equivalent to about 5 cups of coffee consumed within a few hours before testing). Urine tests that detect more caffeine than this disqualify athletes from competition.

Creatine

Interest in—and use of—**creatine** supplements to enhance performance during intense activity has grown dramatically in the past few years. Power athletes such as weightlifters use creatine supplements to enhance stores of the high-energy compound creatine phosphate (CP) in muscles. Theoretically, the more creatine phosphate in muscles, the higher the intensity at which an athlete can train. High-intensity training stimulates the muscles to adapt, which in turn, improves performance.

Research suggests that creatine supplementation does enhance performance of short-term, repetitive, high-intensity activity such as weightlifting or sprinting.[6] Creatine may improve performance by increasing muscle strength and size, cell hydration, or glycogen loading capacity. In contrast, creatine supplementation has not been shown to benefit endurance activity.

The question of whether short-term use (up to a year) of creatine supplements (up to 5 grams per day) is safe continues to be studied, but so far, the supplements are considered safe for healthy adults.[7] More research is needed, however, to confirm the safety of larger doses and long-term use. One side effect of creatine supplementation that no one disputes is weight gain. For some athletes, weight gain, especially muscle gain, is beneficial, but for others, it is not.

Some medical and fitness experts voice concern that, like many performance supplements before it, creatine is being taken in huge doses (up to 30 *grams* per day) before evidence of its value has been ascertained. Even people who eat red meat, which is a creatine-rich food, do not consume nearly the amount supplements provide. (Creatine content varies, but on average, pork, chicken, and beef provide 65 to 180 *milligrams* per ounce.) Despite the uncertainties, creatine supplements are not illegal in international competition. The American Academy of Pediatrics strongly discourages the use of creatine supplements, as well as the use of any performance-enhancing substance in adolescents younger than 18 years old.

Sodium Bicarbonate

During short-term, high-intensity activity, acid and carbon dioxide accumulate in the blood and muscles. **Sodium bicarbonate** (0.3 gram per kilogram of body weight) ingested prior to high-intensity sports performance buffers the acid and neutralizes the carbon dioxide, thereby maintaining muscle pH levels closer to normal and enhancing exercise capacity.[8] Sodium bicarbonate supplementation may cause unpleasant side effects such as diarrhea in some athletes.

Beta-Alanine

Beta-alanine is a nonessential amino acid that has received much attention from exercise researchers.[9] Beta-alanine is the rate-limiting precursor for the synthesis of the dipeptide carnosine. Carnosine occurs in high concentrations in skeletal muscle and is one of the primary buffering substances available in muscles. Supplementation with beta-alanine has been shown to raise the concentration of muscle carnosine, which enhances the muscles' buffering capacity.[10] This enhanced buffering is especially beneficial to high-intensity exercise performance such as sprinting. The only known adverse side effect of beta-alanine supplementation is a "pins and needles" sensation that occurs with high (more than 800 milligrams) single doses.

Additional research is needed to confirm the safety of beta-alanine supplementation.[11]

Dietary Nitrate

Nitrate is an inorganic compound present in both air and water, as well as in certain vegetables (spinach, beets, celery, radishes, and lettuce). Nitrate is also a common food preservative added to processed meats such as bacon, bologna, hot dogs, and luncheon meats. As a supplement, **dietary nitrate** (either as beetroot juice or sodium nitrate) may improve athletic performance, which has sparked a flurry of intense, ongoing research.[12]

Once ingested, nitrate is converted to nitrite, which circulates in the blood. When oxygen availability is low (as can occur during exercise) nitrite can be converted to nitric oxide. Nitric oxide, an important signaling molecule, improves the muscles' efficiency in using oxygen.[13] By enhancing nitric oxide bioavailability, dietary nitrate supplementation reduces oxygen consumption; improves performance during moderate walking, running, rowing, and cycling; and improves exercise tolerance at more vigorous intensities.[14] Despite such findings, some studies of elite or highly trained athletes fail to show performance benefits following nitrate supplementation; such athletes may already be performing at their maximum oxygen efficiency, or perhaps they require larger doses of nitrate to elicit benefits.[15] Additional research is needed to determine how age, health and fitness status, type of activity, and other factors influence the effects of nitrate supplementation on athletic performance. The safety of long-term nitrate supplementation also needs to be addressed.

Dietary Supplements that May Perform as Claimed

For some dietary supplements, it is just too early to tell whether they deliver on the promises made for them because research thus far is inconclusive. One example of a supplement that may perform as claimed, but for which there is insufficient evidence of efficacy, is beta-hydroxymethylbutyrate.

Beta-hydroxymethylbutyrate (HMB) is a metabolite of the amino acid leucine. Some research suggests that supplementing the diet with HMB during training increases muscle mass, power, and strength.[16] HMB supplementation may also help reduce muscle damage in response to strength training. More research is needed to confirm the effects, if any, of HMB supplementation on strength training and to determine the long-term safety of supplementation.

Dietary Supplements that Do Not Perform as Claimed

Most of the dietary supplements promoted as ergogenic aids fall into the category of "those that do not perform as claimed." Carnitine is one example of an ineffective supplement discussed here, but others include boron, chromium picolinate, coenzyme Q, ginseng, and pyruvate.

In the body, **carnitine** facilitates the transfer of fatty acids across the mitochondrial membrane. Supplement manufacturers suggest that with more carnitine available, fat oxidation will be enhanced, but this does not seem to be the case. Carnitine supplements neither raise muscle carnitine concentrations nor enhance exercise performance. Milk and meat products are good sources of carnitine, and supplements are not needed.

Dangerous, Banned, or Illegal Supplements

The dietary supplements discussed thus far may or may not help athletic performance, but in the doses commonly taken, they seem to cause little harm. The remaining discussion features hormonal preparations that are clearly damaging: anabolic steroids, DHEA (dehydroepiandrosterone), androstenedione, and hGH (human growth hormone). All of these ergogenic aids are dangerous to use and are banned by most professional sports leagues and the World Anti-Doping Agency (WADA) established by the International Olympic Committee. The American Academy of Pediatrics and the American College of Sports Medicine also condemn athletes' use of these substances.

Anabolic Steroids

Among the most dangerous and illegal ergogenic practices is the taking of **anabolic steroids.** These drugs are derived from the male sex hormone testosterone, which promotes the development of male characteristics and lean body mass. Athletes who take steroids do so to stimulate muscle bulking.

The known toxic side effects of steroids include, but are not limited to, extreme aggression and hostility, heart disease, and liver damage. Taking these drugs is a form of cheating. Other athletes are put in the difficult position of either conceding an unfair advantage to competitors who use steroids or taking steroids and accepting the risk of harmful side effects. Athletes, especially young athletes, should not be forced to make such a choice.

The price for the potential competitive edge that steroids confer is high—sometimes it is life itself. Steroids are not simple pills that build bigger muscles. They are complex chemicals to which the body reacts in many ways, particularly when bodybuilders and other athletes take large amounts. The safest, most effective way to build muscle has always been through hard training and a nutritious diet, and—despite popular misconceptions—it still is.

Some manufacturers peddle specific herbs as legal substitutes for steroid drugs. They falsely claim that these herbs contain hormones, enhance the body's hormonal activity, or both. In some cases, an herb may contain plant sterols, such as gamma-oryzanol, but these compounds are poorly absorbed. Even if absorption occurs, the body cannot convert herbal compounds to anabolic steroids. None of these products has any proven anabolic steroid activity, none enhances muscle strength, and some contain natural toxins. In short, "natural" does not mean "harmless."

DHEA and Androstenedione

Some athletes use **DHEA** and **androstenedione** as alternatives to anabolic steroids. DHEA (dehydroepiandrosterone) and androstenedione are hormones made in the adrenal glands that serve as precursors to the male hormone testosterone. Advertisements claim the hormones "burn fat," "build muscle," and "slow aging," but evidence to support such claims is lacking.

Short-term side effects of DHEA and androstenedione may include oily skin, acne, body hair growth, liver enlargement, testicular shrinkage, and aggressive behavior. Long-term effects such as serious liver damage may take years to become evident. The potential for harm from DHEA and androstenedione supplements is great, and athletes, as well as others, should avoid them.

Human Growth Hormone

A wide range of athletes, including weightlifters, baseball players, cyclists, and track and field participants use **hGH (human growth hormone)** to build lean tissue and improve athletic performance. These athletes use hGH, believing the injectable hormone will provide the benefits of anabolic steroids without the dangerous side effects.

Taken in large quantities, hGH causes the disease acromegaly, in which the body becomes huge and the organs and bones overenlarge. Other effects include diabetes, thyroid disorder, heart disease, menstrual irregularities, diminished sexual desire, and shortened life span.

A Final Word of Caution

Sometimes it is difficult to distinguish valid claims from bogus ones. Fitness magazines and Internet websites are particularly troublesome because many of them present both valid and invalid nutrition information along with slick advertisements for nutrition products. Advertisements often feature colorful anatomical figures, graphs, and tables that appear scientific. Some ads even include references, citing or linking to such credible sources as the *American Journal of Clinical Nutrition* and the *Journal of the American Medical Association.* These ads create the illusion of endorsement and credibility to gain readers' trust. Keep in mind, however, that the ads are created not to teach, but to sell. A careful reading of the cited research might reveal that the ads have presented the research findings out of context. For example, an ad might use a research article to conclude that its human growth hormone supplement "increases lean body mass and bone mineral," when in fact, the researchers would conclude that "its general use now or in the immediate future is not justified." Scientific facts are often exaggerated and twisted to promote sales. Highlight 1 (p. 28) describes ways to recognize misinformation and quackery.

The search for a single food, nutrient, drug, or technique that will safely and effectively enhance athletic performance will no doubt continue as long as people strive to achieve excellence in sports. When athletic performance does improve after use of an ergogenic aid, the improvement can often be attributed to the placebo effect, which is strongly at work in athletes. Even if a reliable source reports a performance boost from a newly tried product, give the effect time to fade away. Chances are excellent that it simply reflects the power of the mind over the body.

The overwhelming majority of performance-enhancing aids sold for athletes are not effective. Wishful thinking will not substitute for talent, hard training, adequate diet, and mental preparedness in competition. But don't discount the power of mind over body for a minute—it is formidable, and sports psychologists dedicate their work to harnessing it. You can use it by imagining yourself a winner and visualizing yourself excelling in your sport. You don't have to buy magic to obtain a winning edge; you already possess it—your physically fit mind and body.

CRITICAL THINKING QUESTIONS

A. What are the moral implications of using ergogenic aids?

B. Because of serious doping violations, Lance Armstrong was stripped of his seven Tour de France titles and banned from cycling for life. For him, these actions are "equivalent to a death sentence." What is your opinion of Armstrong's doping violations and the imposed consequences? If you were a member of the International Cycling Union, how would you propose determining which, if any, substances to allow and/or ban?

REFERENCES

1. Position of the Academy of Nutrition and Dietetics, Dietitians of Canada, and the American College of Sports Medicine: Nutrition and athletic performance, *Journal of the Academy of Nutrition and Dietetics* 116 (2016): 501–528.
2. P. A. Cohen, Hazards of hindsight—Monitoring the safety of nutritional supplements, *New England Journal of Medicine* 370 (2014): 1277–1280.
3. C. D. Black, D. E. Waddell, and A. R. Gonglach, Caffeine's ergogenic effects on cycling: Neuromuscular and perceptual factors, *Medicine and Science in Sports and Exercise* 47 (2015): 1145–1158; H. K. Stadheim and coauthors, Caffeine and performance over consecutive days of simulated competition, *Medicine and Science in Sports and Exercise* 46 (2014): 1787–1796; A. B. Hodgson, R. K. Randell, and A. E. Jeukendrup, The metabolic and performance effects of caffeine compared to coffee during endurance exercise, *PLoS One* 8 (2013): e59561.
4. C. Rosenbloom, Energy drinks, caffeine, and athletes, *Nutrition Today* 49 (2014): 49–54.
5. Rosenbloom, Energy drinks, caffeine, and athletes, 2014; R. Meeusen, B. Roelands, and L. L. Spriet, Caffeine, exercise and the brain, *Nestle Nutrition Institute Workshop Series* 76 (2013): 1–12.
6. C. Lanhers and coauthors, Creatine supplementation and lower limb strength performance: A systematic review and meta-analysis, *Sports Medicine* 45 (2015): 1285–1294; M. C. Devries and S. M. Phillips, Creatine supplementation during resistance training in older adults—A meta-analysis, *Medicine and Science in Sports and Exercise* 46 (2014): 1194–1203; C. L. Camic and coauthors, The effects of polyethylene glycosylated

creatine supplementation on anaerobic performance measures and body composition, *Journal of Strength and Conditioning Research* 28 (2014): 825–833.

7. E. Galvan and coauthors, Acute and chronic safety and efficacy of dose dependent creatine nitrate supplementation and exercise performance, *Journal of the International Society of Sports Nutrition*, March 31, 2016, doi:10.1186/s12970-016-0124-0.
8. L. M. Burke, Practical considerations for bicarbonate loading and sports performance, *Nestle' Nutrition Institute Workshop Series* 75 (2013): 15–26.
9. P. M. Bellinger, β-alanine supplementation for athletic performance: An update, *Journal of Strength and Conditioning Research* 28 (2014): 1751–1770; R. C. Harris and T. Stellingwerff, Effect of *b*-alanine supplementation on high-intensity exercise performance, *Nestle Nutrition Institute Workshop Series* 76 (2013): 61–71; C. Sale and coauthors, Carnosine: From exercise performance to health, *Amino Acids* 44 (2013): 1477–1491; W. Derave, Use of β-alanine as an ergogenic aid, *Nestle Nutrition Institute Workshop Series* 75 (2013): 99–108.
10. E. T. Trexler and coauthors, International Society of Sports Nutrition position stand: Beta-alanine, *Journal of the International Society of Sports Nutrition* 12 (2015): 30; L. Junior and coauthors, Nutritional strategies to modulate intracellular and extracellular buffering capacity during high-intensity exercise, *Sports Medicine* 45 (2015): S71–S81; Derave, 2013.
11. J. J. Quesnele and coauthors, The effects of beta alanine supplementation on performance: A systematic review of the literature, *International Journal of Sport Nutrition and Exercise Metabolism* 24 (2014): 14–27; R. Ko and coauthors, Evidence-based evaluation of potential benefits and safety of beta-alanine supplementation for military personnel, *Nutrition Reviews* 72 (2014): 217–225.
12. S. Porcelli and coauthors, Aerobic fitness affects the exercise performance responses to nitrate supplementation, *Medicine and Science in Sports and Exercise* 47 (2015): 1643–1651; R. K. Boorsma, J. Whitfield, and L. L. Spriet, Beetroot juice supplementation does not improve performance of elite 1500-m runners, *Medicine and Science in Sports and Exercise* 46 (2014): 2326–2334; A.M. Jones, Dietary nitrate supplementation and exercise performance, *Sports Medicine* 44 (2014): 35–45; W. T. Clements, S. R. Lee, and R. J. Bloomer, Nitrate ingestion: A review of the health and physical performance effects, *Nutrients* 6 (2014): 5224–5264.
13. A. M. Jones, A. Vanhatalo, and S. J. Bailey, Influence of dietary nitrate supplementation on exercise tolerance and performance, *Nestle Nutrition Institute Workshop Series* 75 (2013): 27–40.
14. Clements, Lee, and Bloomer, 2014.
15. Porcelli and coauthors, 2015; Boorsma, Whitfield, and Spriet, 2014.
16. J. M. Wilson and coauthors, The effects of 12 weeks of beta-hydroxy-beta-methylbutyrate free acid supplementation on muscle mass, strength, and power in resistance-trained individuals: A randomized, double-blind placebo-controlled study, *European Journal of Applied Physiology* 114 (2014): 1217–1227; J. M. Wilson and coauthors, β-hydroxy- β-methylbutyrate free acid reduces markers of exercise-induced muscle damage and improves recovery in resistance-trained men, *British Journal of Nutrition* 110 (2013): 538–544.

15 Life Cycle Nutrition: Pregnancy and Lactation

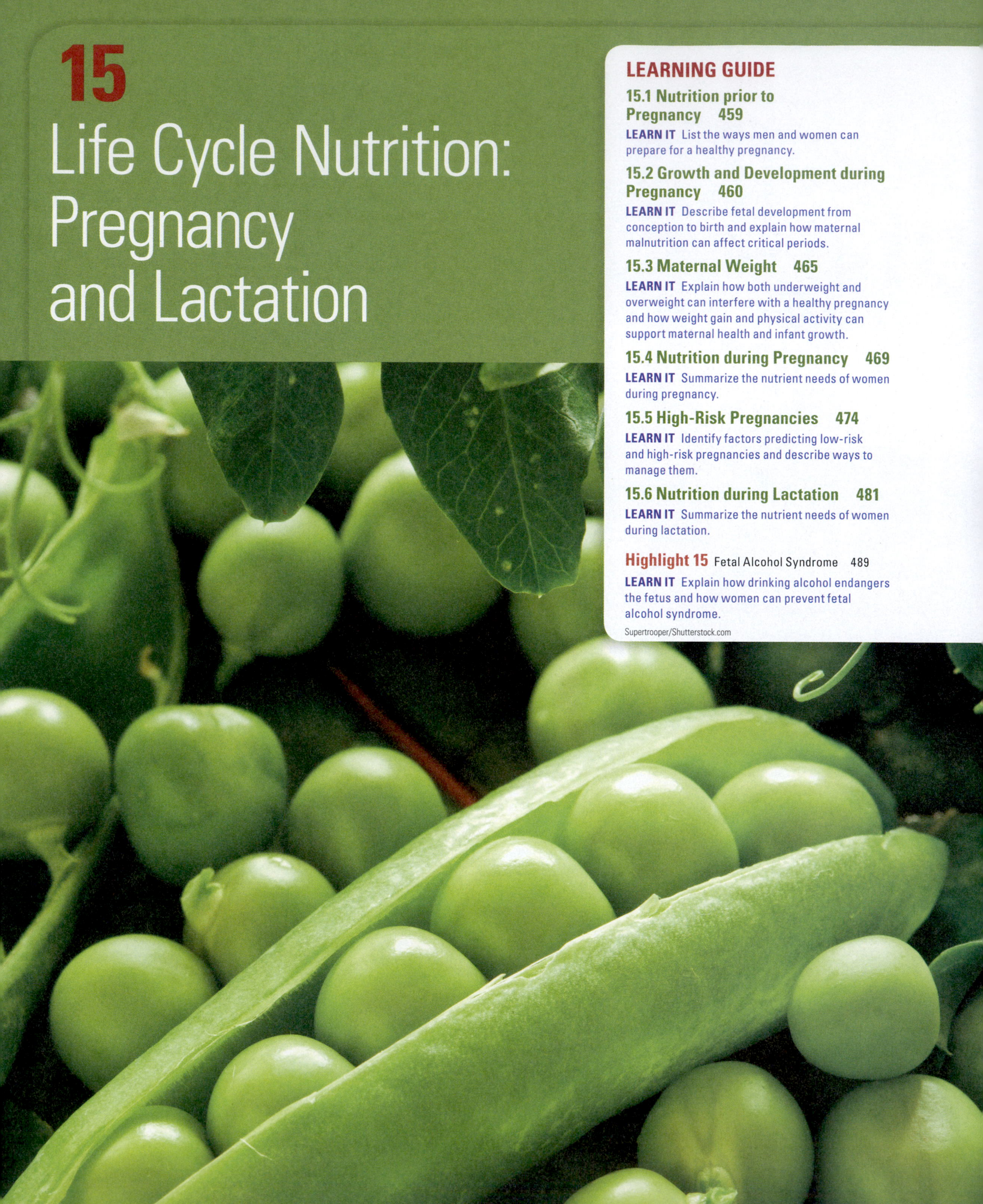

LEARNING GUIDE

Supertrooper/Shutterstock.com

Nutrition in Your Life

Food choices have consequences. Sometimes they are immediate, such as when you get heartburn after eating a pepperoni pizza. Other times they sneak up on you, such as when you gain weight after repeatedly overindulging in hot fudge sundaes. Quite often, they are temporary and easily resolved, such as when hunger pangs strike after you skip lunch. During pregnancy, however, the consequences of a woman's food choices are dramatic. They affect not only her health, but also the growth and development of another human being—and not just for today, but for years to come. Making smart food choices is a huge responsibility, but fortunately, it's fairly simple. As you read this chapter, consider how well your current diet might support the needs of a pregnant woman.

Each person enters this world with a unique genetic map that determines the primary ways that person's physical and mental characteristics will develop throughout life. Some of those characteristics cannot be changed, but others can be influenced within genetically defined limits. One of several ways to ensure the optimal growth, maintenance, and health of the body is through good nutrition. Ideally, a person's diet supplies sufficient amounts of all the nutrients to meet the needs incurred by the physiological demands of pregnancy, lactation, growth, and aging.

All people—pregnant and lactating women, infants, children, adolescents, and adults—need the same nutrients, but the amounts they need vary depending on their stage of life. This chapter focuses on nutrition in preparation for, and support of, pregnancy and lactation. The next two chapters address the needs of infants, children, adolescents, and older adults.

15.1 Nutrition prior to Pregnancy

LEARN IT List the ways men and women can prepare for a healthy pregnancy.

Both a man's and a woman's nutrition may affect **fertility** and possibly the genetic contributions they make to their children, but it is the woman's nutrition that has the most direct influence on the developing fetus.[1] Her body provides the environment for the growth and development of a new human being. Prior to pregnancy, however, both men and women have a unique opportunity to prepare physically, mentally, and emotionally for the many changes to come. In preparation for a healthy pregnancy, they can establish the following habits:

- *Achieve and maintain a healthy body weight.* Both underweight and overweight are associated with infertility.[2] Overweight and obese men have low sperm counts and hormonal changes that reduce fertility; excess body fat in women disrupts menstrual regularity and ovarian hormone production.[3] For obese couples, it just seems to take longer to conceive.[4] Should a pregnancy occur, mothers, both underweight and overweight, and their newborns, face increased risks of complications.
- *Choose an adequate and balanced diet.* Malnutrition reduces fertility and impairs the early development of an infant should a woman become pregnant. In contrast, a healthy diet that includes a full array of vitamins and minerals can favorably influence fertility. Men with healthy diets rich in antioxidant nutrients and low in saturated fats have higher sperm numbers and motility.[5]
- *Be physically active.* A woman who wants to be physically active *when* she is pregnant needs to become physically active *beforehand*.
- *Receive regular medical care.* Regular health-care visits help ensure a healthy start to pregnancy.

fertility: the capacity of a woman to produce a normal ovum periodically and of a man to produce normal sperm; the ability to reproduce.

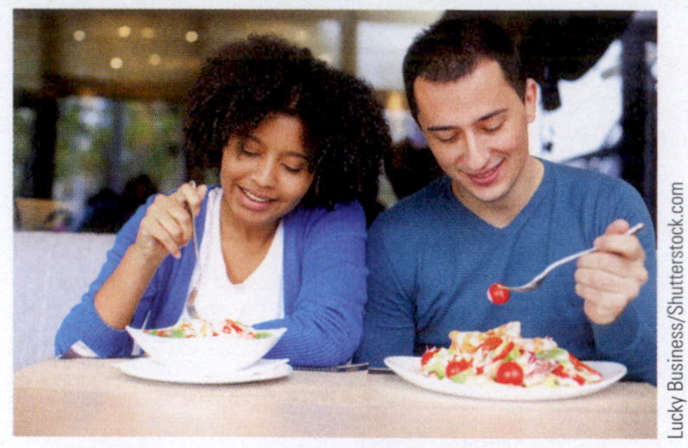
Lucky Business/Shutterstock.com

> **PHOTO 15-1** Young adults can prepare for a healthy pregnancy by taking care of themselves today.

- *Manage chronic conditions.* Conditions such as diabetes, hypertension, HIV/AIDS, phenylketonuria (PKU), and sexually transmitted diseases can adversely affect a pregnancy and need close medical attention to help ensure a healthy outcome.
- *Avoid harmful influences.* Both maternal and paternal ingestion of, or exposure to, harmful substances (such as cigarettes, alcohol, drugs, or environmental contaminants) can cause miscarriage or abnormalities, alter genes or their expression, and interfere with fertility.[6]

Young adults who nourish and protect their bodies do so not only for their own sakes, but also for future generations (see Photo 15-1).

REVIEW IT List the ways men and women can prepare for a healthy pregnancy.
Prior to pregnancy, the health and behaviors of both men and women can influence fertility and fetal development. In preparation, they can achieve and maintain a healthy body weight, choose an adequate and balanced diet, be physically active, receive regular medical care, manage chronic diseases, and avoid harmful influences.

15.2 Growth and Development during Pregnancy

LEARN IT Describe fetal development from conception to birth and explain how maternal malnutrition can affect critical periods.

A whole new life begins at **conception**. Organ systems develop rapidly, and nutrition plays many supportive roles. This section describes placental development and fetal growth, paying close attention to times of intense developmental activity.

Placental Development

In the early days of pregnancy, a spongy structure known as the **placenta** develops in the **uterus.** Two associated structures also form (see Figure 15-1). One is the **amniotic sac,** a fluid-filled balloonlike structure that houses the developing fetus. The other is the **umbilical cord,** a ropelike structure containing fetal blood vessels that extends through the fetus's "belly button" (the umbilicus) to the placenta. These three structures play crucial roles during pregnancy, and then are expelled from the uterus during childbirth.

The placenta develops as an interweaving of fetal and maternal blood vessels embedded in the uterine wall. The maternal blood transfers oxygen and nutrients to the fetus's blood and picks up fetal waste products. By exchanging oxygen, nutrients, and waste products, the placenta performs the respiratory, absorptive, and excretory functions that the fetus's lungs, digestive system, and kidneys will provide after birth.

The placenta is a versatile, metabolically active organ. Like all body tissues, the placenta uses energy and nutrients to support its work. It produces an array of hormones that maintain pregnancy and prepare the mother's breasts for lactation (making milk). A healthy placenta is essential for the developing fetus to attain its full potential.

Fetal Growth and Development

Fetal development begins with the fertilization of an **ovum** by a **sperm.** Three stages follow: the zygote, the embryo, and the fetus (see Figure 15-2).

The Zygote The newly fertilized ovum is called a **zygote.** It begins as a single cell and rapidly divides to become a **blastocyst.** During that first week, the blastocyst floats down into the uterus, where it will embed itself in the inner uterine wall—a process known as **implantation.** Cell division continues at an amazing rate as each set of cells divides into many other cells.

conception: the union of the male sperm and the female ovum; fertilization.

placenta (plah-SEN-tuh): the organ that develops inside the uterus early in pregnancy, through which the fetus receives nutrients and oxygen and returns carbon dioxide and other waste products to be excreted.

uterus (YOU-ter-us): the muscular organ within which the infant develops before birth.

amniotic (am-nee-OTT-ic) **sac:** the "bag of waters" in the uterus, in which the fetus floats.

umbilical (um-BILL-ih-cul) **cord:** the ropelike structure through which the fetus's veins and arteries reach the placenta; the route of nourishment and oxygen to the fetus and the route of waste disposal from the fetus. The scar in the middle of the abdomen that marks the former attachment of the umbilical cord is the *umbilicus* (um-BILL-ih-cus), commonly known as the "belly button."

ovum (OH-vum): the female reproductive cell, capable of developing into a new organism upon fertilization; commonly referred to as an egg.

sperm: the male reproductive cell, capable of fertilizing an ovum.

zygote (ZY-goat): the initial product of the union of ovum and sperm; a fertilized ovum.

blastocyst (BLASS-toe-sist): the developmental stage of the zygote when it is about 5 days old and ready for implantation.

implantation (IM-plan-TAY-shun): the embedding of the blastocyst in the inner lining of the uterus.

> **FIGURE 15-1 The Placenta and Associated Structures**

To understand how placental villi absorb nutrients without maternal and fetal blood interacting directly, think of how the intestinal villi work. The GI side of the intestinal villi is bathed in a nutrient-rich fluid (chyme). The intestinal villi absorb the nutrient molecules and release them into the body via capillaries. Similarly, the maternal side of the placental villi is bathed in nutrient-rich maternal blood. The placental villi absorb the nutrient molecules and release them to the fetus via fetal capillaries.

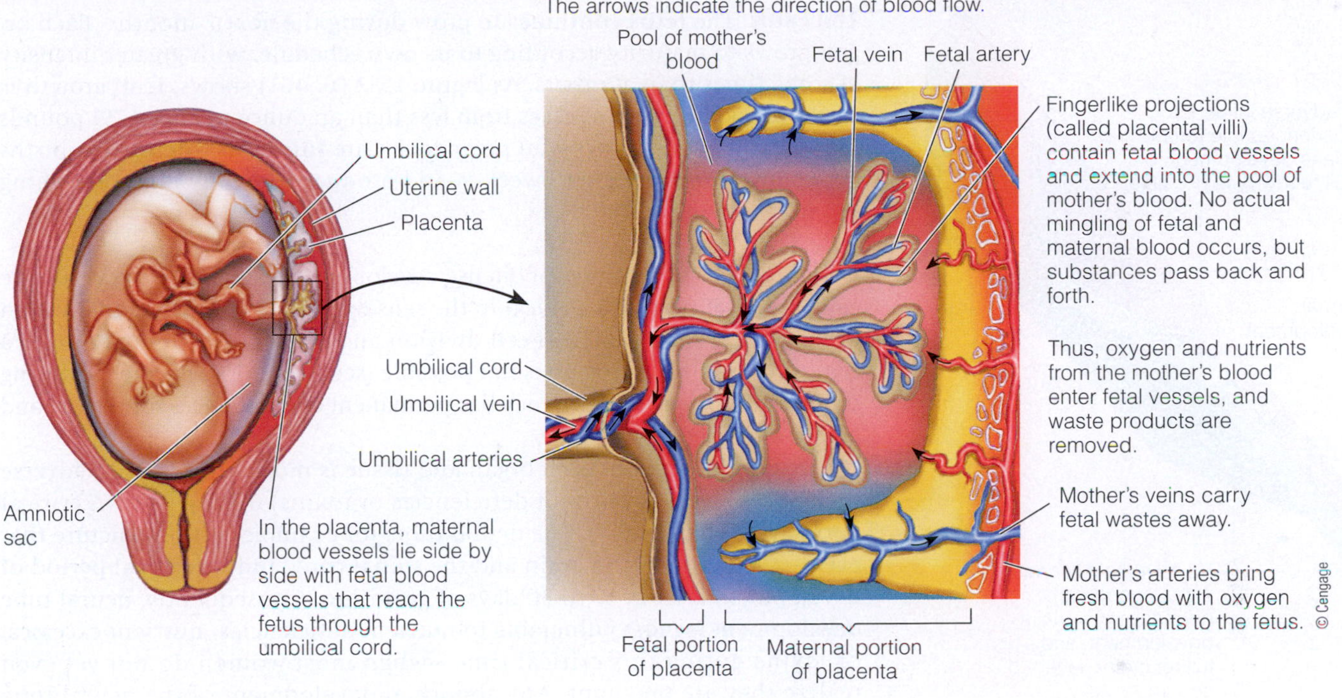

The arrows indicate the direction of blood flow.
Pool of mother's blood
Fetal vein
Fetal artery
Umbilical cord
Uterine wall
Placenta
Fingerlike projections (called placental villi) contain fetal blood vessels and extend into the pool of mother's blood. No actual mingling of fetal and maternal blood occurs, but substances pass back and forth.
Thus, oxygen and nutrients from the mother's blood enter fetal vessels, and waste products are removed.
Umbilical cord
Umbilical vein
Umbilical arteries
Amniotic sac
In the placenta, maternal blood vessels lie side by side with fetal blood vessels that reach the fetus through the umbilical cord.
Mother's veins carry fetal wastes away.
Mother's arteries bring fresh blood with oxygen and nutrients to the fetus.
Fetal portion of placenta
Maternal portion of placenta
© Cengage

> **FIGURE 15-2 Stages of Embryonic and Fetal Development**

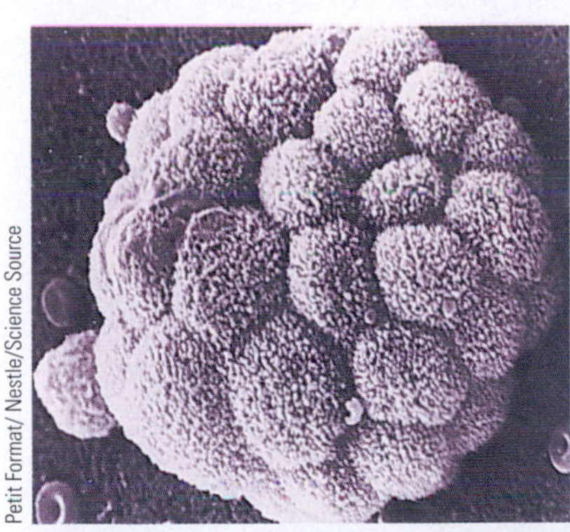
Petit Format/ Nestle/Science Source

1 A newly fertilized ovum is called a **zygote** and is about the size of the period at the end of this sentence. Less than 1 week after fertilization, these cells have rapidly divided multiple times to become a blastocyst ready for implantation.

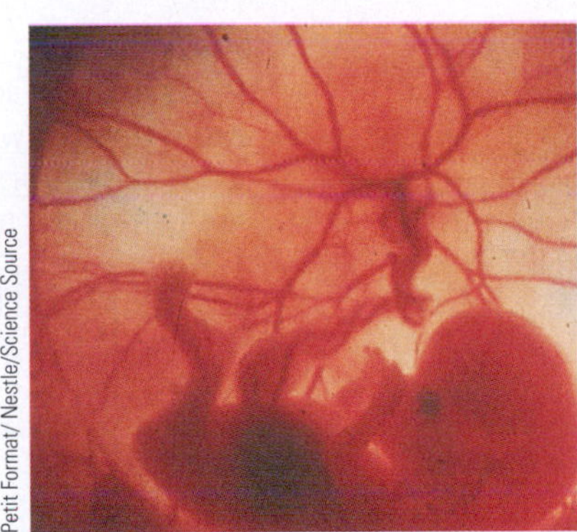
Petit Format/ Nestle/Science Source

3 A **fetus** after 11 weeks of development is just over an inch long. Notice the umbilical cord and blood vessels connecting the fetus with the placenta.

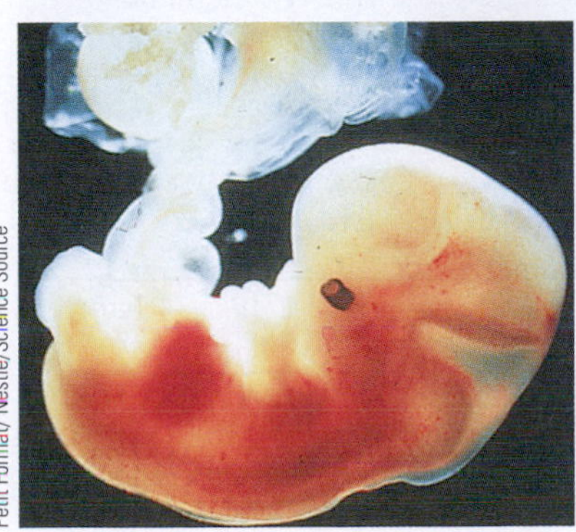
Petit Format/ Nestle/Science Source

2 After implantation, the placenta develops and begins to provide nourishment to the developing embryo. An **embryo** 5 weeks after fertilization is about ½ inch long.

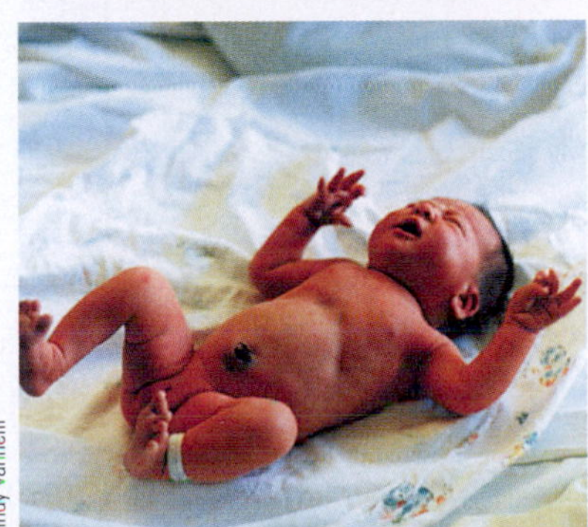
Cindy Vannelli

4 A **newborn infant** after 9 months of development measures close to 20 inches in length. From 8 weeks to term, this infant grew 20 times longer and 50 times heavier.

FIGURE 15-3 The Concept of Critical Periods in Fetal Development

Critical periods occur early in fetal development. An adverse influence felt early in pregnancy can have a much more severe and prolonged impact than one felt later on.

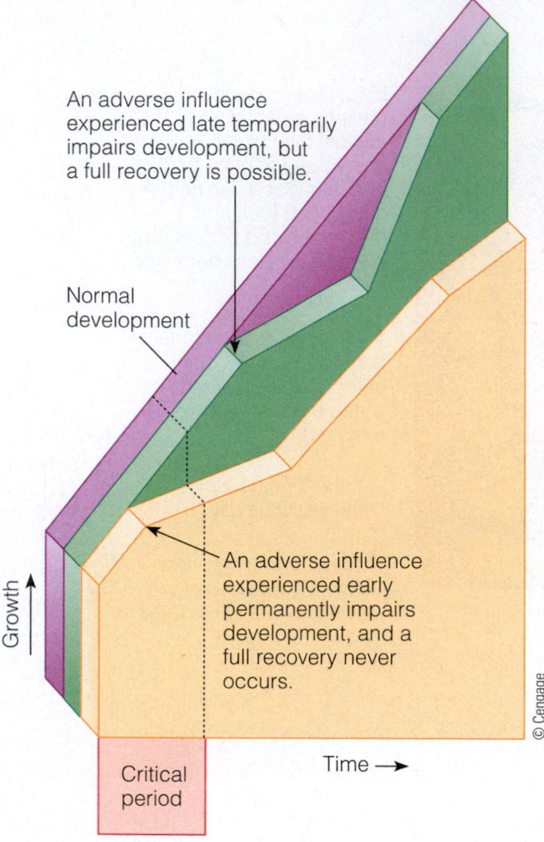

An adverse influence experienced late temporarily impairs development, but a full recovery is possible.
Normal development
An adverse influence experienced early permanently impairs development, and a full recovery never occurs.
Growth
Critical period
Time
© Cengage

The Embryo At first, the number of cells in the **embryo** doubles approximately every 24 hours; later the rate slows, and only one doubling occurs during the final 10 weeks of pregnancy. At 8 weeks, the 1¼-inch embryo has a complete central nervous system, a beating heart, a digestive system, well-defined fingers and toes, and the beginnings of facial features.

The Fetus The **fetus** continues to grow during the next 7 months. Each organ grows to maturity according to its own schedule, with greater intensity at some times than at others. As Figure 15-2 (p. 461) shows, fetal growth is phenomenal: weight increases from less than an ounce to about 7½ pounds (3500 grams). Most successful pregnancies are **full term**—defined as births occurring at 39 through 40 weeks—and produce a healthy infant weighing 6½ to 8 pounds.[7]

Critical Periods

Times of intense development and rapid cell division are called **critical periods**—critical in the sense that those cellular activities can occur only at those times. If cell division and number are limited during a critical period, full recovery is not possible (see Figure 15-3). Damage during these critical times of pregnancy has permanent consequences for the life and health of the fetus.

The development of each organ and tissue is most vulnerable to adverse influences (such as nutrient deficiencies or toxins) during its own critical period (see Figure 15-4). The neural tube, for example, is the structure that eventually becomes the brain and the spinal cord, and its critical period of development is from 17 to 30 days of **gestation**. Consequently, neural tube development is most vulnerable to nutrient deficiencies, nutrient excesses, or toxins during this critical time—when most women do not yet even realize they are pregnant. Any abnormal development of the neural tube or its failure to close completely can cause a major defect in the central nervous system.

Neural Tube Defects Each year in the United States, approximately 3000 pregnancies are affected by **neural tube defects**—malformations of the

FIGURE 15-4 Critical Periods of Development

During embryonic development (from 2 to 8 weeks), many of the tissues are in their critical periods; events occur that will have irreversible effects on the development of those tissues. In the later stages of development, the tissues continue to grow and change, but the events are less critical in that they are relatively minor or reversible.

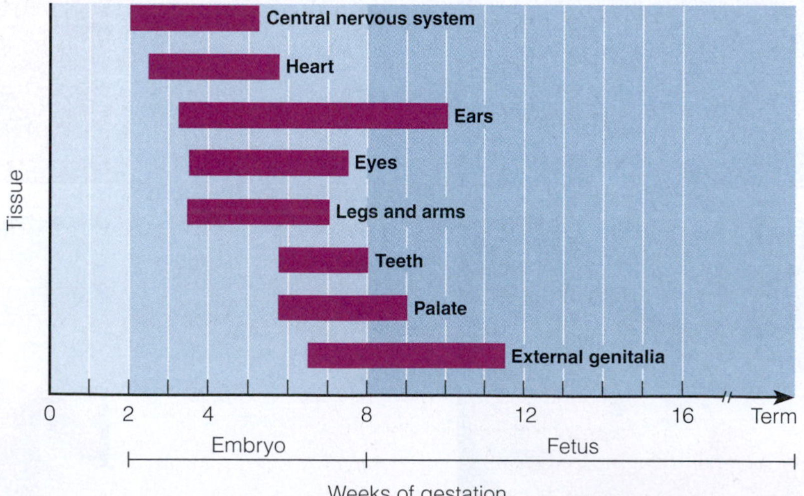

Central nervous system
Heart
Ears
Eyes
Legs and arms
Teeth
Palate
External genitalia
Tissue
0
2
4
8
12
16
Term
Embryo
Fetus
Weeks of gestation

SOURCE: Adapted from *Before We Are Born: Essentials of Embryology and Birth Defects* by K. L. Moore and T.V.N. Persaud (W. B. Saunders, 2003).

embryo (EM-bree-oh): the developing infant from 2 to 8 weeks after conception.

fetus (FEET-us): the developing infant from 8 weeks after conception until term.

full term: births occurring at 39 through 40 weeks of gestation.

critical periods: finite periods during development in which certain events occur that will have irreversible effects on later developmental stages; usually a period of rapid cell division.

gestation (jes-TAY-shun): the period from conception to birth. For human beings, the average length of a healthy gestation is 40 weeks. Pregnancy is often divided into 3-month periods, called *trimesters*.

neural tube defects: malformations of the brain, spinal cord, or both during embryonic development that often result in lifelong disability or death.

> **FIGURE 15-5 Spina Bifida**

Spina bifida, a common neural tube defect, occurs when the vertebrae of the spine fail to close around the spinal cord, leaving it unprotected. The B vitamin folate—consumed prior to and during pregnancy—helps prevent spina bifida and other neural tube defects.

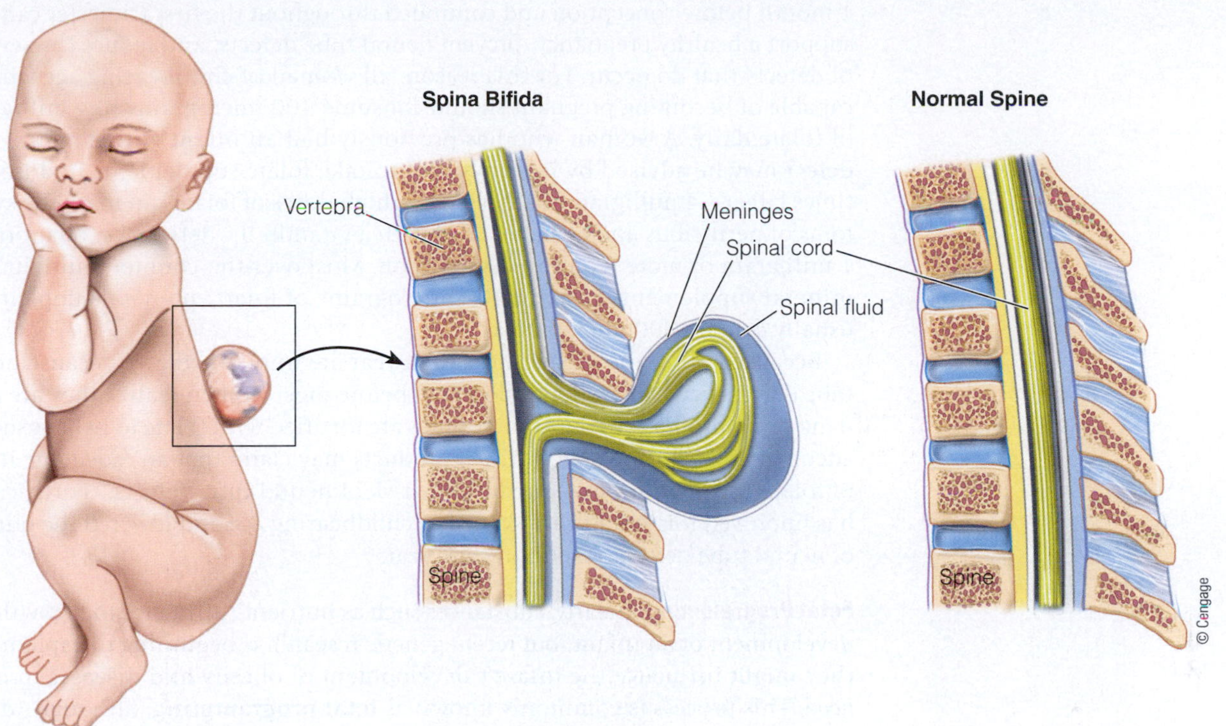
Spina Bifida
Normal Spine
Vertebra
Meninges
Spinal cord
Spinal fluid
Spine
Spine
© Cengage

brain, spinal cord, or both during embryonic development.* The two most common types of neural tube defects are anencephaly (no brain) and spina bifida (split brain). In **anencephaly**, the upper end of the neural tube fails to close. Consequently, the brain is either missing or fails to develop. Pregnancies affected by anencephaly often end in miscarriage; infants born with anencephaly die shortly after birth.

Spina bifida is characterized by incomplete closure of the spinal cord and its bony encasement (see Figure 15-5). The meninges membranes covering the spinal cord often protrude as a sac, which may rupture and lead to meningitis, a life-threatening infection. Spina bifida is accompanied by varying degrees of paralysis, depending on the extent of the spinal cord damage. Mild cases may not even be noticed, but severe cases lead to death. Common problems include clubfoot, dislocated hip, kidney disorders, curvature of the spine, muscle weakness, mental impairments, and motor and sensory losses.

The cause of neural tube defects is unknown, but researchers are examining several gene-gene, gene-nutrient, and gene-environment interactions. A pregnancy affected by a neural tube defect can occur in any woman, but certain factors make it more likely.[8] Risk factors for neural tube defects include:

- A personal or family history of a neural tube defect
- Maternal diabetes or gestational diabetes
- Maternal Hispanic ethnicity
- Maternal use of certain antiseizure medications
- Inadequate folate
- Maternal obesity

*Worldwide, more than 300,000 pregnancies are affected by neural tube defects each year.

anencephaly (AN-en-SEF-a-lee): an uncommon and always fatal type of neural tube defect, characterized by the absence of a brain.

- **an** = not (without)
- **encephalus** = brain

spina (SPY-nah) **bifida** (BIFF-ih-dah): one of the most common types of neural tube defects, characterized by the incomplete closure of the spinal cord and its bony encasement.

- **spina** = spine
- **bifida** = split

Not all cases of neural tube defects can be prevented, but folate supplementation greatly reduces the incidence and severity.

Folate Supplementation Chapter 10 described how folate supplements taken 1 month before conception and continued throughout the first trimester can help support a healthy pregnancy, prevent neural tube defects, and reduce the severity of defects that do occur. For this reason, all women of childbearing age who are capable of becoming pregnant should consume 400 micrograms (0.4 milligram) of folate daily. A woman who has previously had an infant with a neural tube defect may be advised by her physician to take folate supplements in doses ten times larger—4 milligrams daily. Because high doses of folate can mask the symptoms of pernicious anemia associated with a vitamin B_{12} deficiency, quantities of 1 milligram or more require a prescription. Most over-the-counter multivitamin-mineral supplements contain 400 micrograms of folate; prenatal supplements usually contain 800 micrograms.

Because half of the pregnancies each year are unplanned and because neural tube defects occur early in development before most women realize they are pregnant, grain products in the United States are fortified with folate to help ensure an adequate intake. Labels on fortified products may claim that an "adequate intake of folate has been shown to reduce the risk of neural tube defects." Fortification has improved folate status in women of childbearing age and lowered the number of neural tube defects that occur each year.

Fetal Programming Clearly, substances such as nutrients influence the growth and development of an infant, but recent genetic research is beginning to explain how they might influence the infant's development of obesity and diseases in *adulthood.* This process is commonly known as **fetal programming**, although "developmental origins of disease" may more appropriately describe the ever-changing interactions involved in disease development. In the case of pregnancy, the mother's nutrition can change gene expression in the fetus. Such epigenetic changes during pregnancy can affect the infant's development of obesity and chronic diseases later in life.[9] Some research suggests that these epigenetic changes during pregnancy may even influence succeeding generations.[10] (See Highlight 6 for further discussion of epigenetics.)

Chronic Diseases Much research suggests that dietary influences at critical times during fetal development program the infant's bodily functions by permanently changing an organ's structure. For example, undernutrition may limit liver growth and program lipid metabolism in such a way that the infant will develop cardiovascular disease as an adult. Similarly, overnutrition and maternal obesity may program the fetus to develop obesity, heart disease, type 2 diabetes, and asthma later in life.[11] On a positive note, a maternal diet rich in nutrients such as folate can have epigenetic effects that may protect the developing fetus against obesity in childhood and some cancers in adulthood.[12] (See Highlight 6 for a detailed discussion of epigenetics and folate's role in methylation reactions.)

Malnutrition during the critical period of pancreatic cell growth provides an example of how type 2 diabetes may develop in adulthood. The pancreatic cells responsible for producing insulin (the beta cells) normally increase more than 130-fold between 12 weeks of gestation and 5 months after birth. Nutrition is a primary determinant of beta cell growth, and infants who have suffered prenatal malnutrition have significantly fewer beta cells than well-nourished infants. They are also more likely to be low-birthweight infants—and low birthweight correlates with insulin resistance later in life. One hypothesis suggests that diabetes may develop from the interaction of inadequate nutrition early in life (low birthweight) with abundant nutrition later in life (overweight adult): the small mass of beta cells developed in times of undernutrition during fetal development may be insufficient in times of overnutrition during adulthood when the body needs more insulin.

fetal programming: the influence of substances during fetal growth on the development of diseases in later life.

REVIEW IT **Describe fetal development from conception to birth and explain how maternal malnutrition can affect critical periods.**

Maternal nutrition before and during pregnancy affects both the mother's health and the infant's growth. As the infant develops through its three stages—the zygote, embryo, and fetus—its organs and tissues grow, each on its own schedule. Times of intense development are critical periods that depend on nutrients to proceed smoothly. Without folate, for example, the neural tube fails to develop completely during the first month of pregnancy, prompting recommendations that all women of childbearing age take folate daily.

Because critical periods occur throughout pregnancy, a woman should continuously take good care of her health. That care should include achieving and maintaining a healthy body weight prior to pregnancy and gaining sufficient weight during pregnancy to support a healthy infant.

15.3 Maternal Weight

LEARN IT **Explain how both underweight and overweight can interfere with a healthy pregnancy and how weight gain and physical activity can support maternal health and infant growth.**

Birthweight is the most reliable indicator of an infant's health. As a later section of this chapter explains, compared with a normal-weight infant, an underweight infant is more likely to have physical and mental abnormalities, suffer illnesses, and die. In general, higher birthweights present fewer risks for infants. Two characteristics of the mother's weight influence an infant's birthweight: her weight *prior* to conception and her weight gain *during* pregnancy.

Weight prior to Conception

A woman's weight prior to conception influences fetal growth. Even with the same weight gain during pregnancy, underweight women tend to have smaller babies than heavier women. Ideally, before a woman becomes pregnant, she will have established diet and activity habits to support an adequate, and not excessive, weight gain during pregnancy.[13]

Underweight An underweight woman (BMI <18.5) has a high risk of having a low-birthweight infant, especially if she is malnourished or unable to gain sufficient weight during pregnancy. In addition, the rates of **preterm** births and infant deaths are higher for underweight women.[14] An underweight woman improves her chances of having a healthy infant by gaining sufficient weight prior to conception or by gaining extra pounds during pregnancy. To gain weight and ensure nutrient adequacy, an underweight woman can follow the dietary recommendations for pregnant women (described on pp. 469–472).

Overweight and Obesity At least one-half of all pregnant women in the United States are overweight or obese prior to conception, which can create problems related to pregnancy, infancy, and childbirth.[15] Obese women have an especially high risk of medical complications such as gestational hypertension and gestational diabetes. Compared with other women, obese women are also more likely to have other complications of labor and delivery. Complications in women after gastric bypass surgery are lower than in obese women, but their infants are more likely to be small, perhaps because of limited nutrient absorption; stillbirth and infant mortality may also be slightly higher.[16]

Infants of obese women are more likely to be large for gestational age and to continue gaining weight at a rapid rate during the early years of life, setting the stage for childhood obesity.[17] Problems associated with **macrosomia** include increases in the likelihood of a difficult labor and delivery, birth trauma, and **cesarean delivery**, which presents a high risk in obese women.[18] Consequently, these infants have a greater risk of poor health and death than infants of normal weight.

preterm (premature): births occurring before 37 weeks of gestation; births occurring at 37 to 38 weeks of gestation are designated *early term*.

macrosomia (mak-roh-SO-me-ah): abnormally large body size. In the case of infants, a birthweight at the 90th percentile or higher for gestational age (roughly 9 lb—or 4000 g—or more); macrosomia results from prepregnancy obesity, excessive weight gain during pregnancy, or uncontrolled gestational diabetes.

- **macro** = large
- **soma** = body

cesarean (si-ZAIR-ee-un) **delivery:** a surgically assisted birth involving removal of the fetus by an incision into the uterus, usually by way of the abdominal wall.

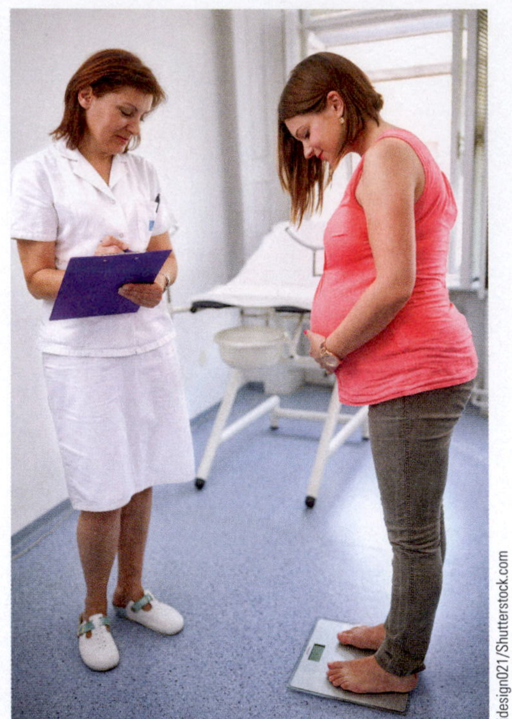

> **PHOTO 15-2** Sufficient weight gain during pregnancy supports fetal growth and maternal health.

didesign021/Shutterstock.com

Of greater concern than infant birthweight is stillbirth and the poor development of infants born to obese mothers.[19] Obesity may increase the risk for neural tube defects, cerebral palsy, heart defects, and other abnormalities.[20]

Even moderate overweight increases the risks for some complications, such as gestational hypertension, gestational diabetes, preterm births, and cesarean deliveries. Risks, including fetal and infant death, tend to increase as BMI increases.[21] Health-care providers have traditionally advised against weight-loss dieting during pregnancy. Limited research, however, suggests that following a well-balanced, kcalorie-restricted diet and regular exercise program can support a healthy pregnancy with little or no weight gain. Ideally, overweight and obese women will achieve a healthier body weight before becoming pregnant and avoid excessive weight gain during pregnancy.[22]

Weight Gain during Pregnancy Fetal growth and maternal health depend on a sufficient weight gain during pregnancy (see Photo 15-2). Maternal weight gain during pregnancy correlates closely with infant birthweight, which is a strong predictor of the health and subsequent development of the infant.

Recommended Weight Gains Table 15-1 presents recommended weight gains for various prepregnancy weights. The recommended gain for a woman who begins pregnancy at a healthy weight and is carrying a single fetus is 25 to 35 pounds. An underweight woman needs to gain between 28 and 40 pounds; an overweight woman, between 15 and 25 pounds; and an obese woman, between 11 and 20 pounds. Table 15-1 also includes weight gain recommendations for twin births; women expecting multiples of three or more need to consult with their health care providers for weight gain guidance.

Almost 50 percent of pregnant women gain more, and about 20 percent gain less, than the recommended amount of weight gain during pregnancy—leaving roughly 30 percent gaining an appropriate amount.[23] Appropriate weight gains reduce complications, help women limit weight retention and gains after pregnancy, and help their infants prevent obesity during childhood.[24] To limit excessive weight gains, pregnant women can select foods with a high nutrient density (nutrient per kcalorie) but a low energy density (kcalorie per gram). Physical activity also plays a key role in preventing excessive weight gains during pregnancy and minimizing weight retention after the birth.

Weight-Gain Patterns For the normal-weight woman, weight gain ideally follows a pattern of 3½ pounds during the first trimester and 1 pound per week thereafter. Health-care professionals monitor weight gain using a prenatal weight-gain grid (see Figure 15-6). Identifying inadequate or excessive weight gains by the second trimester allows sufficient time for adjustments in diet and activity.

Components of Weight Gain Women often express concern about the weight gain that accompanies a healthy pregnancy. They may find comfort by remembering that most of the gain supports the growth and development of the

TABLE 15-1 Recommended Weight Gains Based on Prepregnancy Weight

	Recommended Weight Gain	
Prepregnancy Weight	**For single birth**	**For twin birth**
Underweight (BMI <18.5)	28 to 40 lb	Insufficient data to make recommendation
Healthy weight (BMI 18.5 to 24.9)	25 to 35 lb	37 to 54 lb
Overweight (BMI 25.0 to 29.9)	15 to 25 lb	31 to 50 lb
Obese (BMI ≥30)	11 to 20 lb	25 to 42 lb

SOURCE: American Congress of Obstetricians and Gynecologists, Committee on Obstetric Practice, *Weight Gain during Pregnancy*, January 2013, reaffirmed 2016.

> **FIGURE 15-6 Recommended Prenatal Weight Gain Based on Prepregnancy Weight**

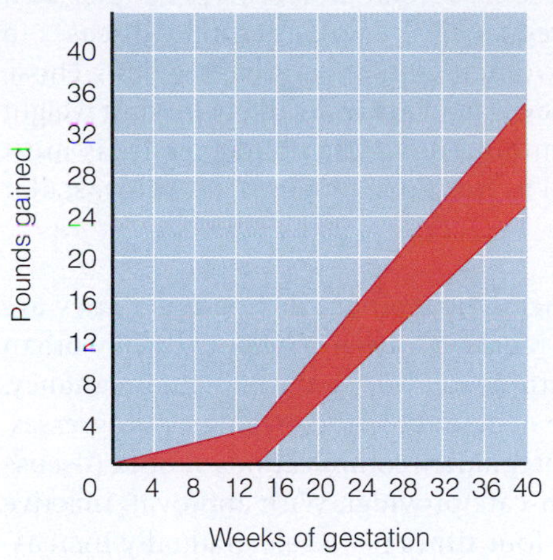

Pounds gained
40
36
32
28
24
20
16
12
8
4
0
4 8 12 16 20 24 28 32 36 40
Weeks of gestation

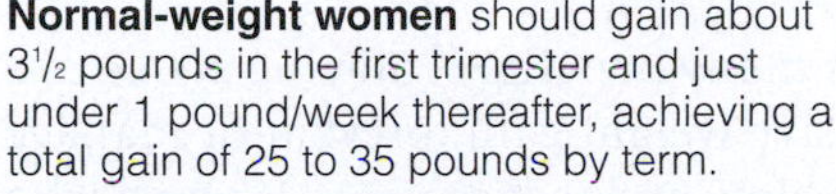

Normal-weight women should gain about 3½ pounds in the first trimester and just under 1 pound/week thereafter, achieving a total gain of 25 to 35 pounds by term.

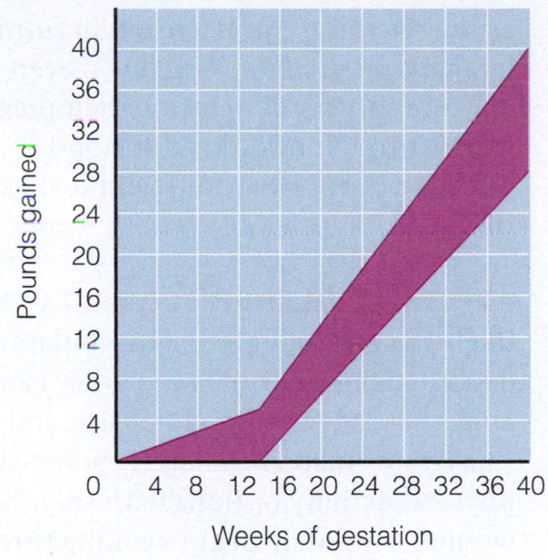

Pounds gained
40
36
32
28
24
20
16
12
8
4
0
4 8 12 16 20 24 28 32 36 40
Weeks of gestation

Underweight women should gain about 5 pounds in the first trimester and just over 1 pound/week thereafter, achieving a total gain of 28 to 40 pounds by term.

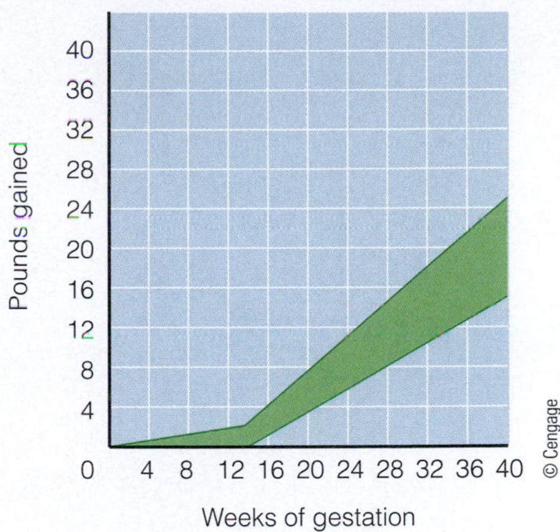

Pounds gained
40
36
32
28
24
20
16
12
8
4
0
4 8 12 16 20 24 28 32 36 40
Weeks of gestation
© Cengage

Overweight women should gain about 2 pounds in the first trimester and ⅔ pound/week thereafter, achieving a total gain of 15 to 25 pounds.

placenta, uterus, blood, and breasts, the increase in blood supply and fluid volume, as well as a healthy 7½-pound infant. A small amount goes into maternal fat stores, and even that fat has a special purpose—to provide energy for growth, labor, and lactation. Figure 15-7 shows the components of a healthy 30-pound weight gain.

Weight Loss after Pregnancy The pregnant woman loses some weight at delivery. In the following weeks, she loses more as her blood volume returns to normal and she sheds accumulated fluids. Quite likely, her goal is to return to her prepregnancy weight, but that may depend in part on whether she stayed within the pregnancy weight gain recommendations. In general, the more weight a woman gains beyond the needs of pregnancy, the more she retains and the more likely she will continue to gain over the next several years. Even with an average weight gain

> **FIGURE 15-7 Components of Weight Gain during Pregnancy**

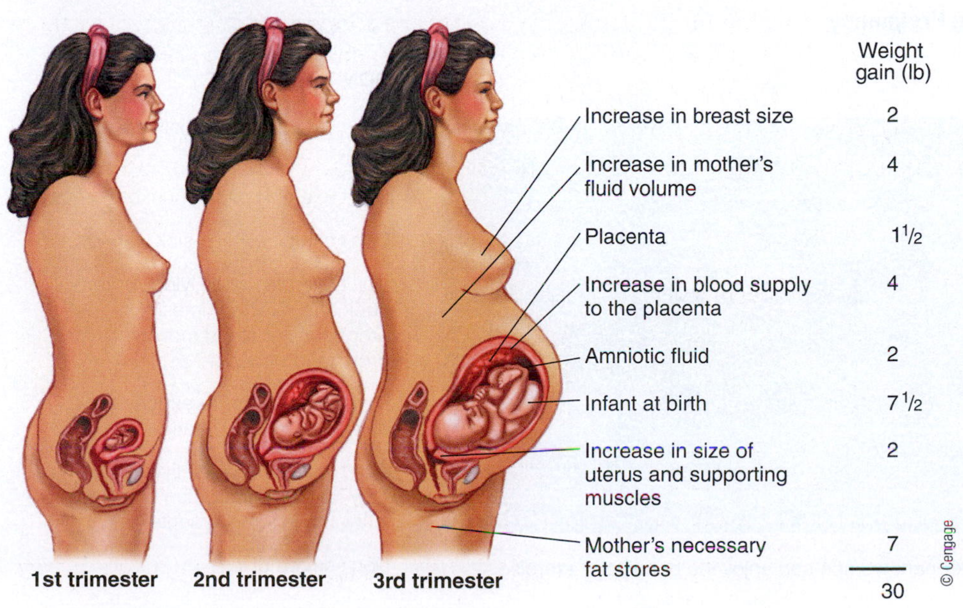

Weight gain (lb)
Increase in breast size 2
Increase in mother's fluid volume 4
Placenta 1½
Increase in blood supply to the placenta 4
Amniotic fluid 2
Infant at birth 7½
Increase in size of uterus and supporting muscles 2
Mother's necessary fat stores 7
30
1st trimester
2nd trimester
3rd trimester
© Cengage

during pregnancy, most women tend to retain a couple of pounds with each pregnancy.[25] When those couple of pounds become several more, complications such as diabetes and hypertension in future pregnancies as well as chronic diseases in later life become more likely—even for women who are not overweight. Those who are successful in losing their pregnancy weight are more likely to limit weight gains through middle adulthood.[26] A combination of diet and exercise is most effective in supporting weight loss as well as improving maternal cardiovascular fitness.[27]

Exercise during Pregnancy Women who exercise during pregnancy are likely to gain enough weight—but not too much.[28] An active, physically fit woman experiencing a normal pregnancy can continue to exercise throughout pregnancy, adjusting the duration, intensity, and type of activity as the pregnancy progresses. Inactive women and those experiencing pregnancy complications should discuss physical activity options with their health-care provider. With approval, inactive women can safely begin walking three to four times per week, gradually increasing from 25 to 40 minutes per session.[29]

Physical activity during pregnancy offers many benefits.[30] Staying active can improve cardiovascular fitness, limit excessive weight gain, prevent or manage gestational diabetes and gestational hypertension, and reduce stress. Women who exercise during pregnancy report fewer discomforts throughout their pregnancies. Regular exercise develops the strength and endurance a woman needs to carry the extra weight through pregnancy and to labor through an intense delivery. It also maintains the habits that help a woman lose excess weight and get back into shape after the birth.

A pregnant woman should participate in low-impact activities and avoid sports in which she might fall or be hit by other people or objects. For example, playing singles tennis with one person on each side of the net is safer than a fast-moving game of racquetball in which the two competitors can collide. Swimming and water aerobics are particularly beneficial because they allow the body to remain cool and move freely with the water's support, thus reducing back pain. Figure 15-8 provides some guidelines for exercise during pregnancy. Several of the guidelines are aimed at preventing excessively high internal body temperature and dehydration, both of which can harm fetal development. To this end, pregnant women should also stay out of saunas, steam rooms, and hot tubs or hot whirlpool baths.

> **FIGURE 15-8 Exercise Guidelines during Pregnancy**

DO

Do begin to exercise gradually.

Do exercise regularly (most, if not all, days of the week).

Do warm up with 5 to 10 minutes of light activity.

Do 30 minutes or more of moderate physical activity.

Do cool down with 5 to 10 minutes of slow activity and gentle stretching.

Do drink water before, after, and during exercise.

Do eat enough to support the needs of pregnancy plus exercise.

Do rest adequately.

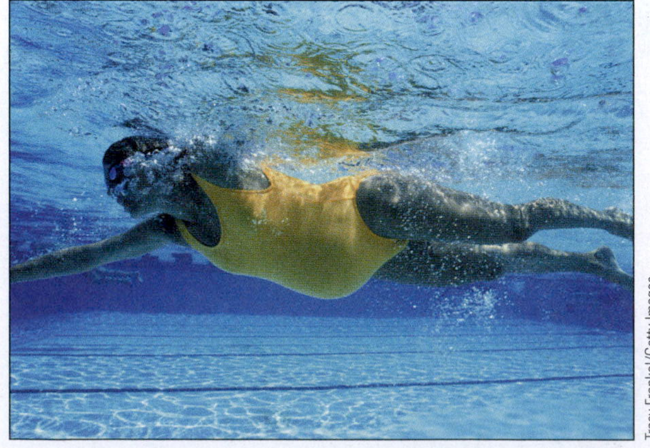

Tracy Frankel/Getty Images

Pregnant women can enjoy the benefits of exercise.

DON'T

Don't exercise vigorously after long periods of inactivity.

Don't exercise in hot, humid weather.

Don't exercise when sick with fever.

Don't exercise while lying on your back after the 1st trimester of pregnancy or stand motionless for prolonged periods.

Don't exercise if you experience any pain, discomfort, or fatigue.

Don't participate in activities that may harm the abdomen or involve jerky, bouncy movements.

Don't scuba dive.

REVIEW IT Explain how both underweight and overweight can interfere with a healthy pregnancy and how weight gain and physical activity can support maternal health and infant growth.

A healthy pregnancy depends on a sufficient weight gain. Women who begin their pregnancies at a healthy weight need to gain about 30 pounds, which covers the growth and development of the placenta, uterus, blood, breasts, and infant. By remaining active throughout pregnancy, a woman can develop the strength she needs to carry the extra weight and maintain habits that will help her lose weight after the birth.

15.4 Nutrition during Pregnancy

LEARN IT Summarize the nutrient needs of women during pregnancy.

A woman's body changes dramatically during pregnancy. Her uterus and its supporting muscles increase in size and strength; her blood volume increases by half to carry the additional nutrients and other materials; her joints become more flexible in preparation for childbirth; her feet swell in response to high concentrations of the hormone estrogen, which promotes water retention and helps ready the uterus for delivery; and her breasts enlarge in preparation for lactation. The hormones that mediate all these changes may influence her mood. She can best prepare to handle these changes given a nutritious diet, regular physical activity, plenty of rest, and caring companions. This section highlights the role of nutrition.

Eating patterns and lifestyle behaviors throughout the course of a pregnancy play key roles in supporting maternal and fetal health.[31] In general, the following guidelines will allow most women to enjoy a healthy pregnancy:

- Strive for good nutrition and health prior to pregnancy and get prenatal care during pregnancy.
- Strive for a healthy prepregnancy weight and gain an appropriate amount of weight during pregnancy.
- Eat a balanced diet, safely prepared, and engage in physical activity regularly.
- Take prenatal vitamin and mineral supplements as prescribed.
- Refrain from cigarettes, alcohol, and drugs (including herbal remedies, unless prescribed by a physician).

An adequate diet may also help a woman manage the challenges and possible depression that can arise *after* the infant arrives. Details follow.

Energy and Nutrient Needs during Pregnancy

From conception to birth, all parts of the infant—bones, muscles, blood cells, skin, and all other tissues—are made from nutrients in the foods the mother eats (see Photo 15-3). For most women, nutrient needs during pregnancy and lactation are higher than at any other time (see Figure 15-9, p. 470). Yet intakes do not consistently meet recommendations for energy and key nutrients. To meet the high nutrient demands of pregnancy, a woman will need to make careful food choices, but her body will also help by maximizing absorption and minimizing losses. The Dietary Reference Intakes (DRI) table on the insert provides separate listings for women during pregnancy and lactation, reflecting their heightened nutrient needs.

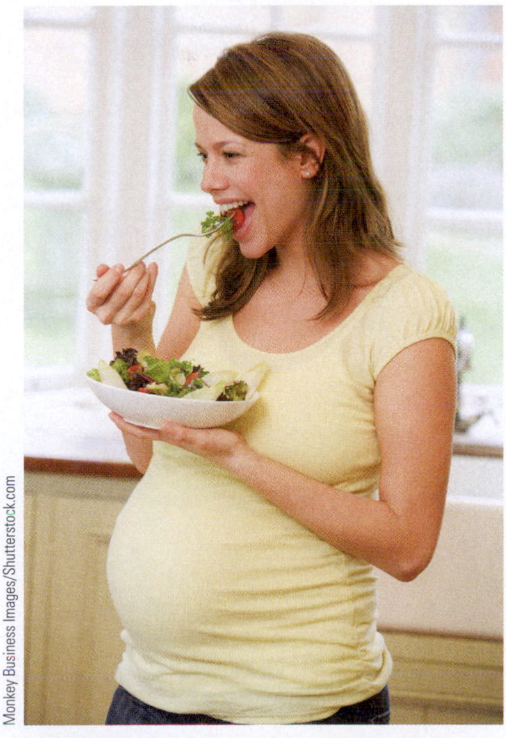
Monkey Business Images/Shutterstock.com

> **PHOTO 15-3** A pregnant woman's food choices support both her health and her infant's growth and development.

Energy The enhanced work of pregnancy raises the woman's basal metabolic rate dramatically and demands extra energy. After the first trimester, energy needs of pregnant women are greater than those of nonpregnant women—an additional 340 kcalories per day during the second trimester and an extra 450 kcalories per day during the third trimester. A woman can easily get these added kcalories with nutrient-dense selections from the five food groups. See Table 2-3 (p. 41) for suggested dietary patterns for several kcalorie levels. A sample menu for pregnant and lactating women is presented in Figure 15-10 (p. 470).

> FIGURE 15-9 Comparison of Nutrient Recommendations for Nonpregnant, Pregnant, and Lactating Women

For actual values, turn to the table on the insert (p. A). For vitamins and minerals not shown here, the values do not change for pregnant and lactating women.

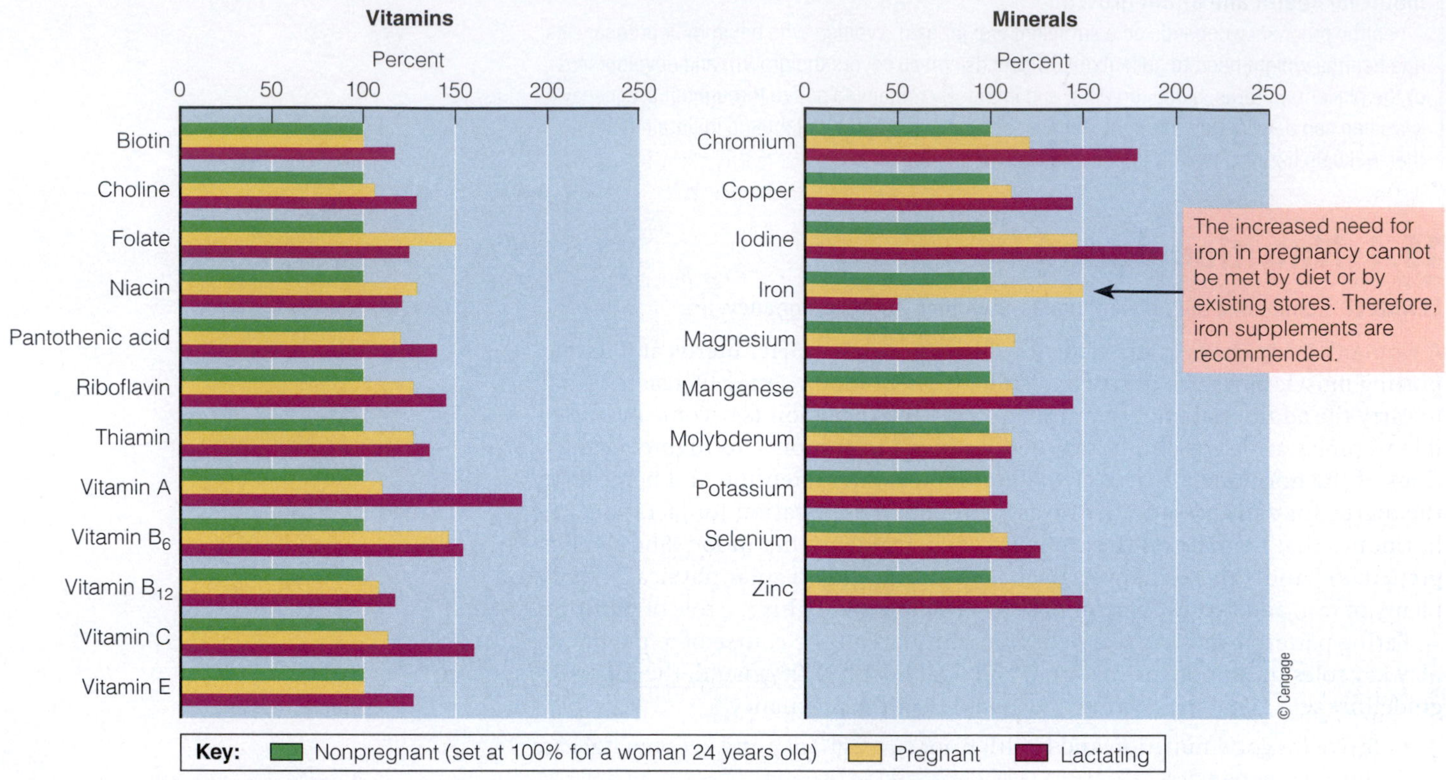

Vitamins
Percent
0
50
100
150
200
250
Biotin
Choline
Folate
Niacin
Pantothenic acid
Riboflavin
Thiamin
Vitamin A
Vitamin B6
Vitamin B12
Vitamin C
Vitamin E
Minerals
Percent
Chromium
Copper
Iodine
Iron
Magnesium
Manganese
Molybdenum
Potassium
Selenium
Zinc
The increased need for iron in pregnancy cannot be met by diet or by existing stores. Therefore, iron supplements are recommended.
© Cengage
Key: Nonpregnant (set at 100% for a woman 24 years old) Pregnant Lactating

For a 2000-kcalorie daily intake, these added kcalories represent about 15 to 20 percent more food energy than before pregnancy. The increase in nutrient needs is often greater than this, so nutrient-dense foods should be chosen to supply the extra kcalories: foods such as whole-grain breads and cereals, legumes, dark green vegetables, citrus fruits, low-fat milk and milk products, and lean meats, fish, poultry, and eggs.

> FIGURE 15-10 Daily Food Choices for Pregnant and Lactating Women

Food Group	Amount
Fruits	2 c
Vegetables	2½–3 c
Grains	6–8 oz
Protein foods	5½–6½ oz
Milk	3 c

SAMPLE MENU

Breakfast
- 1 whole-wheat English muffin
- 2 tbs peanut butter
- 1 c low-fat vanilla yogurt
- ½ c fresh strawberries
- 1 c orange juice

Midmorning snack
- ½ c cranberry juice
- 1 oz pretzels

Lunch
- Sandwich (tuna salad on whole-wheat bread)
- ½ carrot (sticks)
- 1 c low-fat milk

Dinner
- Chicken cacciatore
  - 3 oz chicken
  - ½ c stewed tomatoes
- 1 c rice
- ½ c summer squash
- 1½ c salad (spinach, mushrooms, carrots)
- 1 tbs salad dressing
- 1 slice Italian bread
- 2 tsp soft margarine
- 1 c low-fat milk

© Cengage

NOTE: The range of recommended amounts reflects the differences of the first trimester versus the second and third trimesters. This sample meal plan provides about 2500 kcalories (55% from carbohydrate, 20% from protein, and 25% from fat) and meets most of the vitamin and mineral needs of pregnant and lactating women.

Carbohydrate The RDA for carbohydrate during pregnancy is 175 grams per day to provide adequate fuel for the fetal brain. Sufficient carbohydrate also ensures that the protein needed for growth will not be broken down and used to make glucose.

Protein The protein RDA for pregnancy is an additional 25 grams per day higher than for nonpregnant women. Pregnant women can easily meet their protein needs by selecting meats, milk products, and protein-containing plant foods such as legumes, whole grains, nuts, and seeds. Because use of high-protein supplements during pregnancy may be harmful to the infant's development, it is discouraged unless medically prescribed and carefully monitored.

Essential Fatty Acids The essential long-chain polyunsaturated fatty acids are particularly important to the growth and development of the fetus. The brain is largely made of lipid material, and it depends heavily on the long-chain omega-3 fatty acids for its growth, function, and structure. Research confirms that fish consumption during pregnancy provides a rich source of omega-3 fatty acids and improves brain development and cognition in infants.[32] (See Table 5-4, p. 150, for a list of good food sources of the omega fatty acids.)

Nutrients for Blood Production and Cell Growth New cells are created at a tremendous pace as the fetus grows and develops. At the same time, the mother's red blood cell mass expands. All nutrients are important in these processes, but for folate, vitamin B_{12}, iron, and zinc, the needs are especially great because of their key roles in the synthesis of DNA and new cells.

The requirement for folate increases dramatically during pregnancy (from 400 micrograms to 600 micrograms daily). It is best to obtain sufficient folate from a combination of supplements, fortified foods, and a diet that includes fruits, juices, green vegetables, and whole grains.

The pregnant woman also has a slightly greater need for the B vitamin that activates the folate enzyme—vitamin B_{12}. Generally, even modest amounts of meat, fish, eggs, or milk products together with body stores easily meet the need for vitamin B_{12}. Vegans who exclude all foods of animal origin, however, need daily supplements of vitamin B_{12} or vitamin B_{12}–fortified foods to prevent the neurological complications of a deficiency.

Pregnant women need iron to support their increased blood volume and to provide for placental and fetal needs.[33] The developing fetus draws on maternal iron stores to create sufficient stores of its own to last through the first 4 to 6 months after birth. Ideally, a woman enters pregnancy with adequate iron stores and maintains sufficient iron nutrition throughout the pregnancy. The transfer of significant amounts of iron to the fetus is regulated by the placenta, which gives the iron needs of the fetus priority over those of the mother. Women with inadequate iron stores are left with too little iron to meet their own health needs. In addition, blood losses are inevitable at birth and can further drain the mother's iron supply.

During pregnancy, the body makes several adaptations to help meet the exceptionally high need for iron. Menstruation, the major route of iron loss in women, ceases, and iron absorption improves thanks to an increase in transferrin, the body's iron-absorbing and iron-carrying protein. Without sufficient intake, though, iron stores quickly dwindle. Women with iron-deficiency anemia are likely to give birth to low-birthweight infants.

Few women enter pregnancy with adequate iron stores, so a daily iron supplement is recommended early in pregnancy, if not before. To enhance iron absorption, the supplement should be taken between meals or at bedtime and with liquids other than milk, coffee, or tea, which inhibit iron absorption. Drinking orange juice does not enhance iron absorption from supplements as it does from foods; vitamin C enhances iron absorption by converting iron from ferric to ferrous, but supplemental iron is already in the ferrous form. Vitamin C is helpful, however, in preventing the premature rupture of amniotic membranes.

Zinc is required for DNA and RNA synthesis and thus for protein synthesis and cell development. Typical zinc intakes for pregnant women are lower than recommendations, but fortunately, zinc absorption increases when intakes are low.

Nutrients for Bone Development Vitamin D and the bone-building minerals calcium, phosphorus, magnesium, and fluoride are in great demand during pregnancy. All are needed to produce healthy fetal bones and teeth.

Vitamin D plays a central role in calcium absorption and utilization. Consequently, severe maternal vitamin D deficiency interferes with normal calcium metabolism, resulting in rickets in the infant and osteomalacia in the mother.[34] Regular exposure to sunlight and consumption of vitamin D–fortified milk are usually sufficient to provide the recommended amount of vitamin D during pregnancy, which is the same as for nonpregnant women. Pregnant women who do not receive sufficient dietary vitamin D or enough exposure to sunlight may need a supplement.

Calcium absorption and retention increases dramatically in pregnancy, helping the mother to meet the calcium needs of pregnancy. During the last trimester, as the fetal bones begin to calcify, up to 350 milligrams a day are transferred to the fetus. If the diet is inadequate in calcium, the mother's bones give up their calcium to meet fetal needs and become less dense. Recommendations to ensure an adequate calcium intake during pregnancy help conserve maternal bones while meeting fetal needs.

Calcium intakes for pregnant women typically fall below recommendations. Because bones are still actively depositing minerals until about age 30, adequate calcium is especially important for young women. Pregnant women younger than age 25 who receive less than 600 milligrams of dietary calcium daily need to increase their intake of milk, cheese, yogurt, and other calcium-rich foods. The USDA Food Patterns suggest consuming 3 cups per day of fat-free or low-fat milk or the equivalent in milk products. Alternatively, and less preferably, they may need a daily supplement of 600 milligrams of calcium, taken with meals.

Other Nutrients The nutrients mentioned here are those most intensely involved in blood production, cell growth, and bone development. Of course, other vitamins and minerals are also needed during pregnancy to support the growth and health of both fetus and mother. Even with adequate nutrition, repeated pregnancies within a short time span can deplete nutrient reserves. Short intervals between pregnancies compromise the growth of the fetus and health of the mother. The optimal interval between pregnancies is 18 to 23 months.

Nutrient Supplements A healthy pregnancy and optimal infant development depend on the mother's diet. Pregnant women who make wise food choices can meet most of their nutrient needs, with the possible exception of iron. Even so, physicians routinely recommend daily multivitamin-mineral supplements for pregnant women. Prenatal supplements typically contain greater amounts of folate, iron, and calcium than regular multivitamin-mineral supplements. These supplements are particularly beneficial for women who do not eat adequately and for those in high-risk groups: women carrying multiple fetuses, cigarette smokers, and alcohol and drug abusers.

Common Nutrition-Related Concerns of Pregnancy

Nausea, constipation, heartburn, and food sensitivities are common nutrition-related concerns during pregnancy. A few simple strategies can help alleviate maternal discomforts (see Table 15-2).

Nausea and Vomiting Not all women have queasy stomachs in the early months of pregnancy, but many do. The nausea of "morning sickness" may actually occur anytime and ranges from mild queasiness to debilitating nausea and vomiting. Severe and continued vomiting may require hospitalization if it results in acidosis,

TABLE 15-2 Strategies to Alleviate Maternal Discomforts

To Alleviate the Nausea of Pregnancy	To Prevent or Alleviate Constipation	To Prevent or Relieve Heartburn
• On waking, arise slowly. • Eat dry toast or crackers. • Chew gum or suck hard candies. • Eat small, frequent meals. • Avoid foods with offensive odors. • When nauseated, drink carbonated beverages instead of citrus juice, water, milk, coffee, or tea.	• Eat foods high in fiber (fruits, vegetables, and whole grains). • Exercise regularly. • Drink at least eight glasses of liquids a day. • Respond promptly to the urge to defecate. • Use laxatives only as prescribed by a physician; do not use mineral oil, because it interferes with absorption of fat-soluble vitamins.	• Relax and eat slowly. • Chew food thoroughly. • Eat small, frequent meals. • Drink liquids between meals. • Avoid spicy or greasy foods. • Sit up while eating; elevate the head while sleeping. • Wait 3 hours after eating before lying down. • Wait 2 hours after eating before exercising.

dehydration, or excessive weight loss. Physicians also need to determine whether the nausea and vomiting might be related to other causes.[35]

The hormonal changes of early pregnancy seem to be responsible for a woman's sensitivities to the appearance, texture, or smell of foods. The problem typically peaks at 9 weeks of gestation and resolves within a month or two. Traditional strategies for quelling nausea may be effective and are listed in Table 15-2, but there is little evidence to support such advice.[36] Limited evidence suggests that vitamin B_6 may have an anti-nausea effect.[37] In general, women may benefit most from simply resting when nauseous and eating the foods they want when they feel like eating. They may also find comfort in a clean, quiet, and temperate environment.

Constipation and Hemorrhoids As the hormones of pregnancy alter muscle tone and the growing fetus crowds intestinal organs, an expectant mother may experience constipation. She may also develop hemorrhoids (swollen veins of the rectum). Hemorrhoids can be painful, and straining during bowel movements may cause bleeding. She can gain relief by following the strategies listed in Table 15-2.

Heartburn Heartburn is another common complaint during pregnancy. The hormones of pregnancy relax the digestive muscles, and the growing fetus puts increasing pressure on the mother's stomach. This combination causes gastroesophageal reflux, the painful sensation a person feels when stomach acid splashes back up into the lower esophagus (see Highlight 3, pp. 91–92). Tips to help relieve heartburn are included in Table 15-2.

Food Cravings and Aversions Some women develop cravings for, or aversions to, particular foods and beverages during pregnancy. **Food cravings** and **food aversions** are fairly common, but they do not seem to reflect real physiological needs. In other words, a woman who craves pickles does not necessarily need salt. Similarly, cravings for ice cream are common in pregnancy but do not signify a calcium deficiency. Cravings and aversions that arise during pregnancy are most likely due to hormone-induced changes in sensitivity to taste and smell.

Nonfood Cravings Some pregnant women develop cravings for nonfood items such as freezer frost, laundry starch, clay, soil, or ice—a practice known as **pica**. Pica is a cultural phenomenon that reflects a society's folklore; it is especially common among African American women. Pica is often associated with iron-deficiency anemia, but whether iron deficiency leads to pica or pica leads to iron deficiency is unclear. Eating clay or soil may interfere with iron absorption and displace iron-rich foods from the diet.

REVIEW IT Summarize the nutrient needs of women during pregnancy.

Energy and nutrient needs are high during pregnancy. A balanced diet that includes an extra serving from each of the five food groups can usually meet these needs, with the possible exception of iron and folate (supplements are recommended). The nausea, constipation, and heartburn that sometimes accompany pregnancy can usually be alleviated with a few simple strategies. Food cravings do not typically reflect physiological needs.

food cravings: strong desires to eat particular foods.

food aversions: strong desires to avoid particular foods.

pica (PIE-ka): a craving for and consumption of nonfood substances. Pica is known as *geophagia* (gee-oh-FAY-gee-uh) when referring to eating clay, baby powder, chalk, ash, ceramics, paper, paint chips, or charcoal; *pagophagia* (pag-oh-FAY-gee-uh) when referring to eating large quantities of ice; and *amylophagia* (AM-ee-low-FAY-gee-ah) when referring to eating uncooked starch (flour, laundry starch, or raw rice).

15.5 High-Risk Pregnancies

LEARN IT Identify factors predicting low-risk and high-risk pregnancies and describe ways to manage them.

Some pregnancies jeopardize the life and health of the mother and infant. Each year in the United States, more than 5000 women die during or within a year of pregnancy and more than 20,000 infants die within their first year.[38] Table 15-3 identifies several risk factors for a **high-risk pregnancy.** A woman with none of these risk factors is said to have a **low-risk pregnancy.** The more factors that apply, the higher the risk. All pregnant women, especially those in high-risk categories, need prenatal medical care, including the following nutrition advice:

- Eat well-balanced meals.
- Gain enough weight to support fetal growth.
- Take prenatal supplements as prescribed.
- Stop drinking alcohol.

The Infant's Birthweight

A high-risk pregnancy is likely to produce an infant with **low birthweight (LBW).** Low-birthweight infants, defined as infants who weigh 5½ pounds or less, are classified according to their gestational age. Preterm infants are born before they are fully developed; they are often underweight and have trouble breathing because their lungs are immature. Preterm infants may be small, but if their size and weight are appropriate for their gestational age, they can catch up in growth given adequate nutrition support. In contrast, small-for-gestational-age infants have suffered growth failure in the uterus and do not catch up as well. For the most part, survival improves with increased gestational age and birthweight.

Low-birthweight infants are more likely to experience complications during delivery than normal-weight babies. They also have a statistically greater chance of

TABLE 15-3 High-Risk Pregnancy Factors

Factor	Condition that Raises Risk
Maternal weight	
• Prior to pregnancy	Prepregnancy BMI either <18.5 or ≥ 25
• During pregnancy	Insufficient or excessive pregnancy weight gain (see Table 15-1, p. 466)
Previous pregnancies	
• Number	Many previous pregnancies (3 or more to mothers younger than age 20; 4 or more to mothers age 20 or older)
• Interval	Short or long intervals between pregnancies (<18 months or >59 months)
• Outcomes	Previous history of problems
• Multiple births	Twins or triplets
• Birthweight	Low- or high-birthweight infants
Maternal health	
• High blood pressure	Development of gestational hypertension
• Diabetes	Development of gestational diabetes
• Chronic diseases	Diabetes; heart, respiratory, and kidney disease; certain genetic disorders; special diets and medications
Maternal nutrition	Nutrient deficiencies or toxicities; eating disorders
Socioeconomic status	Poverty, lack of family support, low level of education, limited food availability
Lifestyle habits	Smoking, alcohol or other drug use
Age	Teens, especially 15 years or younger; women 35 years or older

high-risk pregnancy: a pregnancy characterized by risk factors that make it likely the birth will be surrounded by problems such as premature delivery, difficult birth, restricted growth, birth defects, and early infant death.

low-risk pregnancy: a pregnancy characterized by factors that make it likely the birth will be normal and the infant healthy.

low birthweight (LBW): a birthweight of 5½ pounds (2500 grams) or less; indicates probable poor health in the newborn and poor nutrition status in the mother during pregnancy, before pregnancy, or both. Optimal birthweight for a full-term baby is about 6½ to 8 pounds.

having physical and mental birth defects, becoming ill, and dying early in life (see Photo 15-4). Of infants who die before their first birthdays, about two-thirds were low-birthweight newborns. Very-low-birthweight infants (3½ pounds or less) struggle not only for their immediate physical health and survival, but for their future cognitive development and abilities as well.

A strong association is seen between socioeconomic disadvantage and low birthweight. Low socioeconomic status impairs fetal development by causing stress and by limiting access to medical care and nutritious foods. Low socioeconomic status often accompanies teen pregnancies, smoking, and alcohol and drug abuse—all predictors of low birthweight.

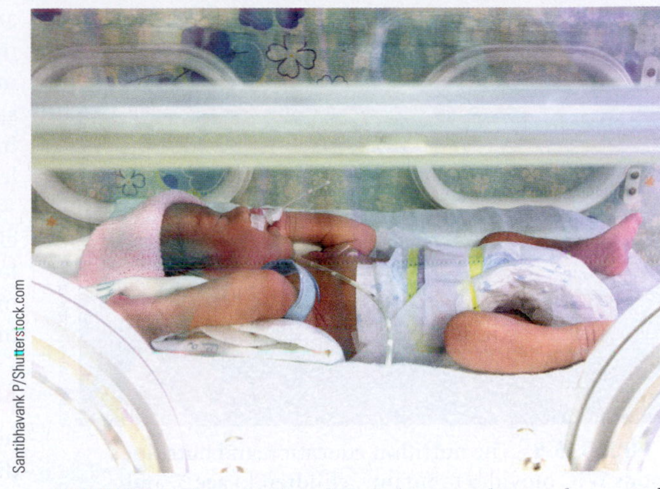

Santibhavank P/Shutterstock.com

> **PHOTO 15-4** Low-birthweight babies need special care and nourishment.

Malnutrition and Pregnancy Good nutrition clearly supports a healthy pregnancy. In contrast, malnutrition interferes with the ability to conceive, the likelihood of implantation, and the subsequent development of a fetus should conception and implantation occur.

Malnutrition and Fertility The nutrition habits and lifestyle choices people make can influence the course of a pregnancy they are not even planning at the time. Inadequate nutrition and food deprivation can reduce fertility. Women may develop amenorrhea—the temporary or permanent absence of menstrual periods.* Men who are poorly nourished may be unable to produce viable sperm. Furthermore, both men and women lose sexual interest during times of starvation. Starvation arises predictably during famines, wars, and droughts, but it can also occur amid peace and plenty. Many young adults with anorexia nervosa are starving and suffering from malnutrition (see Highlight 8, p. 254).

Malnutrition and Early Pregnancy If a poorly nourished woman does become pregnant, she faces the challenge of supporting both the growth of a baby and her own health with inadequate nutrient stores. Inadequate nutrition prior to and around conception prevents the placenta from developing fully. A poorly developed placenta cannot deliver optimal nourishment to the fetus, and the infant will be born small and possibly with physical and cognitive abnormalities. If this small infant is a female, she may develop poorly and have an elevated risk of developing a chronic condition that could impair her ability to give birth to a healthy infant. Thus a woman's poor nutrition status can adversely affect not only her children but also her *grandchildren*.

Malnutrition and Fetal Development Without adequate nutrition during pregnancy, fetal growth and infant health are compromised. In general, consequences of inadequate nutrition during pregnancy include fetal growth restriction, congenital malformations (birth defects), spontaneous abortion and stillbirth, preterm birth, and low infant birthweight. Malnutrition is responsible for almost half of all deaths of children younger than 5 years of age worldwide; almost half of these deaths occur in the first month of life.[39]

Food Assistance Programs Women in high-risk pregnancies can find assistance from the WIC program—a high-quality, cost-effective health-care and nutrition services program for women, infants, and children in the United States. Formally known as the Special Supplemental Nutrition Program for Women, Infants, and Children, WIC provides nutrition education and nutritious foods to infants, children to age 5, and pregnant and breastfeeding women who qualify financially and have a high risk of medical or nutritional problems. The program is both remedial and preventive: services include health-care referrals, nutrition education,

*Amenorrhea is normal before puberty, after menopause, during pregnancy, and during lactation; otherwise it is abnormal.

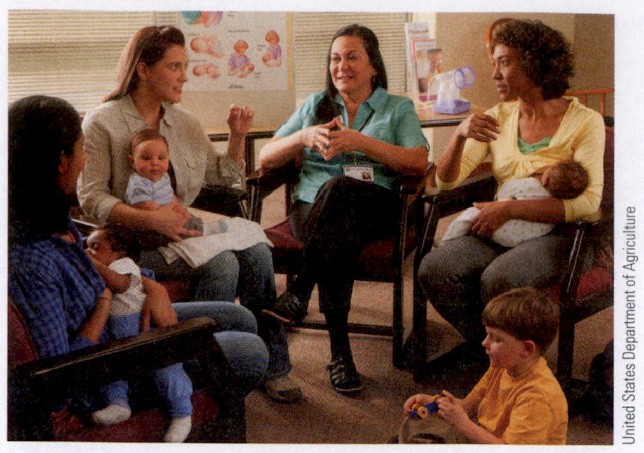
United States Department of Agriculture

> **PHOTO 15-5** The nutrition education and nutritious foods WIC provides to infants, children to age 5, and pregnant and breastfeeding women improves health and saves lives.

and food packages or vouchers for specific foods. These foods supply nutrients known to be lacking in the diets of the target population—most notably, protein, calcium, iron, vitamin A, and vitamin C. WIC-sponsored foods include tuna, tofu, fruits, vegetables, eggs, milk, iron-fortified cereal, whole-grain breads, vitamin C–rich juices, cheeses, legumes, peanut butter, and iron-fortified infant formula and cereal.

More than 8 million mothers and young children receive WIC benefits each month (see Photo 15-5). Prenatal WIC participation can effectively reduce iron deficiency, infant mortality, low birthweight, and maternal and newborn medical costs. Table 15-4 presents some of the many benefits of WIC.

TABLE 15-4 Benefits of WIC

- Earlier prenatal care
- Better diet during pregnancy
- Better weight gain during pregnancy
- Longer duration of pregnancy
- Fewer fetal and infant deaths
- Fewer low-birthweight infants
- Better growth in infants and children
- Less iron-deficiency anemia in children
- Better diet for children
- Better medical care for children
- Better preparation for school
- Improved intellectual development

© Cengage

Maternal Health

Medical disorders can threaten the life and health of both mother and fetus. If diagnosed and treated early, many diseases can be managed to ensure a healthy outcome—another strong argument for early prenatal care. Furthermore, the changes in pregnancy can reveal disease risks, making screening important and early intervention possible.

Preexisting Diabetes The risks of diabetes depend on how well it is managed before and during pregnancy. Without proper management of maternal diabetes, women face high infertility rates, and those who do conceive may experience episodes of severe hypoglycemia or hyperglycemia, preterm labor, and pregnancy-related hypertension. Infants may be large, suffer physical and mental abnormalities, and experience other complications such as severe hypoglycemia or respiratory distress, both of which can be fatal.[40] Signs of fetal health problems are apparent even when maternal glucose is above normal but still below the diagnosis of diabetes. To minimize complications, a woman needs to achieve glucose control before conception and continued glucose control throughout pregnancy.

Gestational Diabetes An estimated 9 percent of pregnancies in the United States are complicated by a condition known as **gestational diabetes.**[41] Gestational diabetes usually develops during the second half of pregnancy, with subsequent return to normal after childbirth. Up to half of the women with gestational diabetes, however, develop type 2 diabetes after pregnancy, especially if they are overweight.[42] For this reason, health-care professionals strongly advise against excessive weight gain during—and after—pregnancy. Weight gains after pregnancy increase the risk of gestational diabetes in the next pregnancy.

The most common consequences of gestational diabetes are complications during labor and delivery and a high birthweight infant. Birth defects associated with gestational diabetes include heart damage, limb deformities, and neural tube defects. To ensure that the problems of gestational diabetes are dealt with promptly, physicians screen for the risk factors listed in Table 15-5 and test high-risk women for glucose intolerance immediately and average-risk women between 24 and 28 weeks gestation.

TABLE 15-5 Risk Factors for Gestational Diabetes

- Age 25 or older
- BMI ≥25 or excessive weight gain
- Complications in previous pregnancies, including gestational diabetes or high-birthweight infant (>9 lb)
- Prediabetes or symptoms of diabetes
- Family history of type 2 diabetes
- Hispanic, African American, Native American, Asian, Pacific Islander

© Cengage

Dietary recommendations should meet the needs of pregnancy and control maternal blood glucose. Diet and moderate exercise may manage gestational diabetes, but if blood glucose fails to normalize, insulin or other drugs may be required. Importantly, treatment reduces preeclampsia, birth complications, large newborns, and infant deaths.[43]

Chronic Hypertension Hypertension complicates pregnancy and affects its outcome in different ways, depending on when the hypertension first develops and on how severe it becomes. In addition to the threats hypertension always carries (such as heart attack and stroke), high blood pressure increases the risks of fetal growth restriction, preterm birth, and separation of the placenta from the wall of the uterus before the birth, resulting in stillbirth. To minimize complications, blood pressure needs to be monitored and managed before and during pregnancy.[44]

gestational diabetes: glucose intolerance with onset or first recognition during pregnancy.

Gestational Hypertension Women with chronic hypertension have a greater likelihood of developing **gestational hypertension**—high blood pressure during the second half of pregnancy.* For some women with gestational hypertension, the rise in blood pressure is mild and does not affect the pregnancy adversely. Blood pressure usually returns to normal during the first few weeks after childbirth. For others, gestational hypertension increases the risks of subsequent hypertension and heart disorders.[45] Gestational hypertension is also an early sign of the most serious maternal complication of pregnancy—preeclampsia.

Preeclampsia **Preeclampsia** is a condition characterized not only by gestational hypertension but also by protein in the urine. Table 15-6 presents the signs and symptoms of preeclampsia. The cause of preeclampsia remains unclear, but it usually occurs with first pregnancies and most often after 20 weeks of gestation. Obesity may increase the risk.[46] Symptoms typically regress within 2 days of delivery. Both men and women who were born of pregnancies complicated by preeclampsia are more likely to have a child born of a pregnancy complicated by preeclampsia, suggesting a genetic predisposition. Black women have a high risk of preeclampsia.

Preeclampsia dramatically affects the mother's body—the circulatory system, liver, kidneys, and brain. Blood flow through the vessels that supply oxygen and nutrients to the placenta diminishes. For this reason, preeclampsia often restricts fetal growth. It also seems to increase the risk of heart defects for the infant.[47] In some cases, the placenta separates from the uterus, resulting in preterm birth or stillbirth.

Preeclampsia can progress rapidly to **eclampsia**—a condition characterized by seizures and coma. Maternal death during pregnancy and childbirth is rare in developed countries, but when it does occur, eclampsia is a common cause. The rate of death for black women with eclampsia is more than two to three times the rate for white women.

Preeclampsia demands prompt medical attention. Treatment focuses on controlling blood pressure and preventing seizures. If preeclampsia develops early and is severe, induced labor or cesarean delivery may be necessary, regardless of gestational age. The infant will be preterm, with all of the associated problems, including poor lung development and special care needs. Several dietary factors have been studied, but none have proved beneficial in preventing preeclampsia.

TABLE 15-6 Signs and Symptoms of Preeclampsia

- Hypertension
- Protein in the urine
- Upper abdominal pain
- Severe headaches
- Swelling of hands, feet, and face
- Vomiting
- Blurred vision
- Sudden weight gain (1 lb/day)
- Fetal growth restriction

The Mother's Age

Maternal age also influences the course of a pregnancy. Compared with women of the physically ideal childbearing age of 20 to 25, both younger and older women face more complications of pregnancy.

Pregnancy in Adolescents About one third of adolescents are sexually active. Almost 250,000 adolescent girls give birth each year in the United States; one out of six of them already have at least one child.[48] Nourishing a growing fetus adds to a teenage girl's nutrition burden, especially if her growth is still incomplete. Simply being young and physically immature increases the risks of pregnancy complications. Pregnant teens are less likely to receive early prenatal care and are more likely to smoke during pregnancy—two factors that predict low birthweight and infant death.

The typical energy-dense, but nutrient-poor diet of pregnant adolescents increases the risk of low-birthweight infants. Common complications among adolescent mothers include iron-deficiency anemia (which may reflect poor diet and inadequate prenatal care) and prolonged labor (which reflects the mother's physical immaturity). On a positive note, maternal death is lowest for mothers younger than age 20.

The rates of stillbirths, preterm births, and low-birthweight infants are high for teenagers—both for teen moms and for teen dads. Many of these infants

*Blood pressure of 140/90 millimeters of mercury or greater during the second half of pregnancy in a woman who has not previously exhibited hypertension indicates high blood pressure.

gestational hypertension: high blood pressure that develops in the second half of pregnancy and resolves after childbirth, usually without affecting the outcome of the pregnancy.

preeclampsia (PRE-ee-KLAMP-see-ah): a condition characterized by high blood pressure and some protein in the urine.

eclampsia (eh-KLAMP-see-ah): a condition characterized by extremely high blood pressure, elevated protein in the urine, seizures, and possibly coma.

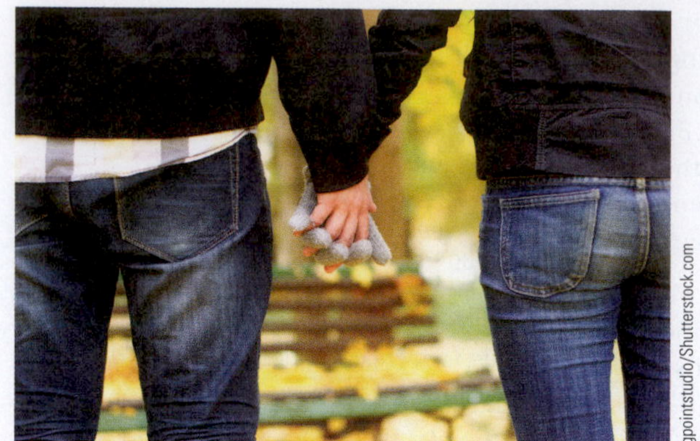
gpointstudio/Shutterstock.com

> **PHOTO 15-6** Pregnancy during the teen years has major health, emotional, social, and financial consequences for young mothers and their children.

suffer physical problems, require intensive care, and die within the first year. The care of teen mothers and their infants costs our society billions of dollars annually. Because teenagers have few financial resources, they cannot pay these costs. Furthermore, their low economic status contributes significantly to the complications surrounding their pregnancies. At a time when prenatal care is most important, it is less accessible. And the pattern of teenage pregnancies continues from generation to generation, with daughters of teenage mothers more likely to become teenage mothers themselves. Clearly, teenage pregnancy is a major public health problem (see Photo 15-6).

To support the needs of both mother and fetus, young teenagers (13 to 16 years old) are encouraged to strive for the highest weight gains recommended for pregnancy (review Table 15-1, p. 466). For a teen who enters pregnancy at a healthy body weight, a weight gain of approximately 35 pounds is recommended; this amount minimizes the risk of delivering a low-birthweight infant. Pregnant and lactating teenagers can use the food patterns presented in Table 2-3 (p. 41), making sure to select a high enough kcalorie level to support adequate weight gain.

Without the appropriate economic, social, and physical support, a young mother will not be able to care for herself during her pregnancy and for her child after the birth. To improve her chances for a successful pregnancy and a healthy infant, she must seek prenatal care. WIC provides health-care referrals and helps pregnant teenagers obtain adequate food for themselves and their infants. (WIC is introduced on pp. 475–476.)

Pregnancy in Older Women In the past several decades, many women have delayed childbearing while they pursue education and careers. As a result, the number of first births to women 35 and older has increased dramatically. Most of these women, even those older than age 50, have healthy pregnancies.

The few complications associated with later childbearing often reflect chronic conditions such as hypertension and diabetes, which can complicate an otherwise healthy pregnancy. These complications may result in a cesarean delivery, which is twice as common in women older than 35 as among younger women. For all these reasons, maternal death rates are higher in women older than 35 than in younger women.

Infants of older mothers face problems of their own, including higher rates of preterm births and low birthweight. Their rates of birth defects are also high. Because 1 out of 50 pregnancies in older women produces an infant with genetic abnormalities, obstetricians routinely screen women older than 35. For a 40-year-old mother, the risk of having a child with **Down syndrome**, for example, is about 1 in 100 compared with 1 in 300 for a 35-year-old and 1 in 10,000 for a 20-year-old. In addition, fetal death is twice as high for women 35 years and older than for younger women. Why this is so remains unclear. One possibility is that the uterine blood vessels of older women may not fully adapt to the increased demands of pregnancy.

Practices Incompatible with Pregnancy

Besides malnutrition, a variety of lifestyle factors can have adverse effects on pregnancy, and some may be **teratogenic**, causing abnormal fetal development and birth defects. By practicing healthy behaviors, people who are planning to have children can reduce the risks.

Alcohol About 10 percent of pregnant women drink alcohol.[49] Alcohol consumption during pregnancy can cause the irreversible mental and physical disorders known as fetal alcohol syndrome (FAS). Of the leading causes of mental disabilities, FAS is the only one that is totally *preventable*. To that end, the surgeon general urges all pregnant women to refrain from drinking alcohol. Fetal alcohol syndrome is the topic of Highlight 15, which includes mention of how alcohol

Down syndrome: a genetic abnormality that causes mental impairment, short stature, and flattened facial features.

teratogenic (ter-AT-oh-jen-ik): causing abnormal fetal development and birth defects.

consumption by men may also affect fertility and fetal development. In addition to fetal alcohol syndrome, maternal alcohol use has been associated with sudden infant death syndrome (SIDS) and other life-threatening disorders.[50]

Medicinal Drugs Drugs other than alcohol can also cause complications in the pregnancy and birth defects in the infant. For these reasons, pregnant women should not take any medicines without consulting their physicians, who must weigh the benefits against the risks.

Herbal Supplements Similarly, pregnant women should seek a physician's advice before using herbal supplements. Women sometimes seek herbal preparations during their pregnancies to quell nausea, induce labor, aid digestion, promote water loss, support restful sleep, and fight depression. As Highlight 18 explains, some herbs may be safe, but others may be harmful.

Illicit Drugs The recommendation to avoid drugs during pregnancy also includes illicit drugs, of course. Unfortunately, use of illicit drugs, such as cocaine, methamphetamine, and marijuana, is common among some pregnant women.[51]

Drugs of abuse, such as cocaine, can damage the placenta and impair fetal growth and development.[52] Furthermore, they are responsible for preterm births, low-birthweight infants, **perinatal** deaths, and sudden infant deaths. If these newborns survive, central nervous system damage is evident: their cries, sleep, and behaviors early in life are abnormal, and their cognitive development later in life is impaired. They may be hypersensitive or underaroused; many suffer the symptoms of withdrawal. Their growth and development throughout childhood and adolescence continues to be delayed.[53]

Smoking and Chewing Tobacco Unfortunately, an estimated 10 percent of pregnant women in the United States smoke.[54] Smoking cigarettes or chewing tobacco at any time exerts harmful effects, and pregnancy dramatically magnifies the hazards of these practices. Smoking restricts the blood supply to the growing fetus and thus limits oxygen and nutrient delivery and waste removal. A mother who smokes is more likely to have a complicated birth and a preterm or low-birthweight infant. Indeed, of all preventable causes of low birthweight in the United States, smoking is at the top of the list. Although most infants born to cigarette smokers are low birthweight, some are not, suggesting that the effect of smoking on birthweight also depends, in part, on genes involved in the metabolism of smoking toxins.

In addition to contributing to low birthweight, smoking interferes with organ growth and arterial structure and function; consequently, it increases the risks of heart, lung, and kidney defects.[55] It can also cause death in an otherwise healthy fetus or newborn. Both cigarette smoking during pregnancy and infant exposure to secondhand smoke increase the risk of **sudden infant death syndrome (SIDS)**.[56] Smoking during pregnancy may reduce brain size and impair the intellectual and behavioral development of the child later in life. Table 15-7 lists complications of smoking during pregnancy.

Alternatives to smoking—such as e-cigarettes and nicotine replacement therapies—still deliver nicotine and can harm the developing fetus.[57] Research on the safety of these products during pregnancy is limited, but why take the risk? No amount of nicotine is known to be safe.[58] Any woman who uses nicotine in any form and is considering pregnancy or who is already pregnant needs to quit. Avoiding secondhand smoke is also advised.

Environmental Contaminants Proving that environmental contaminants cause reproductive damage is difficult, but evidence in wildlife is established and seems likely for human beings. Infants and young children of pregnant women exposed to environmental contaminants such as lead show signs of delayed mental and psychomotor development. During pregnancy, lead readily crosses into the placenta, inflicting severe damage on the developing fetal nervous system. In

TABLE 15-7 Complications Associated with Smoking during Pregnancy

- Fetal growth restriction
- Preterm birth
- Low birthweight
- Premature separation of the placenta
- Miscarriage
- Stillbirth
- Sudden infant death syndrome (SIDS)
- Congenital malformations

perinatal: referring to the time between the twenty-eighth week of gestation and 1 month after birth.

sudden infant death syndrome (SIDS): the unexpected and unexplained death of an apparently well infant; the most common cause of death of infants between the second week and the end of the first year of life; also called *crib death*.

TABLE 15-8 Advice for Pregnant (and Lactating) Women Eating Fish

Best choices Eat 2–3 servings/week	Anchovy, Atlantic croaker, Atlantic mackerel, black sea bass, butterfish, catfish, clam, cod, crab, crawfish, flounder, haddock, hake, herring, lobster, mullet, oyster, Pacific chub mackerel, perch, pickerel, plaice, pollock, salmon, sardine, scallop, shad, shrimp, skate, smelt, sole, squid, tilapia, trout, tuna (canned light), whitefish, whiting
Good choices Eat 1 serving/week	Atlantic tilefish, bluefish, buffalo fish, carp, Chilean sea bass, grouper, halibut, mahi mahi, monkfish, Pacific croaker, rockfish, sablefish, sea trout, sheepshead, snapper, Spanish mackerel, striped bass, tuna (yellowfin and albacore, white tuna, canned and fresh/frozen), white croaker
Poor choices Avoid eating	King mackerel, marlin, orange roughy, shark, swordfish, Gulf of Mexico tilefish, tuna (bigeye)

TABLE 15-9 Tips to Prevent Listeriosis

- Use only pasteurized juices and dairy products; do not eat soft cheeses such as feta, brie, Camembert, Panela, "queso blanco," "queso fresco," and blue-veined cheeses such as Roquefort; do not drink raw (unpasteurized) milk or eat foods that contain it.
- Thoroughly cook meat, poultry, eggs, and seafood.
- Do not eat hot dogs or luncheon meats unless heated until steaming hot.
- Wash all fruits and vegetables.
- Do not eat refrigerated pâtés or meat spreads.
- Do not eat refrigerated smoked seafood such as salmon or trout, or any fish labeled "nova," "lox," or "kippered," unless prepared in a cooked dish.

addition, infants exposed to even low levels of lead during gestation weigh less at birth and consequently struggle to survive. For these reasons, it is particularly important that pregnant women receive foods and beverages grown and prepared in environments free of contamination.

Mercury is another contaminant of concern. As Chapter 5 mentioned, fatty fish are a good source of omega-3 fatty acids, but some fish contain large amounts of the pollutant mercury, which can impair fetal growth and harm the developing brain and nervous system. Because the benefits of seafood consumption seem to outweigh the risks, pregnant (and lactating) women need reliable information on which fish are both high in omega-3 fatty acids and low in mercury (see Table 15-8).

Foodborne Illness As Chapter 19 explains, foodborne illnesses arise when people eat foods that contain infectious microbes or microbes that produce toxins. At best, the vomiting and diarrhea associated with these illnesses can leave a pregnant woman exhausted and dehydrated; at worst, foodborne illnesses can cause meningitis, pneumonia, or even fetal death. Pregnant women are about 20 times more likely than other healthy adults to get the foodborne illness **listeriosis.** Table 15-9 presents tips to prevent listeriosis; Chapter 19 includes precautions to minimize the risks of other common foodborne illnesses.

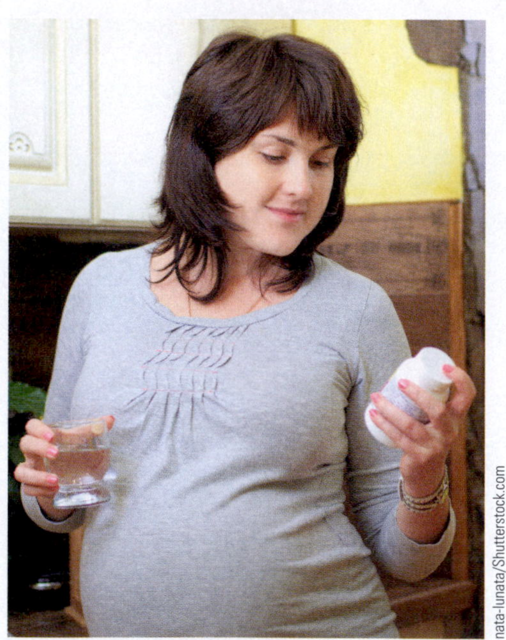

> **PHOTO 15-7** Prenatal dietary supplements may be beneficial, but megadoses can be toxic.

listeriosis (lis-TEAR-ee-OH-sis): an infection caused by eating food contaminated with the bacterium *Listeria monocytogenes,* which can be killed by pasteurization and cooking but can survive at refrigerated temperatures; certain ready-to-eat foods, such as hot dogs and deli meats, may become contaminated after cooking or processing, but before packaging.

Vitamin-Mineral Megadoses Pregnant women who are trying to eat well may mistakenly assume that more is better when it comes to multivitamin-mineral supplements. This is simply not true; excessive vitamin and mineral supplementation during pregnancy can be harmful.[59] Excessive vitamin A is particularly infamous for its role in fetal malformations. Intakes before the seventh week appear to be the most damaging. (Review Figure 15-4, p. 462, to see how many tissues are in their critical periods prior to the seventh week.) For this reason, vitamin A supplements are not given during pregnancy unless there is specific evidence of deficiency, which is rare. A pregnant woman can obtain all the vitamin A and most of the other vitamins and minerals she needs by making wise food choices. She should take supplements only on the advice of a registered dietitian nutritionist or physician (see Photo 15-7).

Caffeine Caffeine crosses the placenta, and the developing fetus has a limited ability to metabolize it. Research studies have not proved that caffeine (even in high doses) causes birth defects or preterm births in human infants (as it does in animals), but limited evidence suggests that heavy use increases the risk of miscarriage and low birthweight.[60] Lower doses of caffeine—say, at levels equivalent to 1 to 2 cups of coffee a day—appear to be compatible with healthy pregnancies.[61]

Restrictive Dieting Restrictive dieting, even for short periods, can be hazardous during pregnancy. Low-carbohydrate diets or fasts that cause ketosis deprive the fetal brain of needed glucose and may impair cognitive development. Such diets are also likely to lack other nutrients vital to fetal growth. Regardless of prepregnancy weight, pregnant women need an adequate diet to support healthy fetal development.

Sugar Substitutes Artificial sweeteners have been approved by the FDA and are generally considered safe to use during pregnancy.[62] Advice to pregnant women includes a caution to use sweeteners in moderation, if at all, and within an otherwise nutritious and well-balanced diet. Women with the inherited disease phenylketonuria (PKU) should not use the artificial sweetener aspartame. Aspartame contains the amino acid phenylalanine, and people with PKU are unable to dispose of any excess phenylalanine. The accumulation of phenylalanine and its by-products is toxic to the developing nervous system, causing irreversible brain damage.

REVIEW IT Identify factors predicting low-risk and high-risk pregnancies and describe ways to manage them.

High-risk pregnancies, especially for teenagers, threaten the life and health of both mother and infant. Proper nutrition and abstinence from smoking, alcohol, and other drugs improve the outcome. In addition, prenatal care includes monitoring pregnant women for gestational diabetes, gestational hypertension, and preeclampsia.

15.6 Nutrition during Lactation

LEARN IT Summarize the nutrient needs of women during lactation.

Childbirth marks the end of pregnancy and the beginning of a new set of parental responsibilities—including feeding the newborn. Before the end of her pregnancy, a woman needs to consider whether to feed her infant breast milk, infant formula, or both. These options are the only recommended foods for an infant during the first 4 to 6 months of life. The current rate of breastfeeding is about 80 percent at birth, but then falls to about 50 percent at 6 months, and 30 percent at 1 year.[63] This section focuses on how the mother's nutrition supports the making of breast milk, and the next chapter describes how the infant benefits from drinking breast milk.

In many countries around the world, a woman breastfeeds her newborn without considering the alternatives or making a conscious decision. In other parts of the world, a woman feeds her newborn formula simply because she knows so little about breastfeeding. She may have misconceptions or feel uncomfortable about a process she doesn't understand.[64] Breastfeeding offers many health benefits to both mother and infant, and every pregnant woman should seriously consider it (see Table 15-10).[65] Even so, women's choices are often influenced by factors other than health and science—factors such as culture, politics, religion, and marketing. In any case, keep in mind that mothers may have valid reasons for not breastfeeding and that formula-fed infants grow and develop into healthy children.

TABLE 15-10 Benefits of Breastfeeding

For Infants

- Provides the appropriate composition and balance of nutrients with high bioavailability
- Provides hormones that promote physiological development
- Improves cognitive development
- Protects against a variety of infections and illnesses, including diarrhea, ear infections, and pneumonia
- May protect against some chronic diseases—such as diabetes (both types), obesity, atherosclerosis, asthma, some cancers, and hypertension—later in life
- Protects against food allergies
- Reduces the risk of SIDS
- Supports healthy weight

For Mothers

- Contracts the uterus
- Delays the return of regular ovulation, thus lengthening birth intervals (this is not, however, a dependable method of contraception)
- Conserves iron stores (by prolonging amenorrhea)
- May protect against breast and ovarian cancer and reduce the risk of type 2 diabetes, hypertension, and heart disease
- Increases energy expenditure, which may contribute to weight loss

Other

- Cost and time savings from not needing medical treatment for childhood illnesses or leaving work to care for sick infants
- Cost and time savings from not needing to purchase and prepare formula (even after adjusting for added foods in the diet of a lactating mother)[a]
- Environmental savings to society from not needing to manufacture, package, and ship formula and dispose of the packaging
- Convenience of not having to shop for and prepare formula

[a]Estimated savings of $1200–$1500 in the first year.

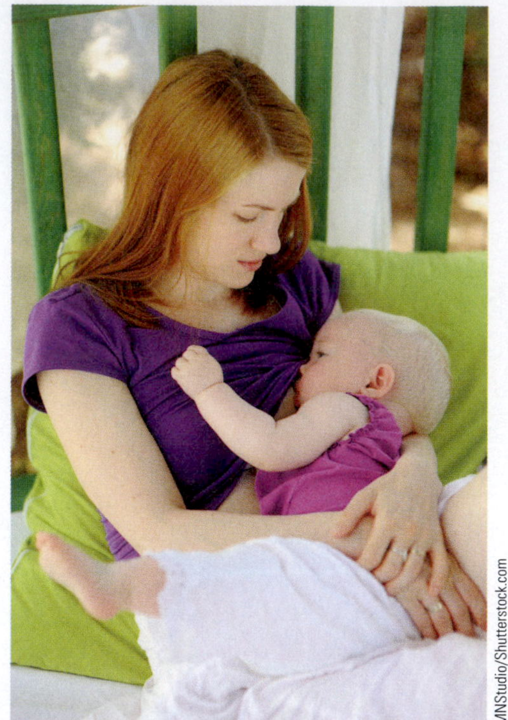

MNStudio/Shutterstock.com

> **PHOTO 15-8** A woman who decides to breastfeed provides her infant with a full array of nutrients and protective factors to support optimal health and development.

Lactation: A Physiological Process **Lactation** naturally follows pregnancy, as the mother's body continues to nourish the infant (see Photo 15-8). The **mammary glands** secrete milk for this purpose. The mammary glands develop during puberty but remain fairly inactive until pregnancy. During pregnancy, hormones promote the growth and branching of a duct system in the breasts and the development of the milk-producing cells.

The hormones **prolactin** and **oxytocin** finely coordinate lactation. The infant's demand for milk stimulates the release of these hormones, which signal the mammary glands to supply milk. Prolactin is responsible for milk production. As long as the infant is nursing, prolactin concentrations remain high, and milk production continues.

The hormone oxytocin causes the mammary glands to eject milk into the ducts, a response known as the **let-down reflex**. The mother may feel this reflex as a contraction of the breast, followed by the flow of milk and the release of pressure. By relaxing and eating well, the nursing mother promotes easy let-down of milk and enhances her ability to successfully breastfeed her infant.

In addition to nourishing the infant, lactation reduces the mother's risks of developing type 2 diabetes, hypertension, and heart disease.[66] Research has yet to explain these associations fully, but one hypothesis suggests that lactation provides a transition time to reset the many metabolic changes that occur during pregnancy. Given these health benefits for mothers and the many well-established benefits for infants, most health care providers readily encourage women to breastfeed.

Breastfeeding: A Learned Behavior Lactation is an automatic physiological process that virtually all mothers are capable of doing. Breastfeeding, on the other hand, is a learned behavior that not all mothers decide to do. Of women who do breastfeed, those who receive early and repeated information and support breastfeed their infants longer than others. Mothers who are confident and committed are most successful in breastfeeding, especially when challenged by obstacles such as a lack of support from friends and family. Health-care professionals play an important role in providing encouragement and accurate information on breastfeeding. Especially helpful are **certified lactation consultants,** who specialize in helping new mothers establish a healthy breastfeeding relationship with their newborn. These consultants are often registered nurses with specialized training. Women who have been successful breastfeeding can also offer advice and dispel misperceptions about lifestyle issues. Table 15-11 lists tips to promote successful breastfeeding among new mothers.

The mother's partner also plays an important role in encouraging breastfeeding. When partners support the decision, mothers are more likely to start and continue breastfeeding.[67] Clearly, educating those closest to the mother could change attitudes and promote breastfeeding.

Most healthy women who want to breastfeed can do so with a little preparation. Physical obstacles to breastfeeding are rare, although most nursing mothers quit within a few months because of perceived difficulties. Overweight and obese mothers seem to have a particularly challenging time because of both psychosocial and biological factors; they tend to be less confident and to have a lower prolactin

TABLE 15-11 Tips for Successful Breastfeeding

- Learn about the benefits of breastfeeding
- Initiate breastfeeding within 1 hour after birth
- Ask a health-care professional to explain how to breastfeed and how to maintain lactation
- Give newborn infants no food or drink other than breast milk, unless medically indicated
- Breastfeed on demand
- Give no artificial nipples or pacifiers to breastfeeding infants[a]
- Find breastfeeding support groups, books, or websites to help troubleshoot breastfeeding problems

[a]Compared with nonusers, infants who use pacifiers breastfeed less frequently and stop breastfeeding at a younger age.

© Cengage

lactation: production and secretion of breast milk for the purpose of nourishing an infant.

mammary glands: glands of the female breast that secrete milk.

prolactin (pro-LAK-tin): a hormone secreted from the anterior pituitary gland that acts on the mammary glands to promote the production of milk. The release of prolactin is mediated by *prolactin-inhibiting hormone (PIH)*.

- **pro** = promote
- **lacto** = milk

oxytocin (OCK-see-TOH-sin): a hormone that stimulates the mammary glands to eject milk during lactation and the uterus to contract during childbirth.

let-down reflex: the reflex that forces milk to the front of the breast when the infant begins to nurse.

certified lactation consultants: health-care providers who specialize in helping new mothers establish a healthy breastfeeding relationship with their newborn. These consultants are often registered nurses with specialized training in breast and infant anatomy and physiology.

response to suckling in the first few days.[68] In general, overweight and obese mothers are more likely to not start breastfeeding or to not continue breastfeeding.[69]

Preparation for breastfeeding includes acquiring and learning how to use a **breast pump**. Most mothers have a need to express milk at some point during their breastfeeding experience. By learning how to use and clean a breast pump—preferably from a person rather than from written or video instructions—a mother can safely collect breast milk.[70] Breast pumps may be purchased or rented; health care insurance policies may cover this expense.

Successful breastfeeding requires adequate nutrition and rest. This, plus the support of all who care, will help enhance the well-being of mother and infant.

Maternal Energy and Nutrient Needs during Lactation

Ideally, the mother who chooses to breastfeed her infant will continue to eat nutrient-dense foods throughout lactation. An adequate diet is needed to support the stamina, patience, and self-confidence that nursing an infant demands.

Energy Intake and Exercise A nursing mother produces about 25 ounces of milk per day, with considerable variation from woman to woman and in the same woman from time to time, depending primarily on the infant's demand for milk. To produce an adequate supply of milk, a woman needs extra energy—almost 500 kcalories a day above her regular need during the first 6 months of lactation. To meet this energy need, she can eat an extra 330 kcalories of food each day during the first 6 months and an extra 400 kcalories each day during the second 6 months and the fat reserves she accumulated during pregnancy can provide the rest. Most women need at least 1800 kcalories a day to receive all the nutrients required for successful lactation. Severe energy restriction may hinder milk production.

After the birth of the infant, many women actively try to lose the extra weight and body fat they accumulated during pregnancy. How much weight a woman retains after pregnancy depends on her gestational weight gain and the duration and intensity of breastfeeding.[71] Many women who follow recommendations for gestational weight gain and breastfeeding can readily return to prepregnancy weight by 6 months. Neither the quality nor the quantity of breast milk is adversely affected by moderate weight loss, and infants grow normally.

Women often exercise to lose weight and improve fitness, and this is compatible with breastfeeding and infant growth (see Photo 15-9).[72] Because intense physical activity can raise the lactate concentration of breast milk and influence the milk's taste, some infants may prefer milk produced prior to exercise. In these cases, mothers can either breastfeed before exercise or express their milk before exercise for use afterward.

Energy Nutrients Recommendations for protein and fatty acids remain about the same during lactation as during pregnancy, but they increase for carbohydrates. Nursing mothers need additional carbohydrate to replace the glucose used to make the lactose in breast milk. The fiber recommendation is 1 gram higher simply because it is based on kcalorie intake, which increases during lactation.

Vitamins and Minerals A question often raised is whether a mother's milk may lack a nutrient if she fails to get enough in her diet. The answer differs from one nutrient to the next, but in general, nutrient inadequacies reduce the *quantity*, not the *quality*, of breast milk. Women can produce milk with adequate protein, carbohydrate, fat, and most minerals, even when their own supplies are limited. For these nutrients and for the vitamin folate as well, milk quality is maintained at the expense of maternal stores. This is most evident in the case of calcium: dietary calcium has no effect on the calcium concentration of breast milk, but maternal bones lose some density during lactation if dietary calcium is inadequate. Exercise may help protect against bone loss during lactation. The nutrients in breast milk that are most likely to decline in response to prolonged inadequate intakes are the vitamins—especially vitamins B_6, B_{12}, A, and D. Review Figure 15-9 (p. 470) to

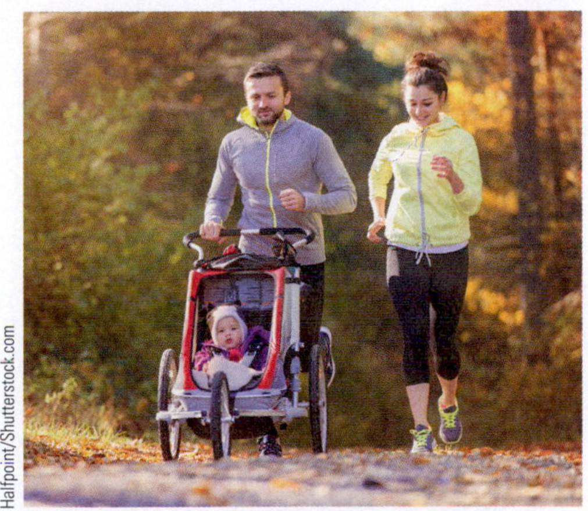

Halfpoint/Shutterstock.com

> **PHOTO 15-9** Physical activity continues to support maternal health after the infant's birth.

breast pump: a device (manual, battery-powered, or electric) that extracts milk from the breast of a lactating woman.

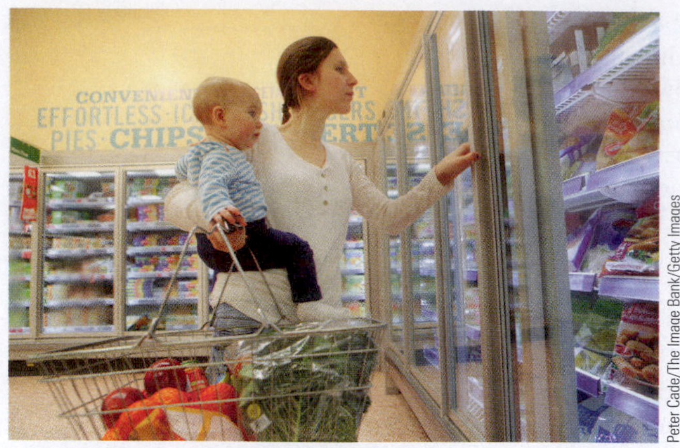
CONVEN
EFFORTLESS
PIES CHIPS
Peter Cade/The Image Bank/Getty Images

> **PHOTO 15-10** Nutritious foods support successful lactation.

compare a lactating woman's nutrient needs with those of pregnant and nonpregnant women.

Water Despite misconceptions, a mother who drinks more fluid does not produce more breast milk. To protect herself from dehydration, however, a lactating woman needs to drink plenty of fluids. The recommendation for *total* water (including drinking water, other beverages, and foods) during lactation is 3.8 liters per day. Because foods provide about 20 percent of total water intake, beverages—including drinking water—should provide about 3.1 liters per day (roughly 13 cups). A sensible guideline is to drink a glass of milk, juice, or water at each meal and each time the infant nurses.

Nutrient Supplements Most lactating women can obtain all the nutrients they need from a well-balanced diet without taking multivitamin-mineral supplements (see Photo 15-10). Nevertheless, some may need iron supplements, not to enhance the iron in breast milk, but to refill their depleted iron stores. The mother's iron stores dwindle during pregnancy as she supplies the developing fetus with enough iron to last through the first 4 to 6 months of the infant's life. In addition, childbirth may have caused blood losses. Thus a woman may need iron supplements during lactation even though, until menstruation resumes, her iron requirement is about half that of other nonpregnant women her age.

Food Assistance Programs In general, women most likely to participate in the food assistance program WIC—those who are poor and have little education—are less likely to breastfeed. Furthermore, WIC provides infant formula at no cost. Because WIC recognizes the many benefits of breastfeeding, efforts are made to overcome this dilemma. In addition to nutrition education and encouragement, breastfeeding mothers receive the following WIC incentives:

- Higher priority in certification into WIC
- Greater quantity and variety of foods
- Longer eligibility to participate in WIC
- Support from peers and experts
- Breast pumps and other support materials

Together, these efforts help provide nutrition support and encourage WIC mothers to breastfeed.

Particular Foods Foods with strong or spicy flavors (such as garlic) may alter the flavor of breast milk. A sudden change in the taste of the milk may annoy some infants. Familiar flavors may enhance enjoyment. Flavors in breast milk from the mother's diet can influence the infant's later food preferences.

A nursing mother can usually eat whatever nutritious foods she chooses. If she suspects a particular food is causing the infant discomfort, her physician may recommend a dietary challenge: eliminate the food from the diet to see if the infant's reactions subside, then return the food to the diet and again monitor the infant's reactions. If a food must be eliminated for an extended time, appropriate substitutions must be made to ensure nutrient adequacy.

Maternal Health

If a woman has an ordinary cold, she can continue nursing without worry. If susceptible, the infant will catch it from her anyway. Thanks to the immunological protection of breast milk, the baby may be less susceptible than a formula-fed baby would be. With appropriate treatment, a woman who has an infectious disease such as tuberculosis or hepatitis can breastfeed; transmission is rare. Women with HIV (human immunodeficiency virus) infections, however, should consider other options.

HIV Infection and AIDS Mothers with HIV infections can transmit the virus (which causes AIDS) to their infants through breast milk, especially during the early months of breastfeeding. In developed countries such as the United States, where safe alternatives are available, HIV-positive women should *not* breastfeed their infants.[73] In developing countries, where the feeding of inappropriate or contaminated formulas causes more than 1 million infant deaths each year, breastfeeding can be critical to infant survival. Thus, in making the decision of whether to breastfeed, HIV-infected women in developing countries must weigh the potential risks and benefits. The World Health Organization (WHO) recommends exclusive breastfeeding for infants of HIV-infected women for the first six months of life unless formula feeding is acceptable, feasible, affordable, sustainable, and safe before that time. In addition, HIV-exposed infants may be protected by receiving antiretroviral treatment while being breastfed.

Diabetes Women with type 1 diabetes may need careful monitoring and counseling to ensure successful lactation. These women need to adjust their energy intakes and insulin doses to meet the heightened needs of lactation. Maintaining good glucose control helps initiate lactation and support milk production.

As mentioned earlier in this chapter, women who have gestational diabetes during pregnancy have an increased risk of subsequently developing type 2 diabetes. During lactation, glucose tolerance and insulin response improve, thereby lowering the risk of type 2 diabetes.[74] Among women with gestational diabetes who later develop type 2 diabetes, the onset is significantly delayed for those who breastfed.[75] This safe and inexpensive intervention adds yet another impressive reason for women to consider breastfeeding their infants.

Postpartum Amenorrhea Women who breastfeed experience prolonged **postpartum amenorrhea.** Absent menstrual periods, however, do not protect a woman from pregnancy. To prevent pregnancy, a couple must use some form of contraception. Breastfeeding women who use oral contraceptives should use progestin-only agents for at least the first 6 months. Estrogen-containing oral contraceptives reduce the volume and the protein content of breast milk.

Breast Health Some women fear that breastfeeding will cause their breasts to sag. The breasts do swell and become heavy and large immediately after the birth, but even when they produce enough milk to nourish a thriving infant, they eventually shrink back to their prepregnancy size. Given proper support, diet, and exercise, breasts often return to their former shape and size when lactation ends. Breasts change their shape as the body ages, but breastfeeding does not accelerate this process.

Whether the physical and hormonal events of pregnancy and lactation protect women from later breast cancer is an area of active research. Some research suggests a protective effect between breastfeeding and breast cancer.[76]

Postpartum Depression An estimated 10 to 15 percent of women experience **postpartum depression**. Several dietary factors—including vitamin D, zinc, selenium, and omega-3 fatty acids—have been studied in an effort to find a nutritional link. Findings have been intriguing, but limited.[77] For example, omega-3 status in pregnant women is inversely associated with postpartum depression, but dietary supplements—of omega-3 fatty acids or any other nutrient—have not proven to be effective.[78] A healthy, well-balanced diet supports a mother's mental and physical health, which can influence her relationships with her children; unfortunately, maternal depression and an unhealthy diet often go hand in hand, and together—as well as independently—contribute to a child's emotional and behavioral problems.[79]

Practices Incompatible with Lactation

Some substances impair milk production or enter breast milk and interfere with infant development. This section discusses practices that a breastfeeding mother should avoid.

Alcohol Alcohol easily enters breast milk, and its concentration peaks within an hour after ingestion. Infants drink less breast milk when their mothers have consumed even small amounts of alcohol (equivalent to a can of beer). Three possible

postpartum amenorrhea (ay-MEN-oh-REE-ah): the normal temporary absence of menstrual periods immediately following childbirth.

postpartum depression: moderate to severe depression in a woman after she has given birth.

reasons, acting separately or together, may explain why. For one, the alcohol may have altered the flavor of the breast milk and thereby the infant's acceptance of it. For another, because an infant metabolizes alcohol inefficiently, even low doses may be potent enough to suppress feeding and cause sleepiness. Third, the alcohol may have interfered with lactation by inhibiting the hormone oxytocin.

In the past, alcohol has been recommended to mothers to facilitate lactation despite a lack of scientific evidence that it does so. The research summarized here suggests that alcohol consumption should be limited while breastfeeding. To minimize the effects of an occasional glass of wine or beer, women should drink after breastfeeding rather than before, eat a meal to decrease alcohol absorption, and wait to breastfeed for several hours after drinking.[80] If breasts are uncomfortably full after excessive drinking, a women can pump and discard the milk.

Medicinal Drugs Most medicines are compatible with breastfeeding, but some are contraindicated, either because they suppress lactation or because they are secreted into breast milk and can harm the infant.[81] As a precaution, a nursing mother should consult with her physician prior to taking any drug, including herbal supplements.

Illicit Drugs Illicit drugs, of course, are harmful to the physical and emotional health of both the mother and the nursing infant. Breast milk can deliver such high doses of illicit drugs as to cause irritability, tremors, hallucinations, and even death in infants. Women whose infants have overdosed on illicit drugs contained in breast milk have been convicted of murder. Women who use methadone to control withdrawal symptoms for opiate addiction can safely breastfeed their infants.

Smoking Many women who quit smoking during pregnancy relapse after delivery. Because cigarette smoking lowers the concentrations of lipids and proteins and reduces milk volume, the breast milk of smokers may not meet their infants' energy needs. The milk they do produce contains nicotine, which alters its smell and flavor. Furthermore, smoking increases the risk for SIDS. Breastfeeding helps protect against SIDS, but infant exposure to passive smoke negates this protective effect.

Environmental Contaminants Chapter 19 discusses environmental contaminants in the food supply. Some of these environmental contaminants can find their way into the food supply and then into breast milk. To limit mercury intake, lactating women should heed the advice for pregnant women eating fish that are presented in Table 15-8 (p. 480).

Caffeine Caffeine enters breast milk and may make an infant irritable and wakeful. As during pregnancy, caffeine consumption should be moderate—the equivalent of 1 to 2 cups of coffee a day. Larger doses of caffeine may interfere with the bioavailability of iron from breast milk and impair the infant's iron status.

REVIEW IT Summarize the nutrient needs of women during lactation.
The lactating woman needs extra fluid and enough energy and nutrients to produce about 25 ounces of milk a day. Breastfeeding is contraindicated for those with HIV/AIDS. Alcohol, other drugs, smoking, and contaminants may reduce milk production or enter breast milk and impair infant development.

This chapter has focused on the nutrition needs of the mother during pregnancy and lactation. The next chapter explores the dietary needs of infants, children, and adolescents.

What's Online

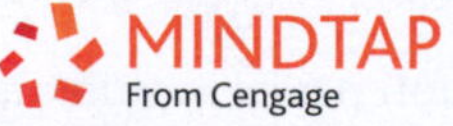
MINDTAP
From Cengage

Visit **www.cengagebrain.com** to access MindTap, a complete digital course that includes Diet & Wellness Plus, interactive quizzes, videos, and more.

REFERENCES

1. R. Sharma and coauthors, Lifestyle factors and reproductive health: Taking control of your fertility, *Reproductive Biology and Endocrinology* 11 (2013): 66.
2. K. L. Rooney and A. D. Domar, The impact of lifestyle behaviors on infertility treatment outcome, *Current Opinion in Obstetrics and Gynecology* 26 (2014): 181–185.
3. J. M. Campbell and coauthors, Paternal obesity negatively affects male fertility and assisted reproduction outcomes: A systematic review and meta-analysis, *Reproductive Biomedicine Online* 31 (2015): 593–604; D. Best and S. Bhattacharya, Obesity and fertility, *Hormone Molecular Biology and Clinical Investigation* 24 (2015): 5–10; T. J. Chambers and R. A. Richard, The impact of obesity on male fertility, *Hormones* 14 (2015): 563–568; N. Sermondade and coauthors, BMI in relation to sperm count: An updated systematic review and collaborative meta-analysis, *Human Reproduction Update* 19 (2013): 221–231; E. S. Jungheim, J. L. Travieso, and M. M. Hopeman, Weighing the impact of obesity on female reproductive function and fertility, *Nutrition Reviews* 71 (2013): S3–S8.
4. R. Sundaram, S. L. Mumford, and G. M. Buck Louis, Couples' body composition and time-to-pregnancy, *Human Reproduction* 32 (2017): 1–7.
5. L. Giahi and coauthors, Nutritional modifications in male infertility: A systematic review covering 2 decades, *Nutrition Reviews* 74 (2016): 118–130.
6. T. K. Jensen and coauthors, Habitual alcohol consumption associated with reduced semen quality and changes in reproductive hormones: A cross-sectional study among 1221 young Danish men, *British Medical Journal* 4 (2014): e005462.
7. C. Y. Spong, Defining "term" pregnancy: Recommendations from the Defining "Term" Pregnancy Workgroup, *Journal of the American Medical Association* 309 (2013): 2445–2446.
8. A. J. Agopian and coauthors, Proportion of neural tube defects attributable to known risk factors, *Birth Defects Research. Part A, Clinical and Molecular Teratology* 97 (2013): 42–46.
9. C. Berti and coauthors, Early-life nutritional exposures and lifelong health: Immediate and long-lasting impacts of probiotics, vitamin D, and breastfeeding, *Nutrition Reviews* 75 (2017): 83–97; J. G. O. Ávila and coauthors, Impact of oxidative stress during pregnancy on fetal epigenetic patterns and early origin of vascular disease, *Nutrition Reviews* 73 (2015): 12–21; J. Zheng and coauthors, DNA methylation: The pivotal interaction between early-life nutrition and glucose metabolism in later life, *British Journal of Nutrition* 112 (2014): 1850–1857.
10. J. L. Saben and coauthors, Maternal metabolic syndrome programs mitochondrial dysfunction via germline changes across three generations, *Cell Reports* 16 (2016): 1–8.
11. K. M. Godfrey and coauthors, Influence of maternal obesity on the long-term health of offspring, *Lancet: Diabetes and Endocrinology* 5 (2017): 53–64.
12. G. Wang and coauthors, Associations of maternal prepregnancy BMI and plasma folate concentrations with child metabolic health, *JAMA Pediatrics* 170 (2016): e160845.
13. Position of the Academy of Nutrition and Dietetics: Obesity, reproduction, and pregnancy outcomes, *Journal of the Academy of Nutrition and Dietetics* 116 (2016): 677–691.
14. A. I. Girsen and coauthors, Women's prepregnancy underweight as a risk factor for preterm birth: A retrospective study, *British Journal of Obstetrics and Gynecology* 123 (2016): 2001–2007; F. Hoellen and coauthors, Does maternal underweight prior to conception influence pregnancy risks and outcome? *In Vivo* 28 (2014): 1165–1170.
15. A. M. Branum, S. E. Kirmeyer, and E. C. W. Gregory, Prepregnancy body mass index by maternal characteristics and state: Data from the birth certificate, 2014, *National Vital Statistics Reports*, August 5, 2016; J. F. Mission, N. E. Marshall, and A. B. Caughey, Obesity in pregnancy: A big problem and getting bigger, *Obstetrical and Gynecological Survey* 68 (2013): 389–399.
16. K. Johansson and coauthors, Outcomes of pregnancy after bariatric surgery, *New England Journal of Medicine* 372 (2015): 814–824.
17. B. F. Fuemmeler and coauthors, Association between prepregnancy body mass index and gestational weight gain with size, temp, and velocity of infant growth: Analysis of the newborn epigenetic study cohort, *Childhood Obesity* 12 (2016): 210–218; A. P. Starling and coauthors, Associations of maternal BMI and gestational weight gain with neonatal adiposity in the Healthy Start study, *American Journal of Clinical Nutrition* 101 (2015): 302–309.
18. B. P. Wispelwey and E. Sheiner, Cesarean delivery in obese women: A comprehensive review, *Journal of Maternal and Fetal Neonatal Medicine* 26 (2013): 547–551.
19. L. M. Bodnar and coauthors, Maternal prepregnancy obesity and cause-specific stillbirth, *American Journal of Clinical Nutrition* 102 (2015): 858–864.
20. I. Forthun and coauthors, Maternal prepregnancy BMI and risk of cerebral palsy in offspring, *Pediatrics* 138 (2016): e20160874.
21. D. Aune and coauthors, Maternal body mass index and the risk of fetal death, stillbirth, and infant death: A systematic review and meta-analysis, *Journal of the American Medical Association* 311 (2014): 1536–1546; S. Cnattingius and coauthors, Maternal obesity and risk of preterm delivery, *Journal of the American Medical Association* 309 (2013): 2362–2370.
22. R. C. Ma and coauthors, Clinical management of pregnancy in the obese mother: Before conception, during pregnancy, and post partum, *Lancet: Diabetes and Endocrinology* 4 (2016): 1037–1049.
23. N. P. Deputy, A. J. Sharma, and S. Y. Kim, Gestational weight gain—United States, 2012 and 2013, *Morbidity and Mortality Weekly Report* 64 (2015): 1215–1220.
24. T. A. Hillier and coauthors, Impact of maternal glucose and gestational weight gain on child obesity over the first decade of life in normal birth weight infants, *Maternal and Child Health Journal* 20 (2016): 1559–1568.
25. M. Mannan, S. A. R. Doi, and A. A. Mamun, Association between weight gain during pregnancy and postpartum weight retention and obesity: A bias-adjusted meta-analysis, *Nutrition Reviews* 71 (2013): 343–352.
26. P. van der Pligt and coauthors, Systematic review of lifestyle interventions to limit postpartum weight retention: Implications for future opportunities to prevent maternal overweight and obesity following childbirth, *Obesity Reviews* 14 (2013): 792–805.
27. S. L. Nascimento and coauthors, The effect of physical exercise strategies on weight loss in postpartum women: A systematic review and meta-analysis, *International Journal of Obesity* 38 (2013): 625–635; A. R. A. Adegboye and Y. M. Linne, Diet or exercise, or both, for weight reduction in women after childbirth, *Cochrane Database of Systematic Reviews* 7 (2013): CD005627.
28. S. T. Harris and coauthors, Exercise during pregnancy and its association with gestational weight gain, *Maternal and Child Health Journal* 19 (2015): 528–537.
29. M. F. Mottola, Physical activity and maternal obesity: Cardiovascular adaptations, exercise recommendations, and pregnancy outcomes, *Nutrition Reviews* 71 (2013): S31–S36.
30. M. Perales, R. Artal, and A. Lucia, Exercise during pregnancy, *Journal of the American Medical Association* 317 (2017): 1113–1114; L. M. Savitsky and coauthors, Cost-effectiveness of exercise for the prevention of preeclampsia and gestational diabetes in obese women, *American Journal of Obstetrics and Gynecology* 216 (2017): S260–S261; L. M. Mudd and coauthors, Health benefits of physical activity during pregnancy: An international perspective, *Medicine and Science in Sports and Exercise* 45 (2013): 268–277.
31. Position of the Academy of Nutrition and Dietetics: Nutrition and lifestyle for a healthy pregnancy outcome, *Journal of the Academy of Nutrition and Dietetics* 114 (2014): 1099–1103.
32. P. M. Emmett, L. R. Jones, and J. Golding, Pregnancy diet and associated outcomes in the Avone Longitudinal Study of Parents and Children, *Nutrition Reviews* 73 (2015): 154–174.
33. C. Cao and K. O. O'Brien, Pregnancy and iron homeostasis: An update, *Nutrition Reviews* 71 (2013): 35–51.
34. C. R. Paterson and D. Ayoub, Congenital rickets due to vitamin D deficiency in the mothers, *Clinical Nutrition* 34 (2015): 793–798.
35. Practice Bulletin No. 153: Nausea and vomiting of pregnancy, *Obstetrics and Gynecology* (2015): e12–e24.
36. A. Matthews and coauthors, Interventions for nausea and vomiting in early pregnancy, *Cochrane Database of Systematic Reviews* (2015): CD007575.
37. I. Matok and coauthors, Studying the antiemetic effect of vitamin B6 for morning sickness: Pyridoxine and pyridoxal are prodrugs, *Journal of Clinical Pharmacology* 54 (2014): 1429–1433.

38. Centers for Disease Control and Prevention, Pregnancy mortality surveillance system, January 31, 2017; M. F. MacDorman and coauthors, Recent increases in the U.S. maternal mortality rate: Disentangling trends from measurement issues, *Obstetrics and Gynecology* 128 (2016): 447–455; Centers for Disease Control and Prevention, Infant health, October 6, 2016.
39. World Health Organization, Children: Reducing mortality, September 2016.
40. G. H. Visser and H. W. deValk, Management of diabetes in pregnancy: Antenatal follow-up and decisions concerning timing and mode of delivery, *Best Practice and Research: Obstetrics and Gynaecology* 29 (2015): 237–243.
41. C. L. DeSisto, S. Y. Kim, and A. J. Sharma, Prevalence estimates of gestational diabetes mellitus in the United States, Pregnancy Risk Assessment Monitoring System (PRAMS), 2007-2010, *Preventing Chronic Disease* 11 (2014): 130415.
42. A. Allalou and coauthors, A predictive metabolic signature for the transition from gestational diabetes to type 2 diabetes, *Diabetes* 65 (2016): 2529–2539; W. Bao and coauthors, Long-term risk of type 2 diabetes mellitus in relation to BMI and weight change among women with a history of gestational diabetes mellitus: A prospective cohort study, *Diabetologia* 58 (2015): 1212–1219.
43. L. Hartling and coauthors, Benefits and harms of treating gestational diabetes mellitus: A systematic review and meta-analysis for the U. S. Preventive Services Task Force and the national Institutes of health Office of Medical Applications of Research, *Annals of Internal Medicine* 159 (2013): 123–129.
44. H. N. Moussa, S. E. Arian, and B. M. Sibai, Management of hypertensive disorders in pregnancy, *Women's Health* 10 (2014): 385–404.
45. I. Behrens and coauthors, Association between hypertensive disorders of pregnancy and later risk of cardiomyopathy, *Journal of the American Medical Association* 315 (2016): 1026–1033.
46. A. Jeyabalan, Epidemiology of preeclampsia: Impact of obesity, *Nutrition Reviews* 71 (2013): S18–S25.
47. N. Auger and coauthors, Association between preeclampsia and congenital heart defects, *Journal of the American Medical Association* 314 (2015): 1588–1598.
48. Trends in teen pregnancy and childbearing, www.hhs.gov/ash/oah/adolescent-health-topics/reproductive-health/teen-pregnancy/trends.html, June 2, 2016.
49. C. H. Tan and coauthors, Alcohol use and binge drinking among women of childbearing age—the United States, 2011–2013, *Morbidity and Mortality Weekly Report* 64 (2015): 1042–1046.
50. C. M. O'Leary and coauthors, Maternal alcohol-use and sudden infant death syndrome and infant mortality excluding SIDS, *Pediatrics* 131 (2013): e770–e778.
51. M. Behnke, V. C. Smith, Committee on Substance Abuse and Committee on Fetus and Newborn, Prenatal substance abuse: Short- and long-term effects on the exposed fetus, *Pediatrics* 131 (2013): e1009–e1024.
52. A. M. Cressman and coauthors, Cocaine abuse during pregnancy, *Journal of Obstetrics and Gynaecology Canada* 36 (2014): 628–631.
53. S. Buckingham-Howes and coauthors, Systematic review of prenatal cocaine exposure and adolescent development, *Pediatrics* 131 (2013): e1917–e1936.
54. S. C. Curtin and T. J. Mathews, Smoking prevalence and cessation before and during pregnancy: Data from the birth certificate, 2014, Centers for Disease Control and Prevention, February 10, 2016.
55. M. N. Kooijman and coauthors, Fetal smoke exposure and kidney outcomes in school-aged children, *American Journal of Kidney Disease* 66 (2015): 412–420.
56. Center for Disease Control and Prevention, Tobacco use and pregnancy, July 20, 2016.
57. M. K. Wong and coauthors, Adverse effects of perinatal nicotine exposure on reproductive outcomes, *Reproduction* 150 (2015): 185–193.
58. M. A. Suter and coauthors, Is there evidence for potential harm of electronic cigarette use in pregnancy? *Birth Defects Research* 103 (2015): 186–195.
59. E. Pannia and coauthors, Role of maternal vitamins in programming health and chronic disease, *Nutrition Reviews* 74 (2016): 166-180.
60. L. W. Chen and coauthors, Maternal caffeine intake during pregnancy and risk of pregnancy loss: A categorical and dose-response meta-analysis of prospective studies, *Public Health Nutrition* 19 (2016): 1233–1244; J. Li and coauthors, A meta-analysis of risk of pregnancy loss and caffeine and coffee consumption during pregnancy, *International Journal of Gynaecology and Obstetrics* 130 (2015): 116–122; J. Rhee and coauthors, Maternal caffeine consumption during pregnancy and risk of low birth weight: A dose-response meta-analysis of observational studies, *PLoS One* 10 (2015): e0132334; L. W. Chen and coauthors, Maternal caffeine intake during pregnancy is associated with risk of low birth weight: A systematic review and dose-response meta-analysis, *BMC Medicine* 12 (2014): 174.
61. S. Morgan, G. Koren, and P. Bozzo, is caffeine consumption safe during pregnancy? *Canadian Family Physician* 59 (2013): 361–362.
62. Position of the Academy of Nutrition and Dietetics: Use of nutritive and nonnutritive sweeteners, *Journal of the Academy of Nutrition and Dietetics* 112 (2012): 739–758.
63. Centers for Disease Control and Prevention, Breastfeeding rates continue to rise, August 22, 2016.
64. R. L. Dunn and coauthors, Engaging field-based professionals in a qualitative assessment of barriers and positive contributors to breastfeeding using the social ecological model, *Maternal and Child Health Journal* 19 (2015): 6–16.
65. Position of the Academy of Nutrition and Dietetics: Promoting and supporting breastfeeding, *Journal of the Academy of Nutrition and Dietetics* 115 (2015): 444–449.
66. C. G. Perrine and coauthors, Lactation and maternal cardio-metabolic health, *Annual Review of Nutrition* 36 (2016): 627–645.
67. J. Abbass-Dick and coauthors, Coparenting breastfeeding support and exclusive breastfeeding: A randomized controlled trial, *Pediatrics* 135 (2015): 102–110.
68. L. E. Hauff, S. A. Leonard, and K. M. Rasmussen, Associations of maternal obesity and psychosocial factors with breastfeeding intention, initiation, and duration, *American Journal of Clinical Nutrition* 99 (2014): 524–534.
69. A. H. Garcia and coauthors, Maternal weight status, diet, and supplement use as determinants of breastfeeding and complementary feeding: A systematic review and meta-analysis, *Nutrition Reviews* 74 (2016): 490–516; J. Verret-Chalifour and coauthors, Breastfeeding initiation: Impact of obesity in a large Canadian perinatal cohort study, *PLoS One* 10 (2015): e0117512; J. Mäkelä and coauthors, Maternal overweight impacts infant feeding patterns—The STEPS Study, *European Journal of Clinical Nutrition* 68 (2014): 43–49.
70. A. Eglash and M. L. Malloy, Breastmilk expression and breast ump technology, *Clinical Obstetrics and Gynecology* 58 (2015): 855–867; Y. Qi and coauthors, Maternal and breast pump factors associated with breast pump problems and injuries, *Journal of Human Lactation* 30 (2014): 62–72.
71. R. Sámano and coauthors, Effects of breastfeeding on weight loss and recovery of pregestational weight in adolescent and adult mothers, *Food and Nutrition Bulletin* 34 (2013): 123–130.
72. A. Zourladani and coauthors, The effect of physical exercise on postpartum fitness, hormone and lipid levels: A randomized controlled trial in primiparous, lactating women, *Archives of Gynecology and Obstetrics* 291 (2015): 525–530.
73. Committee on Pediatric AIDS, Infant feeding and transmission of human immunodeficiency virus in the United States, *Pediatrics* 131 (2013): 391–396.
74. S. Chouinard-Castonguay and coauthors, Relationship between lactation duration and insulin and glucose response among women with prior gestational diabetes, *European Journal of Endocrinology* 168 (2013): 515–523.
75. A. G. Ziegler and coauthors, Long-term protective effect of lactation on the development of type 2 diabetes in women with recent gestational diabetes mellitus, *Diabetes* 61 (2012): 3167–3171.
76. C. G. Victora and coauthors, Breastfeeding in the 21st century: Epidemiology, mechanisms, and lifelong effect, *Lancet* 387 (2016): 475–490.
77. E. R. Ellsworth-Bowers and E. J. Corwin, Nutrition and the psychoneuroimmunology of postpartum depression, *Nutrition Research Reviews* 25 (2012): 180–192.
78. M. W. Markhus and coauthors, Low omega-3 index in pregnancy is a possible biological risk factor for postpartum depression, *PLoS One* 8 (2013): e67617; B. J. Miller and coauthors, Dietary supplements for preventing postnatal depression, *Cochrane Database of Systematic Reviews* (2013): CD009104.
79. L. Pina-Camacho and coauthors, Maternal depression symptoms, unhealthy diet and child emotional-behavioural dysregulation, *Psychological Medicine* 45 (2015): 1851–1860.
80. American Academy of Pediatrics, *New Mother's Guide to Breastfeeding* (New York: Bantam Books, 2011), p. 31.
81. H. C. Sachs and Committee on Drugs, The transfer of drugs and therapeutics into human breast milk: An update on selected topics, *Pediatrics* 132 (2013): e796–e809.

 LEARN IT Explain how drinking alcohol endangers the fetus and how women can prevent fetal alcohol syndrome.

Fetal Alcohol Syndrome

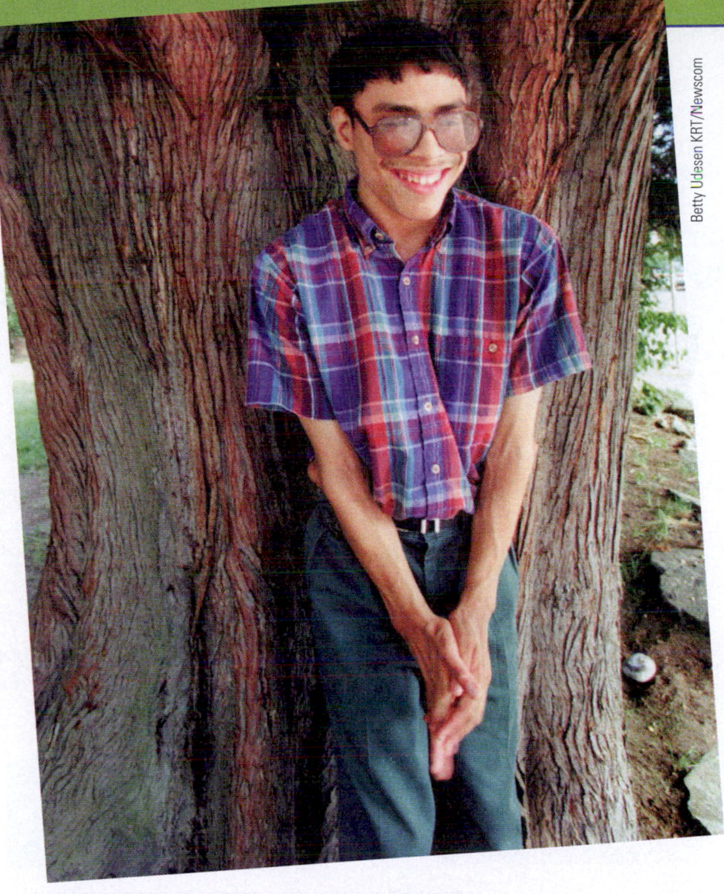
Betty Udesen KRT/Newscom

As Chapter 15 mentions, drinking alcohol during pregnancy endangers the fetus. Alcohol crosses the placenta freely and deprives the developing fetus of both nutrients and oxygen. The damaging effects of alcohol on the developing fetus cover a range of abnormalities referred to as **fetal alcohol spectrum disorder** (see Glossary H15-1). Diagnosis is based on specific criteria of physical, mental, and neurobehavioral symptoms.[1] Those at the most severe end of the spectrum are described as having **fetal alcohol syndrome (FAS),** a cluster of symptoms that includes:

- Prenatal and postnatal growth restriction
- Abnormalities of the brain and central nervous system, with consequent impairment in cognition and behavior
- Physical abnormalities of the face and skull that alter normal patterns of symmetry (see Figure H15-1, p. 490)
- Increased frequency of major birth defects such as cleft palate, heart defects, and defects in ears, eyes, genitals, and urinary system

Tragically, the damage evident at birth persists: children with FAS never fully recover (see Photo H15-1, p. 490).

It is difficult to estimate how many infants are born in the United States each year with problems caused by their mothers' drinking too much alcohol during pregnancy. Thousands of infants have had enough **prenatal alcohol exposure** to result in symptoms that fall somewhere along the spectrum. The cluster of *mental* problems associated with prenatal alcohol exposure is known as **alcohol-related neurodevelopmental disorder (ARND),** and the *physical* malformations are referred to as **alcohol-related birth defects (ARBD).** Some children with ARBD and ARND have no outward signs; others may be short or have only minor facial abnormalities.

Diagnosis is often missed. One study of more than 150 children who met the criteria for diagnosis within the spectrum reported that 80 percent had not been previously diagnosed and more than 5 percent had been misdiagnosed.[2] Children commonly go undiagnosed even when they develop learning difficulties in the early school years. Mood disorders and behavior problems, such as aggression, are common. These children typically need support and guidance to function and participate in daily activities. Early diagnosis can help ensure early intervention; although treatment cannot correct the abnormalities, limited research suggests that some interventions (such as choline supplementation) may benefit some functions (such as memory).[3]

The surgeon general states that pregnant women should abstain from alcohol. Abstinence from alcohol is the best policy for pregnant women both because alcohol consumption during pregnancy has such severe consequences and because FAS can only be prevented—it cannot be treated. Further, because the most severe damage occurs around the time of conception—*before a woman may even realize that she is pregnant*—the warning to abstain includes women who may become pregnant.

Drinking during Pregnancy

As mentioned in Chapter 15, 1 out of 10 pregnant women drinks alcohol; 1 out of 33 admits to binge drinking.[4] When a woman drinks during pregnancy, she causes damage in two ways: directly, by intoxication, and indirectly, by malnutrition. Prior to the complete formation of the

GLOSSARY H15-1

alcohol-related birth defects (ARBD): malformations in the skeletal and organ systems (heart, kidneys, eyes, ears) associated with prenatal alcohol exposure.

alcohol-related neurodevelopmental disorder (ARND): abnormalities in the central nervous system and cognitive development associated with prenatal alcohol exposure.

fetal alcohol spectrum disorder (FASD): an umbrella term used to describe a range of physical, behavioral, and cognitive abnormalities resulting from prenatal alcohol exposure.

fetal alcohol syndrome (FAS): a clinical diagnosis based on specific physical, behavioral, and cognitive abnormalities resulting from prenatal alcohol exposure, including facial malformations, stunted growth, and central nervous disorders.

prenatal alcohol exposure: subjecting a fetus to a pattern of excessive alcohol intake characterized by substantial regular use or heavy episodic drinking.

NOTE: See Highlight 7 for other alcohol-related terms and information.

> FIGURE H15-1 Typical Facial Characteristics of FAS

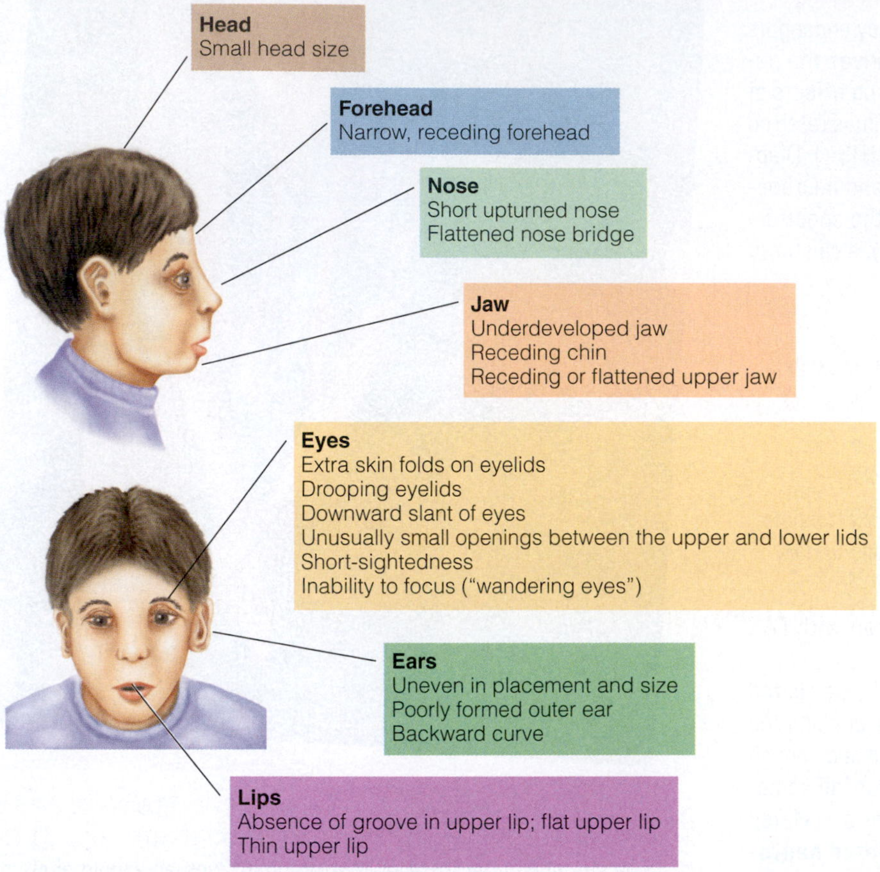

Head
Small head size
Forehead
Narrow, receding forehead
Nose
Short upturned nose
Flattened nose bridge
Jaw
Underdeveloped jaw
Receding chin
Receding or flattened upper jaw
Eyes
Extra skin folds on eyelids
Drooping eyelids
Downward slant of eyes
Unusually small openings between the upper and lower lids
Short-sightedness
Inability to focus ("wandering eyes")
Ears
Uneven in placement and size
Poorly formed outer ear
Backward curve
Lips
Absence of groove in upper lip; flat upper lip
Thin upper lip

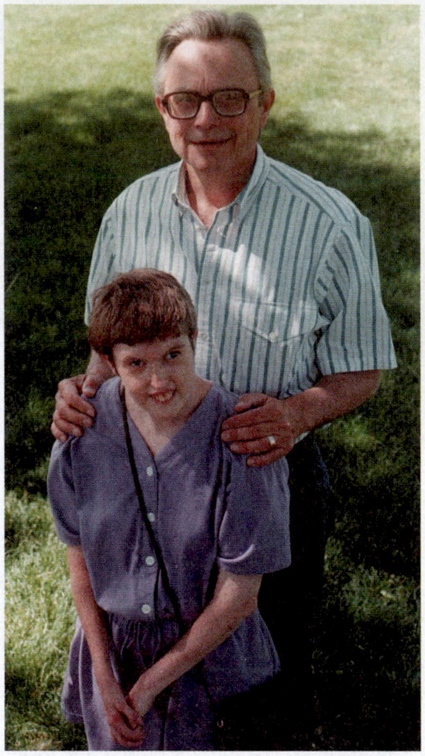

> PHOTO H15-1 As can be seen from this 25-year-old woman with FAS, the characteristic facial features may diminish with time, but physical impairments continue, resulting in short height.

placenta (approximately 12 weeks), alcohol diffuses directly into the tissues of the developing embryo, causing incredible damage. (Review Figure 15-4, p. 462, and note that the critical periods for most tissues occur during this time of embryonic development.) Alcohol interferes with the orderly development of tissues during critical periods, reducing the number of cells and damaging those that are produced. The damage of alcohol toxicity during brain development is apparent in its reduced size and impaired function.

When alcohol crosses the placenta, fetal blood alcohol rises until it reaches equilibrium with maternal blood alcohol. The mother may not even appear drunk, but the fetus may be poisoned. The fetus's body is small, its detoxification system is immature, and alcohol remains in fetal blood long after it has been cleared from maternal blood (see Photo H15-2).

A pregnant woman harms her unborn child not only by consuming alcohol but also by not consuming food. This combination enhances the likelihood of malnutrition and a poorly developed infant. It is important to realize, however, that malnutrition is not the cause of FAS. It is true that mothers of FAS children often have unbalanced diets and nutrient deficiencies. It is also true that nutrient deficiencies may exacerbate the clinical signs seen in these children, but it is the *alcohol* that causes the damage. An adequate diet alone will not prevent FAS if alcohol use continues.

How Much Is Too Much?

A pregnant woman need not have an alcohol-abuse problem to give birth to a baby with FAS. She need only drink in excess of her liver's capacity to detoxify alcohol. The damaging effects on the developing fetus are dose-dependent, becoming greater as the dose increases. Even one drink a day threatens neurological development and behaviors. Four drinks a day dramatically increase the risk of having an infant with physical malformations.

In addition to total alcohol intake, drinking patterns play an important role. Most FAS studies report their findings in terms of average intake per day, but people often drink more heavily on some days than on others. For example, a woman who drinks an *average* of 1 ounce of alcohol (2 drinks) a day may not drink at all during the week, but then have 10 drinks on Saturday night, exposing the fetus to extremely toxic quantities of alcohol. Whether various drinking patterns incur damage depends on the frequency of consumption, the quantity consumed, and the stage of fetal development at the time of each drinking episode.

An occasional drink may be innocuous, but researchers are unable to say how much alcohol is safe to consume during pregnancy. For this reason, health-care professionals urge women to stop drinking alcohol as soon as they realize they are pregnant, or better, as soon as they *plan* to become pregnant. Why take any risk? The only sure way to protect an infant from alcohol damage is for the mother to abstain.[5]

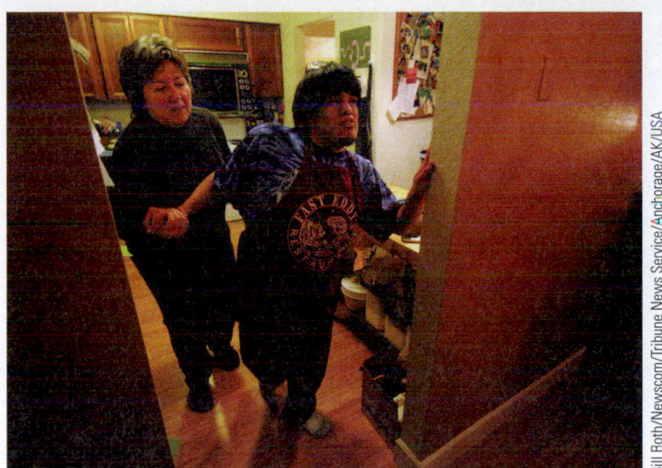

Bill Roth/Newscom/Tribune News Service/Anchorage/AK/USA

> **PHOTO H15-2** Children born with FAS must live with the long-term consequences of alcohol damage. This 20-year-old man was born 3 months preterm with a 0.237 blood alcohol level, which took his 2-pound body 4 days to clear from his system.

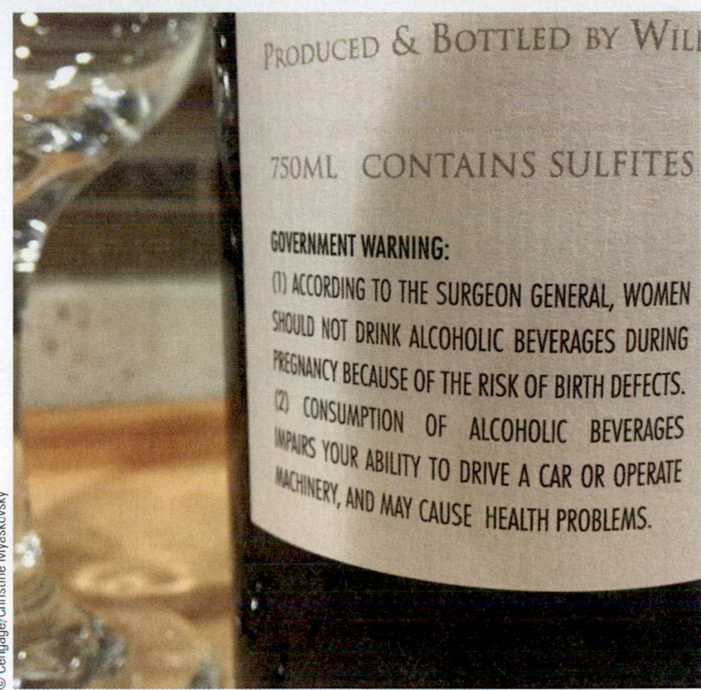
PRODUCED & BOTTLED BY WIL
750ML CONTAINS SULFITES
GOVERNMENT WARNING:
(1) ACCORDING TO THE SURGEON GENERAL, WOMEN SHOULD NOT DRINK ALCOHOLIC BEVERAGES DURING PREGNANCY BECAUSE OF THE RISK OF BIRTH DEFECTS.
(2) CONSUMPTION OF ALCOHOLIC BEVERAGES IMPAIRS YOUR ABILITY TO DRIVE A CAR OR OPERATE MACHINERY, AND MAY CAUSE HEALTH PROBLEMS.

© Cengage/Christine Myaskovsky

> **PHOTO H15-3** All containers of beer, wine, and liquor warn women not to drink alcoholic beverages during pregnancy because of the risk of birth defects.

When Is the Damage Done?

The type of abnormality observed in an FAS infant depends on the developmental events occurring at the times of alcohol exposure. During the first trimester, developing organs such as the brain, heart, and kidneys may be malformed. During the second trimester, the risk of spontaneous abortion increases. During the third trimester, body and brain growth may be impaired. Quite simply, the risk begins with any use.

The father's alcohol ingestion may also affect fertility and fetal development. Animal studies have found smaller litter sizes, lower birthweights, reduced survival rates, and impaired learning ability in the offspring of males consuming alcohol prior to conception. An association between paternal alcohol intake 1 month prior to conception and low infant birthweight has been reported in human beings. Alcohol use creates epigenetic changes in sperm DNA that may alter gene expression and result in features of fetal alcohol spectrum disorders.

In view of the damage caused by FAS, prevention efforts focus on educating women not to drink during pregnancy. Public service announcements and alcohol beverage warning labels help raise awareness (see Photo H15-3). Everyone should hear the message loud and clear: don't drink alcohol during pregnancy.

CRITICAL THINKING QUESTIONS

A. What are the moral implications of using alcohol during pregnancy?
B. Clearly, drinking alcohol during pregnancy endangers the developing fetus, yet controversy surrounds the questions as to how much alcohol causes damage and when the damage is done. What difficulties might researchers encounter in trying to determine the exact amount of alcohol and the timing during pregnancy that might be reasonably safe for fetal development?

REFERENCES

1. H. E. Hoyme and coauthors, Updated clinical guidelines for diagnosing fetal alcohol spectrum disorders, *Pediatrics* 138 (2016): e20154256.
2. I. J. Chasnoff, A. M. Wells, and L. King, Misdiagnosis and missed diagnoses in foster and adopted children with prenatal alcohol exposure, *Pediatrics* 135 (2015): 264–270.
3. J. R. Wozniak and coauthors, Choline supplementation in children with fetal alcohol spectrum disorders: A randomized, double-blind, placebo-controlled trial, *American Journal of Clinical Nutrition* 102 (2015): 1113–1125.
4. C. H. Tan and coauthors, Alcohol use and binge drinking among women of childbearing age—the United States, 2011–2013, *Morbidity and Mortality Weekly Report* 64 (2015): 1042–1046.
5. J. F. Williams, V. C. Smith, and the Committee on Substance Abuse, Fetal alcohol spectrum disorders, *Pediatrics* 136 (2015): e1395–e1406.

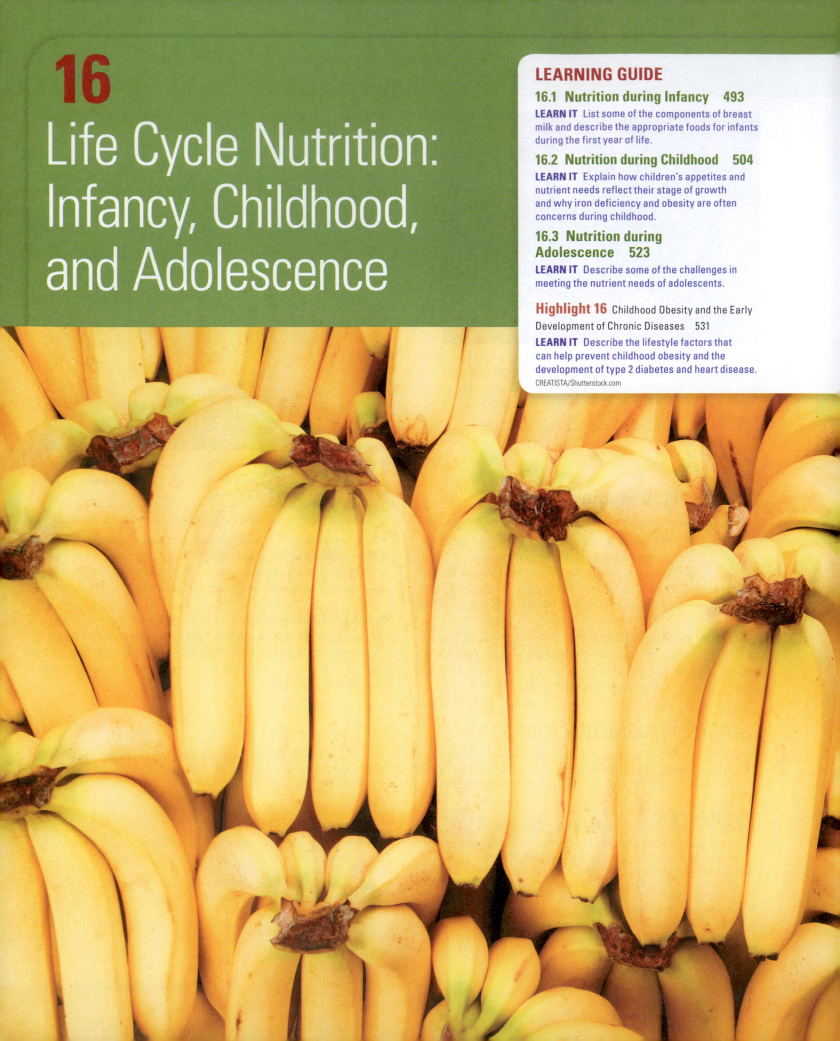

16 Life Cycle Nutrition: Infancy, Childhood, and Adolescence

LEARNING GUIDE

CREATISTA/Shutterstock.com

Nutrition in Your Life

Much of this book has focused on you—your food choices and how they might affect your health. This chapter shifts the focus from you the recipient to you the caregiver. One day (if not already), children may depend on you to feed them well and teach them wisely. The responsibility of nourishing children can seem overwhelming at times, but the job is fairly simple. Offer children a variety of nutritious foods to support their growth and teach them how to make healthy food and activity choices. Presenting foods in a relaxed and supportive environment nourishes both physical and emotional well-being. As you read this chapter, consider how you might plan a day's menu for a child and determine whether it meets nutrient requirements to support healthy growth but not so much as to promote obesity.

Nutrient needs change throughout the growing years and vary from individual to individual. The first year of life (infancy) is a time of phenomenal growth and development. The infant's high nutrient needs and developing maturity determine which foods are most appropriate to meet the needs for each stage of the first year. After the first year, a child continues to grow and change, but more slowly. Still, the cumulative effects over the next decade are remarkable. Then as the child enters the teen years, the pace toward adulthood accelerates dramatically. The physical changes of adolescents make their nutrient needs high, and their emotional, intellectual, and social changes make meeting those needs a challenge. Sound nutrition throughout infancy, childhood, and adolescence promotes normal growth and development, facilitates academic and physical performance, and may help prevent the development of obesity, diabetes, heart disease, some cancers, and other chronic diseases in adulthood. This chapter examines the special nutrient needs of infants, children, and adolescents.

16.1 Nutrition during Infancy

LEARN IT List some of the components of breast milk and describe the appropriate foods for infants during the first year of life.

Initially, the infant drinks only breast milk or formula but later begins to eat some foods, as appropriate. Common sense in the selection of infant foods—along with a nurturing, relaxed environment—supports an infant's health and well-being.

Energy and Nutrient Needs An infant grows fast during the first year, as Figure 16-1 shows. Growth directly reflects nutrient intake and is an important factor in assessing the nutrition status of infants and children. Health-care professionals measure the height and weight of an infant or child at intervals and compare the measurements with standard growth charts for gender and age and with previous measures of that infant or child (see How To 16-1, p. 494).

Energy Intake and Activity A healthy infant's birthweight doubles by about 5 months of age and triples by 1 year, typically reaching 20 to 25 pounds. The infant's length changes more slowly than weight, increasing about 10 inches from birth to 1 year. By the end of the first year, infant growth slows considerably; during the second year, an infant typically gains less than 10 pounds and grows about 5 inches in length. At the age of 2, healthy children have attained approximately half of their adult height.

Not only do infants grow rapidly, but their energy requirement is remarkably high—about twice that of an adult, based on body weight. A newborn baby requires about 450 kcalories per day, whereas most adults require about 2000 kcalories per day.

> **FIGURE 16-1 Weight Gain of Infants in Their First Five Years of Life**

In the first year, an infant's birthweight may triple, but over the following several years, the rate of weight gain gradually diminishes.

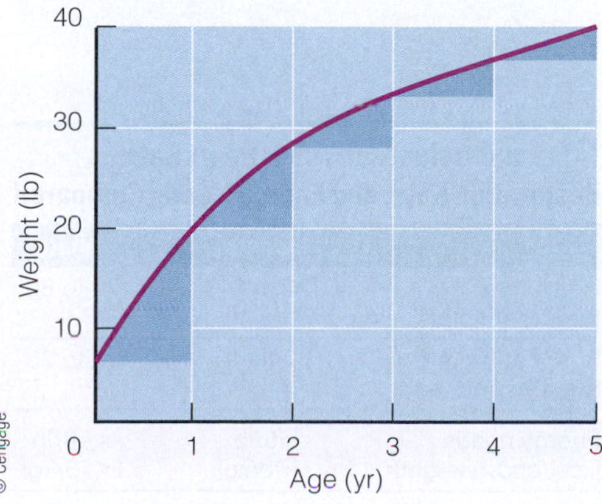
40
30
20
10
Weight (lb)
0
1
2
3
4
5
Age (yr)
© Cengage

>How To 16-1 Plot Measures on a Growth Chart

You can assess the growth of infants and children by plotting their measurements on a percentile graph. Percentile graphs divide the measures of a population into 100 equal divisions so that half of the population falls at or above the 50th percentile and half falls below. Using percentiles allows for comparisons among people of the same age and gender.

To plot measures on a growth chart, follow these steps:

- Select the appropriate chart based on age and gender. For this example, use the accompanying chart, which gives percentiles for weight for girls from birth to 36 months. (Appendix E provides other growth charts for both boys and girls of various ages.)
- Locate the infant's age along the horizontal axis at the bottom of the chart (in this example, 6 months).
- Locate the infant's weight in pounds or kilograms along the vertical axis of the chart (in this example, 17 pounds or 7.7 kilograms).
- Mark the chart where the age and weight lines intersect (shown here with a red dot), and follow the curved line to find the percentile.

This 6-month-old infant is at the 75th percentile. Her pediatrician will weigh her again over the next few months and expect the growth curve to follow the same percentile throughout the first year. In general, dramatic changes or measures much above the 80th percentile or much below the 10th percentile may be cause for concern.

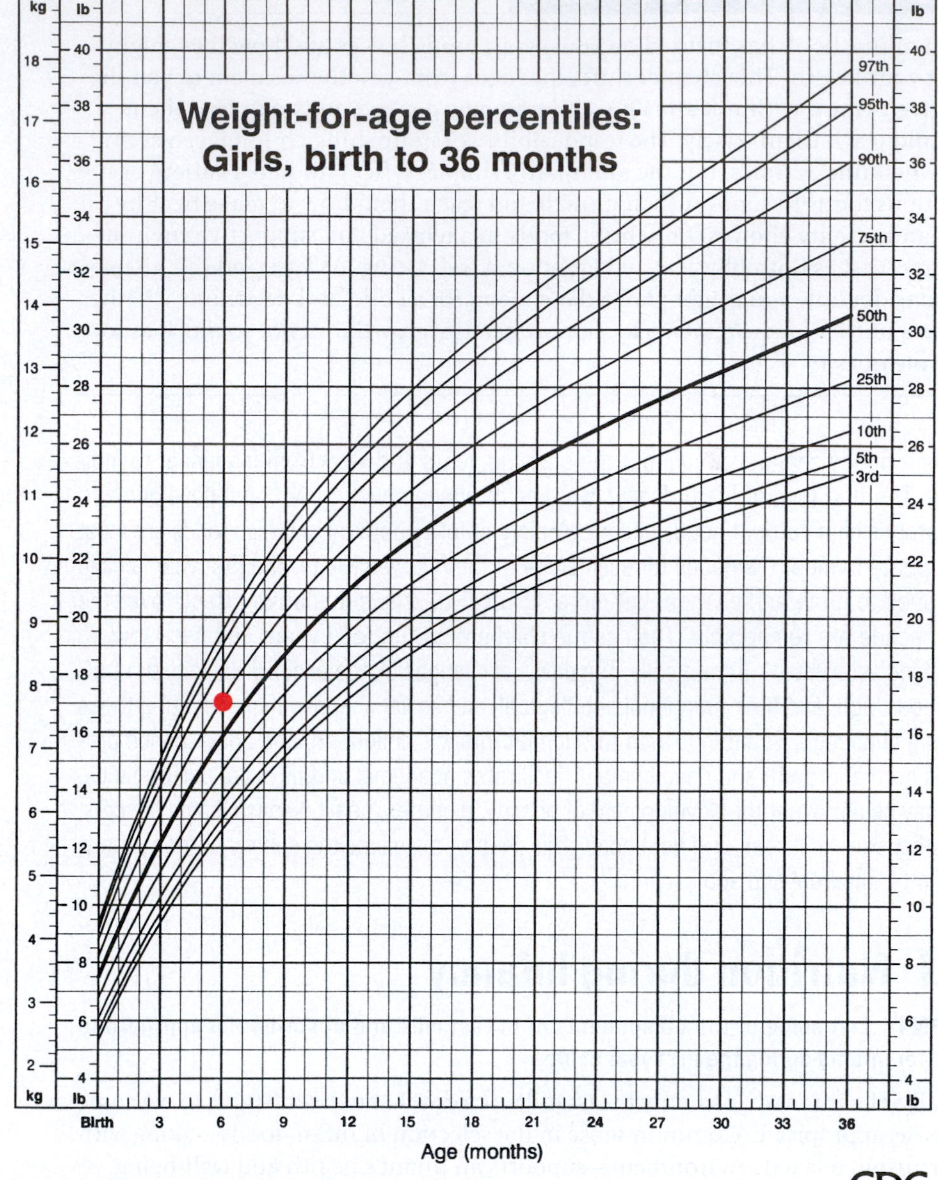
Weight-for-age percentiles:
Girls, birth to 36 months
kg
lb
97th
95th
90th
75th
50th
25th
10th
5th
3rd
Birth 3 6 9 12 15 18 21 24 27 30 33 36
Age (months)
SOURCE: Developed by the National Center for Health Statistics in collaboration with
the National Center for Chronic Disease Prevention and Health Promotion (2000).
CDC

> TRY IT Determine the percentile for a 12-month-old girl who weighs 21 pounds.

TABLE 16-1 Infant and Adult Heart Rate, Respiration Rate, and Energy Needs Compared

	Infants	Adults
Heart rate (beats/minute)	120 to 140	70 to 80
Respiration rate (breaths/minute)	20 to 40	15 to 20
Energy needs (kcal/body weight)	45/lb (100/kg)	<18/lb (<40/kg)

In terms of body weight, the difference is remarkable. Infants require about 100 kcalories per kilogram of body weight per day, whereas most adults need fewer than 40 (see Table 16-1). If an infant's energy needs were applied to an adult, a 170-pound adult would require more than 7000 kcalories a day. After 6 months, the infant's energy needs decline as the growth rate slows, but some of the energy saved by slower growth is spent in increased activity (see Photo 16-1).

Energy Nutrients Recommendations for the energy nutrients—carbohydrate, fat, and protein—during the first 6 months of life are based on the average intakes of healthy, full-term infants fed breast milk. During the second 6 months of life, recommendations reflect typical intakes from **complementary foods** as well as breast milk.

As Chapter 4 discussed, carbohydrates provide energy to all the cells of the body, but those in the brain depend primarily on glucose to fuel activities. Relative to the size of the body, the size of an infant's brain is greater than that of an adult's. An infant's brain weight is about 12 percent of body weight, whereas an adult's brain weight is about 2 percent. Thus, an infant's brain uses *relatively* more glucose—about 60 percent of the day's total energy intake.

Fat provides most of the energy in breast milk and standard infant formula. Its high energy density supports the rapid growth of early infancy. Fat also provides the essential fatty acids needed for normal growth and development. As Chapter 5 mentioned, DHA (docosahexaenoic acid) is the most abundant fatty acid in the brain and is also present in the retina of the eye, contributing to neural and visual development. DHA accumulation in the brain is greatest during fetal development and early infancy.[1]

No single nutrient is more essential to growth than protein; it is the basic building material of the body's tissues. All of the body's cells and most of its fluids contain protein. Consequently, inadequate protein intake has widespread effects, limiting brain function, weakening immune defenses, and disrupting digestion and absorption. The term *failure to thrive* is sometimes used to describe the many problems associated with infants and children suffering from protein deficiency. Excess dietary protein can cause problems, too, especially in a small infant. Too much protein stresses the liver and kidneys, which have to metabolize and excrete the excess nitrogen. Signs of protein overload include acidosis, dehydration, diarrhea, elevated blood ammonia, elevated blood urea, and fever. Such problems are not common, but they have been observed in infants fed inappropriate foods, such as fat-free milk or concentrated formula.

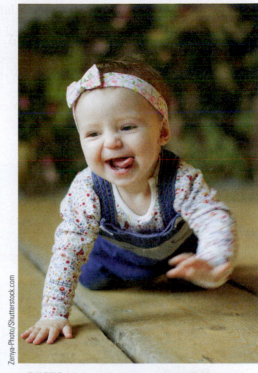

Zenya-Photo/Shutterstock.com

> **PHOTO 16-1** After 6 months, energy saved by slower growth is spent in increased activity.

Vitamins and Minerals An infant's needs for most nutrients, in proportion to body weight, are more than double those of an adult. Figure 16-2 (p. 496) illustrates this by comparing a 5-month-old infant's needs per unit of body weight with those of an adult man. Some of the differences are extraordinary. Infant recommendations are based on the average amount of nutrients consumed by thriving infants breastfed by well-nourished mothers.

Water One of the most essential nutrients for infants, as for everyone, is water. The younger the infant, the greater the percentage of body weight is water. During early infancy, breast milk or infant formula normally provides enough water to replace fluid losses in a healthy infant. If the environmental temperature is extremely high, however, infants need supplemental water.[2] Because much of the fluid in an infant's body is located *outside* the cells—between the cells and within the blood vessels—rapid fluid losses and the resulting dehydration can be life-threatening. Conditions that cause rapid fluid loss, such as diarrhea or vomiting, require prompt treatment with an electrolyte solution designed for infants.

Breast Milk

In the United States, the two dietary practices that have the most significant effect on an infant's nutrition are the milk the infant receives and the age at which complementary foods are introduced. A later section discusses the introduction of complementary foods, but as to the milk, the American Academy of Pediatrics strongly recommends breastfeeding for healthy full-term infants, except where specific contraindications exist. The Academy of Nutrition and Dietetics also advocates breastfeeding for the nutritional health of the infant as well as for the many other benefits it provides both infant and mother (review Table 15-10, p. 481).[3]

Breast milk excels as a source of nutrients for infants. Its unique nutrient composition and protective factors promote optimal infant health and development throughout the first year of life. Ideally, infants will receive exclusive breastfeeding

complementary foods: nutrient- and energy-containing solid or semisolid foods (or liquids) fed to infants in addition to breast milk or infant formula.

> FIGURE 16-2 Recommended Intakes of an Infant and an Adult Compared on the Basis of Body Weight

Because infants are small, they need smaller total amounts of the nutrients than adults do, but when comparisons are based on body weight, infants need more than twice as much of many nutrients. Infants use large amounts of energy and nutrients, in proportion to their body size, to keep all their metabolic processes going.

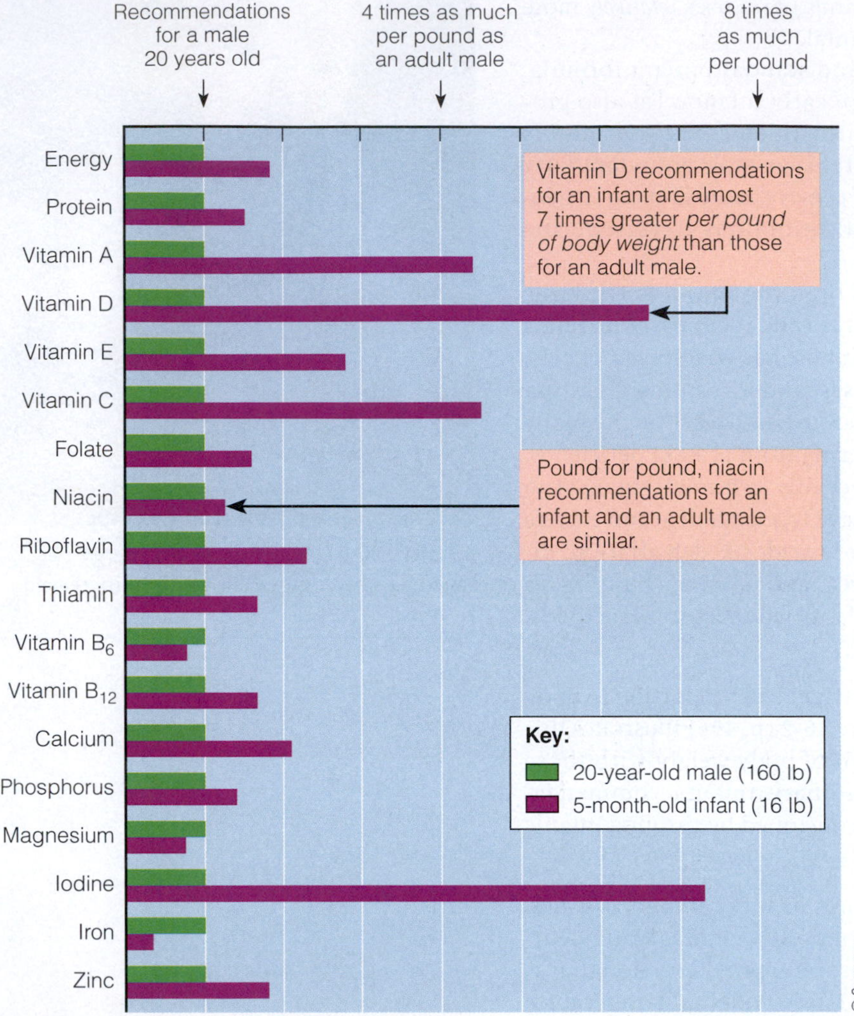

Recommendations for a male 20 years old
4 times as much per pound as an adult male
8 times as much per pound
Energy
Protein
Vitamin A
Vitamin D
Vitamin E
Vitamin C
Folate
Niacin
Riboflavin
Thiamin
Vitamin B6
Vitamin B12
Calcium
Phosphorus
Magnesium
Iodine
Iron
Zinc
Vitamin D recommendations for an infant are almost 7 times greater *per pound of body weight* than those for an adult male.
Pound for pound, niacin recommendations for an infant and an adult male are similar.
Key:
20-year-old male (160 lb)
5-month-old infant (16 lb)
© Cengage

for 6 months, and breastfeeding with complementary foods for at least 12 months.[4] Experts add, though, that iron-fortified formula, which imitates the nutrient composition of breast milk, is an acceptable alternative. After all, the primary goal is to provide the infant nourishment in a relaxed and loving environment. Chapter 15 discussed maternal nutrition to support successful breastfeeding; this section focuses on infants.

Frequency and Duration of Breastfeeding Breast milk is more easily and completely digested than formula, so breastfed infants usually need to eat more frequently than formula-fed infants do. During the first few weeks, approximately 8 to 12 feedings a day, on demand, as soon as the infant shows early signs of hunger such as increased alertness, activity, or suckling motions. Such a schedule promotes optimal milk production and infant growth. Crying is a late indicator of hunger. An infant who nurses every 2 to 3 hours and sleeps contentedly between feedings is adequately nourished. As the infant gets older, stomach capacity enlarges and the mother's milk production increases, allowing for longer intervals between feedings.

Even though the infant obtains about half the milk from the breast during the first 2 to 3 minutes of suckling, the infant should be encouraged to breastfeed on the first breast for as long as he or she is actively suckling, before being offered the second breast. The next feeding begins on the breast offered last. The infant's suckling, as well as the complete removal of milk from the breast, stimulates milk production.

Energy Nutrients The energy-nutrient composition of breast milk differs dramatically from that recommended for adult diets (see Figure 16-3). Yet for infants, breast milk is nature's most nearly perfect food, providing the clear lesson that people at different stages of life have different nutrient needs (see Photo 16-2).

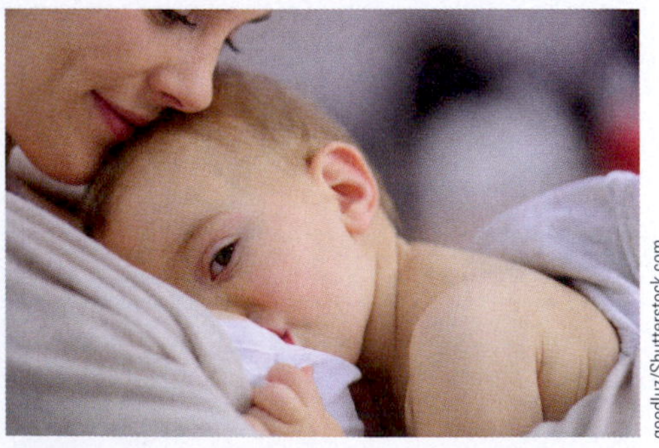

goodluz/Shutterstock.com

> PHOTO 16-2 Women are encouraged to breastfeed whenever possible because breast milk provides infants with many nutrient and health advantages.

alpha-lactalbumin (lact-AL-byoo-min): a major protein in human breast milk, as opposed to *casein* (CAY-seen), a major protein in cow's milk.

The main carbohydrate in breast milk (and standard infant formula) is the disaccharide lactose. In addition to being easily digested, lactose enhances calcium absorption. The carbohydrate component of breast milk also contains abundant oligosaccharides, which are present only in trace amounts in cow's milk and infant formula made from cow's milk.[5] Breast milk oligosaccharides help protect the infant from infection by preventing the binding of pathogens to the infant's intestinal cells.[6]

The amount of protein in breast milk is less than in cow's milk, but this quantity is actually beneficial because it places less stress on the infant's immature kidneys to excrete urea, the major end product of protein metabolism. Much of the protein in breast milk is **alpha-lactalbumin,** which is efficiently digested and absorbed.

As for the lipids, breast milk contains a generous proportion of the essential fatty acids linoleic acid and linolenic acid, as well as their longer-chain derivatives arachidonic acid and DHA. DHA accumulation in the brain is higher in breastfed infants than in formula-fed infants.[7] Research has focused on the mental and visual development of breastfed infants and infants fed standard formula with and without DHA added.[8] Results of studies for visual acuity are mixed, perhaps because of factors such as the amount of DHA provided, the source of the DHA, and the sensitivity of different measures for visual acuity.[9] Some evidence from studies examining the effects of DHA status during fetal and infant development on cognitive function suggests that DHA supplementation can make a positive difference.[10] Adding DHA to standard infant formulas has no adverse effects; most standard formulas are currently fortified with both DHA and arachidonic acid.

Vitamins With the exception of vitamin D, the vitamins in breast milk are ample to support infant growth. The vitamin D in breast milk is low, however, and vitamin D deficiency impairs bone mineralization.[11] Vitamin D deficiency is most likely in infants who are not exposed to sunlight daily, have darkly pigmented skin, and receive breast milk without vitamin D supplementation. Reports of infants in the United States developing the vitamin D–deficiency disease rickets and recommendations to limit sun exposure in infants younger than 6 months of age prompted revisions in vitamin D guidelines. The American Academy of Pediatrics recommends a vitamin D supplement for all infants who are breastfed exclusively and for all infants who do not receive at least 1 liter (1000 milliliters, roughly 1 quart or 32 ounces) of vitamin D–fortified formula daily.[12]

Minerals The calcium content of breast milk is ideal for infant bone growth, and the calcium is well absorbed. Breast milk contains relatively small amounts of iron, but the iron has a high bioavailability. Zinc also has a high bioavailability, thanks to the presence of a zinc-binding protein. Breast milk is low in sodium, another benefit for the infant's immature kidneys. Fluoride promotes the development of strong teeth, but breast milk is not a good source.

Supplements Many pediatricians routinely prescribe liquid supplements containing vitamin D, iron, and fluoride as outlined in Table 16-2. In addition, infants receive a single dose of vitamin K at birth to protect them from bleeding to death. (See Chapter 11 for a description of vitamin K's role in blood clotting.)

Immunological Protection In addition to its nutritional benefits, breast milk offers immunological protection. Not only is breast milk sterile, but it also actively fights disease and protects infants from illnesses.[13] Such protection is most valuable during the first year, when the infant's immune system is not fully prepared to mount a response against infections.

During the first 2 to 3 days after delivery, the breasts produce **colostrum**, a premilk substance containing mostly serum with antibodies and white blood cells. Colostrum (like breast milk) helps protect the newborn from infections against which the mother has developed immunity. The maternal antibodies in the breast milk inactivate disease-causing bacteria within the infant's digestive tract before they can start infections.[14] This explains, in part, why breastfed infants have fewer infections than formula-fed infants.[15] In addition to antibodies, colostrum and breast milk provide other protective factors that help fight against bacterial and viral infection (see Table 16-3, p. 498).

Allergy and Disease Protection In addition to protection against infections, breast milk may offer protection against the development of allergies.[16] Compared with formula-fed infants, breastfed infants have a lower incidence of allergic reactions,

FIGURE 16-3 Percentages of Energy-Yielding Nutrients in Breast Milk and in Recommended Adult Diets

The proportions of energy-yielding nutrients in human breast milk differ from those recommended for adults.

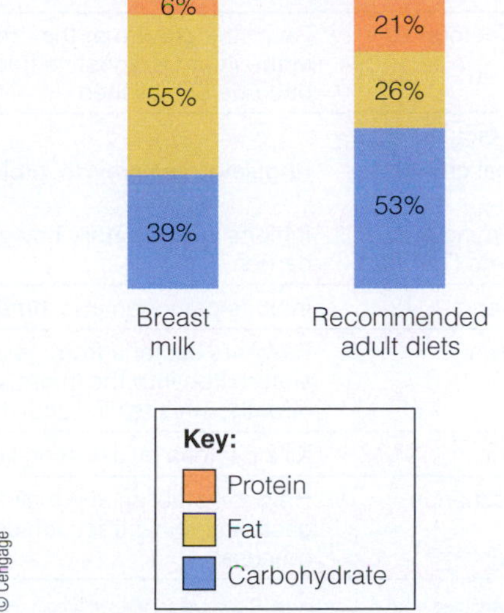
6%
55%
39%
21%
26%
53%
Breast milk
Recommended adult diets
Key:
Protein
Fat
Carbohydrate
© Cengage

NOTE: The values listed for adults represent approximate midpoints of the acceptable ranges for protein (10 to 35 percent), fat (20 to 35 percent), and carbohydrate (45 to 65 percent).

TABLE 16-2 Supplements for Full-Term Breastfed Infants

Birth	4 months of Age	6 months of Age
Vitamin D[a]	Iron[b]	Fluoride[c]

[a] Vitamin D supplements are recommended for all infants who are exclusively breastfed and for all infants who do not receive at least 1 liter (1000 milliliters) or 1 quart (32 ounces) of vitamin D–fortified formula per day.

[b] At 4 months of age, 1 mg per kilogram of body weight per day of supplemental iron is recommended for all infants who are exclusively breastfed and for all infants who are receiving more than one half of their daily feedings as breast milk and no iron-containing complementary foods. Once iron-containing foods are introduced, iron supplements may not be needed.

[c] At 6 months of age, breastfed infants and formula-fed infants who receive ready-to-use formulas (which are made with water low in fluoride) or formula mixed with water that contains little or no fluoride (less than 0.3 ppm) may need supplements, depending on the health care provider's assessment of the infant's fluoride exposure.

SOURCE: Adapted from Committee on Nutrition, American Academy of Pediatrics, *Pediatric Nutrition*, 7th ed., ed., R. E. Kleinman (Elk Grove Village, IL.: American Academy of Pediatrics, 2014).

colostrum (ko-LAHS-trum): a milklike secretion from the breast, present during the first few days after delivery before milk appears; rich in protective factors.

TABLE 16-3 Protective Factors in Breast Milk

Factor(s)	Action(s)
Antibodies	Offer protection in the upper respiratory tract and gastrointestinal tract by inhibiting pathogen attachment to the mucosa and protecting against invasive infections; may stimulate the infant's immune system
Bifidus factors	Favor the growth of the "friendly" bacterium *Lactobacillus bifidus* in the infant's digestive tract so that other, harmful bacteria cannot become established
Growth factors:	
Epidermal growth factor	Regulates cell growth, proliferation, and differentiation
Transforming growth factor-beta (TGF-β)	Inhibits inflammatory bowel diseases; supports a healthy epithelial barrier
Lactadherin	Inhibits pathogen attachment to the intestinal mucosa
Lactoferrin	Prevents bacteria from getting the iron needed to grow; helps absorb iron into the infant's bloodstream; kills some bacteria directly; inhibits viral activity
Lysozyme	Kills bacteria by assisting lactoferrin
Oligosaccharides	Help to establish and maintain growth of desired bacteria in gastrointestinal tract; inhibit pathogen attachment to the intestinal mucosa

SOURCE: Adapted from B. Lonnerdal, Bioactive proteins in breast milk, *Journal of Paediatrics and Child Health* (Supplement S1) 49 (2013): 1–7; D. E. W. Chatterton and coauthors, Anti-inflammatory mechanisms of bioactive milk proteins in the intestine of newborns, *International Journal of Biochemistry and Cell Biology* 45 (2013): 1730–1747; P. V. Jeurink and coauthors, Mechanisms underlying immune effects of dietary oligosaccharides, *American Journal of Clinical Nutrition* 98 (2013): 572S–577S; A. Walker, Breast milk as the gold standard for protective nutrients, *Journal of Pediatrics* 156 (2010): 53–57.

such as recurrent wheezing and skin rashes. This protection is especially noticeable among infants with a family history of allergies.[17] Breastfeeding may also reduce the risk of sudden infant death syndrome (SIDS).[18] The protective effect against SIDS is stronger when infants are exclusively breastfed, but breastfeeding to any extent for any duration offers some protection. Similarly, breast milk may offer protection against the development of cardiovascular disease in adulthood, but additional research, using consistent and precise definitions of breastfeeding, is needed to confirm this effect.[19]

Other Potential Benefits Breastfeeding may offer some protection against excessive weight gain later, although findings are inconsistent.[20] Researchers note that many other factors—socioeconomic status, other infant and child feeding practices, and especially the mother's weight—strongly predict a child's body weight.[21]

Many studies suggest a beneficial effect of breastfeeding on intelligence, but when subjected to strict standards of methodology (for example, large sample size and appropriate intelligence testing), the evidence is less than convincing.[22] Nevertheless, the possibility that breastfeeding may positively affect later intelligence is intriguing. It may be that some specific component of breast milk, such as DHA, stimulates brain development or that certain factors associated with the feeding process itself promote intellect. Most likely, a combination of factors is involved. More large, well-controlled studies are needed to confirm the effects, if any, of breastfeeding on brain development and intelligence.

Breast Milk Banks Similar to blood banks that collect blood from individuals to give to others in need, **breast milk banks** receive milk from lactating women who have an abundant supply to give to infants whose own mothers' milk is unavailable or insufficient. The women who donate breast milk are carefully screened to exclude those who smoke cigarettes, use illicit drugs, take medications (including high doses of dietary supplements), drink more than two alcoholic beverages a day, or have communicable diseases. The breast milk from several donors is pooled to ensure an even distribution of all components, pasteurized to destroy bacteria, checked for contamination, and frozen before being shipped overnight to hospitals, where it is dispensed by physician prescription. In the absence of a mother's own breast milk, donor milk may be the life-saving solution for fragile infants, most notably those with very low birthweight or unusual medical conditions.[23]

The Food and Drug Administration (FDA) recommends against purchasing breast milk from online sources. Research shows that some of the milk sold online may be diluted with cow's milk or infant formula.[24] Such milk can be dangerous to infants who are allergic to cow's milk.

Infant Formula

A woman who breastfeeds for a year can **wean** her infant to cow's milk, bypassing the need for infant formula. A woman who decides to feed her infant formula from birth, to wean to formula after less than a year of breastfeeding, or to substitute formula for breastfeeding on occasion must select an appropriate infant formula and learn to prepare it. Cow's milk is inappropriate during the first year of life.

breast milk bank: a service that collects, screens, processes, and distributes donated human milk.

wean: to gradually replace breast milk with infant formula or other foods appropriate to an infant's diet.

Infant Formula Composition Formula manufacturers attempt to copy the nutrient composition of breast milk as closely as possible. Figure 16-4 illustrates the energy-nutrient balance of breast milk, infant formula, and cow's milk. All formula-fed infants should be given iron-fortified infant formulas.[25] The increasing use of iron-fortified formulas over the past few decades is responsible for the decline in iron-deficiency anemia among infants in the United States.

Risks of Formula Feeding Infant formulas contain no protective antibodies for infants, but in general, vaccinations, purified water, and clean environments in developed countries help protect infants from infections. Formulas can be prepared safely by following the rules of proper food handling and by using water that is free of contamination. Of particular concern is lead-contaminated water, a major source of lead poisoning in infants. Because the first water drawn from the tap each day is highest in lead, a person living in a house with old, lead-soldered plumbing should let the water run a few minutes before drinking or using it to prepare formula or food.

Water supplies contain variable concentrations of minerals, including fluoride. As mentioned in Chapter 13, optimal levels of fluoride protect against dental caries, but too much fluoride during tooth development can cause defects in the teeth known as fluorosis. Inadequate fluoride after 6 months of age may also be a concern. Thus, health experts urge caregivers to have their well water analyzed for mineral contents and to check with the local health department to determine the fluoride content of the community water supply. Caregivers should reconstitute powdered or concentrated liquid formulas with optimally fluoridated water (0.7 to 1.2 parts per million).[26] If fluoride levels are excessive, ready-to-feed formulas or formulas prepared with fluoride-free or low-fluoride water can be used. Such waters are labeled "purified," "demineralized," "deionized," or "distilled." If fluoride levels are inadequate, formulas may need to be prepared with fluoridated bottled water once the infant is 6 months of age.

In developing countries and in poor areas of the United States, formula may be unavailable, prepared with contaminated water, or overdiluted in an attempt to save money. Contaminated formulas may cause infections, leading to diarrhea, dehydration, and malabsorption. Without sterilization and refrigeration, formula is an ideal breeding ground for bacteria. Whenever such risks are present, breastfeeding can be a life-saving option: breast milk is sterile, and its antibodies enhance an infant's resistance to infections.

Infant Formula Standards National and international standards have been set for the nutrient contents of infant formulas. In the United States, the standard developed by the American Academy of Pediatrics reflects "human milk taken from well-nourished mothers during the first or second month of lactation, when the infant's growth rate is high." The Food and Drug Administration (FDA) mandates the safety and nutritional quality of infant formulas. Formulas meeting these standards have similar nutrient compositions. Small differences among formulas are sometimes confusing, but they are usually unimportant; all support infant growth and health (see Photo 16-3).

Recently, the FDA issued new quality-control procedures to further ensure that infant formulas are safe and support healthy growth.[27] These new standards specify how and when manufacturers must inform the FDA about new formulas and changes to formulas, and require testing for contamination with harmful bacteria such as *Salmonella*.

Special Formulas Standard formulas are inappropriate for some infants. Special formulas have been designed to meet the dietary needs of infants with specific conditions such as prematurity or inherited diseases. Most infants allergic to milk protein can drink formulas based on soy protein.[28] Soy formulas also use cornstarch and sucrose instead of lactose and so are recommended for infants with lactose intolerance as well. They are also useful as an alternative to milk-based

> **FIGURE 16-4 Percentages of Energy-Yielding Nutrients in Breast Milk, Infant Formula, and Cow's Milk**

The average proportions of energy-yielding nutrients in human breast milk and formula differ slightly. In contrast, cow's milk provides too much protein and too little carbohydrate.

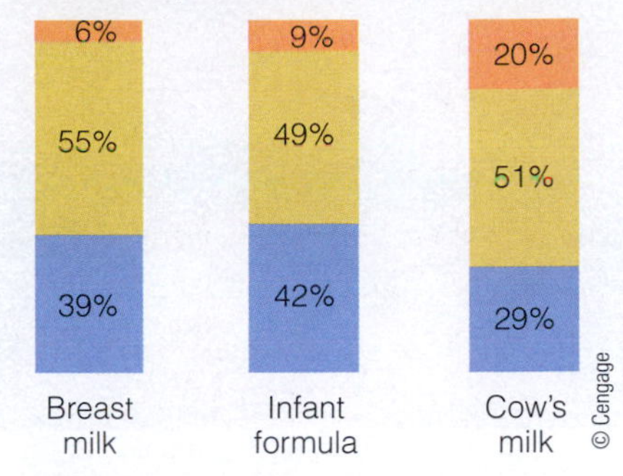
6%
55%
39%
Breast milk
9%
49%
42%
Infant formula
20%
51%
29%
Cow's milk
© Cengage

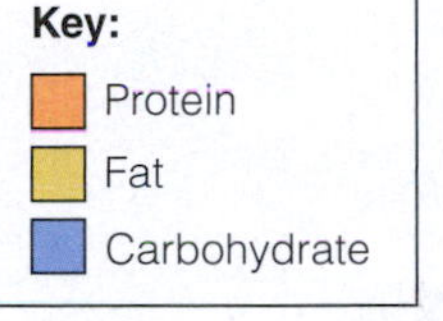
Key:
Protein
Fat
Carbohydrate

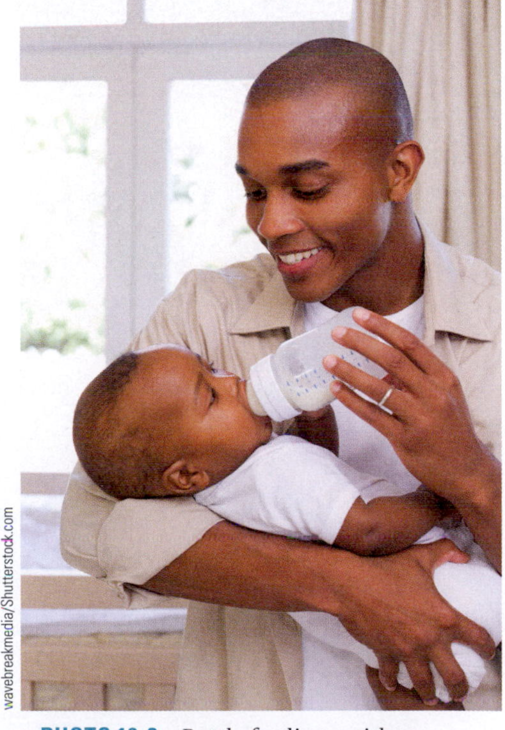
wavebreakmedia/Shutterstock.com

> **PHOTO 16-3** Bottle feeding—either expressed breast milk or infant formula—offers fathers and other caregivers an opportunity to feed infants.

> **FIGURE 16-5 Nursing Bottle Tooth Decay**
This child was frequently put to bed sucking on a bottle filled with apple juice, so the teeth were bathed in carbohydrate for long periods of time—a perfect medium for bacterial growth. The upper teeth show signs of decay.

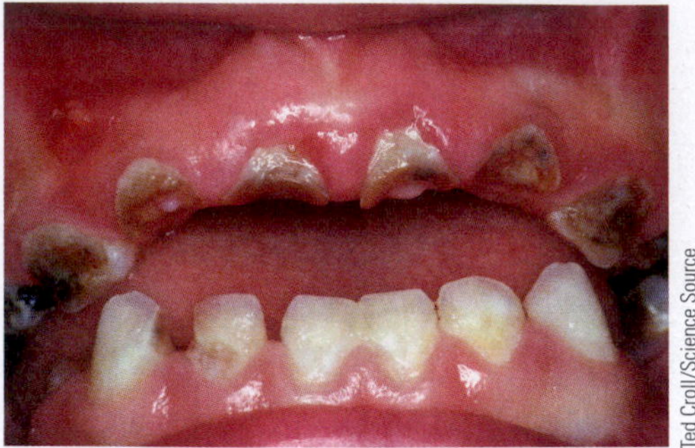
Ted Croll/Science Source

formulas for vegan families. Despite these limited uses, soy formulas account for about 15 percent of the infant formulas sold today. Although soy formulas support the normal growth and development of infants, for infants who don't need them, they offer no advantage over milk formulas.

Some infants who are allergic to cow's milk protein may also be allergic to soy protein.[29] For these infants, special formulas based on hydrolyzed protein are available. The protein in these formulas is a mixture of free amino acids, dipeptides, tripeptides, and short-chain peptides that do not elicit an allergic reaction in most infants.

Inappropriate Formulas Caregivers must use only products designed for infants; soy *beverages,* for example, are nutritionally incomplete and inappropriate for infants. Goat's milk is also inappropriate for infants in part because of its low folate content.[30] An infant receiving goat's milk is likely to develop "goat's milk anemia," an anemia characteristic of folate deficiency.

Nursing Bottle Tooth Decay An infant cannot be allowed to sleep with a bottle because of the potential damage to developing teeth. Salivary flow, which normally cleanses the mouth, diminishes as the infant falls asleep. Prolonged sucking on a bottle of formula, milk, or juice bathes the upper teeth in a carbohydrate-rich fluid that nourishes decay-producing bacteria. (The tongue covers and protects most of the lower teeth, but they, too, may be affected.) The result is extensive and rapid tooth decay (see Figure 16-5). To prevent **nursing bottle tooth decay**, no infant should be put to bed with a bottle of nourishing fluid.

Special Needs of Preterm Infants

An estimated one out of nine pregnancies in the United States results in a preterm birth.[31] The terms *preterm* and *premature* imply incomplete fetal development, or immaturity, of many body systems. As might be expected, preterm birth is a leading cause of infant deaths. Preterm infants face physical independence from their mothers before some of their organs and body tissues are ready. The rate of weight gain in the fetus is greater during the last trimester of gestation than at any other time. Therefore, a preterm infant is most often a low-birthweight infant as well. A premature birth deprives the infant of the nutritional support of the placenta during a time of maximal growth.

The last trimester of gestation is also a time of building nutrient stores. Being born with limited nutrient stores intensifies the already precarious situation for the infant. The physical and metabolic immaturity of preterm infants further compromises their nutrition status. Nutrient absorption, especially of fat and calcium, from an immature GI tract is limited. Consequently, preterm, low-birthweight infants are candidates for nutrient imbalances. Deficiencies of the fat-soluble vitamins, and the minerals calcium, iron, and zinc are common.

Preterm breast milk is well suited to meet a preterm infant's needs. During early lactation, preterm breast milk contains higher concentrations of protein and is lower in volume than term breast milk. The low milk volume is advantageous because preterm infants consume small quantities of milk per feeding, and the higher protein concentration allows for better growth. In many instances, supplements of nutrients specifically designed for preterm infants are added to the mother's expressed breast milk and fed to the infant from a bottle. When fortified with a preterm supplement, preterm breast milk supports growth at a rate that approximates the growth rate that would have occurred within the uterus.[32]

Introducing Cow's Milk

The age at which cow's milk should be introduced to the infant's diet has long been a source of controversy. The American Academy of Pediatrics advises that cow's milk is not appropriate during the first year.[33] For some infants, particularly those younger than 6 months of age, cow's milk may cause intestinal bleeding, which can lead to iron deficiency. Cow's milk is also a poor source of iron. Consequently, it both causes iron loss and fails to replace iron. Furthermore, the bioavailability of iron from infant cereal and other

nursing bottle tooth decay: extensive tooth decay due to prolonged tooth contact with formula, milk, fruit juice, or other carbohydrate-rich liquid offered to an infant in a bottle.

foods is reduced when cow's milk replaces breast milk or iron-fortified formula during the first year. Compared with breast milk or iron-fortified formula, cow's milk is higher in calcium and lower in vitamin C, characteristics that further reduce iron absorption. In addition, the higher protein concentration of cow's milk can stress the infant's kidneys. In short, infants need breast milk or iron-fortified infant formula, *not* cow's milk.

Ideally, by 1 year, the infant is obtaining at least two thirds of the total daily food energy from a balanced mixture of protein foods, cereals, vegetables, fruits, and other foods. At this time, reduced-fat or low-fat cow's milk is an acceptable and recommended beverage to accompany a diet that supplies 30 percent of kcalories from fat.[34] After the age of 2, a transition to fat-free milk can take place, but care should be taken to avoid excessive restriction of dietary fat.

Introducing First Foods

The high nutrient needs of infancy are met first by breast milk or formula only and then by the limited addition of selected foods over time. Infants gradually develop the ability to chew, swallow, and digest the wide variety of foods available to adults. The caregiver's selection of appropriate foods at the appropriate stages of development supports the infant's optimal growth and health.

When to Begin In addition to breast milk or formula, an infant can begin eating complementary foods between 4 and 6 months.[35] The American Academy of Pediatrics supports exclusive breastfeeding for 6 months but recognizes that infants are often developmentally ready to accept complementary foods between 4 and 6 months of age. The main purpose of introducing complementary foods is to provide needed nutrients that are no longer supplied adequately by breast milk or formula alone. The foods chosen must be those that the infant is developmentally capable of handling both physically and metabolically. As digestive secretions gradually increase throughout the first year of life, the digestion of complementary foods becomes more efficient. The exact timing depends on the individual infant's needs and developmental readiness (see Table 16-4), which vary from infant to

TABLE 16-4 Infant Development and Recommended Foods

Because each stage of development builds on the previous stage, the foods from an earlier stage continue to be included in all later stages.

Age (mo)	Feeding Skill	Appropriate Foods Added to the Diet
0–4	Turns head toward any object that brushes cheek. Initially swallows using back of tongue; gradually begins to swallow using front of tongue as well. Strong reflex to push food out (extrusion) during first 2 to 3 months.	Feed breast milk or infant formula.
4–6	Extrusion reflex diminishes, and the ability to swallow nonliquid foods develops. Indicates desire for food by opening mouth and leaning forward. Indicates satiety or disinterest by turning away and leaning back. Sits erect with support at 6 months. Begins chewing action. Brings hand to mouth. Grasps objects with palm of hand.	Begin iron-fortified cereal mixed with breast milk, formula, or water. Begin pureed meats, legumes, vegetables, and fruits.
6–8	Able to self-feed finger foods. Develops pincer (finger to thumb) grasp. Begins to drink from cup.	Begin textured vegetables and fruits. Begin unsweetened, diluted fruit juices from cup.
8–10	Begins to hold own bottle. Reaches for and grabs food and spoon. Sits unsupported.	Begin breads and cereals from table. Begin yogurt. Begin pieces of soft, cooked vegetables and fruit from table. Gradually begin finely cut meats, fish, casseroles, cheese, eggs, and mashed legumes.
10–12	Begins to master spoon, but still spills some.	Add variety. Gradually increase portion sizes.[a]

[a]Portion sizes for infants and young children are smaller than those for an adult. For example, a grain serving might be ½ slice of bread instead of 1 slice, or ¼ cup rice instead of ½ cup.

SOURCE: Adapted in part from Committee on Nutrition, American Academy of Pediatrics, *Pediatric Nutrition*, 7th ed., ed. R. E. Kleinman (Elk Grove Village, Ill.: American Academy of Pediatrics, 2014), pp. 113–142.

infant because of differences in growth rates, activities, and environmental conditions. In addition to the infant's nutrient needs and physical readiness to handle different forms of foods, the need to detect and control allergic reactions should also be considered when introducing complementary foods. With respect to nutrient needs, the nutrients needed earliest are iron and zinc, then vitamin C.

Food Allergies To prevent allergies and to facilitate prompt identification should they occur, experts recommend introducing single-ingredient foods, one at a time, in small portions, and waiting 3 to 5 days before introducing the next new food.[36] For example, rice cereal is usually the first cereal introduced because it is the least allergenic. When it is clear that rice cereal is not causing an allergy, another grain, perhaps barley or oat is introduced. Wheat cereal is offered last because it is the most common offender. If a cereal causes an allergic reaction such as a skin rash, digestive upset, or respiratory discomfort, it should be discontinued before introducing the next food.

Food allergies in the United States have increased over the past few decades, especially allergy to peanuts. New guidelines recommend introducing peanut-based foods early (between 4 and 11 months), rather than later (between 12 and 36 months) to prevent peanut allergy. Infants at high risk—those with severe skin rash or egg allergies—need medical approval and oversight, but for most other infants, parents may start adding peanut-containing foods such as watered down peanut butter or peanut puffs to the diet in the same way oatmeal and mashed vegetables are introduced.[37]

Choice of Infant Foods Infant foods should be selected to provide variety, balance, and moderation. Commercial baby foods offer a wide variety of palatable, nutritious foods in a safe and convenient form. Parents or caregivers should not feed directly from the jar; instead, spoon the needed portion into a dish and feed from there, leaving the leftovers in the jar uncontaminated by a used spoon. Homemade infant foods can be as nutritious as commercially prepared ones, so long as the cook minimizes nutrient losses during preparation. Ingredients for homemade foods should be fresh, whole foods without added salt, sugar, or seasonings. Pureed food can be frozen in ice cube trays, providing convenient-size blocks of food that can be thawed, warmed, and fed to the infant. To guard against foodborne illnesses, hands and equipment must be kept clean.

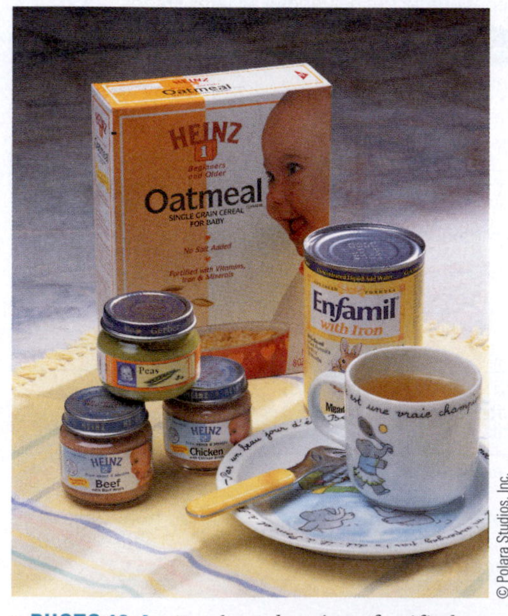
HEINZ
Oatmeal
Enfamil
with Iron
Peas
HEINZ
Chicken
HEINZ
Beef

> **PHOTO 16-4** Foods such as iron-fortified cereals and formulas, mashed legumes, and strained meats provide iron.

Foods to Provide Iron and Zinc Rapid growth demands iron. At about 4 to 6 months of age, the infant begins to need more iron than body stores plus breast milk or iron-fortified formula can provide. In addition to breast milk or iron-fortified formula, infants can receive iron from iron-fortified cereals and, once they readily accept complementary foods, from meats or legumes (see Photo 16-4). Iron-fortified cereals contribute a significant amount of iron to an infant's diet, but the iron's bioavailability is poor.[38] Caregivers can enhance iron absorption from iron-fortified cereals by serving vitamin C–rich foods with meals.

The concentration of zinc in breast milk is initially high, but decreases sharply over the first few months of lactation. The high efficiency of zinc absorption does not compensate for its low concentration over time. Infant formulas are fortified with zinc at levels higher than those found in breast milk. Thus, breastfed infants depend more on complementary foods to provide adequate zinc intakes than formula-fed infants do.[39] Infant cereals are not routinely fortified with zinc, so the best sources are protein foods such as meats, poultry, seafood, eggs, and legumes. Zinc is not as well absorbed from legumes as it is from other protein foods, however.

Foods to Provide Vitamin C The best sources of vitamin C are fruits and vegetables (see Chapter 10, pp. 321–322). It has been suggested that infants who are introduced to fruits before vegetables may develop a preference for sweets and find the vegetables less palatable, but there is no evidence to support offering these foods in a particular order.

Fruit juice is a good source of vitamin C, but excessive juice intake can lead to diarrhea in infants and young children.[40] Furthermore, too much fruit juice contributes excessive kcalories and displaces other nutrient-rich foods. The American Academy of Pediatrics recommends no fruit juice in the first year and limiting juice for young children (1 to 6 years of age) to 4 to 6 ounces per day. Fruit juices should be served in a cup, not a bottle.

Foods to Omit Concentrated sweets, including baby food "desserts," have no place in an infant's diet. They convey no nutrients to support growth, and the extra food energy can promote obesity. Products containing sugar alcohols such as sorbitol should also be limited because they may cause diarrhea. Canned vegetables are also inappropriate for infants because they often contain too much sodium. Honey and corn syrup should never be fed to infants because of the risk of **botulism.*** Infants and young children are vulnerable to foodborne illnesses. Foodborne illnesses and their prevention are topics in Chapter 19.

Infants and even young children cannot safely chew and swallow any of the foods listed in Table 16-5; they can easily choke on these foods, a risk not worth taking. Nonfood items may present even greater choking hazards to infants and young children. Parents and caregivers must pay careful attention to eliminate choking hazards in children's environments.

TABLE 16-5 Examples of Common Choking Items

Foods	
• Gum • Hard or gel-type candies • Hot dog slices • Large raw apple slices • Marshmallows • Nuts • Peanut butter • Popcorn, chips, or pretzel nuggets	• Raw carrots • Raw celery • Sausage sticks or slices • Whole beans • Whole cherries • Whole grapes
Nonfood items	
• Balloons • Coins • Pen tops	• Small balls and marbles • Other items of similar size

Vegetarian Diets during Infancy The newborn infant is a lacto-vegetarian. As long as the infant has access to sufficient quantities of either iron-fortified infant formula or breast milk (plus a vitamin D supplement) from a mother who eats an adequate diet, the infant will thrive during the early months. "Health-food beverages," such as rice milk, are inappropriate choices because they lack the protein, vitamins, and minerals infants and toddlers need; in fact, their use can lead to nutrient deficiencies.

Infants older than about 6 months of age present a greater challenge in terms of meeting nutrient needs by way of vegetarian and, especially, vegan diets. Continued breastfeeding or formula feeding is recommended, but supplementary feedings are necessary to ensure adequate energy and iron intakes. Infants and young children in vegetarian families should be given iron-fortified infant cereals well into the second year. Mashed or pureed legumes, tofu, and cooked eggs can be added to their diets in place of meats.

Infants who receive a well-balanced vegetarian diet that includes milk products and a variety of other foods can easily meet their nutritional requirements for growth. This is not always true for vegan infants; the growth of vegan infants slows significantly when weaning from breast milk to complementary foods. Deficiencies of protein, vitamin D, vitamin B_{12}, iron, zinc, and calcium have been reported in infants fed vegan diets. Vegan diets that are high in fiber, other complex carbohydrates, and water will fill infants' stomachs before meeting energy needs. This problem can be partially alleviated by providing more energy-dense foods, such as mashed legumes, tofu, and avocado. Using soy formulas (or milk) fortified with calcium, vitamin B_{12}, and vitamin D and including vitamin C–containing foods at meals to enhance iron absorption will help prevent some nutrient deficiencies in vegan diets. Parents or caregivers who choose to feed their infants vegan diets should consult with their pediatrician and a registered dietitian nutritionist frequently to ensure a nutritionally adequate diet that will support growth.

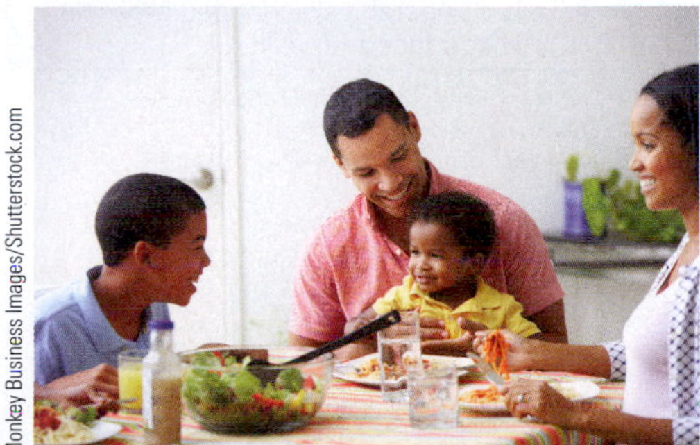

> **PHOTO 16-5** Ideally, a 1-year-old is able to eat many of the same foods as the rest of the family.

Foods at 1 Year Ideally, a 1-year-old will sit at the table, eat many of the same foods everyone else eats, and drink liquids from a cup, not a bottle (see Photo 16-5). At 1 year of age, reduced-fat or low-fat cow's milk can become a primary source of most of the nutrients an infant needs; 2 to 3 cups a day meets those needs

*In infants, but not in older individuals, ingestion of *Clostridium botulinum* spores can cause illness when the spores germinate in the intestine and produce a toxin, which is absorbed. Symptoms include poor feeding, constipation, loss of tension in the arteries and muscles, weakness, and respiratory compromise. Infant botulism has been implicated in 5 percent of cases of sudden infant death syndrome (SIDS).

botulism (BOT-chew-lism): an often fatal foodborne illness caused by the ingestion of foods containing a toxin produced by bacteria that grow without oxygen. (See Chapter 19 for details.)

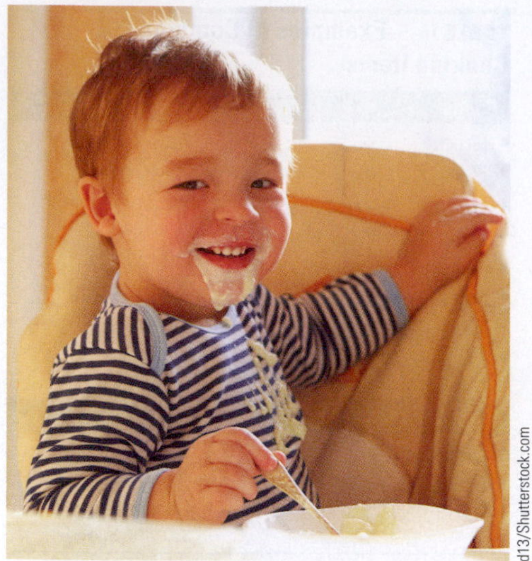

d13/Shutterstock.com

> **PHOTO 16-6** For a toddler, eating may involve touching, smelling, and playing with foods before tasting them.

> **FIGURE 16-6 Sample Meal Plan for a 1-Year-Old**

SAMPLE MENU	
Breakfast	1 scrambled egg 1 slice whole-wheat toast ½ c reduced-fat milk
Morning snack	½ c yogurt ¼ c fruit[a]
Lunch	½ grilled cheese sandwich: 1 slice whole-wheat bread with ½ slice cheese ½ c vegetables[b] (steamed carrots) ¼ c 100% fruit juice (diluted)
Afternoon snack	½ c fruit[a] ½ c toasted oat cereal
Dinner	1 oz chopped meat or ¼ c well-cooked mashed legumes ½ c rice or pasta ½ c vegetables[b] (chopped broccoli) ½ c reduced-fat milk

© Cengage

NOTE: This sample menu provides about 1000 kcalories.
[a]Include citrus fruits, melons, and berries.
[b]Include dark-green, leafy, and deep-yellow vegetables.

sufficiently. Ingesting more milk than this can displace iron-rich foods, which can lead to **milk anemia**. If powdered milk is used, it should contain some fat.

Other foods—meats, other protein foods, iron-fortified cereals, enriched or whole-grain breads, fruits, and vegetables—should be supplied in variety and in amounts sufficient to round out total energy needs. Figure 16-6 shows a meal plan that meets a 1-year-old's requirements.

Mealtimes with Toddlers The nurturing of a young child involves more than nutrition. Those who care for young children are responsible not only for providing nutritious foods, milk, and water, but also a safe, loving, secure environment in which the children may grow and develop. In light of toddlers' developmental and nutrient needs and their often contrary and willful behavior, a few feeding guidelines may be helpful:

- *Discourage unacceptable behavior, such as standing at the table or throwing food.* Be consistent and firm, not punitive. For example, instead of saying "You make me mad when you don't sit down," say "The fruit salad tastes good; please sit down and eat some with me." The child will soon learn to sit and eat.
- *Let toddlers explore and enjoy food, even if this means eating with fingers for a while.* Learning to use a spoon will come in time. Children who are allowed to touch, mash, and smell their food while exploring it are more likely to accept it (see Photo 16-6).
- *Don't force food on children.* Rejecting new foods is normal, and acceptance is more likely as children become familiar with new foods through repeated opportunities to taste them. Instead of saying "You cannot go outside to play until you taste your carrots," say "You can try the carrots again another time."
- *Provide nutritious foods and let children choose which ones, and how much, they will eat.* Gradually, they will acquire a taste for different foods.
- *Limit sweets.* Infants and young children have little room for empty-kcalorie foods in their daily energy allowance. Do not use sweets as a reward for eating meals.
- *Don't turn the dining table into a battleground.* Make mealtimes enjoyable. Teach healthy food choices and eating habits in a pleasant environment. Mealtimes are not the time to fight, argue, or scold.

REVIEW IT List some of the components of breast milk and describe the appropriate foods for infants during the first year of life.

The primary food for infants during the first 12 months is either breast milk or iron-fortified formula. In addition to nutrients, breast milk also offers immunological protection. At about 4 to 6 months of age, infants should gradually begin eating complementary foods. By 1 year, they are drinking from a cup and eating many of the same foods as the rest of the family.

16.2 Nutrition during Childhood

LEARN IT Explain how children's appetites and nutrient needs reflect their stage of growth and why iron deficiency and obesity are often concerns during childhood.

Each year from age 1 to adolescence, a child typically grows taller by 2 to 3 inches and heavier by 5 to 6 pounds. Growth charts provide valuable clues to a child's health. Weight gains out of proportion to height gains may reflect overeating and inactivity, whereas measures significantly less than the standard suggest inadequate nutrition.

Increases in height and weight are only two of the many changes growing children experience (see Figure 16-7). At age 1, children can stand alone and are beginning to toddle; by 2, they can walk and are learning to run; and

milk anemia: iron-deficiency anemia that develops when an excessive milk intake displaces iron-rich foods from the diet.

by 3, they can jump and climb with confidence. Bones and muscles increase in mass and density to make these accomplishments possible. Thereafter, lengthening of the long bones and increases in musculature proceed unevenly and more slowly until adolescence.

> **FIGURE 16-7 Body Shape of 1-Year-Old and 2-Year-Old Compared**

The body shape of a 1-year-old (left) changes dramatically by age 2 (right). The 2-year-old has lost much of the baby fat; the muscles (especially in the back, buttocks, and legs) have firmed and strengthened; and the leg bones have lengthened.

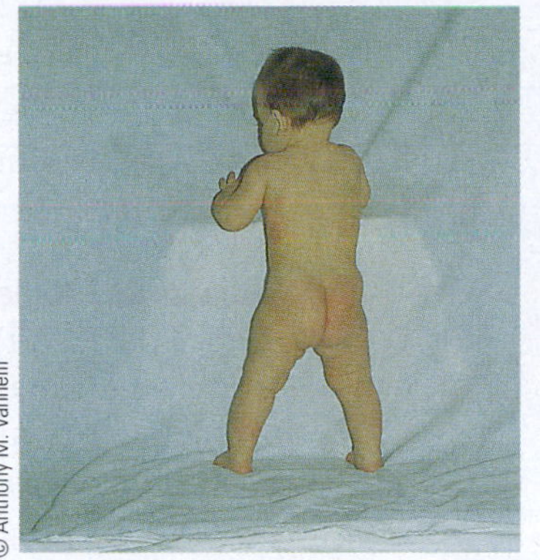

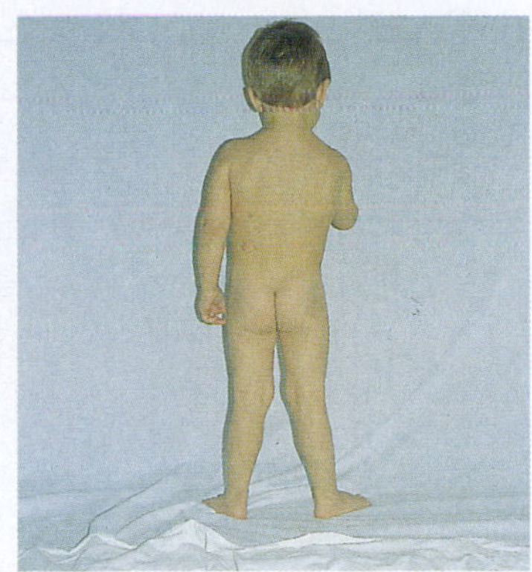

© Anthony M. Vannelli

Energy and Nutrient Needs Children's appetites begin to diminish around 1 year, consistent with the slowing growth. Thereafter, children spontaneously vary their food intakes to coincide with their growth patterns; they demand more food during periods of rapid growth than during slow growth. Sometimes they seem insatiable, and other times they seem to live on air and water.

Children's energy intakes also vary widely from meal to meal. Even so, their total daily intakes remain remarkably constant. If children eat less at one meal, they typically eat more at the next, and vice versa. Overweight children do not always adjust their energy intakes appropriately, however, and may eat in response to external cues such as television commercials, disregarding hunger and satiety signals.[41]

Energy Intake and Activity As mentioned, children's energy needs vary widely, depending on their growth and physical activity. A 1-year-old child needs about 800 kcalories a day; an active 6-year-old child needs twice as many kcalories a day. By age 10, an active child needs about 2000 kcalories a day. Total energy needs increase slightly with age, but energy needs per kilogram of body weight actually decline gradually.

Physically active children of any age need more energy because they expend more, and inactive children can become obese even when they eat less food than the average. Unfortunately, our nation's children are becoming less and less active; child care programs and schools would serve our children well by offering more activities to promote physical fitness.[42] Children who learn to enjoy physical play and exercise, both at home and at school, are best prepared to maintain active lifestyles as adults.

Some children, notably those adhering to a vegan diet, may have difficulty meeting their energy needs. Grains, vegetables, and fruits provide plenty of fiber, adding bulk, but may provide too little energy to support growth. Soy products, other legumes, and nut or seed butters offer more concentrated sources of energy to support optimal growth and development.[43]

Carbohydrate and Fiber Carbohydrate recommendations are based on the brain's glucose needs. After 1 year of age, the brain's use of glucose remains fairly constant and is within the adult range. Carbohydrate recommendations for children older than 1 year are therefore the same as for adults (see the insert).

Fiber recommendations derive from adult intakes shown to reduce the risk of heart disease and are based on energy intakes. Consequently, fiber recommendations for younger children with low energy intakes are less than those for older ones with high energy intakes (see the insert).

Fat and Fatty Acids No RDA for total fat has been established, but the DRI Committee recommends a fat intake of 30 to 40 percent of energy for children 1 to 3 years of age and 25 to 35 percent for children 4 to 18 years of age. As long as children's energy intakes are adequate, however, fat intakes less than 30 percent of total energy do not impair growth. Children who eat low-fat diets, however, tend to have low intakes of some vitamins and minerals. Recommended intakes of the essential fatty acids are based on average intakes (see the insert).

TABLE 16-6 USDA Food Patterns: Recommended Daily Amounts from Each Food Group (1000 to 1800 kCalories)

Food Group	1000 kcal	1200 kcal	1400 kcal	1600 kcal	1800 kcal
Fruits	1 c	1 c	1½ c	1½ c	1½ c
Vegetables	1 c	1½ c	1½ c	2 c	2½ c
Grains	3 oz	4 oz	5 oz	5 oz	6 oz
Protein foods	2 oz	3 oz	4 oz	5 oz	5 oz
Milk	2 c	2½ c	2½ c	3 c	3 c

Protein Like energy needs, total protein needs increase slightly with age, but when the child's body weight is considered, the protein requirement actually declines slightly (see the insert). Protein recommendations must consider the requirements for maintaining nitrogen balance, the quality of protein consumed, and the added needs of growth. Protein needs of children are well covered by typical US diets and well-planned vegetarian diets.

Vitamins and Minerals The vitamin and mineral needs of children increase with age (see the insert). A balanced diet of nutritious foods can meet children's needs for these nutrients, with the notable exception of iron, and possibly vitamin D. Iron-deficiency anemia is a major problem worldwide and is prevalent among US children, especially toddlers 1 to 3 years of age.[44] During the second year of life, toddlers progress from a diet of iron-rich infant foods such as breast milk, iron-fortified formula, and iron-fortified infant cereal to a diet of adult foods and iron-poor cow's milk. In addition, their appetites often fluctuate—some become finicky about the foods they eat, and others prefer milk and juice to solid foods. These situations can interfere with children eating iron-rich foods at a critical time for brain growth and development.

To prevent iron deficiency, children's foods must deliver 7 to 10 milligrams of iron per day. To achieve this goal, snacks and meals should include iron-rich foods, and milk intake should be reasonable so that it will not displace lean meats, fish, poultry, eggs, legumes, and whole-grain or enriched products. (Chapter 13 described iron-rich foods and ways to maximize iron absorption.)

According to the DRI committee, children's intakes of vitamin D–fortified foods—including milk, ready-to-eat cereals, and juices—should provide 15 micrograms of vitamin D each day to maximize calcium absorption and ensure normal, healthy bone growth.[45] Children who do not meet their RDA from these sources should receive a vitamin D supplement. Remember that sunlight is also a source of vitamin D, especially in tropical climates and warm seasons.

Supplements With the exception of specific recommendations for fluoride, iron, and vitamin D during infancy and childhood, the American Academy of Pediatrics and other professional groups agree that well-nourished children do not need vitamin and mineral supplements. Despite this, many children and adolescents take supplements.[46] Researchers are still studying the safety of supplement use by children. The Federal Trade Commission has warned parents about giving supplements advertised to prevent or cure childhood illnesses such as colds, ear infections, or asthma. Dietary supplements on the market today include many herbal products that have not been tested for safety and effectiveness in children.

TABLE 16-7 Estimated Daily Energy Needs for Sedentary Children and Adolescents

Males (age)	Energy (kcal/day)	Females (age)	Energy (kcal/day)
2–3 yr	1000	2–3 yr	1000
4–5 yr	1200	4–7 yr	1200
6–8 yr	1400	8–10 yr	1400
9–10 yr	1600	11–13 yr	1600
11–12 yr	1800	14–18 yr	1800
13–14 yr	2000		
15 yr	2200		
16–18 yr	2400		

NOTE: Sedentary describes a lifestyle that includes only the activities typical of independent living; individuals who are more physically active may need more kcalories per day.

Planning Children's Meals To provide all the needed nutrients, children's meals should include a variety of foods from each food group—in amounts suited to their appetites and needs. Table 16-6 provides USDA Food Patterns for several kcalorie levels. Estimated daily kcalorie needs for active and sedentary children of various ages are shown in Table 16-7. MyPlate online resources for preschoolers (2 to 5 years) translate the eating patterns into messages that can help parents ensure that the foods they provide meet their child's needs. For older children (6 to 11 years), the site provides an interactive "Blast Off" nutrition teaching game and other resources for teachers, parents, and children themselves (Figure 16-8). These guidelines and resources also stress the importance of balancing kcalorie intake with kcalorie expenditure through adequate physical activity to promote growth without increasing

> **FIGURE 16-8** MyPlate Resources for Children

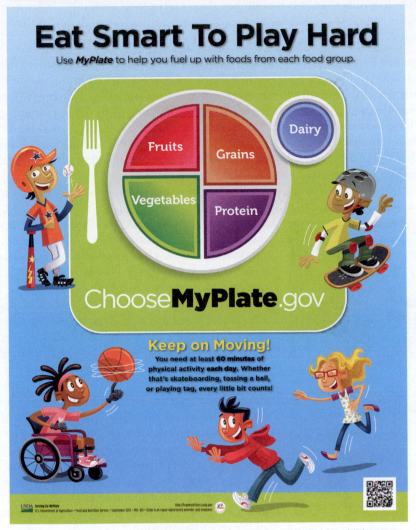
Eat Smart To Play Hard
Use MyPlate to help you fuel up with foods from each food group.
Fruits
Grains
Dairy
Vegetables
Protein
ChooseMyPlate.gov
Keep on Moving!
You need at least 60 minutes of physical activity each day. Whether that's skateboarding, tossing a ball, or playing tag, every little bit counts!

NOTE: Abundant MyPlate resources for preschool children and older children can be found at www.choosemyplate.gov.

the risks of developing obesity. Childhood obesity is the topic of a later section in this chapter.

Children whose diets follow the patterns presented in Table 16-6 can meet their nutrient needs fully, but few children eat according to these recommendations.[47] One analysis of the quality of young (2 to 6 years of age) children's diets found an increase in the proportion of foods that contribute solid fat, added sugar, and sodium between 1989 and 2008.[48] Preschool children today consume more salty snack foods, pizza, sweet snacks, candy, and fruit juices than in previous decades. On a positive note, children consume slightly more fruit than before. Overall, many children between the ages of 2 and 11 do not meet recommendations for fruits, vegetables, grains, and milk. Parents and caregivers of young children thus need to offer a much greater variety of nutrient-dense foods at meals and snacks to help ensure adequate nutrition. Among other nutrition concerns for US children are inadequate intakes of vitamin E, potassium, and fiber, and excessive intakes of sodium.[49]

Hunger and Malnutrition in Children Most children in the United States have access to regular meals, but hunger and malnutrition are not uncommon, especially among children in very low-income families. More than 16 million US children live in households that do not always have food available.[50] Chapter 20 examines the causes and consequences of hunger in the United States and around the world.

Hunger and Behavior Both short-term and long-term hunger exert negative effects on behavior and health. Short-term hunger, such as when a child misses a meal, impairs the child's ability to pay attention and be productive. Hungry children are irritable, apathetic, and uninterested in their environment. Long-term hunger impairs growth and immune defenses. Food assistance programs such as the WIC program (discussed in Chapter 15) and the School Breakfast and National School Lunch Programs (discussed later in this chapter) are designed to protect against hunger and improve children's health.[51]

A nutritious breakfast is a central feature of a diet that meets the needs of children and supports their healthy growth and development (see Photo 16-7).[52] Children who skip breakfast typically do not make up the deficits at later meals—they simply have lower intakes of energy, vitamins, and minerals than those who eat breakfast. Poorly nourished children are particularly vulnerable.

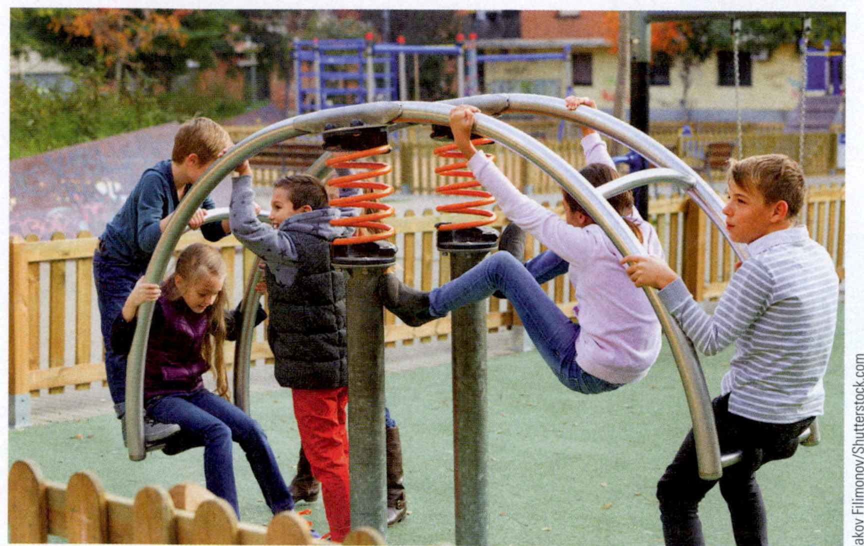
Iakov Filimonov/Shutterstock.com

> **PHOTO 16-7** Healthy, well-nourished children are alert in the classroom and energetic at play.

Compared to their well-fed peers, children who eat no breakfast may have shorter attention spans and may be more likely to perform poorly in tasks requiring concentration, but more research is needed to substantiate these findings.[53] Common sense dictates that it is unreasonable to expect anyone to learn and perform without fuel. For the child who hasn't had breakfast, the morning's lessons may be lost altogether. Even if a child has eaten breakfast, discomfort from hunger may become distracting by late morning. Teachers aware of the late-morning slump in their classrooms wisely request that midmorning snacks be provided; snacks improve classroom performance all the way to lunchtime.[54]

Iron Deficiency and Behavior Iron deficiency has well-known and widespread effects on children's behavior and intellectual performance.[55] In addition to carrying oxygen in the blood, iron transports oxygen within cells, which use it during energy metabolism. Iron is also used to make neurotransmitters—most notably, those that regulate the ability to pay attention, which is crucial to learning. Consequently, iron deficiency not only causes an energy crisis, but also directly impairs attention span and learning ability.

Iron deficiency is often diagnosed by a quick, easy, inexpensive hemoglobin or hematocrit test that detects a deficit of iron in the *blood.* A child's *brain,* however, is sensitive to low iron concentrations long before the blood effects appear. Iron deficiency lowers the motivation to persist in intellectually challenging tasks and impairs overall intellectual performance. Anemic children perform poorly on tests and are disruptive in the classroom; iron supplementation improves learning and memory. When combined with other nutrient deficiencies, iron-deficiency anemia has synergistic effects that are especially detrimental to learning. Furthermore, children who had iron-deficiency anemia *as infants* continue to perform poorly as they grow older, even if their iron status improves.[56] The long-term damaging effects on mental development make prevention and treatment of iron deficiency during infancy and early childhood a high priority.

Other Nutrient Deficiencies and Behavior A child with any of several nutrient deficiencies may be irritable, aggressive, and disagreeable, or sad and withdrawn.

TABLE 16-8 Physical Signs of Malnutrition in Children

	Well-Nourished	Malnourished	Possible Nutrient Deficiencies
Hair	Shiny, firm in the scalp	Dull, brittle, dry, loose; falls out	Protein
Eyes	Bright, clear pink membranes; adjust easily to light	Pale membranes; spots; redness; adjust slowly to darkness	Vitamin A, the B vitamins, zinc, and iron
Teeth and gums	No pain or caries, gums firm, teeth bright	Missing, discolored, decayed teeth; gums bleed easily and are swollen and spongy	Minerals and vitamin C
Face	Clear complexion without dryness or scaliness	Off-color, scaly, flaky, cracked skin	Protein, vitamin A, and iron
Glands	No lumps	Swollen at front of neck, cheeks	Protein and iodine
Tongue	Red, bumpy, rough	Sore, smooth, purplish, swollen	B vitamins
Skin	Smooth, firm, good color	Dry, rough, spotty; "sandpaper" feel or sores; lack of fat under skin	Protein, essential fatty acids, vitamin A, B vitamins, and vitamin C
Nails	Firm, pink	Spoon-shaped, brittle, ridged	Iron
Internal systems	Regular heart rhythm, heart rate, and blood pressure; no impairment of digestive function, reflexes, or mental status	Abnormal heart rate, heart rhythm, or blood pressure; enlarged liver, spleen; abnormal digestion; burning, tingling of hands, feet; loss of balance, coordination; mental confusion, irritability, fatigue	Protein and minerals
Muscles and bones	Muscle tone; posture, long bone development appropriate for age	"Wasted" appearance of muscles; swollen bumps on skull or ends of bones; small bumps on ribs; bowed legs or knock-knees	Protein, minerals, and vitamin D

Such a child may be labeled "hyperactive," "depressed," or "unlikable," when in fact these traits may be due to simple, even marginal, malnutrition. Parents and medical practitioners often overlook the possibility that malnutrition may account for abnormalities of appearance and behavior. Any departure from normal healthy appearance and behavior is a sign of possible poor nutrition (see Table 16-8). In any such case, inspection of the child's diet by a registered dietitian nutritionist or other qualified health-care professional is in order. Any suspicion of dietary inadequacies, no matter what other causes may be implicated, should prompt steps to correct those inadequacies immediately.

The Malnutrition-Lead Connection Children who are malnourished are vulnerable to lead poisoning. They absorb more lead if their stomachs are empty; if they have low intakes of calcium, zinc, vitamin C, or vitamin D; and, of greatest concern because it is so common, if they have an iron deficiency. Iron deficiency weakens the body's defenses against lead absorption, and lead poisoning can cause iron deficiency.[57] Common to both iron deficiency and lead poisoning are a low socioeconomic background and a lack of immunizations against infectious diseases. Another common factor is pica—a craving for nonfood items. Many children with lead poisoning eat dirt or chips of old paint, two common sources of lead (see Photo 16-8).

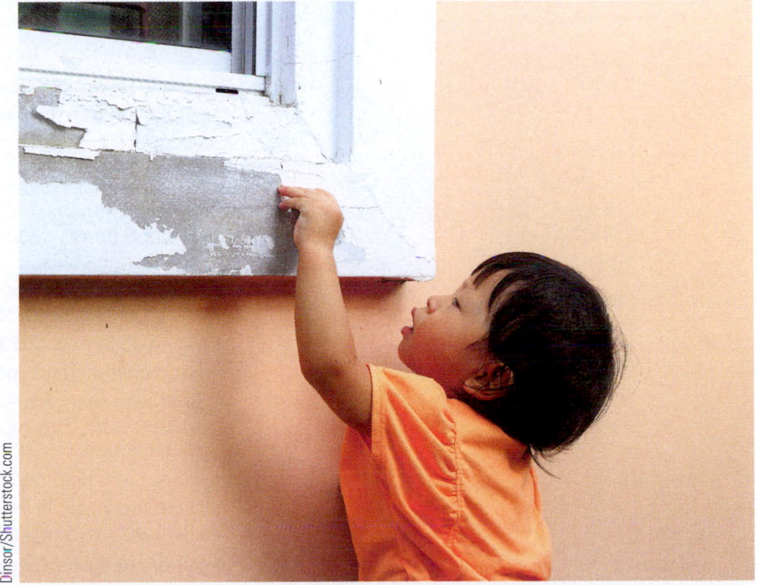

> **PHOTO 16-8** Old, lead-based paint threatens the health of an exploring child.

The anemia brought on by lead poisoning may be mistaken for a simple iron deficiency and therefore may be incorrectly treated. Like iron deficiency, mild lead toxicity has nonspecific symptoms, including diarrhea, irritability, and fatigue. Adding iron to the diet does not reverse the symptoms; exposure to lead must stop and treatment for lead poisoning must begin. With further exposure, the symptoms become more pronounced, and children develop learning disabilities and behavioral problems. Still more severe lead toxicity can cause irreversible nerve damage, paralysis, mental impairment, and death.

Approximately half a million children between the ages of 1 and 5 in the United States have blood lead concentrations above 5 micrograms per deciliter, the level at which the Centers for Disease Control and Prevention recommend public health actions be initiated.[58] Sometimes lead toxicity in young children comes from their own behaviors and activities—putting their hands in their mouths, playing in dirt and dust, and chewing on nonfood items. Unfortunately, the body readily absorbs lead during times of rapid growth and hoards it possessively thereafter. Lead is not easily excreted and accumulates mainly in the bones, but also in the brain, teeth, and kidneys. Tragically, a child's neuromuscular system is also maturing during these first few years of life. No wonder children with elevated lead levels experience impairment of balance, motor development, and the relaying of nerve messages to and from the brain. Deficits in intellectual development are only partially reversed when blood lead levels decline.

Federal laws mandating reductions in leaded gasoline, lead-based solder, and other products over the past four decades have helped reduce the amounts of lead in food and in the environment in the United States. As a consequence, the prevalence of lead toxicity in children has declined dramatically for most of the United States, but lead exposure is still a threat in certain communities. Table 16-9 presents strategies for defending children against lead toxicity. Unfortunately, regulations and precautions to protect people from lead contamination sometimes fail. In Flint, Michigan, dangerous levels of lead and other toxins in the water supply occurred when the city switched water sources to cut costs. Residents of Flint, including many children, were exposed to the contamination and the health risks posed by high concentrations of lead in the water.

Hyperactivity and "Hyper" Behavior

All children are naturally active, and many of them become overly active on occasion—for example, in anticipation of a birthday party. Such behavior is markedly different from true **hyperactivity**.

Hyperactivity

Hyperactive children have trouble sleeping, cannot sit still for more than a few minutes at a time, act impulsively, and have difficulty paying attention. These behaviors interfere with social development and academic progress. The cause of hyperactivity remains unknown, but it affects about 11 percent of young school-age children.[59] To resolve the problems surrounding hyperactivity, physicians often recommend specific behavioral strategies, special educational programs, and

TABLE 16-9 Strategies to Protect against Lead Toxicity

- Ask a pediatrician whether your child should be tested for lead poisoning.
- Prevent small children from putting dirty or old painted objects in their mouths, and make sure children wash their hands before eating. Similarly, keep small children from eating any nonfood items. Lead poisoning has been reported in young children who have eaten crayons or pool cue chalk.
- Wash floors, window sills, and other surfaces regularly. Use a mop or sponge with warm water and a general all-purpose cleaner.
- Wash children's bottles, pacifiers, and toys often.
- Feed children balanced, timely, meals with ample iron and calcium.
- Be aware that other countries do not have the same regulations protecting consumers against lead. Children have been poisoned by eating crayons made in China and drinking fruit juice canned in Mexico.
- Do not use lead-contaminated water to make infant formula.
- Have the water in your home tested by a competent laboratory.
- Use only cold water for drinking, cooking, and making formula (cold water absorbs less lead).
- When water has been standing in pipes for more than 2 hours, flush the coldwater pipes by running water through them for 30 seconds before using it for drinking, cooking, or mixing formulas.

By taking these steps, parents can protect their children from this preventable danger.

hyperactivity: inattentive and impulsive behavior that is more frequent and severe than is typical of others a similar age; professionally called *attention-deficit/hyperactivity disorder (ADHD).*

psychological counseling. If these interventions are ineffective, they may prescribe medication.

Research on hyperactivity has focused on several nutritional factors as possible causes or treatments.[60] Parents often blame sugar. They hopefully believe that simply eliminating candy and other sweet treats will solve the problem. Studies have found no convincing evidence that sugar causes hyperactivity or worsens behavior but dietary changes may still be helpful. Sugar-sweetened foods and beverages displace more nutritious choices from the diet, and, as stated previously, nutrient deficiencies are known to cause behavioral problems.

Food additives have also been blamed for hyperactivity and other behavior problems in children, but scientific evidence to substantiate the connection has been elusive.[61] Limited research suggests that food additives such as artificial colors or sodium benzoate preservative (or both) may exacerbate hyperactive symptoms such as inattention and impulsivity in some children. Additional studies are needed to confirm the findings and to determine which additives might be responsible for specific negative behaviors.

Misbehaving Even a child who is not truly hyperactive can be difficult to manage at times. Michael may act unruly out of a desire for attention, Jessica may be cranky because of a lack of sleep, Christopher may react violently after watching too much television, and Ashley may be unable to sit still in class because of a lack of exercise. All of these children may benefit from more consistent care—regular hours of sleep, regular mealtimes, and regular outdoor activity.

Food Allergy and Intolerance

Food allergy is frequently blamed for physical and behavioral abnormalities in children, but only 4 to 8 percent of children younger than 4 years of age are diagnosed with true food allergies.[62] Food allergies diminish with age, until in adulthood they affect less than 4 percent of the population. The prevalence of food allergy, especially peanut allergy, is on the rise, however.[63] Reasons for an increase in peanut allergy are not yet clear, but possible contributing factors include genetics, composition and diversity of GI microbiota during infancy, food preparation methods (roasting peanuts at very high temperatures makes them more allergenic), and exposure to medicinal skin creams containing peanut oil.[64]

A true food allergy occurs when fractions of a food protein or other large molecule are absorbed into the blood and elicit an immunologic response. (Recall that proteins are normally dismantled in the digestive tract to amino acids that are absorbed without such a reaction.) The body's immune system reacts to these large food molecules as it does to other antigens—by producing antibodies, histamines, and other defensive agents.

Detecting Food Allergy Allergies may have one or two components. They always involve antibodies, but they may or may not involve symptoms. Therefore, allergies cannot be diagnosed from symptoms alone. Physicians use clinical guidelines to diagnose and manage food allergy. Even symptoms exactly like those of an allergy may not be caused by an allergy. Food allergy should be considered when an individual, especially a young child, experiences symptoms such as skin rash, respiratory difficulties, vomiting, diarrhea, or anaphylactic shock (described later) within minutes to hours of eating.

Diagnosis of food allergy requires medical testing and food challenges. Once a food allergy has been diagnosed, the required treatment is strict elimination of the offending food. Children with allergies, like all children, need all their nutrients, so it is important to include other foods that offer the same nutrients as the omitted foods. Nutritional counseling and growth monitoring are recommended for all children with food allergies.[65]

Allergic reactions to food may be immediate or delayed. In either case, the antigen interacts immediately with the immune system, but the timing of symptoms varies from minutes to 24 hours after consumption of the antigen.

food allergy: an adverse reaction to food that involves an immune response; also called *food-hypersensitivity reaction.*

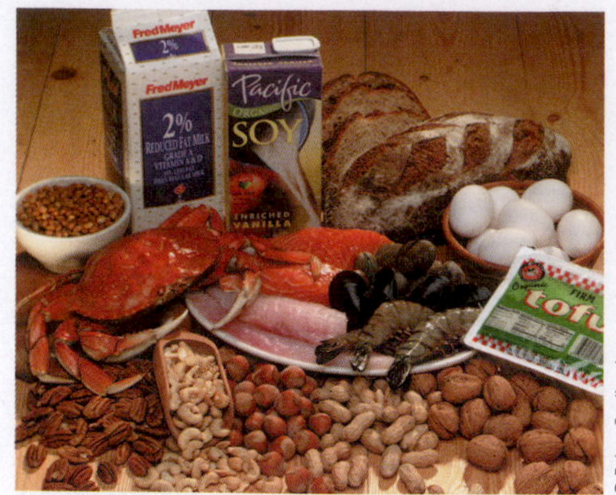
Fred Meyer
2%
Pacific
SOY
ENRICHED VANILLA
tofu
© Polara Studios, Inc.

> **PHOTO 16-9** These normally wholesome foods—peanuts, tree nuts, milk, eggs, wheat, soy, fish, and shellfish—may cause life-threatening symptoms in people with allergies.

Identifying the food that causes an immediate allergic reaction is fairly easy because the symptoms appear shortly after the food is eaten. Identifying the food that causes a delayed reaction is more difficult because the symptoms may not appear until much later. By this time, many other foods may have been eaten, complicating the picture.

Anaphylactic Shock The life-threatening food allergy reaction of **anaphylactic shock** is most often caused by peanuts, tree nuts, milk, eggs, wheat, soy, fish, or shellfish (see Photo 16-9). Among these foods, eggs, milk, soy, and peanuts most often cause problems in children. Children are more likely to outgrow allergies to eggs, milk, and soy than allergies to peanuts. Peanuts cause more life-threatening reactions than do all other food allergies combined. Research is currently under way to help people with peanut allergies tolerate small doses, thus saving lives and minimizing reactions.[66] Families of children with a life-threatening food allergy and the school personnel who supervise those children must guard them against any exposure to the allergen. The child must learn to identify which foods pose a problem and then learn and use refusal skills for all foods that may contain the allergen.

Parents of children with allergies can pack safe lunches and snacks and ask school officials to strictly enforce a "no swapping" policy in the lunchroom. The child and caregivers must be able to recognize symptoms of impending anaphylactic shock:

- Tingling sensation in mouth
- Swelling of the tongue and throat
- Irritated, reddened eyes
- Difficulty breathing, asthma
- Hives, swelling, rashes
- Vomiting, abdominal cramps, diarrhea
- Drop in blood pressure
- Loss of consciousness

Any person with food allergies severe enough to cause anaphylactic shock should wear a medical alert bracelet or necklace. Finally, the responsible child and the school staff should be prepared with injections of epinephrine, which prevents anaphylactic shock after exposure to the allergen by opening the airways and maintaining the heartbeat and blood pressure. Many preventable deaths occur each year when people with food allergies accidentally ingest the allergen but have no epinephrine available.

Food Labeling As discussed in Chapter 2, food labels must list the presence of common allergens in plain language. For example, a food containing "textured vegetable protein" must say "soy" on its label. People with food allergies rely heavily on the accuracy of food labels.

Technology may soon offer new solutions. New drugs are being developed that may interfere with the immune response that causes allergic reactions. Also, through genetic engineering, scientists may one day create allergen-free peanuts, soybeans, and other foods to make them safer.

Food Intolerances Not all **adverse reactions** to foods are food allergies, although even physicians may describe them as such. Signs of adverse reactions to foods include stomachaches, headaches, rapid pulse rate, nausea, wheezing, hives, bronchial irritation, coughs, and other such discomforts. Among the causes may be reactions to chemicals in foods, such as the flavor enhancer monosodium glutamate (MSG), the natural laxative in prunes, or the mineral sulfur; digestive diseases, obstructions, or injuries; enzyme deficiencies, such as lactose intolerance; and even psychological aversions. These reactions involve symptoms but no antibody production. Therefore, they are **food intolerances**, not allergies.

anaphylactic (ana-fill-LAC-tic) **shock:** a life-threatening, whole-body allergic reaction to an offending substance.

adverse reactions: unusual responses to food (including intolerances and allergies).

food intolerances: adverse reactions to foods that do not involve the immune system.

Pesticides on produce may also cause adverse reactions. Pesticides that were applied in the fields may linger on foods. Health risks from pesticide exposure may be low for healthy adults, but children are vulnerable. Therefore, government agencies have set a **tolerance level** for each pesticide by first identifying foods that children commonly eat in large amounts and then considering the effects of pesticide exposure during each stage of development. Chapter 19 revisits the issues surrounding the use of pesticides on food crops.

Hunger, lead poisoning, hyperactivity, and allergic reactions can all adversely affect a child's nutrition status and health. Fortunately, each of these problems has solutions. They may not be easy solutions, but programs are in place and improvements are evident. As for the most pervasive health problem for children in the United States today—obesity—health experts and researchers understand much about the causes, the consequences, and even the solutions, but putting this knowledge into action that meets with success is an ongoing challenge.

Childhood Obesity The number of overweight children has increased dramatically over the past four decades.[67] Like their parents, children in the United States are becoming fatter. An estimated 32 percent of US children and adolescents 2 to 19 years of age are either overweight or obese.[68] Based on data from the BMI-for-age growth charts, children and adolescents are categorized as *overweight* at the 85th percentile and above and as *obese* at the 95th percentile and above.[69] There are exceptions to the use of the 85th and 95th percentile cutoff points. For older adolescents, a BMI at the 95th percentile is higher than a BMI of 30, the adult obesity cutoff point. Therefore, obesity is defined as a BMI at the 95th percentile or a BMI of 30 or greater, whichever is lower. For children younger than 2 years of age, BMI values are not available. For this age group, weight-for-height values above the 95th percentile are classified as overweight. How To 16-2 (p. 514) presents the BMI for children and adolescents, indicating cutoff points for obesity and overweight.

A third cutoff point (using the 97th percentile or a BMI of 35 or greater, whichever is lower) defines severe obesity in childhood.[70] Unfortunately, severe obesity in children is becoming more prevalent. Many of these children have multiple risk factors for cardiovascular disease and a high risk of severe obesity in adulthood.[71] The special risks and treatment needs of severely obese children need to be recognized.

The problem of obesity in children is especially troubling because overweight children have the potential of becoming obese adults with all the social, economic, and medical ramifications that often accompany obesity. They have additional problems, too, arising from differences in their growth, physical health, and psychological development. In trying to explain the rise in childhood obesity, researchers point to both genetic and environmental factors.

Genetic and Environmental Factors Parental obesity predicts an early increase in a young child's BMI, and it more than doubles the chances that a young child will become an obese adult.[72] Children with neither parent obese have a less than 10 percent chance of becoming obese in adulthood, whereas overweight teens with at least one obese parent have a greater than 80 percent chance of being obese adults. The chances of an obese child becoming an obese adult grow greater as the child grows older.[73] The link between parental and child obesity reflects both genetic and environmental factors (as described in Chapter 9).

Diet and physical inactivity are the two strongest environmental factors explaining why children are heavier today than they were 40 or so years ago. In that time, the prevalence of childhood obesity throughout the United States more than doubled for young children and more than tripled for children 6 to 11 years of age and adolescents. As a society, our eating and activity patterns changed considerably. In many families, both parents work outside the home and work longer hours; more emphasis is placed on convenience foods and foods eaten away from

tolerance level: the maximum amount of residue permitted in a food when a pesticide is used according to the label directions.

>How To 16-2 Determine Weight Status for Children and Adolescents

To determine the weight status of children and adolescents, follow these steps:

- Select the appropriate chart based on gender.
- Locate the age along the horizontal axis at the bottom of the chart.
- Locate the BMI along the vertical axis at the left of the chart.
- Note the color of the chart where the age and BMI lines intersect and use the key to determine the weight status; follow the curved line to the right to find the percentile.

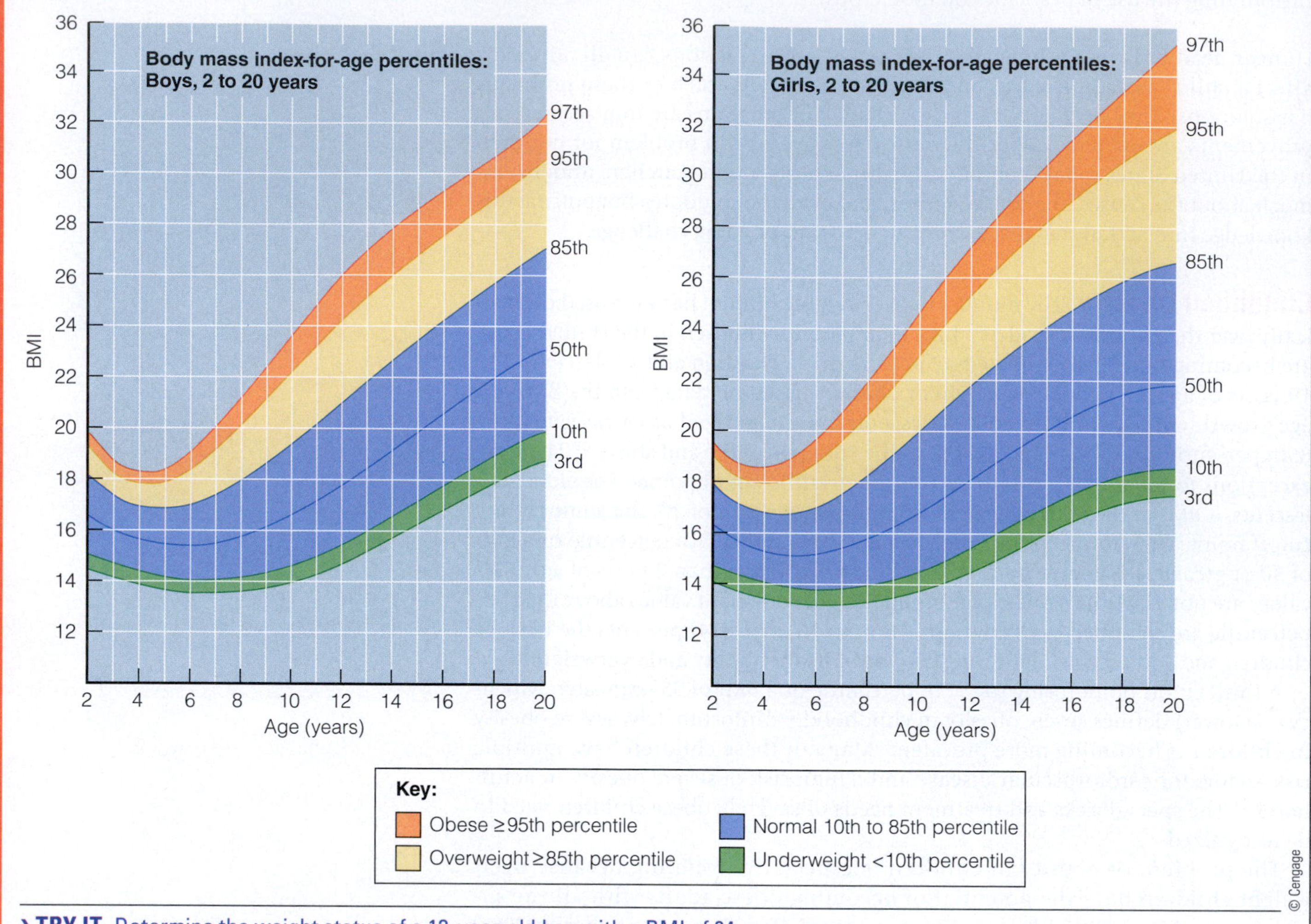

Body mass index-for-age percentiles: Boys, 2 to 20 years
Body mass index-for-age percentiles: Girls, 2 to 20 years
BMI
Age (years)
97th
95th
85th
50th
10th
3rd
Key:
Obese ≥95th percentile
Overweight ≥85th percentile
Normal 10th to 85th percentile
Underweight <10th percentile

> TRY IT Determine the weight status of a 13-year-old boy with a BMI of 24.

home; meal choices at school are more diverse and often less nutritious; sedentary activities such as watching television and playing video or computer games occupy much of children's free time; and opportunities for physical activity and outdoor play both during and after school have declined.[74] All of these factors—and many others—influence children's eating and activity patterns.

Children learn food behaviors from their families, and research confirms the significant roles parents play in teaching their children about healthy food choices, providing nutrient-dense foods, and serving as role models.[75] When parents eat fruits and vegetables frequently, their children do too. The more fruits and vegetables children eat, the more vitamins, minerals, and fiber, and the less saturated fat, in their diets.[76]

In children 2 to 18 years of age, about one third of total energy intake comes from solid fats and added sugars—in other words—empty kcalories.[77] The top contributors of these empty kcalories are sugar-sweetened beverages, dairy desserts (ice cream, frozen yogurt, sorbet, sherbet, pudding, and custard), grain desserts (cakes, cookies, pies, cobblers, donuts, and granola bars), pizza, and whole milk. Not surprisingly, when researchers ask "Are today's children eating more kcalories than those of 40 years ago?" the answer is, "Yes."

As Highlight 4 (p. 124) discussed, as the prevalence of obesity among both children and adults has surged over the past four decades, so has the consumption of added sugars and, especially, high-fructose corn syrup—the easily consumed, energy-dense liquid sugar added to soft drinks.[78] Each 12-ounce can of soft drink provides the equivalent of about 10 teaspoons of sugar and 150 kcalories. More than half of school-age children consume at least one soft drink each day at school; adolescent males consume the most—two or more cans daily. Research shows that soft drink consumption is associated with increased energy intake and body weight.[79]

No doubt, the tremendous increase in soft drink consumption plays a role, but much of the obesity epidemic can be explained by lack of physical activity. Children have become more sedentary, and sedentary children are more often overweight.[80] Television watching may contribute most to physical inactivity. Children 8 to 18 years of age spend an average of 4.5 hours per day watching television. Longer television time is linked with overweight in children.[81] Television fosters overweight and obesity because it:

- Requires no energy beyond basal metabolism
- Replaces vigorous activities
- Encourages snacking
- Promotes a sedentary lifestyle

A child who spends more than an hour or two each day in front of a television, computer monitor, or other media can become overweight even while eating fewer kcalories than a more active child. Too much screen time and not enough activity time also contributes to a child's psychological distress.

Children who have television sets in their bedrooms spend more time watching TV, less time being physically active, less time sleeping, and are more likely to be overweight than children who do not have televisions in their rooms.[82] Watching television influences food intake as well as physical activity (see Photo 16-10).[83] Children who watch a great deal of television are most likely to be overweight and least likely to eat family meals or fruits and vegetables.[84] They often snack on the nutrient-poor, energy-dense foods that are advertised.[85]

Child-targeted food ads on television peddle foods high in sugar, saturated fat, and salt such as sugar-coated breakfast cereals, candy bars, chips, fast foods, and carbonated beverages.[86] More than half of all food advertisements are aimed specifically at children and market products as fun and exciting, oftentimes using sports heroes. Not surprisingly, the more time children spend watching television, the more they request these advertised foods and beverages—and they get their requests about half of the time. The most popular foods and beverages are marketed to children and adolescents on the Internet as well, using "advergaming" (advertised product as part of a game), cartoon characters or "spokes-characters," and designated children's areas.[87] Food marketing to children, including TV ads and Internet ads, as well as marketing to children in their local communities by way of store giveaways, restaurant promotions, school activities, and sporting events has a profound effect on children's nutrition and health.[88] Despite initiatives by the food industry to answer public health concerns about child-targeted advertising, much remains to be done to reduce the marketing of unhealthy foods to children.[89]

The physically inactive time spent watching television is second only to time spent sleeping. Children also spend more time playing computer and video games. In most cases, these activities use no more energy than resting, displace participation in more vigorous activities, and foster snacking on high-fat foods.[90] Compared to sedentary screen-time activities, playing active video games does expend a little more energy, but more research is needed to ascertain whether playing

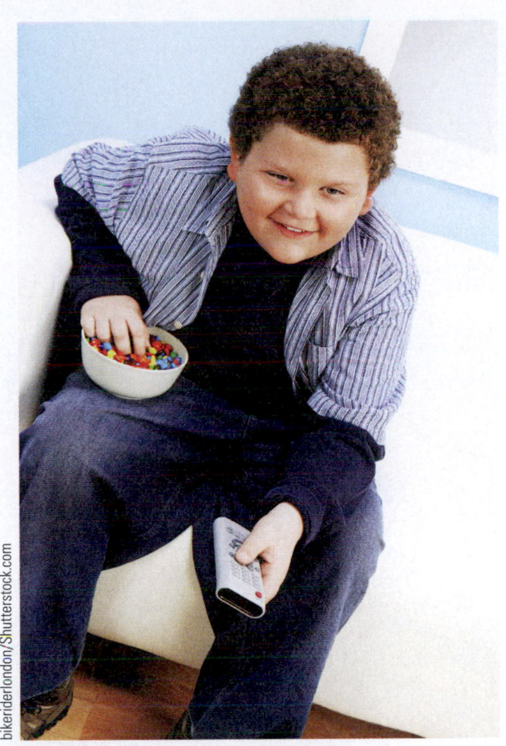
bikeriderlondon/Shutterstock.com

> **PHOTO 16-10** Excessive television watching promotes physical inactivity and poor snacking habits.

active video games increases habitual physical activity or decreases sedentary behaviors.[91] Simply reducing the amount of time spent watching television (and playing sedentary video games) can improve a child's BMI. The American Academy of Pediatrics recommends no television viewing before 2 years of age, and limiting daily screen time to one hour between 2 and 5 years of age and 2 hours for older children to help prevent childhood obesity.[92]

Growth Overweight children develop a characteristic set of physical traits. They typically begin puberty earlier and so grow taller than their peers at first, but then they stop growing at a shorter height. They develop greater bone and muscle mass in response to the demand of having to carry more weight—both fat and lean weight. Consequently, they appear "stocky" even when they lose their excess fat.

Physical Health Like overweight adults, overweight and obese children display a blood lipid profile indicating that atherosclerosis is beginning to develop—high levels of total cholesterol, triglycerides, and LDL cholesterol. Overweight and obese children also tend to have high blood pressure; in fact, obesity is a leading cause of pediatric hypertension.[93] Their risks for developing type 2 diabetes and respiratory diseases (such as asthma) are also exceptionally high.[94] These relationships between childhood obesity and chronic diseases are discussed fully in Highlight 16.

Psychological Development In addition to the physical consequences, childhood obesity brings a host of emotional and social problems.[95] Because people frequently judge others on appearance more than on character, overweight and obese children are often victims of prejudice and bullying. Many suffer discrimination by adults and rejection by their peers. They may have poor self-images, a sense of failure, and a passive approach to life. Television shows, which are a major influence in children's lives, often portray the fat person as the bumbling misfit. Overweight children may come to accept this negative stereotype in themselves and in others, which can lead to additional emotional and social problems. Researchers investigating children's reactions to various body types find that both normal-weight and underweight children respond unfavorably to overweight bodies.

Prevention and Treatment of Obesity Medical science has worked wonders in preventing or curing many of even the most serious childhood diseases, but obesity remains a challenge. Once excess fat has been stored, it is difficult to lose. In light of all this, parents are encouraged to make major efforts to prevent childhood obesity, starting at birth, or to begin treatment early—before adolescence. Table 16-10 presents specific eating and physical activity behaviors to prevent obesity, for all children.

The main goal of obesity treatment is to improve long-term physical health through permanent changes in lifestyle habits. The most successful approach integrates diet, physical activity, psychological support, and behavioral changes.[96] As a first step, overweight and obese children and their families are advised to adopt the same healthy eating and activity behaviors presented in Table 16-10 for obesity prevention. The goal for overweight and obese children is to improve BMI. If the child's BMI does not improve after several months, the intensity of the treatment is increased. The level of intensity depends on treatment response, age, degree of obesity, health risks, and the family's readiness to change.[97] Advanced treatment

TABLE 16-10 Recommended Eating and Physical Activity Behaviors to Prevent Obesity

The following healthy habits are recommended for children 2 to 18 years of age to help prevent childhood obesity:

- Limit or avoid consumption of sugar-sweetened beverages, such as soft drinks and fruit-flavored punches.
- Eat the recommended amounts of fruits and vegetables every day.
- Learn to eat age-appropriate portions of foods.
- Eat foods low in energy density such as those high in fiber and/or water and modest in fat.
- Eat a nutritious breakfast every day.
- Eat foods rich in calcium every day.
- Choose a dietary pattern balanced in recommended proportions for carbohydrate, fat, and protein.
- Eat foods high in fiber every day.
- Eat together as a family as often as possible.
- Limit the frequency of restaurant meals.
- Limit television watching or other screen time to no more than 2 hours per day and do not have televisions or computers in bedrooms.
- Engage in at least 60 minutes of moderate to vigorous physical activity every day.

TABLE 16-11 Examples of Aerobic, Muscle-Strengthening, and Bone-Strengthening Physical Activities for Children and Adolescents

Moderate-to-Vigorous Aerobic Activities	Muscle-Strengthening Activities	Bone-Strengthening Activities
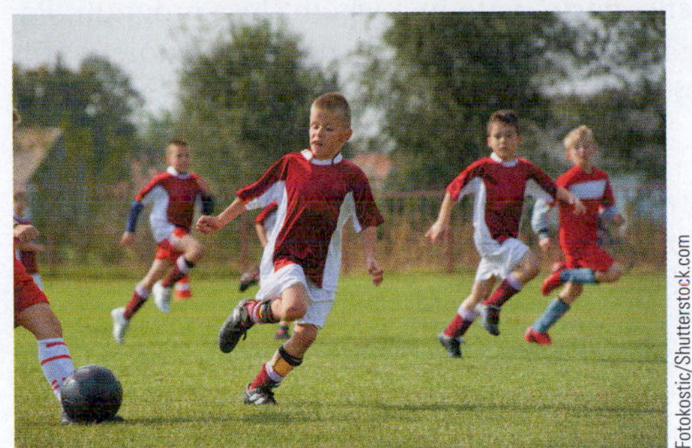 Fotokostic/Shutterstock.com	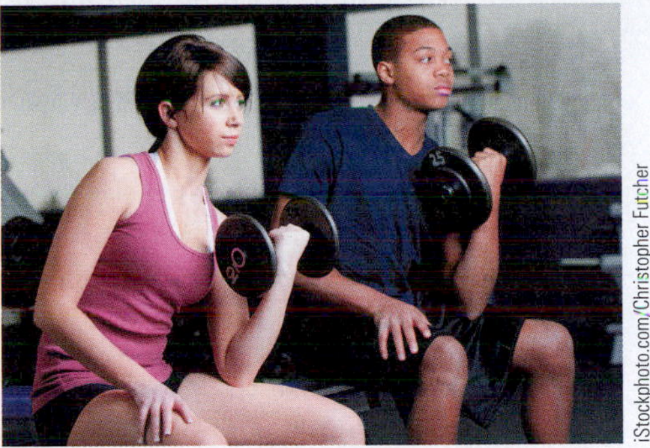 iStockphoto.com/Christopher Futcher	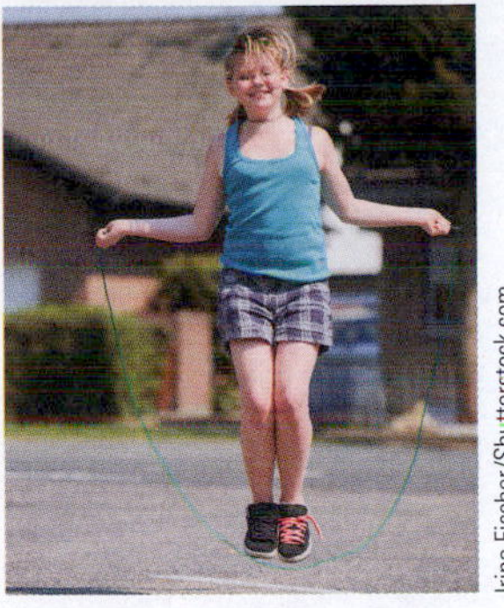 Irina Fischer/Shutterstock.com
Moderate Active recreation such as hiking, skateboarding, rollerblading Bicycle riding[a] Brisk walking **Vigorous** Active games involving running and chasing, such as tag Bicycle riding[a] Cross-country skiing Jumping rope Martial arts Running Sports such as soccer, ice or field hockey, basketball, swimming, tennis	Games such as tug-of-war Modified push-ups (with knees on the floor) Resistance exercises using body weight, free weights, or resistance bands Rope or tree climbing Sit-ups (curl-ups or crunches) Swinging on playground equipment/bars	Games such as hopscotch Hopping, skipping, jumping Jumping rope Running Sports such as gymnastics, basketball, volleyball, tennis

[a]Some activities, such as bicycling, can be moderate or vigorous, depending on level of effort.

involves close follow-up monitoring by a health care provider and greater support and structure for the child.

Diet The initial goal for overweight children is to reduce the rate of weight gain; that is, to maintain weight as the child grows taller. Continued growth will then accomplish the desired change in BMI. Weight loss is usually not recommended because diet restriction can interfere with growth and development. Intervention for some overweight children with accompanying medical conditions may warrant weight loss, but this treatment requires an individualized approach based on the degree of overweight and severity of the medical conditions. Dietary strategies begin with those listed in Table 16-10 and progress to more structured family meal plans when necessary. For example, the child or the parent may be instructed to keep detailed records of dietary intake and physical activity.

Physical Activity The many benefits of physical activity are well known but often are not enough to motivate overweight people, especially children. Yet regular vigorous activity can improve a child's weight, body composition, and physical fitness.[98] Ideally, parents will limit sedentary activities and encourage at least 1 hour of daily physical activity to promote strong skeletal, muscular, and cardiovascular development and instill in their children the desire to be physically active throughout life. Opportunities to be physically active can include team, individual, and recreational activities (see Table 16-11). Most importantly, parents need to set a good example (see Photo 16-11). Physical activity is a natural and lifelong behavior of healthy living. It can be as simple as riding a bike, playing tag, jumping rope, or doing chores. The American Academy of Pediatrics supports the efforts of schools to include more physical activity in the curriculum and encourages parents to support their children's participation.

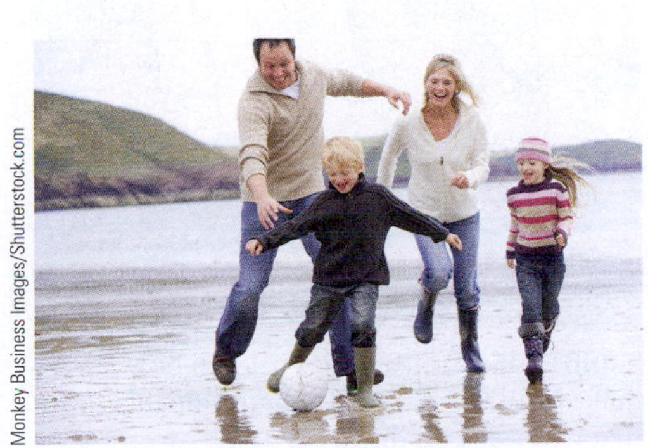

Monkey Business Images/Shutterstock.com

> **PHOTO 16-11** Physical activity is fun play time for children—climb monkey bars in the park, build a sandcastle or a snowman, row a boat, toss a Frisbee, run with the dog, or plant a garden.

Psychological Support Weight-loss programs that involve parents and other caregivers in treatment report greater success than those without parental involvement. Because obesity in parents and their children tends to be positively correlated, both benefit when parents participate in a weight-loss program. Parental attitudes about food greatly influence children's eating behavior, so it is important that the influence be positive. Otherwise, eating problems may become exacerbated.

Behavioral Changes In contrast to traditional weight-loss programs that focus on *what* to eat, behavioral programs focus on *how* to eat. These techniques involve learning new habits that lead a child to make healthy choices.

Drugs The use of weight-loss drugs to treat obesity in children merits special concern because the long-term effects of these drugs on growth and development have not been studied. The drugs may be used in addition to structured lifestyle changes for carefully selected children or adolescents who are at high risk for severe obesity in adulthood. Orlistat (see Chapter 9) is the only prescription weight-loss medication that has been approved for use in adolescents 12 years of age and older.[99] Alli, the over-the-counter version of orlistat, should not be given to anyone younger than age 18.

Surgery The use of surgery to treat severe obesity in adults (see Chapter 9) has created interest in its use for adolescents. Limited research shows that after surgery extremely obese adolescents lose significant weight and experience improvements in type 2 diabetes and cardiovascular risk factors.[100] The selection criteria for surgery to treat obesity in adolescents are based on recommendations of a panel of pediatricians and surgeons and include the following:

- Physically mature
- BMI ≥40 or BMI >35 with significant weight-related health problems
- Limited success in a formal, 6-month weight-loss program
- Capable of adhering to the long-term lifestyle changes required after surgery

Obesity is prevalent in our society. Because treatment of obesity is frequently unsuccessful, it is most important to prevent its onset. Above all, be sensible in teaching children how to maintain appropriate body weight. Children can easily get the impression that their worth is tied to their body weight. Parents and the media are most influential in shaping self-concept, weight concerns, and dieting practices.[101] Some parents fail to realize that society's ideal of slimness can be perilously close to starvation and that a child encouraged to "diet" cannot obtain the energy and nutrients required for normal growth and development. Weight loss in obese children can be managed without compromising growth, but it should be overseen by a health-care professional.

Mealtimes at Home

Traditionally, parents served as **gatekeepers**, determining what foods and activities were available in their children's lives. Then the children made their own selections. Gatekeepers who wanted to promote nutritious choices and healthful habits provided access to nutrient-dense foods and opportunities for active play at home.

In today's consumer-oriented society, children have greater influence over family decisions concerning food—the fast-food restaurant the family chooses when eating out, the snacks the family eats at home, and the specific brands the family purchases at the grocery store. Parental guidance in food choices is still necessary, but teaching children consumer skills to help them make informed choices is equally important (see Photo 16-12).

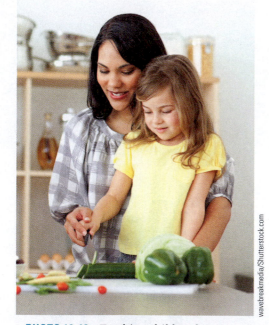

wavebreakmedia/Shutterstock.com

> **PHOTO 16-12** Teaching children how to make healthy meals gives them valuable skills that will last a lifetime.

gatekeepers: with respect to nutrition, key people who control other people's access to foods and thereby exert profound impacts on their nutrition. Examples are the spouse who buys and cooks the food, the parent who feeds the children, and the caregiver in a day-care center.

Honoring Children's Preferences Researchers attempting to explain children's food preferences encounter contradictions. Children say they like colorful foods, yet they most often reject green and yellow vegetables in favor of brown peanut butter and white potatoes, apple wedges, and bread. They seem to like raw vegetables better than cooked ones, so it is wise to offer vegetables that are raw or slightly undercooked, served separately, and easy to eat. Foods should be warm, not hot, because a child's mouth is much more sensitive than an adult's. The flavor should be mild because a child has more taste buds, and smooth foods such as mashed potatoes or split-pea soup should contain no lumps (a child, may wonder what the lumps might be).

Make mealtimes fun for children. Young children like to eat at little tables and to be served small portions of food. They like sandwiches cut in different geometric shapes and common foods called silly names. They also like to eat with other children, and they tend to eat more when in the company of their friends (see Photo 16-13). Children are also more likely to give up their prejudices against foods when they see their peers eating them.

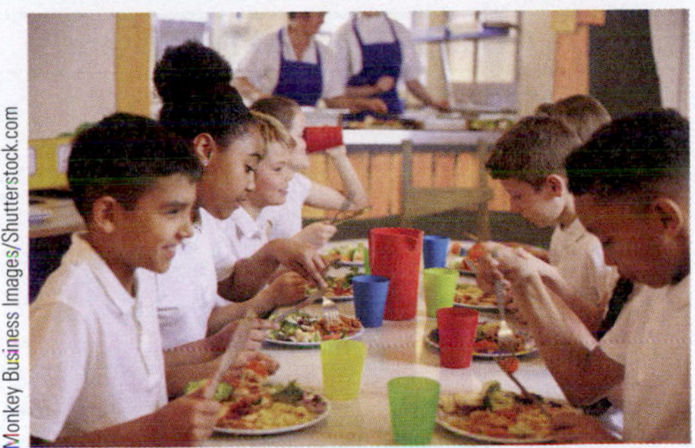
Monkey Business Images/Shutterstock.com

> **PHOTO 16-13** Children tend to eat more and try new flavors when friends are there.

Learning through Participation Allowing children to help plan and prepare the family's meals provides enjoyable learning experiences and encourages children to eat the foods they have prepared. Vegetables are attractive, especially when fresh, and provide opportunities for children to learn about color, seeds, growing vegetables, and shapes and textures—all of which are fascinating to young children. Measuring, stirring, washing, and arranging foods are skills that even a young child can practice with enjoyment and pride (see Table 16-12).

Avoiding Power Struggles Problems over food often arise during the second or third year, when children begin asserting their independence. For example, very young children may suddenly refuse foods they once liked, but as they get a little older, these same children will begin to request favorite foods and make simple choices when given the opportunity. Many food choice problems stem from the conflict between children's developmental stages and capabilities and parents who, in attempting to do what they think is best for their children, try to control every aspect of eating. Such conflicts can disrupt children's abilities to regulate their own food intakes and to determine their own likes and dislikes. For example, many people share the misconception that children must be persuaded or coerced to try new foods. In fact, the opposite is true. When children are forced to try new foods, even by way of rewards, they are less likely to try those foods again than are children who are left to decide for themselves. Similarly, when children are restricted from eating their favorite foods, they are more likely to want those foods. Wise parents provide healthful foods and allow their child to determine *how much* and even *whether* to eat.

When introducing new foods, offer them one at a time and only in small amounts such as a small bite at first. The more often a food is presented to a young child, the more likely the child will accept that food.[102] Offer the new food at the beginning of the meal, when the child is hungry, and allow the child to make the

TABLE 16-12 Food Skills of Preschool Children

Age 2 years, when large muscles develop:
- Uses a spoon
- Helps feed self
- Lifts and drinks from a cup
- Helps scrub fruits and vegetables, tear lettuce or greens, snap green beans, or dip foods
- Wipes table
- Places items in recycle bin or trash

Age 3 years, when medium hand muscles develop:
- Spears food with a fork
- Feeds self independently
- Adds ingredients to pancake batters, cookie recipes, salads or other mixed dishes
- Helps wrap, pour, mix, shake, stir, or spread foods
- Helps crack nuts with supervision
- Follows simple instructions

Age 4 years, when small finger muscles develop:
- Uses all utensils and napkin
- Helps roll, juice, or mash foods
- Helps measure dry ingredients
- Cracks egg shells
- Helps make sandwiches and toss salads
- Peels foods such as hard-boiled eggs and bananas
- Learns table manners

Age 5 years, when fine coordination of fingers and hands develops:
- Measures liquids
- Helps grind, grate, and cut (soft foods with dull knife)
- Uses hand mixer with supervision

NOTE: These ages are approximate. Healthy children develop at their own pace.

TABLE 16-13 Tips for Feeding Picky Eaters

Get Them Involved

- Encourage children to help with meal planning.
- Take children grocery shopping.
- Ask children to help with cooking.
- Help children garden and harvest foods they will eat.

Be Creative

- Try serving vegetables as finger foods with dips or spreads.
- Use cookie cutters to cut breads, fruits, and vegetables into fun shapes.
- Put healthy snacks in ice cube trays or muffin pans where children can easily reach them and graze as they play.
- Serve traditional meals out of order (for example, breakfast for dinner).
- Use healthy foods such as vegetables and whole grains in craft projects to help kids become familiar with them and encourage their interest in and enthusiasm for these foods.

Enhance Favorite Recipes

- Include sliced or shredded vegetables in sauces, casseroles, pancakes, and muffins.
- Serve fruit over cereal, yogurt, or ice cream.
- Bake brownies with black beans or cookies with lentils as an ingredient.

Model and Share

- Be a role model to children by eating healthy foods alongside them and offer to share your healthy snack with them.
- Make healthy options readily available and don't give up on repeatedly offering foods in which your child might not seem interested.
- Encourage your child to taste at least one bite of each food served at a meal.

Respect and Relax

- Remember that it is not uncommon for children to eat sporadically. They have smaller stomachs, and therefore are likely to feel full faster and become hungry again not long after a snack or meal.
- Focus on your child's overall weekly intake of foods and nutrients rather than daily consumptions.
- Discuss concerns with your child's doctor. It might be helpful to maintain a 3-day food record to review at the next appointment.

SOURCE: Adapted from Mayo Clinic Staff, Children's nutrition: 10 tips for picky eaters, 2011, www.mayoclinic.com/health/childrens-health/HQ01107.

decision to accept or reject it. Never make an issue of food acceptance. Table 16-13 offers tips for feeding picky eaters.

Choking Prevention Parents must always be alert to the dangers of choking. A choking child is silent, so an adult should be present whenever a child is eating. Make sure the child sits when eating; choking is more likely when a child is running or falling. See Table 16-5 (p. 503) for foods and nonfood items most likely to cause choking.

Playing First Children may be more relaxed and attentive during meals if outdoor play or other fun activities are scheduled before, rather than immediately after, mealtimes. Otherwise children "hurry up and eat" so that they can go play.

Snacking Parents may find that when children snack, they aren't hungry at mealtimes. Instead of teaching children *not* to snack, parents are wise to teach them *how* to snack. Provide snacks that are as nutritious as the foods served at mealtime. Snacks can even be mealtime foods served individually over time, instead of all at once on one plate. When providing snacks to children, think of the five food groups and offer such snacks as pieces of cheese, tangerine slices, and egg salad on whole-wheat crackers (see Table 16-14). Replacing nutrient-poor, high-kcalorie snacks such as potato chips with nutrient-rich, low-kcalorie snacks such as vegetables not only reduces children's energy intakes, but improves their nutrient intakes as well.[103] Snacks that are easy to prepare should be readily available to children, especially if they arrive home from school before their parents.

To ensure that children have healthy appetites and plenty of room for nutritious foods when they are hungry, parents and teachers must limit access to candy, soft drinks, and other concentrated sweets. Limiting access includes limiting the amount of pocket money children have to buy such foods themselves. If these foods are permitted in large quantities, the only possible outcomes are nutrient deficiencies, obesity, or both. The preference for sweets is innate; most children do not naturally select nutritious foods on the basis of taste. When children are allowed to create meals freely from a variety of foods, they typically select foods that provide a lot of sugar. When their parents are watching, or even when they only think their parents are watching, children improve their selections.

Sweets need not be banned altogether. Children who are exceptionally active can enjoy high-kcalorie foods such as ice cream or pudding from the milk group or pancakes from the bread group. Sedentary children need to become more active so they can also enjoy some of these foods without unhealthy weight gain.

Preventing Dental Caries Children frequently snack on sticky, sugary foods that stay on the teeth and provide an ideal environment for the growth of bacteria that cause dental caries. Teach children to brush and floss after meals, to brush or rinse after eating snacks, to avoid sticky foods, and to select crisp or fibrous foods frequently.

Serving as Role Models In an effort to practice these many tips, parents may overlook perhaps the single most important influence on their children's food habits—themselves. Parents who don't eat carrots shouldn't be surprised when their children refuse to eat carrots. Likewise, parents who comment negatively on the smell of brussels sprouts may not be able to persuade children to try them. Children learn much through imitation. It is not surprising that children prefer the foods other family members enjoy and dislike foods that are never offered to them. Parents, older siblings, and other caregivers set an irresistible example by sitting with younger children, eating the same foods, and having pleasant conversations during mealtimes.

While serving and enjoying food, caregivers can promote both physical and emotional growth at every stage of a child's life. They can help their children develop both a positive self-concept and a positive attitude toward food. With good beginnings, children will grow without the conflicts and confusions about food that can lead to nutrition and health problems.

TABLE 16-14 Healthful Snack Ideas—Think Food Groups, Alone and in Combination

Selecting two or more foods from different food groups adds variety and nutrient balance to snacks. The combinations are endless, so be creative. Whenever possible, choose whole grains, low-fat or reduced-fat milk products, and lean meats.

Grains

Grain products are filling snacks, especially when combined with other foods:

- Cereal with fruit and milk
- Crackers and cheese
- Whole-grain toast with peanut butter
- Popcorn with grated cheese
- Oatmeal raisin cookies with milk

Vegetables

Cut-up, fresh, raw vegetables make great snacks alone or in combination with foods from other food groups:

- Celery with peanut butter
- Broccoli, cauliflower, and carrot sticks with hummus or a flavored cottage cheese dip

Fruits

Fruits are delicious snacks and can be eaten alone—fresh, dried, or juiced—or combined with other foods:

- Apples and cheese
- Bananas and peanut butter
- Peaches with yogurt
- Raisins mixed with sunflower seeds or nuts

Protein Foods

Seafood, meat, poultry, eggs, legumes, nuts, seeds, and soy products add protein to snacks:

- Refried beans with nachos and cheese
- Tuna on crackers
- Luncheon meat on whole-grain bread

Milk and Milk Products

Milk can be used as a beverage with any snack, and many other milk products, such as yogurt and cheese, can be eaten alone or with other foods as listed above.

Nutrition at School

While parents are doing what they can to establish good eating habits in their children at home, others are preparing and serving foods to their children at day-care centers and schools. In addition, children begin to learn about food and nutrition in the classroom. Meeting the nutrition and education needs of children is critical to supporting their healthy growth and development.[104]

The Academy of Nutrition and Dietetics has set nutrition standards for child-care programs. Among them, meal plans should:

- Be nutritionally adequate and consistent with the *Dietary Guidelines for Americans.*
- Emphasize fresh fruit, fresh and frozen vegetables, whole grains, and low-fat milk and milk products.
- Limit foods and beverages high in energy, added sugars, solid fats, and sodium, and low in vitamins and minerals.
- Provide foods and beverages in quantities and meal patterns appropriate to ensure optimal growth and development.
- Involve parents in planning.
- Provide furniture and eating utensils that are age appropriate and developmentally suitable to encourage children to accept and enjoy mealtime.

In addition, child-care providers can encourage active play for children by creating opportunities for children to engage in both structured and unstructured activity throughout the day.

Meals at School The US government assists schools financially so that every student can receive nutritious meals at school. Both the School Breakfast Program

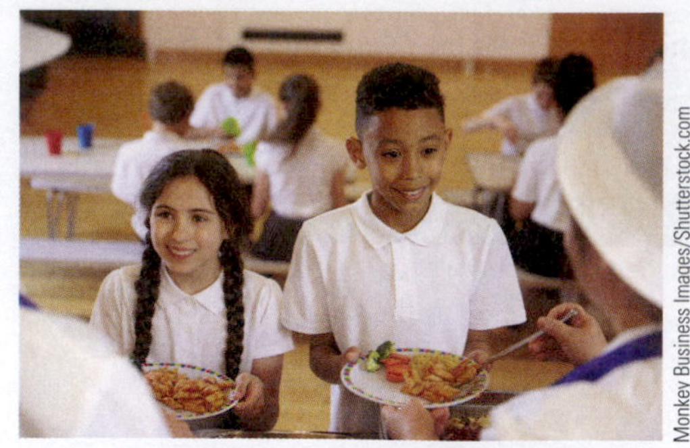
Monkey Business Images/Shutterstock.com

> **PHOTO 16-14** School lunches provide children with nourishment at little or no charge.

and the National School Lunch Program provide meals free or at reduced cost to children from low-income families. In addition, schools can obtain food commodities. Nationally, the US Department of Agriculture (USDA) administers the programs; on the state level, state departments of education operate them.

More than 31 million children receive lunches through the National School Lunch Program—more than half of them free or at a reduced price (see Photo 16-14).[105] School lunches offer a variety of food choices and help children meet at least one third of their recommended intakes for energy, protein, vitamin A, vitamin C, iron, and calcium. Table 16-15 shows school lunch patterns for children of different ages and specifies the numbers of servings of milk, protein-rich foods (meat, poultry, fish, cheese, eggs, legumes, or peanut butter), vegetables, fruits, and whole grains. In an effort to help reduce disease risk, all government-funded meals served at schools must follow the *Dietary Guidelines for Americans*. Recent changes to school meal patterns and nutrition standards have resulted in greater availability of fruits, vegetables, whole grains, and fat-free and low-fat milk; decreased levels of sodium, saturated fat, and *trans* fat; and guidelines for meeting nutrient needs within specified kcalorie ranges based on age/grade groups for school children.

Parents often rely on school lunches to meet a significant part of their children's nutrient needs on school days. Indeed, students who regularly eat school lunches have higher intakes of many nutrients and fiber than students who do not. Children don't always like what they are served, however, and school lunch programs must strike a balance between what children want to eat and what will nourish them and guard their health. Interestingly, research shows many more students will self-serve fruits and vegetables from a salad bar located inside the serving line compared with one located outside the line.[106]

TABLE 16-15 School Lunch Patterns

	Grades		
	K–5	6–8	9–12
Food Group	Amount per week (minimum per day)		
Fruits[a] (cups)	2½ (½)	2½ (½)	5 (1)
Vegetables[a] (cups)	3¾ (¾)	3¾ (¾)	5 (1)
Dark green	≥½	≥½	≥½
Red and orange	≥¾	≥¾	≥1¼
Legumes	≥½	≥½	≥½
Starchy	≥½	≥½	≥½
Other	≥½	≥½	≥¾
Any additional vegetables to meet total requirement	1	1	1½
Grains (oz equivalents)	8–9 (1)	8–10 (1)	10–12 (2)
Protein foods (oz equivalents)	8–10 (1)	9–10 (1)	10–12 (2)
Fluid milk[b] (cups)	5 (1)	5 (1)	5 (1)
Other			
kCalories	550–650	600–700	750–850
Saturated fat (% of total kcalories)	<10	<10	<10
Sodium (mg)	≤640	≤710	≤740
Trans fat (g per serving)	0	0	0

[a]No more than half of the fruit or vegetable servings may be in the form of juice. All juice must be 100% full strength.
[b]Fluid milk must be low-fat (unflavored) or fat-free (flavored or unflavored).
SOURCE: US Department of Agriculture, *Nutrition Standards in the National School Lunch and School Breakfast Programs*, January 25, 2012.

The School Breakfast Program is available in more than 80 percent of the nation's schools that offer school lunch, and more than 12 million children participate in it.[107] At a minimum, the school breakfast must contain:

- One serving of fluid milk (either unflavored low-fat or flavored or unflavored fat-free)
- One serving of fruit or vegetable (no more than half of the servings may be 100% full-strength juice)
- One to two servings of whole grains; or one serving of whole grains and one serving of meat or meat alternatives

Unfortunately, for many children who need it, the School Breakfast Program is either unavailable or the children do not participate in it.[108] The majority of children who eat school breakfasts are from low-income families. As research results continue to emphasize the positive impact breakfast has on school performance and health, vigorous campaigns to expand and improve school breakfast programs are under way.

Another federal program, the Child and Adult Care Food Program (CACFP), operates similarly and provides funds to organized child-care programs. All eligible children, centers, and family day-care homes may participate. Sponsors are reimbursed for most meal costs and may also receive USDA commodity foods.

Competing Influences at School Serving healthful lunches is only half the battle; students need to eat them too. Short lunch periods and long waiting lines prevent some students from eating a school lunch and leave others with too little time to finish their meals.[109] Nutrition efforts at schools are also undermined when students can buy what the USDA labels "competitive" or "nonreimbursable" foods—meals from fast-food restaurants or a la carte foods such as pizza or snack foods and carbonated beverages from snack bars, school stores, and vending machines. When students have access to competitive foods, participation in the school lunch program decreases, nutrient intake from lunch declines, and more food is discarded.[110]

TABLE 16-16 USDA Smart Snacks in Schools

Foods must:	Beverages must be:
• Be a "whole grain–rich" grain product; or • Have a fruit, vegetable, dairy product, or protein food as the first ingredient; or • Be a combination food that contains at least ¼ cup of fruit, vegetable, or both • Limit kcalories, sodium, fat, *trans* fat, and sugar	• Plain or carbonated water • Unflavored low-fat milk • Unflavored or flavored fat-free milk or milk alternative • 100% fruit or vegetable juice with no added sugars

SOURCE: Healthier school day, tools for schools: Focus on smart snacks, www.fns.usda.gov/healthierschoolday/tools-schools-focusing-smart-snacks, October 3, 2016.

Increasingly, school-based nutrition issues are being addressed by legislation. Nationwide, USDA's Smart Snacks in Schools regulations now require that competitive foods and beverages, including those sold in vending machines, offer students healthier options with more fruit, vegetables, dairy products, and whole grains (see Table 16-16). The foods and beverages must also meet standards for kcalories, sodium, fat, saturated fat, *trans* fat, and added sugars.

Today's school food environment continues to improve, and the changes promise a generation of healthier children. Realizing this goal demands the full participation and cooperation of all those involved in feeding children at schools—legislators, food vendors, school district officials, administrators, and parents.

REVIEW IT Explain how children's appetites and nutrient needs reflect their stage of growth and why iron deficiency and obesity are often concerns during childhood.

Children's appetites and nutrient needs reflect their stage of growth. Those who are chronically hungry and malnourished suffer stunted growth; when hunger is temporary and nutrient deficiencies are mild, the problems are usually more subtle—such as poor academic performance. Iron deficiency is widespread and has many physical and behavioral consequences. Hyperactivity is not caused by poor nutrition; misbehavior may be due to lack of sleep, too little physical activity, or too much television, among other factors. Childhood obesity has become a major health problem. Adults at home and at school need to provide children with nutrient-dense foods and teach them how to make healthful diet and activity choices

16.3 Nutrition during Adolescence

LEARN IT Describe some of the challenges in meeting the nutrient needs of adolescents.

As children pass through **adolescence** on their way to becoming adults, they change in many ways. Their physical changes make their nutrient needs high, and their emotional, intellectual, and social changes make meeting those needs a challenge.

Teenagers make many more choices for themselves than they did as children. They are not fed, they eat. Food choices made during the teen years profoundly affect present and future health. At the same time, social pressures thrust choices at them, such as whether to drink alcoholic beverages and whether to develop their bodies to meet extreme ideals of slimness or athletic prowess. Their interest in nutrition—both valid information and misinformation—derives from personal, immediate experiences. They are concerned with how their dietary choices can improve their lives now—they engage in fad dieting in order to fit into a new bathing suit, avoid greasy foods in an effort to clear acne, or eat a plate of spaghetti to prepare for a big sporting event. In presenting information on the nutrition and health of adolescents, this section includes many topics of interest to teens.

Growth and Development With the onset of adolescence, the steady growth of childhood speeds up abruptly and dramatically, and the growth patterns of females and males become distinct. Hormones direct the intensity of the adolescent

adolescence: the period from the beginning of puberty until maturity.

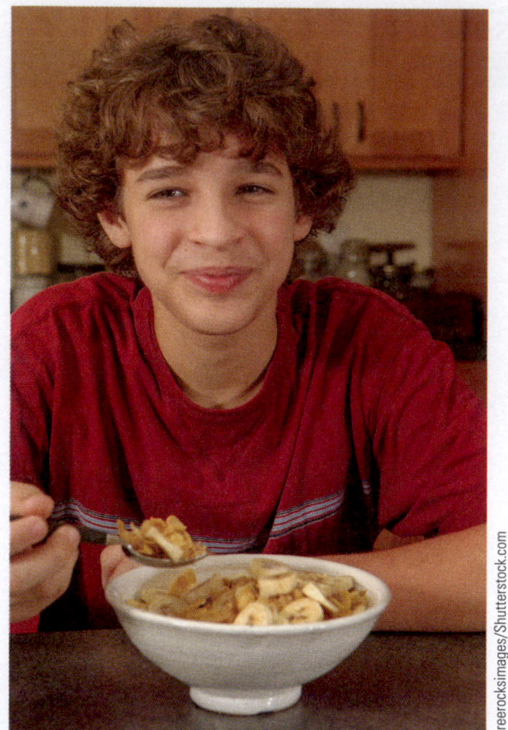

threerocksimages/Shutterstock.com

> **PHOTO 16-15** Nutritious snacks contribute valuable nutrients and energy to an active teen's diet.

growth spurt, profoundly affecting every organ of the body, including the brain. After 2 to 3 years of intense growth and a few more at a slower pace, physically mature adults emerge.

In general, the adolescent growth spurt begins at age 10 to 11 for females and at 12 to 13 for males. It lasts about 2½ years. Before **puberty**, male and female body compositions differ only slightly, but during the adolescent spurt, differences between the genders become apparent in the skeletal system, lean body mass, and fat stores. In females, fat assumes a larger percentage of total body weight, and in males, the lean body mass—principally muscle and bone—increases much more than in females (review Figure 1-1, p. 7). During adolescence, males grow an average of 8 inches taller, and females, 6 inches taller. Males gain approximately 45 pounds, and females, about 35 pounds.

Energy and Nutrient Needs

Energy and nutrient needs are greater during adolescence than at any other time of life (see Photo 16-15), except pregnancy and lactation. In general, nutrient needs rise throughout childhood, peak in adolescence, and then level off or even diminish as the teen becomes an adult.

Energy Intake and Activity

The energy needs of adolescents vary greatly, depending on the current rate of growth, gender, body composition, and physical activity. Boys' energy needs may be especially high; they typically grow faster than girls and, as mentioned, develop a greater proportion of lean body mass. An exceptionally active boy of 15 may need 3500 kcalories or more a day just to maintain his weight. Girls start growing earlier than boys and attain shorter heights and lower weights, so their energy needs peak sooner and decline earlier than those of their male peers. A sedentary girl of 15 whose growth is nearly at a standstill may need fewer than 1800 kcalories a day if she is to avoid excessive weight gain. Thus adolescent girls need to pay special attention to being physically active and selecting foods of high nutrient density so as to meet their nutrient needs without exceeding their energy needs.

The problems of obesity become ever more apparent in adolescence and often continues into adulthood. Without intervention, overweight adolescents face numerous physical and emotional consequences. The consequences of obesity are so dramatic and our society's attitude toward thin people is so intense that even healthy-weight or underweight teens may perceive a need to lose weight. When taken to extremes, restrictive diets bring dramatic physical consequences of their own, as Highlight 8 explained.

Vitamins

The RDA (or AI) for most vitamins increases during the adolescent years (see the insert). Several of the vitamin recommendations for adolescents are similar to those for adults, including recommendations for vitamin D. Vitamin D is essential for bone growth and development. Recent studies of vitamin D status in adolescents show that many adolescents are vitamin D deficient; blacks, females, and overweight adolescents are most at risk.[111] Adolescents who do not receive enough vitamin D from fortified foods such as milk and cereals, or from sun exposure each day, may need a vitamin D supplement.[112]

Iron

The need for iron increases during adolescence for both females and males, but for different reasons. Iron needs increase for females as they start to lose blood through menstruation and for males as their lean body mass develops. Hence the RDA increases at age 14 for both males and females. For females, the RDA remains high into late adulthood. For males, the RDA returns to preadolescent values in early adulthood.

In addition, iron needs increase when the adolescent growth spurt begins, whether that occurs before or after age 14. Therefore, boys in a growth spurt need an additional 2.9 milligrams of iron per day above the RDA for their age; girls need an additional 1.1 milligrams per day.

puberty: the period in life in which a person becomes physically capable of reproduction.

Furthermore, iron recommendations for girls before age 14 do not reflect the iron losses of menstruation. The average age of menarche (first menstruation) in the United States is 12.5 years. Therefore, for girls younger than the age of 14 who have started to menstruate, an additional 2.5 milligrams of iron per day is recommended. Thus the RDA for iron depends not only on age and gender but also on whether the individual is in a growth spurt or has begun to menstruate, as listed in Table 16-17.

Iron intakes often fail to keep pace with increasing needs, especially for females, who typically consume fewer iron-rich foods such as meat and fewer total kcalories than males. Not surprisingly, iron deficiency is most prevalent among adolescent girls. Iron-deficient children and teens score lower on standardized tests than those who are not iron deficient.

TABLE 16-17 Iron Recommendations for Adolescents

Males	Females
9–13 yr: 8 mg/day	9–13 yr: 8 mg/day
9–13 yr in growth spurt: 10.9 mg/day	9–13 yr in menarche: 10.5 mg/day
	9–13 yr in menarche and growth spurt: 11.6 mg/day
14–18 yr: 11 mg/day	14–18 yr: 15 mg/day
14–18 yr in growth spurt: 13.9 mg/day	14–18 yr in growth spurt: 16.1 mg/day

Calcium Adolescence is a crucial time for bone development, and the requirement for calcium reaches its peak during these years.[113] Unfortunately, many adolescents, especially females, have calcium intakes below recommendations. Low calcium intakes during times of active growth, especially if paired with physical inactivity, can compromise the development of peak bone mass, which is considered the best protection against adolescent fractures and adult osteoporosis. Increasing milk and milk products in the diet to meet calcium recommendations greatly increases bone density.[114] Once again, however, teenage girls are most vulnerable because their milk—and therefore their calcium—intakes begin to decline at the time when their calcium needs are greatest.[115] Furthermore, women have much greater bone losses than men in later life. In addition to dietary calcium, physical activity causes bones to grow stronger (see Photo 16-16). Because some high schools do not require students to participate in physical education classes, however, many adolescents are not as physically active as healthy bones demand.

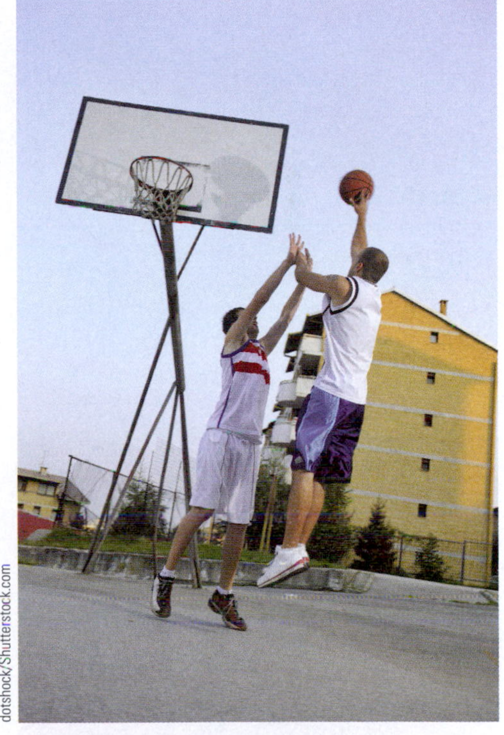

> **PHOTO 16-16** Bones grow stronger with physical activity.

Food Choices and Health Habits

Teenagers like the freedom to come and go as they choose. They eat what they want if it is convenient and if they have the time. With a multitude of after school, social, and job activities, they almost inevitably fall into irregular eating habits. At any given time on any given day, a teenager may be skipping a meal, eating a snack, preparing a meal, or consuming food prepared by a parent or restaurant. Adolescents who frequently help prepare and eat meals with their families, however, eat more fruits, vegetables, grains, and calcium-rich foods, and drink fewer soft drinks, than those who seldom eat with their families.[116] Many adolescents also begin to skip breakfast on a regular basis, missing out on important nutrients that are not made up at later meals during the day. Compared with those who skip breakfast, teenagers who do eat breakfast have higher intakes of vitamin A, vitamin C, and riboflavin, as well as calcium, iron, and zinc.[117] Teenagers who eat breakfast are therefore more likely to meet their nutrient recommendations.

Breakfast skipping may also lead to weight gain in adolescents. Eating breakfast each day, especially a breakfast rich in fiber and protein, improves satiety and reduces hunger and the desire to eat throughout the day.[118] As adolescents make the transition to adulthood, not only do they skip breakfast more often, but they also eat fast food more often. Both skipping breakfast and eating fast foods lead to weight gain.[119]

Ideally, parents continue to play the role of gatekeepers, providing nutritious, easy-to-grab foods in the refrigerator (meats for sandwiches; low-fat cheeses; fresh, raw vegetables and fruits; fruit juices; and milk) and more in the cabinets (whole-grain breads and crackers, peanut butter, nuts, popcorn, and cereal). In many households today, adults work outside the home and teenagers help with some of the gatekeepers' tasks, such as shopping for groceries or choosing fast or prepared foods.

Snacks Snacks typically provide about 25 percent of the average teenager's daily food energy intake. If chosen carefully, snacks can contribute some needed nutrients (see Table 16-14, p. 521). Energy-dense, nutrient-poor snack foods are readily available in settings where teens spend their time, however, and frequent snacking on these foods can contribute to higher total energy intakes as well as higher energy intakes from added sugars.[120]

Beverages Most frequently, adolescents drink soft drinks instead of fruit juice or milk with lunch, supper, and snacks. About the only time they select fruit juice is at breakfast. When teens drink milk, they are more likely to consume it with a meal (especially breakfast) than as a snack. Because of their greater food intakes, boys are more likely than girls to drink enough milk to meet their calcium needs.[121]

Soft drinks, when chosen as the primary beverage, may affect bone density, partly because they displace milk from the diet. Over the past three decades, teens (especially girls) have been drinking more soft drinks and less milk. Adolescents who drink soft drinks regularly have a higher energy intake and a lower calcium intake than those who do not.[122]

Soft drinks containing caffeine present another problem if caffeine intake becomes excessive. Many adolescents consume energy drinks on a regular basis and these beverages contain much more caffeine than soft drinks.* Caffeine seems to be relatively harmless when used in *moderate* doses (less than 100 milligrams per day, roughly the equivalent of fewer than three 12-ounce cola beverages a day). In greater amounts, however, caffeine can cause symptoms associated with anxiety, such as sweating, tenseness, and inability to concentrate. Teens with certain diseases such as diabetes, heart abnormalities, and mood disorders and those taking certain medications may encounter more severe consequences such as seizures, heart failure, and death.

Eating Away from Home Adolescents eat about one-third of their meals away from home, and their nutritional welfare is enhanced or hindered by the choices they make.[123] A lunch consisting of a hamburger, a chocolate shake, and french fries supplies substantial quantities of many nutrients at a kcalorie cost of about 800, an energy intake some adolescents can afford. When they eat this sort of lunch, teens can adjust their breakfast and dinner choices to include fruits and vegetables for vitamin A, vitamin C, folate, and fiber and lean meats and legumes for iron and zinc (see Photo 16-17). Fortunately, many fast-food restaurants are now offering more nutritious choices than the standard hamburger meal.

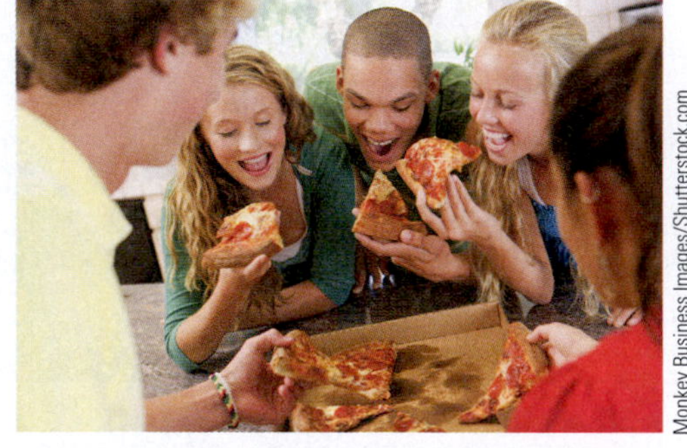

Monkey Business Images/Shutterstock.com

> **PHOTO 16-17** Because their lunches rarely include fruits, vegetables, or milk, many teens fail to get all the vitamins and minerals they need each day.

Peer Influence Physical maturity and growing independence present adolescents with new choices. The consequences of those choices will influence their health and nutrition status both today and throughout life. Many of the food and health choices adolescents make reflect the opinions and actions of their peers. When others perceive milk as "babyish," a teen may choose soft drinks instead; when others skip lunch and hang out in the parking lot, a teen may join in for the camaraderie, regardless of hunger. Some teenagers begin using drugs, alcohol, and tobacco; others wisely refrain. Adults can set up the environment so that nutritious foods are available and can stand by with reliable information and advice about health and nutrition, but the rest is up to the adolescents. Ultimately, they make the choices. (Highlight 8 examined the influence of social pressures on the development of eating disorders.)

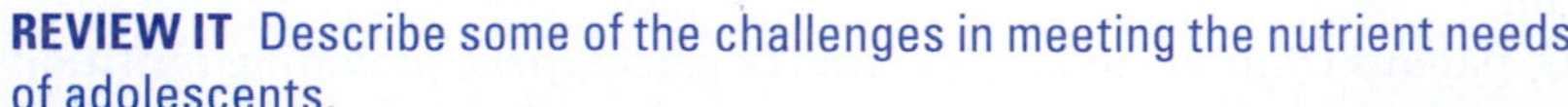

REVIEW IT Describe some of the challenges in meeting the nutrient needs of adolescents.

Nutrient needs rise dramatically as children enter the rapid growth phase of adolescence. Teenagers' busy lifestyles add to the challenge of meeting their nutrient needs, especially for iron and calcium.

The nutrition and lifestyle choices people make as children and adolescents have long-term, as well as immediate, effects on their health. Highlight 16 (p. 531) describes how sound choices and good habits during childhood and adolescence can help prevent chronic diseases later in life.

*Caffeine-containing soft drinks typically deliver about 30 mg of caffeine per 12-ounce can; energy drinks typically deliver about 100 mg of caffeine for equivalent amounts. A pharmacologically active dose of caffeine is defined as 200 mg.

What's Online

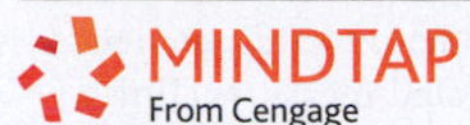

MINDTAP
From Cengage

Visit **www.cengagebrain.com** to access MindTap, a complete digital course that includes Diet & Wellness Plus, interactive quizzes, videos, and more.

REFERENCES

1. J. T. Brenna and S. E. Carlson, Docosahexaenoic acid and human brain development: Evidence that a dietary supply is needed for optimal development, *Journal of Human Evolution* 77 (2014): 99–106.
2. Formula feeding of term infants, in *Pediatric Nutrition*, 7th ed., ed. R. E. Kleinman (Elk Grove Village, Ill.: American Academy of Pediatrics, 2014), pp. 61–81.
3. Position of the Academy of Nutrition and Dietetics: Promoting and supporting breastfeeding, *Journal of the Academy of Nutrition and Dietetics* 115 (2015): 444–449.
4. Breastfeeding, in *Pediatric Nutrition*, 7th ed., ed. R. E. Kleinman (Elk Grove Village, Ill.: American Academy of Pediatrics, 2014), pp. 41–59; American Academy of Pediatrics, Policy statement: Breastfeeding and the use of human milk, *Pediatrics* 129 (2012): e827–e841, available at www.pediatrics.org/content/129/3/e827.full.
5. T. Jost and coauthors, Impact of human milk bacteria and oligosaccharides on neonatal gut microbiota establishment and gut health, *Nutrition Reviews* 73 (2015): 426–437; J. T. Smilowitz and coauthors, Breast milk oligosaccharides: Structure-function relationships in the neonate, *Annual Review of Nutrition* 34 (2014): 143–169; P. V. Jeurink and coauthors, Mechanisms underlying immune effects of dietary oligosaccharides, *American Journal of Clinical Nutrition* 98 (2013): 572S–577S.
6. B. M. Jakaitis and P. W. Denning, Human breast milk and the gastrointestinal innate immune system, *Clinics in Perinatology* 41 (2014): 423–435; E. Castanys-Munoz, M. J. Martin, and P. A. Prieto, 2′-Fucosyllactose: An abundant, genetically determined soluble glycan present in human milk, *Nutrition Reviews* 71 (2013): 773–789; Jeurink and coauthors, 2013.
7. P. Willatts and coauthors, Effects of long-chain PUFA supplementation in infant formula on cognitive function in later childhood, *American Journal of Clinical Nutrition* 98 (2013): 536S–542S.
8. S. M. Innis, Impact of maternal diet on human milk composition and neurological development of infants, *American Journal of Clinical Nutrition* 99 (2014): 734S–741S; Brenna and Carlson, 2014; A. Qawasmi, A. Landeros-Weisenberger, and M. H. Bloch, Meta-analysis of LCPUFA supplementation of infant formula and visual acuity, *Pediatrics* 131 (2013): e262–e272; Willatts and coauthors, 2013.
9. C. S. Molloy and coauthors, Long-term effect of high-dose supplementation with DHA on visual function at school age in children born at <33 wk gestational age: Results from a follow-up of a randomized controlled trial, *American Journal of Clinical Nutrition* 103 (2016): 268–275; Qawasmi and Landeros-Weisenberger, 2013.
10. J. J. Qingqing and coauthors, Effect of n-3 PUFA supplementation on cognitive function throughout the life span from infancy to old age: A systematic review and meta-analysis of randomized controlled trials, *American Journal of Clinical Nutrition* 100 (2014): 1422–1436; Willatts and coauthors, 2013.
11. Fat-soluble vitamins, in *Pediatric Nutrition*, 7th ed., ed. R. E. Kleinman (Elk Grove Village, Ill.: American Academy of Pediatrics, 2014), pp. 495–515.
12. Breastfeeding, 2014; S. Gallo and coauthors, Effect of different dosages of oral vitamin D supplementation on vitamin D status in healthy, breastfed infants, *Journal of the American Medical Association* 309 (2013): 1785–1792.
13. Jost and coauthors, 2015; Smilowitz and coauthors, 2014; E. W. Chatterton and coauthors Anti-inflammatory mechanisms of bioactive milk proteins in the intestine of newborns, *International Journal of Biochemistry and Cell Biology* 45 (2013): 1730–1747; B. Lonnerdal, Bioactive proteins in breast milk, *Journal of Paediatrics and Child Health* (Supplement S1) 49 (2013): 1–7.
14. Jost and coauthors, 2015; Jakaitis and Denning, 2014.
15. G. Bowatte and coauthors, Breastfeeding and childhood acute otitis media: A systematic review and meta-analysis, *Acta Paediatrica* 104 (2015): 85-95.
16. K. Grimshaw and coauthors, Modifying the infant's diet to prevent food allergy, *Archives of Disease in Childhood* 2016, doi:10.1136/archdischild-2015-309770; V. Bion and coauthors, Evaluating the efficacy of breastfeeding guidelines on long-term outcomes for allergic disease, *Allergy* 71 (2016): 661–670; C. J. Lodge and coauthors, Breastfeeding and asthma and allergies: A systematic review and meta-analysis, *Acta Paediatrica* 104 (2015): 38–53; A. von Berg, Dietary interventions for primary allergy prevention—What is the evidence? *World Review of Nutrition and Dietetics* 108 (2013): 71–78; American Academy of Pediatrics, 2012.
17. American Academy of Pediatrics, 2012.
18. R. A. Danall and coauthors, American Academy of Pediatrics' Task Force on SIDS fully supports breastfeeding, *Breastfeeding Medicine* 9 (2014): 486–487.
19. I. Ramirez-Silva and coauthors, Breastfeeding status at age 3 months is associated with adiposity and cardiometabolic markers at age 4 years in Mexican children, *Journal of Nutrition* 145 (2015): 1295–1302; T. W. McDade and coauthors, Long-term effects of birth weight and breastfeeding duration on inflammation in early adulthood, *Proceedings. Biological Sciences* 281 (2014): 20133116; S. Pirilä and coauthors, Breast-fed infants and their later cardiovascular health: A prospective study from birth to age 32 years, *British Journal of Nutrition* 111 (2014): 1069–1076.
20. W. Liang and coauthors, Breastfeeding reduces childhood obesity risks, *Childhood Obesity* (2017) doi:10.1089/chi.2016.0210; R. J. Hancox and coauthors, Association between breastfeeding and body mass index at age 6-7 years in an international survey, *Pediatric Obesity* 10 (2015): 283–287; C. M. Lefebvre and R. M. John, The effect of breastfeeding on childhood overweight and obesity: A systematic review of the literature, *Journal of the American Association of Nurse Practitioners* 26 (2014): 386–401.
21. Lefebvre and John, 2014.
22. S. Bar, R. Milanaik, and A. Adesman, Long-term neurodevelopmental benefits of breastfeeding, *Current Opinion in Pediatrics* 28 (2016): 559–566; S. Cai and coauthors, Infant feeding effects on early neurocognitive development in Asian children, *American Journal of Clinical Nutrition* 101 (2015): 326–336; M. B. Belfort and coauthors, Infant feeding and childhood cognition at ages 3 and 7 years: Effects of breastfeeding duration and exclusivity, *JAMA Pediatrics* 167 (2013): 836–844.
23. A. Kantorowska and coauthors, Impact of donor milk availability on breast milk use and necrotizing enterocolitis rates, *Pediatrics* 137 (2016): e20153123.
24. S. A. Keim and coauthors, Cow's milk contamination of human milk purchased via the internet, *Pediatrics* 135 (2015): e1157–e1162.
25. Formula feeding of term infants, in *Pediatric Nutrition*, 7th ed., ed. R. E. Kleinman (Elk Grove Village, Ill.: American Academy of Pediatrics, 2014), pp. 61–81.
26. Position of the Academy of Nutrition and Dietetics: The impact of fluoride on health, *Journal of the Academy of Nutrition and Dietetics* 112 (2012): 1443–1453.
27. U. S. Food and Drug Administration, FDA sets standards for infant formula, www.fda.gov/food/newsevents/constituentupdates/ucm384911.htm, updated June 6, 2014.
28. Formula feeding of term infants, 2014.
29. Formula feeding of term infants, 2014.
30. D. Turck, Cow's and goat's milk, *World Review of Nutrition and Dietetics* 108 (2013): 56–62.

31. M. J. K. Osterman and coauthors, Annual summary of vital statistics: 2012-2013, *Pediatrics* 135 (2015): 1115–1125.
32. B. E. Cormack and F. H. Bloomfield, Early nutrition for preterm babies, *Nutrition Today* 50 (2015): 230–239; Nutritional needs of the preterm infant, in *Pediatric Nutrition*, 7th ed., ed. R. E. Kleinman (Elk Grove Village, Ill.: American Academy of Pediatrics, 2014), pp. 83–121.
33. Formula feeding of term infants, 2014.
34. Complementary feeding, in *Pediatric Nutrition*, 7th ed., ed. R. E. Kleinman (Elk Grove Village, Ill.: American Academy of Pediatrics, 2014), pp. 123–139; Expert Panel on Integrated Guidelines for Cardiovascular Health and Risk Reduction in Children and Adolescents: Summary report, *Pediatrics* 128 (2011): S213–S256.
35. Complementary feeding, 2014.
36. Complementary feeding, 2014.
37. P. J. Turner and D. E. Campbell, Implementing primary prevention for peanut allergy at a population level, *Journal of the American Medical Association* 317 (2017): 1111-1112; A. Togias and coauthors, Addendum guidelines for the prevention of peanut allergy in the United States: Report of the National Institute of Allergy and Infectious Diseases–sponsored expert panel, *Annals of Allergy, Asthma, and Immunology*, 118 (2017): 166.e7–173.e7; G. Du Toit and coauthors, Randomized trial of peanut consumption in infants at risk for peanut allergy, *New England of Medicine* 372 (2015): 803–813; D. M. Fleischer and coauthors, Consensus communication on early peanut introduction and the prevention of peanut allergy in high-risk infants, *Pediatrics* 136 (2015): 600–604.
38. Complementary feeding, 2014.
39. Complementary feeding, 2014.
40. Feeding the child, in *Pediatric Nutrition*, 7th ed., ed. R. E. Kleinman (Elk Grove Village, Ill.: American Academy of Pediatrics, 2014), pp. 143–173.
41. Position of the Academy of Nutrition and Dietetics: Nutrition guidance for healthy children ages 2 to 11 years, *Journal of the Academy of Nutrition and Dietetics* 114 (2014): 1257–1276; D. M. Hoelscher and coauthors, Position of the Academy of Nutrition and Dietetics: Interventions for the prevention and treatment of pediatric overweight and obesity, *Journal of the Academy of Nutrition and Dietetics* 113 (2013): 1375–1394.
42. Position of the Academy of Nutrition and Dietetics, 2014.
43. Nutritional aspects of vegetarian diets, in *Pediatric Nutrition*, 7th ed., ed. R. E. Kleinman (Elk Grove Village, Ill.: American Academy of Pediatrics, 2014), pp. 241–264.
44. M. Domellöf and coauthors, Iron requirements of infants and toddlers, *Journal of Pediatric Gastroenterology* 58 (2014): 119-129; G. Paoletti, D. L. Bogen, and A. K. Ritchey, Severe iron-deficiency anemia still an issue in toddlers, *Clinical Pediatrics* 53 (2014): 1352–1358.
45. C. Mortensen and coauthors, Estimation of the dietary requirement for vitamin D in white children aged 4-8 y: A randomized, controlled, dose-response trial, *American Journal of Clinical Nutrition*, 2016, doi:10.3945/ajcn.116.136697; Committee on Dietary Reference Intakes, *Dietary Reference Intakes for Calcium and Vitamin D* (Washington, D.C.: National Academies Press, 2011), pp. 345–402.
46. J. Dwyer and coauthors, Prevalence and predictors of children's dietary supplement use: The 2007 National Health Interview Survey, *American Journal of Clinical Nutrition* 97 (2013): 1331–1337.
47. Position of the Academy of Nutrition and Dietetics, 2014; C. N. Ford, M. M. Slining, and B. M. Popkin, Trends in dietary intake among US 2- to 6-year-old children, 1989–2008, *Journal of the Academy of Nutrition and Dietetics* 113 (2013): 35–42.
48. Ford, Slining, and Popkin, 2013.
49. Position of the Academy of Nutrition and Dietetics, 2014; N. Tian and coauthors, Sodium and potassium intakes among US infants and preschool children, 2003–2010, *American Journal of Clinical Nutrition* 98 (2013): 1113–1122.
50. Bread for the World, About hunger, www.bread.org/where-does-hunger-exist, accessed October 26, 2016.
51. Position of the Academy of Nutrition and Dietetics, 2014.
52. S. S. Pineda Vargas and coauthors, Eating ready-to-eat cereal for breakfast is positively associated with daily nutrient intake, but not weight, in Mexican-American children and adolescents, *Nutrition Today* 51 (2016): 206–215; S.I. Barr, L. DiFrancesco, and V. L. Fulgoni, Breakfast consumption is positively associated with nutrient adequacy in Canadian children and adolescents, *British Journal of Nutrition* 112 (2014): 1373–1383.
53. I. Iovino and coauthors, Breakfast consumption has no effect on neuropsychological functioning in children: A repeated-measures clinical trial, *American Journal of Clinical Nutrition* 104 (2016): 715–721; V. Edefonti and coauthors, The effect of breakfast composition and energy contribution on cognitive and academic performance: A systematic review, *American Journal of Clinical Nutrition* 100 (2014): 626–656.
54. F. Koohdani and coauthors, Midmorning snack programs have a beneficial effect on cognitive performance of students from high socioeconomic background, *Nutrition Today*, 2014, doi:10.1097/NT.0b013e318298e7dd.
55. P. M. Gupta and coauthors, Iron, anemia, and iron deficiency anemia among young children in the United States, *Nutrients*, 2016, doi:10.3390/nu8060330; J. R. Doom and M. K. Georgieff, Striking while the iron is hot: Understanding the biological and neurodevelopmental effects of iron deficiency to optimize intervention in early childhood, *Current Pediatric Reports* 2 (2014): 291–298.
56. Doom and Georgieff, 2014.
57. B. P. Lanphear and Council on Environmental Health, American Academy of Pediatrics Policy Statement, Prevention of childhood lead toxicity, *Pediatrics* 138 (2016): 146–160; C. S. Sim and coauthors, Iron deficiency increases blood lead levels in boys and pre-menarche girls surveyed in KNHANES 2010-2011, *Environmental Research* 130 (2014): 1–6.
58. Centers for Disease Control and Prevention, Lead, www.cdc.gov/nceh/lead, updated September 7, 2016.
59. Centers for Disease Control and Prevention, Attention-Deficit/Hyperactivity Disorder, Data and Statistics, www.cdc.gov/ncbddd/adhd/data.html, updated October 5, 2016.
60. S. Cruchet, Y. Lucero, and V. Cornejo, Truths, myths, and needs of special diets: Attention-deficit/hyperactivity disorder, autism, non-celiac gluten sensitivity, and vegetarianism, *Annals of Nutrition and Metabolism* 68 (2016): 43–50.
61. J. Stevenson and coauthors, Research review: The role of diet in the treatment of attention-deficit/hyperactivity disorder—An appraisal of the evidence on efficacy and recommendations on the design of future studies, *Journal of Child Psychology and Psychiatry* 55 (2014): 416–427; L. J. Stevens and coauthors, Mechanisms of behavioral, atopic, and other reactions to artificial food colors in children, *Nutrition Reviews* 71 (2013): 268–281.
62. Food and Drug Administration, Food allergies: Reducing the risks, https://www.fda.gov/forconsumers/consumerupdates/ucm089307.htm; updated September 10, 2015.
63. S. Benedè and coauthors, The rise of food allergy: Environmental factors and emerging treatments, *EBioMedicine* 7 (2016): 27–34; D. M. Fleischer and coauthors, Consensus communication on early peanut introduction and the prevention of peanut allergy in high-risk infants, *Pediatrics* 136 (2015): 600–604; Food and Drug Administration, Food allergies: Reducing the risks, https://www.fda.gov/forconsumers/consumerupdates/ucm089307.htm; updated September 10, 2015.
64. Benedé and coauthors, 2016.
65. S. C. Collins, Practice paper of the Academy of Nutrition and Dietetics: Role of the registered dietitian nutritionist in the diagnosis and management of food allergies, *Journal of the Academy of Nutrition and Dietetics* 116 (2016): 1621-1631; R. B. Canani and coauthors, The effects of dietary counseling on children with food allergy: A prospective, multicenter intervention study, *Journal of the Academy of Nutrition and Dietetics* 114 (2014): 1432–1439.
66. B. P. Vickery and coauthors, Early oral immunotherapy in peanut-allergic preschool children is safe and highly effective, *Journal of Allergy and Clinical Immunology* 139 (2016): 183–181; K. Anagnostou and coauthors, Assessing the efficacy of oral immunotherapy for the desensitization of peanut allergy in children (STOPII): A phase 2 randomised controlled trial, *Lancet* 383 (2014): 1297–1304.
67. C. L. Ogden and coauthors, Trends in obesity prevalence among children and adolescents in the United State, 1988-1994 through 2013-2014, *Journal of the American Medical Association* 315 (2016): 2292–2299.
68. C. L. Ogden, M. D. Carroll, and K. M. Flegal, Prevalence of childhood and adult obesity in the United States, 2011–2012, *Journal of the American*

Medical Association 311 (2014): 806–814; S. A. Cunningham, M. R. Kramer, and K. M. Venkat Narayan, Incidence of childhood obesity in the United States, *New England Journal of Medicine* 370 (2014): 403–411.
69. Ogden, Carroll, and Flegal, 2014; Expert Panel on Integrated Guidelines for Cardiovascular Health and Risk Reduction in Children and Adolescents, Summary Report, *Pediatrics* 128 (2011): S213–S256.
70. A. C. Skinner and J. A. Skelton, Prevalence and trends in obesity and severe obesity among children in the United States, 1999-2012, *JAMA Pediatrics* 168 (2014): 561–566.
71. A. C. Skinner and coauthors, Cardiometabolic risks and severity of obesity in children and young adults, *New England Journal of Medicine* 373 (2015): 1307–1317; A. S. Kelly and coauthors, Severe obesity in children and adolescents: Identification, associated health risks, and treatment approaches: A Scientific Statement from the American Heart Association, *Circulation* 128 (2013): 1689–1712.
72. P. Dolton and M. Xiao, The intergenerational transmission of body mass index across countries, *Economics and Human Biology* 24 (2017): 140–152; K. Silventoinen and coauthors, Genetic and environmental effects on body mass index from infancy to the onset of adulthood: An individual-based pooled analysis of 45 twin cohorts participating in the Collaborative project of Development of Anthropometrical measures in Twins (CODATwins) study, *American Journal of Clinical Nutrition* 104 (2016): 371–379; M. G. Hohenadel and coauthors, The impact of genetic variants on BMI increase during childhood versus adulthood, *International Journal of Obesity* 40 (2016): 1301–1309; A. L. Thompson, Intergenerational impact of maternal obesity and postnatal feeding practices on pediatric obesity, *Nutrition Reviews* 71(2013): S55–S61.
73. Skinner and Skelton, 2014.
74. Centers for Disease Control and Prevention, Childhood obesity causes & consequences, www.cdc.gov/obesity/childhood/causes.html, updated June 19, 2015.
75. J. Martin-Biggers and coauthors, Translating it into real life: A qualitative study of the cognitions, barriers and supports for key obesogenic behaviors of parents of preschoolers, *BMC Public Health* 15 (2015): 189; S. C. couch and coauthors, Home food environment in relation to children's diet quality and weight status, *Journal of the Academy of Nutrition and Dietetics* 114 (2014): 1569–1579; A. W. Watts and coauthors, Parent-child associations in selected food group and nutrient intakes among overweight and obese adolescents, *Journal of the Academy of Nutrition and Dietetics* 114 (2014): 1580–1586; L. McGowan and coauthors, Healthy feeding habits: Efficacy results from a cluster-randomized, controlled exploratory trial of a novel, habit-based intervention with parents, *American Journal of Clinical Nutrition* 98 (2013): 769–777.
76. Position of the Academy of Nutrition and Dietetics, 2014; C. R. McGill and coauthors, Improved diet quality and increased nutrient intakes associated with grape product consumption by U.S. children and adults: National Health and Nutrition Examination Survey 2003–2008, *Journal of Food Science* (Suppl 1) 78 (2013): A1–A4.
77. J. M. Poti, M. M. Slining, and B.M. Popkin, Where are kids getting their empty calories? Stores, schools, and fast-food restaurants each played an important role in empty calorie intake among US children during 2009-2010, *Journal of the Academy of Nutrition and Dietetics* 114 (2014): 908–917.
78. M. B. Vos and coauthors, Added sugars and cardiovascular disease risk in children: A Scientific Statement from the American Heart Association, *Circulation*, 2016, http://dx.doi.org/10.1161/CIR.0000000000000439; L. Tappy and K. A. Lê, Health effects of fructose and fructose-containing caloric sweeteners: Where do we stand 10 years after the initial whistle blowings? *Current Diabetes Reports* 15 (2015): 54; G. A. Brady and B. M. Popkin, Dietary sugar and body weight: Have we reached a crisis in the epidemic of obesity and diabetes? *Diabetes Care* 37 (2014): 950–956; S. C. Bundrick and coauthors, Soda consumption during ad libitum food intake predicts weight change, *Journal of the Academy of Nutrition and Dietetics* 114 (2014): 444–449.
79. S. D. Poppitt, Beverage consumption: Are alcoholic and sugary drinks tipping the balance toward overweight and obesity? *Nutrients* 7 (2015): 6700–6718; The Obesity Society, Position statement: Reduced consumption of sugar-sweetened beverages can reduce total caloric intake, 2014, www.obesity.org/obesity/publications/position-and-policies/sugar-sweetened; Bray and Popkin, 2014; Bundrick and coauthors, 2014.
80. A. Marques and coauthors, Association between physical activity, sedentary time, and healthy fitness in youth, *Medicine* and *Science in Sports and Exercise* 47 (2015): 575–580; T. Remmers and coauthors, Relationship between physical activity and the development of body mass index in children, *Medicine and Science in Sports and Exercise* 46 (2014): 177–184; C. Lees and J. Hopkins, Effect of aerobic exercise on cognition, academic achievement, and psychosocial function in children: A systematic review of randomized control trials, *Preventing Chronic Disease* 10 (2013): 130010.
81. V. Carson and coauthors, Systematic review of sedentary behavior and health indicators in school-aged children and youth: An update, *Applied Physiology, Nutrition, and Metabolism* 41 (2016): S240–S265; A. G. LeBlanc and coauthors, Correlates of total sedentary time and screen time in 9-11 year-old children around the world: The International Study of Childhood Obesity, Lifestyle and the Environment, *PLoS One* 10 (2015): e0129622; M. Govindan and coauthors, Gender differences in physiologic markers and health behaviors associated with childhood obesity, *Pediatrics* 132 (2013): 468–474; J. Falbe and coauthors, Adiposity and different types of screen time, *Pediatrics* 132 (2013): e1497–e1505.
82. M. M. Borghese and coauthors, Mediating role of television time, diet patterns, physical activity and sleep duration in the association between television in the bedroom and adiposity in 10 year-old children, *International Journal of Behavioral Nutrition and Physical Activity* 13 (2015): 60; E. M. Cespedes and coauthors, Television viewing, bedroom television, and sleep duration from infancy to mid-childhood, *Pediatrics* 133 (2014): e1163–1171; J. Owens, Insufficient sleep in adolescents and young adults: An update on causes and consequences, *Pediatrics* 134 (2014): e921–e932; A. E. Staiano and coauthors, Television, adiposity, and cardiometabolic risk in children and adolescents, *American Journal of Preventive Medicine* 44 (2013): 40–47.
83. Carson and coauthors, 2016; Borghese and coauthors, 2015; J. Falbe and coauthors, Longitudinal relations of television, electronic games, and digital versatile discs with changes in diet in adolescents, *American Journal of Clinical Nutrition* 100 (2014): 1173–1181.
84. Carson and coauthors, 2016; Borghese and coauthors, 2015; M. M. Borghese and coauthors, Independent and combined associations of total sedentary time and television viewing time with food patterns of 9- to 11-year-old Canadian children, *Applied Physiology, Nutrition, and Metabolism* 39 (2014): 937–943; Falbe and coauthors, 2014.
85. Carson and coauthors, 2014; Borghese and coauthors, 2014.
86. M. R. Longacre and coauthors, Child-targeted TV advertising and preschoolers' consumption of high-sugar breakfast cereals, *Appetite* 108 (2016): 295–302; E. J. Boyland and R. Whalen, Food advertising to children and its effects on diet: Review of recent prevalence and impact data, *Pediatric Diabetes* 16 (2015): 331–337.
87. F. Folkvord and coauthors, The effect of playing advergames that promote energy-dense snacks or fruit on actual food intake among children, *American Journal of Clinical Nutrition* 97 (2013): 239–245.
88. M. Nestle, WHO Europe takes on food marketing to children, November 7, 2016, www.foodpolitics.com/2016/11/who-europe-takes-on-food-marketing-to-children; Boyland and Whalen, 2015.
89. M. D. Hingle and coauthors, Alignment of children's food advertising with proposed Federal Guidelines, *American Journal of Preventive Medicine* 48 (2015): 707–713; A. M. Bernhardt and coauthors, Children's recall of fast food television advertising—Testing the adequacy of food marketing regulation, *PLoS One* 10 (2015): e0119300.
90. Falbe and coauthors, 2014.
91. M. Simmons and coauthors, Associations between active video gaming and other energy-balance related behaviours in adolescents: A 24-hour recall diary study, *International Journal of Behavioral Nutrition and Physical Activity* 12 (2015): 32; A. G. LeBlanc and coauthors, Active video games and health indicators in children and youth: A systematic review, *PLoS One* 8 (2013): e65351.
92. American Academy of Pediatrics, Policy statement, Council on Communications and Media, Media and young minds, *Pediatrics* 138 (2016): e20162592; American Academy of Pediatrics, Policy statement, Council on Communications and media, Media use in school-aged children and adolescents, *Pediatrics* 138 (2016): e20162592.

93. A. C. Skinner and coauthors, Cardiometabolic risks and severity of obesity in children and young adults, *New England Journal of Medicine* 373 (2015): 1307–1317; K. R. Armstrong and coauthors, Childhood obesity, arterial stiffness, and prevalence and treatment of hypertension, *Current Treatment Options in Cardiovascular Medicine* 16 (2014): 339.
94. G. Twig and coauthors, BMI at age 17 years and diabetes mortality in midlife: A nationwide cohort of 2.3 million adolescents, *Diabetes Care,* 2016, http://dx.doi.org/10.2337/dc16-1203; B. Tobisch, L. Blatniczky, and L. Barkai, Cardiometabolic risk factors and insulin resistance in obese children and adolescents: Relation to puberty, *Pediatric Obesity* 10 (2015): 37–44.
95. A. W. Harrist and coauthors, The social and emotional lives of overweight, obese, and severely obese children, *Child Development* 87 (2016): 1564–1580; S. A. Taylor and coauthors, A qualitative study of the day-to-day lives of obese Mexican-American adolescent females, *Pediatrics* 131 (2013): 1132–1138.
96. D. M. Styne and coauthors, Pediatric obesity—assessment, treatment, and prevention: An Endocrine Society Clinical Practice Guideline, *Journal of Clinical Endocrinology and Metabolism* (2017): jc2016–jc2573; P. T. Katzmarzyk and coauthors, An evolving scientific basis for the prevention and treatment of pediatric obesity, *International Journal of Obesity* 38 (2014): 887–905; D. M. Hoelscher and coauthors, Position of the Academy of Nutrition and Dietetics: Interventions for the prevention and treatment of pediatric overweight and obesity, *Journal of the Academy of Nutrition and Dietetics* 113 (2013): 1375–1394.
97. Katzmarzyk and coauthors, 2014; Hoelscher and coauthors, 2013.
98. J. Bangsbo and coauthors, The Copenhagen Consensus Conference 2016: Children, youth, and physical activity in schools and during leisure time, *British Journal of Sports Medicine* 50 (2016): 1177–1178; P. T. Katzmarzyk and coauthors, Physical activity, sedentary time, and obesity in an international sample of children, *Medicine and Science in Sports and Exercise* 47 (2015): 2062–2069; A. Marques and coauthors, Association between physical activity, sedentary time, and healthy fitness in youth, *Medicine and Science in Sports and Exercise* 47 (2015): 575–580; P. J. Colllings and coauthors, Physical activity intensity, sedentary time, and body composition in preschoolers, *American Journal of Clinical Nutrition* 97 (2013): 1020–1028.
99. Hoelscher and coauthors, 2013.
100. T. H. Inge and coauthors, Weight loss and health status 3 years after bariatric surgery in adolescents, *New England Journal of Medicine* 374 (2016): 113–123; Katzmarzyk and coauthors, 2014.
101. A. Ek and coauthors, Associations between parental concerns about preschoolers' weight and eating and parental feeding practices: Results from analyses of the Child Eating Behavior Questionnaire, the Child Feeding Questionnaire, and the Lifestyle Behavior Checklist, *PLoS One* 11 (2016): e0147257; S. R. Damiano, L. M. Hart, and S. J. Paxton, Correlates of parental feeding practices with pre-schoolers: Parental body image and eating knowledge, attitudes, and behaviours, *Appetite* 101 (2016): 192–198; A. J. Jeffers and coauthors, BMI and depressive symptoms: The role of media pressures, *Eating Behaviors* 14 (2013): 468–471.
102. Position of the Academy of Nutrition and Dietetics, 2014.
103. B. Wansink, M. Shimizu, and A. Brumberg, Association of nutrient dense snack combinations with calories and vegetable intake, *Pediatrics* 131 (2013): 22–29.
104. Position of the American Dietetic Association: Benchmarks for nutrition in child care, *Journal of the American Dietetic Association* 111 (2011): 607–615, reaffirmed 2016.
105. National School Lunch Program, www.fns.usda.gov/nslp/national-school-lunch-program-nslp, August 18, 2016; Position of the American Dietetic Association: Local support for nutrition integrity in schools, *Journal of the American Dietetic Association* 110 (2010): 1244–1254, reaffirmed 2016.
106. M. A. Adams and coauthors, Location of school lunch salad bars and fruit and vegetable consumption in middle schools: A cross-sectional plate waste study, *Journal of the Academy of Nutrition and Dietetics* 116 (2016): 407–416.
107. The School Breakfast Program, https://www.fns.usda.gov/sbp/school-breakfast-program-sbp, August 10, 2016; Position of the American Dietetic Association: Local support for nutrition integrity in schools, *Journal of the American Dietetic Association* 110 (2010): 1244–1254, reaffirmed 2016.
108. Position of the American Dietetic Association: Local support for nutrition integrity in schools, *Journal of the American Dietetic Association* 110 (2010): 1244–1254, reaffirmed 2016.
109. J. F. W. Cohen and coauthors, Amount of time to eat lunch is associated with children's selection and consumption of school meal entrée, fruits, vegetables, and milk, *Journal of the Academy of Nutrition and Dietetics* 116 (2016): 123–128; Position of the American Dietetic Association, Local support for nutrition integrity in schools, *Journal of the American Dietetic Association* 110 (2010): 1244–1254, reaffirmed 2016.
110. Position of the Academy of Nutrition and Dietetics, 2014; Position of the American Dietetic Association: Local support for nutrition integrity in schools, *Journal of the American Dietetic Association* 110 (2010): 1244–1254, reaffirmed 2016.
111. The Society for Adolescent Health and Medicine, Recommended vitamin D intake and management of low vitamin D status in adolescents: A position statement of the Society for Adolescent Health and Medicine, *Journal of Adolescent Health* 52 (2013): 801–803; L. E. Au and coauthors, Associations of vitamin D intake with 25-hydroxyvitamin D in overweight and racially/ethnically diverse US children, *Journal of the Academy of Nutrition and Dietetics* 113 (2013): 1511–1516.
112. The Society for Adolescent Health and Medicine, 2013.
113. C. M. Weaver and coauthors, The National Osteoporosis Foundation's position statement on peak bone mass development and lifestyle factors: A systematic review and implementation recommendations, *Osteoporosis International* 27 (2016): 1281–1386.
114. D. K. Dror and L. H. Allen, Dairy product intake in children and adolescents in developed countries: Trends, nutritional contribution, and a review of association with health outcomes, *Nutrition Reviews* 72 (2014): 68–81.
115. Dror and Allen, 2014.
116. J. M. Berge and coauthors, Family food preparation and its effects on adolescent dietary quality and eating patterns, *Journal of Adolescent Health* 59 (2016): 530–536; J. M. Berge and coauthors, Structural and interpersonal characteristics of family meals: Associations with adolescent body mass index and dietary patterns, *Journal of the Academy of Nutrition and Dietetics* 113 (2013): 816–822.
117. S. I. Barr, L. DiFrancesco, and V. L. Fulgone, Breakfast consumption is positively associated with nutrient adequacy in Canadian children and adolescents, *British Journal of Nutrition* 112 (2014): 1373–1383.
118. H. J. Leidy and coauthors, Beneficial effects of a higher-protein breakfast on the appetitive, hormonal, and neural signals controlling energy intake regulation in overweight/obese, "breakfast-skipping" late-adolescent girls, *American Journal of Clinical Nutrition* 97 (2013): 677–688; L. W. Jackson, The most important meal of the day: Why children skip breakfast and what can be done about it, *Pediatric Annals* 42 (2013): 184–187.
119. J. M. Poti, K. J. Duffey, and B. M. Popkin, The association of fast food consumption with poor dietary outcomes and obesity among children: Is it the fast food or the remainder of the diet? *American Journal of Clinical Nutrition* 99 (2014): 162–171.
120. E. W. Evans and coauthors, The role of eating frequency on total energy intake and diet quality in a low-income, racially diverse sample of schoolchildren, *Public Health Nutrition* 18 (2015): 474–481; F. Bellisle, Meals and snacking, diet quality and energy balance, *Physiology and Behavior* 134 (2014): 38–43.
121. Dror and Allen, 2014.
122. S. D. Poppitt, Beverage consumption: Are alcoholic and sugary drinks tipping the balance toward overweight and obesity? *Nutrients* 7 (2015): 6700–6715; Obesity Society, Position statement: Reduced consumption of sugar-sweetened beverages can reduce total caloric intake, April, 2014, www.obesity.org/publications/position-and-policies/sugar-sweetened; Dror and Allen, 2014; E. Han and L. M. Powell, Consumption patterns of sugar-sweetened beverages in the United States, *Journal of the Academy of Nutrition and Dietetics* 113 (2013): 43–53.
123. Poti, Duffey, and Popkin, 2014.

LEARN IT Describe the lifestyle factors that can help prevent childhood obesity and the development of type 2 diabetes and heart disease.

Childhood Obesity and the Early Development of Chronic Diseases

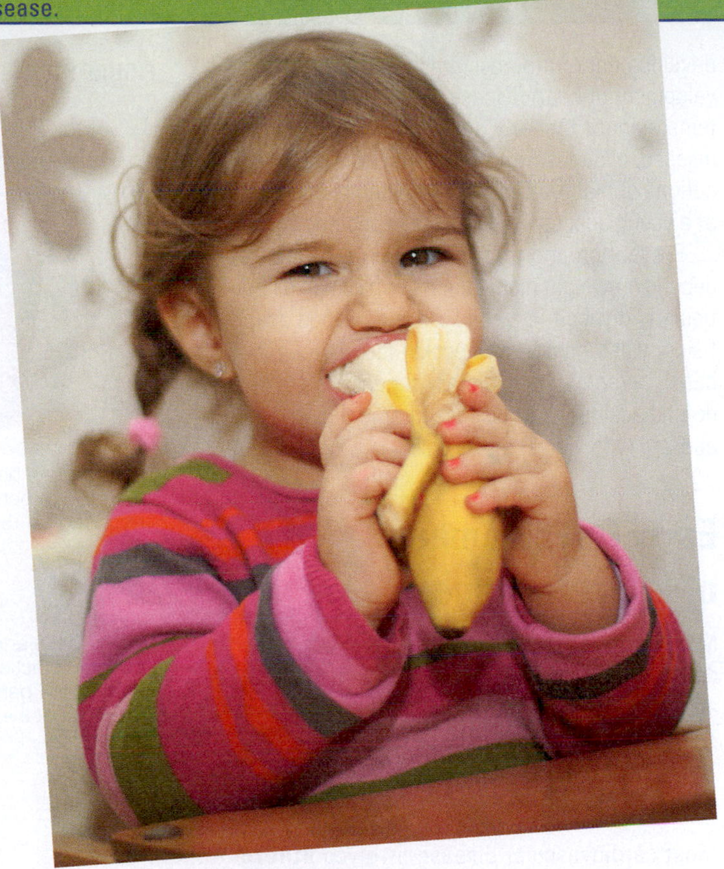
Mica81/Shutterstock.com

When people think about the health problems of children and adolescents, they typically think of ear infections, colds, and acne—not heart disease, diabetes, or hypertension. Today, however, unprecedented numbers of US children are being diagnosed with obesity and serious "adult diseases," such as **type 2 diabetes**, that accompany overweight.[1] When type 2 diabetes develops before the age of 20, the incidence of diabetic kidney disease and death in middle age increases dramatically, largely because of the long duration of the disease. For children born in the United States in the year 2000, the risk of developing type 2 diabetes sometime in their lives is estimated to be 30 percent for boys and 40 percent for girls. US children are not alone—rapidly rising rates of obesity threaten the health of an alarming number of children around the globe.[2] Without immediate intervention, millions of children are destined to develop type 2 diabetes and hypertension in childhood followed by **cardiovascular disease (CVD)** in early adulthood.[3] (See Glossary H16-1 for this and related terms.)

This highlight focuses on efforts to prevent childhood obesity and the development of heart disease and type 2 diabetes, but the benefits extend to other obesity-related diseases as well. The years of childhood (ages 2 to 18) are emphasized here because the earlier in life health-promoting habits become established, the better they will stick. Chapter 18 fills in the rest of the story of nutrition's role in reducing chronic disease risk.

Invariably, questions arise as to what extent genetics is involved in disease development. For heart disease and type 2 diabetes, genetics does not appear to play a *determining* role; that is, a person is not simply destined at birth to develop these diseases. Instead, genetics appears to play a *permissive* role—the potential is inherited and will develop if given a push by poor health choices such as excessive weight gain, poor diet, sedentary lifestyle, and cigarette smoking (review Figure H6-4, p. 194).[4]

Many experts agree that preventing or treating obesity in childhood will reduce the rate of chronic diseases in adulthood. Without intervention, most obese children become obese adolescents who become obese adults, and being obese exacerbates every chronic disease that adults face.[5] Fatty liver, a condition that correlates directly with BMI, was not even recognized in pediatric research until recently. Today, fatty liver disease has a high prevalence in obese children.[6]

Early Development of Type 2 Diabetes

In recent years, type 2 diabetes, a chronic disease closely linked with obesity, has been on the rise among children and adolescents as the prevalence of obesity in US youth has increased.[7] Obesity is the most important risk factor for type 2 diabetes; it is most likely to occur in those who are obese and sedentary and have a family history of diabetes. Diagnoses typically are made during puberty, but as younger children become more obese and less active, the trend is shifting to younger ages.

In type 2 diabetes, the cells become insulin-resistant—that is, the cells become less sensitive to insulin, reducing the amount of glucose entering the cells from the blood. The combination of obesity and insulin resistance produces a cluster of symptoms, including high blood cholesterol and high blood pressure, which, in turn, promotes the

GLOSSARY H16-1

atherosclerosis (ATH-er-oh-scler-OH-sis): a type of artery disease characterized by plaques (accumulations of lipid-containing material) on the inner walls of the arteries (see Chapter 18).
- **athero** = porridge or soft
- **scleros** = hard
- **osis** = condition

cardiovascular disease (CVD): diseases of the heart and blood vessels throughout the body. Atherosclerosis is the main cause of CVD. When the arteries that carry blood to the heart muscle become blocked, the heart suffers damage known as *coronary heart disease (CHD).*
- **cardio** = heart
- **vascular** = blood vessels

fatty streaks: accumulations of cholesterol and other lipids along the walls of the arteries.

plaque (PLACK): an accumulation of fatty deposits, smooth muscle cells, and fibrous connective tissue that develops in the artery walls in atherosclerosis. Plaque associated with atherosclerosis is known as *atheromatous* (ATH-er-OH-ma-tus) *plaque.*

type 2 diabetes: the more common type of diabetes in which the cells fail to respond to insulin. Type 2 diabetes usually accompanies obesity and results from insulin resistance coupled with insufficient insulin secretion.

development of atherosclerosis and the early development of heart disease.[8] Other common problems evident by early adulthood include kidney disease, blindness, and miscarriages. The complications of diabetes, especially when encountered at a young age, can shorten life expectancy.

Prevention and treatment of type 2 diabetes depend on weight management, which can be particularly difficult in a child's world of food advertising, video games, and pocket money for candy bars. The activity and dietary suggestions to help defend against heart disease later in this highlight apply to type 2 diabetes as well.

> FIGURE H16-1 The Formation of Plaques in Atherosclerosis

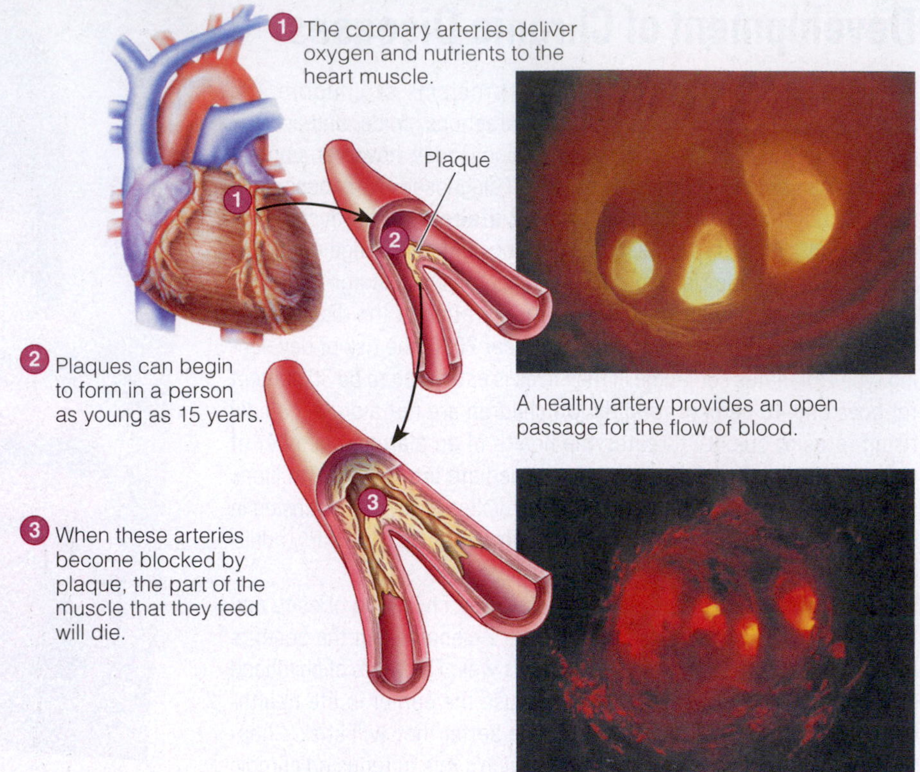
1 The coronary arteries deliver oxygen and nutrients to the heart muscle.
Plaque
2 Plaques can begin to form in a person as young as 15 years.
3 When these arteries become blocked by plaque, the part of the muscle that they feed will die.
A healthy artery provides an open passage for the flow of blood.
Plaques form along the artery's inner wall, reducing blood flow. Clots can form, aggravating the problem.
Courtesy of Zeneca Pharmaceutical Division, Cheshire, England

Early Development of Heart Disease

Most people consider heart disease to be an adult disease because its incidence rises with advancing age, and symptoms rarely appear before age 30. The disease process actually begins much earlier.

Atherosclerosis

Most cardiovascular disease involves **atherosclerosis**. Atherosclerosis develops when regions of an artery's walls become progressively thickened with **plaque**—an accumulation of fatty deposits, smooth muscle cells, and fibrous connective tissue. If it progresses, atherosclerosis may eventually block the flow of blood to the heart and cause a heart attack or cut off blood flow to the brain and cause a stroke. Infants are born with healthy, smooth, clear arteries, but within the first decade of life, **fatty streaks** may begin to appear (see Figure H16-1). During adolescence, these fatty streaks may begin to accumulate fibrous connective tissue. By early adulthood, the fibrous plaques may begin to calcify and become raised lesions, especially in boys and young men. As the lesions grow more numerous and enlarge, the heart disease rate begins to rise, most dramatically at about age 45 in men and 55 in women. From this point on, arterial damage and blockage progress rapidly, and heart attacks and strokes threaten life. In short, the consequences of atherosclerosis, which become apparent only in adulthood, have their beginnings in the first decades of life.[9]

Atherosclerosis is not inevitable; people can grow old with relatively clear arteries. Early lesions may either progress or regress, depending on several factors, many of which reflect lifestyle behaviors. Smoking, for example, is strongly associated with the prevalence of fatty streaks and raised lesions, even in young adults.

Blood Cholesterol

As blood cholesterol rises, atherosclerosis worsens. Cholesterol values at birth are similar in all populations; differences emerge in early childhood. Standard values for cholesterol in children and adolescents (ages 2 to 18 years) are listed in Table H16-1. Cholesterol concentrations change with age in children and adolescents, however, and are especially variable during puberty. Thus, use of a single cut-off point for all pediatric age groups has limitations.

In general, blood cholesterol tends to rise as dietary saturated fat intakes increase. Blood cholesterol also correlates with childhood obesity, especially abdominal obesity; LDL cholesterol rises and HDL declines. These relationships are apparent throughout childhood, and their magnitude increases with age.

Parents who develop heart disease early are likely to have children who are both overweight or obese and have high blood cholesterol. For this reason, selective screening is recommended for children and

TABLE H16-1 **Cholesterol Values for Children and Adolescents**

Disease Risk	Total Cholesterol (mg/dL)	LDL Cholesterol (mg/dL)
Acceptable	<170	<110
Borderline	170–199	110–129
High	≥200	≥130

NOTE: Adult values appear in Chapter 18.

adolescents of any age who are overweight or obese; those whose parents (or grandparents) have premature heart disease (≤55 years of age for men and ≤65 years of age for women); those whose parents have elevated blood cholesterol; those who have other risk factors for heart disease such as hypertension, cigarette smoking, or diabetes; and those whose family history is unavailable. Because blood cholesterol in children is a good predictor of adult values, some experts recommend universal screening for all children aged 9 to 11.[10] The US Preventive Services Task Force, however, concludes there is insufficient evidence of the benefits and harms of lipid screening in children and adolescents to make a recommendation.[11]

Early—but not advanced—atherosclerotic lesions are reversible, making screening and education a high priority. Both those with family histories of heart disease and those with multiple risk factors need intervention. Children with the highest risks of developing heart disease are sedentary and obese, with high blood pressure and high blood cholesterol.[12] In contrast, children with the lowest risks of heart disease are physically active and of normal weight, with low blood pressure and favorable lipid profiles. Routine pediatric care should identify these known risk factors and provide intervention when needed.

Blood Pressure

Pediatricians routinely monitor blood pressure in children and adolescents. High blood pressure may signal an underlying disease or the early onset of hypertension. Childhood hypertension, left untreated, can accelerate the development of atherosclerosis.

Like atherosclerosis and high blood cholesterol, hypertension may develop in the first decades of life, especially among obese children, and worsen with time. Children can control their hypertension by participating in regular aerobic activity and by losing weight or maintaining their weight as they grow taller. Restricting dietary sodium also causes an immediate drop in most children's and adolescents' blood pressure.[13]

Physical Activity

Research has also confirmed an association between blood lipids and physical activity in children, similar to that seen in adults. Physically active children have a better lipid profile and lower blood pressure than physically inactive children, and these positive findings often persist into adulthood.[14] Table 16-11 (p. 517) provides examples of aerobic, muscle-strengthening, and bone-strengthening physical activities for children.

Just as blood cholesterol and obesity track over the years, so does a child's level of physical activity. Those who are inactive now are likely to still be inactive years later. Similarly, those who are physically active now tend to remain so. Compared with inactive teens, those who are physically active weigh less, smoke less, eat a diet lower in saturated fats, and have better blood lipid profiles. Both obesity and blood cholesterol correlate with the inactive pastime of watching television. The message is clear: physical activity offers numerous health benefits, and children who are active today are most likely to be active for years to come.

Dietary Recommendations for Children

Regardless of family history, experts agree that all children older than age 2 should eat a variety of foods and maintain a desirable weight (see Table H16-2). For heart health, children older than 2 years of age benefit from the same dietary pattern recommended for older individuals—that is, a diet limited in saturated fat, *trans* fat, sodium, and added sugars, while rich in nutrients and age-appropriate in kcalories. Such a diet benefits blood lipids without compromising nutrient adequacy, physical growth, or neurological development.

Moderation, Not Deprivation

Healthy children older than age 2 can begin the transition to eating according to recommendations by selecting more fruits and vegetables and fewer foods high in saturated fat, sodium, and added sugars. Like saturated fat and sodium, excessive intake of added sugars may increase the risk of obesity, heart disease, and hypertension.[15] Healthy meals can occasionally include moderate amounts of a child's favorite food, such as ice cream, even if it is high in saturated fat and added sugars. A steady diet from the children's menus in some

TABLE H16-2 American Heart Association Dietary Guidelines and Strategies for Children

- Balance dietary kcalories with physical activity to maintain normal growth.
- Every day, engage in 60 minutes of moderate to vigorous play or physical activity.
- Eat a variety of vegetables and fruits daily while limiting juice intake. Serve fresh, frozen, or canned vegetables and fruits at every meal; limit those with added fats, salt, and sugar.
- Eat foods low in saturated fat, *trans* fat, sodium, and added sugars.
- Use vegetable oils (canola, soybean, olive, safflower, or other unsaturated oils) and soft margarines low in saturated fat and *trans*-fatty acids instead of butter or most other animal fats in the diet.
- Choose whole-grain breads and cereals rather than refined products; read labels and make sure that "whole grain" is the first ingredient.
- Limit or avoid the intake of sugar-sweetened beverages; encourage water.
- Consume low-fat and nonfat milk and milk products daily.
- Include two servings of fish per week, especially fatty fish such as broiled or baked salmon.
- Choose legumes and tofu in place of meat for some meals.
- Choose only lean cuts of meat and reduced-fat meat products; remove the skin from poultry.
- Serve age-appropriate portion sizes on appropriately sized plates and bowls.

NOTE: These guidelines are for children 2 years of age and older.
SOURCE: Adapted from American Heart Association, Dietary recommendations for healthy children, http://www.heart.org/HEARTORG/HealthyLiving/Dietary-Recommendations-for-Healthy-Children_UCM_303886_Article.jsp#.WMR_FBLyuF0 Expert Panel on Integrated Guidelines for Cardiovascular Health and Risk Reduction in Children and Adolescents, Summary report, *Pediatrics* 128 (2011): S213–S256.

restaurants—which feature chicken nuggets, hot dogs, french fries, and sugar-sweetened beverages—easily exceeds a prudent intake of saturated fat, *trans* fat, sodium, added sugars, and kcalories (see Photo H16-1), however, and invites both nutrient shortages and weight gains. Fortunately, most restaurant chains are changing children's menus to include steamed vegetables, fruit cups, low-fat milk, and broiled or grilled chicken—additions welcomed by busy parents who often dine out or purchase take-out foods.

Other fatty foods, such as nuts, vegetable oils, and some varieties of fish such as tuna or salmon, contribute essential fatty acids. Low-fat milk and milk products also deserve special attention in a child's diet for the needed calcium and other nutrients they supply. In addition, some research suggests that children who eat or drink fermented milk products such as yogurt may lower their risk of obesity and cardiovascular disease.[16]

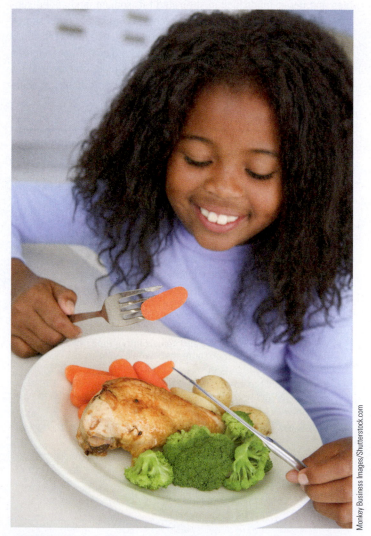

Monkey Business Images/Shutterstock.com

> **PHOTO H16-1** Adopting lifelong healthy eating patterns and regular physical activity habits at an early age help prevent chronic diseases later in life.

Parents and caregivers play a key role in helping children establish healthy eating habits. Balanced meals need to provide lean meat, poultry, fish, and legumes; fruits and vegetables; whole grains; and low-fat milk products. Such meals can provide enough energy and nutrients to support growth and maintain blood cholesterol within a healthy range.

Pediatricians warn parents to avoid extremes. Although intentions may be good, excessive food restriction may create nutrient deficiencies and impair growth. Furthermore, parental control over eating may instigate battles and foster attitudes about foods that can lead to inappropriate eating behaviors.

Diet First, Drugs Later

Experts agree that children with high blood cholesterol should first be treated with diet ary changes. If high blood cholesterol persists despite dietary intervention in children 10 years of age and older, then drugs may be necessary to lower blood cholesterol. Drugs can effectively lower blood cholesterol without interfering with adolescent growth or development.

Smoking

Even though the focus of this text is nutrition, another risk factor for heart disease that starts in childhood and carries over into adulthood must also be addressed—cigarette smoking. Each day more than 3000 young people between the ages of 12 and 18 light up for the first time, and an additional 2000 become daily cigarette smokers.[17] Among high school students, about 25 percent use some type of tobacco product (electronic cigarettes, cigars, smokeless tobacco, pipes). Approximately 90 percent of all adult smokers began smoking before the age of 18.

Of those teenagers who continue smoking, half will eventually die of smoking-related causes. Efforts to teach children about the dangers of smoking need to be aggressive. Children are not likely to consider the long-term health consequences of tobacco use. They are more likely to be struck by the immediate health consequences, such as shortness of breath when playing sports, or social consequences, such as having bad breath. Whatever the context, the message to all children and teens should be clear: don't start smoking. If you've already started, quit.

In conclusion, *adult* heart disease is a major *pediatric* problem. Without intervention, some 60 million children are destined to suffer its consequences within the next 30 years. Optimal prevention efforts focus on children, especially on those who are obese. Just as young children receive vaccinations against infectious diseases, they need screening for, and education about, chronic diseases. Many health education programs have been implemented in schools around the country. These programs are most effective when they include education in the classroom, heart-healthy meals in the lunch room, fitness activities on the playground, and parental involvement at home.[18]

CRITICAL THINKING QUESTIONS

A. How does childhood obesity influence a person's health and a country's health care system?

B. Child abuse is defined as either action or neglect that damages a child or puts the child at risk of injury. If found guilty of child abuse, parents can lose their parental rights and face criminal charges. Recently, the mother of a 14-year-old was arrested and charged with criminal neglect because her son weighed more than 500 pounds. Is severe childhood obesity a life-threatening form of abuse that justifies removing a child from his or her parents?

REFERENCES

1. C. L. Ogden and coauthors, Trends in obesity prevalence among children and adolescents in the United States, 1988-1994 through 2013-2014, *Journal of the American Medical Association* 315 (2016): 2292–2299; C. L. Ogden, M. D. Carroll, and K. M. Flegal, Prevalence of childhood and adult obesity in the United States, 2011–2012, *Journal of the American Medical Association* 311 (2014): 806–814; D. Dabelea and coauthors, Prevalence of type 1 and type 2 diabetes among children and adolescents from 2001 to 2009, *Journal of the American Medical Association* 311 (2014): 1778–1786; N. K. Güngor, Overweight and obesity in children and adolescents, *Journal of Clinical Research in Pediatric Endocrinology* 6 (2014): 129–143; Position of the Academy of Nutrition and Dietetics: The role of nutrition in health promotion and chronic disease prevention, *Journal of the Academy of Nutrition and Dietetics* 113 (2013): 972S–979S; S. Saydah and coauthors, Cardiometabolic risk factors among US adolescents and young adults and risk of early mortality, *Pediatrics* 131 (2013): e679–e686; J. P. Reiss and coauthors, Association between duration of overall and abdominal obesity beginning in young adulthood and coronary artery calcification in middle age, *Journal of the American Medical Association* 310 (2013): 280–288.
2. World Health Organization, Global strategy on diet, physical activity and health, Childhood overweight and obesity, www.who.int/dietphysicalactivity/childhood/en/, 2016; M. Ng and coauthors, Global, regional, and national prevalence of overweight and obesity in children and adults during 1980-2013: A systematic analysis for the Global Burden of Disease Study 2013, *Lancet* 384 (2014): 766–781.
3. T. Lobstein and R. Jackson-Leach, Planning for the worst: Estimates of obesity and comorbidities in school-age children in 2025, *Pediatric Obesity* 11 (2016): 321–325; G. Twig and coauthors, BMI at age 17 years and diabetes mortality in midlife: A nationwide cohort of 2.3 million adolescents, *Diabetes Care*, September 2016, http://dx.doi.org/10.2337/dc16-1203; A. C. Skinner and coauthors, Cardiometabolic risks and severity of obesity in children and young adults, *New England Journal of Medicine* 373 (2015): 1307–1317; N. Mangner and coauthors, Childhood obesity: Impact on cardiac geometry and function, *JACC Cardiovascular Imaging*, 2014, doi:10.1016/j.jcmg.2014.08.006; K. R. Armstrong and coauthors, Childhood obesity, arterial stiffness, and prevalence and treatment of hypertension, *Current Treatment Options in Cardiovascular Medicine* 16 (2014): 339; T. H. Inge and coauthors, The effect of obesity in adolescence on adult health status, *Pediatrics* 132 (2013): 1098–1104.
4. R. D. Telford and coauthors, Sensitivity of blood lipids to changes in adiposity, exercise, and diet in children, *Medicine and Science in Sports and Exercise* 47 (2015): 974–982; Skinner and coauthors, 2015; R. N. H. Touwslager and coauthors, Genetic and environmental factors in associations between infant growth and adult cardiometabolic risk profile in twins, *American Journal of Clinical Nutrition* 98 (2013): 994–1001; L. Brazionis and coauthors, Diet spanning infancy and toddlerhood is associated with child blood pressure at age 7.5 y, *American Journal of Clinical Nutrition* 97 (2013): 1375–1386.
5. W. H. Dietz, C. E. Douglas, and R. C. Brownson, Chronic Disease Prevention: Tobacco avoidance, physical activity, and nutrition for a healthy start, *Journal of the American Medical Association* 316 (2016): 1645–1646; A. Llewellyn and coauthors, Childhood obesity as a predictor of morbidity in adulthood: A systematic review and meta-analysis, *Obesity Reviews* 17 (2016): 56–67; C. Y. Lee and coauthors, Association of parental overweight and cardiometabolic diseases and pediatric adiposity and lifestyle factors with cardiovascular risk factor clustering adolescents, *Nutrients* 8 (2016): 567; Mangner and coauthors, 2014; Güngor, 2014; Reiss and coauthors, 2013.
6. M. G. Clemente and coauthors, Pediatric nonalcoholic fatty liver disease: Recent solutions, unresolved issues, and future research directions, *World Journal of Gastroenterology* 22 (2016): 8078–8093.
7. Llewellyn and coauthors, 2016; B. Tobisch, L. Blatniczky, and L. Barkai, Cardiometabolic risk factors and insulin resistance in obese children and adolescents: Relation to puberty, *Pediatric Obesity* 10 (2015): 37–44.
8. Tobisch, Blatniczky, and Barkai, 2015; N. F. Butte and coauthors, Global metabolomics profiling targeting childhood obesity in the Hispanic population, *American Journal of Clinical Nutrition* 102 (2015): 256–267.
9. T. Lobstein and R. Jackson-Leach, Planning for the worst: Estimates of obesity and comorbidities in school-age children in 2025, *Pediatric Obesity* 11 (2016): 321–325; Llewelllyn and coauthors, 2016; K. A. LaBresh and coauthors, Adoption of cardiovascular risk reduction guidelines: A cluster-randomized trial, *Pediatrics* 134 (2014): e732–e738.
10. S. S. Gidding and coauthors, American Heart Association Atherosclerosis, Hypertension, and Obesity in Young Committee of Council on Cardiovascular Disease in Young, Council on Cardiovascular and Stroke Nursing, Council on Functional Genomics and Translational Biology, and Council on Lifestyle and Cardiometabolic Health, The agenda for familial hypercholesterolemia: A Scientific Statement from the American Heart Association, *Circulation* 132 (2015): 2167–2192; Expert Panel on Integrated Guidelines for Cardiovascular Health and Risk Reduction in Children and Adolescents, Summary report, *Pediatrics* 128 (2011): S213–S256.
11. US Preventive Services Task Force, Screening for lipid disorders in children and adolescents, US Preventive Services Task Force Recommendation Statement, *Journal of the American Medical Association* 316 (2016): 625–633.
12. Telford and coauthors, 2015.
13. L. J. Appel and coauthors, Reducing sodium intake in children: A public health investment, *Journal of Clinical Hypertension* 17 (2015): 657–662.
14. B. Gopinath and coauthors, Activity behaviors in schoolchildren and subsequent 5-yr change in blood pressure, *Medicine and Science in Sports and Exercise* 46 (2014): 724–729; R. Telama and coauthors, Tracking of physical activity from early childhood through youth into adulthood, *Medicine and Science in Sports and Exercise* 46 (2014): 955–962; J. P. Chaput and coauthors, Combined associations between moderate to vigorous physical activity and sedentary behavior with cardiometabolic risk factors in children, *Applied Physiology, Nutrition, and Metabolism* 38 (2013): 477–483.
15. M. B. Vos and coauthors, Added sugars and cardiovascular disease risk in children, A Scientific Statement from the American Heart Association, *Circulation*, 2016, doi.org/10.1161/CIR.0000000000000439; K. P. Kell and coauthors, Added sugars in the diet are positively associated with diastolic blood pressure and triglycerides in children, *American Journal of Clinical Nutrition* 100 (2014): 46–52.
16. L. A. Moreno and coauthors, Dairy products, yogurt consumption, and cardiometabolic risk in children and adolescents, *Nutrition Reviews* 73 (2015): 8–14.
17. Centers for Disease Control and Prevention, Youth and tobacco use, www.cdc.gov/tobacco/data_statistics/fact_sheets/youth_data/tobacco_use/index.htm, April 14, 2016.
18. D. M. Hoelscher and coauthors, Position of the Academy of Nutrition and Dietetics: Interventions for the prevention and treatment of pediatric overweight and obesity, *Journal of the Academy of Nutrition and Dietetics* 113 (2013): 1375–1394.

17 Life Cycle Nutrition: Adulthood and the Later Years

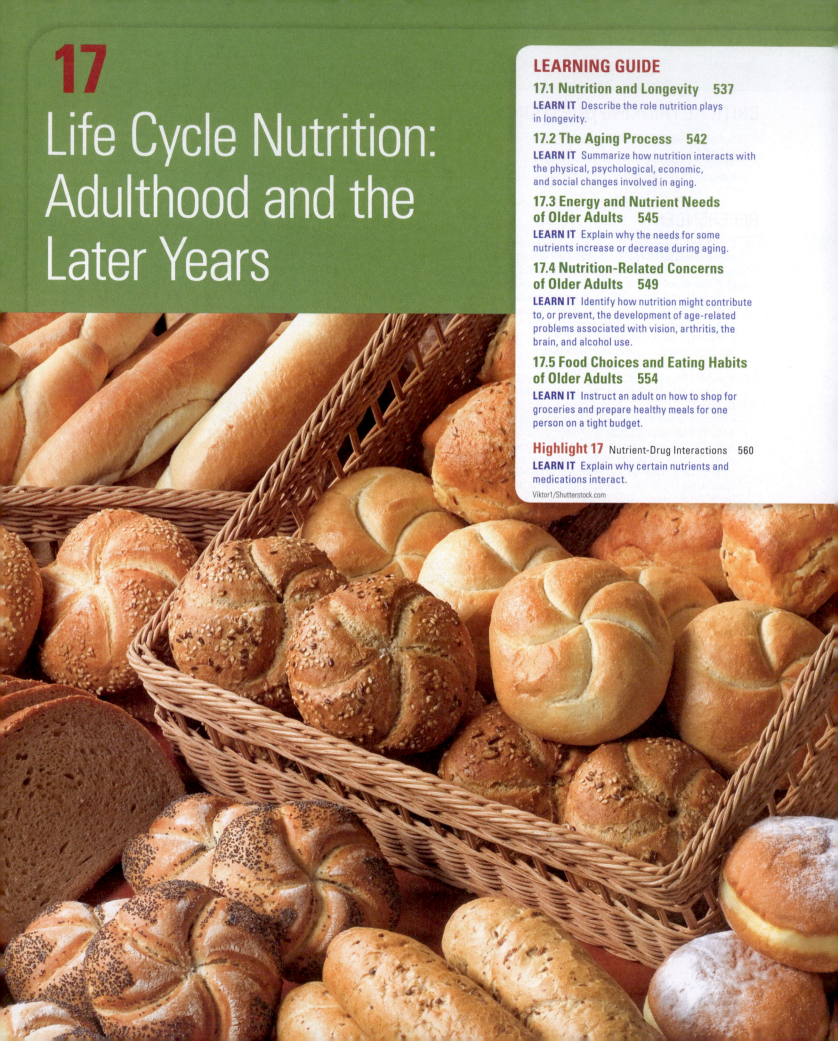

LEARNING GUIDE

Viktor1/Shutterstock.com

Nutrition in Your Life

Take a moment to envision yourself at age 60, 75, or even 90. Are you physically fit and healthy? Can you see yourself walking on the beach with friends or tossing a ball with children? Are you able to climb stairs and carry your own groceries? Importantly, are you enjoying life? If you're lucky, you will enjoy old age in good health. Making nutritious foods and physical activities a priority in your life can help bring rewards of continued health and enjoyment throughout the later years. As you this chapter, consider the nutritional health and concerns of an older adult.

Much of this text has focused on nutrition to support health, and Chapter 18 features prevention of chronic diseases such as cancer and heart disease. This chapter focuses on aging and the nutrition needs of older adults. As you will see, the same diet and behaviors that reduce disease risks also slow aging.

Our society uses the arbitrary age of 65 years to define the transition point between middle age and old age, but growing "old" happens day by day, with changes occurring gradually over time. Since 1950 the population of those older than 65 has almost tripled—and it is expected to double again by 2050.[1] Remarkably, the fastest-growing age group has been people older than 85 years; since 1950 their numbers have increased sevenfold. The number of people in the United States age 100 or older has doubled in the past decade. Similar trends are occurring in populations worldwide. Interestingly, there are places around the world where people live long and, importantly, healthy and active lives even after the age of 100 years. These places have been called *Blue Zones,* and include Sardinia, Italy; Okinawa, Japan; Loma Linda, California; Nicoya, Costa Rica; and Ikaria Island, Greece. The "secrets" of these peoples' **longevity** are presented on p. 539.

17.1 Nutrition and Longevity

LEARN IT Describe the role nutrition plays in longevity.

Figure 17-1 (p. 538) shows how the US population is growing older and the ratio of old people to young is increasing. In 1900, only 1 out of 25 people was 65 or older. In 2010, 1 out of 8 had reached age 65. Projections for 2030 are 1 out of 5. **Life expectancy** in the United States is 79 years: 81 years for white women and 78 years for black women, 77 years for white men and 73 years for black men.[2] All of these record highs are much higher than the average life expectancy of 47 years in 1900. Women who live to 85 can expect to survive an additional 7 years, on average; men, an additional 6 years. As these statistics reveal, women tend to live longer than men, not only in the United States, but in populations around the world.[3]

Advances in medical science—antibiotics and other treatments—are largely responsible for almost doubling the life expectancy in the 20th century. Improved nutrition and an abundant food supply have also contributed to lengthening life expectancy. Ironically, an abundant food supply has also jeopardized life expectancy as obesity rates increase.

The **life span** has not lengthened as dramatically; human longevity appears to have an upper limit. The maximum potential human life span is currently about 130 years. The verifiably oldest person died in 1997 at age 122. As medical technology and genetic knowledge advance, researchers may one day be able to extend the life span even further by slowing, or perhaps preventing, aging and its accompanying diseases.

longevity: long duration of life.

life expectancy: the average number of years lived by people in a given society.

life span: the maximum number of years of life attainable by a member of a species.

> FIGURE 17-1 The Aging of the US Population

In general, the percentage of older people in the population has increased over the decades whereas the percentage of younger people has decreased

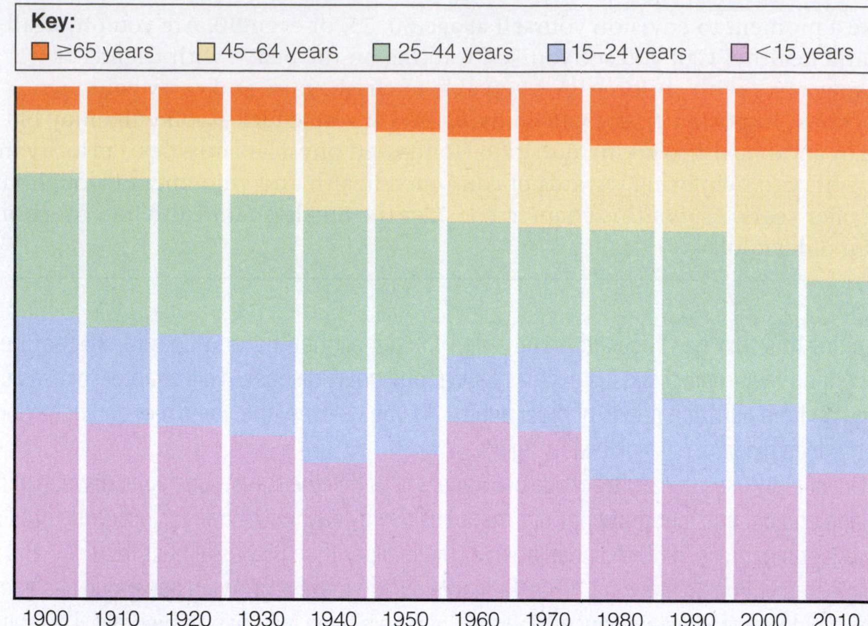

Key:
≥65 years
45–64 years
25–44 years
15–24 years
<15 years
1900
1910
1920
1930
1940
1950
1960
1970
1980
1990
2000
2010

NOTE: Data for 2010 split age groups slightly differently. Blue represents 18–24 years and purple represents <18 years.
SOURCE: US Census Bureau.

Research in the field of aging is active—and difficult. Researchers are challenged by the diversity of older adults. When older adults experience health problems, it is hard to know whether to attribute these problems to genetics, aging, or environmental factors such as nutrition. The idea that nutrition can influence the aging process is particularly appealing because people can control and change their eating habits. The questions being asked include:

- To what extent is aging inevitable, and can it be slowed through changes in lifestyle and environment?
- What role does nutrition play in the aging process, and what role can it play in slowing aging?

With respect to the first question, it seems that aging is an inevitable, natural process, programmed into the genes at conception. People can, however, slow the process within genetic limits by adopting healthy lifestyle habits such as eating nutritious foods and engaging in physical activities. In fact, a person's life expectancy depends on both individual health-related behaviors and genes.

With respect to the second question, good nutrition helps maintain a healthy body and can therefore ease the aging process in many significant ways. Clearly, nutrition can improve the **quality of life** in the later years.

Observation of Older Adults

The strategies adults use to meet two goals that motivate them to make changes—promoting health and slowing aging—are actually very much the same. What to eat, how physically active to be, and other lifestyle choices greatly influence both physical health and the aging process.

Healthy Habits

A person's **physiological age** reflects his or her health status and may or may not reflect the person's **chronological age.** Quite simply, some people seem younger, and others older, than their years. While most young adults age at a normal pace, others age more slowly or more quickly. One study reported that the physiological age of 38-year-old adults ranged from 30 to 60 years.[4] These young adults who were aging at a rapid pace were not as physically able, mentally sharp,

quality of life: a person's perceived physical and mental well-being.

physiological age: a person's age as estimated from her or his body's health and probable life expectancy.

chronological age: a person's age in years from his or her date of birth.

or youthful looking as their peers. Some behaviors seem to have the greatest influence on people's health and therefore on their physiological age:

- Following a healthy plant-based eating pattern, such as the Mediterranean diet (rich in fruits, vegetables, whole grains, poultry, fish, and low fat milk products)
- Engaging in physical activity daily
- Not smoking
- Not using alcohol, or using it in moderation
- Maintaining a healthy body weight
- Sleeping regularly and adequately
- Having a sense of purpose
- Relieving stress (through meditation, prayer, naps, or other calming activity)
- Belonging to a community of loving family and friends (home, church, or other social networks)

Over the years, the effects of these lifestyle choices accumulate—that is, people who follow most of these practices live longer and have a better quality of life as they age.[5] They are in better health, even when older in chronological age, than people who do not adopt these behaviors. Even though people cannot change their birth dates, they may be able to add years to, and enhance the quality of, their lives. Physical activity seems to be most influential in preventing or slowing the many changes that define a stereotypical "old" person; active older adults are younger physiologically than inactive ones.[6] After all, many of the physical limitations that accompany aging occur because people become inactive, not simply because they become older.

Physical Activity The many remarkable benefits of regular physical activity outlined in Chapter 14 are not limited to the young. Compared with those who are inactive, older adults who are active weigh less; have greater strength and flexibility, reduced inflammation, increased bone density, more endurance, and better balance; and they live longer.[7] Perhaps most importantly, they enjoy better overall health. They reap additional benefits from various activities as well: aerobic activities improve cardiorespiratory endurance, blood pressure, and blood lipid concentrations; moderate-endurance activities improve the quality of sleep; and strength training improves posture and mobility. In fact, regular physical activity is the most powerful predictor of a person's mobility in the later years. Mobility, in turn, is closely associated with longevity. Physical activity also increases blood flow to the brain, thereby preserving mental ability, alleviating depression, supporting independence, and improving quality of life.[8]

Muscle mass and muscle strength tend to decline with aging, making older people vulnerable to falls and immobility. Falls are a major cause of fear, injury, disability, and even death among older adults. Many lose their independence as a result of falls. Regular physical activity tones, firms, and strengthens muscles, helping to improve balance, restore confidence, reduce the risk of falling, and lessen the risk of injury should a fall occur (see Photo 17-1).[9]

Even without a fall, older adults may become so weak that they can no longer perform life's daily tasks, such as climbing stairs, carrying packages, and opening jars. Resistance training helps older adults to maintain independence by improving mobility and muscle strength to perform these tasks.[10] Even in frail, elderly people older than 85 years of age, strength training not only improves balance, muscle strength, and mobility, but it also increases energy expenditure and energy intake, thereby enhancing nutrient intakes. This finding highlights another reason to be physically active: a person who is committed to an ongoing fitness program can benefit from higher energy and nutrient intakes and still maintain a healthy body weight.

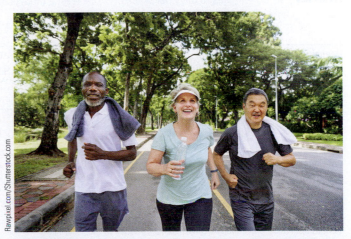
Rawpixel.com/Shutterstock.com

> **PHOTO 17-1** Regular physical activity promotes a healthy, independent lifestyle.

Ideally, physical activity should be part of each day's schedule and should be intense enough to prevent muscle atrophy and to speed the heartbeat and respiration rate. Although aging reduces both speed and endurance to some degree, older adults can still train and achieve exceptional performances. Some older adults may enjoy pumping iron and running marathons, but such activities are not essential to good health. Daily activities can be as simple as growing gardens and doing household chores.

Healthy older adults who have not been active can ease into a suitable routine, becoming as physically active as their abilities allow. They can start by walking short distances until they are walking at least 10 minutes continuously, and then gradually increase their distance to a 30- to 60-minute workout at least 5 days a week. Table 17-1 provides exercise goals and guidelines for older adults. Relatively few older adults meet these goals. People with medical conditions should check with a physician before beginning an exercise routine, as should sedentary men older than 40 and sedentary women older than 50 who want to participate in a vigorous program.

Manipulation of Diet

In their efforts to understand longevity, researchers have not only observed people, but they have also studied animals. This research has given rise to some interesting findings.

Energy Restriction in Animals Decades of research has revealed that animals live longer and have fewer age-related diseases when their energy intakes are restricted.[11] These life-prolonging benefits become evident when the diet provides enough food to prevent malnutrition and an energy intake of about 70 percent

TABLE 17-1 Exercise Guidelines for Older Adults

	Aerobic	Strength	Balance	Flexibility
Examples	Purestock/Jupiter Images	Polka Dot Images/Jupiter Images	IT Stock Free/PictureQuest/Jupiter Images	Thinkstock/Stockbyte (RF)/Jupiter Images
Start easy and progress gradually	Be active 5 minutes on most or all days	Using no weights or weights up to 2 pounds, do 1 set of 8–12 repetitions twice a week	Hold onto table or chair with one hand, then with one finger	Hold stretch for 10 seconds; do each stretch three times
Frequency	At least 5 days per week of moderate activity or at least 4 days per week of vigorous activity	At least 2 (nonconsecutive) days per week	2 to 3 days each week	At least 2 days per week; preferably on all days that aerobic or strength activities are performed
Intensity[a]	Moderate, vigorous, or combination	Moderate to high; 10 to 15 repetitions per exercise; gradually increase weights		Moderate
Duration	At least 30 minutes of moderate activity in bouts of at least 10 minutes each or at least 20 minutes of continuous vigorous activity	8 to 10 exercises involving the major muscle groups	At least 20 to 30 minutes	Stretch major muscle groups for 10–30 seconds, repeating each stretch three or four times
Cautions and comments	Stop if you are breathing so hard you can't talk or if you feel dizziness or chest pain	Breathe out as you contract and in as you relax (do not hold breath); use smooth, steady movements	Incorporate balance techniques with strength exercises as you progress	Stretch after strength and endurance exercises for 20 minutes, three times a week; use slow, steady movements; bend joints slightly

[a]On a 10-point scale, where sitting = 0 and maximum effort = 10, moderate intensity = 5 to 6 and vigorous intensity = 7 to 8.
NOTE: Activity recommendations are in addition to routine activities of daily living (such as getting dressed, cooking, grocery shopping) and moderate activities lasting less than 10 minutes.
SOURCE: Centers for Disease Control and Prevention, Division of Nutrition Physical Activity and Obesity, National Center for Chronic Disease prevention and Health Promotion, 2011, www.cdc.gov/physicalactivity/everyone/guidelines/olderadults.html; C. E. Garber and coauthors, Quantity and quality of exercise for developing and maintaining cardiorespiratory, musculoskeletal, and neuromotor fitness in apparently healthy adults: Guidance for prescribing exercise, *Medicine & Science in Sports & Exercise* 43 (2011): 1334–1359.

of normal; benefits decline as the age of starting the energy restriction is delayed. Exactly how energy restriction prolongs life remains under investigation, although gene activity appears to play a key role. The genetic activity of old mice differs from that of young mice, with some genes becoming more active with age and others less active. With an energy-restricted diet, many of the genetic activities of older mice parallel those of younger mice. These "slow-aging" genetic changes are apparent in as little as 1 month on an energy-restricted, but still nutritionally adequate, diet.

The consequences of energy restriction in animals include a delay in the onset, or prevention, of chronic diseases such as cancer and atherosclerosis and age-related conditions such as neuron degeneration. In addition, energy metabolism slows and body temperature drops—indications of a reduced rate of oxygen consumption. As Highlight 11 (p. 353) explained, the use of oxygen during energy metabolism produces free radicals, which have been implicated in the aging process. Restricting energy intake in animals not only produces fewer free radicals, but also increases antioxidant activity and enhances DNA repair. Reducing oxidative stress may at least partially explain how restricting energy intake lengthens life expectancy.

Interestingly, longevity appears to depend on restricting energy intake and not on energy balance or body composition. Genetically obese rats live longer when given a restricted diet even though their body fat is similar to that of other rats allowed to eat freely.

Energy Restriction in Human Beings Research on a variety of species—including mice, rats, monkeys, spiders, and fish—confirms the relationship between energy restriction and longevity.[12] Applying the results of animal studies to human beings is problematic, however, and conducting studies on human beings raises numerous questions—beginning with how to define *energy restriction.* Does it mean eating less or weighing less? Is it less than you want or less than the average? Does eating less have to result in weight loss? Does it matter whether weight loss results from more exercise or from less food? Or whether weight loss is intentional or unintentional? Answers await additional research.

Extreme starvation to extend life, like any extreme, is rarely, if ever, worth the price. Hunger is persistent when energy is restricted by 30 percent. Furthermore, using animal data to extrapolate to humans, researchers estimate that it would take 30 years of such energy-restricted dieting to increase life expectancy by less than 3 years.

Moderation, on the other hand, may be valuable. Many of the physiological responses to energy restriction seen in animals also occur in people whose intakes are *moderately* restricted. When people cut back on their usual energy intake by 10 to 20 percent, body weight, body fat, inflammatory proteins, growth factors, and blood pressure drop, and blood lipids and insulin response improve—favorable changes for preventing chronic diseases such as some cancers, type 2 diabetes, hypertension, and heart disease. (For perspective, a person with a usual energy intake of 2000 kcalories might cut back to 1600 to 1800 kcalories.) Some research suggests that intermittent fasting may provide similar benefits (see Chapter 7, p. 217).[13]

The reduction in oxidative damage that occurs with energy restriction in animals also occurs in people whose diets include antioxidant nutrients and phytochemicals. Diets, such as the Mediterranean diet that include an abundance of fruits, vegetables, olive oil, and moderate amounts of red wine—with their array of phytochemicals that have antioxidant activity—support good health and long life.[14] Clearly, nutritional adequacy is essential to living a long and healthy life.

REVIEW IT Describe the role nutrition plays in longevity

Life expectancy in the United States increased dramatically in the 20th century. Factors that enhance longevity include well-balanced meals, regular physical activity, abstinence from smoking, limited or no alcohol use, healthy body weight, adequate sleep, and strong social relationships. Energy restriction in animals seems to lengthen their lives. Whether such dietary intervention in human beings is beneficial remains unknown. At the very least, nutrition—especially when combined with regular physical activity—can influence aging and longevity in human beings by supporting good health and preventing disease.

17.2 The Aging Process

LEARN IT Summarize how nutrition interacts with the physical, psychological, economic, and social changes involved in aging.

As people get older, each person becomes less and less like anyone else. The older people are, the more time has elapsed for such factors as nutrition, genetics, physical activity, and everyday **stress** to influence physical and psychological aging.

Stress contributes to a variety of age-related conditions. Both physical **stressors** (such as alcohol abuse, other drug abuse, smoking, pain, and illness) and psychological stressors (such as exams, divorce, moving, and the death of a loved one) elicit the body's **stress response.** The body responds to such stressors with an elaborate series of physiological reactions, as the nervous and hormonal systems bring about defensive readiness in every body part. These effects favor physical action—the classic fight-or-flight response. Prolonged or severe stress can drain the body of its reserves and leave it weakened, aged, and vulnerable to illness, especially if physical action is not taken. As people age, they lose their ability to adapt to both external and internal disturbances. When disease strikes, the reduced ability to adapt makes the aging individual more vulnerable to death than a younger person. Strategies to preserve health forestall disease, disability, and death.

Because the stress response is mediated by hormones, it differs between men and women. The fight-or-flight response may be more typical of men than of women. Women's reactions to stress more typically follow a pattern of "tend-and-befriend." Women *tend* by nurturing and protecting themselves, their children, and other loved ones. These actions promote safety and reduce stress. Women *befriend* by creating and maintaining a social group that can help in the process.

Highlight 11 described the oxidative stresses and cellular damage that occur when free radicals exceed the body's ability to defend itself. Increased free-radical activity and decreased antioxidant protection are common features of aging—and foods rich in antioxidants may help slow the aging process and improve cognition. Such findings seem to suggest that the fountain of youth may actually be a cornucopia of fruits and vegetables rich in antioxidants. (Return to Highlight 11 for more details on the antioxidant action of fruits and vegetables in defending against oxidative stress.)

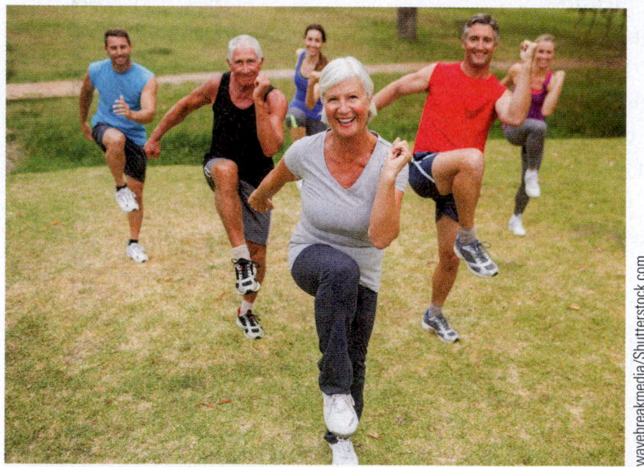
wavebreakmedia/Shutterstock.com

> **PHOTO 17-2** Growing old can be enjoyable for people who take care of their health and live each day fully.

Physiological Changes

As aging progresses, inevitable changes in each of the body's organ systems contribute to the body's declining function. These physiological changes influence nutrition status, just as growth and development do in the earlier stages of the life cycle. In general, older adults who follow healthy eating patterns have fewer physical impairments (see Photo 17-2).[15]

Body Weight An estimated 35 percent of older adults in the United States are obese. Chapter 8 presented the many health problems that accompany obesity and the BMI guidelines for a healthy body weight (18.5 to 24.9). These guidelines apply to all adults, regardless of age, but they may be inappropriate for older adults. The importance of body weight in defending against chronic diseases differs for older adults. Being *moderately overweight* may not be harmful. For adults older than 65, the lowest mortality correlates with a slightly higher BMI (23.5 to 27.5). Older adults who are *obese,* however, may still face serious medical complications, at least until age 85.

For older adults, a low body weight is more detrimental than a high one; the risk of mortality increases for older adults with a BMI below 23.[16] Low body weight often reflects malnutrition and the trauma associated with a fall. Many older adults experience unintentional weight loss, in large part because of inadequate food intake. Without adequate body fat and nutrient reserves, an underweight person's body may be unprepared to fight against diseases. For underweight people, even a

stress: any threat to a person's well-being; a demand placed on the body to adapt.

stressors: environmental elements, physical or psychological, that cause stress.

stress response: the body's response to stress, mediated by both nerves and hormones.

slight weight loss (5 percent) increases the likelihood of disease and death, making every meal a life-saving event. Drinking liquid nutritional supplements and snacking between meals can help older adults obtain needed nutrients and energy.[17]

Body Composition In general, older people tend to lose bone and muscle and gain body fat. Many of these changes occur because some hormones that regulate appetite and metabolism become less active with age, whereas others become more active.

Loss of muscle, known as **sarcopenia**, can be significant in the later years, and its consequences can be quite dramatic (see Figure 17-2). As muscles diminish and weaken, people lose the ability to move and maintain balance—making falls likely. The limitations that accompany the loss of muscle mass and strength play a key role in the diminishing health that often accompanies aging. Optimal nutrition with sufficient protein at each meal along with regular strength-building physical activity can help maintain muscle mass and strength and minimize the changes in body composition associated with aging. Supplements of omega-3 fatty acids, amino acids, and vitamin D may also stimulate muscle protein synthesis in older adults and help prevent sarcopenia.[18]

> FIGURE 17-2 Sarcopenia

These cross sections of two women's thighs may appear to be about the same size from the outside, but the 20-year-old woman's thigh (left) is dense with muscle tissue. The 64-year-old woman's thigh (right) has lost muscle and gained fat, changes that would be significantly less dramatic with good nutrition and strength-building physical activities.

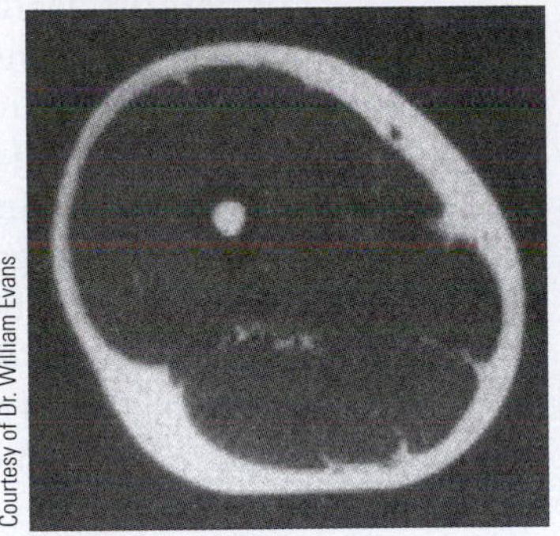

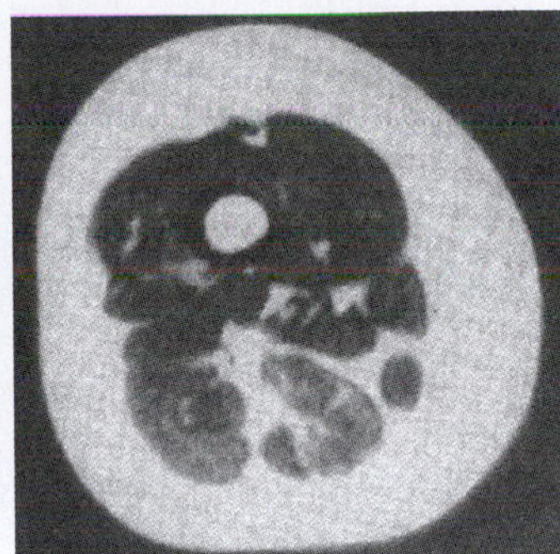

Courtesy of Dr. William Evans

Immunity and Inflammation As people age, the immune system loses function. As they become ill, the immune system becomes overstimulated. The combination of an inefficient and overactive response in aging—known as "inflammaging"—results in a chronic inflammation that accompanies frailty, illness, and death.

Most diseases common in older adults—such as atherosclerosis, Alzheimer's disease, obesity, and rheumatoid arthritis—are different in obvious ways, but they all reflect an underlying inflammatory process. Because of this association with diseases, inflammation is often perceived as a harmful process, yet it is critical in supporting health as the immune system destroys invading organisms and repairs damaged tissues. Thus, inflammation presents a challenge to identify factors that will both protect the beneficial effects and limit the harmful consequences.

In addition to aging and diseases, the immune system is compromised by nutrient deficiencies. Thus, the combination of age, illness, and poor nutrition makes older people particularly vulnerable to infectious diseases. Adding insult to injury, antibiotics often are not effective against infections in people with compromised immune systems. Consequently, infectious diseases are a major cause of death in older adults. Older adults may lower inflammation and slow aging by following an eating pattern such as the Mediterranean diet that is rich in whole grains, fish, fruits, and vegetables and low in red meats and butter.[19]

GI Tract In the GI tract, numerous changes take place, contributing to poor appetite, early satiety, and malnutrition. The intestinal wall loses strength and elasticity with age, and GI hormone secretions change. All of these actions slow GI motility. Constipation is much more common in the elderly than in the young. Changes in GI hormone secretions also diminish appetite, leading to decreased energy intake and unintentional weight loss.

Atrophic gastritis, a relatively prevalent condition that affects older adults, is characterized by an inflamed stomach, bacterial overgrowth, and a lack of hydrochloric acid and intrinsic factor. All of these factors can impair the digestion and absorption of nutrients, most notably, vitamin B_{12}, but also biotin, folate, calcium, iron, and zinc.

Difficulty swallowing, medically known as **dysphagia**, occurs in all age groups, but especially in the elderly. Being unable to swallow a mouthful of food can be scary, painful, and dangerous. Even swallowing liquids can be a problem for some people. Consequently, the person may eat less food and drink fewer beverages, resulting in weight loss, malnutrition, and dehydration.[20] Dietary intervention for

sarcopenia (SAR-koh-PEE-nee-ah): loss of skeletal muscle mass, strength, and quality.
- **sarco** = flesh
- **penia** = loss or lack

dysphagia (dis-FAY-jah): difficulty swallowing.

dysphagia is critical to survival and highly individualized based on the person's abilities and tolerances.[21] The diet typically provides moist, soft-textured, tender-cooked, or pureed foods and thickened liquids.

Tooth Loss Regular dental care over a lifetime protects against tooth loss and gum disease, which are common in old age. These conditions make chewing difficult or painful. Dentures, even when they fit properly, are less effective than natural teeth, and inefficient chewing can cause choking. Chewing crushes foods into smaller pieces in preparation for digestion. Inefficient chewing leaves larger pieces of food moving from the stomach into the small intestine, thus limiting enzyme accessibility. Simple changes in food texture might improve chewing efficiency and benefit digestion. For example, chopped beef is more rapidly digested and absorbed than beef steak, resulting in increased amino acid availability.[22]

People with tooth loss, gum disease, and ill-fitting dentures tend to limit their food selections to soft foods.* If foods such as corn on the cob and apples are replaced by creamed corn and applesauce, then nutrition status may not be greatly affected. However, when food groups are eliminated and variety is limited, poor nutrition follows. People without teeth typically eat fewer fruits and vegetables and have less variety in their diets. Consequently, they have low intakes of fiber and vitamins, which exacerbates their dental and overall health problems. The following conditions help determine whether a visit to the dentist is needed:

- Dry mouth
- Eating difficulty
- No dental care within 2 years
- Tooth or mouth pain
- Altered food selections
- Lesions, sores, or lumps in mouth

Sensory Losses and Other Physical Problems Sensory losses and other physical problems can also interfere with an older person's ability to obtain adequate nourishment. Failing eyesight, for example, can make driving to the grocery store impossible and shopping for food a frustrating experience. It may become so difficult to read food labels and count money that the person doesn't buy needed foods. Carrying bags of groceries may be an unmanageable task. Similarly, a person with limited mobility may find cooking and cleaning up too hard to do. Not too surprisingly, the prevalence of undernutrition is high among those who are home-bound.

Sensory losses can also interfere with a person's ability or willingness to eat. Taste and smell sensitivities tend to diminish with age and may make eating less enjoyable. If a person eats less, then weight loss and nutrient deficiencies may follow. Loss of vision and hearing may contribute to social isolation, and eating alone may lead to poor intake.

Other Changes

In addition to the physiological changes that accompany aging, adults change in many other ways that influence their nutrition status. Psychological, economic, and social factors play major roles in a person's ability and willingness to eat.

Psychological Changes Although not an inevitable component of aging, depression is common among older adults, especially among those in poor health and those living in long-term nursing homes. Relatively few receive adequate treatment from either antidepressant medication or mental health counseling.

Depressed people, even those without physical frailties, lose their ability to perform simple physical tasks. They frequently lose their appetite and the motivation to cook or even to eat. An overwhelming sense of grief and sadness at the death of

*The medical term for lack of teeth is *edentulous* (ee-DENT-you-lus).

a spouse, friend, or family member may leave a person, especially an elderly person, feeling powerless to overcome depression. When a person is suffering the heartache and loneliness of bereavement, cooking meals may not seem worthwhile. The support and companionship of family and friends, especially at mealtimes, can help overcome depression and enhance appetite (see Photo 17-3).

Several nutrient interventions to relieve depression have been studied, but evidence of effectiveness is inconclusive. A balanced, healthy diet may be the best nutritional approach to reducing symptoms of depression and improving quality of life.

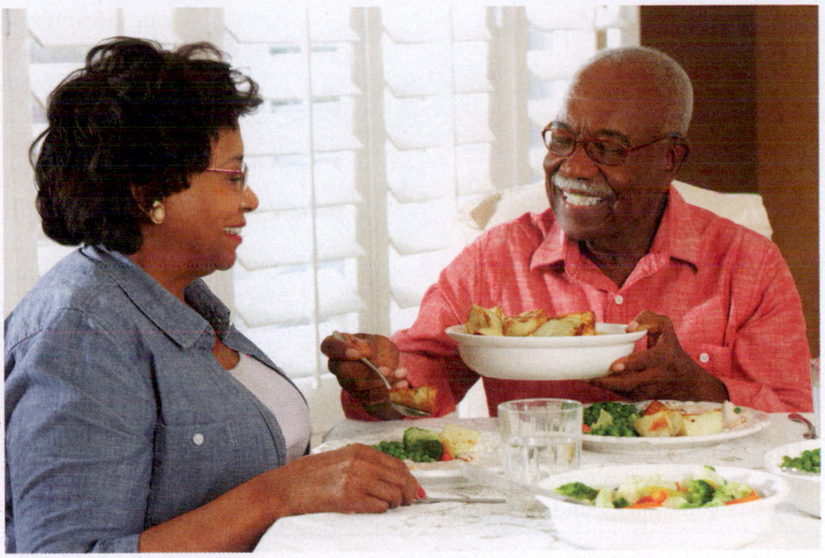

Monkey Business Images/Shutterstock.com

> **PHOTO 17-3** Shared meals can brighten the day and enhance the appetite.

Economic Changes Overall, older adults today have higher incomes than their cohorts of previous generations. Still, 9 percent of the people older than age 65 live in poverty; without the help of Social Security, it would be 40 percent.[23] Factors such as living arrangements and income make significant differences in the food choices, eating habits, and nutrition status of older adults, especially those older than age 80. People of low socioeconomic means are likely to have inadequate food and nutrient intakes. Only about one-third of eligible seniors participate in the Supplemental Nutrition Assistance Program (SNAP).

Social Changes Malnutrition is most likely to occur among those living alone, especially men; those with the least education; those living in federally funded housing (an indicator of low income); and those who have recently experienced a change in lifestyle (such as getting a divorce or becoming widowed). Adults who live alone do not necessarily make poor food choices, but they often consume too little food or not enough variety, especially of fruits and vegetables.[24] Loneliness is directly related to nutritional inadequacies, especially of energy intake. Feeling lonely is also associated with a decline in activities of daily living and mobility as well as an increased risk of death.

REVIEW IT Summarize how nutrition interacts with the physical, psychological, economic, and social changes involved in aging.

Many changes that accompany aging can impair nutrition status. Among physiological changes, hormone activity alters body composition, immune system changes raise the risk of infections, atrophic gastritis interferes with digestion and absorption, and tooth loss limits food choices. Psychological changes such as depression, economic changes such as loss of income, and social changes such as loneliness contribute to poor food intake.

17.3 Energy and Nutrient Needs of Older Adults

LEARN IT Explain why the needs for some nutrients increase or decrease during aging.

Knowledge about the nutrient needs and nutrition status of older adults has grown considerably in recent years. The Dietary Reference Intakes (DRI) cluster people older than 50 into two age categories—one group of 51 to 70 years and one of 71 and older.

Setting standards for older people is difficult because individual differences become more pronounced as people grow older. People start out with different genetic predispositions and ways of handling nutrients, and the effects of these differences become magnified with years of unique dietary habits. For example,

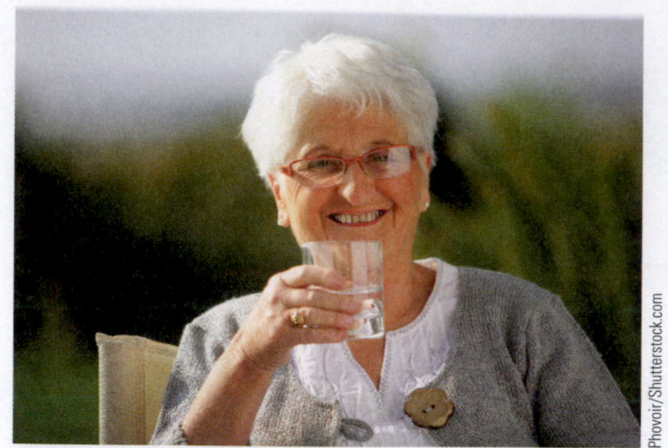
Phovoir/Shutterstock.com

> PHOTO 17-4 To ensure adequate hydration, keep a glass of water next to you at home, drink from water fountains whenever you walk by, and put a bottle of water in your car.

one person may tend to omit fruits and vegetables from his diet, and by the time he is old, he may have a set of nutrition problems associated with a lack of fiber and antioxidants. Another person may have omitted milk and milk products all her life—her nutrition problems may be related to a lack of calcium. Also, as people age, they suffer different chronic diseases and take various medicines—both of which will affect nutrient needs. For all of these reasons, researchers have difficulty even defining *healthy aging*, a prerequisite to developing recommendations to meet the "needs of practically all healthy persons." The following discussion gives special attention to the nutrients of greatest concern.

Water Despite real fluid needs, many older people do not seem to feel thirsty or notice mouth dryness. Many nursing home employees say it is hard to persuade their elderly clients to drink enough water and fruit juices. Older adults may find it difficult and bothersome to get a drink or to get to a bathroom. Those who have lost bladder control may avoid drinking too much water.

Dehydration is a common problem for many older adults.[25] Total body water decreases as people age, so even mild stresses such as fever or hot weather can precipitate rapid dehydration in older adults. Dehydrated older adults seem to be more susceptible to urinary tract infections, pneumonia, **pressure ulcers,** and confusion and disorientation. To prevent dehydration, older adults need to drink *at least* six glasses of water or other beverages every day (see Photo 17-4). Emphasizing foods with high-water content, such as melons and soups, can also be helpful.

Energy and Energy Nutrients On average, energy needs decline an estimated 5 percent per decade. One reason is that people usually reduce their physical activity as they age, although they need not do so. Another reason is that the basal metabolic rate declines 1 to 2 percent per decade in part because lean body mass and thyroid hormones diminish.

The lower energy expenditure of older adults means that they need to eat less food to maintain their weight. Accordingly, the estimated energy requirements for adults decrease steadily after age 19 (see Appendix F).

While older adults need fewer kcalories as they age, their nutrient needs remain high. For this reason, it is important that they select mostly nutrient-dense foods. There is little leeway for added sugars, solid fats, or alcohol; such nutrient-poor selections can easily lead to weight gain and malnutrition. The USDA Food Patterns (see Table 2-3, p. 41) offer a dietary framework for adults of all ages.

Protein Because energy needs decrease, protein must be obtained from low-kcalorie sources of high-quality protein, such as lean meats, poultry, fish, and eggs; fat-free and low-fat milk products; and legumes. Protein is especially important for the elderly to support a healthy immune system, prevent muscle wasting, and optimize bone mass.[26] Some research suggests that the optimal protein intake for older adults is greater than the current recommendations that apply to all adults.[27]

Carbohydrate and Fiber As always, abundant carbohydrate is needed to protect protein from being used as an energy source. Carbohydrate-rich foods such as legumes, vegetables, whole grains, and fruits are also rich in fiber and essential vitamins and minerals. High-fiber diets support good physical, mental, and social health.[28] Average fiber intakes among older adults are lower than current recommendations (14 grams per 1000 kcalories). Eating high-fiber foods and drinking water can alleviate constipation—a condition common among older adults, especially nursing home residents. (Physical inactivity and medications also contribute to the high incidence of constipation.)

pressure ulcers: damage to the skin and underlying tissues as a result of compression and poor circulation; commonly seen in people who are bedridden or chair-bound.

Fat As is true for people of all ages, polyunsaturated fats provide valuable nutrients, and saturated fats raise the risks of atherosclerosis and other degenerative diseases. Limiting fat too severely may lead to nutrient deficiencies and weight loss—two problems that carry greater health risks in the elderly than being overweight.

Vitamins and Minerals

Most people can achieve adequate vitamin and mineral intakes simply by including foods from all food groups in their diets (see Photo 17-5), but older adults often omit fruits and vegetables. Similarly, few older adults consume the recommended amounts of milk or milk products.

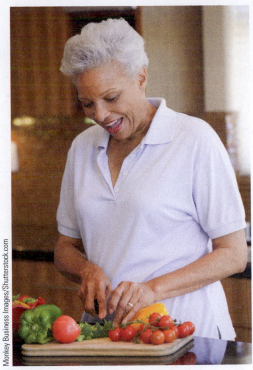

Monkey Business Images/Shutterstock.com

> **PHOTO 17-5** Taking time to nourish your body well can have long-lasting health benefits.

Vitamin B_{12} An estimated 10 to 30 percent of adults older than 50 have **atrophic gastritis;** as Chapter 10 explained, people with atrophic gastritis are particularly vulnerable to vitamin B_{12} deficiency. The bacterial overgrowth that accompanies this condition uses up the vitamin, and without hydrochloric acid and intrinsic factor, digestion and absorption of vitamin B_{12} are inefficient. Given the poor cognition, anemia, and devastating neurological effects associated with a vitamin B_{12} deficiency, an adequate intake is imperative. The RDA for older adults is the same as for younger adults, but with the added suggestion to obtain most of a day's intake from vitamin B_{12}–fortified foods and supplements. The bioavailability of vitamin B_{12} from these sources is better than from foods.

Vitamin D Vitamin D deficiency is associated with two common problems of aging—osteoporosis and dementia.[29] Getting enough vitamin D poses a problem for many older adults. Vitamin D–fortified milk is the most reliable source of vitamin D, but many older adults drink little or no milk. Further compromising the vitamin D status of many older people, especially those in nursing homes, is their limited exposure to sunlight. Finally, aging reduces the skin's capacity to make vitamin D and the kidneys' ability to convert it to its active form. Not only are older adults not getting enough vitamin D, but they may actually need more to improve both muscle and bone strength. To maintain vitamin D status, especially in those who engage in minimal outdoor activity, adults 51 to 70 years old need 15 micrograms daily, and those 71 and older need 20 micrograms. Supplements may be needed to achieve adequate levels of vitamin D.

Folate As is true of vitamin B_{12}, folate intakes of older adults typically fall short of recommendations. The elderly are also more likely to have medical conditions or to take medications that can compromise folate status (see Highlight 17, p. 560).

Calcium Chapter 12 emphasized the importance of adequate dietary calcium throughout life, especially for women after menopause, to protect against osteoporosis. The DRI Committee recommends 1200 milligrams of calcium daily for women older than 50 and men older than 70, but the calcium intakes of older people in the United States are well below recommendations. Some older adults avoid milk and milk products because they dislike these foods or associate them with stomach discomfort. Simple solutions include using calcium-fortified juices, adding powdered milk to recipes, and taking supplements. Chapter 12 offered many other strategies for including nonmilk sources of calcium for those who do not drink milk.

Iron The iron needs of men remain unchanged throughout adulthood. For women, iron needs decrease substantially at menopause when blood loss through menstruation ceases. Consequently, iron-deficiency anemia is less common in older adults than in younger people. In fact, elevated iron stores are more likely than deficiency in older people, especially for those who take iron supplements, eat red meat regularly, and include vitamin C–rich fruits in their daily diet.

Nevertheless, iron deficiency may develop in older adults, especially when their food intakes are low. Aside from an inadequate diet, two other factors may lead to iron deficiency in older people: chronic blood loss from diseases and

atrophic (a-TRO-fik) **gastritis** (gas-TRY-tis): chronic inflammation of the stomach accompanied by a diminished size and functioning of the mucous membranes and glands. This condition is also characterized by inadequate hydrochloric acid and intrinsic factor—two substances needed for vitamin B_{12} absorption.

medicines and poor iron absorption due to reduced stomach acid secretion and antacid use. Iron deficiency impairs immunity and leaves older adults vulnerable to infectious diseases. Anyone concerned with older people's nutrition should keep these possibilities in mind.

Zinc Zinc intake is commonly low in older people. Zinc deficiency can depress the appetite and blunt the sense of taste, thereby reducing food intake and worsening zinc status. Many medications that older adults commonly use can impair zinc absorption or enhance its excretion and thus lead to deficiency. Low zinc status impairs immune function and increases the risk of pneumonia and death.

Dietary Supplements

People decide for themselves how to manage their nutrition, and more than half of older adults turn to dietary supplements. When recommended by a physician or registered dietitian nutritionist, vitamin D and calcium supplements for osteoporosis or vitamin B_{12} for pernicious anemia may be beneficial. Many health-care professionals recommend a daily multivitamin-mineral supplement that provides 100 percent or less of the Daily Value for the listed nutrients. They reason that such a supplement is more likely to be beneficial than to cause harm. Supplement use may help older adults obtain enough of some nutrients, but it may also lead to excessive intakes of others.

Supplements are just that—supplements to foods, not substitutes for them. Foods are the best source of nutrients for everybody. For anyone who is motivated to obtain the best possible health, it is never too late to learn to eat well, drink water, exercise regularly, and adopt other lifestyle habits such as quitting smoking and moderating alcohol use.

REVIEW IT Explain why the needs for some nutrients increase or decrease during aging.

Table 17-2 provides a summary of the nutrient concerns of aging. Although some nutrients need special attention in the diet, supplements are not routinely recommended. The ever-growing number of older people creates an urgent need to learn more about how their nutrient requirements differ from those of others and how such knowledge can enhance their health.

TABLE 17-2 Nutrient Concerns of Aging

Nutrient	Effect of Aging	Comments
Water	Lack of thirst and decreased total body water make dehydration likely.	Mild dehydration is a common cause of confusion. Difficulty obtaining water or getting to the bathroom may compound the problem.
Energy	Need decreases as muscle mass decreases (sarcopenia).	Physical activity moderates the decline.
Fiber	Likelihood of constipation increases with low intakes and changes in the GI tract.	Inadequate water intakes and lack of physical activity, along with some medications, compound the problem.
Protein	Needs may stay the same or increase slightly.	Low-fat, high-fiber legumes and grains meet both protein and other nutrient needs.
Vitamin B_{12}	Atrophic gastritis is common.	Deficiency causes neurological damage; supplements may be needed.
Vitamin D	Increased likelihood of inadequate intake; skin synthesis declines.	Daily sunlight exposure in moderation or supplements may be beneficial.
Calcium	Intakes may be low; osteoporosis is common.	Stomach discomfort commonly limits milk intake; calcium substitutes or supplements may be needed.
Iron	In women, status improves after menopause; deficiencies are linked to chronic blood losses and low stomach acid output.	Adequate stomach acid is required for absorption; antacid or other medicine use may aggravate iron deficiency; vitamin C and meat increase absorption.
Zinc	Intakes are often inadequate and absorption may be poor, but needs may also increase.	Medications interfere with absorption; deficiency may depress appetite and sense of taste.

17.4 Nutrition-Related Concerns of Older Adults

LEARN IT Identify how nutrition might contribute to, or prevent, the development of age-related problems associated with vision, arthritis, the brain, and alcohol use.

Nutrition may play a greater role than has been realized in preventing many changes once thought to be inevitable consequences of growing older. The following discussions of vision, arthritis, the aging brain, and alcohol use show how nutrition interacts with these conditions.

Vision

One key aspect of healthy aging is maintaining good vision. Age-related eye diseases that impair vision, such as cataracts and macular degeneration, correlate with poor survival that cannot be explained by other risk factors.

Cataracts **Cataracts** are age-related cloudy areas in the lenses of the eyes that impair vision (see Figure 17-3). If not surgically removed, they ultimately lead to blindness. Cataracts may develop as a result of ultraviolet light exposure, oxidative stress, injury, viral infections, toxic substances, and genetic disorders. Most cataracts, however, are vaguely called senile cataracts—meaning "caused by aging." In the United States, half of all adults have a cataract by age 75.[30]

Oxidative stress appears to play a significant role in the development of cataracts, but supplements of the antioxidant nutrients (vitamin C, vitamin E, selenium, and carotenoids) do not seem to prevent or slow the progression.[31] By comparison, a healthy diet that includes plenty of fruits and vegetables rich in these antioxidant nutrients does seem to slow the progression or reduce the risk of developing cataracts.[32] A word of caution: vitamin C supplements in high doses (1000 milligrams) and long duration (several years) may *increase* the risk of cataracts.

One other diet-related factor may play a role in the development of cataracts—obesity. Obesity appears to be associated with cataracts, but its role has not been identified. Risk factors that typically accompany obesity, such as inactivity, diabetes, or hypertension, do not explain the association.

Macular Degeneration The leading cause of visual loss among older people is age-related **macular degeneration,** a deterioration of the macular region of the retina. As with cataracts, risk factors for age-related macular degeneration include oxidative stress from sunlight. Preventive factors may include supplements of the omega-3 fatty acids, some B vitamins (folate, vitamin B_6, and vitamin B_{12}), antioxidants (vitamin C, vitamin E, and beta-carotene), zinc, and the carotenoids lutein and zeaxanthin.[33]

cataracts (KAT-ah-rakts): clouding of the eye lenses that impairs vision and can lead to blindness.

macular (MACK-you-lar) **degeneration:** deterioration of the macular area of the eye that can lead to loss of central vision and eventual blindness. The *macula* is a small, oval, yellowish region in the center of the retina that provides the sharp, straight-ahead vision so critical to reading and driving.

> FIGURE 17-3 Healthy Lens and Cataract Lens Compared

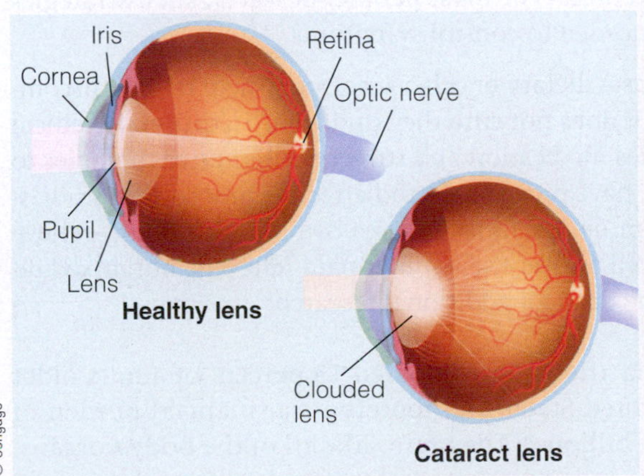
Iris
Retina
Cornea
Optic nerve
Pupil
Lens
Healthy lens
Clouded lens
Cataract lens
© Cengage

The healthy lens (on the left) focuses light, producing clear, sharp images on the retina. A lens affected by cataracts (on the right) scatters the light, resulting in blurred vision.

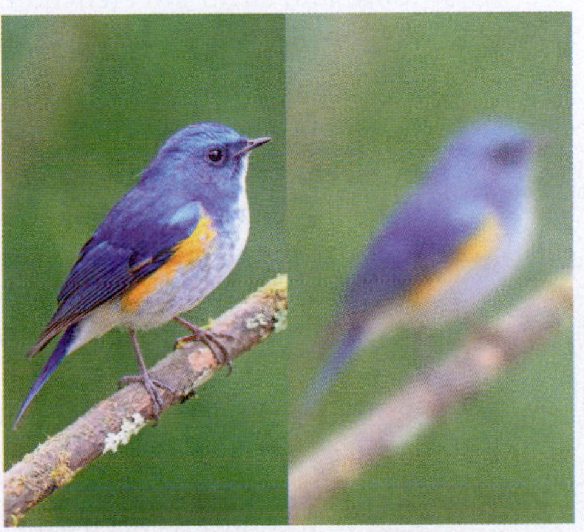
Panu Ruangjan/Shutterstock.com

Vision through a healthy lens (on the left) is crisp and clear, whereas vision through cataracts (on the right) is cloudy.

Arthritis

More than 50 million people in the United States are diagnosed with some form of **arthritis** each year.[34] As the population ages, it is expected that the prevalence will increase to 78 million by 2040. Arthritis pain and fear of further damage limit physical activity.

Osteoarthritis

The most common type of arthritis that disables older people is **osteoarthritis,** a painful deterioration of the cartilage in the joints. During movement, the ends of bones are normally protected from wear by cartilage and by small sacs of fluid that act as a lubricant. With age, cartilage begins to deteriorate, and the joints may become malformed and painful to move.

Obesity increases the risk of arthritis.[35] Weight loss may relieve some of the pain for overweight persons with osteoarthritis, partly because the joints affected are often weight-bearing joints that are stressed and irritated by having to carry excess pounds. Interestingly, though, weight loss often relieves much of the pain of arthritis in the hands as well, even though they are not weight-bearing joints. Importantly, walking and other weight-bearing exercises do not worsen arthritis. In fact, low-impact aerobic activity and resistance strength training offer improvements in physical performance and pain relief, especially when accompanied by even modest weight loss.

Rheumatoid Arthritis

Another type of arthritis known as **rheumatoid arthritis** has possible links to diet through the immune system. In rheumatoid arthritis, the immune system mistakenly destroys bone and cartilage as if they were made of foreign tissue.

The omega-3 fatty acids commonly found in fatty fish reduce joint tenderness and improve mobility in some people with rheumatoid arthritis. The same diet recommended for heart health—a Mediterranean-type diet low in saturated fat from meats and milk products and high in vegetables, olive oil, and omega-3 fats from fish—helps prevent or reduce the inflammation in the joints that makes rheumatoid arthritis so painful.

Another possible link between nutrition and rheumatoid arthritis involves the oxidative damage to the membranes within joints that causes inflammation and swelling. The antioxidant vitamins C and E and the carotenoids defend against oxidation, and increased intakes of these nutrients may help prevent or relieve the pain of rheumatoid arthritis.

Gout

Another form of arthritis, which most commonly affects men, is **gout,** a condition characterized by deposits of uric acid crystals in the joints. Uric acid derives from the breakdown of **purines,** primarily from those made by the body but also from those found in foods. Recommendations to lower uric acid levels and the risk of gout include limiting alcohol and excessive amounts of meat, seafood, and sugar-sweetened beverages. For most people, however, such strategies are insufficient, and drugs are needed to control symptoms.

Treatment

Treatment for arthritis—dietary or otherwise—may help relieve discomfort and improve mobility, but it does not cure the condition. Traditional medical intervention for arthritis includes medication and surgery. Alternative therapies to treat arthritis abound, but none have proved safe and effective in scientific studies. Popular supplements—glucosamine, chondroitin, or a combination—may relieve pain and improve mobility as well as over-the-counter pain relievers, but mixed reports from studies emphasize the need for additional research.

The Aging Brain

Dementia affects an estimated 15 percent of adults older than 70 years of age in the United States and represents a financial burden of between $157 billion and $215 billion.[36] The brain, like all of the body's organs, ages in response to both genetic and environmental factors—such as physical activities, intellectual challenges, social interactions, and nutritious diets—that enhance or diminish its amazing capacities (see Photo 17-6).[37] One of the challenges researchers face when studying the human brain is to distinguish among normal

arthritis: inflammation of a joint, usually accompanied by pain, swelling, and structural changes.

osteoarthritis: a painful, degenerative disease of the joints that occurs when the cartilage in a joint deteriorates; joint structure is damaged, with loss of function; also called *degenerative arthritis.*

rheumatoid (ROO-ma-toyd) **arthritis:** a disease of the immune system involving painful inflammation of the joints and related structures.

gout (GOWT)**:** a common form of arthritis characterized by deposits of uric acid crystals in the joints.

purines: compounds of nitrogen-containing bases such as adenine, guanine, and caffeine. Purines that originate from the body are *endogenous* and those that derive from foods are *exogenous.*

age-related physiological changes, changes caused by diseases, and changes that result from cumulative, environmental factors such as diet.

The brain normally changes in some characteristic ways as it ages. For one thing, its blood supply decreases. For another, the number of **neurons,** the brain cells that specialize in transmitting information, diminishes as people age. When the number of neurons in one part of the cerebral cortex diminishes, hearing and speech are affected. Losses of neurons in other parts of the cortex can impair memory and cognitive function. When the number of neurons in the cerebellum diminishes, balance and posture are affected. Losses of neurons in other parts of the brain affect still other functions. Some of the cognitive loss and forgetfulness generally attributed to aging may be due in part to environmental, and therefore controllable, factors—including obesity and nutrient deficiencies.

Obesity and Brain Structure Being overweight or obese may accelerate the onset and progression of brain shrinkage that naturally occurs as a person ages. Adults who are overweight or obese have significantly reduced white brain matter compared with those of normal weight. Brain scans indicate that the volume of white brain matter of overweight or obese adults is similar to those of normal weight adults who are 10 years older.[38] In other words, the brain degeneration of an overweight 50-year-old adult is comparable to that of a 60-year-old adult. Maintaining a healthy body weight and participating in regular physical activity may be the best way to slow the brain's natural aging process and degeneration.[39]

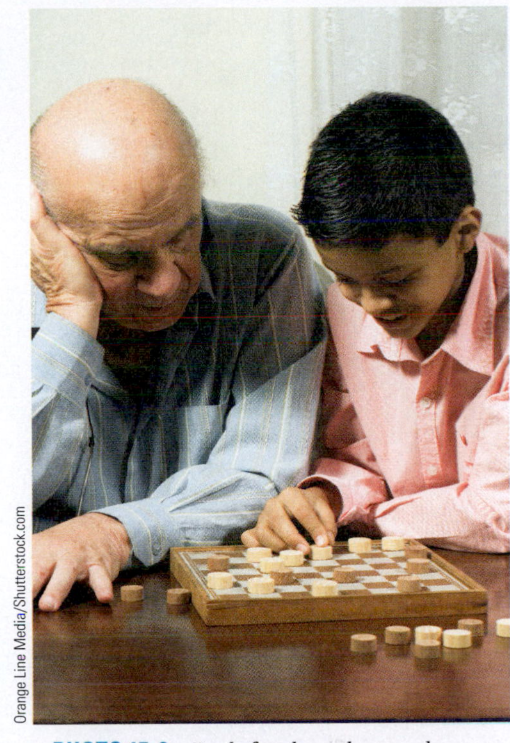

> **PHOTO 17-6** Both foods and mental challenges nourish the brain.

Orange Line Media/Shutterstock.com

Nutrient Deficiencies and Brain Function Nutrients influence the development and activities of the brain. The ability of neurons to synthesize specific neurotransmitters depends in part on the availability of precursor nutrients that are obtained from the diet. The neurotransmitter serotonin, for example, derives from the amino acid tryptophan. To function properly, the enzymes involved in neurotransmitter synthesis require vitamins such as vitamin C and pantothenic acid. The B vitamins folate, vitamin B_6, and vitamin B_{12} slow brain atrophy and improve cognition and memory; seafood and their essential fatty acid DHA counteract the cognitive decline commonly seen in elderly adults.[40] Thus the lack of key nutrients may contribute to the loss of memory and cognition that some older adults experience. Such losses may be preventable or at least diminished or delayed through diet and exercise. Healthy eating patterns, such as the Mediterranean diet, seem to slow cognitive decline and lower the risk of dementia.[41]

In some instances, the degree of cognitive loss is extensive. Some **senile dementia** may be attributable to a specific disorder such as a brain tumor or Alzheimer's disease.

Alzheimer's Disease Much attention has focused on the *abnormal* deterioration of the brain called **Alzheimer's disease,** which affects one out of eight US adults older than age 65 and almost half of adults aged 85 and older. Nerve cells in the brain die, and communication between the cells breaks down. Diagnosis of Alzheimer's disease depends on its characteristic symptoms: the victim gradually loses memory and reasoning, the ability to communicate, physical capabilities, and eventually life itself. Alzheimer's disease is the sixth leading cause of death in the United States overall, but ranks third (behind heart disease and cancer) as a cause of death for older people.[42] Table 17-3 (p. 552) compares the signs of Alzheimer's disease with typical age-related changes.

The primary risk factor for Alzheimer's disease is age, but the exact cause remains unknown. Clearly, genetic factors are involved. Free radicals and oxidative stress also seem to be involved. Nerve cells in the brains of people with Alzheimer's disease show evidence of free-radical attack—damage to DNA, cell membranes, and proteins. They also show evidence of the minerals that trigger free-radical attacks—iron, copper, zinc, and aluminum. Increasing evidence also suggests that obesity and inflammation are associated with cognitive decline and dementia in general, and with Alzheimer's disease in particular.[43]

neurons: nerve cells; the structural and functional units of the nervous system. Neurons initiate and conduct nerve impulse transmissions.

senile dementia: the loss of brain function beyond the normal loss of physical adeptness and memory that occurs with aging.

Alzheimer's (AHLZ-high-merz) **disease:** a degenerative disease of the brain involving memory loss and major structural changes in neuron networks; also known as *senile dementia of the Alzheimer's type (SDAT), primary degenerative dementia of senile onset,* or *chronic brain syndrome.*

TABLE 17-3 Signs of Alzheimer's and Typical Age-Related Changes Compared

Signs of Alzheimer's	Typical Age-Related Changes
Memory loss that disrupts daily life such as asking for the same information repeatedly or asking others to handle tasks of daily living	Forgetting a name or missing an appointment
Challenges in planning or solving problems such as following a recipe or paying monthly bills	Missing a monthly payment or making an error when balancing the checkbook
Difficulty completing familiar tasks at home such as using the microwave, at work such as preparing a report, or at leisure such as playing a game	Needing help recording a television program
Confusion with time or place including current season and location	Not knowing today's date
Trouble understanding visual images and spatial relationships such as judging distances and recognizing self in a mirror	Experiencing visual changes due to cataracts
New problems with words in speaking or writing such as knowing the name of a common object	Being unable to find the right word to use
Misplacing things and losing the ability to retrace steps such as putting the milk in the closet and having no idea when or where the milk was last seen	Misplacing a pair of glasses or the car keys
Decreased or poor judgment such as giving large sums of money to strangers	Making a bad decision on occasion
Withdrawal from work projects or social activities	Feeling too tired to participate in work, family, or social activities
Changes in mood and personality such as confusion, suspicion, depression, and anxiety especially when in unfamiliar places or with unfamiliar people	Becoming irritable when routines are disrupted

SOURCE: Adapted from Alzheimer's Association, www.alz.org/alzheimers_disease_10_signs_of_alzheimers.asp.

In Alzheimer's disease, the brain develops **senile plaques** and **neurofibrillary tangles** (see Figure 17-4). Senile plaques are clumps of a protein fragment called beta-amyloid, whereas neurofibrillary tangles are snarls of the fibers that extend from the nerve cells. Biochemical markers of beta-amyloid deposits and impaired brain metabolism are apparent decades before the onset of symptoms. Oxidative stress seems to be a contributing factor, but antioxidant supplements do not seem to be effective in preventing the progression of the disease. The accumulation of beta-amyloid seems to be a problem of impaired clearance more than excessive production. Much treatment research focuses on lowering beta-amyloid levels. Interestingly, the fat cell hormone leptin that decreases appetite and increases energy expenditure also promotes beta-amyloid clearance and lowers the risk of Alzheimer's disease.[44]

Late in the course of the disease there is a decline in the activity of the enzyme that assists in the production of the neurotransmitter acetylcholine from choline and acetyl CoA. Acetylcholine is essential to memory, but supplements of choline (or of lecithin, which contains choline) have no effect on memory or on the progression of the disease. Drugs that inhibit the breakdown of acetylcholine, on the other hand, have proved beneficial.

Research suggests that cardiovascular disease risk factors such as high blood pressure, diabetes, obesity, smoking, and physical inactivity may be related to the development of dementia and Alzheimer's disease. Heart healthy diets that include the omega-3 fatty acid DHA and vitamin E may benefit brain health as well, although supplements may not be beneficial in treating Alzheimer's, given that they are often initiated "too late" in the disease process.[45] Similarly, physical

senile plaques: clumps of the protein fragment beta-amyloid on the nerve cells, commonly found in the brains of people with Alzheimer's dementia.

neurofibrillary tangles: snarls of the threadlike strands that extend from the nerve cells, commonly found in the brains of people with Alzheimer's dementia.

> FIGURE 17-4 Alzheimer's and Healthy Brains Compared

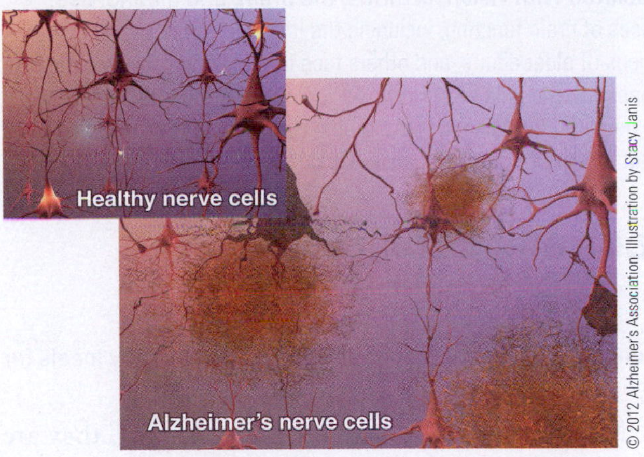

Healthy nerve cells
Alzheimer's nerve cells
© 2012 Alzheimer's Association. Illustration by Stacy Janis

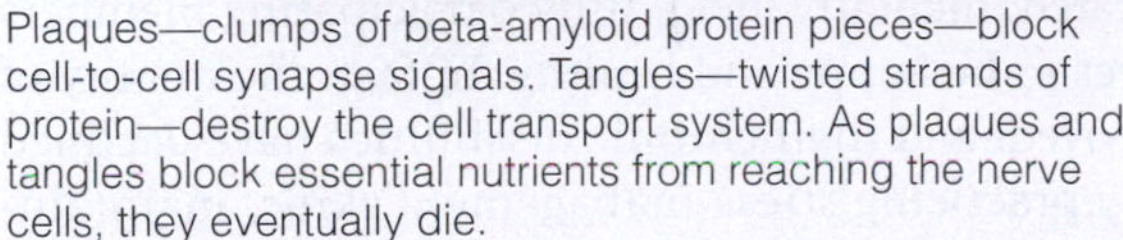

Plaques—clumps of beta-amyloid protein pieces—block cell-to-cell synapse signals. Tangles—twisted strands of protein—destroy the cell transport system. As plaques and tangles block essential nutrients from reaching the nerve cells, they eventually die.

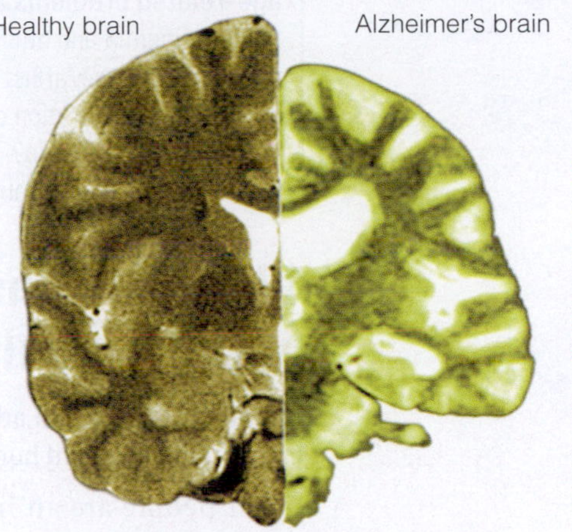

Healthy brain
Alzheimer's brain
Jessica Wilson/Medical Body Scans/Science Source

As nerve cells die, the brain shrinks and loses its ability to think, plan, remember, and form new memories. The fluid-filled spaces within the brain grow larger.

SOURCE: Alzheimer's Association, www.alz.org/research/science/alzheimers_brain_tour.asp.

activity supports heart health and slows cognitive decline. Just as saturated fatty acids contribute to heart disease, they also worsen cognition and memory and contribute to Alzheimer's disease.[46]

Treatment for Alzheimer's disease includes providing care to clients and support to their families. Drugs may be used to improve or at least to slow the loss of short-term memory and cognition, but they do not cure the disease. Other drugs may be used to control depression, anxiety, and behavior problems.

Maintaining appropriate body weight may be the most important nutrition concern for the person with Alzheimer's disease. Depression and forgetfulness can lead to changes in eating behaviors and poor food intake. Perhaps the best that a caregiver can do nutritionally for a person with Alzheimer's disease is to supervise food planning and mealtimes. Providing well-liked and well-balanced meals and snacks in a cheerful atmosphere encourages food consumption. To minimize confusion, offer a few ready-to-eat foods, in bite-size pieces, with seasonings and sauces. To avoid mealtime disruptions, control distractions such as music, television, children, and the telephone. One study reported that simply having an aquarium in the dining area increased food intake and helped maintain body weight, perhaps because it provided a naturally attractive and calming environment.[47]

Alcohol Highlight 7 (p. 219) presented information on alcohol metabolism and some of the health consequences of excessive use. Among the consequences of chronic alcohol use are impaired memory and cognition, which can complicate the diagnosis and treatment of age-related dementia.

A variety of tools can be used to diagnose alcohol abuse, but simply asking a question or two can identify hazardous drinking behaviors and potential problems in the elderly. "In the past year, how often did you drink four (for women, and five for men) or more drinks? What is the maximum number of drinks you consumed on any given day?" Such questions help identify regular heavy use of alcohol and binge drinking.

Although the age group with the most binge drinkers is adults younger than 35, the age group that binge drinks most often is adults 65 and older.[48] Excessive alcohol use among elderly adults is associated with other risk factors as well, including illicit drug use, tobacco use, and misuse of prescription medications—all factors exacerbating overall health, independence, and health-care costs.

REVIEW IT Identify how nutrition might contribute to, or prevent, the development of age-related problems associated with vision, arthritis, the brain, and alcohol use.

Senile dementia and other losses of brain function, including the impaired memory and cognition of alcohol use, afflict millions of older adults, and others face loss of vision due to cataracts or macular degeneration or cope with the pain of arthritis. As the number of people older than age 65 continues to grow, the need for solutions to these problems becomes urgent. Some problems may be inevitable, but others are preventable, and good nutrition may play a key role.

17.5 Food Choices and Eating Habits of Older Adults

LEARN IT Instruct an adult on how to shop for groceries and prepare healthy meals for one person on a tight budget.

Older people are an incredibly diverse group, and for the most part, they are independent, socially sophisticated, mentally lucid, fully participating members of society who report themselves to be happy and healthy. In fact, the quality of life among the elderly has improved, and their chronic disabilities have declined dramatically in recent years. By practicing stress-management skills, maintaining physical fitness, participating in activities of interest, and cultivating spiritual health, as well as obtaining adequate nourishment, people can support a high quality of life into old age (see Table 17-4 for some strategies).

Compared with other age groups, older people spend more money per person on foods to eat at home and less money on foods away from home. Manufacturers would be wise to cater to the preferences of older adults by providing good-tasting, nutritious foods in easy-to-open, single-serving packages with labels that are easy to read. Such services enable older adults to maintain their independence and to feel a sense of control and involvement in their own lives. Another way older adults can take care of themselves is by remaining or becoming physically active. As mentioned earlier, physical activity helps preserve one's ability to perform daily tasks and so promotes independence.

Familiarity, taste, and health beliefs are most influential on older people's food choices. Eating foods that are familiar, especially ethnic foods that recall family meals and pleasant times, can be comforting. Older adults are less likely to diet to lose weight than younger people are, but they are more likely to diet in pursuit of medical goals such as controlling blood glucose and cholesterol.

TABLE 17-4 Strategies for Growing Old Healthfully

- Choose nutrient-dense foods.
- Be physically active. Walk, run, dance, swim, bike, or row for aerobic activity. Lift weights, do calisthenics, or pursue some other activity to tone, firm, and strengthen muscles. Practice balancing on one foot or doing simple movements with your eyes closed. Modify activities to suit changing abilities and preferences.
- Maintain appropriate body weight.
- Reduce stress—cultivate self-esteem, maintain a positive attitude, manage time wisely, know your limits, practice assertiveness, release tension, and take action.
- For women, discuss with a physician the risks and benefits of estrogen replacement therapy.
- For people who smoke, discuss with a physician strategies and programs to help you quit.
- Expect to enjoy sex, and learn new ways of enhancing it.
- Use alcohol only moderately, if at all; use drugs only as prescribed.
- Take care to prevent accidents.
- Expect good vision and hearing throughout life; obtain glasses and hearing aids if necessary.
- Take care of your teeth; obtain dentures if necessary.
- Be alert to confusion as a disease symptom, and seek diagnosis.
- Take medications as prescribed; see a physician before self-prescribing medicines or herbal remedies and a registered dietitian nutritionist before self-prescribing supplements.
- Control depression through activities and friendships; seek professional help if necessary.
- Drink six to eight glasses of water every day.
- Practice mental skills. Keep on solving math problems and crossword puzzles, playing cards or other games, reading, writing, imagining, and creating.
- Make financial plans early to ensure security.
- Accept change. Work at recovering from losses; make new friends.
- Cultivate spiritual health. Cherish personal values. Make life meaningful.
- Go outside for sunshine and fresh air as often as possible.
- Be socially active—play bridge, join an exercise or dance group, take a class, teach a class, eat with friends, volunteer time to help others.
- Stay interested in life—pursue a hobby, spend time with grandchildren, take a trip, read, grow a garden, or go to the movies.
- Enjoy life.

TABLE 17-5 Risk Factors for Malnutrition in Older Adults

These questions help *determine* the risk of malnutrition in older adults.

Disease	Do you have an illness or condition that changes the types or amounts of foods you eat?
Eating poorly	Do you eat fewer than two meals a day? Do you eat fruits, vegetables, and milk products daily?
Tooth loss or mouth pain	Is it difficult or painful to eat?
Economic hardship	Do you have enough money to buy the food you need?
Reduced social contact	Do you eat alone most of the time?
Multiple medications	Do you take three or more different prescribed or over-the-counter medications daily?
Involuntary weight loss or gain	Have you lost or gained 10 pounds or more in the last 6 months?
Needs assistance	Are you physically able to shop, cook, and feed yourself?
Elderly person	Are you older than 80?

Malnutrition As mentioned, most older adults are adequately nourished, but the risk of malnutrition increases with age as chronic illnesses, medications, depression, and social isolation become factors.[49] Malnutrition limits a person's ability to function and diminishes quality of life by:

- Impairing muscle function
- Decreasing bone mass
- Limiting immune defenses
- Reducing cognitive abilities
- Delaying wound healing
- Slowing recovery from falls, illness, and surgery
- Increasing hospitalizations

Healthy snacks or liquid nutrition supplements between meals enhance energy and nutrient intakes, which improves body weight and body composition as well as physical and cognitive functioning.

The Nutrition Screening Initiative is part of a national effort to identify and treat nutrition problems in older adults; it uses a screening checklist to *determine* the risk of malnutrition (see Table 17-5). Providing access to safe, adequate food and nutrition programs and services can help ensure healthful aging.

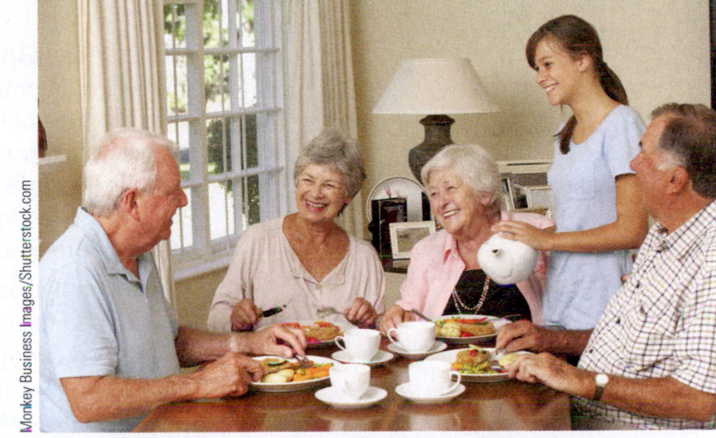

> **PHOTO 17-7** Social interactions at an assisted living facility or a congregate meal site for seniors can be as nourishing as the foods served.

Food Assistance Programs An integral component of the Older Americans Act (OAA) is the OAA Nutrition Program. Its services are designed to improve older people's nutrition status and enable them to avoid medical problems, continue living in communities of their own choice, and stay out of institutions. Its specific goals are to provide low-cost, nutritious meals; opportunities for social interaction; homemaker education and shopping assistance; counseling and referral to social services; and transportation. The program's mission has always been to provide "more than a meal."

The OAA Nutrition Program provides for **congregate meals** at group settings such as community centers. Administrators try to select sites for congregate meals where as many eligible people as possible can participate (see Photo 17-7). Volunteers may also deliver meals to those who are home-bound either permanently or temporarily; these home-delivered meals are known as **Meals on Wheels.** Home-delivered meals help older adults live independently in the community.[50] Although the home-delivery program ensures nutrition, its recipients miss out on the social benefits of the congregate meals. Therefore, every effort is made to persuade older

congregate meals: nutrition programs that provide food for the elderly in conveniently located settings such as community centers.

Meals on Wheels: a nutrition program that delivers food for the elderly to their homes.

people to come to the shared meals, if they can. All persons aged 60 years and older and their spouses are eligible to receive meals from these programs, regardless of their income. Priority is given to those who are economically and socially needy. An estimated 3 million of our nation's older adults benefit from these meals.

These programs provide at least one meal a day that meets one-third of the RDA for this age group, and they operate five or more days a week. Many programs voluntarily offer additional services designed to appeal to older adults: provisions for special diets (to meet medical needs or religious preferences), food pantries, ethnic meals, and delivery of meals to the homeless. Adding breakfast to the service increases energy and nutrient intakes, which helps relieve hunger and depression.

Older adults can also take advantage of the Senior Farmers Market Nutrition Program, which provides low-income older adults with coupons that can be exchanged for fresh fruits, vegetables, and herbs at community-supported farmers' markets and roadside stands. This program increases fresh fruit and vegetable consumption, provides nutrition information, and even reaches the home-bound elderly, a group of people who normally do not have access to farmers' markets.

Older adults can learn about the available programs in their communities by contacting the Eldercare section of the Department of Health and Human Services.* In addition, the local senior center and hospital can usually direct people to programs that provide nutrition and other health-related services.

In addition to programs designed specifically for older adults, the Supplemental Nutrition Assistance Program (SNAP) offers services to eligible people of all ages. As mentioned earlier, though, the participation rate for eligible seniors is only about 30 percent.

Meals for Singles

Many older adults live alone, and singles of all ages face challenges in purchasing, storing, and preparing food. Large packages of meat and vegetables are often intended for families of four or more, and even a head of lettuce can spoil before one person can use it all. Many singles live in small dwellings and have little storage space for foods. A limited income presents additional obstacles. This section offers suggestions that can help solve some of the problems singles face, beginning with a special note about the dangers of foodborne illnesses.

Foodborne Illnesses The risk of foodborne illness is greater for older adults than for other adults. The consequences of an upset stomach, diarrhea, fever, vomiting, abdominal cramps, and dehydration are oftentimes more severe, sometimes leading to paralysis, meningitis, or even death. For these reasons, older adults need to carefully follow the food safety suggestions presented in Chapter 19.

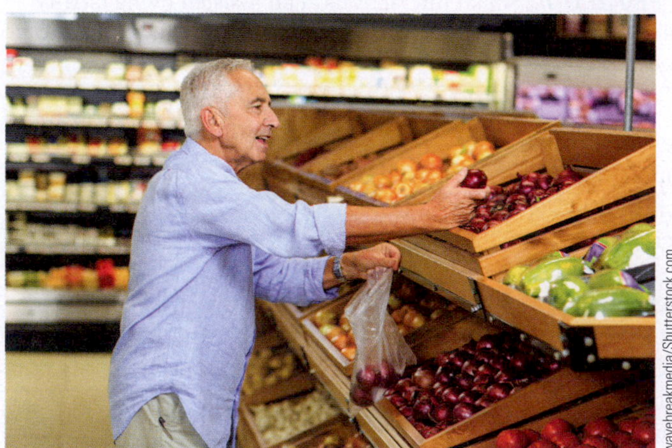
wavebreakmedia/Shutterstock.com

> **PHOTO 17-8** To save money and reduce food waste, buy only what you will use.

Spend Wisely People who have the means to shop and cook for themselves can cut their food bills simply by being wise shoppers. Large supermarkets are usually less expensive than convenience stores. Shopping when not hungry and having a grocery list helps reduce impulse buying, and specials and coupons can save money when the items featured are those that the shopper needs and uses.

Buying the right amount so as not to waste any food is a challenge for people eating alone (see Photo 17-8). They can buy fresh milk in the size best suited for personal needs. Boxes of milk that have been exposed to temperatures above those of pasteurization just long enough to sterilize the milk—a process called *ultrahigh temperature (UHT)*—are available and can be stored unopened on a shelf for several months without refrigeration.

Foods in bulk are usually less expensive than packaged items. Staples such as rice, pastas, oatmeal, dry powdered milk, and dried legumes can be purchased in bulk and stored for months at room temperature.

*Call Eldercare Locator at (800) 677-1116 or search www.eldercare.gov.

A person who has ample freezer space can buy large packages of meat or whole chickens when they are on sale. Then the meat or chicken can be portioned and immediately wrapped into individual servings for the freezer. All the individual servings can be put in a bag marked appropriately with the contents and the date.

Frozen vegetables are more economical in large bags than in small boxes. After the amount needed is taken out, the bag can be closed tightly with a twist tie or rubber band. If the package is returned quickly to the freezer each time, the vegetables will stay fresh for a long time.

Finally, breads and cereals usually must be purchased in larger quantities. Again the amount needed for a few days can be taken out and the rest stored in the freezer. Consider buying day-old bread and baked goods for added savings.

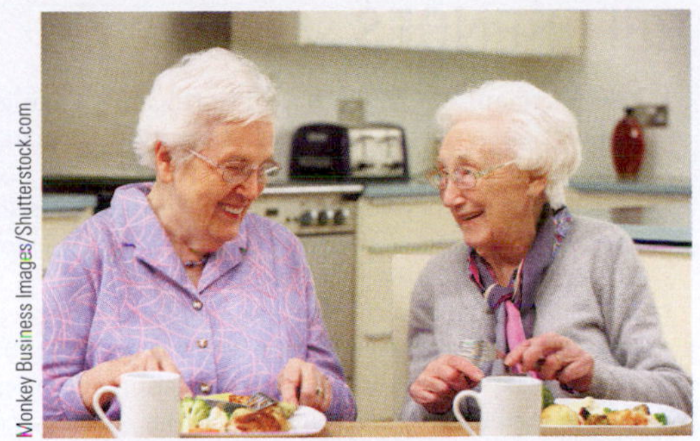
Monkey Business Images/Shutterstock.com

> **PHOTO 17-9** Invite guests to share a meal.

Grocers will break open a package of wrapped meat and rewrap the portion needed. Similarly, eggs can be purchased by the half-dozen. Eggs do keep for long periods, though, if stored properly in the refrigerator.

Fresh fruits and vegetables generally cost less when they are in season. A person can buy individual pieces of fresh fruit at various stages of ripeness: a ripe one to eat right away, a semiripe one to eat soon after, and a green one to ripen on the windowsill. If vegetables are packaged in large quantities, the grocer can divide the package so that a smaller amount can be purchased. Small cans of fruits and vegetables, even though they are more expensive per unit, are a reasonable alternative, considering that it is expensive to buy a regular-size can and let the unused portion spoil.

Be Creative Creative chefs think of various ways to use foods when only large amounts are available. For example, a head of cauliflower can be divided into thirds. Then one-third is cooked and eaten hot. Another third is put into a vinegar and oil marinade for use in a salad. And the last third can be used in a casserole or stew.

A variety of vegetables and meats can be enjoyed stir-fried; inexpensive vegetables such as cabbage, celery, and onion are delicious when sautéed in a little oil with herbs or lemon added. A variety of frozen vegetable mixtures are also available in larger grocery stores. Cooked, leftover vegetables can be dropped in at the last minute. A bonus of a stir-fried meal is that there is only one pan to wash. Similarly, a microwave oven allows a chef to use fewer pots and pans. Meals and leftovers can also be frozen or refrigerated in microwavable containers to reheat as needed.

Many frozen dinners offer nutritious options. Adding a fresh salad, a whole-wheat roll, and a glass of milk can make a nutritionally balanced meal.

Finally, single people might want to invite someone to share meals with them whenever there is enough food (see Photo 17-9). It's likely that the person will return the invitation, and both parties will get to enjoy companionship and a meal prepared by others.

REVIEW IT Instruct an adult on how to shop for groceries and prepare healthy meals for one person on a tight budget.

Older people can benefit from both the nutrients provided and the social interaction available at congregate meals. Other government programs deliver meals to those who are home-bound. With creativity and careful shopping, those living alone can prepare nutritious, inexpensive meals.

Healthy meal patterns throughout adulthood support good health and long life. Physical activity, mental challenges, stress management, and social activities can also help people grow old comfortably. The next chapter describes how similar lifestyle choices help prevent chronic diseases as well.

What's Online

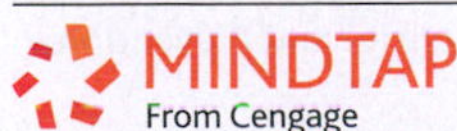
MINDTAP
From Cengage

Visit **www.cengagebrain.com** to access MindTap, a complete digital course that includes Diet & Wellness Plus, interactive quizzes, videos, and more.

REFERENCES

1. J. M. Ortman, V. A. Velkioff, and H. Hogan, An aging nation: The older population in the United States: Population estimates and projections. *Current Population Reports*, P25-1140 (2014).
2. Federal Interagency Forum on Aging Related Statistics, *2016 Older Americans: Key indicators of well-being* (Washington, DC: Government Printing Office), August 2016.
3. F. Colchero and coauthors, The emergence of longevous populations, *Proceedings of the National Academy of Sciences* 113 (2016): E7681–E7690.
4. D. W. Belsky and coauthors, Quantification of biological aging in young adults, *Proceedings of the National Academy of Sciences of the United States of America* 112 (2015): E4104–E4110.
5. A. M. May and coauthors, The impact of a healthy lifestyle in disability-adjusted life years: A prospective cohort study, *BMC Medicine* 13 (2015): 39.
6. R. D. Pollock and coauthors, An investigation into the relationship between age and physiological function in highly active older adults, *Journal of Physiology* 593 (2015): 657–680.
7. E. A. Marques and coauthors, Response of bone mineral density, inflammatory cytokines, and biochemical bone markers to a 32-week combined loading exercise programme in older men and women, *Archives of Gerontology and Geriatrics* 57 (2013): 226–233.
8. D. P. Gill and coauthors, The healthy mind, healthy mobility trial: A novel exercise program for older adults, *Medicine and Science in Sports and Exercise* 48 (2016): 297–306.
9. K. Uusi-Rasi and coauthors, Exercise and vitamin D in fall prevention among older women: A randomized clinical trial, *JAMA Internal Medicine* 175 (2015): 703–711.
10. L. Krist, F. Dimeo, and T. Keil, Can progressive resistance training twice a week improve mobility, muscle strength, and quality of life in a very elderly nursing-home residents with impaired mobility? A pilot study, *Clinical Interventions in Aging* 8 (2013): 443–448.
11. S. Brandhorst and coauthors, A periodic diet that mimics fasting promotes multi-system regeneration, enhanced cognitive performance, an healthspan, *Cell Metabolism* 22 (2015): 86–99.
12. L. Fontana and L. Partridge, Promoting health and longevity through diet: From model organisms to humans, *Cell* 161 (2015): 106–118.
13. R. V. Seimon and coauthors, Do intermittent diets provide physiological benefits over continuous diets for weight loss? A systematic review of clinical trials, *Molecular and Cellular Endocrinology* 418 (2015): 153–172.
14. C. Samieri and coauthors, The association between dietary patterns at midlife and health in aging: An observational study, *Annals of Internal Medicine* 159 (2013): 584–591.
15. K. A. Hagan, Greater adherence to the Alternative Healthy Eating Index is associated with lower incidence of physical function impairment in the Nurses' Health Study, *Journal of Nutrition* 146 (2016): 1341–1347.
16. Z. Chen and coauthors, Body mass index, waist circumference, and mortality in a large multiethnic postmenopausal cohort: Results from the Women's Health Initiative, *Journal of the American Geriatrics Society* (2017): doi: 10.1111/jgs.14790; J. E. Winter and coauthors, BMI and all-cause mortality in older adults: A meta-analysis, *American Journal of Clinical Nutrition* 99 (2014): 875–890.
17. J. Trabal and A. Farran-Codina, Effects of dietary enrichment with conventional foods on energy and protein intake in older adults: A systematic review, *Nutrition Reviews* 73 (2015): 624–633.
18. A. M. Martone and coauthors, Treating sarcopenia in older and oldest old, *Current Pharmaceutical Design* 21 (2015): 1715–1722; A. M. Verreijen and coauthors, A high whey protein-, leucine-, and vitamin D-enriched supplement preserves muscle mass during intentional weight loss in obese older adults: A double-blind randomized controlled trial, *American Journal of Clinical Nutrition* 101 (2015): 279–286; G. I. Smith and coauthors, Fish oil-derived n-3 PUFA therapy increases muscle mass and function in healthy older adults, *American Journal of Clinical Nutrition* 102 (2015): 115–122.
19. S. García-Calzón and coauthors, Dietary inflammatory index and telomere length in subjects with a high cardiovascular disease risk from the PREDIMED-NAVARRA study: Cross-sectional and longitudinal analyses over 5 y, *American Journal of Clinical Nutrition* 102 (2015):897–904; J. C. Mathers, Impact of nutrition on the ageing process, *British Journal of Nutrition* 113 (2015): S18–S22.
20. K. Takeuchi and coauthors, Nutritional status and dysphagia risk among community-dwelling frail older adults, *Journal of Nutrition, Health, and Aging* 18 (2014): 352–357.
21. M. Iwamoto and coauthors, Swallowing rehabilitation with nutrition therapy improves clinical outcome in patients with dysphagia at an acute care hospital, *Journal of Medical Investigation* 61 (2014): 353–360.
22. B. Pennings and coauthors, Minced beef is more rapidly digested and absorbed than beef steak, resulting in greater postprandial protein retention in older men, *American Journal of Clinical Nutrition* 98 (2013): 121–128.
23. K. Romig and A. Sherman, Social Security keeps 22 million Americans out of poverty: A state-by-state analysis, Center on Budget and Policy Priorities, www.cbpp.org, October 25, 2016.
24. J. L. Vinther and coauthors, Marital transitions and associated changes in fruit and vegetable intake: Findings from the population-based prospective EPIC-Norfolk cohort, UK, *Social Science and Medicine* 157 (2016): 120–126; K. L. Hanna and P. F. Collins, Relationship between living alone and food and nutrient intake, *Nutrition Reviews* 73 (2015): 594–611.
25. L. Hooper, Why, oh why, are so many older adults not drinking enough fluid? *Journal of the Academy of Nutrition and Dietetics* 116 (2016): 774–778.
26. J. I. Baum, I. Y. Kim, and R. R. Wolfe, Protein consumption and the elderly: What is the optimal level of intake? *Nutrients* 8 (2016): E359; R. R. Deer and E. Volpi, Protein intake and muscle function in older adults, *Current Opinion in Clinical Nutrition and Metabolic Care* 18 (2015): 248–253; R. R. Wolfe, Update on protein intake: Importance of milk proteins for health status of the elderly, *Nutrition Reviews* 73 (2015): 41–47.
27. J. Bauer and coauthors, Evidence-based recommendations for optimal dietary protein intake in older people: A position paper from the PROT-AGE Group, *Journal of the American Medical Directors Association* 14 (2013): 542–559.
28. B. Gopinath and coauthors, Association between carbohydrate nutrition and successful aging over 10 years, *Journal of Gerontology* 71 (2016): 1335–1340.
29. L. Shen and H. F. Ji, Vitamin D deficiency is associated with increased risk of Alzheimer's disease and dementia: Evidence from meta-analysis, *Nutrition Journal* 14 (2015): 76; T. J. Littlejohns and coauthors, Vitamin D and the risk of dementia and Alzheimer disease, *Neurology* 83 (2014): 920–928; S. M. Hudec and P. M. Camacho, Secondary causes of osteoporosis, *Endocrine Practice* 19 (2013): 120–128.
30. National Eye Institute, Cataracts, www.nei.nih.gov/eyedata/cataract, accessed February 2017.
31. W. G. Christen and coauthors, Age-related cataract in men in the Selenium and Vitamin E Cancer Prevention Trial eye endpoints study, *JAMA Ophthalmology* 133 (2015): 17–24.
32. J. Mares, Food antioxidants to prevent cataract, *Journal of the American Medical Association* 313 (2015): 1048–1049; K. A. Weikel and coauthors, Nutritional modulation of cataract, *Nutrition Reviews* 72 (2014): 30–47; Y. Cui, C. Jing, and H. Pan, Association of blood antioxidants and vitamin with risk of age-related cataract: A meta-analysis of observational studies, *American Journal of Clinical Nutrition* 98 (2013): 778–786.
33. B. Gopinath and coauthors, Homocysteine, folate, vitamin B-12, and 10-y incidence of age-related macular degeneration, *American Journal of Clinical Nutrition* 98 (2013): 129–135; The Age-Related Eye Disease Study 2 (AREDS2) Research Group, Lutein 1 zeaxanthin and omega-3 fatty acids for Age-Related Eye Disease Study 2 (AREDS2) randomized clinical trial, *Journal of the American Medical Association* 309 (2013): 2005–2015.
34. Arthritis-related statistics, Centers for Disease Control and Prevention, www.cdc.gov/arthritis, November 9, 2016.
35. C. Reyes and coauthors, Association between overweight and obesity and risk of clinically diagnosed knee, hip, and hand osteoarthritis: A

population-based cohort study, *Arthritis and Rheumatology* 68 (2016): 1869–1875; G. Musumeci and coauthors, Osteoarthritis in the XXIst century: Risk factors and behaviours that influence disease onset and progression, *International Journal of Molecular Sciences* 16 (2015): 6093–6112.

36. M. D. Hurd and coauthors, Monetary costs of dementia in the United States, *New England Journal of Medicine* 368 (2013): 1326–1334.
37. D. G. Blazer, K. Yaffe, and J. Karlawish, Cognitive aging: A report from the Institute of Medicine, *Journal of the American Medical Association* 313 (2015): 2121–2122; M. P. Mattson, Lifelong brain health is a lifelong challenge: From evolutionary principles to empirical evidence, *Ageing Research Reviews* 20C (2015): 37-45.
38. L. Ronan and coauthors, Obesity associated with increased brain-age from mid-life, *Neurobiology of Aging* 47 (2016): 63–70.
39. C. P. Boyle and coauthors, Physical activity, body mass index, and brain atrophy in Alzheimer's disease, *Neurobiology of Aging* 36 (2015): S194–S202.
40. Y. Zhang and coauthors, Intakes of fish and polyunsaturated fatty acids and mild-to-severe cognitive impairment risks: A dose-response meta-analysis of 21 cohort studies, *American Journal of Clinical Nutrition* 103 (2016): 330–340; M. C. Morris and coauthors, Association of seafood consumption, brain mercury level, and *APOE ε4* status with brain neuropathology in older adults, *Journal of the American Medical Association* 315 (2016): 489–497; J. C. Agnew-Blais and coauthors, Folate, vitamin B-6, and vitamin B-12 intake and mild cognitive impairment and probable dementia in the Women's Health Initiative Memory Study, *Journal of the Academy of Nutrition and Dietetics* 115 (2015): 231–241; F. Jernerén and coauthors, Brain atrophy in cognitively impaired elderly: The importance of long-chain ω-3 fatty acids and B vitamin status in a randomized controlled trial, *American Journal of Clinical Nutrition* 102 (2015): 215–221; C. McGarel and coauthors, Emerging roles for folate and related B-vitamins in brain health across the lifecycle, *Proceedings of the Nutrition Society* 74 (2015): 46–55.
41. C. Valls-Pedret and coauthors, Mediterranean diet and age-related cognitive decline: A randomized clinical trial, *JAMA Internal Medicine* 175 (2015): 1094-1103; A. Smith and coauthors, Healthy eating and reduced risk of cognitive decline, *Neurology* 84 (2015): 2258-2265; I. Lourida and coauthors, Mediterranean diet, cognitive function, and dementia: A systematic review, *Epidemiology* 24 (2013): 479–489; M. Ozawa and coauthors, Dietary patterns and risk of dementia in an elderly Japanese population: The Hisayama Study, *American Journal of Clinical Nutrition* 97 (2013): 1076–1082.
42. National Institute on Aging, Alzheimer's disease fact sheet, www.nia.nih.gov/alzheimers, August 18, 2016.
43. M. T. Heneka and coauthors, Neuroinflammation in Alzheimer's disease, *Lancet: Neurology* 14 (2015): 388–405.
44. M. J. McGuire and M. Ishii, Leptin dysfunction and Alzheimer's disease: Evidence from cellular, animal, and human studies, *Cellular and Molecular Neurobiology* 36 (2016): 203–217; C. A. Magalhães and coauthors, Leptin in Alzheimer's disease, *International Journal of Clinical* Chemistry 450 (2015): 162–168.
45. H. N. Yassine and coauthors, Association of serum docosahexaenoic acid with cerebral amyloidosis, *JAMA Neurology* 73 (2016): 1208–1216; M. W. Dysken and coauthors, Effect of vitamin E and memantine on functional decline in Alzheimer disease, *Journal of the American Medical Association* 311 (2014): 33–44.
46. A. J. Hanson and coauthors, Effect of apolipoprotein E genotype and diet on apolipoprotein E lipidation and amyloid peptides, *JAMA Neurology* 70 (2013): 972–980.
47. N. E. Edwards and A. M. Beck, The influence of aquariums on weight in individuals with dementia, *Alzheimer Disease and Associated Disorders* 27 (2013): 379–383.
48. Centers for Disease Control and Prevention, Binge drinking, *Vital Signs* (January 2012), http://www.cdc.gov/vitalsigns/BingeDrinking/index.html
49. S. Guyonnet and Y. Rolland, Screening for malnutrition in older people, *Clinical Geriatric Medicine* 31 (2015): 429-437.
50. K. S. Thomas and V. Mor, Providing more home-delivered meals is one way to keep older adults with low care needs out of nursing homes, *Health Affairs* 32 (2013): 1796–1802.

LEARN IT Explain why certain nutrients and medications interact.

Nutrient-Drug Interactions

As people age, their likelihood of taking medicines increases. Up to 90 percent of adults aged 65 years and older take at least one prescription medicine; almost 40 percent use five or more daily.[1] They take a variety of over-the-counter medicines and dietary supplements, such as glucosamine, as well.

Most often, older adults take multiple drugs and supplements for heart disease, but also to treat arthritis, respiratory problems, and gastrointestinal disorders. They often go to different doctors for each condition and receive different prescriptions from each. Furthermore, physiologic changes associated with aging may alter drug metabolism and excretion, which may in turn, diminish drug effectiveness or create potential toxicities. For all these reasons, physicians need to "start low and go slow" when prescribing for older adults.

To avoid harmful drug interactions, consumers need to inform all of their physicians and pharmacists of all the medicines being taken. These medicines enable people of all ages to enjoy better health, but they also bring side effects and risks.

This highlight focuses on some of the nutrition-related consequences of medical drugs, both prescription drugs and over-the-counter drugs. Highlight 7 described the relationships between nutrition and alcohol, and Highlight 18 presents information on herbal supplements and other alternative therapies.

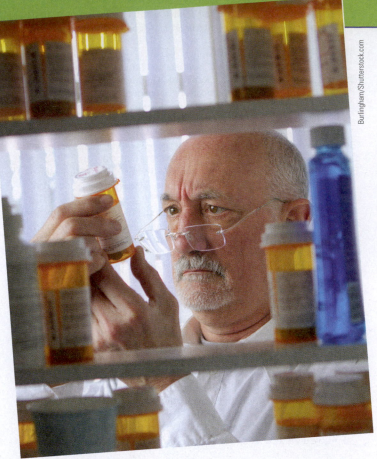

Burlingham/Shutterstock.com

The Actions of Drugs

Most people think of drugs either as medicines that help them recover from illnesses or as illegal substances that lead to bodily harm and addiction. Actually, both uses of the term *drug* are correct because any substance that modifies one or more of the body's functions is, technically, a drug. Even medical drugs have both desirable and undesirable consequences within the body.

Consider aspirin. One action of aspirin is to limit the production of certain prostaglandins (biologically active compounds derived from the omega-3 fatty acid EPA). Some prostaglandins help produce fevers, some sensitize pain receptors, some cause contractions of the uterus, some stimulate GI motility, some control nerve impulses, some regulate blood pressure, some promote blood clotting, and some cause inflammation. By interfering with prostaglandin actions, aspirin reduces fever and inflammation, relieves pain, and slows blood clotting, among other actions.

A person cannot use aspirin to produce one of its effects without producing all of its other effects. Someone who is prone to strokes and heart attacks might take aspirin to prevent blood clotting, but it will also ease that person's sense of pain. Another person who takes aspirin only for pain will also experience slow blood clotting. The anticlotting effect might be dangerous if it causes abnormal bleeding. A single two-tablet dose of aspirin doubles the bleeding time of wounds, an effect that lasts from 4 to 7 hours. For this reason, physicians instruct clients to refrain from taking aspirin before surgery.

The Interactions between Drugs and Nutrients

Hundreds of drugs and nutrients interact, and these interactions can lead to nutrient imbalances or interfere with drug effectiveness. Adverse nutrient-drug interactions are most likely if drugs are taken over long periods, if several drugs are taken, or if nutrition status is poor or deteriorating. Understandably, then, elderly people with chronic diseases are most vulnerable.

Nutrients and medications may interact in the following ways:

- Drugs can alter food intake and the absorption, metabolism, and excretion of nutrients.
- Foods and nutrients can alter the absorption, metabolism, and excretion of drugs.
- Combinations can be toxic.

The following paragraphs describe these interactions, and Table H17-1 summarizes this information and provides specific examples.[2]

Drugs Alter Food Intake

Some medications can make eating difficult or unpleasant. They may suppress appetite, alter taste sensations, induce nausea or vomiting, cause mouth dryness, or create inflammation or lesions in the mouth, stomach, or intestinal lining. Side effects, such as abdominal

TABLE H17-1 Examples of Diet-Drug Interactions

Drugs May Alter Food Intake by

- Altering the appetite (Amphetamines suppress appetite; corticosteroids increase appetite.)
- Interfering with taste or smell (Amphetamines change taste perceptions.)
- Inducing nausea or vomiting (Digitalis may do both.)
- Interfering with oral function (Some antidepressants may cause dry mouth.)
- Causing sores or inflammation in the mouth (Methotrexate may cause painful mouth ulcers.)

Drugs May Alter Nutrient Absorption by

- Changing the acidity of the digestive tract (Antacids may interfere with iron and folate absorption.)
- Damaging mucosal cells (Cancer chemotherapy may damage mucosal cells.)
- Binding to nutrients (Bile acid binders bind to fat-soluble vitamins.)

Foods and Nutrients May Alter Drug Absorption by

- Stimulating secretion of gastric acid (The antifungal agent ketoconazole is absorbed better with meals because of increased acid secretion.)
- Altering rate of gastric emptying (Intestinal absorption of drugs may be delayed when they are taken with food.)
- Binding to drugs (Calcium binds to tetracycline, reducing both drug and calcium absorption.)
- Competing for absorption sites in the small intestine (Dietary amino acids interfere with levodopa absorption.)

Drugs and Nutrients May Interact and Alter Metabolism by

- Acting as structural analogs (Warfarin and vitamin K are structural analogs.)
- Using similar enzyme systems (Phenobarbital induces liver enzymes that increase metabolism of folate, vitamin D, and vitamin K.)
- Competing for transport on serum proteins (Fatty acids and drugs may compete for the same sites on the serum protein albumin.)

Drugs May Alter Nutrient Excretion by

- Altering nutrient reabsorption in the kidneys (Some diuretics increase the excretion of sodium and potassium.)
- Causing diarrhea or vomiting (Diarrhea and vomiting may cause electrolyte losses.)

Foods May Alter Medication Excretion by

- Inducing activities of liver enzymes that metabolize drugs, increasing drug excretion (Components of charcoal-broiled meats increase metabolism of warfarin, theophylline, and acetaminophen.)

Diet and Drug Interactions May Cause Toxicity

- Increasing side effects of the drug (Caffeine in beverages can increase adverse effects of stimulants.)
- Increasing drug action to excessive levels (Grapefruit components inhibit the enzymes that degrade certain drugs, increasing drug concentrations in the body.)

discomfort, constipation, and diarrhea may worsen when food is eaten. Medications that cause drowsiness may make a person too tired to eat. All of these complications limit food intake and can lead to weight loss and malnutrition if not resolved.

Some medications stimulate appetite and cause weight gain. Unintentional weight gain may result from the use of some antipsychotics, antidepressants, and corticosteroids (for example, prednisone). People using these drugs do not feel satiated and sometimes gain 40 to 60 pounds in just a few months. For many adults, fear of weight gain is a common reason for avoiding treatment. For patients with diseases that cause wasting, such as cancer or AIDS, weight gain may be desirable. They may be prescribed appetite enhancers, such as megestrol acetate (Megace), a progesterone analog, or dronabinol (Marinol), which is derived from the active ingredient in marijuana.

Drugs Alter Nutrient Absorption

Nutrient malabsorption is most likely to occur with medications that upset GI function or damage the intestinal mucosa. Antineoplastic and antiretroviral drugs are especially detrimental, whereas nonsteroidal anti-inflammatory drugs (NSAIDs) and some antibiotics can have similar, though milder, effects.

Some medications bind to nutrients in the GI tract, preventing their absorption. For example, bile acid binders (such as cholestyramine, or Questran), which are used to reduce cholesterol levels, also bind to the fat-soluble vitamins A, D, E, and K. Some antibiotics, notably tetracycline and ciprofloxacin (Cipro), bind to the calcium in foods and supplements, reducing the absorption of both the drug and the calcium. Other minerals, such as iron, magnesium, and zinc, may also bind to antibiotics. For this reason, pharmacists advise consumers to use dairy products and all mineral supplements at least 2 hours before or after taking these medications.

Medications that reduce stomach acidity may interfere with the absorption of vitamin B_{12}, folate, and iron. Examples include antacids, which neutralize stomach acid by acting as weak bases, and antiulcer drugs (such as proton pump inhibitors and H2 blockers), which interfere with acid secretion.

Several drugs impede nutrient absorption by interfering with the intestinal metabolism or transport into mucosal cells. For example, the antibacterial drug trimethoprim and the antimalarial drug pyrimethamine compete with folate for absorption into intestinal cells. The anti-inflammatory medication colchicine, a treatment for gout, inhibits vitamin B_{12} absorption. These drug-induced interactions commonly result in megaloblastic anemia.[3]

Diets Alter Drug Absorption

Major influences on drug absorption include the stomach-emptying rate, level of acidity in the stomach, and direct interactions with dietary components. The drug's formulation may also influence its absorption, and pharmacists often provide instructions advising whether the medication should be taken with food or on an empty stomach.

Drugs reach the small intestine more quickly when the stomach is empty. Therefore, taking a medication with meals may delay its absorption, even though the total amount absorbed may not be lower. As an example, aspirin works faster when taken on an empty stomach, but taking it with food is often encouraged to reduce stomach irritation. Slow stomach emptying can sometimes enhance drug absorption because the drug's absorption sites in the small intestine are less likely to become saturated. A slow drug absorption rate due to slow stomach emptying can be a problem if high drug concentrations are needed for effectiveness, as when a hypnotic is given to induce sleep.

Some drugs are better absorbed in an acidic environment, whereas others are better absorbed in alkaline conditions. For example, reduced stomach acidity (due to disorders or antacid medications) may reduce the absorption of ketoconazole (Nizoral, an antifungal medication) and atazanavir (an antiretroviral medication), but increase the absorption of digoxin (Lanoxin, which treats heart failure) and alendronate (Fosamax, which treats osteoporosis). Some drugs can be damaged by acid and are available in coated forms that resist the action of the stomach's acidity.

Nutrients and other dietary substances may bind to drugs and inhibit their absorption. For example, high-fiber meals may decrease the absorption of some tricyclic antidepressants. Conversely, the absorption of many lipophilic drugs is improved when the drugs are taken with a fat-contaning meal. As mentioned earlier, minerals may bind to some antibiotics, reducing absorption of both the minerals and the drugs.

> **FIGURE H17-1 Folate and Methotrexate**

By competing for the enzyme that activates folate, methotrexate prevents cancer cells from obtaining the folate they need to multiply. This interference with folate metabolism creates a secondary deficiency of folate that deprives normal cells of the folate they need as well. Notice the similarities in their chemical structures.

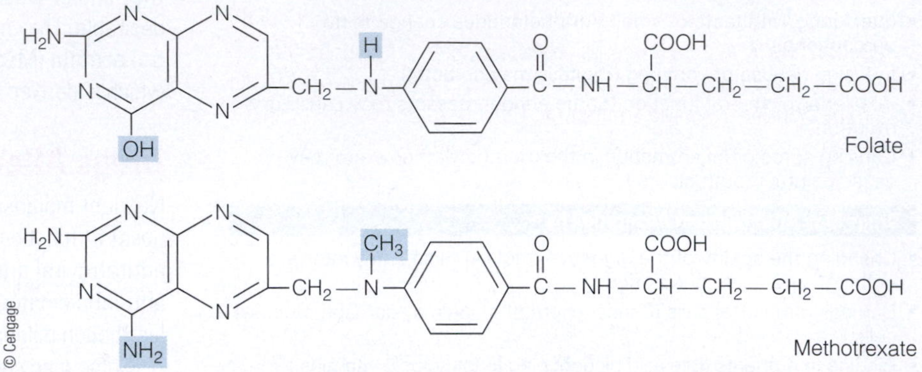

Folate

Methotrexate

TABLE H17-2 Grapefruit Juice–Drug Interactions—Selected Examples

Drug Category	Drugs Affected by Grapefruit Juice	Drugs Unaffected by Grapefruit Juice
Anticoagulants	—	Acenocoumarol Warfarin
Anti-diabetic drugs	Repaglinide Saxagliptin	Glyburide Metformin
Anti-infective drugs	Erythromycin Saquinavir	Clarithromycin Indinavir
Cardiovascular drugs	Amiodarone Felodipine Nicardipine	Amlodipine Digoxin Diltiazem
Central nervous system drugs	Buspirone Carbamazepine Diazepam	Haloperidol Lorazepam Risperidone
Cholesterol-lowering drugs	Atorvastatin Lovastatin Simvastatin	Fluvastatin Pravastatin Rosuvastatin
Immunosuppressants	Cyclosporine Tacrolimus	Prednisone

Drugs Alter Nutrient Metabolism

Drugs and nutrients share similar enzyme systems in the small intestine and the liver. Consequently, some drugs may enhance or inhibit the activities of enzymes that are needed for nutrient metabolism. For example, the anticonvulsants phenobarbital and phenytoin increase levels of the liver enzymes that metabolize folate, vitamin D, and vitamin K; therefore, persons using these drugs may require supplements of these vitamins.

The drug methotrexate, used to treat cancer and some inflammatory conditions, acts by interfering with folate metabolism and thus depriving rapidly dividing cancer cells of the folate they need to multiply. Methotrexate resembles folate in structure (see Figure H17-1) and competes with folate for the enzyme that converts folate to its active form. The adverse effects of using methotrexate therefore include symptoms of folate deficiency. These adverse effects can be reduced by using a pre-activated form of folate (called leucovorin or folinic acid), which is often prescribed along with methotrexate to ensure that the body's rapidly dividing cells (such as cells of the digestive tract, skin cells, and red blood cells) receive adequate folate.

Isoniazid, an antibacterial agent used to treat and prevent tuberculosis, inhibits the conversion of vitamin B_6 to its coenzyme form (pyridoxal phosphate), which is involved in neurotransmitter synthesis. To prevent the peripheral neuropathy that commonly develops from a vitamin B_6 deficiency, supplements of vitamin B_6 are routinely given during the course of isoniazid treatment.

Diet Alters Drug Metabolism

Some foods affect the activities of enzymes that metabolize drugs or may counteract the drugs' effects in other ways. For example, compounds in grapefruit and grapefruit juice interfere with enzymes that metabolize a number of drugs. As a result of reduced enzyme action, blood concentrations of the drugs increase, leading to stronger physiological effects. The effect of the grapefruit juice lasts for a substantial period, possibly as long as several days after the juice is consumed; thus, the interaction cannot be avoided by simply separating grapefruit juice consumption from drug usage. Table H17-2 provides examples of drugs that interact with grapefruit juice, as well as some drugs that are not affected.

A number of dietary factors affect the activity of the anticoagulant drug warfarin (Coumadin). One important interaction is with vitamin K, which is structurally similar to warfarin. Warfarin acts by blocking the enzyme that activates vitamin K, thereby preventing the synthesis of blood-clotting factors. The amount of warfarin prescribed is dependent, in part, on how much vitamin K is in the diet. If vitamin K consumption from foods or supplements changes substantially, it can alter the effect of the drug. Individuals using warfarin are advised to consume similar amounts of vitamin K daily to keep warfarin activity stable. The dietary sources highest in vitamin K are dark-green, leafy vegetables. Several popular herbs contain natural compounds that affect blood coagulation or warfarin metabolism and therefore should be avoided during warfarin treatment. These herbs include St. John's wort, garlic, ginseng, ginkgo, dong quai, and others.[4]

Drugs Alter Nutrient Excretion

Drugs that increase urine production may reduce nutrient reabsorption in the kidneys, resulting in greater urinary losses of the nutrients. For example, some diuretics accelerate the losses of calcium, potassium, magnesium, and thiamin; thus, dietary supplements may be needed to avoid deficiency. Risk of nutrient depletion is higher if multiple drugs with the same effect are used, if kidney function is impaired, or if medications are used for a long time. Note that some diuretics may cause certain minerals to be retained, rather than excreted.

Corticosteroids, which are used as anti-inflammatory agents and immunosuppressants, promote sodium and water retention and increase urinary potassium excretion.[5] Long-term use of corticosteroids can have multiple adverse effects, which include muscle wasting, bone loss, weight gain, and hyperglycemia, with eventual development of osteoporosis and diabetes.

Diets Alter Drug Excretion

Inadequate excretion of medications can cause toxicity, whereas excessive losses may reduce the amount available for therapeutic effect. Some food components influence drug excretion by altering the amount of drug reabsorbed by the kidneys. For example, the amount of lithium (a mood stabilizer) reabsorbed by the kidneys correlates with the amount of sodium reabsorbed. Consequently, both dehydration and sodium depletion, which increase sodium reabsorption, may result in lithium retention. Similarly, a person with a high sodium intake will excrete more sodium in the urine, and therefore more lithium. Individuals using lithium are advised to maintain a consistent sodium intake from day to day in order to maintain stable blood concentrations of lithium.

Urine acidity can also affect drug excretion because of the effects of pH on a compound's chemistry. The medication quinidine, used to treat arrhythmias, is excreted more readily in acidic urine. Foods or drugs that cause urine to become more alkaline may reduce quinidine excretion and raise its blood levels.

Diet-Drug Toxicities

Some interactions between foods and drugs can cause toxicity or exacerbate a drug's side effects. The combination of tyramine, a compound in some foods, and monoamine oxidase (MAO) inhibitors, which treat depression and Parkinson's disease, can be fatal. MAO inhibitors block an enzyme that normally inactivates tyramine, as well as the hormones epinephrine and norepinephrine. When people who take MAO inhibitors consume excessive tyramine, the increased tyramine in the blood can cause a sudden release of accumulated norepinephrine. This surge in norepinephrine results in severe headaches, rapid heartbeat, and a dangerous increase in blood pressure. For this reason, people taking MAO inhibitors are advised to restrict their intakes of foods rich in tyramine (see Table H17-3). Tyramine occurs naturally in foods and is also formed when bacteria degrade the protein in foods. Thus, the tyramine content of a food usually increases when a food ages or spoils. Individuals at risk of tyramine toxicity are advised to buy mainly fresh foods and consume them promptly.

TABLE H17-3 Examples of Foods with a High Tyramine Content

- Aged cheeses (cheddar, Gruyère)
- Aged or cured meats (sausage, salami)
- Beer
- Fermented vegetables (sauerkraut, kimchi)
- Fish or shrimp sauce
- Prepared soy foods (miso, tempeh, tofu)
- Soy sauce
- Yeast extract (Marmite, Vegemite)

NOTE: The tyramine content of foods depends on storage conditions and processing; thus the amounts in similar products can vary substantially.

The Inactive Ingredients in Drugs

Besides the active ingredients, medicines may contain other substances such as sugar, sorbitol, lactose, and sodium. For most people who use medicines on occasion and in small amounts, such ingredients pose no problem. When medicines are taken regularly or in large doses, however, people on special diets may need to be aware of these additional ingredients and their effects.

Sugar, Sorbitol, and Lactose

Many liquid preparations contain sugar or sorbitol to make them taste better. For people who must regulate their intakes of carbohydrates, such as people with diabetes, the amount of sugar in these medicines may need to be considered. Large doses of liquids containing sorbitol may cause diarrhea. The lactose added as filler to some medications may cause problems for people who are lactose intolerant.

Sodium

Antibiotics and antacids often contain sodium. People who take Alka Seltzer, for example, may not realize that a single two-tablet dose may exceed their recommended sodium intake for a whole day. In addition, antacids neutralize stomach acid, and many nutrients depend on acid for their digestion. Taking any antacid regularly will reduce the absorption of many nutrients.

Nutrient interactions and risks are not unique to prescription drugs. People who buy over-the-counter drugs also need to protect themselves. The increasing availability of over-the-counter drugs allows people to treat themselves for many ailments from arthritis to yeast infections. Consumers need to ask their physicians about potential interactions and check with their pharmacists for instructions on taking drugs with foods. If problems arise, they should seek professional care without delay.

CRITICAL THINKING QUESTIONS

A. What could be done to minimize the risks associated with nutrient-drug interactions?

B. Drug packaging commonly includes an oversized sheet of paper with small writing that includes a description of the many possible side effects, including possible nutrient-drug interactions. Unfortunately, few people take the time to carefully read and follow these instructions. How might you improve patient education and compliance with these instructions?

REFERENCES

1. E. D. Kantor and coauthors, Trends in prescription drug use among adults in the United States from 1999–2012, *Journal of the American Medical Association* 314 (2015): 1818–1831.
2. L. N. Chan, Drug-nutrient interactions, in A. C. Ross and coeditors, eds., *Modern Nutrition in Health and Disease* (Baltimore: Lippincott Williams & Wilkins, 2014), pp. 1440–1452.
3. C. S. Hesdorffer and D. L. Longo, Drug-induced megaloblastic anemia, *New England Journal of Medicine* 373 (2015): 1649–1658.
4. C. E. Dennehy and C. Tsourunis, Dietary supplements and herbal medications, in B. G. Katzung, ed., *Basic and Clinical Pharmacology* (New York: Lange Medical Books/McGraw-Hill, 2015).
5. G. W. Cannon, Immunosuppressing drugs including corticosteroids, in L. Goldman and A. I. Schafer, ed., *Goldman-Cecil Medicine* (Philadelphia: Saunders, 2016), pp. 162–169.

18 Diet and Health

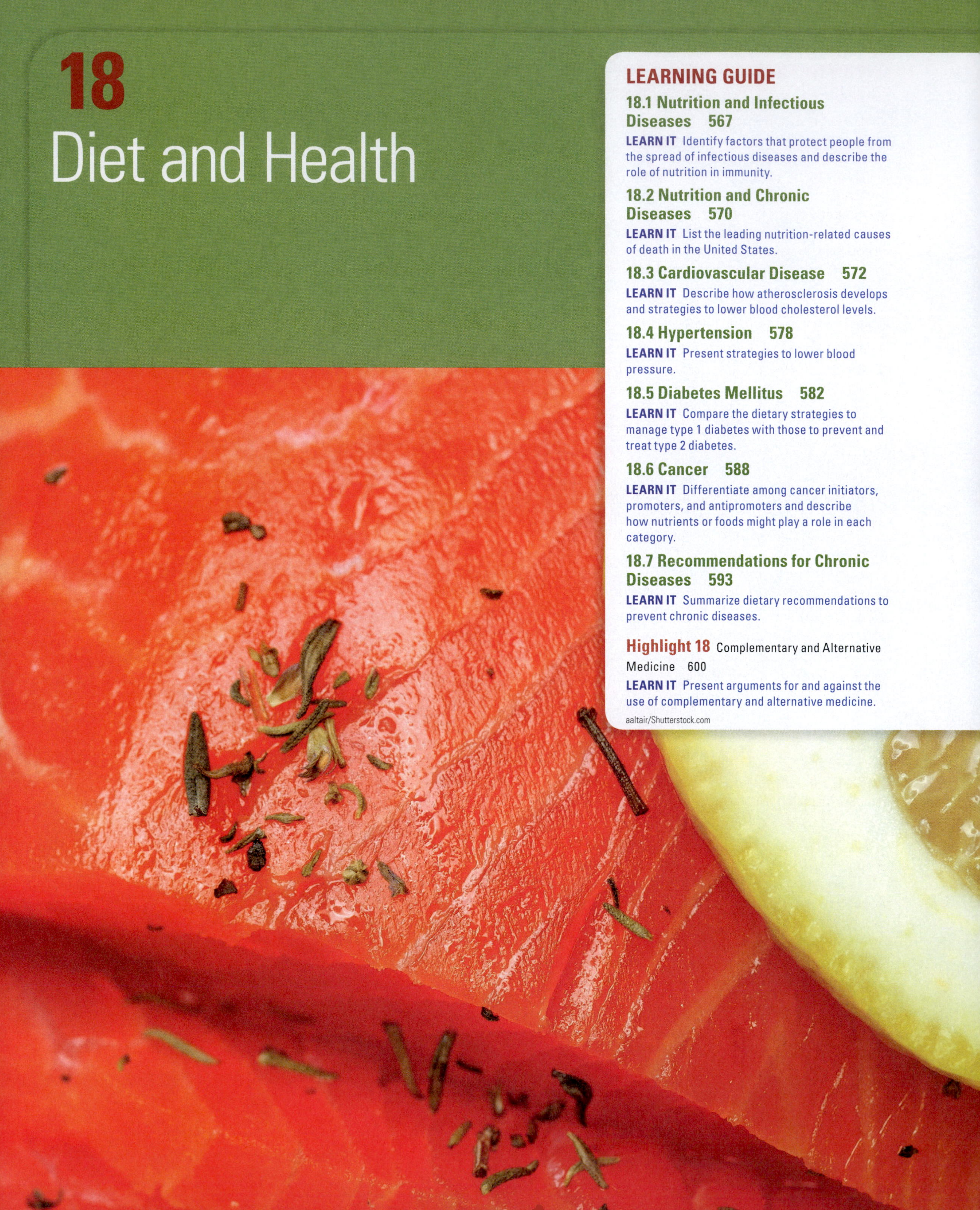

LEARNING GUIDE

aaltair/Shutterstock.com

Nutrition in Your Life

No doubt, you're familiar with the recommendations. Eat more veggies. Eat more fiber. Eat more fish. Put down the saltshaker. Limit saturated fats and added sugars. Be active. Don't smoke. And don't drink too much alcohol. What's the deal? If you follow this advice, will it really make a difference in how well or how long you live? In a word, yes. You can bet your life on it. If you could grow old in good health without having a heart attack or stroke, or getting diabetes, hypertension, or cancer, wouldn't you be willing to do just about anything—including improving your diet and activity habits? Of course, you would. And you can start today. As you read this chapter, examine your risk factors for chronic diseases and learn how to minimize those risks.

Much of this text has described how good nutrition supports good health. This chapter examines some of the relationships between nutrition and disease—exploring how poor nutrition may promote the progression of diseases and how good nutrition may guard against the development of diseases. The bulk of this chapter focuses on the chronic diseases that pose the greatest threat to the lives of most people in developed countries, but it begins with a description of the immune system and its inflammatory response. As you will see, inflammation underlies many chronic diseases. Chronic diseases develop over a lifetime as a result of metabolic abnormalities induced by such factors as genetics, age, gender, and lifestyle. As you have learned, several dietary factors influence the development of chronic diseases—most notably, high intakes of sodium, processed and red meats, and sugar-sweetened beverages and low intakes of nuts and seeds, seafood, vegetables, fruits, whole grains, and polyunsaturated fats.[1]

In their efforts to prevent and treat chronic diseases, many people in the United States turn to complementary and alternative medicine—which includes products such as herbs and practices such as acupuncture. Because complementary and alternative approaches range from useful folk medicine to dangerous frauds, consumers need to become informed about the products and practices they are considering and discuss their decisions with their health care providers. Highlight 18 explores the usefulness and safety of complementary and alternative medicine and its role in health care.

18.1 Nutrition and Infectious Diseases

LEARN IT Identify factors that protect people from the spread of infectious diseases and describe the role of nutrition in immunity.

Infectious diseases such as smallpox once claimed the lives of many children and limited the average life expectancy of adults. Thanks to medical science's ability to identify disease-causing microorganisms and develop preventive strategies, most people now live well into their later years, and the average life expectancy far exceeds that of our ancestors. In developed nations, improved diagnostic techniques, purification of water, and safe handling of foods help prevent the spread of infection. Antibiotics and immunizations provide additional protection for individuals.[2]

Despite these advances, some infectious diseases still endanger many lives today. Disease strains such as tuberculosis and some foodborne infections, for example, have become resistant to antibiotics, while other diseases such as measles and pertussis, despite vaccine availability, have resurged periodically.[3] Public health strategies help the entire country defend against the spread of infection, and each individual's immune system provides a personal line of defense. A strong immune system depends on adequate nutrition. Poor nutrition weakens the immune system, which increases susceptibility to infections.[4]

infectious diseases: diseases caused by bacteria, viruses, parasites, or other microorganisms that can be transmitted from one person to another through air, water, or food; by contact; or through vector organisms such as mosquitoes.

The Immune System The **immune system** defends the body so diligently that people do not even notice the thousands of enemy attacks mounted against them every day (Glossary 18-1 defines immune system terms). If the immune system fails, though, the body suddenly becomes vulnerable to every wayward disease-causing agent that comes its way. Infectious disease invariably follows.

The body's first lines of defense—the skin, mucous membranes, and GI tract—normally deter foreign substances. If these barriers fail, then the organs (spleen, lymph nodes, and thymus) and cells of the immune system race into action. Foreign substances that gain entry into the body and elicit such a response—the **immune response**—are called **antigens.** Examples include bacteria, viruses, toxins, and food proteins that cause allergies.

Of the 100 trillion cells that make up the human body, one in every hundred is a white blood cell. Two types of white blood cells, the phagocytes and lymphocytes, defend the body against infectious diseases.

Phagocytes: Neutrophils and Macrophages **Phagocytes,** the scavengers of the immune system, are the first to arrive at the scene if an invader, such as a microorganism, gains entry. Upon recognizing the foreign invader, the phagocyte engulfs and digests it, if possible, in a process called **phagocytosis**. Two types of immune system cells ingest and destroy foreign antigens by phagocytosis: **neutrophils** and **macrophages**. Neutrophils are the most common type of white blood cell and are responsible for much of the body's protection against infection. Macrophages move and kill bacteria more slowly than neutrophils, but they are larger and can engulf larger targets, including the body's dead and damaged cells. Phagocytes also secrete special proteins called **cytokines** that activate the metabolic and immune responses to infection.

Lymphocytes: B-cells There are two distinct types of **lymphocytes:** B-cells and T-cells. **B-cells** respond to infection by rapidly dividing and producing large proteins known as **antibodies.** Antibodies travel in the bloodstream to the site of infection. There they stick to the surfaces of antigens and kill or otherwise inactivate them, making them easy for phagocytes to ingest.

The antibodies are members of a class of proteins known as **immunoglobulins**—literally, large globular proteins that provide immunity. Antibodies react selectively to a specific foreign organism, and the B-cells retain a memory of how to make them. Consequently, the immune system can respond with greater speed the next time it encounters the same foreign organism. By doing so, B-cells play a major role in resistance to infection.

Lymphocytes: T-cells The **T-cells** travel directly to the invasion site to battle the invaders. T-cells recognize the antigens displayed on the surfaces of phagocyte cells and multiply in response. Then they release powerful cytokines to destroy all the foreign particles that have this antigen on their surfaces. As the T-cells begin to win the battle against infection, they release signals to slow down the immune response.

GLOSSARY 18-1
IMMUNE SYSTEM TERMS

antibodies: large proteins of the blood and body fluids, produced by the immune system in response to the invasion of the body by foreign molecules (usually proteins called *antigens*). Antibodies combine with and inactivate the foreign invaders, thus protecting the body.

antigens: substances that elicit the formation of antibodies or an inflammation reaction from the immune system. Examples of antigens include viruses, bacteria, and toxins.

B-cells: lymphocytes that produce antibodies. *B* stands for *bone marrow,* where the B-cells develop and mature.

cytokines (SIGH-toe-kines): special proteins that direct immune and inflammatory responses.

immune response: the body's reaction to foreign antigens, which neutralizes or eliminates them, thus preventing damage.

immune system: the body's natural defense against foreign materials that have penetrated the skin or mucous membranes.

immunoglobulins (IM-you-noh-GLOB-you-linz): proteins capable of acting as antibodies.

lymphocytes (LIM-foh-sites): white blood cells that participate in acquired immunity; B-cells and T-cells.

macrophages (mak-roe-fay-jez): large phagocytic cells that serve as scavengers of the blood, clearing it of old or abnormal cells, cellular debris, and antigens.

neutrophils (new-tro-fills): the most common type of white blood cell. Neutrophils destroy antigens by phagocytosis.

phagocytes (FAG-oh-sites): white blood cells (neutrophils and macrophages) that have the ability to ingest and destroy foreign substances.

- **phagein** = to eat

phagocytosis (FAG-oh-sigh-TOH-sis): the process by which phagocytes engulf and destroy foreign materials.

T-cells: lymphocytes that attack antigens. *T* stands for the *thymus gland,* where the T-cells mature.

Unlike the phagocytes, which are capable of inactivating many different types of invaders, T-cells are highly specific. Each T-cell can attack only one type of antigen. This specificity is remarkable, for nature creates millions of antigens. After destroying a particular antigen, some T-cells retain the necessary information to serve as memory cells so that the immune system can rapidly produce the same type of T-cells again if the identical infection recurs.

T-cells actively defend the body against fungi, viruses, parasites, and a few types of bacteria; they can also destroy cancer cells. In organ transplant patients, T-cells participate in the rejection of newly transplanted tissues, which is why physicians prescribe immunosuppressive drugs following such surgery.

Each of the immune system cells plays a key role in fighting infectious disease. The differentiation and multiplication of these cells depends on a full array of nutrients.

Nutrition and Immunity The immune system is sensitive to subtle changes in nutrition status. Malnutrition—whether undernutrition or overnutrition—compromises both immune system tissues and immune responses.[5] From day to day, the immune system requires adequate amounts of protein, fat, carbohydrate, vitamins, and minerals to maintain its tissues and mount a response. Immune cells in tissues, lymph, and blood constantly survey their surroundings to detect foreign invaders and destroy those invaders before any symptoms of illness set in. If some of these foreign invaders escape destruction, then the immune system initiates a response. The immune response demands greater amounts of nutrients for the synthesis of antibodies and cytokines, for cell multiplication, for free radical generation, and for the active process of ending the response.[6] Exactly which nutrients are needed in greater quantities, and how much, is not yet fully known, but Table 18-1 lists several nutrients known to play key roles in immunity.

Impaired immunity opens the way for infectious diseases, which typically raise nutrient needs and reduce food intake. Consequently, nutrition status suffers further. Thus disease and malnutrition create a **synergistic** downward spiral that must be broken for recovery to occur.

synergistic (SIN-er-JIS-tick): multiple factors operating together in such a way that their combined effects are greater than the sum of their individual effects.

TABLE 18-1 Selected Nutrients in Immune Function

The immune system requires all nutrients for optimal functioning. The nutrients listed here have well-known, specific roles in immunity.

Nutrient	Key Role(s) in Immune Function
Protein	Maintains healthy skin and other epithelial tissues (barriers to infection); participates in the synthesis and function of the organs and cells of the immune system and antibody production
Omega-3 fatty acids	Help resolve inflammation when it is no longer needed for the immune response through production of lipid mediators known as resolvins and protectins, which also play a role in enhancing host defense
Vitamin A	Maintains healthy skin and other epithelial tissues (barriers to infection); participates in the cell replication and specialization that supports immune-cell and antibody production and the anti-inflammatory response
Vitamin D	Regulates immune cell (T-cell) responses; participates in antibody production
Vitamins C and E	Protect against oxidative damage
Vitamin B_6	Helps maintain an effective immune response; participates in antibody production
Vitamin B_{12} and folate	Assist in cell replication and specialization that support immune cell and antibody production
Selenium	Protects against oxidative damage
Zinc	Helps maintain an effective immune response; participates in antibody production

Quite simply, optimal immunity depends on optimal nutrition—enough, but not too much, of each of the nutrients. People with weakened immune systems, such as the elderly, benefit from a nutritious diet and supplements of selected nutrients.

Inflammation and Chronic Diseases The immune system's response to infection or injury results in inflammation. The blood supply to the infected area increases and the blood vessels become permeable, which allows the white blood cells to rush to the site. As phagocytes engulf the offending microbes, they release oxidative molecules, such as hydrogen peroxide, that kill the microbes. In this acute phase, inflammation fights off the infection or injury, removes damaged tissue, heals wounds, and promotes recovery from external stressors. In this way, acute inflammation and oxidative stress are beneficial.

When the inflammatory process persists, however, chronic inflammation is harmful. Cells of chronically inflamed tissues produce cytokines, oxidative molecules, blood clotting factors, and other bioactive chemicals that sustain the inflammatory response.[7] Chronic inflammation is apparent in obesity, and helps explain why obesity underlies so many of the chronic diseases discussed in the remainder of this chapter.

REVIEW IT Identify factors that protect people from the spread of infectious diseases and describe the role of nutrition in immunity.

Public health measures such as purification of water and safe handling of food help prevent the spread of infection in developed nations, and immunizations and antibiotics protect individuals. Nevertheless, some infectious diseases still endanger people today. Nutrition cannot prevent or cure infectious diseases, but adequate intakes of all the nutrients can help support the immune system as the body defends against disease-causing agents. If the immune system is impaired because of malnutrition or disease, a person becomes vulnerable to infectious disease. Inflammation underlies obesity and many chronic diseases.

18.2 Nutrition and Chronic Diseases

LEARN IT List the leading nutrition-related causes of death in the United States.

Figure 18-1 shows the 10 leading causes of death in the United States.[8] Many of these deaths reflect chronic diseases that developed in response to lifestyle factors such as diet, physical inactivity, overweight, tobacco use, and alcohol and

> FIGURE 18-1 The 10 Leading Causes of Death in the United States

Many deaths have multiple causes, but diet influences the development of several chronic diseases—notably, heart disease, some cancers, stroke, and diabetes.

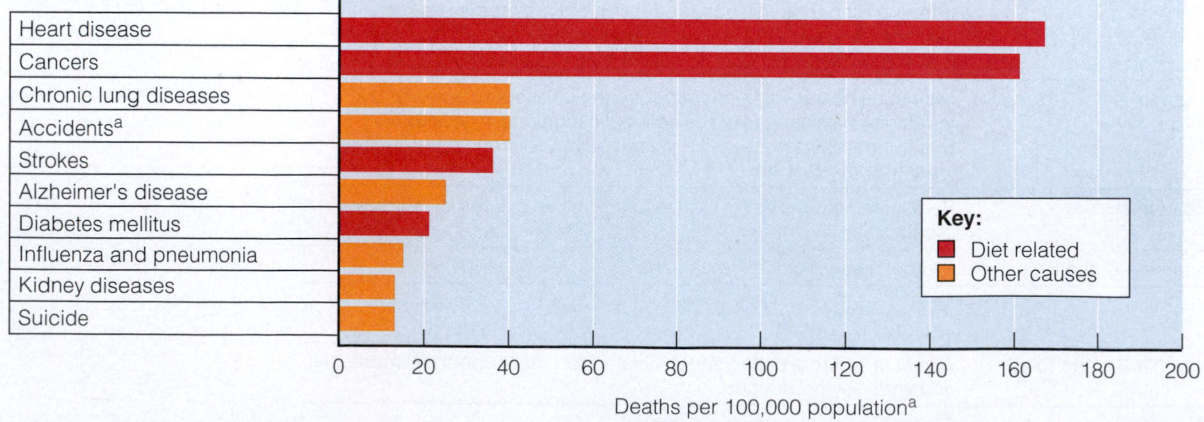
Heart disease
Cancers
Chronic lung diseases
Accidents[a]
Strokes
Alzheimer's disease
Diabetes mellitus
Influenza and pneumonia
Kidney diseases
Suicide
Key:
Diet related
Other causes
0
20
40
60
80
100
120
140
160
180
200
Deaths per 100,000 population[a]

NOTE: Rates are age adjusted to allow relative comparisons of mortality among groups and over time.
[a]Motor vehicle and other accidents are the leading cause of death among people aged 15–24, followed by homicide, suicide, cancer, and heart disease. Alcohol contributes to many accident fatalities.
SOURCE: Data from K. D. Kochanek and coauthors, Deaths: Final data for 2014, *National Vital Statistics Reports*, June 30, 2016.

drug abuse. Note that four of these causes of death, including the top two, have some relationship with diet (see Photo 18-1). Taken together, these four conditions account for over 50 percent of the nation's more than 2 million deaths each year. Worldwide, statistics are similar, with developing nations sharing many of the same chronic diseases as developed nations.[9]

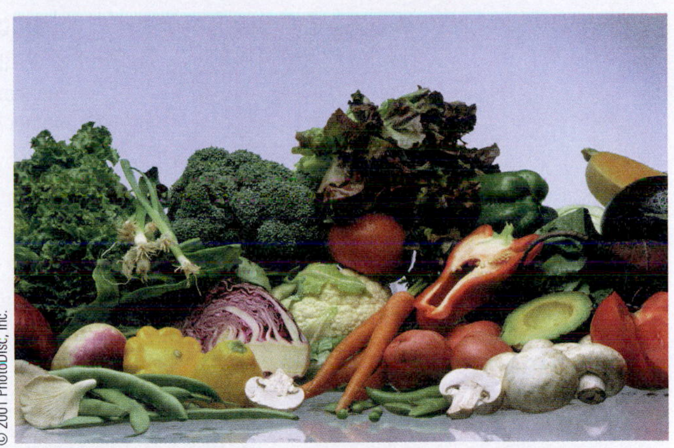
© 2001 PhotoDisc, Inc.

> **PHOTO 18-1** Vegetables rich in fiber, phytochemicals, and the antioxidant nutrients (beta-carotene, vitamin C, and vitamin E) help protect against chronic diseases.

This chapter explains how the major chronic diseases develop and summarizes their most important links with nutrition. Earlier chapters that described the connections between individual nutrients and diseases may have left the mistaken impression of "one disease–one nutrient" relationships. Indeed, valid links do exist between saturated fat and heart disease, calcium and osteoporosis, and antioxidant nutrients and cancer, but focusing only on these links oversimplifies the story. In reality, each nutrient may have connections with several diseases because its role in the body is not specific to a disease but to a body function. Furthermore, each of the chronic diseases develops in response to multiple risk factors, including many nondietary factors such as genetics, physical inactivity, and smoking. This chapter presents an integrated and balanced approach to disease prevention, paying careful attention to all of the factors involved. Table 18-2 presents some of the relationships between risk factors and chronic diseases. Figure 18-2 (p. 572) shows how many of the diseases themselves are risk factors for other chronic diseases. Notice that obesity is a gateway disease that contributes to several other diseases.

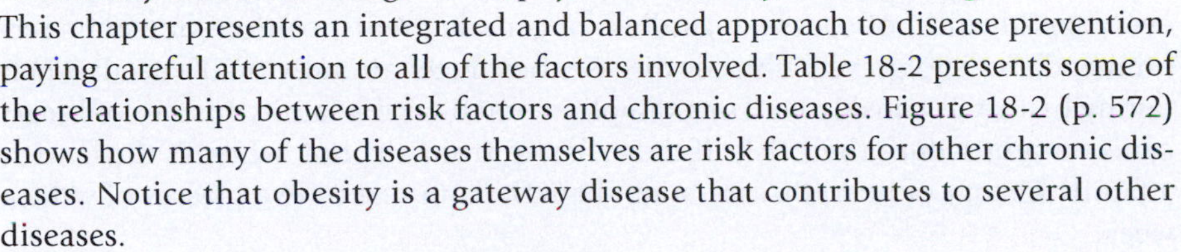

All of the diseases listed in Table 18-2 have a genetic component. A family history of a certain disease is a powerful indicator of a person's tendency to contract that disease.[10] Still, lifestyle factors are often pivotal in determining whether that tendency will be expressed.[11] Genetics and lifestyle often work synergistically; for instance, cigarette smoking is especially likely to bring on heart disease in people who are genetically predisposed to develop it. Not smoking would benefit

TABLE 18-2 Risk Factors and Chronic Diseases

	Cancers	Hypertension	Diabetes (type 2)	Atherosclerosis	Obesity	Stroke
Dietary Risk Factors						
Diets high in added sugars (beverages)					✓	
Diets high in salty or pickled foods	✓	✓				
Diets high in saturated and/or *trans* fat	✓	✓	✓	✓	✓	✓
Diets low in fruits, vegetables, and other foods rich in fiber and phytochemicals	✓			✓	✓	✓
Diets low in vitamins and/or minerals	✓	✓		✓		
Excessive alcohol intake	✓	✓		✓	✓	✓
Other Risk Factors						
Age	✓	✓	✓	✓		✓
Environmental contaminants	✓					
Genetics	✓	✓	✓	✓	✓	✓
Sedentary lifestyle	✓	✓	✓	✓	✓	✓
Smoking and tobacco use	✓	✓		✓		✓
Stress		✓		✓		✓

© Cengage

> **FIGURE 18-2 Interrelationships among Chronic Diseases**

Notice that many chronic diseases are themselves risk factors for other chronic diseases and that all of them are linked to obesity. The risk factors highlighted in blue define the metabolic syndrome.

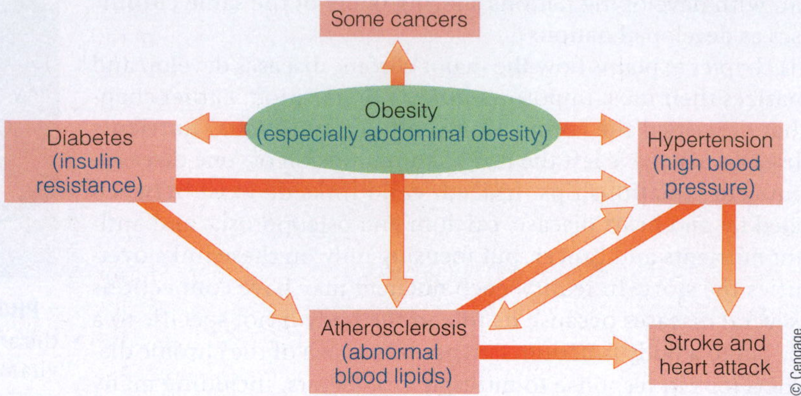
Some cancers
Obesity
(especially abdominal obesity)
Diabetes
(insulin
resistance)
Hypertension
(high blood
pressure)
Atherosclerosis
(abnormal
blood lipids)
Stroke and
heart attack
© Cengage

everyone's health, of course, regardless of genetic predisposition, but some recommendations to prevent chronic diseases best meet an individual's needs when family history is considered. For example, women with a family history of breast cancer might reduce their risks if they abstain from alcohol, whereas those with a family history of heart disease might benefit from one or two glasses of wine a week.

REVIEW IT List the leading nutrition-related causes of death in the United States.
Heart disease and cancers are the two leading causes of death in the United States, and strokes and diabetes also rank among the top 10. All four of these chronic diseases have significant links with nutrition. Other lifestyle risk factors and genetics are also important.

18.3 Cardiovascular Disease

LEARN IT Describe how atherosclerosis develops and strategies to lower blood cholesterol levels.

The major causes of death around the world today are diseases of the heart and blood vessels, collectively known as **cardiovascular disease (CVD).** (Glossary 18-2 defines this and other heart disease terms.) In the United States, cardiovascular disease claims the lives of more than 800,000 people each year.[12] CVD not only exacts a huge burden on the health of people in the United States (and around the world), but the economic burden is enormous. In the United States, the cost of CVD is more than $550 billion a year; by the year 2035, the cost is expected to soar to over $1 trillion.[13]

Coronary heart disease (CHD) is the most common form of cardiovascular disease and is usually caused by **atherosclerosis** in the **coronary arteries** that supply blood to the heart muscle. Atherosclerosis is the accumulation of lipids and other materials in the arteries.

How Atherosclerosis Develops

As Highlight 16 (p. 531) pointed out, no one is free of the fatty streaks that may one day become the **plaques** of atherosclerosis.* For most adults, the question is not whether you have plaques, but how advanced they are and what you can do to slow or reverse their progression.

*Plaque associated with atherosclerosis is known as *atheromatous* (ATH-er-OH-ma-tus) *plaque.*

Atherosclerosis or "hardening of the arteries" usually begins with the accumulation of soft fatty streaks along the inner arterial walls, especially at branch points (review Figure H16-1, p. 532). These fatty streaks gradually enlarge and harden as they fill with cholesterol, other lipids, and calcium, and they become encased in fibrous connective tissue, forming plaques. Plaques stiffen the arteries and narrow the passages through them. Most people have well-developed plaques by the age of 30. As Chapter 5 pointed out, dietary patterns high in saturated and *trans* fats contribute to the development of plaques and the progression of atherosclerosis.[14] But atherosclerosis is much more than the simple accumulation of lipids within the artery wall—it is a complex inflammatory response to tissue damage. Indeed, extensive evidence confirms that inflammation is centrally involved in all stages of atherosclerosis.[15]

Inflammation The cells lining the blood vessels may incur damage from high LDL cholesterol, hypertension, toxins from cigarette smoking, obesity, elevated homocysteine, or some viral and bacterial infections.[16] Such damage increases the permeability of the blood vessel walls and elicits an inflammatory response. The immune system sends in macrophages (the large, phagocytic cells of the immune system mentioned earlier), and the smooth muscle cells of the artery wall try to repair the damage. Particles of LDL cholesterol become trapped in the blood vessel walls. Free radicals produced during inflammatory responses oxidize the LDL cholesterol, and the macrophages engulf it. The macrophages swell with large quantities of oxidized LDL cholesterol and eventually become the cells of plaque. Arterial damage and the inflammatory response also favor the formation of blood clots and allow minerals to harden plaque and form the fibrous connective tissue that encapsulates it.

The inflammatory response of atherosclerosis weakens the walls of the arteries and may cause an **aneurysm**—the abnormal bulging of a blood vessel wall. Aneurysms can rupture and lead to massive bleeding and death, particularly when a large blood vessel such as the aorta is affected. The central role of the inflammatory response in atherosclerosis has led researchers to look for signs or markers of inflammation in the blood vessel walls. One of these markers is a protein known as **C-reactive protein (CRP)**. High levels of CRP have proved to more accurately predict future heart attack than high LDL cholesterol, which has a strong

C-reactive protein (CRP): a protein released during the acute phase of infection or inflammation that enhances immunity by promoting phagocytosis and activating platelets. Its presence may be used to assess a person's risk of an impending heart attack or stroke.

GLOSSARY 18-2
HEART DISEASE TERMS

aneurysm (AN-you-rizm): an abnormal enlargement or bulging of a blood vessel (usually an artery) caused by damage to or weakness in the blood vessel wall.

angina (an-JYE-nah or AN-ji-nah): a painful feeling of tightness or pressure in and around the heart, often radiating to the back, neck, and arms; caused by a lack of oxygen to an area of heart muscle.

atherosclerosis (ATH-er-oh-scler-OH-sis): a type of artery disease characterized by plaques (accumulations of lipid-containing material) on the inner walls of the arteries.

cardiovascular disease (CVD): diseases of the heart and blood vessels throughout the body. Atherosclerosis is the main cause of CVD. When the arteries that carry blood to the heart muscle become blocked, the heart suffers damage known as *coronary heart disease (CHD)*.

CHD risk equivalents: disorders that raise the risk of heart attacks, strokes, and other complications associated with cardiovascular disease to the same degree as existing CHD. These disorders include symptomatic carotid artery disease, peripheral arterial disease, abdominal aortic aneurysm, and diabetes mellitus.

coronary arteries: blood vessels that supply blood to the heart.

coronary heart disease (CHD): the damage that occurs when the blood vessels carrying blood to the heart (the *coronary arteries*) become narrow and occluded.

embolism (EM-boh-lizm): the obstruction of a blood vessel by an *embolus* (EM-boh-luss), or traveling clot, causing sudden tissue death.

- **embol** = to insert, plug

heart attack: sudden tissue death caused by blockages of vessels that feed the heart muscle; also called *myocardial* (my-oh-KAR-dee-al) *infarction* (in-FARK-shun) or *cardiac arrest*.

- **myo** = muscle
- **cardial** = heart
- **infarct** = tissue death

hypertension: consistently higher-than-normal blood pressure. Hypertension that develops without an identifiable cause is known as *essential* or *primary hypertension*; hypertension that is caused by a specific disorder such as kidney disease is known as *secondary hypertension*.

plaques (PLACKS): an accumulation of fatty deposits, smooth muscle cells, and fibrous connective tissue that develops in the artery walls in atherosclerosis. Plaque associated with atherosclerosis is known as *atheromatous* (ATH-er-OH-ma-tus) *plaque*.

prehypertension: blood pressure slightly higher than normal, but below the diagnosis of hypertension (see Table 18-4, p. 575).

stroke: an event in which the blood flow to a part of the brain is cut off; also called *cerebrovascular accident (CVA)*.

- **cerebro** = brain
- **vascular** = blood vessels

thrombosis (throm-BOH-sis): the formation of a *thrombus* (THROM-bus), or a blood clot, that may obstruct a blood vessel, causing gradual tissue death.

- **thrombo** = clot

transient ischemic (is-KEY-mik) **attack (TIA):** a temporary reduction in blood flow to the brain, which causes temporary symptoms that vary depending on the part of the brain affected. Common symptoms include light-headedness, visual disturbances, paralysis, staggering, numbness, and inability to swallow.

relationship with atherosclerosis, as a later section explains.[17] Another important inflammatory marker, **lipoprotein-associated phospholipase A(2)** or **Lp-PLA(2)**, appears to be a highly specific marker for plaque inflammation and the formation of plaques that are most susceptible to rupture.[18]

Plaques Once plaque has formed, a sudden spasm or surge in blood pressure in an artery can tear away part of its fibrous coat, causing it to rupture. Some plaques are more unstable than others and are therefore more vulnerable to rupture.[19]* Such plaques have a thin fibrous cap, a large lipid core, and an abundance of macrophages—characteristics that undermine plaque stability. Researchers now know that the *composition* of plaques—rather than the *size* of plaques—is a key predictor of plaque rupture and subsequent clot formation. When plaques rupture, the immune system responds to the damage as it would to other tissue injuries.

Blood Clots Blood clots form when **platelets** and other factors cover an injured or damaged area. Abnormal blood clotting can trigger life-threatening events. For example, a blood clot may gradually grow large enough to restrict or close off a blood vessel **(thrombosis)**. A *coronary thrombosis* blocks blood flow through an artery that feeds the heart muscle. A *cerebral thrombosis* blocks blood flow through an artery that feeds the brain. A clot may also break free from an artery wall and travel through the circulatory system until it lodges in a small artery and suddenly shuts off blood flow to the tissues **(embolism)**.

The action of platelets is under the control of certain eicosanoids, known as prostaglandins and thromboxanes, which are made from the 20-carbon omega-6 and omega-3 fatty acids (introduced in Chapter 5). Each eicosanoid plays a specific role in helping to regulate many of the body's activities, including the regulation of blood pressure, blood clot formation, blood vessel contractions, immune response, and nerve impulse transmissions. Sometimes their actions oppose each other.[20] For example, one eicosanoid prevents clot formation, and another promotes it. Similarly, one dilates the blood vessels, and another constricts them. When omega-3 fatty acids are abundant in the diet, they make more of the kinds of eicosanoids that favor heart health.[21] (Table 5-4 on p. 150 includes good sources of omega-3 fatty acids.)

Blood Pressure The stress of blood flow along artery walls can cause physical damage to arteries. High blood pressure intensifies the stress of blood flow on arterial tissue, provoking a low-grade inflammatory state that may stimulate plaque formation and progression.[22]

The Result: Heart Attacks and Strokes When atherosclerosis in the coronary arteries becomes severe enough to restrict blood flow and deprive the heart muscle of oxygen, CHD develops. The person with CHD often experiences pain and pressure in the area around the heart **(angina)**. A **heart attack** occurs when blood flow to the heart is cut off and that area of the heart muscle dies. Restricted blood flow to the brain causes a **transient ischemic attack (TIA)** or **stroke.** Coronary heart disease and strokes are the first and fifth leading causes of death, respectively, for adults in the United States.

Risk Factors for Coronary Heart Disease

Although atherosclerosis can develop in any blood vessel, the coronary arteries are most often affected, leading to CHD. Table 18-3 lists the major risk factors for CHD. Notice that some risk factors, such as diet and physical activity, are *modifiable*, meaning that they can be changed; others, such as age, gender, and family history are not modifiable. The criteria for defining blood lipids, blood pressure, and obesity in relation to CHD risk are shown in Table 18-4; Table H16-1 (p. 532) presents cholesterol standards for children and adolescents.

*Plaque that is susceptible to rupture because it has only a thin fibrous barrier between its lipid-rich core and the artery lining is called *vulnerable plaque*.

lipoprotein-associated phospholipase A(2) or **Lp-PLA(2):** a lipoprotein-bound enzyme that generates potent proinflammatory and proatherogenic products such as oxidized free fatty acids and lysophosphatidylcholine. Lp-PLA(2) is a specific marker of plaque inflammation.

platelets: tiny, disc-shaped bodies in the blood, important in blood clot formation.

TABLE 18-3 Risk Factors for CHD

Risk Factors for CHD
Major Risk Factors for CHD (not modifiable)
• Increasing age
• Male gender
• Family history of premature heart disease
Major Risk Factors for CHD (modifiable)
• High blood LDL cholesterol
• Low blood HDL cholesterol
• High blood triglycerides (VLDL)
• High blood pressure (hypertension)
• Diabetes
• Obesity (especially abdominal obesity)
• Physical inactivity
• Cigarette smoking
• An "atherogenic" diet (high in saturated fats and low in vegetables, fruits, and whole grains)

NOTE: Risk factors highlighted in yellow have relationships with diet.
SOURCE: D. Mozaffarian and coauthors, Heart disease and stroke statistics—2016 update: A report from the American Heart Association, *Circulation* 133 (2016): e38–e360.

TABLE 18-4 Standards for CHD Risk Factors

Risk Factors	Desirable	Borderline	High Risk
Total blood cholesterol (mg/dL)	<200	200–239	≥240
LDL cholesterol (mg/dL)	<100[a]	130–159	160–189[b]
HDL cholesterol (mg/dL)	≥60	59–40	<40
Triglycerides, fasting (mg/dL)	<150	150–199	200–499[c]
Body mass index (BMI)[d]	18.5–24.9	25–29.9	≥30
Blood pressure (systolic and/or diastolic pressure)[e]	<120/<80	120–139/80–89[f]	≥140/≥90[g]

[a]100–129 mg/dL LDL indicates a near or above optimal level.
[b]≥190 mg/dL LDL indicates a very high risk.
[c]≥500 md/dL triglycerides indicates a very high risk.
[d]Body mass index (BMI) was defined in Chapter 8; BMI standards are found on the insert.
[e]Blood pressure is measured in millimeters of mercury (mm Hg). Blood pressure is measured both when the heart muscle contracts (systolic blood pressure) and when it relaxes (diastolic blood pressure).
[f]These values indicate prehypertension.
[g]These values indicate stage one hypertension; ≥160/≥100 indicates stage two hypertension. Physicians use these classifications to determine medical treatment.

By age 20, half of the adults in the United States have at least one major risk factor for CHD, and many have more than one. Public health officials in the United States recommend screening to identify risk factors in individuals and offer preventive advice for the population.[23] Regular screening and early detection have proved successful: since 1960, both blood cholesterol levels and deaths from cardiovascular disease among US adults have shown a continuous and substantial downward trend. These trends also reflect behavior changes in individuals.[24] As adults grow older, many of them stop smoking, limit alcohol consumption, and become mindful that their food choices can improve their cardiovascular health.

Age, Gender, and Family History A review of Table 18-3 shows that three of the major risk factors for CHD cannot be modified by diet or otherwise: age, gender, and family history. As men and women grow older, the risk of CHD rises. The increasing risk of CHD with advancing age reflects the steady progression of atherosclerosis. On average, older people have more atherosclerosis than younger people do.

In men, aging becomes a significant risk factor at age 45 and older. CHD occurs about 10 to 15 years later in women than in men. Women younger than 45 tend to have lower LDL cholesterol than men of the same age, but women's blood cholesterol typically begins to rise between ages 45 and 55. Thus, aging becomes a significant risk factor for women who are 55 and older. The speed at which atherosclerosis progresses, however, depends more on the presence or absence of risk factors such as hypertension, high blood cholesterol, diabetes, and smoking than on age alone.[25] Ultimately, CHD kills as many women as men—and kills more women in the United States than any other disease.[26]

Nonetheless, at every age, men have a greater risk of CHD than women do. The reasons for this gender difference are not completely understood, but they can be partly explained by the earlier onset of risk factors such as elevated LDL cholesterol and blood pressure in men. Levels of the amino acid homocysteine, which damages artery walls and increases oxidative stress, rise with age and are generally higher in men. Researchers have not determined whether the damage is caused by homocysteine itself or by an associated factor.[27]

A history of early CHD in immediate family members is an independent risk factor even when other risk factors are considered. The more family members affected and the earlier the age of onset, the greater the risk.[28]

Important research shows that even people with a high genetic risk for heart disease can improve their odds of staying healthy by way of lifestyle factors such as regular physical activity, not smoking, not being obese, and having a healthy diet.[29] Each one these four lifestyle factors reduces the risk of heart disease independently, but together, their synergistic effect is dramatic. Adhering to three of the four factors cuts heart attack risk in half. Clearly, lifestyle choices can make a powerful difference to heart health.

High LDL and Low HDL Cholesterol In population studies, the relationship between total blood cholesterol and atherosclerosis is strong—and most of the total cholesterol is made up of LDL cholesterol. The higher the LDL cholesterol, the greater the risk of CHD. In contrast, the lower the LDL cholesterol and blood pressure, the slower the progression of atherosclerosis.[30]

The LDL are clearly the most **atherogenic** lipoproteins. As Chapter 5 explained, HDL also carry cholesterol, but HDL are helpfully returning the cholesterol from the cells to the liver, where it will be used to make bile and excreted in the GI tract. Because HDL remove cholesterol from circulation and contain proteins that inhibit inflammation, LDL oxidation, and plaque accumulation, *low* HDL levels can contribute to the development of atherosclerosis as well.[31] Having adequate levels of HDL is beneficial, but high levels of HDL do not necessarily confer additional benefit.[32]

Any LDL cholesterol that remains in the blood after the body's cells take up the amount they need becomes vulnerable to oxidation. High blood levels of LDL cholesterol, especially oxidized LDL, trigger a series of events that promote plaque formation and contribute to plaque instability.[33] Oxidized LDL cholesterol stimulates production of atherogenic signaling molecules. These signaling molecules attract immune cells and allow them to adhere to, and penetrate, the innermost layer of the arterial wall. Within the arterial wall, these immune cells become macrophages that form the lipid-rich foam cells characteristic of fatty streaks. Macrophages within the arterial wall perpetuate chronic inflammation by releasing inflammatory cytokines that contribute to plaque rupture. When plaques rupture, a heart attack or stroke may occur. In the early stages of atherosclerosis, the goal of treatment is to slow plaque development. In the later stages, the goal of treatment is to stabilize plaques.

LDL vary in size and density, and these LDL subtypes have differing effects on heart disease risk. The smallest, most dense LDL can slip into the artery walls easily and are therefore more atherogenic than the larger, less dense LDL.[34]

High Blood Triglycerides High blood triglycerides (found in VLDL) also promote atherosclerosis, either by influencing the production of other atherogenic lipoproteins or by causing molecular changes in endothelial cells and macrophages that promote inflammation and plaque development.[35] About one-third of adults in the United States have high blood triglyceride levels. High blood triglyceride levels are associated with a sedentary lifestyle, overweight and obesity (especially abdominal obesity), and type 2 diabetes.

High Blood Pressure (Hypertension) Atherosclerosis is frequently accompanied by chronic high blood pressure (**hypertension**). The higher blood pressure is above normal, the greater the risk of heart disease. However, even values only slightly higher than desirable—classified as **prehypertension** in Table 18-4—increase the risk of heart attack and stroke.[36] This relationship between hypertension and heart disease risk holds true for men and women, young and old. High blood pressure injures the artery walls and accelerates plaque formation, thus initiating or worsening the progression of atherosclerosis. Then the plaques and reduced blood flow raise blood pressure further, and hypertension and atherosclerosis become mutually aggravating conditions.

Diabetes Diabetes is a major independent risk factor for cardiovascular disease and substantially increases the risk of death from CHD.[37] In diabetes, blood vessels often become blocked and circulation diminishes. Atherosclerosis progresses rapidly. For many people with diabetes, the risk of heart attack is similar to that for people with CHD. In fact, physicians describe diabetes and other disorders that have risks similar to CHD as **CHD risk equivalents.** Treatment to lower LDL cholesterol in diabetes follows the same recommendations as for CHD.

atherogenic: able to initiate or promote atherosclerosis.

Obesity and Physical Inactivity Obesity, especially abdominal obesity, and physical inactivity significantly increase risk factors for CHD, contributing to high LDL cholesterol, low HDL cholesterol, high triglycerides, hypertension, and diabetes.[38] Conversely, weight loss and physical activity protect against CHD by lowering LDL, raising HDL, lowering triglycerides, improving insulin sensitivity, and lowering blood pressure (see Photo 18-2).[39]

Table 14-2 in Chapter 14 (p. 427) presents guidelines for developing and maintaining cardiorespiratory fitness. Cardiorespiratory fitness reflects the health of the heart and circulatory system and strongly relates to health outcomes—low levels of cardiorespiratory fitness predict high risks of heart disease and other chronic diseases.[40] In fact, cardiorespiratory fitness is as strong a predictor of mortality as smoking, hypertension, and diabetes, but it is not routinely assessed by health care providers. Many experts believe that assessment of, and improvement in, cardiorespiratory fitness should be included in routine clinical care.

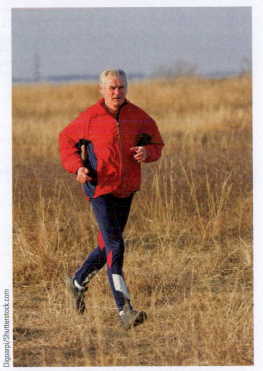

Digoarpi/Shutterstock.com

> **PHOTO 18-2** Regular aerobic exercise can help defend against heart disease by strengthening the heart muscle, promoting weight loss, and improving blood lipids and blood pressure.

Cigarette Smoking Cigarette smoking is a powerful risk factor for CHD and other forms of cardiovascular disease.[41] The risk increases the more a person smokes and is the same for men and women. Smoking damages the heart directly by increasing blood pressure and the heart's workload. It deprives the heart of oxygen and damages platelets, making blood clot formation likely. Toxins in cigarette smoke damage blood vessels, setting the stage for atherosclerosis. When people quit smoking, their risk of CHD begins to decline within a few months.

Atherogenic Diet Diet also influences the risk of CHD. An "atherogenic" diet—high in saturated fats and *trans* fats and low in vegetables, fruits, and whole grains—elevates LDL cholesterol.[42] Fortunately, a well-chosen eating pattern such as the the Healthy Vegetarian Eating Pattern (Highlight 2, p. 64), the Healthy Mediterranean-Style Eating Pattern (Highlight 5, p. 164), and the DASH eating pattern (discussed in a later section) can often lower the risk of CVD.[43] A number of beneficial factors share the credit, including vitamins, minerals, fibers, phytochemicals, and omega-3 fatty acids.

As Table 18-3 (p. 574) shows, most of the modifiable risk factors for CHD are directly related to diet. Several of these diet-related risk factors—low HDL, high blood triglycrides, high blood pressure, elevated fasting blood glucose, and abdominal obesity—comprise a cluster of health risks known as **metabolic syndrome.** As Figure 18-2 (p. 572) shows, the risks that define metabolic syndrome underlie several chronic diseases and increase the risks of CHD and type 2 diabetes.[44] Abdominal obesity and **insulin resistance** are both considered primary factors contributing to the metabolic syndrome.[45] Metabolic syndrome, like the chronic diseases associated with it, also includes markers of inflammation and thrombosis.[46] Overeating and physical inactivity play major roles in the development of metabolic syndrome. The prevalence of metabolic syndrome among US adults is high, and treatment to reduce these risk factors for heart disease and diabetes should begin early and focus on changes in lifestyle.

Recommendations for Reducing Cardiovascular Disease Risk

Recommendations to reduce cardiovascular disease (CVD) risk, including CHD, comprise both screening and intervention. The American Heart Association, together with the American College of Cardiology, developed guidelines for the assessment of CVD risk, the treatment of elevated blood cholesterol, and the management of lifestyle factors that reduce risk.[47]

Screening for Cardiovascular Disease Risk The American Heart Association has developed an online calculator and downloadable spreadsheet to estimate risk for heart attack or stroke.* The risk factors included in the assessment are age, sex, race, total cholesterol, HDL cholesterol, blood pressure, blood pressure medication use,

metabolic syndrome: a combination of risk factors—insulin resistance, high blood pressure, abnormal blood lipids, and abdominal obesity—that greatly increase a person's risk of developing coronary heart disease; also called *Syndrome X, insulin resistance syndrome,* or *dysmetabolic syndrome.*

insulin resistance: the condition in which a normal amount of insulin produces a subnormal effect in muscle, adipose, and liver cells, resulting in an elevated fasting glucose; a metabolic consequence of obesity that precedes type 2 diabetes.

*To calculate your risk for CVD, visit http://my.americanheart.org/cvriskcalculator.

TABLE 18-5 Recommendations and Strategies for Reducing CVD Risk

Recommendation	Strategy
Dietary patterns: Choose a dietary pattern that emphasizes vegetables, fruits, and whole grains; includes low-fat dairy products, poultry, fish, legumes, nontropical vegetable oils, and nuts; and limits intake of sweets, sugar-sweetened beverages, and red meats.	Adopt a heart-healthy eating pattern such as DASH, the USDA Healthy US-Style Eating Pattern, the Healthy Mediterranean-Style Eating Pattern, the Vegetarian Eating Pattern, or other well-planned plant-based dietary patterns.
Energy: Balance energy intake and physical activity to prevent weight gain and to achieve or maintain a healthy body weight.	Engage in at least 30 minutes of moderate-intensity endurance activity or 15 minutes of vigorous-intensity endurance activity on most days of the week.
Saturated fat and *trans* fat: Limit saturated fat to less than 10 percent of total kcalories and *trans* fat to less than 1 percent of total kcalories. For those who have been advised to lower LDL cholesterol or those who have diabetes, limit saturated fat to 5 to 6 percent of total kcalories.	Replace solid fats (saturated and *trans* fats) with food or oils containing unsaturated fatty acids such as omega-3 fatty fish, avocado, nuts, olive oil, canola oil, safflower oil, corn oil, and soybean oil.
Sodium: Limit sodium intake to 1500 milligrams per day.	Choose and prepare foods with little or no salt.
Alcohol: If alcohol is consumed, practice moderation.	Limit alcohol intake to no more than one drink daily for women and two drinks daily for men.
Tobacco: Avoid exposure to any form of tobacco or tobacco smoke.	Do not smoke or use tobacco in any form and avoid exposure to second-hand smoke.

SOURCE: R. H. Eckel and coauthors, 2013 AHA/ACC Guidelines on lifestyle management to reduce cardiovascular risk: A report of the American College of Cardiology/American Heart Association Task Force on Practice Guidelines, *Circulation* 129 (2014): S76–S99.

diabetes, and smoking. Once risks have been assessed, the guidelines define when physicians should prescribe the use of cholesterol-lowering medications (statins), with cautions to use clinical judgments with each individual.[48] Thus, health care providers are encouraged to discuss options with their patients and to consider personal preferences, possible harms, costs, and inconveniences of taking medications. In this way, the assessment guidelines focus on patient-centered care. In addition to medications, treatment plans include major lifestyle changes in diet, physical activity, and smoking cessation.

Lifestyle Interventions To reduce the risk of CVD, people are encouraged to increase physical activity, lose weight (if necessary), implement dietary changes, and reduce exposure to tobacco smoke either by quitting smoking or by avoiding secondhand smoke. Altering one's lifestyle is challenging, and instruction and guidance are critical for success. Health professionals can explain the reasons for change, set obtainable goals, and offer practical suggestions. If lifestyle changes fail to lower LDL or blood pressure to acceptable levels, then medications are prescribed. Table 18-5 summarizes strategies to reduce the risk of heart disease. How To 18-1 offers suggestions for implementing a heart-healthy diet.

REVIEW IT Describe how atherosclerosis develops and strategies to lower blood cholesterol levels.

Atherosclerosis is characterized by plaque build-up in artery walls. Plaques rupturing or blood clotting can cause heart attacks and strokes. Dietary recommendations to lower the risks of cardiovascular disease are summarized in Table 18-5. Quitting smoking and engaging in regular physical activity also improve heart health.

18.4 Hypertension

LEARN IT Present strategies to lower blood pressure.

Anyone concerned about atherosclerosis and the risk it presents must also be concerned about hypertension. Together, the two are a life-threatening combination. The higher the blood pressure is above normal, the greater the risk. Low blood pressure is generally a sign of long life expectancy and low heart disease risk.

> How To 18-1 Implement a Heart-Healthy Diet

Following a heart-healthy diet can require major changes in dietary choices. It helps to make a few changes at a time and to focus on positive choices (what to eat) first, rather than negative ones (what not to eat).

Grains

- Choose whole-grain breads and cereals that list "whole wheat" as the first ingredient on labels and provide at least 1.1 grams of dietary fiber per 10 grams of carbohydrate.
- Limit foods that list any *trans* fat in the Nutrition Facts panel or "hydrogenated oil" in the ingredients list.
- Limit products that contain tropical oils (coconut, palm, and palm kernel oil), which are high in saturated fat.

Fruits and Vegetables

- Consume fruits and vegetables frequently. Keep the refrigerator stocked with a variety of colorful fruits and vegetables (carrots, grapes, blueberries, melon).
- Incorporate at least one or two servings of fruits and vegetables into each meal.
- Choose canned products carefully. Canned vegetables (especially tomato-based products) may be high in sodium. Canned fruits may be high in added sugars.
- Limit high-sodium foods such as pickles, olives, sauerkraut, and kimchee.
- Limit french fries from fast-food restaurants, which are often loaded with *trans* fats.

Lunch and Dinner Entrées

- Limit meat, fish, and poultry servings to 5 ounces per day.
- Include at least two 3.5-ounce servings of fish rich in omega-3 fatty acids (salmon, mackerel, herring, trout) each week.
- Select lean cuts of beef, such as sirloin tip, round steak, and arm roast, and lean cuts of pork, such as center-cut ham, loin chops, and tenderloin. Trim visible fat before cooking.
- Select extra-lean ground meat and drain well after cooking. Use lean ground turkey, without skin added, in place of ground beef.
- Include more vegetarian entrées or legume dishes to reduce meat intake and boost vegetable, soluble fiber, and soy protein intakes.
- Restrict these high-sodium foods:
  - Cured or smoked meats such as beef jerky, bologna, corned or chipped beef, frankfurters, ham, luncheon meats, salt pork, and sausage
  - Salty or smoked fish, such as anchovies, caviar, salted or dried cod, herring, sardines, and smoked salmon
  - Packaged, canned, or frozen soups, sauces, and entrées

Milk Products

- To obtain two to three servings of milk daily, include a portion of fat-free or low-fat milk, yogurt, or cottage cheese in each meal.
- Use yogurt or fat-free sour cream to make dips or salad dressings. Substitute evaporated fat-free milk for heavy cream.
- Limit foods high in saturated fat or sodium, such as cheese, processed cheeses, ice cream, and other milk-based desserts.

Fats and Oils

- Add nuts (not salted) and avocados to meals to increase monounsaturated fat intakes and make meals more appetizing.
- Include unsaturated vegetable oils such as canola, corn, olive, peanut, safflower, sesame, soybean, and sunflower oils, in salad dressings and recipes.
- Use margarines with added plant sterols or stanols regularly.
- Select soft margarines in tubs or liquid form; limit stick margarines and solid vegetable shortenings.

Spices and Seasonings

- Use salt only at the end of cooking and you will need to add much less. Use salt substitutes at the table.
- Spices and herbs improve the flavor of foods without adding sodium. Try using more garlic, ginger, basil, curry or chili powder, cumin, pepper, lemon, mint, oregano, rosemary, and thyme.
- Check the sodium content on labels. Flavorings and sauces that are usually high in sodium include bouillon cubes, soy sauce, steak and barbecue sauces, relishes, mustard, and catsup.

Snacks and Desserts

- Select low-sodium and low-saturated fat choices such as unsalted pretzels, nuts, popcorn, chips, and crackers.
- Choose canned or dried fruits and some raw vegetables to boost fruit and vegetable intake.
- Enjoy angel food cake, which is made without egg yolks and added fat.
- Select low-fat frozen desserts such as sherbet, sorbet, fruit bars, and some low-fat ice creams.

> TRY IT Plan heart-healthy meals for a day and analyze them using your personal profile. Discuss whether these meals meet the strategies listed in Table 18-5 and how to improve any shortcomings.

Hypertension affects about one out of three adults in the United States.[49] It contributes to, or is a primary cause of, more than 400,000 deaths each year.[50] People usually do not feel the physical effects of high blood pressure, but it can impair life's quality and end life prematurely.

How Hypertension Develops The underlying causes of most cases of hypertension are not fully understood, but much is known about the physiological factors that affect blood pressure. Blood pressure arises from contractions in the heart muscle that pump blood away from the heart (**cardiac output**) and the resistance blood encounters in the arterioles (**peripheral resistance**). When either cardiac output or peripheral resistance increases, blood pressure rises. Cardiac output is raised when heart rate or blood volume increases; peripheral resistance is affected mostly by the diameters of the arterioles. Blood pressure is therefore influenced by the nervous system, which regulates heart muscle contractions and the arteriole's diameters, and hormonal signals, which may cause fluid retention or blood vessel constriction. The kidneys play a key role in regulating blood pressure by controlling the secretion of the hormones involved in vasoconstriction and retention of sodium and water (review Figure 12-6, p. 364).

Risk Factors for Hypertension Several major risk factors predicting the development of hypertension have been identified, including:

- *Aging.* Hypertension risk increases with age. An estimated two-thirds of persons 65 and older have hypertension.[51] Individuals who have normal blood pressure at age 55 still have a 90 percent risk of developing high blood pressure during their lifetimes.
- *Genetics.* Hypertension risk is similar among family members. It is also more prevalent and severe in certain ethnic groups: for African Americans in the United States, the prevalence of high blood pressure is among the highest in the world.[52] Compared with others, African Americans typically develop high blood pressure earlier in life, and their average blood pressure is much higher.
- *Obesity.* Most people with hypertension—an estimated 70 percent—are overweight or obese.[53] Obesity is recognized as a major cause of high blood pressure, and the combination of obesity and hypertension greatly increases the risk for CVD. Obesity raises blood pressure by altering kidney function, increasing blood volume, and promoting blood vessel damage through insulin resistance.[54]
- *Salt intake.* Excess intake of salt plays a major role in hypertension.[55] Reducing salt intake lowers blood pressure in people with or without hypertension and also diminishes the age-related rise in blood pressure.
- *Alcohol.* Alcohol consumption, especially if consumed regularly in amounts greater than two drinks per day, is strongly associated with hypertension.[56] Alcohol is also associated with strokes independently of hypertension, and its use may interfere with medications.

Treatment of Hypertension The single most effective step people can take against hypertension is to find out whether they have it (see Photo 18-3). At checkup time, a health-care professional can provide an accurate resting blood pressure reading. Under normal conditions, blood pressure fluctuates continuously in response to a variety of factors, including stress, and such actions as talking or shifting position. Some people react emotionally to the procedure, which raises the blood pressure reading. For these reasons, if the resting blood pressure is above normal, the reading should be repeated before confirming the diagnosis of hypertension (see Table 18-4, p. 575, for blood pressure standards). Thereafter, blood pressure should be checked regularly. Both lifestyle modifications and medications are used to treat hypertension. Recently, new guidelines for initiating medication in the treatment of hypertension in adults have been issued.[57]

cardiac output: the volume of blood discharged by the heart each minute; determined by multiplying the stroke volume by the heart rate. The stroke volume is the amount of oxygenated blood the heart ejects toward the tissues at each beat. Cardiac output (volume/minute) = stroke volume (volume/beat) × heart rate (beats/minute).

peripheral resistance: the resistance to pumped blood in the small arterial branches (arterioles) that carry blood to the tissues.

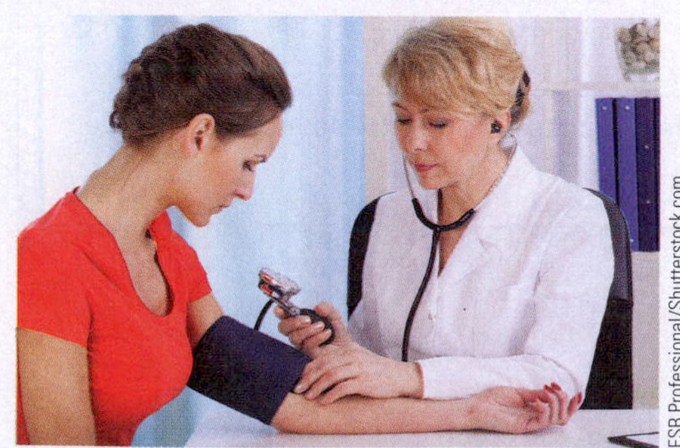

ESB Professional/Shutterstock.com

> PHOTO 18-3 To guard against hypertension, have your blood pressure checked regularly.

TABLE 18-6 Lifestyle Modifications to Reduce Blood Pressure

Modification	Recommendation	Expected Reduction in Systolic Blood Pressure
Weight reduction	Maintain healthy body weight (BMI 18.5–24.9).	10 mm Hg/10 kg lost
DASH Eating Plan	Adopt a diet that includes abundant fruits, vegetables, and whole grains; moderate low-fat milk products, poultry, fish, legumes, nontropical vegetable oils, and nuts; and minimal sweets, sugar-sweetened beverages, and red meats.	5–6 mm Hg
Sodium restriction	Reduce dietary sodium intake to less than 2300 mg sodium (less than 6 g salt) per day, and further reduce intake to 1500 mg among people who have prehypertension or hypertension.	2–7 mm Hg
Physical activity	Perform aerobic physical activity for at least 40 minutes per day, most days of the week.	2–5 mm Hg
Moderate alcohol consumption	Men: Limit to two drinks per day. Women and lighter-weight men: Limit to one drink per day.	2–4 mm Hg

SOURCE: Adapted from US Department of Health and Human Services and US Department of Agriculture, *2015–2020 Dietary Guidelines for Americans*, 8th ed. (2015): health.gov/dietaryguidelines/2015/guidelines; R. H. Eckel and coauthors, 2013 AHA/ACC Guidelines on lifestyle management to reduce cardiovascular risk: A report of the American College of Cardiology/American Heart Association Task Force on Practice Guidelines, *Circulation* 129 (2014): S76–S99; L. Landberg and coauthors, Obesity-related hypertension: Pathogenesis, cardiovascular risk, and treatment, A position paper of The Obesity Society and the American Society of Hypertension, *Journal of Clinical Hypertension* 15 (2013): 14–33.

Table 18-6 describes the lifestyle changes that reduce blood pressure and the expected reduction in systolic blood pressure for each change.

Weight Control Efforts to lower blood pressure focus on weight control. Weight loss alone is one of the most effective nondrug treatments for hypertension.[58] Those who are using drugs to control their blood pressure can often reduce or discontinue the drugs when they lose weight. Even a modest weight loss of 5 to 10 percent of body weight can lower blood pressure significantly.

The DASH Eating Pattern Results of the Dietary Approaches to Stop Hypertension (DASH) trials show that an eating pattern rich in fruits, vegetables, low-fat milk products, whole grains, and nuts, and low in total fat and saturated fat can significantly lower blood pressure. In addition to lowering blood pressure, DASH lowers total cholesterol and LDL cholesterol, and reduces inflammation.[59] Compared to the typical American diet, DASH provides more fiber, potassium, magnesium, and calcium and less red meat, sweets, and sugar-containing beverages. Table 18-7

TABLE 18-7 DASH and USDA Healthy US-Style Eating Patterns Compared

Food Group	DASH	USDA
Grains	6–8 oz	6 oz
Vegetables	2–2½ c	2½ c
Fruits	2–2½ c	2 c
Milk (fat-free/low-fat)	2–3 c	3 c
Lean meats, poultry, fish	6 oz or less	5½ oz
Nuts, seeds, legumes	4–5 oz per week	—[a]

NOTE: These diet plans are based on 2000 kcalories per day. Both DASH and USDA Food Patterns recommend that fats and sugars be used sparingly and with discretion.
[a]The USDA Food Patterns combine nuts, seeds, and legumes with meat, poultry, and fish.

shows how DASH compares to the USDA Healthy US-Style Eating Pattern (introduced in Chapter 2). Both eating patterns meet the goals specified in the *Dietary Guidelines for Americans*.[60]

Salt/Sodium Intake Strong evidence supports the important role restricting sodium and/or salt plays in preventing and reducing hypertension. Lowering sodium intake reduces blood pressure regardless of gender or race, presence or absence of hypertension, or whether people follow the DASH eating pattern or a typical American diet. The combination of DASH with a limited intake of sodium, however, improves blood pressure better than either strategy alone.[61] Furthermore, the lower the sodium intake, the greater the drop in blood pressure. (See How To 12-1, p. 371, for suggestions to limit sodium intake.)

Physical Activity The higher the blood pressure and the less active a person is to begin with, the greater the effect physical activity has in reducing blood pressure. Physical activity helps with weight control, of course, but moderate aerobic activity, such as 30 to 60 minutes of brisk walking most days, along with resistance training on 2 to 3 days per week, also helps lower blood pressure directly.[62] Those who engage in regular physical activity may be able to control mild hypertension without medication.

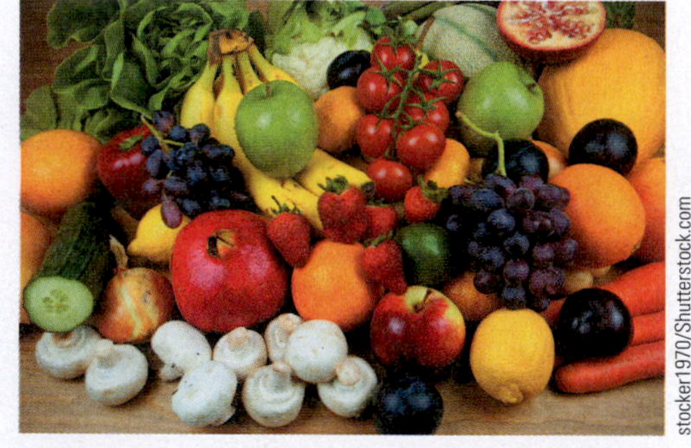

stocker1970/Shutterstock.com

> **PHOTO 18-4** Increasing potassium in the diet helps lower blood pressure and defend against losses caused by some hypertension medicines. The richest sources of potassium are fresh fruits and vegetables of all kinds.

Medications When diet and physical activity fail to reduce blood pressure, diuretics and antihypertensive drugs may be prescribed. Diuretics lower blood pressure by increasing fluid loss and lowering blood volume.

Some diuretics can lead to a potassium deficiency (see Photo 18-4). People taking these diuretics need to include rich food sources of potassium or supplements daily and watch for signs of potassium imbalances such as weakness (particularly of the legs), unexplained numbness or tingling sensation, cramps, irregular heartbeats, and excessive thirst and urination. Blood potassium should be monitored regularly. Although some diuretics can lead to a potassium deficiency, others spare potassium. A combination of these two types of diuretics may be prescribed to prevent potassium deficiency.

Most people with hypertension use two or more medications to meet their blood pressure goals. Using a combination of drugs with different modes of action can reduce the doses needed and minimize side effects.

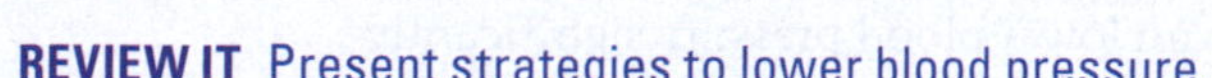

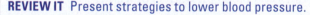

REVIEW IT Present strategies to lower blood pressure.
The most effective dietary strategy for preventing hypertension is weight control. Also beneficial are diets rich in fruits, vegetables, nuts, and low-fat milk products and low in fat, saturated fat, and sodium.

18.5 Diabetes Mellitus

LEARN IT Compare the dietary strategies to manage type 1 diabetes with those to prevent and treat type 2 diabetes.

The incidence of diabetes among children and adults has risen dramatically in recent years (see Figure 18-3). An estimated 29 million people in the United States have been diagnosed with diabetes.[63] As many as 86 million adults have **prediabetes**—their blood glucose is elevated but not to such an extent as to be classified as diabetes. People with prediabetes have a high risk of developing diabetes. Glossary 18-3 (p. 584) defines diabetes terms.

Diabetes ranks seventh among the leading causes of death (review Figure 18-1, p. 570). In addition, diabetes underlies, or contributes to, several other major diseases, including heart disease, stroke, hypertension, blindness, and kidney failure. Cardiovascular disease is a leading cause of diabetes-related deaths. People with diabetes are twice as likely to have heart disease or a stroke as people without diabetes, and at a younger age.[64]

How Diabetes Develops **Diabetes mellitus** includes several metabolic disorders characterized by high blood glucose concentrations and disturbed insulin metabolism. People with diabetes may have insufficient insulin, ineffective insulin, or a combination of the two. The result is **hyperglycemia,** a marked elevation in blood glucose that can ultimately damage blood vessels, nerves, and tissues.

To appreciate the problems presented by an absolute or relative lack of insulin, consider insulin's normal action. After a meal, insulin signals the body's cells to receive the energy nutrients from the blood—amino acids, glucose, and fatty acids. Insulin helps maintain blood glucose within normal limits and stimulates protein synthesis, glycogen synthesis in liver and muscle, and fat synthesis. Without insulin, glucose regulation falters, and metabolism of the energy-yielding nutrients changes.

Diagnosis of Diabetes Diabetes can be diagnosed by one of several tests, including a **fasting plasma glucose** or a nonfasting **A1C.**[65] A fasting plasma glucose test measures plasma glucose after a person has fasted for at least 8 hours to determine whether current glucose levels are within the normal range (see Table 18-8, p. 584). The A1C test measures the percentage of a person's hemoglobin that has glucose attached to it. The higher the percentage, the higher a person's blood glucose levels have been over time. Because red blood cells typically live for about 3 months, the A1C test provides a long-term evaluation of glucose control. Table 18-8 includes A1C values.

Types of Diabetes Mellitus Table 18-9 (p. 584) shows the distinguishing features of the two main forms of diabetes, type 1 diabetes and type 2 diabetes. As the following pages explain, the development of type 1 and type 2 diabetes differs, but some of their complications are similar.

Type 1 Diabetes In **type 1 diabetes,** the less common type of diabetes (about 5 to 10 percent of all diagnosed cases), the pancreas loses its ability to synthesize the hormone insulin. Type 1 diabetes is an **autoimmune disorder.** In most cases, the individual inherits a defect in which immune cells mistakenly attack and destroy the insulin-producing beta cells of the pancreas. The rate of beta cell destruction in type 1 diabetes varies. In some people (mainly infants and children), destruction is rapid; in others (mainly adults), it is slow. Type 1 diabetes commonly occurs in childhood and adolescence, but it can occur at any age, even late in life.

Without insulin, the body's energy metabolism changes, with such severe consequences as to threaten survival. The cells must have insulin to take up the needed fuels from the blood. People with type 1 diabetes must receive insulin either by injection or external pumps; insulin cannot be taken orally because it is a protein, and the enzymes of the GI tract would digest it.

Type 2 Diabetes **Type 2 diabetes** is the most prevalent form of diabetes, accounting for 90 to 95 percent of cases.[66] The primary defect in type 2 diabetes is insulin resistance, a reduced sensitivity to insulin. Consequently, muscle and adipose cells cannot remove glucose from the blood, and blood glucose remains elevated. To compensate, the pancreas secretes larger amounts of insulin, and plasma insulin concentrations can rise to abnormally high levels (hyperinsulinemia). Over time, the pancreas becomes less able to compensate for the cells' reduced sensitivity to insulin, and hyperglycemia worsens. The high demand for insulin can eventually exhaust the beta cells of the pancreas and lead to impaired insulin secretion and reduced plasma insulin concentrations. Type 2 diabetes is therefore associated both with insulin resistance and with relative insulin deficiency; that is, the amount of insulin is insufficient to compensate for its diminished action in cells.

Although the actual causes of type 2 diabetes are unknown, the risk is substantially increased by obesity (especially abdominal obesity), poor dietary habits, smoking, excessive alcohol consumption, aging, and physical inactivity. When

> **FIGURE 18-3 Prevalence of Diabetes among Adults in the United States**

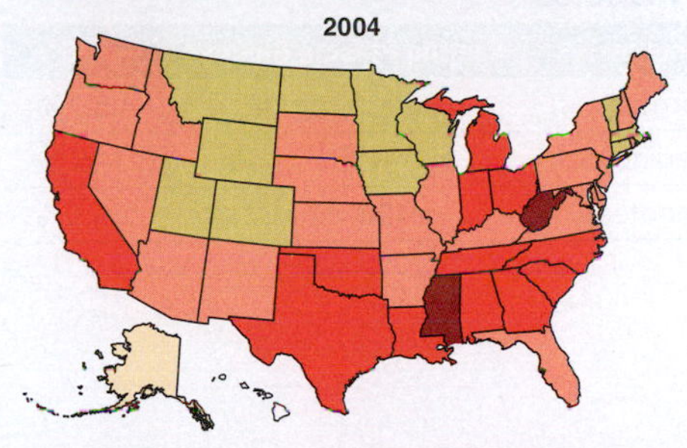
2004

<4.5%	4.5%–5.9%	6.0%–7.4%	7.5%–8.9%	≥9.0%
1 state	11 states	23 states	12 states	2 states

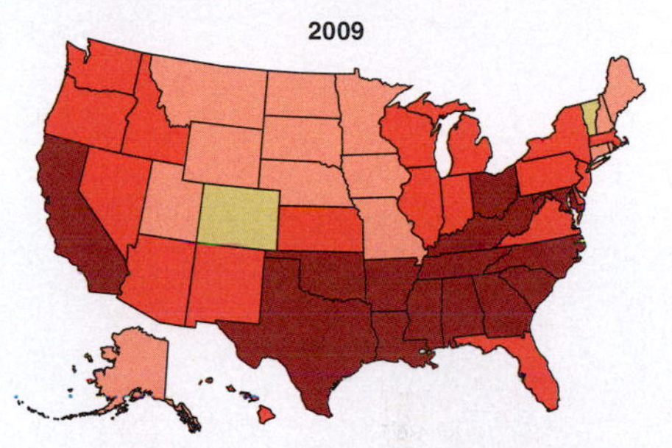
2009

<4.5%	4.5%–5.9%	6.0%–7.4%	7.5%–8.9%	≥9.0%
0 state	2 states	14 states	19 states	15 states

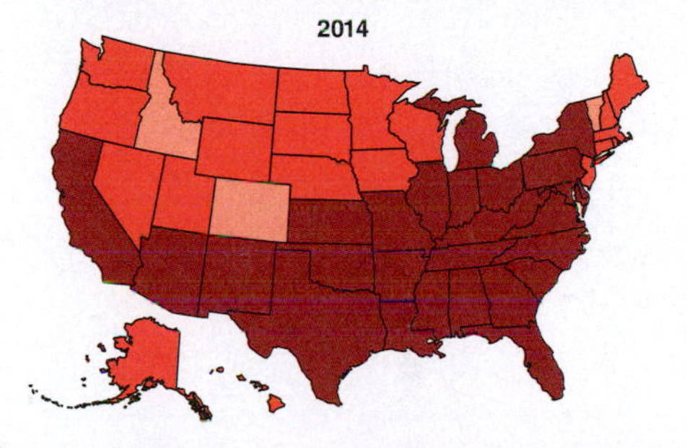
2014

4.5%–5.9%	6.0%–7.4%	7.5%–8.9%	≥9.0%
0 states	3 states	20 states	27 states

hyperglycemia: elevated blood glucose concentrations.

fasting plasma glucose: a test that measures plasma glucose after a person has fasted (no food or kcaloric beverages) for at least 8 hours.

A1C: a test that measures the percentage of hemoglobin that has glucose attached, which helps diagnose diabetes and evaluate long-term glycemic control.

autoimmune disorder: a condition in which the body develops antibodies to its own proteins and then proceeds to destroy cells containing these proteins. In type 1 diabetes, the body develops antibodies to its insulin and destroys the pancreatic cells that produce the insulin, creating an insulin deficiency.

TABLE 18-8 Criteria for the Diagnosis of Diabetes

Diagnosis	Fasting Plasma Glucose	A1C
Normal	70–99 mg/dL	<5.7%
Prediabetes	100–125 mg/dL	5.7–6.4%
Diabetes	≥126 mg/dL	≥6.5%

TABLE 18-9 Features of Type 1 and Type 2 Diabetes

	Type 1	Type 2
Prevalence in diabetic population	5–10% of cases	90–95% of cases
Age of onset	<30 years	>40 years[a]
Associated conditions	Autoimmune diseases, viral infections, inherited factors	Obesity, aging, inactivity, inherited factors
Major defect	Destruction of pancreatic beta cells; insulin deficiency	Insulin resistance; insulin deficiency (relative to needs)
Insulin secretion	Little or none	Varies; may be normal, increased, or decreased
Requirement for insulin therapy	Always	Sometimes
Older names	Juvenile-onset diabetes Insulin-dependent diabetes mellitus (IDDM)	Adult-onset diabetes Noninsulin-dependent diabetes mellitus (NIDDM)

[a]Incidence of type 2 diabetes is increasing in children and adolescence; in more than 90 percent of these cases, it is associated with overweight or obesity and a family history of type 2 diabetes.

people take action to control their lifestyle choices, prevention of type 2 diabetes is not only possible, but likely.[67]

Most people with type 2 diabetes are obese, and obesity itself can directly cause some degree of insulin resistance.[68] As discussed in Highlight 16 (p. 531), obesity has led to a dramatic rise in the incidence of type 2 diabetes among children and adolescents during the past two decades.[69] Inherited factors also strongly influence risk, and type 2 diabetes is more common in certain ethnic populations, including Native Americans, Hispanic Americans, Mexican Americans, African Americans, Asian Americans, and Pacific Islanders.

Inflammation contributes to insulin resistance, and its many links with obesity, metabolic syndrome, and CVD make inflammation central to the development of diabetes as well.[70] Chronic inflammation correlates with increases in blood glucose and decreases in insulin effectiveness.

Complications of Diabetes

In both types of diabetes, glucose fails to gain entry into the cells and consequently accumulates in the blood. These two problems lead to both acute and chronic complications. Figure 18-4 summarizes the metabolic changes and acute complications that can arise in uncontrolled diabetes. Notice that when some glucose enters the cells, as in type 2 diabetes, many of the symptoms of type 1 diabetes do not occur.

Over the long term, the person with diabetes suffers not only from the acute complications shown in Figure 18-4, but also from its chronic effects. Chronically elevated blood glucose alters glucose metabolism in virtually every cell of the body. Some cells begin to convert excess glucose to sugar alcohols, for example, causing toxicity and cell distention—distended cells in the lenses of the eyes cause blurry vision. Some cells produce glycoproteins by attaching excess glucose to an amino acid in a protein; the altered proteins cannot function normally, which leads to a

GLOSSARY 18-3
DIABETES TERMS

diabetes (DYE-uh-BEE-teez): metabolic disorder characterized by elevated blood glucose resulting from insufficient insulin, ineffective insulin, or both; the complete medical term is *diabetes mellitus* (meh-LIE-tus). When blood glucose levels are higher than normal but below the diagnosis of diabetes, the condition is called *prediabetes*.

- **mellitus** = honey-sweet (sugar in urine)

prediabetes: condition in which blood glucose levels are higher than normal but below the diagnosis of diabetes; formerly called *impaired glucose tolerance*. Prediabetes is considered a major risk factor for future diabetes and cardiovascular diseases.

type 1 diabetes: the less common type of diabetes in which the pancreas produces little or no insulin. Type 1 diabetes usually results from autoimmune destruction of pancreatic beta cells.

type 2 diabetes: the more common type of diabetes in which the cells fail to respond to insulin. Type 2 diabetes usually accompanies obesity and results from insulin resistance coupled with insufficient insulin secretion.

> FIGURE 18-4 Metabolic Consequences of Untreated Diabetes

The metabolic consequences of type 1 diabetes differ from those of type 2. In type 1, no insulin is available to allow any glucose to enter the cells. When glucose cannot enter the cells, a cascade of metabolic changes quickly follows. In type 2 diabetes, some glucose enters the cells. Because the cells are not "starved" for glucose, the body does not shift into the metabolism of fasting (losing weight and producing ketones).

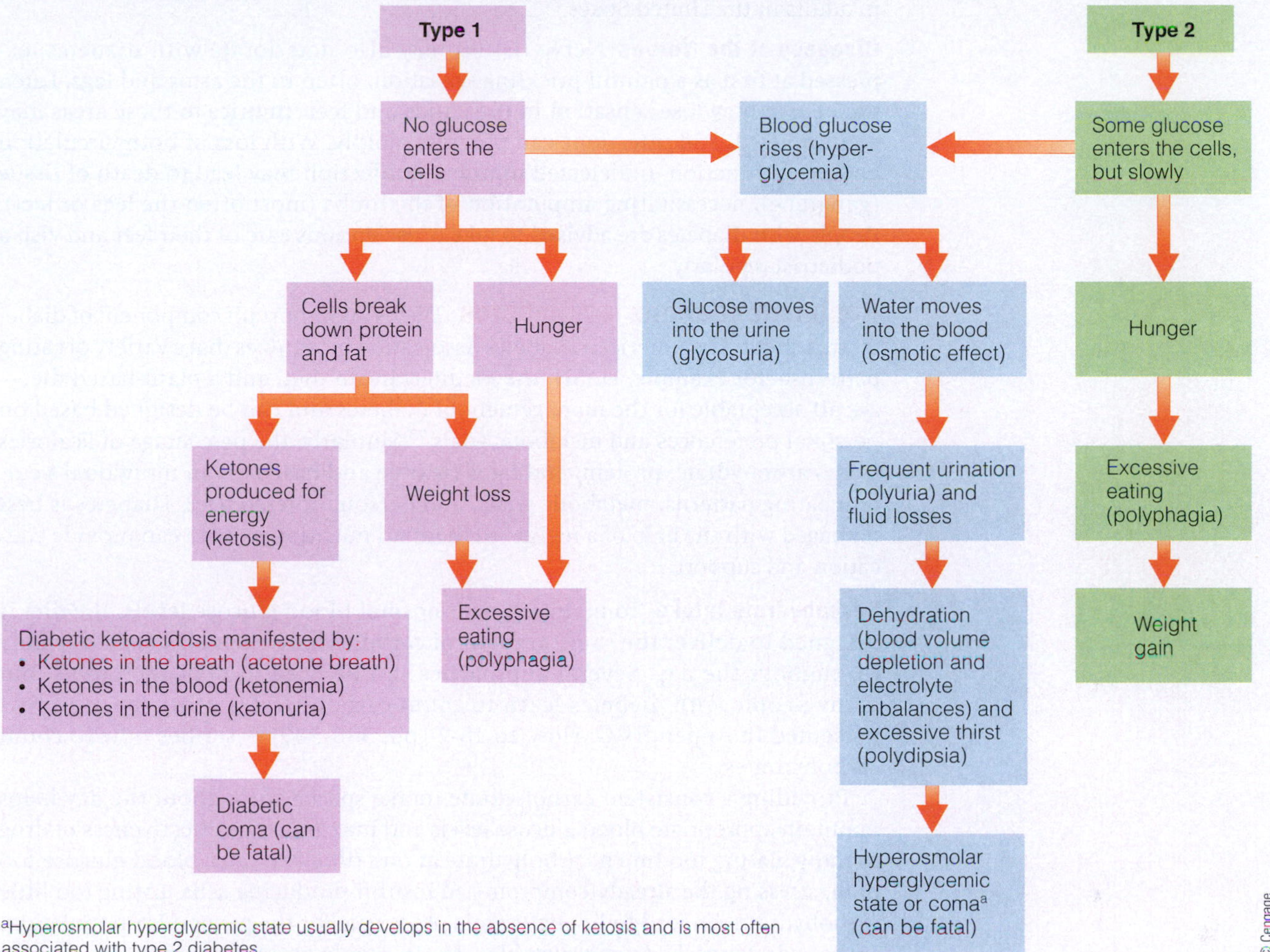

Type 1
Type 2
No glucose enters the cells
Blood glucose rises (hyperglycemia)
Some glucose enters the cells, but slowly
Cells break down protein and fat
Hunger
Glucose moves into the urine (glycosuria)
Water moves into the blood (osmotic effect)
Hunger
Ketones produced for energy (ketosis)
Weight loss
Frequent urination (polyuria) and fluid losses
Excessive eating (polyphagia)
Excessive eating (polyphagia)
Dehydration (blood volume depletion and electrolyte imbalances) and excessive thirst (polydipsia)
Weight gain
Diabetic ketoacidosis manifested by:
• Ketones in the breath (acetone breath)
• Ketones in the blood (ketonemia)
• Ketones in the urine (ketonuria)
Diabetic coma (can be fatal)
Hyperosmolar hyperglycemic state or coma[a] (can be fatal)
© Cengage

[a]Hyperosmolar hyperglycemic state usually develops in the absence of ketosis and is most often associated with type 2 diabetes.

host of other problems. (Attachment of glucose to the hemoglobin protein is the basis of the A1C test for diabetes diagnosis mentioned earlier.) The structures of the blood vessels and nerves become damaged, leading to loss of circulation and nerve function. Poor circulation coupled with glucose-rich blood and urine readily lead to infections. People with diabetes must pay special attention to hygiene and keep alert for early signs of infection. Early, aggressive treatment to control blood glucose significantly reduces the risk of long-term diabetes-related complications.

Diseases of the Large Blood Vessels As mentioned earlier, atherosclerosis tends to develop early, progress rapidly, and be more severe in people with diabetes. The interrelationships among insulin resistance, obesity, hypertension, and atherosclerosis help explain why about 75 percent of people with diabetes die as a consequence of cardiovascular diseases, especially heart attacks. Intensive diabetes treatment that keeps blood glucose levels tightly controlled can reduce the risk of cardiovascular disease among some people with diabetes.[71]* Although intensive therapy is associated with some risks, including an increased risk of abnormally low blood glucose (hypoglycemia), benefits usually outweigh these disadvantages.

*Intensive treatment may be inappropriate for some individuals with diabetes; examples include individuals with limited life expectancy, a history of hypoglycemia, or previous heart disease or multiple heart disease risk factors.

Diseases of the Small Blood Vessels For people with diabetes, disorders of the small blood vessels (capillaries)—called **microangiopathies**—may also develop and lead to loss of kidney function and retinal degeneration with accompanying loss of vision. Diabetes is the leading cause of both kidney failure and blindness in adults in the United States.[72]

Diseases of the Nerves Nerve tissues may also deteriorate with diabetes, expressed at first as a painful prickling sensation, often in the arms and legs. Later, the person may lose sensation in the hands and feet. Injuries to these areas may go unnoticed, and infections can progress rapidly. With loss of both circulation and nerve function, undetected injury and infection may lead to death of tissue (gangrene), necessitating amputation of the limbs (most often the legs or feet). People with diabetes are advised to take conscientious care of their feet and visit a podiatrist regularly.

Recommendations for Diabetes

Diet is an important component of diabetes treatment. The American Diabetes Association recognizes that a variety of eating patterns—for example, DASH, the Mediterranean diet, and a plant-based diet—are all acceptable for the management of diabetes and can be designed based on personal preferences and metabolic goals.[73] Similarly, the percentage of kcalories from carbohydrate, protein, and fat is flexible and based on an individual's current eating patterns, metabolic goals, and personal preferences. Diabetes is best managed with the help of a registered dietitian nutritionist, who can provide education and support.

Carbohydrate Intake To maintain near-normal blood glucose levels, the diet is designed to deliver the same amount of carbohydrate each day, spaced evenly throughout the day. Several approaches can be used to plan such diets, but many people with diabetes learn to count carbohydrates using the food lists presented in Appendix G. How To 18-2 (pp. 588-589) describes how to count carbohydrates.

Providing a consistent carbohydrate intake spaced throughout the day helps maintain appropriate blood glucose levels and maximize the effectiveness of drug therapy. Eating too much carbohydrate at one time can raise blood glucose too high, stressing the already-compromised insulin-producing cells. Eating too little carbohydrate can lead to hypoglycemia. As is true for the general US population, carbohydrate intake from vegetables, fruits, whole grains, legumes, and low-fat or nonfat dairy products is recommended over other carbohydrate sources, especially those that have added fats, sugars, or sodium.[74]

Carbohydrate Sources Different carbohydrate-containing foods have varying effects on blood glucose levels; for example, consuming a portion of white rice may cause blood glucose to rise higher and quicker than would a similar portion of barley. As Chapter 4 described, this *glycemic effect* of foods is influenced by a food's fiber content, the preparation method, the other foods included in a meal, and individual tolerances. For individuals with diabetes, using the glycemic index may provide some additional benefit for achieving glucose control as compared with that obtained by considering only the amount of carbohydrate consumed. In addition, high-fiber, minimally processed foods—which typically have more moderate effects on blood glucose than do highly processed, starchy foods—are among foods frequently recommended for people with diabetes.

Sugar recommendations for people with diabetes are similar to those for the general population, which suggests limiting foods and beverages with added sugars. Of course, sugars and sugary foods must be counted as part of the daily carbohydrate allowance.

Sugar alcohols (such as sorbitol) have lower glycemic effects than glucose or sucrose and may be used as sugar substitutes. Artificial sweeteners (such as aspartame, saccharin, and sucralose) contain no digestible carbohydrate and can also be used in place of sugar.

microangiopathies: disorders of the small blood vessels.

- **micro** = small
- **angeion** = vessel
- **pathos** = disease

Dietary Fat People with diabetes are advised to follow the *Dietary Guidelines for Americans* regarding saturated fat and *trans* fat intake.[75] These recommendations include reducing saturated fat intake to less than 10 percent of kcalories and limiting *trans* fat as much as possible. As is true for the general population, foods rich in omega-3 fatty acids are recommended for those with diabetes because such foods have beneficial effects on lipoproteins and the prevention of heart disease.[76]

Protein An ideal protein intake to control blood glucose or to improve CVD risk factors in diabetes has not been determined.[77] Protein intake goals should therefore be individualized.

Alcohol Adults with diabetes can drink alcohol in moderation. Guidelines are similar to those for the general population, which advise a daily limit of one drink for women and two drinks for men.

Recommendations for Type 1 Diabetes Normally, the body secretes a constant baseline amount of insulin at all times and secretes more as blood glucose rises following meals. People with type 1 diabetes, however, produce little or no insulin. They must learn to adjust the amount and schedule of their insulin doses to accommodate meals, physical activity, and health status. To maintain blood glucose within a fairly normal range requires a lifelong commitment to a carefully coordinated program of diet, physical activity, and insulin.

Nutrition therapy for type 1 diabetes focuses on maintaining optimal nutrition status, controlling blood glucose, achieving a desirable blood lipid profile, controlling blood pressure, and preventing and treating the complications of diabetes. In addition to meeting basic nutrient requirements, the diet must provide a fairly consistent carbohydrate intake from day to day and at each meal and snack to help minimize fluctuations in blood glucose. Further alterations in diet may be necessary for a person with chronic complications such as cardiovascular or kidney disease.

Participation in all levels of physical activity is possible for people with type 1 diabetes who have good blood glucose control and no complications, but they should check with their physician first (see Photo 18-5). One potential problem is hypoglycemia, which can occur during, immediately after, or many hours after physical activity. To avoid hypoglycemia, the person must monitor blood glucose before and after activity to identify when adjustments in insulin or food intake are needed. Carbohydrate-rich foods should be readily available during and after activity to prevent hypoglycemia. Because dietary protein increases the insulin response, but does not increase blood glucose concentrations, carbohydrates rich in protein should not be used to treat or prevent hypoglycemia.

Recommendations for Type 2 Diabetes In overweight people with type 2 diabetes, even moderate weight loss (5 to 10 percent of body weight) can help improve insulin resistance, blood lipids, and blood pressure. Together with diet, a regular routine of moderate physical activity not only supports weight loss, but also improves blood glucose control, blood lipid profiles, and blood pressure. Thus the benefits of regular, long-term physical activity for the treatment and prevention of type 2 diabetes are substantial.[78]

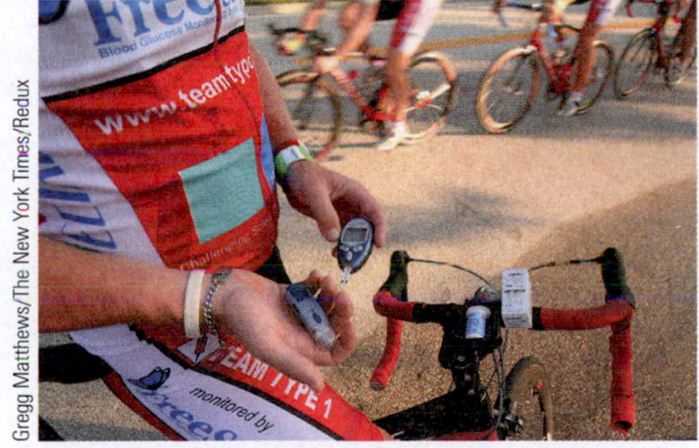
TEAM TYPE 1
monitored by

Gregg Matthews/The New York Times/Redux

> **PHOTO 18-5** Phil Southerland has raced his bicycle across America and checks his blood glucose regularly. With appropriate diet, regular physical activity, frequent glucose checks, and treatment as needed, people with diabetes can achieve their dreams (www.teamtype1.org).

REVIEW IT Compare the dietary strategies to manage type 1 diabetes with those to prevent and treat type 2 diabetes.

Diabetes is characterized by high blood glucose and insufficient insulin, ineffective insulin, or a combination of the two. People with type 1 diabetes coordinate diet, insulin, and physical activity to help control their blood glucose. Those with type 2 diabetes benefit most from a diet and physical activity program that controls glucose fluctuations and promotes weight loss.

>How To 18-2 Count Carbohydrates

Success with carbohydrate counting requires knowledge about the food sources of carbohydrates and an understanding of portion control. Chapter 2 introduced *Choose Your Foods* (p. 47), a food lists approach to diet planning that facilitates carbohydrate counting. Table 18-10 presents food groups from the food lists that contain about 15 grams of carbohydrate; all of these selections are interchangeable. The portion sizes, however, may vary substantially, even among foods within a single food group.

1. The first step in carbohydrate counting is to determine an appropriate carbohydrate allowance. A registered dietitian nutritionist can assess your current carbohydrate intake and help you make adjustments as needed. Carbohydrate allowance may be described in terms of grams or as a percentage of total kcalories. If the allowance is stated as a percentage of total kcalories, you can calculate the carbohydrate allowance in grams. Consider, for example, a person consuming 2000 kcalories a day, with a carbohydrate allowance of 50 percent of total kcalories:

TABLE 18-10 Carbohydrate-Containing Food Groups and Sample Portion Sizes

Bread, cereal, rice, and pasta: 1 portion = 15 g carbohydrate • 1 slice of bread or 1 tortilla • ½ English muffin • ¾ c unsweetened, ready-to-eat cereal • ½ c cooked oatmeal • ⅓ c cooked rice or pasta	**Milk products:** 1 portion = 12 g carbohydrate; may be rounded up to 15 g for ease in counting carbohydrate portions • 1 c milk (whole, low-fat, or nonfat) • 1 c buttermilk • 6 oz plain yogurt
Starchy vegetables: 1 portion = 15 g carbohydrate • 1 small (3 oz) potato • ½ c canned or frozen corn • ½ c cooked beans • 1 c winter squash, cubed	**Sweets and desserts[a]:** Carbohydrate content varies; portions listed contain approximately 15 g • ½ c ice cream • 2 sandwich cookies (with cream filling) • 1 small (¾ oz) granola bar • 5 chocolate kisses • 1 tbs honey
Fruit: 1 portion = 15 g carbohydrate • 1 small (4 oz) apple • 1 medium (6 oz) peach • ¾ c blueberries • ½ c apple juice or orange juice	**Nonstarchy vegetables:** 1 portion = approximately 5 g carbohydrate; 3 servings are equivalent to 1 carbohydrate portion; can be disregarded if fewer than 3 servings are consumed • ½ c cooked cauliflower • ½ c cooked cabbage, collards, or kale • ½ c cooked okra • ½ c diced or raw tomatoes

NOTE: Unprocessed meats, fish, and poultry contain negligible amounts of carbohydrate.

[a]Products sweetened with artificial sweeteners or sugar alcohols contain fewer grams of carbohydrate than products sweetened with sugar or honey.

18.6 Cancer

LEARN IT Differentiate among cancer initiators, promoters, and antipromoters and describe how nutrients or foods might play a role in each category.

Cancer, the growth of **malignant** tissue, ranks just below cardiovascular disease as a cause of death in the United States (see Glossary 18-4). As with cardiovascular disease, the prognosis for cancer today is far brighter than in the past. Identification of risk factors, new detection techniques, and innovative therapies offer hope and encouragement (see Photo 18-6).

GLOSSARY 18-4
CANCER TERMS

antipromoters: factors that oppose the development of cancer.

cancers: malignant growths or tumors that result from abnormal and uncontrolled cell division.

carcinogenesis (CAR-sin-oh-JEN-eh-sis): the process of cancer development.

carcinogen (CAR-sin-oh-jen or car-SIN-oh-jen): a substance that can cause cancer; the adjective is *carcinogenic*.

- **carcin** = cancer
- **gen** = gives rise to

initiators: factors that cause mutations that give rise to cancer, such as radiation and carcinogens.

malignant (ma-LIG-nant): describes a cancerous cell or tumor, which can injure healthy tissue and spread cancer to other regions of the body.

metastasize (me-TAS-tah-size): the spread of cancer from one part of the body to another.

promoters: factors that favor the development of cancers once they have begun.

tumor: an abnormal tissue mass with no physiological function; also called a *neoplasm* (NEE-oh-plazm).

Cancers are classified by the tissues or cells from which they develop:

Adenomas (ADD-eh-NOH-mahz) arise from glandular tissues.

Carcinomas (KAR-see-NOH-mahz) arise from epithelial tissues.

Gliomas (gly-OH-mahz) arise from glial cells of the central nervous system.

Leukemias (loo-KEE-mee-ahz) arise from white blood cell precursors.

Lymphomas (lim-FOH-mahz) arise from lymph tissue.

Melanomas (MEL-ah-NOH-mahz) arise from pigmented skin cells.

Sarcomas (sar-KOH-mahz) arise from connective tissues, such as muscle or bone.

$$2000 \text{ kcal} \times 0.50 = 1000 \text{ kcal of carbohydrate/day}$$
$$1000 \text{ kcal carbohydrate} \div 4 \text{ kcal/g carbohydrate} = 250 \text{ g carbohydrate/day}$$

2. The second step in carbohydrate counting is to distribute the carbohydrate allowance throughout the day's meals and snacks. Knowing that the typical carbohydrate serving equivalent is 15 grams, you can determine how many portions are allowed in a day:

$$250 \text{ g carbohydrate/day} \div 15\text{g/carbohydrate portion} = 16.7 \text{ carbohydrate portions/day (rounded to 17)}$$

3. To maintain steady glucose control, the meal pattern should provide roughly the same amount of carbohydrate each day, spaced evenly throughout the day. Table 18-11 provides a meal pattern that distributes these 17 portions among three meals and two snacks. Now instead of counting carbohydrate grams, you can count the number of portions for each meal or snack. An afternoon snack, for example, would need 2 portions—either a glass of milk with two cookies or a small apple with a granola bar.

TABLE 18-11 Sample Carbohydrate Distribution for a 2000-kCalorie Diet

	Carbohydrate Allowance	
Meals	**Grams**	**Portions[a]**
Breakfast	60	4
Lunch	60	4
Afternoon snack	30	2
Dinner	75	5
Evening snack	30	2
Totals	**255 g**	**17**

NOTE: The carbohydrate allowance in this example is approximately 50% of total kcalories.

[a]1 portion = 15 g carbohydrate = 1 portion of starchy food, milk, or fruit.

Alternatively, some people simply count the grams of carbohydrate provided by foods. When using packaged foods, you can check the Nutrition Facts panel of food labels to find the total carbohydrate content of a serving. If the fiber content is more than 5 grams per serving, it should be subtracted from the total carbohydrate value, as fiber does not contribute to blood glucose. If the sugar alcohol content is greater than 5 grams per serving, half of the grams of sugar alcohol can be subtracted from the *total carbohydrate* value.

Once you have learned the basic carbohydrate-counting method, you can select whatever foods you wish as long as you do not exceed your carbohydrate goals. Although carbohydrate counting focuses on a single macronutrient, it is important to follow a healthy eating pattern that meets other dietary needs as well. Accurate carbohydrate counting often requires instruction and practice in portion control using measuring cups, spoons, and a food scale. Foods lists that indicate the carbohydrate content of common foods are provided in Appendix G.

› TRY IT Using the food listings in Table 18-10, create a 1-day menu of four meals and snacks that provides about 230 grams of carbohydrate. Make sure the carbohydrate intake is spread out fairly evenly throughout the day.

Cancer is not a single disorder. There are many **cancers**; that is, many different kinds of malignant growths. They have different characteristics, occur in different locations in the body, take different courses, and require different treatments.

How Cancer Develops

The development of cancer, called **carcinogenesis,** begins as a single cell that loses control of its normal growth and replication processes. A cancer arises from mutations in the genes that control cell division in a single cell. These mutations may promote cellular replication, interfere with growth restraint, or prevent cellular death.[79] The affected cell thereby loses its built-in capacity for halting cell division, and it produces daughter cells with the same genetic defects. As the abnormal mass of cells, called a **tumor,** grows, a network of blood vessels develops to supply the tumor with the nutrients it needs to support its growth.* The tumor can disrupt the functioning of the normal tissue around it, and some tumor cells may **metastasize** to other regions of the body. Figure 18-5 (p. 590) illustrates cancer development. In leukemia (cancer affecting the white blood cells) the cells do not form a tumor, but rather accumulate in blood and other tissues.

The reasons cancers develop are numerous and varied. Vulnerability to cancer is sometimes inherited, such as when a person is born with a genetic defect that

Steve Bridge/Shutterstock.com

› PHOTO 18-6 People with cancer take comfort from the support of others and from the knowledge that medical science is waging an unrelenting battle in their defense.

*An abnormal mass of cells that is noncancerous is called a *benign* tumor.

> **FIGURE 18-5 Cancer Development**

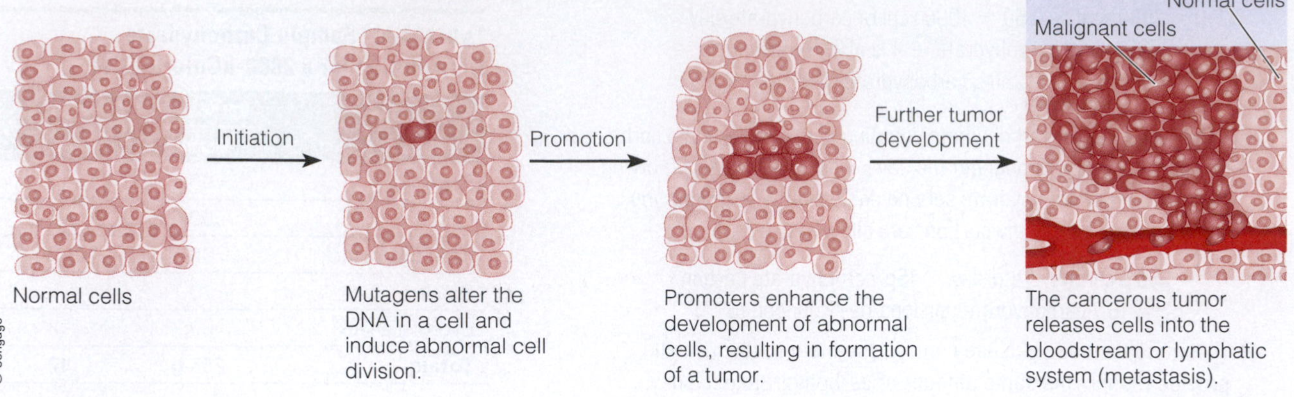

Initiation
Promotion
Further tumor development
Normal cells
Malignant cells
Normal cells
Mutagens alter the DNA in a cell and induce abnormal cell division.
Promoters enhance the development of abnormal cells, resulting in formation of a tumor.
The cancerous tumor releases cells into the bloodstream or lymphatic system (metastasis).

alters DNA structure, function, or repair. A few cancers are linked with microbial infections.[80]* Certain metabolic processes may initiate carcinogenesis, as when phagocytes of the immune system produce oxidants that cause DNA damage or when chronic inflammation enhances the rate of cell division and the risk of a damaging mutation. More often, cancers are caused by interactions between a person's genes and the environment. Exposure to a cancer-causing substance, or **carcinogen,** may either induce genetic mutations that lead to cancer or promote proliferation of cancerous cells.

Environmental Factors Among environmental factors, exposure to radiation and sun, water and air pollution, and smoking are known to cause cancer. Lack of physical activity may also play a role in the development of some cancers.[81] Men and women whose lifestyles include regular, vigorous physical activity have the lowest risk of colon cancer, for example. Physical activity may also protect against breast cancer by reducing body weight and by other mechanisms, such as changes in hormone levels and immune functions not related to body weight.[82]

Obesity itself is clearly a risk factor for certain cancers (such as colon, breast in postmenopausal women, endometrial, pancreas, kidney, and esophageal) and possibly for other types (such as gallbladder) as well.[83] Because different cancers have various causes, obesity's influence on cancer development depends on the site as well as other factors such as hormonal interactions. In the case of breast cancer in postmenopausal women, for example, the hormone estrogen is implicated. Obese postmenopausal women have much higher levels of estrogen than lean women do because fat tissue produces estrogen. Researchers believe that the extended exposure to estrogen in obese women is linked to the increased risk of breast cancer after menopause.[84] The relationships between excessive body weight and certain cancers provide yet another reason to adopt a lifestyle that embraces physical activity and good nutrition.[85]

As Table 18-12 shows, specific dietary constituents are associated with an increased risk of certain cancers. Some dietary factors may initiate cancer development (**initiators**), others may promote cancer development once it has started (**promoters**), and still others may protect against the development of cancer (**antipromoters**).

Dietary Factors—Cancer Initiators Some experts estimate that diet may be linked to as many as one-third of all cancer cases. Consequently, many people think that certain foods are carcinogenic, especially those that contain additives or pesticides. As Chapter 19 explains, our food supply is one of the safest in the world. Additives that have been approved for use in foods are not carcinogens.

---

*Examples include viral hepatitis and liver cancer, human papillomavirus and cervical cancer, and *Helicobacter pylori* bacterium (the ulcer bacterium) and stomach cancer.

TABLE 18-12 Factors Associated with Cancer at Specific Sites

Cancer Sites	Risk Factors	Protective Factors
Breast (postmenopause)	Alcoholic drinks, body fatness, adult attained height,[a] abdominal fatness, adult weight gain	Lactation, physical activity
Breast (premenopause)	Alcoholic drinks, adult attained height,[a] greater birth weight	Lactation, body fatness
Colon and rectum	Red meat, processed meat, alcoholic drinks, body fatness, abdominal fatness, adult attained height[a]	Physical activity, foods containing dietary fiber, garlic, milk, calcium
Endometrium	Body fatness, abdominal fatness	Physical activity
Esophagus	Alcoholic drinks, body fatness, maté[b]	Nonstarchy vegetables, fruits, foods containing beta-carotene, foods containing vitamin C
Gallbladder	Body fatness	
Kidney	Body fatness	
Liver	Aflatoxins,[c] alcoholic drinks	
Lung	Arsenic in drinking water, beta-carotene supplements[d]	Fruits, foods containing carotenoids
Mouth, pharynx, and larynx	Alcoholic drinks	Nonstarchy vegetables, fruits, foods containing carotenoids
Nasopharynx	Cantonese-style salted fish	
Ovary	Adult attained height[a]	
Pancreas	Body fatness, abdominal fatness, adult attained height[a]	Foods containing folate
Prostate	Diets high in calcium	Foods containing lycopene, foods containing selenium, selenium[e]
Skin	Arsenic in drinking water	
Stomach	Salt, salty and salted foods	Nonstarchy vegetables, allium vegetables,[f] fruits

[a]Adult attained height is unlikely to directly modify the risk of cancer. It is a marker for genetic, environmental, hormonal, and also nutritional factors affecting growth during the period from preconception to completion of linear growth.
[b]As drunk traditionally in parts of South America, scalding hot through a metal straw. Any increased risk of cancer is judged to be caused by epithelial damage resulting from the heat, and not by the herb itself.
[c]Aflatoxins are toxins produced by molds or fungi. The main foods that may be contaminated are all types of grains (wheat, rye, rice, corn, barley, oats) and legumes, notably peanuts.
[d]The evidence is derived from studies using high-dose supplements (20 mg/day for beta-carotene; 25,000 IU/day for retinol) in smokers.
[e]The evidence is derived from studies using supplements at a dose of 200 μg/day. Selenium is toxic at higher doses.
[f]This includes vegetables such as garlic, onions, leeks, and shallots.
NOTE: Strength of evidence for all these factors is either "convincing" or "probable."
SOURCES: W. C. Willett, T. Key, and I. Romieu, Diet, obesity, and physical activity, in B. W. Stewart and C. P. Wild (eds.), *World Cancer Report 2014* (Lyon, France: International Agency for Research on Cancer, 2014), pp. 124–133; World Cancer Research Fund/American Institute for Cancer Research, *Food, Nutrition, Physical Activity and the Prevention of Cancer: A Global Perspective* (Washington, DC: AICR, 2007).

Some pesticides are carcinogenic at high doses, but not at the concentrations commonly found on fruits and vegetables. The benefits of eating fruits and vegetables are far greater than the current risks. In fact, results of population studies suggest that fruits and vegetables offer protection against multiple cancers.[86]

Cancers of the head and neck correlate strongly with the combination of alcohol and tobacco use and with low intakes of fruits and vegetables. Alcohol intake alone is associated with cancers of the mouth, throat, breast, and colon, and alcoholism often damages the liver and precedes the development of liver cancer.[87]

Cooking meats at high temperatures (frying, broiling, grilling) causes amino acids and creatine in the meats to react together and form carcinogens.* Grilling meat, fish, poultry, or other foods over a direct flame causes fat and added oils to splash on the fire, creating carcinogens that vaporize onto the food.** Eating grilled food introduces these carcinogens to the digestive system, where they may damage the stomach and intestinal lining. Once these compounds are absorbed into the blood, however, they are detoxified by the liver. To minimize carcinogen formation when grilling, line the grill with foil or wrap the food in foil, take care not to burn foods, and marinate meats beforehand. Research shows that marinades made of beer, especially dark ales, significantly reduce the levels of potential carcinogens in meats.[88]

*These carcinogens are *heterocyclic amines.*
**These carcinogens are *polycyclic aromatic hydrocarbons.*

Evidence from population studies spanning the globe for more than 30 years strongly suggests that diets high in red meat and processed meat (meat preserved by smoking, curing, or salting, or by the addition of preservatives) are a cause of colon cancer.[89] Processed meats are listed among human carcinogens by the World Health Organization (WHO).[90] Compounds that may be carcinogenic are formed during meat processing or cooking. Based on such evidence, replacing most servings of processed meat or red meat with poultry, fish, or legumes and choosing only occasional servings of grilled, fried, blackened, or smoked foods is in the best interest of health.

Another reason to moderate consumption of fried foods such as french fries and potato chips is the presence of acrylamide, a potential carcinogen. Acrylamide is produced when certain starches such as potatoes are fried or baked at high temperatures. In the body, some acrylamide is metabolized to a substance that may mutate or damage genetic material. As such, acrylamide is classified as a "probable human carcinogen." Chapter 19 also discusses acrylamide in foods.

Dietary Factors—Cancer Promoters Unlike carcinogens, which initiate cancers, some dietary components promote cancers. That is, once the initiating step has taken place, these components may accelerate cancer development.

Although studies in animals suggest that high-fat diets may promote cancer, studies in human beings have not proved that the effects of fat are independent of the effects of energy intake and physical inactivity. Overall, the evidence associating fats and oils with cancer risk is limited.[91]

The type of fat in the diet, however, may influence cancer promotion or prevention. Studies of colon cancer implicate animal fats but not vegetable fat, and although a number of studies suggest that omega-3 fatty acids from fish may protect against some cancers, other studies do not support such findings.[92] Researchers note that factors such as total fat intake, the ratio of dietary omega-3 fatty acids to omega-6 fatty acids, an individual's genetic risk of cancer, body fatness, and gender, as well as the specific cancer studied, may all influence the relationship between omega-3 fatty acids and cancer. Such findings underscore the importance of consulting with a health care provider before taking fish oil or other supplements to prevent disease.

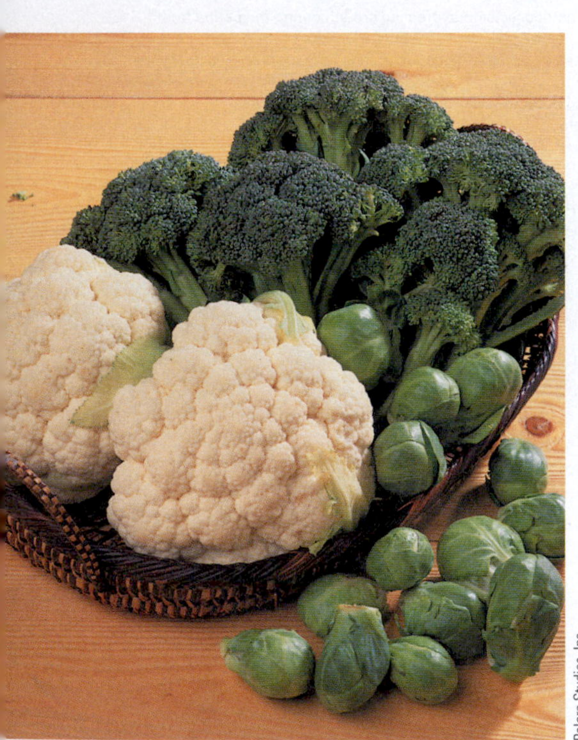

Polara Studios, Inc.

> **PHOTO 18-7** Cruciferous vegetables, such as cauliflower, broccoli, and brussels sprouts, contain nutrients and phytochemicals that may inhibit cancer development.

Dietary Factors—Antipromoters Some foods may contain antipromoters—dietary compounds that defend against cancer. Table 18-12 (p. 591) includes these protective dietary factors. Research on dietary patterns of populations has led to recommendations aimed at reducing cancer risks.

Recommendations for Reducing Cancer Risks

As noted earlier, a diet rich in fruits and vegetables may provide protection against the development of some cancers.[93] Fruits and vegetables contain both nutrients and phytochemicals with antioxidant activity, and antioxidants may prevent or reduce the oxidative reactions in cells that damage DNA. Phytochemicals may also enhance immune functions that protect against cancer development and promote enzyme reactions that inactivate carcinogens. The nutrients and phytochemicals in fruits and vegetables may also reduce the risk of some cancers by way of epigenetic actions such as DNA methylation and gene silencing.[94] For example, the **cruciferous vegetables**—cabbage, cauliflower, broccoli, and brussels sprouts—contain a variety of phytochemicals that defend against certain cancers (see Photo 18-7). Further knowledge and understanding of the roles and interactions among environmental, genetic, and epigenetic factors will help explain cancer development, predict a person's susceptibility, and provide specific treatment recommendations.

Fruits and vegetables, as well as legumes and whole grains, are rich in fiber. As Chapter 4 explained, fiber may protect against cancer by binding, diluting, and rapidly removing potential carcinogens from the GI tract. High-fiber and whole-grain foods also help a person maintain a healthy body weight—another

cruciferous vegetables: vegetables of the cabbage family, including cauliflower, broccoli, and brussels sprouts.

TABLE 18-13 Recommendations and Strategies for Reducing Cancer Risk

Recommendation	Strategy
Body fatness: Achieve and maintain a healthy body weight throughout life.	Follow the USDA Healthy US-Style Eating Pattern for your appropriate energy level. Engage in regular physical activity. Limit consumption of energy-dense foods and avoid beverages with added sugars. Consume "fast foods" sparingly, if at all.
Physical activity: Adopt a physically active lifestyle.	Engage in at least 150 minutes of moderate-intensity physical activity or 75 minutes of vigorous-intensity activity or an equivalent combination throughout the week. Limit sedentary behaviors such as sitting, lying down, watching television, or other forms of screen-based recreation.
Plant foods: Consume a healthy diet with an emphasis on plant foods.	Eat at least the daily amounts of vegetables and fruits recommended by the USDA food patterns. Choose whole grains instead of refined grain products. Limit intake of red meat. Limit refined starchy foods.
Alcoholic drinks: If you drink alcoholic beverages, limit consumption.	Drink no more than two drinks a day for men and one drink a day for women.
Preservation, processing, preparation: Limit consumption of salt-cured foods and processed meats.	Avoid salt-preserved, salted, or salty foods. Limit consumption of processed foods with added salt to ensure an intake of less than 6 grams of salt (2.4 grams of sodium) a day. Avoid processed meats.
Dietary supplements: Aim to meet nutritional needs through diet.	Dietary supplements are not recommended for cancer prevention.

SOURCE: L. H. Kushi and coauthors, American Cancer Society Guidelines on Nutrition and Physical Activity for Cancer Prevention, CA: *Cancer Journal for Clinicians* 62 (2012): 30–67; World Cancer Research Fund/American Institute for Cancer Research, *Food, nutrition, physical activity and the prevention of cancer: A global perspective* (Washington, D.C.: AICR, 2007), pp. 373–390.

preventive measure against cancer. Physical activity also helps maintain a healthy body weight and reduce the risk of some cancers. Table 18-13 summarizes dietary and lifestyle recommendations for reducing cancer risk.

> **REVIEW IT** Differentiate among cancer initiators, promoters, and antipromoters and describe how nutrients or foods might play a role in each category.
>
> Some dietary factors, such as alcohol and heavily smoked foods, may initiate cancer development; others, such as animal fats, may promote cancer once it has gotten started; and still others, such as fiber, antioxidant nutrients, and phytochemicals, may act as antipromoters that protect against the development of cancer. By eating many fruits, vegetables, legumes, and whole grains and reducing saturated fat intake, people obtain the best possible nutrition at the lowest possible risk. Minimizing weight gain through regular physical activity and a healthy diet is also beneficial.

18.7 Recommendations for Chronic Diseases

LEARN IT Summarize dietary recommendations to prevent chronic diseases.

This chapter's discussion of chronic diseases described cardiovascular diseases, hypertension, diabetes, and cancer—four different conditions with distinct sets of causes. Yet dietary excesses, particularly excess food energy and saturated fat intakes, increase the likelihood of all of them.[95] Similarly, all are responsive to diet, and in most cases, the beneficial foods are similar.

Not all diet recommendations apply equally to all of the diseases or to all people with a particular disease, but fortunately for the consumer, dietary recommendations do not contradict one another. In fact, they support one another. Most people can gain some disease-prevention benefits by making dietary changes. To that end, the recommendations presented earlier for reducing the risks of heart disease (Table 18-5, p. 578), hypertension (Table 18-6, p. 581), and cancer (Table 18-13) describe the kinds of foods people should include or limit.

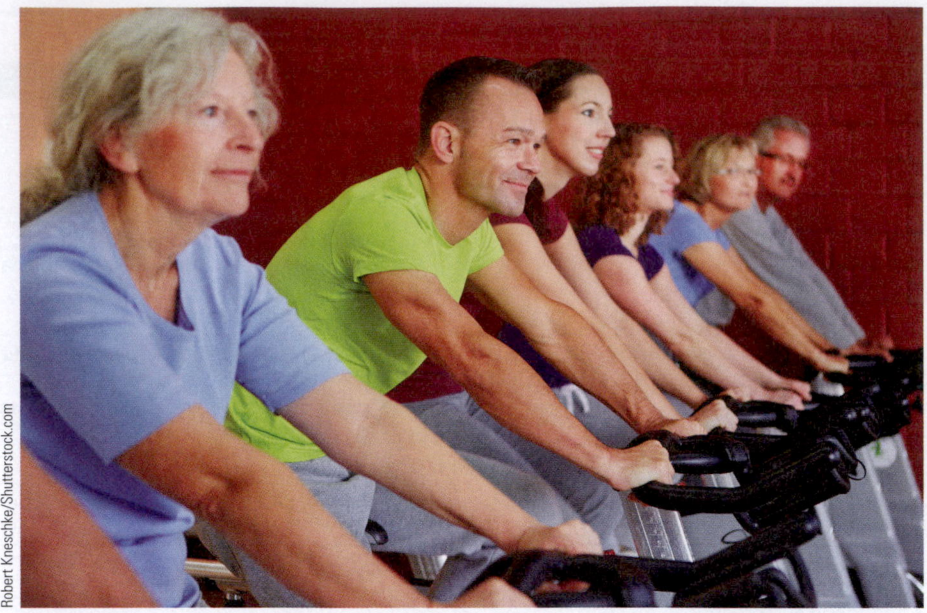

Robert Kneschke/Shutterstock.com

> **PHOTO 18-8** Physical activity and a moderate weight loss of even 10 to 20 pounds can help improve blood glucose, blood lipids, and blood pressure.

(A summary of the *Diet, Nutrition, and Prevention of Chronic Diseases* report from the World Health Organization is presented in Appendix I.)

Several recommendations are aimed at weight control (see Photo 18-8). Obesity is common in the United States, and it is linked with most of the chronic diseases that threaten life (review Figure 18-2, p. 572).[96] The problems of obesity multiply when medical conditions develop. For example, obese people readily develop diabetes, which is often accompanied by high blood pressure and high blood cholesterol. Such a combination of problems may require only one treatment: adopting a healthful diet and regular exercise program.

The USDA Food Patterns and MyPlate offer guidance on selecting a healthy diet, but as Chapter 2 discussed, critics have noted several shortcomings. An alternative plate was created by the nutrition faculty from the Harvard School of Public Health.[97] The *Healthy Eating Plate* (Figure 18-6) is based on their critical review of links between diet and health.

Recommendations for the Population Recommendations to prevent chronic diseases take a population approach and urge all people to make dietary changes believed to forestall or prevent diseases. Such a strategy is similar to national efforts to vaccinate to prevent measles, fluoridate water to prevent dental caries, and fortify grains with folate to prevent neural tube defects.

Recommendations for Individuals Unlike nutrient-deficiency diseases, which develop when nutrients are lacking and disappear when the nutrients are provided, chronic diseases are neither caused nor prevented by diet alone. Many people have followed dietary advice and developed heart disease or cancer anyway; others have ignored all advice and lived long and healthy lives. For many people, though, diet does influence the time of onset and course of some chronic diseases.

To determine whether dietary recommendations are important to you personally, look at your family history to see which diseases are common to your relatives. In addition, examine your personal history, taking note of your body weight, blood pressure, blood lipid profile, and lifestyle habits such as smoking and physical activity.

> **FIGURE 18-6 The Healthy Eating Plate—An Alternative to USDA MyPlate**

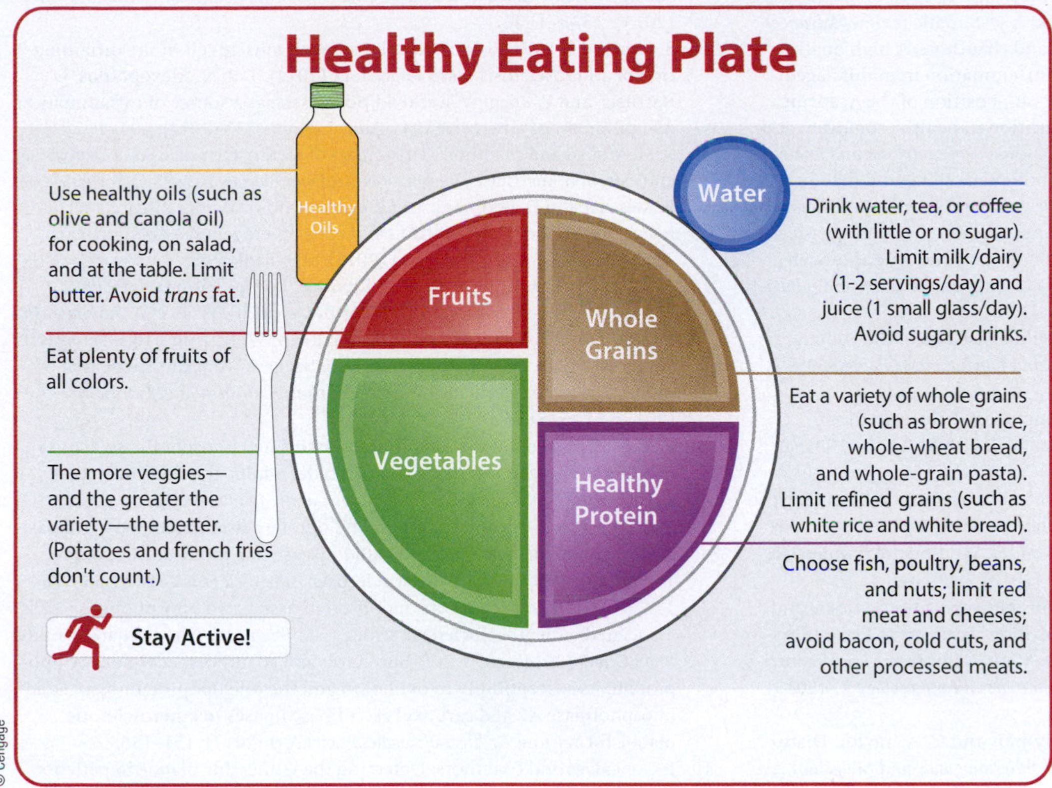

Healthy Eating Plate
Healthy Oils
Use healthy oils (such as olive and canola oil) for cooking, on salad, and at the table. Limit butter. Avoid trans fat.
Eat plenty of fruits of all colors.
The more veggies—and the greater the variety—the better. (Potatoes and french fries don't count.)
Stay Active!
Water
Drink water, tea, or coffee (with little or no sugar). Limit milk/dairy (1-2 servings/day) and juice (1 small glass/day). Avoid sugary drinks.
Fruits
Whole Grains
Vegetables
Healthy Protein
Eat a variety of whole grains (such as brown rice, whole-wheat bread, and whole-grain pasta). Limit refined grains (such as white rice and white bread).
Choose fish, poultry, beans, and nuts; limit red meat and cheeses; avoid bacon, cold cuts, and other processed meats.

REVIEW IT Summarize dietary recommendations to prevent chronic diseases.

Clearly, optimal nutrition plays a key role in keeping people healthy and reducing the risk of chronic diseases. To have the greatest impact possible, dietary recommendations are aimed at the entire population, not just at the individuals who might benefit most. Recommendations focus on weight control and urge people to limit saturated and *trans* fat; increase fiber-rich fruits, vegetables, legumes, and whole grains; and balance food intake with physical activity.

Not all diseases can be prevented through good nutrition, but many can. This chapter has presented the eating and activity patterns that can help people reduce the risk of chronic diseases and promote overall health. In addition to promoting health and preventing chronic diseases, a healthy eating pattern should also prevent foodborne illnesses, as described in the next chapter.

What's Online

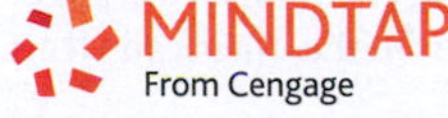

MINDTAP
From Cengage

Visit **www.cengagebrain.com** to access MindTap, a complete digital course that includes Diet & Wellness Plus, interactive quizzes, videos, and more.

REFERENCES

1. R. Micha and coauthors, Association between dietary factors and mortality from heart disease, stroke, and type 2 diabetes in the United States, *Journal of the American Medical Association* 317 (2017): 912–924; S. Onvani and coauthors, Adherence to the Healthy Eating Index and Alternative Healthy Eating Index dietary patterns and mortality from all causes, cardiovascular disease and cancer: A meta-analysis of observational studies, *Journal of Human Nutrition and Dietetics*, September 13, 2016, doi:10.1111/jhn.12415; W. H. Dietz, C. E. Douglas, and R. C. Brownson, Chronic disease prevention: Tobacco avoidance, physical activity, and nutrition for a healthy start, *Journal of the American Medical Association* 316 (2016): 1645–1646; D. Yu and coauthors, Healthy eating and risks of total and cause-specific death among low-income populations of African-Americans and

other adults in the southeastern United States: A prospective cohort study, *PLoS Medicine* 12 (2015): e1001830; S. E. Steck and coauthors, Index-based dietary patterns and colorectal cancer risk: A systematic review, *Advances in Nutrition* 6 (2015): 763–773; J. A. Dias and coauthors, A high quality diet is associated with reduced systemic inflammation in middle-aged individuals, *Atherosclerosis* 238 (2015): 38–44; Position of the Academy of Nutrition and Dietetics: The role of nutrition in health promotion and chronic disease prevention, *Journal of the Academy of Nutrition and Dietetics* 113 (2013): 972–979; M. Ezzati and E. Riboli, Behavioral and dietary risk factors for noncommunicable diseases, *New England Journal of Medicine* 369 (2013): 954–964; A. Fardet and Y. Boirie, Associations between diet-related diseases and impaired physiological mechanisms: A holistic approach based on meta analyses to identify targets for preventive nutrition, *Nutrition Reviews* 71 (2013): 643–656.

2. W. G. van Panhuis and coauthors, Contagious diseases in the United States from 1888 to the present, *New England Journal of Medicine* 369 (2013): 2152–2158.
3. D. F. Warner and V. Mizrahi, Complex genetics of drug resistance in Mycobacterium tuberculosis, *Nature Genetics* 45 (2013): 1107–1108; van Panhuis and coauthors, 2013.
4. V. De Rosa and coauthors, Nutritional control of immunity: Balancing the metabolic requirements with an appropriate immune function, *Seminars in Immunology* 27 (2015): 300–309; P. C. Calder, Feeding the immune system, *Proceedings of the Nutrition Society* 72 (2013): 299–309.
5. F. M. Wensveen and coauthors, Interactions between adipose tissue and the immune system in health and malnutrition, *Seminars in Immunology* 27 (2015): 322–333; J. R. DiSpirito and D. Mathis, Immunological contributions to adipose tissue homeostasis, *Seminars in Immunology* 27 (2015): 315–321; De Rosa and coauthors, 2015.
6. De Rosa and coauthors, 2015; D. E. Berryman and C. A. Taylor, Disturbances in energy balance, in *Biochemical, Physiological, and Molecular Aspects of Human Nutrition*, 3rd ed., eds. M. H. Stipanuk and M. A. Caudill (St. Louis, MO: Elsevier Saunders, 2013), pp. 519–535; B. H. Maskrey and coauthors, Emerging importance of omega-3 fatty acids in the innate immune response: Molecular mechanisms and lipidomic strategies for their analysis, *Molecular and Food Research* 57 (2013): 1390–1400; M. Spite, Deciphering the role of n-3 polyunsaturated fatty acid-derived lipid mediators in health and disease, *Proceedings of the Nutrition Society* 72 (2013): 441–450; L. Paul, P. M. Ueland, and J. Selhub, Mechanistic perspective on the relationship between pyridoxal 5′-phosphate and inflammation, *Nutrition Reviews* 71 (2013): 239–244.
7. DeRosa and coauthors, 2015.
8. K. D. Kochanek and coauthors, Deaths: Final data for 2014, *National Vital Statistics Reports*, June 30, 2016.
9. World Health Organization, 2017, Chronic diseases and health promotion, www.who.int/chp/en
10. B. M. Welch, W. Dere, and J. D. Schiffman, Family health history, *Journal of the American Medical Association* 313 (2015): 1711–1712.
11. A. V. Khera and coauthors, Genetic risk, adherence to a healthy lifestyle, and coronary disease, *New England Journal of Medicine* 375 (2016): 2349–2358; E. Incalcaterra and coauthors, Pro-inflammatory genetic markers of atherosclerosis, *Current Atherosclerosis Reports* 15 (2013): 329–335.
12. D. Mozaffarian and coauthors, Heart disease and stroke statistics—2016 update: A report from the American Heart Association, *Circulation* 133 (2016): e38–e360.
13. American Heart Association, American Stroke Association, *Cardiovascular Disease: A Costly Burden for America, Projections through 2015* (Washington DC: American Heart Association Office of Federal Advocacy, 2017).
14. R. P. Mensink, Effects of saturated fatty acids on serum lipids and lipoproteins: A systematic review and regression analysis, Geneva: World Health Organization, 2016; D. D. Wang and coauthors, Association of specific dietary fats with total and cause-specific mortality, *JAMA Internal Medicine* 176 (2016): 1134–1145; G. Zong and coauthors, Intake of individual saturated fatty acids and risk of coronary heart disease in US men and women: Two prospective longitudinal cohort studies, *BMJ* 355 (2016): i5796; L. Hooper and coauthors, Reduction in saturated fat intake for cardiovascular disease, *Cochrane Database Systematic Reviews* 10 (2015): CD011737; Y. Li and coauthors, Saturated fats compared with unsaturated fats and sources of carbohydrates in relation to risk of coronary heart disease, *Journal of the American College of Cardiology* 66 (2015): 1538–1548.
15. S. Lim and S. Park, Role of vascular smooth muscle cell in the inflammation of atherosclerosis, *BMB Reports* 47 (2014): 1–7; N. Alexopoulos, D. Katritsis, and P. Raggi, Visceral adipose tissue as a source of inflammation and promoter of atherosclerosis, *Atherosclerosis* 233 (2014): 104–112.
16. S. M. Afonso and coauthors, The impact of dietary fatty acids on macrophage cholesterol homeostasis, *Journal of Nutritional Biochemistry* 25 (2014): 95–103; B. Messner and D. Bernhard, Smoking and cardiovascular disease: Mechanisms of endothelial dysfunction and early atherogenesis, *Arteriosclerosis, Thrombosis and Vascular Biology* 34 (2014): 509–515.
17. A. Agrawal, T. B. Gang, and A. E. Rusiñol, Recognition functions of pentameric C-reactive protein in cardiovascular disease, *Mediators of Inflammation*, 2014, doi:10.1155/2014/319215; W. Koenig, High-sensitivity C-reactive protein and atherosclerotic disease: From improved risk prediction to risk-guided therapy, *International Journal of Cardiology* 168 (2013): 5126–5134.
18. P. K. Garg and coauthors, Lipoprotein-associated phospholipase A2 and incident peripheral arterial disease in older adults: the Cardiovascular Health Study, *Atherosclerosis, Thrombosis, and Vascular Biology* 36 (2016): 750–756; P. K. Garg and coauthors, Lipoprotein-associated phospholipase A2and risk of incident cardiovascular disease in a multi-ethnic cohort: The multi ethnic study of atherosclerosis, *Atherosclerosis* 241 (2015): 176–182; M. Katan and coauthors, Lipoprotein-associated phospholipase A2 is associated with atherosclerotic stroke risk: The northern Manhattan study, *PLoS One* 9 (2014): e83393; P. Burchardt and coauthors, Low-density lipoprotein, its susceptibility to oxidation and the role lipoprotein-associated phospholipase A2 and carboxyl ester lipase lipases in atherosclerotic plaque formation, *Archives of Medical Science* 9 (2013): 151–158.
19. I. Goncalves and coauthors, Detecting the vulnerable plaque in patients, *Journal of Internal Medicine* 278 (2015): 520–530; G. Niccoli and coauthors, Advances in mechanisms, imaging and management of the unstable plaque, *Atherosclerosis* 233 (2014): 467–477.
20. E. A. Dennis and P. C. Norris, Eicosanoid storm in infection and inflammation, *Nature Reviews. Immunology* 15 (2015): 511–523.
21. J. Jiang and coauthors, Effect of marine-derived n-3 polyunsaturated fatty acids on major eicosanoids: A systematic review and meta-analysis from 18 randomized controlled trials, *PLoS One* 11 (2016): e0147351; C. Dawczynski and coauthors, Randomized placebo-controlled intervention with n-3 LC-PUFA-supplemented yoghurt: Effects on circulating eicosanoids and cardiovascular risk factors, *Clinical Nutrition* 32 (2013): 686–696.
22. E. L. Schiffrin, Immune mechanisms in hypertension and vascular injury, *Clinical Science* 126 (2014): 267–274; M. van Rooy and E. Pretorius, Obesity, hypertension, and hypercholesterolemia as risk factors for atherosclerosis leading to ischemic events, *Current Medicinal Chemistry* 21 (2014): 2121–2129.
23. S. Sidney and coauthors, Recent trends in cardiovascular mortality in the United States and public health goals, *JAMA Cardiology* 1 (2016): 594–599; D. J. Hunter and K. S. Reddy, Noncommunicable diseases, *New England Journal of Medicine* 369 (2013): 1336–1343.
24. A. Rosinger and coauthors, Trends in total cholesterol, triglycerides, and low-density lipoprotein in US adults, 1999-2014, *JAMA Cardiology* 2016, doi:10.001/jamacardio.2016.4396; Mozaffarian and coauthors, Heart disease and stroke statistics—2016 update: A report from the American Heart Association, 2016, e147–e166.
25. J. D. Berry and coauthors, Lifetime risks of cardiovascular disease, *New England Journal of Medicine* 366 (2012): 323–329.
26. J. T. Cox, K. Chapman-Novakofski, and C.A. Thomson, Practice paper of the Academy of Nutrition and Dietetics Abstract: Nutrition and Women's Health, *Journal of the Academy of Nutrition and Dietetics* 113 (2013): 1544.
27. P. Ganguly and S. F. Alam, Role of homocysteine in the development of cardiovascular disease, *Nutrition Journal* 14 (2015): 6; A. Schaffer and coauthors, Relationship between homocysteine and coronary artery disease. Results from a large prospective cohort study, *Thrombosis Research* 134 (2014): 288–293; B. Debreceni and L. Debreceni, The role of homocysteine-lowering B-vitamin in the primary prevention of cardiovascular disease, *Cardiovascular Therapeutics* 32 (2014): 130–138.

28. Mozaffarian and coauthors, Heart disease and stroke statistics—2016 update: A report from the American Heart Association, 2016, e84–e89.
29. A. V. Khera and coauthors, Genetic risk, adherence to a healthy lifestyle, and coronary disease, *New England Journal of Medicine* 375 (2016): 2349–2358.
30. R. C. Hooqeveen and coauthors, Small dense low-density lipoprotein cholesterol concentrations predict risk for coronary heart disease: The Atherosclerosis Risk in Communities (ARIC) Study, *Arteriosclerosis, Thrombosis, and Vascular Biology* 34 (2014): 1069–1077; N. B. Allen and coauthors, Blood pressure trajectories in early adulthood and subclinical atherosclerosis in middle age, *Journal of the American Medical Association* 311 (2014): 490–497.
31. A. Ramirez and P. P. Hu, Low high-density lipoprotein and risk of myocardial infarction, *Clinical Medicine Insights: Cardiology* 9 (2015): 113–117; H. K. Siddiqi, D. Kiss, and D. Rader, HDL-cholesterol and cardiovascular disease: Rethinking our approach, *Current Opinion in Cardiology* 30 (2015): 536–542; G. K. Hovingh, D. J. Rader, and R. A. Hegele, HDL re-examined, *Current Opinion in Lipidology* 26 (2015): 127–132.
32. Ramirez and Hu, 2015; Siddiqi, Kiss, and Rader, 2015.
33. A. Trpkovic and coauthors, Oxidized low-density lipoprotein as a biomarker of cardiovascular diseases, *Critical Reviews in Clinical Laboratory Sciences* 52 (2015): 70–85; P. Burchardt and coauthors, Low-density lipoprotein, its susceptibility to oxidation and the role of lipoprotein-associated phospholipase A2 and carboxyl ester lipase lipases in atherosclerotic plaque formation, *Archives of Medical Science* 9 (2013): 151–158; A. A. Kalanuria, P. Nyquist, and G. Ling, The prevention and regression of atherosclerotic plaques: Emerging treatments, *Vascular Health and Risk Management* 8 (2012): 549–561.
34. Hoogeveen and coauthors, 2014.
35. A. Tenenbaum, R. Klempfner, and E. Z. Fisman, Hypertriglyceridemia: A too long unfairly neglected major cardiovascular risk factor, *Cardiovascular Diabetology* 13 (2014): 159.
36. Mozaffarian and coauthors, Heart disease and stroke statistics—2016 update: A report from the American Heart Association, 2016, e98–e110; P. A. James and coauthors, 2014 Evidence-based guidelines for the management of high blood pressure in adults: Report from the panel members appointed to the Eighth Joint National Committee (JNC8), *Journal of the American Medical Association* 311 (2014): 507–520.
37. Mozaffarian and coauthors, Heart disease and stroke statistics—2016 update: A report from the American Heart Association, 2016, e111–e124; Y. Huang and coauthors, Association between prediabetes and risk of cardiovascular disease and all-cause mortality: Systematic review and meta-analysis, *BMJ* 355 (2016): i5953.
38. R. V. Same and coauthors, Relationship between sedentary behavior and cardiovascular risk, *Current Cardiology Reports* 18 (2016): 6; Mozaffarian and coauthors, Heart disease and stroke statistics—2016, e41–51; e110–e120; C. K. Roberts and coauthors, Strength, fitness, and body weight status on markers of cardiometabolic health, *Medicine and Science in Sports and Exercise* 47 (2015): 1211–1218; M. Bastien and coauthors, Overview of epidemiology and contribution of obesity to cardiovascular disease, *Progress in Cardiovascular Diseases* 56 (2014): 369–381; M. Hamer, E. Stamatakis, and A. Steptoe, Effects of substituting sedentary time with physical activity on metabolic risk, *Medicine and Science in Sports and Exercise* 46 (2014): 1946–1950; A. Fardet and Y. Boirie, Association between diet-related diseases and impaired physiological mechanisms: A holistic approach based on meta-analyses to identify targets for preventive nutrition, *Nutrition Reviews* 71 (2013): 643–656.
39. G. N. Healy and coauthors, Replacing sitting time with standing or stepping: Associations with cardio-metabolic risk biomarkers, *European Heart Journal* 36 (2015): 2643–2649; C. H. Lin and coauthors, Moderate physical activity level as a protective factor against metabolic syndrome in middle-aged and older women, *Journal of Clinical Nursing* 24 (2015): 1234–1245; Hamer, Stamatakis, and Steptoe, 2014.
40. R. Ross and coauthors, Importance of assessing cardiorespiratory fitness in clinical practice: A case for fitness as a clinical vital sign: A Scientific Statement from the American Heart Association, *Circulation* 134 (2016): e653–e699; J. P. Despres, Physical activity, sedentary behaviours, and cardiovascular health: When will cardiorespiratory fitness become a vital sign? *Canadian Journal of Cardiology* 32 (2016): 505–513.
41. Mozaffarian and coauthors, Heart disease and stroke statistics—2016, e68–e77.
42. G. Zong and coauthors, Intake of individual saturated fatty acids and risk of coronary heart disease in US men and women, two prospective longitudinal cohort studies, *BMJ* 355 (2016): i5796.
43. A. M. Freeman and coauthors, Trending cardiovascular nutrition controversies, *Journal of the American college of Cardiology* 69 (2017): doi: 10.1016/j.jacc.2016.10.086; Mozaffarian and coauthors, Heart disease and stroke statistics—2016, e89–e109; US Department of Health and Human Services and US Department of Agriculture, 2015-2020 Dietary Guidelines for Americans, 8th ed. (2015), health.gov/dietaryguidelines/2015/guidelines/; D. P. Reidlinger and coauthors, How effective are current dietary guidelines for cardiovascular disease prevention in healthy middle-aged and older men and women? A randomized controlled trial, *American Journal of Clinical Nutrition* 101 (2015): 922–930;
P. L. B. Hollaender, A. B. Ross, and M. Kristensen, Whole-grain and blood lipid changes in apparently healthy adults: A systematic review and meta-analysis of randomized controlled studies, *American Journal of Clinical Nutrition* 102 (2015): 556–572; R. G. M. Souza and coauthors, Nuts and legume seeds for cardiovascular risk reduction: Scientific evidence and mechanisms of action, *Nutrition Reviews* 73 (2015): 335–347; R. H. Eckel and coauthors, 2013 HAH/ACC guideline on lifestyle management to reduce cardiovascular risk: A report of the American College of Cardiology/American Heart Association Task Force on Practice Guidelines, *Circulation* 129 (2014): S76–S99.
44. Mozaffarian and coauthors, Heart disease and stroke statistics—2016 update, 2016, e162–e177; A. R. Aroor and coauthors, Maladaptive immune and inflammatory pathways lead to cardiovascular insulin resistance, *Metabolism* 62 (2013): 1543–1552.
45. M. Santaniemi and coauthors, Metabolic syndrome in the prediction of cardiovascular events: The potential additive role of hsCRP and adiponectin, *European Journal of Preventive Cardiology* 21 (2014): 1242–1248.
46. M. Al Rifai and coauthors, The association of nonalcoholic fatty liver disease, obesity, and metabolic syndrome, with systemic inflammation and subclinical atherosclerosis: The Multi-Ethnic Study of Atherosclerosis (MESA), *Atherosclerosis* 239 (2015): 629–633; F. Bonomini, L. F. Rodella, and R. Rezzani, Metabolic syndrome, aging and involvement of oxidative stress, *Aging and Disease* 10 (2015): 109–120; Santaniemi and coauthors, 2014.
47. D. C. Goff and coauthors, 2013 ACC/AHA guideline on the assessment of cardiovascular risk: A report of the American College of Cardiology/American Heart Association Task Force on Practice Guidelines, *Circulation* 129 (2014): S49–S73; N. J. Stone and coauthors, ACC/AHA guideline on the treatment of blood cholesterol to reduce atherosclerotic cardiovascular risk in adults: A report of the American College of Cardiology/American Heart Association Task Force on Practice Guidelines, *Circulation* 129 (2014): S1–S45; R. H. Eckel and coauthors, 2013 AHA/ACC Guideline on lifestyle management to reduce cardiovascular risk: A report of the American College of Cardiology/American Heart Association Task Force on Practice Guidelines, *Circulation* 129 (2014): S76–S99.
48. V. M. Montori, J. P. Brito, and H. H. Ting, Patient-centered and practical application of new high cholesterol guidelines to prevent cardiovascular disease, *Journal of the American Medical Association* 311 (2014): 464–466; J. F. Keaney, G.D. Curfman, and J. A. Jarcho, A pragmatic view of the new cholesterol treatment guidelines, *New England Journal of Medicine* 370 (2014): 275–278.
49. Centers for Disease Control and Prevention, High blood pressure facts, www.cdc.gov/bloodpressure/facts.htm, updated November 30, 2016.
50. Centers for Disease Control and Prevention, High blood pressure fact sheet, www.cdc.gov/dhdsp/data_statistics/fact_sheets/fs_bloodpressure.htm, updated November 30, 2016.
51. Centers for Disease Control and Prevention, High blood pressure facts, www.cdc.gov/bloodpressure/facts.htm, updated November 30, 2016.
52. Mozaffarian and coauthors, Heart disease and stroke statistics—2016 update, 2016, e135–e147.
53. L. Landsberg and coauthors, Obesity-related hypertension: Pathogenesis, cardiovascular risk, and treatment: A position paper of The Obesity Society and the American Society of Hypertension, *Journal of Clinical Hypertension* 15 (2013): 14–33.

54. Landsberg and coauthors, 2013.
55. C. Koliaki and N. Katsilambros, Dietary sodium, potassium, and alcohol: Key players in the pathophysiology, prevention, and treatment of human hypertension, *Nutrition Reviews* 71 (2013): 402–411;T. A. Kotchen, A. W. Cowley, and E. D. Frohlich, Salt in health and disease—A delicate balance, *New England Journal of Medicine* 368 (2013): 1229–1237.
56. Koliaki and Katsilambros, 2013.
57. P. A. James and coauthors, 2014 Evidence-based guidelines for the management of high blood pressure in adults, Report from the panel members appointed to the Eighth Joint National Committee (JNC 8), *Journal of the American Medical Association* 311 (2014): 507–520.
58. Landsberg and coauthors, 2013.
59. M. Siervo and coauthors, Effects of the Dietary Approach to Stop Hypertension (DASH) diet on cardiovascular risk factors: A systematic review and meta-analysis, *British Journal of Nutrition* 113 (2015): 1–15; Eckel and coauthors, 2014.
60. US Department of Health and Human Services and US Department of Agriculture, 2015-2020 Dietary Guidelines for Americans, 8th ed. (2015): health.gov/dietaryguidelines/2015/guidelines/.
61. Eckel and coauthors, 2014.
62. Z. S. Zeigler and coauthors, Effects of standing and light-intensity activity on ambulatory blood pressure, *Medicine and Science in Sports and Exercise* 48 (2016): 175–181; J. E. Sharman, A. LaGerche, and J. S. Coombes, Exercise and cardiovascular risk in patients with hypertension, *American Journal of Hypertension* 28 (2015): 147–158; Eckel and coauthors, 2014.
63. Centers for Disease Control and Prevention, *Diabetes: Working to reverse the US epidemic, at a glance, 2016*, https://www.cdc.gov/chronicdisease/resources/publications/aag/diabetes.htm.
64. Centers for Disease Control and Prevention, *Diabetes: Working to reverse the US epidemic, at a glance, 2016*, https://www.cdc.gov/chronicdisease/resources/publications/aag/diabetes.htm.
65. American Diabetes Association, Classification and diagnosis of diabetes, *Diabetes Care* 40 (2017): S11–S24.
66. American Diabetes Association, Classification and diagnosis of diabetes, *Diabetes Care* 40 (2017): S11–S24.
67. A. L. Feldman and coauthors, Impact of weight maintenance and loss on diabetes risk and burden: A population-based study in 33,184 participants, *BMC Public Health* 17 (2017): 170; J. J. Joseph and coauthors, Physical activity, sedentary behaviors and the incidence of type 2 diabetes mellitus: The Multi-Ethnic Study of Atherosclerosis (MESA), *BMJ Open Diabetes Research and Care* 4 (2016): e000185; A. B. Evert and coauthors, Nutrition therapy recommendations for management of adults with diabetes, *Diabetes Care* 37 (2014): S120–S143.
68. American Diabetes Association, Classification and diagnosis of diabetes, *Diabetes Care* 40 (2017): S11–S24.
69. G. Twig and coauthors, Body mass index at age 17 and diabetes mortality in midlife: A nationwide cohort of 2.3 million adolescents, *Diabetes Care* 39 (2016): 1996–2003; D. Dabelea and coauthors, Prevalence of type 1 and type 2 diabetes among children and adolescents from 2001 to 2009, *Journal of the American Medical Association* 311 (2014): 1778–1786.
70. M. Y. Donath, Multiple benefits of targeting inflammation in the treatment of type 2 diabetes, *Diabetologia* 59 (2016): 679–682; V. R. Richardson, K. A. Smith, and A. M. Carter, Adipose tissue inflammation: Feeding the development of type 2 diabetes mellitus, *Immunobiology* 218 (2013): 1497–1504.
71. American Diabetes Association, Glycemic targets, *Diabetes Care* 39 (2016): S39–S46; M. Teleb and coauthors, Glycemic control and excess cardiovascular mortality in type 1 diabetes, *Current Cardiology Reports* 18 (2016): 29; A. Saremi and coauthors, The effect of intensive glucose lowering therapy among major racial/ethnic groups in the Veterans Affairs Diabetes Trial, *Metabolism* 64 (2015): 218–225; R. A. Hayward and coauthors, Follow-up of glycemic control and cardiovascular outcomes in type 2 diabetes, *New England Journal of Medicine* 372 (2015): 2197–2206.
72. Centers for Disease Control and Prevention, *Diabetes: Working to reverse the US epidemic, at a glance, 2016*, https://www.cdc.gov/chronicdisease/resources/publications/aag/diabetes.htm.
73. A. B. Evert and coauthors, Nutrition therapy recommendations for the management of adults with diabetes, A position statement from the American Diabetes Association, *Diabetes Care* 37 (2014): S120–S143.
74. Evert and coauthors, 2014.
75. Evert and coauthors, 2014.
76. A. Wallin and coauthors, Fish consumption in relation to myocardial infarction, stroke and mortality among women and men with type 2 diabetes: A prospective study, *Clinical Nutrition*, 2017, doi.org/10.1016/j.clnu.2017.01.012.
77. Evert and coauthors, 2014.
78. S. Fan and coauthors, Physical activity level and incident type 2 diabetes among Chinese adults, *Medicine and Science in Sports and Exercise* 47 (2015): 751–756; D. T. Lackland and J. H. Voeks, Metabolic syndrome and hypertension: Regular exercise as part of lifestyle management, *Current Hypertension Reports* 16 (2014): 492; C. P. Earnest and coauthors, Aerobic and strength training in concomitant metabolic syndrome and type 2 diabetes, *Medicine and Science in Sports and Exercise* 46 (2014): 1293–1301; C. K. Roberts , J. P. Little, and J. P. Thyfault, Modification of insulin sensitivity and glycemic control by activity and exercise, *Medicine and Science in Sports and Exercise* 45 (2013): 1868–1877.
79. K. Brinkmann and H. Kashkar, Targeting the mitochondrial apoptotic pathway: A preferred approach in hematologic malignancies? *Cell Death and Disease* 5 (2014): e1098; D. T. Fisher, M. M. Appenheimer, and S. S. Evans, The two faces of IL-6 in the tumor microenvironment, *Seminars in Immunology* 26 (2014): 38–47.
80. American Cancer Society, Infections that can lead to cancer, https://old.cancer.org/acs/groups/cid/documents/webcontent/002782-pdf.pdf, 2016; S. Franceschi and R. Herrero, Infections, in *World Cancer Report 2014*, eds. B. W. Stewart and C. P. Wild (Lyon, France, International Agency for Research on Cancer, 2014), pp. 105–114.
81. S.C. Moore and coauthors, Association of leisure-time physical activity with risk of 26 types of cancer in 1.44 million adults, JAMA Internal Medicine 176 (2016): 816–825; F. T. Frajacomo and coauthors, Aerobic training activates interleukin 10 for colon anticarcinogenic effects, *Medicine and Science in Sports and Exercise* 47 (2015): 1806–1813; W. C. Willett, T. Key, and I. Romieu, Diet, obesity, and physical activity in *World Cancer Report 2014*, eds. B. W. Stewart and C. P. Wild (Lyon, France, International Agency for Research on Cancer, 2014), pp. 124–133; L. H. Kushi and coauthors, American Cancer Society Guidelines on Nutrition and Physical Activity for Cancer Prevention, *CA: Cancer Journal for Clinicians* 62 (2012): 30–67.
82. Willett, Key, and Romieu, 2014.
83. M. Arnold and coauthors, Duration of adulthood overweight, obesity, and cancer risk in the Women's Health Initiative: A longitudinal study from the United States, *PLoS Medicine* 13 (2016): e1002081; M. Song and E. Giovannucci, Preventable incidence and mortality of carcinoma associated with lifestyle factors among white adults in the United States, *JAMA Oncology* 2 (2016): 1154–1161; M. L. Neuhouser and coauthors, Overweight , obesity, and postmenopausal invasive breast cancer risk: A secondary analysis of the Women's Health Initiative Randomized Clinical Trials, *JAMA Oncology* 1 (2015): 611–621; Y. Chen, C. Yu, and Y. Li, Physical activity and risks of esophageal and gastric cancers: A meta-analysis, *PLoS One* 9 (2014): e88082.
84. Willett, Key, and Romieu, 2014; S. Ghosh and coauthors, Association of obesity and circulating adipose stromal cells among breast cancer survivors, *Molecular Biology Reports* 41 (2014): 2907–2916.
85. L. N. Kohler and coauthors, Adherence to diet and physical activity Cancer prevention guidelines and cancer outcomes: A systematic review, *Cancer Epidemiology Biomarkers and Prevention* 25 (2016): 1018–1028; M. Song and E. Giovannucci, Preventable incidence and mortality of carcinoma associated with lifestyle factors among white adults in the United States, *JAMA Oncology* 2 (2016): 1154–1161.
86. M. Stepien, V. Chajes, and I. Romieu, The role of diet in cancer: The epidemiologic link, *Salud Publica de Mexico* 58 (2016): 261–273.
87. C. Scoccianti and coauthors, European Code against Cancer 4th Edition: Alcohol drinking and cancer, *Cancer Epidemiology* 39 (2015): S67–S74; J. Rehm and K. Shield, Alcohol consumption, in *World Cancer Report 2014*,

eds. B. W. Stewart and C. P. Wild (Lyon, France, International Agency for Research on Cancer, 2014), pp. 96–104.

88. O. Viegas and coauthors, Effect of beer marinades on formation of polycyclic aromatic hydrocarbons in charcoal-grilled port, Journal of Agricultural and Food Chemistry 62 (2014): 2638–2643.

89. U. Hammerling and coauthors, Consumption of red/processed meat and colorectal carcinoma: Possible mechanisms underlying the significant association, *Critical Reviews in Food Science and* Nutrition 56 (2016): 614–634; D. Demeyer and coauthors, Mechanisms linking colorectal cancer to the consumption of (processed) red meat: A review, *Critical Reviews in Food Science and Nutrition*, 2015, doi:10.1080/10408398.2013.873886; D. Aune and coauthors, Red and processed meat intake and risk of colorectal adenomas: A systematic review and meta-analysis of epidemiological studies, *Cancer Causes and Control:* CCC 24 (2013): 611–627; M. Di Maso and coauthors, Red meat and cancer risk in a network of case-control studies focusing on cooking practices, *Annals of Oncology* 24 (2013): 3107–3112.

90. Known and probable carcinogens, https://www.cancer.org/cancer/cancer-causes/general-info/known-and-probable-human-carcinogens.html, updated November 3, 2016.

91. Stepien, Chajes, and Romieu, 2016; Kushi and coauthors, 2012.

92. T. M. Brasky and coauthors, Long-chain ω-3 fatty acid intake and endometrial cancer risk in the Women's Health Initiative, *American Journal of Clinical Nutrition* 101 (2015): 824–834; T. M. Brasky and coauthors, Associations of long-chain v-3 fatty acids and fish intake with endometrial cancer risk in the VITamins And Lifestyle cohort, *American Journal of Clinical Nutrition* 99 (2014): 599–608; E. D. Kantor and coauthors, Long-chain omega-3 polyunsaturated fatty acid intake and risk of colorectal cancer, *Nutrition and Cancer* 66 (2014): 716–727. N. M. Iyengar, C. A. Hudis, and A. Gucalp, Omega-3 fatty acids for the prevention of breast cancer: An update and state of the science, *Current Breast Cancer Reports* 5 (2013): 247–254; N. Makarem and coauthors, Dietary fat in breast cancer survival, *Annual Review of Nutrition* 33 (2013): 319–348.

93. Stepien, Chajes, and Romieu, 2016; O. Oyebode and coauthors, Fruit and vegetable consumption and all-cause, cancer, and CVD mortality: Analysis of Health Survey for England data, *Journal of Epidemiology and Community Health* 68 (2014): 856–862; T. Norat and coauthors, Fruits and vegetables: Updating the epidemiologic evidence for the WCRF/AICR lifestyle recommendations for cancer prevention, *Cancer Treatment and Research* 159 (2014): 35–50; L. B. Link and coauthors, Dietary patterns and breast cancer risk in the California Teachers Study cohort, *American Journal of Clinical Nutrition* 98 (2013): 1524–1532.

94. A. M. Jankowska, C. L. Millward, and C. W. Caldwell, The potential of DNA modifications as biomarkers and therapeutic targets in oncology, *Expert Review of Molecular Diagnostics* 15 (2015): 1325–1337; G. Supic, M. Jagodic, and Z. Magic, Epigenetics: A new link between nutrition and cancer, *Nutrition and Cancer* 65 (2013): 781–792.

95. Eckel and coauthors, 2014; Evert and coauthors, 2013; Kushi and coauthors, 2012.

96. S. B. Heymsfield and T. A. Wadden, Mechanisms, pathophysiology, and management of obesity, *New England Journal of Medicine* 376 (2017): 254–266; A. Fardet and Y. Boirie, Associations between diet-related diseases and impaired physiological mechanisms: A holistic approach based on meta-analyses to identify targets for preventive nutrition, *Nutrition Reviews* 71 (2013): 643–656.

97. Harvard School of Public Health The Nutrition Source, Healthy Eating Plate and Healthy Eating Pyramid, https://www.hsph.harvard.edu/nutritionsource/healthy-eating-plate/, 2017.

LEARN IT Present arguments for and against the use of complementary and alternative medicine.

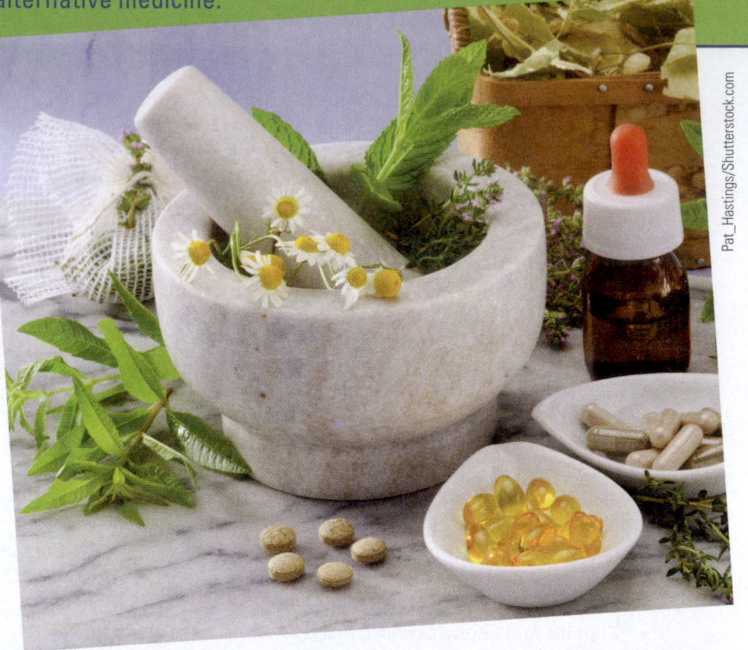
Pat_Hastings/Shutterstock.com

Complementary and Alternative Medicine

If you suffered from migraine headaches or severe joint pain, where would you turn for relief? Would you visit a physician? Or are you more likely to go to an herbalist or an acupuncturist? Most physicians diagnose and treat medical conditions in ways that are accepted by the established medical community; herbalists and acupuncturists, among others, offer alternatives to standard medical practice. Instead of taking two aspirin, for example, you might be advised to chew two fresh leaves of the herb feverfew or to swallow a tincture of white willow bark. Or you might receive a massage and several acupuncture needles.

Complementary and alternative medicine (CAM) has become increasingly popular in recent decades (see Glossary H18-1 for this and related terms).[1] People use these therapies for a variety of reasons. Some want to take more responsibility for both maintaining their own health and finding cures for their own diseases, especially when traditional medical therapies prove ineffective. Others have become distrustful of, and feel overwhelmed by, the high-tech diagnostic tests and costly treatments that **conventional medicine** offers. This highlight explores alternative therapies in search of their possible benefits and with an awareness of their potential harms.

Defining Complementary and Alternative Medicine

By definition, complementary and alternative medicine is not conventional medicine because there is insufficient scientific evidence that it is safe and effective. It includes a variety of approaches, philosophies, and treatments, some of which are defined in Glossary H18-2. When these therapies are used instead of conventional medicine, they are called *alternative;* when used together with conventional medicine, they are called *complementary.* **Integrative medicine** combines conventional medicine and CAM treatments for which there is some high-quality scientific evidence of safety and effectiveness.[2]

A growing number of health-care professionals are learning about alternative therapies; many US medical schools now offer elective courses in alternative medicine or include discussions of these therapies in their required courses. More than ever before, health-care professionals are incorporating some of the beneficial alternative therapies into their practices, thus the gap between conventional medicine and CAM is narrowing.[3]

For some alternative therapies, preliminary and limited scientific evidence suggests some effectiveness; but for most, well-designed scientific studies have yet to determine safety and effectiveness. If proved safe and effective, an alternative therapy may be adopted by conventional medicine. Cancer radiation therapy, for example, was once considered an unconventional therapy, but it proved its clinical value and became part of accepted medical practice. In some cases, a therapy that is accepted by conventional medicine for a specific ailment is used for a different purpose in an alternative therapy. For example, chelation therapy, the preferred medical treatment for lead poisoning, is a common alternative therapy for cardiovascular disease.[4]

Sound Research, Loud Controversy

Much information on alternative therapies comes from folklore, tradition, and testimonial accounts. Relatively few clinical trials have been conducted. Consequently, scientific evidence proving the safety and effectiveness of many alternative therapies is lacking. Some say that alternative therapies simply do not work; others suggest that these therapies have not been given a fair trial. In an effort to "explore complementary and alternative healing practices through vigorous science," the National

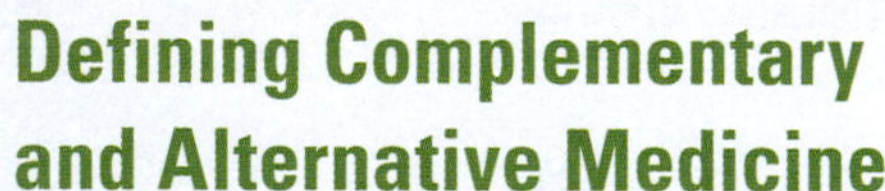

GLOSSARY H18-1

complementary and alternative medicine (CAM): diverse medical and health-care systems, practices, and products that are not currently considered part of conventional medicine; also called *adjunctive, unconventional,* or *unorthodox therapies.*

conventional medicine: diagnosis and treatment of diseases as practiced by medical doctors (MD), doctors of osteopathy (DO), and allied health professionals such as physical therapists and registered nurses; also called *allopathy; Western, mainstream, orthodox,* or *regular medicine;* and *biomedicine.*

integrative medicine: care that combines conventional and complementary therapies for which there is some high-quality scientific evidence of safety and effectiveness. Integrative medicine emphasizes the importance of the relationship between the practitioner and the patient and focuses on wellness, healing, and the whole person.

Center for Complementary and Integrative Health supports clinical trials of these therapies. Articles reporting the results of these clinical trials are available at their website (nccih.nih.gov/research).

Sound research would answer two important questions. First, does the treatment offer better results than either doing nothing or giving a placebo? Second, do the benefits clearly outweigh the risks? Each of these points is worthy of elaboration.

Placebo Effect

Stories abound that credit alternative therapies with miraculous cures. Without scientific research to determine effectiveness, however, one is left to wonder whether it is the therapies or the placebo effect that produces the cure. Recall from Chapter 1 that giving a placebo often brings about a healing effect in people who believe they are receiving the treatment.[5] Conventional medicine tends to neglect this powerful remedy, whereas many alternative therapies embrace it.

Risks versus Benefits

Ideally, a therapy provides benefits with little or no risk. Figure H18-1 (p. 602) presents several examples of herbal remedies that appear to be generally safe and possibly effective in treating various conditions.[6] Such findings, if replicated, hold promise that these alternative therapies may one day be integrated into conventional medicine.

Some alternative therapies are innocuous, providing little or no benefit for little or no risk. Sipping a cup of warm tea with a pleasant aroma, for example, won't cure heart disease, but it may improve one's mood and help relieve tension. Given no physical hazard and little financial risk, such therapies are acceptable.

In contrast, other products and procedures are downright dangerous, posing great risks while providing no benefits. One example is the folk practice of geophagia (eating earth or clay), which can cause GI impaction and impair iron absorption. Another is the taking of laetrile to treat cancer, which can cause cyanide poisoning. Clearly, such therapies are too harmful to be used.

Perhaps most controversial are alternative therapies that may provide benefits, but also carry significant, unknown, or debatable risks. Smoking or ingesting marijuana is an example of such an alternative therapy.[7] The compounds in marijuana seem to provide relief from symptoms such as nausea, vomiting, and pain that commonly accompany cancer, AIDS, and other diseases, but marijuana use also poses risks that some people consider acceptable whereas others deem them intolerable. Figure H18-2 (p. 602) summarizes the relationships between risks and benefits.

Nutrition-Related Alternative Therapies

Most alternative therapies fall outside the field of nutrition, but nutrition itself can be an alternative therapy. Furthermore, many alternative therapies prescribe specific dietary regimens even though most practitioners are not registered dietitian nutritionists (see Highlight 1, p. 28). Nutrition-related alternative therapies include the use of foods, vitamin and mineral supplements, and herbs to prevent and treat illnesses.

GLOSSARY H18-2

CAM TERMS

acupuncture (AK-you-PUNK-cher): a technique that involves piercing the skin with long thin needles at specific anatomical points to relieve pain or illness. Acupuncture sometimes uses heat, pressure, friction, suction, or electromagnetic energy to stimulate the points.

aroma therapy: a technique that uses oil extracts from plants and flowers (usually applied by massage or baths) to enhance physical, psychological, and spiritual health.

ayurveda (AH-your-VAY-dah): a traditional Hindu system of improving health by using herbs, diet, meditation, massage, and yoga to stimulate the body, mind, and spirit to prevent and treat disease.

bioelectromagnetic medical applications: the use of electrical energy, magnetic energy, or both to stimulate bone repair, wound healing, and tissue regeneration.

biofeedback: the use of special devices to convey information about heart rate, blood pressure, skin temperature, muscle relaxation, and other body functions to enable a person to learn how to consciously control these medically important activities.

biofield therapeutics: a manual healing method that directs a healing force from an outside source (commonly God or another supernatural being) through the practitioner and into the client's body; commonly known as "laying on of hands."

cartilage therapy: the use of cleaned and powdered connective tissue, such as collagen, to improve health.

chelation (kee-LAY-shun) therapy: the use of ethylene diamine tetraacetic acid (EDTA) to bind with metallic ions, thus healing the body by removing toxic metals.

chiropractic (KYE-roh-PRAK-tik) **manipulation:** a manual healing method of adjusting the spine to restore health.

faith healing: healing by invoking divine intervention without the use of medical, surgical, or other traditional therapy.

herbal (ERB-al) **medicine:** the use of plants to treat disease or improve health; also known as *botanical medicine* or *phytotherapy*.

homeopathy (hoh-me-OP-ah-thee): a practice based on the theory that "like cures like," that is, that substances that cause symptoms in healthy people can cure those symptoms when given in very dilute amounts.

- **homeo** = like
- **pathos** = suffering

hydrotherapy: the use of water (in whirlpools, as douches, or packed as ice, for example) to promote relaxation and healing.

hypnotherapy: a technique that uses hypnosis and the power of suggestion to improve health behaviors, relieve pain, and heal.

imagery: a technique that guides clients to achieve a desired physical, emotional, or spiritual state by visualizing themselves in that state.

iridology: the study of changes in the iris of the eye and their relationships to disease.

macrobiotic diet: a philosophical eating pattern based on mostly plant foods such as whole grains, legumes, and vegetables, with small amounts of fish, fruits, nuts, and seeds.

- **macro** = large, great
- **biotic** = life

massage therapy: a healing method in which the therapist manually kneads muscles to reduce tension, increase blood circulation, improve joint mobility, and promote healing of injuries.

meditation: a self-directed technique of relaxing the body and calming the mind.

naturopathic (nay-chur-oh-PATH-ick) **medicine:** a system that taps the natural healing forces within the body by integrating several practices, including traditional medicine, herbal medicine, clinical nutrition, homeopathy, acupuncture, East Asian medicine, hydrotherapy, and manipulative therapy.

orthomolecular medicine: the use of large doses of vitamins to treat chronic disease.

ozone therapy: the use of ozone gas to enhance the body's immune system.

qi gong (chee GUNG): a Chinese system that combines movement, meditation, and breathing techniques to enhance the flow of *qi* (vital energy) in the body.

> **FIGURE H18-1 Examples of Herbal Remedies**

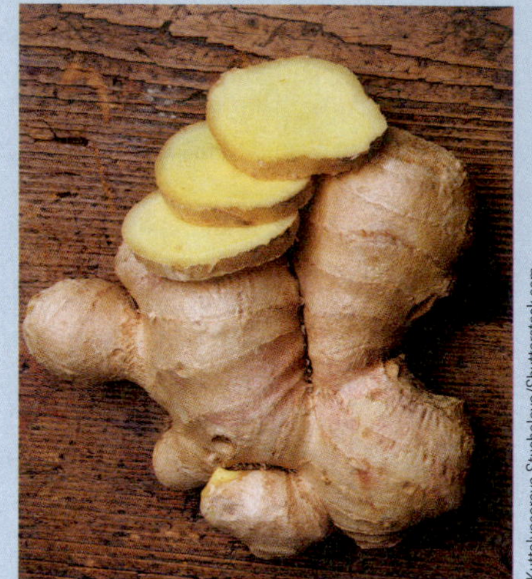

Kuttelvaserova Stuchelova/Shutterstock.com

Ginger may relieve nausea and vomiting due to motion sickness or pregnancy.

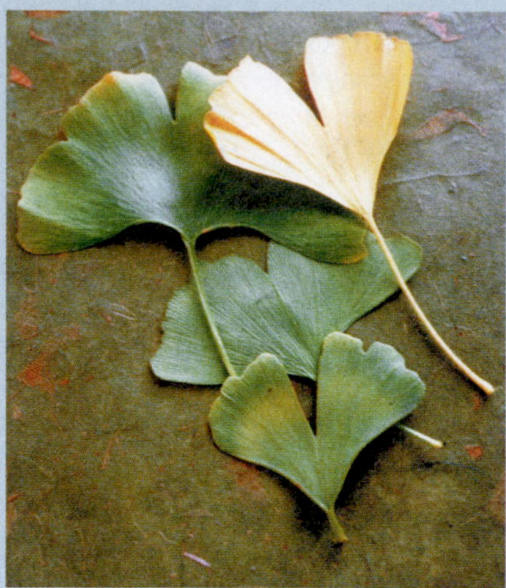

James Worrell/Getty Images

Ginkgo may slow the loss of cognitive function associated with aging.

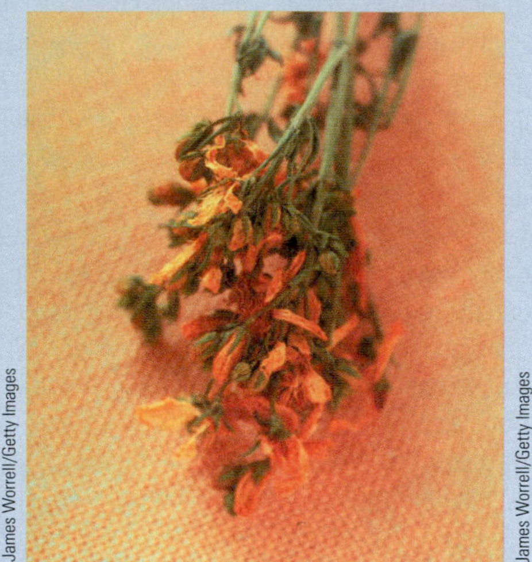

James Worrell/Getty Images

St. John's wort may be effective in treating mild depression.

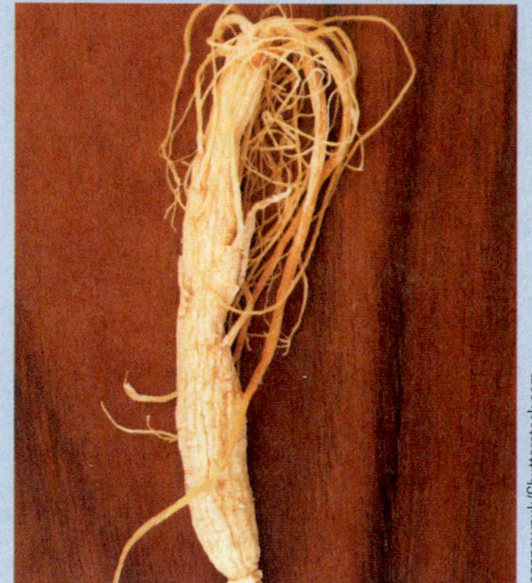

joannawnuk/Shutterstock.com

American ginseng may improve glucose control in people with type 2 diabetes.

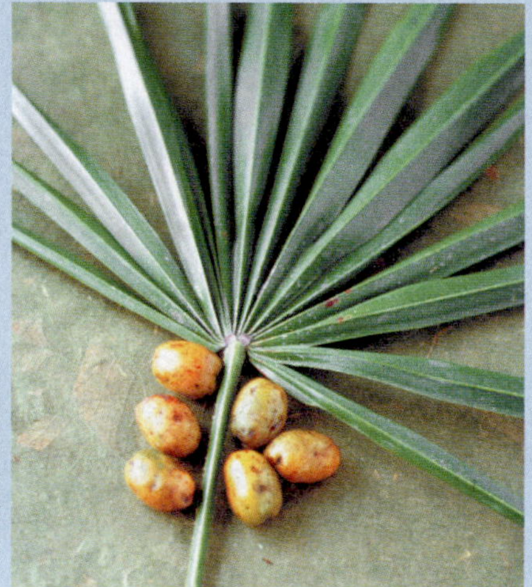

James Worrell/Getty Images

Saw palmetto may improve the symptoms associated with an enlarged prostate.

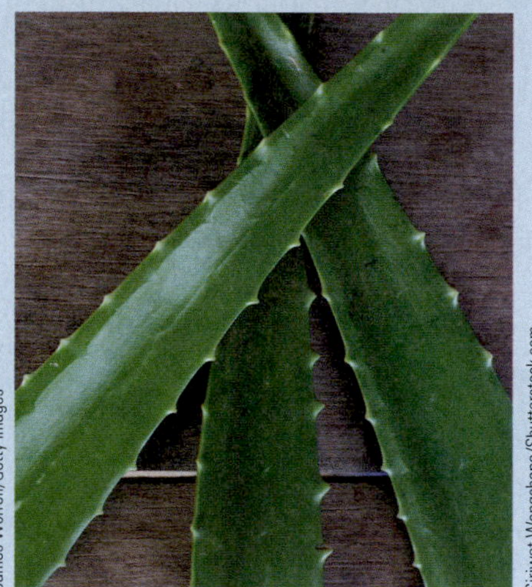

Siriwat Wongchana/Shutterstock.com

The gel of an aloe vera plant soothes a minor burn.

> **FIGURE H18-2 Risk-Benefit Relationships**

RISK: No (or little) → Much

BENEFIT: No (or little) → Much

BENEFIT \ RISK	No (or little)	Much
Much	**Ideal situation** Benefits with little or no risk (Accept)	**Cautionary situation** Possible benefits with great or unknown risks (Consider carefully)
No (or little)	**Neutral situation** Little or no benefit with little or no risk (Accept or reject as preferred)	**Dangerous situation** No benefits with great risks (Reject)

Foods

The many dietary recommendations presented throughout this text are based on scientific evidence and do *not* fall into the alternative therapies category; strategies that are still experimental, however, do. For example, alternative therapists may recommend macrobiotic diets to help prevent chronic diseases, whereas most registered dietitian nutritionists would advise people to eat a balanced diet that includes servings from each of the five food groups. Similarly, enough scientific evidence is available to recommend including soy foods in the diet to protect against heart disease—but not to determine whether the phytoestrogens of soy supplements are safe or beneficial in managing the symptoms of menopause.[8]

Highlight 13 explored the potential health benefits of soy and many other functional foods and concludes that no one food is magical. As part of a balanced diet, these foods can support good health and protect against disease. Importantly, the benefits derive from a variety of *foods.* More research is needed to determine the safety and effectiveness of taking supplements of the nutrients and phytochemicals found in these foods.

Vitamin and Mineral Supplements

Like foods, vitamin and mineral supplements may fall into either the conventional or the alternative realm of medicine. For example, conventional advice recommends consuming 400 micrograms of folate to prevent neural tube defects, but not the taking of 1000 milligrams of vitamin C to prevent the common cold. Highlight 10 examined the appropriate use of supplements and potential dangers of excessive intakes.

As research on nutrition and chronic diseases has revealed many of the roles played by the vitamins and minerals in supporting health, conventional medicine has warmed up to the possibility that vitamin and mineral supplements might be an appropriate preventive therapy.[9] Some vitamin and mineral supplements appear to be in transition from alternative medicine to conventional medicine; that is, they have begun to prove their safety and effectiveness. Herbal remedies, however, still remain clearly in the realm of complementary and alternative medicine.

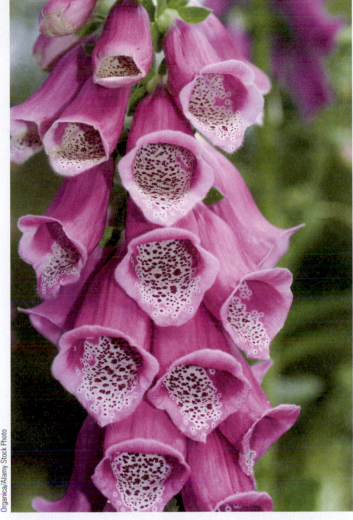

Organica/Alamy Stock Photo

> **PHOTO H18-1** Digoxin, the most commonly prescribed heart medication, derives from the leaves of the foxglove plant *(Digitalis purpurea).*

Herbal Remedies

From earliest times, people have used myriad herbs and other plants to cure aches and ills with varying degrees of success (review Figure H18-1). In fact, today's pharmaceutical industry originated from the use of plant-derived products for human health.[10] Upon scientific study, dozens of these folk remedies reveal their secrets (see Photo H18-1). For example, myrrh, a plant resin used as a painkiller in ancient times, does indeed have an analgesic effect. The herb valerian, which has long been used as a tranquilizer, contains oils that have a sedative effect. Senna leaves, brewed as a laxative tea, produce compounds that act as a potent cathartic drug. Green tea, brewed from the dried leaves of *Camellia sinensis,* contains phytochemicals that induce cancer cells to self-destruct. Naturally occurring salicylates provide the same protective effects as low doses of aspirin. Salicylates are found in spices such as curry, paprika, and thyme; fruits; vegetables; teas; and candies flavored with wintergreen (methylsalicylate).

Beneficial compounds from wild species contribute to about half of our modern medicines. By analyzing these compounds, pharmaceutical labs can synthesize pure forms of the drugs. Unlike herbs and wild species, which vary from batch to batch, synthesized medicines deliver exact dosages. By synthesizing drugs, we are also able to conserve endangered species. Consider that it took all of the bark from one 40-foot-tall, 100-year-old Pacific yew tree to produce one 300 milligram dose of the anticancer drug paclitaxel (Taxol), until scientists learned how to synthesize it. Many yet undiscovered cures may be forever lost as wild species are destroyed, long before their secrets are revealed to medicine.

Herbal Precautions

Plants are "natural," but that does not mean all plants are beneficial or even safe.[11] Nothing could be more natural—and deadly—than the poisonous herb hemlock. Several herbal remedies have toxic effects. The popular Chinese herbal potion jin bu huan, which is used as a pain and insomnia remedy, has been linked with several cases of acute hepatitis. Lead poisoning and anemia have been associated with popular herbal medications made in India.[12] Germanium, a nonessential mineral commonly found in many herbal products, has been associated with chronic kidney failure. Paraguay tea produces symptoms of agitation, confusion, flushed skin, and fever. Kombucha tea, commonly used in the hopes of preventing cancer, relieving arthritis, curing insomnia, and stimulating hair regrowth, can cause severe metabolic acidosis. Table H18-1 provides an overview of selected herbs.[13]

Although some people use herbs to treat or prevent disease, herbs are not regulated as drugs; they are considered dietary supplements. The Food and Drug Administration (FDA) does not evaluate dietary supplements for safety or effectiveness, nor does it monitor their contents. Under the Dietary Supplement Health and Education Act, rather than the herb manufacturers having to prove the safety of their products, the FDA has the burden of proving that a product is not safe. Consequently, consumers may lack information about or find discrepancies regarding:

- *True identification of herbs.* Most mint teas are safe, for instance, but some varieties contain the highly toxic pennyroyal oil. Mistakenly used to soothe a colicky baby, mint tea laden with pennyroyal has been blamed for the liver and neurological injuries of at least two infants, one of whom died.
- *Purity of herbal preparations.* A young child diagnosed with lead poisoning had been given an herbal vitamin that contained large quantities of lead and mercury for 4 years. Twelve cases of lead poisoning among adults using ayurvedic remedies were reported to the Centers for Disease Control and Prevention in recent years. In New York, investigators found six cases of lead poisoning in pregnant women who had taken ayurvedic medications made in India. Some of the medications also contained mercury or arsenic.
- *Appropriate uses and contraindications of herbs.* Herbal remedies alone may be appropriate for minor ailments—a cup of chamomile tea to ease gastric discomfort or the gel of an aloe vera plant to soothe a sunburn, for example—but not for major health problems such as cancer or AIDS.
- *Effectiveness of herbs.* Herbal remedies may claim to work wonders without having to prove effectiveness. Research studies often report conflicting findings, with some suggesting a benefit and others indicating no effectiveness.
- *Variability of herbs.* Not all species are created equal. The various species of coneflower provide an example. *Echinacea purpurea,* for example, may help in the early treatment of colds, but *Echinacea augustifolia* may not. Similarly, not all parts of a plant provide the same compounds. Leaves, roots, and oils contain different compounds and extracts, and the temperatures used during manufacturing may affect their potency. Consumers are not always aware of such differences, and manufacturers do not always make such distinctions when preparing and labeling supplements.
- *Accuracy of labels.* Supplements may contain none of an herb or mixed species, and labels are often inaccurate. More often than not, supplements do not contain the species or the quantities of active ingredients stated on their labels.[14] In several cases, supplements do not even contain herbs, but drugs that are known to interact with prescription medicines and lower blood pressure to dangerous levels. Such discrepancies in the contents of supplements can be dangerous to the consumer, interfere with scientific research, and make it difficult to interpret the findings. Consumers may want to shop for supplements bearing a logo from either US Pharmacopeia or Consumer Lab indicating that the contents have been analyzed and found to contain the ingredients and quantities listed on the label.
- *Safe dosages of herbs.* Herbs may contain active ingredients—compounds that affect the body. Each of these active ingredients has a different potency, time of onset, duration of activity, and consequent effects, making the plant itself too unpredictable to be useful. Foxglove leaves, for example, contain dozens of compounds that have an effect on the heart; digoxin, a drug derived from foxglove, offers a standard dosage that allows for a more predictable cardiac response. Even when herbs are manufactured into capsules or liquids, their concentrations of active ingredients differ dramatically from batch to batch and from the quantities stated on the labels.
- *Interactions of herbs with medicines and other herbs.* Like drugs, herbs may interfere with, or potentiate, the effects of other herbs and drugs (see Table H18-2, p. 606).[15] A person taking both cardiac medication and the herb foxglove may be headed for disaster from the combined effect on the heart. Similarly, taking St. John's wort with medicines used to treat heart disease, depression, seizures, and certain cancers might diminish or exaggerate the intended effects.[16] Because *Ginkgo biloba* impairs blood clotting, it can cause bleeding problems for people taking aspirin or other blood-thinning medicines regularly.[17]
- *Adverse reactions and toxicity levels of herbs.* Herbs may produce undesirable reactions. The herbal root kava, commonly used to treat anxiety and insomnia, can cause liver abnormalities and may have such a sedating effect as to impair driving. Chinese herbal treatments containing *Aristolochia fangchi* are known to cause kidney damage and cancers. Table H18-1 includes risks associated with commonly used herbs. To ensure the safety and standardization of herbal remedies, Congress may need to establish new regulations.

Because herbal medicines are sold as dietary supplements, their labels cannot claim to cure a disease, but they can make various other claims. Not surprisingly, when a label claims that an herbal product may strengthen immunity, improve memory, support

TABLE H18-1 Overview of Selected Herbs

Common and Scientific Names	Claims	Research Findings	Risks[a]
Aloe (gel) *Aloe vera*	Promote wound healing	May help heal minor burns and abrasions; may cause infections in severe wounds	Generally considered safe
Black cohosh (stems and roots) *Actaea racemosa, Cimifuga racemosa*	Ease menopause symptoms	Conflicting evidence	May cause headaches, stomach discomfort, liver damage
Chamomile (flowers) *Matricaria recutita, Chamomilla recutita*	Relieve indigestion	Little evidence available	Generally considered safe
Chaparral (leaves and twigs) *Larrea tridentata*	Slow aging, "cleanse" blood, heal wounds, cure cancer, treat acne	No evidence available	Acute, toxic hepatitis; liver damage
Cinnamon (bark) *Cinnamomum zeylanicum, C. cassia*	Relieve indigestion, lower blood glucose and blood lipids	May lower blood glucose in type 2 diabetes	May have a blood-thinning effect; not safe for pregnant women or those taking diabetes medication
Comfrey (leafy plant) *Symphytum officinale, S. asperum, S. x uplandicum*	Soothe nerves	No evidence available	Liver damage
Echinacea (roots) *Echinacea angustifolia, E. pallida, E. purpurea*	Alleviate symptoms of colds, flus, and infections; promote wound healing; boost immunity	Ineffective in preventing colds or other infections	Generally considered safe; may cause headache, dizziness, nausea
Ephedra (stems) *Ephedra sinica*	Promote weight loss	Little evidence available; FDA has banned the sale of ephedra-containing products	Rapid heart rate, tremors, seizures, insomnia, headaches, hypertension
Feverfew (leaves) *Tanacetum parthenium*	Prevent migraine headaches	May prevent migraine headaches	Generally considered safe; may cause mouth irritation, swelling, ulcers, and GI distress
Garlic (bulbs) *Allium sativum*	Lower blood lipids and blood pressure	May lower blood cholesterol slightly; conflicting evidence on blood pressure	Generally considered safe; may cause garlic breath, body odor, gas, and GI distress; inhibits blood clotting
Ginger (roots) *Zingiber officinale*	Prevent motion sickness, nausea	May relieve pregnancy-induced nausea; conflicting evidence on nausea caused by motion, chemotherapy, or surgery	Generally considered safe
Ginkgo (tree leaves) *Ginkgo biloba*	Improve memory, relieve vertigo	Little evidence available	Generally considered safe; may cause headache, GI distress, dizziness; may inhibit blood clotting
Ginseng (roots) *Panax ginseng* (Asian), *P. quinquefolius* (American)	Boost immunity, increase endurance	Little evidence available	Generally considered safe; may cause insomnia, headaches, and high blood pressure
Goldenseal (roots) *Hydrastis canadensis*	Relieve indigestion, treat urinary infections	Little evidence available	Generally considered safe; not safe for people with hypertension or heart disease
Kava (roots) *Piper methysticum*	Relieves anxiety, promotes relaxation	Little evidence available	Liver failure
Saw palmetto (ripe fruits) *Serenoa repens*	Relieve symptoms of enlarged prostate; diuretic; enhance sexual vigor	Little evidence available	Generally considered safe; may cause nausea, vomiting, diarrhea
St. John's wort (leaves and tops) *Hypericum perforatum*	Relieve depression and anxiety	May relieve mild depression	Generally considered safe; may cause fatigue, increased sensitivity to sunlight, and GI distress
Turmeric (roots) *Curcuma longa*	Reduces inflammation; relieves heartburn; prevents or treats cancer	No evidence available	Generally considered safe; may cause indigestion; not safe for people with gallbladder disease
Valerian (roots) *Valeriana officinalis*	Calm nerves, improve sleep	Little evidence available	Long-term use associated with liver damage
Yohimbe (tree bark) *Pausinystalia yohimbe*	Enhance "male performance"	No evidence available	Kidney failure, seizures

[a]Allergies are always a possible risk; see Table H18-2 (p. 606) for drug interactions. Pregnant women should not use herbal supplements.

TABLE H18-2 Herb and Drug Interactions

Herb	Drug	Interaction
American ginseng	Estrogens, corticosteroids	Enhances hormonal response
American ginseng	Breast cancer therapeutic agent	Synergistically inhibits cancer cell growth
American ginseng, karela	Blood glucose regulators	Affect blood glucose levels
Echinacea (possible immunostimulant)	Cyclosporine and corticosteroids (immunosuppressants)	May reduce drug effectiveness
Evening primrose oil, borage	Anticonvulsants	Lower seizure threshold
Feverfew	Aspirin, ibuprofen, and other nonsteroidal anti-inflammatory drugs	Negates the effect of the herb in treating migraine headaches
Feverfew, garlic, ginkgo, ginger, and Asian ginseng	Warfarin, coumarin (anticlotting drugs, "blood thinners")	Prolong bleeding time; increase likelihood of hemorrhage
Garlic	Protease inhibitor (HIV drug)	May reduce drug effectiveness
Kava, valerian	Anesthetics	May enhance drug action
Kelp (iodine source)	Synthroid or other thyroid hormone replacers	Interferes with drug action
Kyushin, licorice, plantain, uzara root, hawthorn, Asian ginseng	Digoxin (cardiac antiarrhythmic drug derived from the herb foxglove)	Interfere with drug action and monitoring
St. John's wort, saw palmetto, black tea	Iron supplements	Tannins in herbs inhibit iron absorption
St. John's wort	Protease inhibitors (HIV drugs), warfarin (anticlotting drug), digoxin (cardiac antiarrhythmic drug), oral contraceptives, tamoxifen (breast cancer drug)	May enhance or reduce drug effectiveness
Valerian	Barbiturates	Causes excessive sedation

eyesight, or maintain heart health, consumers believe that taking the product will provide those benefits. Beware. Manufacturers need not prove effectiveness; they need only state on the product label that this claim "Has not been evaluated by the FDA." Consumers who decide to use herbs need to become informed of the possible risks.

Internet Precautions

As Highlight 1 pointed out, just because something appears on the Internet, "it ain't necessarily so." Keep in mind that the thousands of websites touting the benefits of herbal medicines and other dietary supplements are marketing their products. Most product advertisements claim to prevent or treat specific diseases, but few include the FDA disclaimer statement. Many of the websites promote products by quoting researchers or physicians. Such quotations lend an air of authority to advertisements, but be aware that these sources may not even exist—and if they do, their comments may have been taken out of context. When asked, these experts may not agree at all with the claims attributed to them by the manufacturer.

Other deceits and dangers lurk in cyberspace as well. Potentially toxic substances, illegal and unavailable in many countries, are now easy to obtain via the Internet. Electronic access to products such as absinthe and oil of wormwood could be deadly. When the FDA discovers websites selling unapproved drugs, such as laetrile, it can order the business to shut down. But consumers need to remain vigilant because other similar businesses pop up quickly.

The Consumer's Perspective

Some health-care professionals may dismiss alternative therapies as ineffective and perhaps even dangerous, but many consumers think otherwise. About 4 out of 10 adults have used at least one alternative therapy for a variety of medical symptoms ranging from back pain and anxiety to heart disease and cancer. Interestingly, those who seek alternative therapies seem to do so not so much because they are dissatisfied with conventional medicine as because they find these alternatives more in line with their beliefs about health and life.

Most often, people use alternative therapies in addition to, rather than in place of, conventional therapies. Few consult an alternative therapist without also seeing a physician. In fact, most people seek alternative therapies for nonserious medical conditions or for health promotion. They simply want to feel better and access is easy. Sometimes their symptoms are chronic and subjective, such as pain and fatigue, and difficult to treat. In these cases, the chances of finding relief are often as good with a placebo, standard medical intervention, or even nonintervention.

Consumers spend tens of billions of dollars on alternative health services and related products such as herbs, crystals, and aromas. As Highlight 1 pointed out, selecting a reliable practitioner depends on finding out about training, qualifications, and licenses. (To review how a person can identify health fraud and quackery, and for a list of credible sources of nutrition information, see p. 31.)

In addition, consumers should inform their physicians about the use of any alternative therapies so that a comprehensive treatment plan can be developed and potential problems can be averted. Remember to include supplements, teas, and garden plants. Sometimes herbal products may need to be discontinued, especially before surgery when interactions with anesthesia or normal blood clotting can be life-threatening.

Alternative therapies come in a variety of shapes and sizes. Both their benefits and their risks may be small, none, or great. Wise consumers and health-care professionals accept the beneficial, or even neutral, practices with an open mind and reject those practices known to cause harm. Making healthful choices requires understanding all the choices.

CRITICAL THINKING QUESTIONS

A. How would you judge the accuracy or validity of complementary and alternative medicine practices?

B. A friend of yours was recently diagnosed with cancer. His physician discussed surgery, radiation, and possibly chemotherapy as recommended treatment options. His sister suggested that in *addition* to the physician's treatment, your friend might also benefit from a few acupuncture sessions and yoga classes. His roommate disagreed, suggesting that *instead* of following the physician's recommendations, your friend should start taking high doses of dietary supplements and doing colonic enemas daily. At this point, your friend is confused. What advice might you offer to help him make an informed decision?

REFERENCES

1. R. L. Nahin, P. M. Barnes, and B. J. Stussman, Expenditures on complementary health approaches: United States, 2012, *National Health Statistics Reports* 95, June 22, 2016; T. C. Clarke and coauthors, Trends in the use of complementary health approaches among adults: United States, 2002–2012, *National Health Statistics Reports* 79, February 10, 2015.
2. National Center for Complementary and Integrative Health, Complementary, alternative, or integrative health: What's in a name? https://nccih.nih.gov/health/integrative-health, updated June, 2016.
3. E. F. Myers, Herbal/botanical medicine: Where's the evidence? *Nutrition Today* 50 (2015): 194–206.
4. G. A. Lamas and coauthors, effect of disodium eDTA chelation regimen on cardiovascular events in patients with previous myocardial infarction: The TACT randomized trial, *Journal of the American Medical Association* 309 (2013): 1241–1250.
5. T. J. Kaptchuk and F. G. Miller, Placebo effects in medicine, *New England Journal of Medicine* 373 (2015): 8–9.
6. W. Marx and coauthors, Ginger—mechanism of action in chemotherapy-induced nausea and vomiting: A review, *Critical Reviews in Food Science and Nutrition* 57 (2017): 141–146; E. A. Apaydin and coauthors, A *systematic review* of St. John's wort for major depressive disorder, *Systematic Reviews* 5 (2016): 148; N. A. Qureshi and A. M. Al-Bedah, Mood disorders and complementary and alternative medicine: A literature review, *Neuropsychiatric Disease and Treatment* 9 (2013): 639–658; C. M. Luberto and coauthors, Integrative medicine for treating depression: A update on the latest evidence, *Current Psychiatric Reports* 15 (2013): 391–392.
7. K. P. Hill, Medical marijuana for treatment of chronic pain and other medical and psychiatric problems: A clinical review, *Journal of the American Medical Association* 313 (2015): 2474–2483; P. F. Whiting and coauthors, Cannabinoids for medical use: A systematic review and meta-analysis, *Journal of the American Medical Association* 313 (2015): 2456–2473.
8. O. H. Franco and coauthors, Use of plant-based therapies and menopausal symptoms, *Journal of the American Medical Association* 315 (2016): 2554–2563; The North American Menopause Society, 2015 position statement: Nonhormonal management of menopause-associated vasomotor *symptoms, Menopause* 22 (2015): 1155–1172; E. Poluzzi and coauthors, Phytoestrogens in postmenopause: The state of the art from a chemical, pharmacological and regulatory perspective, *Current medicinal Chemistry* 21 (2014): 417–436.
9. G. Angelo, V. J. Drake, and B. Frei, Efficacy of multivitamin/mineral supplementation to reduce chronic disease risk: A critical review of the evidence from observational studies and randomized trials, *Critical Review in Food Science and Nutrition* 55 (2015): 1968–1991; S. Rautiainen and coauthors, Multivitamin use and cardiovascular disease in a prospective study of women, *American Journal of Clinical Nutrition* 101 (2015): 144–152; R. L. Bailey and coauthors, Multivitamin-mineral use is associated with reduced risk of cardiovascular disease mortality among women in the United States, *Journal of Nutrition* 145 (2015): 572–578.
10. L. E. Grivetti, Herbs, spices, and flavoring agents, Part 1: Old world contributions, *Nutrition Today* 51 (2016): 139–150.
11. G. Onder and R. Liperoti, Herbal medications, *Journal of the American Medical Association* 315 (2016): 1068.
12. J. Meiman, R. Thiboldeaux, and H. Anderson, Lead poisoning and anemia associated with use of Ayurvedic medications purchased on the Internet—Wisconsin, 2015, *Morbidity and Mortality Weekly Report* 64 (2015): 883.
13. National Institutes of Health, National Center for Complementary and Alternative Medicine, Herbs at a glance, http://nccam.nih.gov/health, updated September 19, 2016.
14. S. G. Newmaster and coauthors, DNA barcoding detects contamination and substitution in North American herbal products, *BMC medicine* 11 (2013): 222.
15. Onder and Liperoti, 2016.
16. National Institutes of Health, National Center for Complementary and Alternative Medicine, Herbs at a glance, St. John's wort, https://nccih.nih.gov/health/stjohnswort/ataglance.htm#hed4, updated December 1, 2016.
17. National Institutes of Health, National Center for Complementary and Alternative Medicine, Herbs at a glance: Ginkgo, https://nccih.nih.gov/health/ginkgo/ataglance.htm#hed4, updated November 30, 2016.

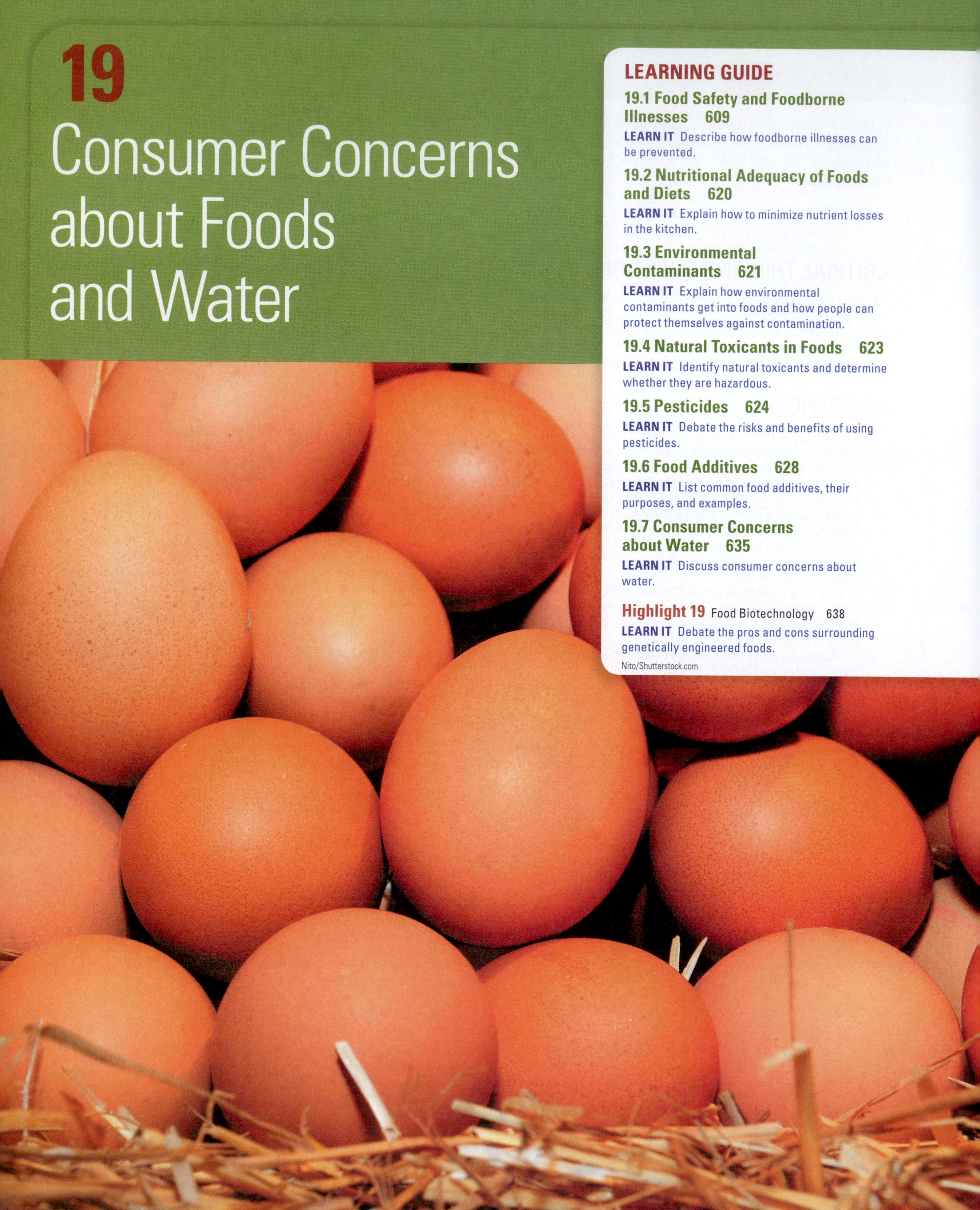

19 Consumer Concerns about Foods and Water

LEARNING GUIDE

Nito/Shutterstock.com

Nutrition in Your Life

Do you know what causes food poisoning and how to protect yourself against it? Were you alarmed to learn that french fries contain acrylamide or that fish contain mercury? Are you concerned about the pesticides that might linger on fruits and vegetables—or the hormones and antibiotics that remain in beef and chicken? Do you wonder whether foods contain enough nutrients—or too many additives? Making informed choices and practicing a few food safety tips will allow you to enjoy a variety of foods while limiting your risks of experiencing food-related illnesses. As you read this chapter, consider whether your food-handling practices are safe.

Take a moment to consider the task of supplying food to almost 325 million people in the United States (and millions more in all corners of the world). To feed this nation, farmers grow and harvest crops; dairy producers supply milk products; ranchers raise livestock; shippers deliver foods to manufacturers by land, sea, and air; manufacturers prepare, process, preserve, and package products for refrigerated food cases and grocery-store shelves; and grocers store the food and supply it to consumers. After much time, much labor, and extensive transport, an abundant supply of a large variety of safe foods finally reaches consumers at reasonable market prices.

The **Food and Drug Administration (FDA)** is a large federal agency with a multitude of global responsibilities. Its primary mission is to protect consumers from unsafe foods and drugs, which it does by using a network of people and sophisticated equipment. More than 2000 FDA inspectors process more than 24 million shipments from more than 300,000 facilities representing more than 150 countries. (Glossary 19-1, p. 610, identifies the various food regulatory agencies by their abbreviations.)

19.1 Food Safety and Foodborne Illnesses

LEARN IT Describe how foodborne illnesses can be prevented.

Government agencies focus on the potential **hazard** of foods, which differs from the **toxicity** of a substance—a distinction worth understanding. Anything can be toxic. Toxicity simply means that a substance *can* cause harm *if* enough is consumed. We consume many substances that are toxic, without **risk**, because the amounts are so small. The term *hazard*, on the other hand, is more relevant to our daily lives because it refers to the harm that is *likely* under real-life conditions. Consumers rely on government monitoring agencies to set **safety** standards and can learn to protect themselves from food-related illnesses by taking a few preventive measures.

This chapter focuses on the actions of individuals to promote food safety (see Photo 19-1). It addresses the following food safety concerns:

- Foodborne illnesses
- Nutritional adequacy of foods
- Environmental contaminants
- Naturally occurring toxicants
- Pesticides
- Food additives
- Water safety

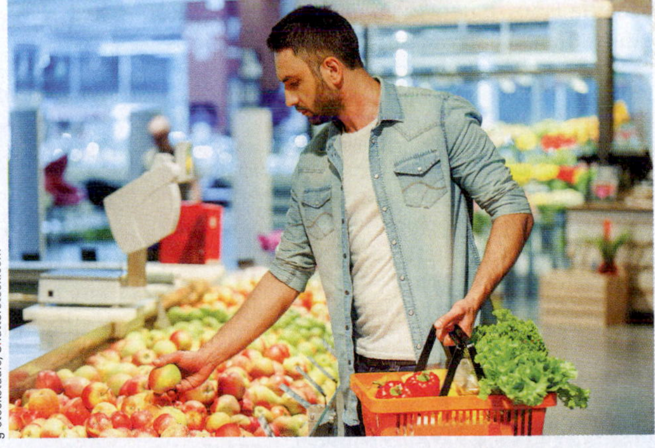

g-stockstudio/Shutterstock.com

> **PHOTO 19-1** With the benefits of a safe and abundant food supply comes the responsibility to select, prepare, and store foods safely.

hazard: a source of danger; used to refer to circumstances in which harm is possible under normal conditions of use.

toxicity: the ability of a substance to harm living organisms. All substances are toxic if high enough concentrations are used.

risk: a measure of the probability and severity of harm.

safety: the condition of being free from harm or danger.

The chapter begins with the FDA's highest priority—the serious and prevalent threat of foodborne illnesses. The highlight that follows looks at genetically engineered foods.

Foodborne illness is the leading food safety concern because **outbreaks** of food poisoning far outnumber episodes of any other kind of food contamination. The **CDC** estimates 48 million cases of foodborne illnesses occur each year in the United States.[1] An estimated 128,000 people become so sick as to need hospitalization. For some 3000 people each year, the symptoms are so severe as to cause death. The following symptoms demand medical attention:

- Bloody diarrhea or diarrhea lasting more than 3 days
- Difficulty breathing or swallowing
- Double vision
- Fever lasting more than 24 hours
- Headache, muscle stiffness, and fever
- Numbness, muscle weakness, and tingling sensations in the skin
- Rapid heart rate, fainting, and dizziness

Most vulnerable are pregnant women; very young, very old, sick, or malnourished people; and those with a weakened immune system (as in AIDS). By taking the proper precautions, people can minimize their chances of contracting foodborne illnesses.

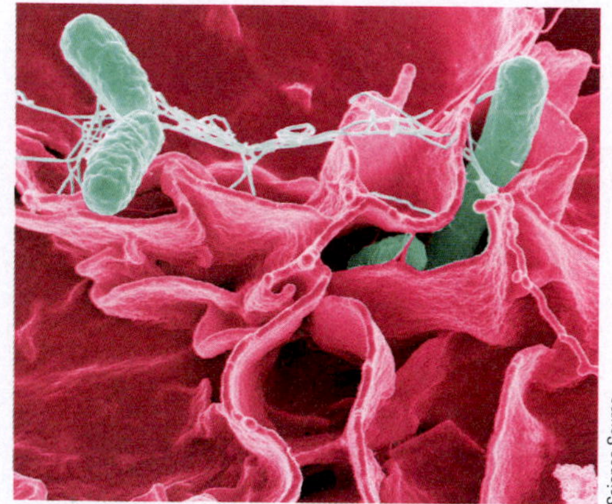

Science Source

> **PHOTO 19-2** An infection with *Salmonella* bacteria (shown here in green) typically causes diarrhea, fever, and abdominal cramps.

Foodborne Infections and Food Intoxications

Foodborne illness can be caused by either an infection or an intoxication. Table 19-1 summarizes the foodborne illnesses responsible for 90 percent of illnesses, hospitalizations, and deaths, along with their food sources, general symptoms, and prevention methods.

Foodborne Infections

Foodborne infections are caused by eating foods contaminated by infectious microbes. Among foodborne infections, *Salmonella* (see Photo 19-2) is the leading cause of illnesses and hospitalizations; *Listeria* is responsible for the most deaths.[2] **Pathogens** commonly enter the GI tract in contaminated foods such as undercooked poultry and unpasteurized milk. Symptoms generally include abdominal cramps, fever, vomiting, and diarrhea.

Food Intoxications

Food intoxications are caused by eating foods containing natural toxins or, more likely, microbes that produce toxins. The most common food toxin in the United States is produced by *Staphylococcus aureus;* it affects more than 1 million people each year. Less common, but more infamous, is *Clostridium botulinum,* an organism that produces a deadly toxin in anaerobic conditions such as improperly canned (especially home-canned) foods and improperly stored foods (such as homemade herb-flavored oils shown in Photo 19-3 or commercially made, chilled foods stored at room temperature). The botulinum toxin paralyzes muscles,

foodborne illness: an illness transmitted to human beings through food and water, caused by either an infectious agent (foodborne infection) or a poisonous substance (food intoxication); commonly known as *food poisoning.*

outbreaks: two or more cases of a similar illness resulting from the ingestion of a common food.

pathogens (PATH-oh-jenz): microorganisms capable of producing disease.

GLOSSARY 19-1 REGULATORY AGENCY TERMS

CDC (Centers for Disease Control and Prevention): a branch of the Department of Health and Human Services that is responsible for, among other things, monitoring foodborne diseases.
www.cdc.gov

EPA (Environmental Protection Agency): a federal agency that is responsible for, among other things, regulating pesticides and establishing water quality standards.
www.epa.gov

FAO (Food and Agriculture Organization): an international agency (part of the United Nations) that has adopted standards to regulate pesticide use, among other responsibilities.
www.fao.org

FDA (Food and Drug Administration): a part of the an agency within the US Department of Health and Human Services that is responsible for ensuring the safety and wholesomeness of all dietary supplements and foods processed and sold in interstate commerce except meat, poultry, and eggs (which are under the jurisdiction of the USDA); inspecting food plants and imported foods; and setting standards for food composition and product labeling, among other responsibilities.
www.fda.gov

USDA (US Department of Agriculture): the federal agency responsible for enforcing standards for the wholesomeness and quality of meat, poultry, and eggs produced in the United States; conducting nutrition research; and educating the public about nutrition, among other responsibilities.
www.usda.gov

WHO (World Health Organization): an international agency concerned with promoting health and eradicating disease.
www.who.int

TABLE 19-1 Foodborne Illnesses

Organism Name	Most Frequent Food Sources	Onset and General Symptoms	Prevention Methods[a]
Foodborne Infections			
Campylobacter (KAM-pee-loh-BAK-ter) bacterium	Raw and undercooked poultry, unpasturized milk, contaminated water	Onset: 2 to 5 days. Diarrhea, vomiting, abdominal cramps, fever; sometimes bloody stools; lasts 2 to 10 days.	Cook foods thoroughly; use pasteurized milk; use sanitary food-handling methods.
Clostridium (klo-STRID-ee-um) ***perfringens*** (per-FRINGE-enz) bacterium	Meats and meat products stored at between 120°F and 130°F	Onset: 8 to 16 hours. Abdominal pain, diarrhea, nausea; lasts 1 to 2 days.	Use sanitary food-handling methods; use pasteurized milk; cook foods thoroughly; refrigerate foods promptly and properly.
Escherichia (esh-uh-RIK-ee-uh) ***coli*** (KOH-lie); commonly called ***E.coli*** bacterium	Undercooked ground beef, unpasteurized milk and juices, raw dough, raw fruits and vegetables, contaminated water, and person-to-person contact	Onset: 1 to 8 days. Severe bloody diarrhea, abdominal cramps, vomiting; lasts 5 to 10 days.	Cook ground beef thoroughly; use pasteurized milk; use sanitary food-handling methods; use treated, boiled, or bottled water.
Listeria (lis-TER-ee-AH) bacterium	Unpasteurized milk; fresh soft cheeses; luncheon meats, hot dogs	Onset: 1 to 21 days. Fever, muscle aches; nausea, vomiting, blood poisoning, complications in pregnancy, and meningitis (stiff neck, severe headache, and fever).	Use sanitary food-handling methods; cook foods thoroughly; use pasteurized milk.
Norovirus	Person-to-person contact; raw foods, salads, sandwiches	Onset: 1 to 2 days. Vomiting; lasts 1 to 2 days.	Use sanitary food-handling methods.
Salmonella (sal-moh-NEL-ah) bacteria (>2300 types)	Raw or undercooked eggs, meats, poultry, raw milk and other dairy products, shrimp, frog legs, yeast, coconut, pasta, and chocolate	Onset: 1 to 3 days. Fever, vomiting, abdominal cramps, diarrhea; lasts 4 to 7 days; can be fatal.	Use sanitary food-handling methods; use pasteurized milk; cook foods thoroughly; refrigerate foods promptly and properly.
Toxoplasma (TOK-so-PLAZ-ma) ***gondii*** (GONE-dee-eye) parasite	Raw or undercooked meat; unwashed fruits and vegetables; contaminated water	Onset: 7 to 21 days. Swollen glands, fever, headache, muscle pain, stiff neck.	Use sanitary food-handling methods; cook foods thoroughly.
Food Intoxications			
Clostridium (claw-STRID-ee-um) ***botulinum*** (bot-chew-LINE-um) bacterium produces the ***botulinum toxin*** responsible for causing botulism	Anaerobic environment of low acidity (canned corn, peppers, green beans, soups, beets, asparagus, mushrooms, ripe olives, spinach, tuna, chicken, chicken liver, liver pâté, luncheon meats, ham, sausage, stuffed eggplant, lobster, and smoked and salted fish)	Onset: 4 to 36 hours. Nervous system symptoms, including double vision, inability to swallow, speech difficulty, and progressive paralysis of the respiratory system; often fatal; leaves prolonged symptoms in survivors.	Use proper canning methods for low-acid foods; refrigerate homemade garlic and herb oils; avoid commercially prepared foods with leaky seals or with bent, bulging, or broken cans. Do not give infants honey because it may contain spores of *Clostridium botulinum,* which is a common source of infection for infants.
Staphylococcus (STAF-il-oh-KOK-uhs) ***aureus*** (AWR-ee-uhs) bacterium produces staphylococcal toxin	Toxin produced in improperly refrigerated meats; egg, tuna, potato, and macaroni salads; cream-filled pastries	Onset: 1 to 6 hours. Diarrhea, nausea, vomiting, abdominal cramps, fever; lasts 1 to 2 days.	Use sanitary food-handling methods; cook food thoroughly; refrigerate foods promptly and properly; use proper home-canning methods.

NOTE: Travelers' diarrhea is most commonly caused by *E. coli, Campylobacter jejuni, Shigella,* and *Salmonella.*
[a]How To 19-1 (pp. 616–617) provides more details on the proper handling, cooking, and refrigeration of foods.

making it difficult to see, speak, swallow, and breathe. Because death can occur within 24 hours of onset, botulism demands immediate medical attention. Even then, survivors may suffer the effects for months or years.

Other microbial toxins—called aflatoxins—are not common in the United States, but threaten the health of more than half the world's population. Aflatoxins contaminate corn, grains, and nuts in tropical countries where foods are stored in warm, humid conditions that promote fungal growth. Strategies to reduce exposure in vulnerable populations is a global health priority.

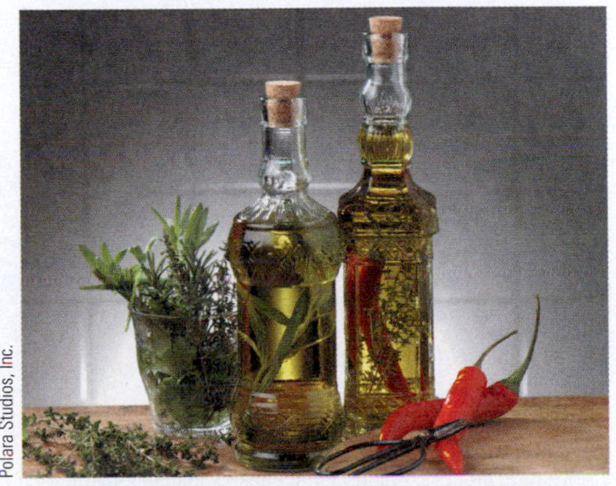

> **PHOTO 19-3** To prevent food intoxication from homemade flavored oils, wash and dry the herbs before adding them to the oil and keep the oil refrigerated. Discard after a week to 10 days.

Food Safety in the Marketplace Transmission of foodborne illness has changed as our food supply and lifestyles have changed. In the past, foodborne illness was caused by one person's error in a small setting, such as improperly refrigerated egg salad at a family picnic, and affected only a few victims. Today, we eat more foods that have been prepared and packaged by others. Consequently, when a food manufacturer or cruise ship chef makes an error, foodborne illness can quickly affect many people. An estimated 80 percent of reported foodborne illnesses are caused by errors in a commercial setting, such as the improper **pasteurization** of milk at a large dairy.

In 2013, *Cyclospora* in salads and fresh cilantro from Mexico infected more than 600 people in 25 states. In 2014, a *Salmonella* outbreak led to the recall of almost 34,000 pounds of chicken after people from more than a dozen states became ill. In 2015, a major ice cream company recalled all of its products after 3 people died from *Listeria* contamination. In 2016, 10 million pounds of flour contaminated with *E. coli* was recalled. These incidents and others focus the national spotlight on two important safety issues: disease-causing organisms are commonly found in a variety of foods, and safe food-handling practices can minimize harm from most of these foodborne pathogens.

Industry Controls All food producers use a **Hazard Analysis Critical Control Point (HACCP)** plan to help prevent foodborne illnesses at their source. Each slaughterhouse, packer, distributor, and transporter of susceptible foods must identify "critical control points" that pose a risk of contamination and then devise and implement verifiable ways to eliminate or minimize the risk. The HACCP system has proved a remarkable success for domestic products, but such programs do not apply to imported foods.

An estimated 15 to 20 percent of all food consumed in the United States is imported from 300,000 facilities located in more than 150 countries each year. As the number of imports have increased over the years, so has the number of foodborne illnesses associated with imported foods, most commonly fish and produce.[3] Many countries cooperate with the FDA and have adopted many of the safe food-handling practices used in the United States, but some imported foods come from countries with little or no regulatory oversight. To help consumers distinguish between imported and domestic foods, certain foods—including fish, shellfish, meats, fruits, vegetables, and some nuts—must display the country of origin on the label, specifying where they were produced.

Consumer Awareness Canned and packaged foods sold in grocery stores are easily controlled, but rare accidents do happen. Batch numbering makes it possible to recall contaminated foods through public announcements via the Internet, newspapers, television, and radio. In the grocery store, consumers can buy items before the expiration date and inspect the safety seals and wrappers of packages. A broken seal, bulging can lid, or mangled package fails to protect the consumer against microbes, insects, spoilage, or even vandalism.

Speaking of dates, consumers find a variety of dates on food products—"sell by," "use by," "best before," and "expires on." None of these messages has been legally defined, which has resulted in consumers being confused and wasting food. Only infant formulas are required to follow national guidelines for "use by" dates. All other dates on food products currently reflect the food producer's recommendations for peak quality and freshness—not for safety. Consumers may think the food has gone bad, but in reality, the "sell by" date is designed to help retailers manage their inventory. For all these reasons, manufacturers have recently joined together to adopt standard date-labeling recommendations.

Of course, whether a food is safe also depends on how it was stored, cooked, refrigerated, or frozen after the purchase—regardless of the date on the package. Foods that are not properly handled can cause foodborne illnesses even if the expiration date has not yet been reached. Likewise, foods that are handled properly may still be safe and wholesome even after the "sell by" or "best by" date passes.

State and local health regulations provide guidelines on the cleanliness of facilities and the safe preparation of foods for restaurants, cafeterias, and fast-food establishments. Even so, consumers can also take the following actions to help prevent foodborne illnesses when dining out:

pasteurization: heat processing of food that inactivates some, but not all, microorganisms in the food; not a sterilization process. Bacteria that cause spoilage are still present.

Hazard Analysis Critical Control Points (HACCP): a systematic plan to identify and correct potential microbial hazards in the manufacturing, distribution, and commercial use of food products; commonly referred to as "HASS-ip."

> **FIGURE 19-1 Food Safety from Farm to Table**

FARM
Workers must use safe methods of growing, harvesting, sorting, packing, and storing food to minimize contamination hazards.

PROCESSING
Processors must follow FDA guidelines concerning contamination, cleanliness, and education and training of workers and must monitor for safety at critical control points.

TRANSPORTATION
Containers and vehicles transporting food must be clean. Cold food must be kept cold at all times.

RETAIL
Employees in grocery stores and restaurants must follow the FDA's Food Code on how to prevent foodborne illnesses. Establishments must pass local health inspections and train staff in sanitation.

TABLE
Consumers must learn and use sound principles of food safety as taught in this chapter. Be mindful that foodborne illness is a real possibility, and take steps to prevent it.

© Cengage

- Wash hands with hot, soapy water before meals.
- Expect clean tabletops, dinnerware, utensils, and food preparation areas.
- Expect cooked foods to be served piping hot and salads to be fresh and cold.
- Refrigerate take-home items within 2 hours and use leftovers within 3 to 4 days.

Improper handling of foods can occur anywhere along the line from commercial farms and manufacturers to supermarkets and restaurants to private homes. Maintaining a safe food supply requires everyone's efforts (see Figure 19-1).

Food Safety in the Kitchen

Whether microbes multiply and cause illness depends, in part, on a few key food-handling behaviors in the kitchen—whether the kitchen is in your home, a school cafeteria, a gourmet restaurant, or a commercial canning facility. Figure 19-2 summarizes the four simple things that can help most to prevent foodborne illness:

- *Clean.* Keep a clean, safe kitchen by washing hands and surfaces often. Wash countertops, cutting boards, sponges, and utensils in hot, soapy water before and after each step of food preparation. To reduce bacterial contamination on hands, wash hands with soap and warm water (see Photo 19-4); if soap and water are not available, use an alcohol-based sanitizing gel.[4]
- *Separate.* Avoid foodborne infections by keeping raw eggs, meat, poultry, and seafood separate from other foods. Wash all utensils and surfaces (such as cutting boards or platters) that have been in contact with these foods with hot, soapy water before using them again. Bacteria inevitably left on the surfaces from the raw meat can recontaminate the cooked meat or other foods—a problem known as **cross-contamination.** Washing raw eggs, meat, and poultry is not recommended because the extra handling increases the risk of cross-contamination.
- *Cook.* Keep hot foods hot by cooking to proper temperatures (see Figure 19-3, p. 614). Foods need to cook long enough to reach internal temperatures that will kill microbes and maintain adequate temperatures to prevent bacterial growth until the foods are served.
- *Chill.* Keep cold foods cold by refrigerating promptly. Go directly home upon leaving the grocery store and immediately place foods in the refrigerator or freezer. After a meal, refrigerate any leftovers immediately.

Unfortunately, consumers commonly fail to follow these simple food-handling recommendations.[5] Anyone believing that food dropped on the floor for less than

> **FIGURE 19-2 Fight Bac!**

The FightBac! website (www.fightbac.org) describes four ways to keep food safe.

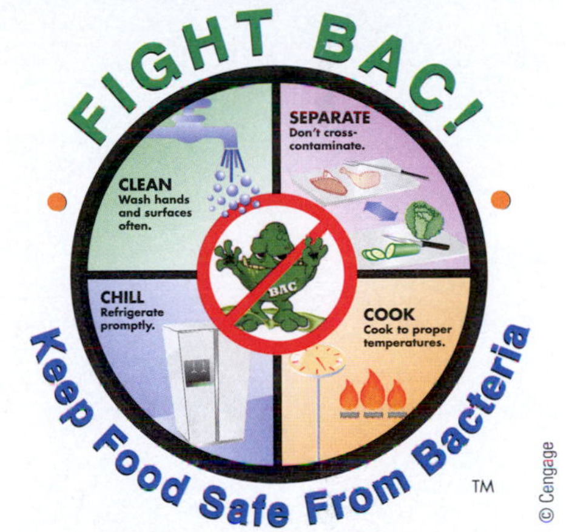
FIGHT BAC!
SEPARATE
Don't cross-contaminate.
CLEAN
Wash hands and surfaces often.
CHILL
Refrigerate promptly.
COOK
Cook to proper temperatures.
BAC
Keep Food Safe From Bacteria
TM

© Cengage

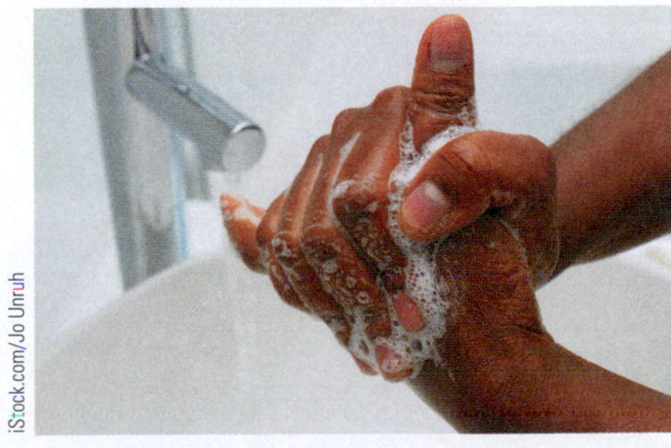

iStock.com/Jo Unruh

> **PHOTO 19-4** Wash your hands with warm water and soap for at least 20 seconds before preparing or eating food to reduce the chance of microbial contamination.

cross-contamination: the contamination of food by bacteria that occurs when the food comes into contact with surfaces previously touched by raw meat, poultry, or seafood.

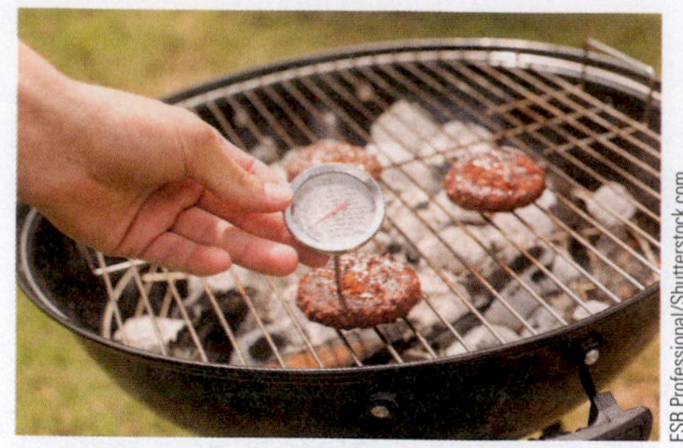
ESB Professional/Shutterstock.com

> **PHOTO 19-5** Cook hamburgers to 160°F; color alone cannot determine doneness. Some burgers will turn brown before reaching 160°F, whereas others may retain some pink color, even when cooked to 175°F.

> **FIGURE 19-3 Recommended Safe Temperatures (Fahrenheit)**

Bacteria multiply rapidly at temperatures in the danger zone—between 40°F and 140°F. Cook foods to the minimum internal temperatures shown on this thermometer and hold them at 140°F or higher. Place the thermometer in the thickest part of the meat; for whole cuts of meat, allow the meat to rest for 3 minutes before carving or consuming. Refrigerate foods to below 40°F.

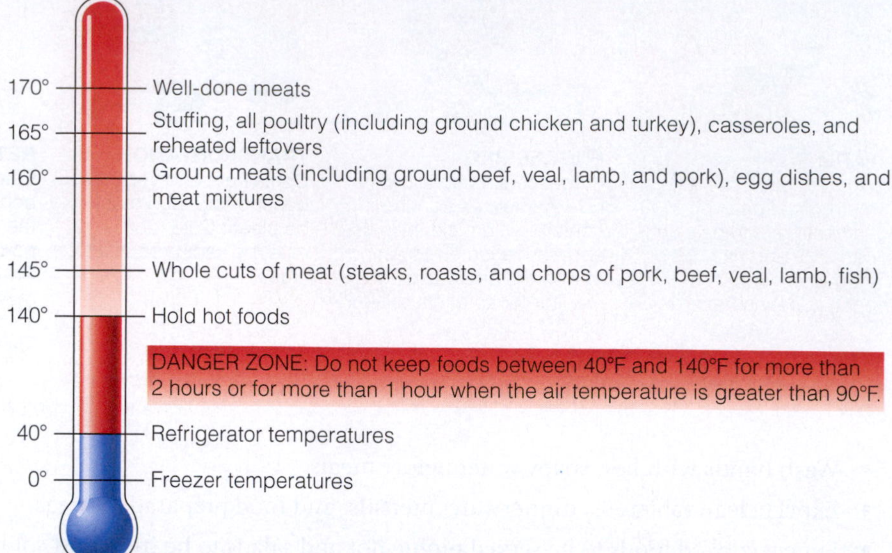
170° Well-done meats
165° Stuffing, all poultry (including ground chicken and turkey), casseroles, and reheated leftovers
160° Ground meats (including ground beef, veal, lamb, and pork), egg dishes, and meat mixtures
145° Whole cuts of meat (steaks, roasts, and chops of pork, beef, veal, lamb, fish)
140° Hold hot foods
DANGER ZONE: Do not keep foods between 40°F and 140°F for more than 2 hours or for more than 1 hour when the air temperature is greater than 90°F.
40° Refrigerator temperatures
0° Freezer temperatures
© Cengage

NOTE: To reduce the risk of foodborne illnesses, the *Dietary Guidelines for Americans* suggest that consumers heed this temperature danger zone. Professionals in the food industry must adhere to more specific guidelines as published in the FDA Food Code, available at www.fda.gov/FoodCode.

five seconds is safe to eat should know that, depending on the food and the surface, bacterial contamination can occur instantaneously, thus disproving the "five second rule."[6] See How To 19-1 (pp. 616–617) for additional food safety tips.

Safe Handling of Meats and Poultry Figure 19-4 presents label instructions for the safe handling of meat and poultry and two types of USDA seals. Meats and poultry contain bacteria and provide a moist, nutrient-rich environment that favors microbial growth. Ground meat and mechanically tenderized beef are especially susceptible because they receive more handling than other meats and have more surface area exposed to bacterial contamination. Consumers cannot detect the harmful bacteria in or on meat. For safety's sake, cook meat thoroughly, using a thermometer to test the internal temperature (see Photo 19-5).

Unrelated to safe handling practices, **bovine spongiform encephalopathy (BSE)** is a slowly progressive, fatal disease that affects the central nervous system of cattle and wild game such as deer and elk. A similar disease develops in people who have eaten contaminated beef from infected cows (milk products appear to be safe).* The USDA has taken numerous steps to prevent the transmission of BSE in cattle, and consequently, the risks from US cattle are extremely low.

Safe Handling of Seafood Most seafood available in the United States is safe, but eating it undercooked or raw can cause severe illnesses—hepatitis, worms, parasites, viral intestinal disorders, and other diseases.** Rumor has it that freezing fish will make it safe to eat raw, but this is only partly true. Commercial freezing kills mature parasitic worms, but only cooking can kill all worm eggs and other microorganisms that can cause illness. For safety's sake, all seafood should be cooked until it is opaque.

bovine spongiform encephalopathy (BOH-vine SPON-jih-form in-SEF-eh-LOP-eh-thee) or **BSE:** an often fatal illness of cattle and wild game that affects the nervous system and is transmitted to people by eating infected meats; commonly called *mad cow disease.*

*The human form of BSE is called *variant Creutzfeldt-Jakob disease (vCJD)*.
**Diseases caused by toxins from the sea include ciguatera poisoning, scombroid poisoning, and paralytic and neurotoxic shellfish poisoning.

> FIGURE 19-4 Meat and Poultry Safety, Grading, and Inspection Seals

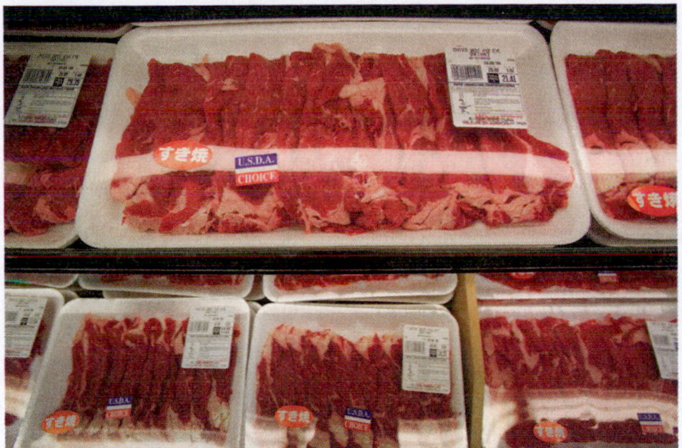
U.S.D.A.
CHOICE

James Leynse/Getty Images

Neither inspection nor grading guarantees that the product will not cause foodborne illnesses, but consumers can help prevent foodborne illnesses by following the safe handling instructions.

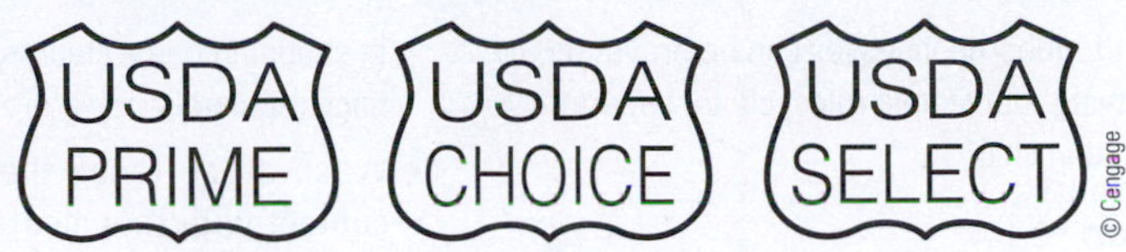
USDA
PRIME
USDA
CHOICE
USDA
SELECT

© Cengage

The voluntary "Graded by USDA" seal indicates that the product has been graded for tenderness, juiciness, and flavor. Beef is graded Prime (abundant marbling of the meat muscle), Choice (less marbling), or Select (lean). Similarly, poultry is graded A, B, or C.

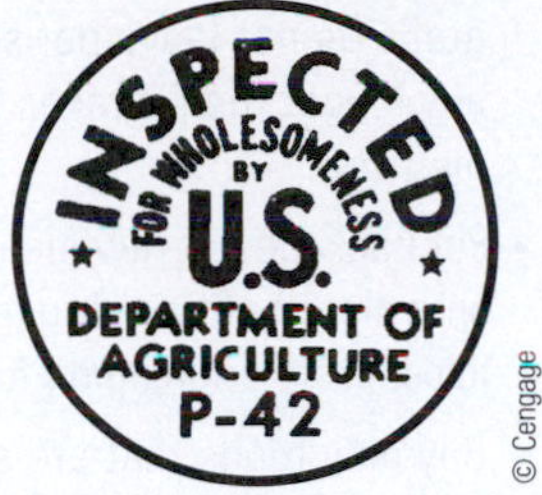
INSPECTED
FOR WHOLESOMENESS
BY
U.S.
DEPARTMENT OF
AGRICULTURE
P-42

© Cengage

The mandatory "Inspected and Passed by the USDA" seal ensures that meat and poultry products are safe, wholesome, and correctly labeled. Inspection does not guarantee that the meat is free of potentially harmful bacteria.

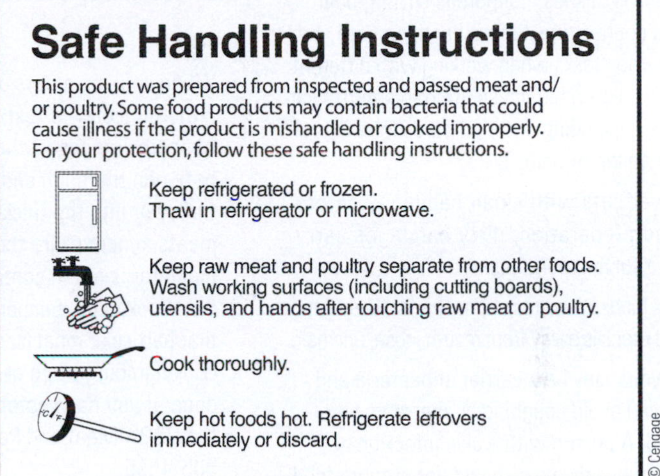

Safe Handling Instructions

This product was prepared from inspected and passed meat and/or poultry. Some food products may contain bacteria that could cause illness if the product is mishandled or cooked improperly. For your protection, follow these safe handling instructions.

Keep refrigerated or frozen. Thaw in refrigerator or microwave.

Keep raw meat and poultry separate from other foods. Wash working surfaces (including cutting boards), utensils, and hands after touching raw meat or poultry.

Cook thoroughly.

Keep hot foods hot. Refrigerate leftovers immediately or discard.

© Cengage

The USDA requires that safe handling instructions appear on all packages of meat and poultry.

As for **sushi**, even a master chef cannot detect harmful microbes that may occur in even the best-quality, freshest fish (see Photo 19-6). The marketing term *sushi grade* implies wholesomeness, but is not legally defined and does not guarantee quality, purity, or freshness. Sushi can be safe to eat when chefs combine cooked seafood and other ingredients into these delicacies.

Eating raw oysters can be dangerous for anyone, but people with liver disease and weakened immune systems are most vulnerable. At least 10 species of bacteria found in raw oysters can cause serious illness and even death. Raw oysters may also carry the hepatitis A virus, which can cause liver disease. Some hot sauces can kill many of these bacteria, but not the virus; alcohol inactivates some bacteria, but not enough to guarantee protection (or to recommend drinking alcohol). Pasteurization of raw oysters—holding them at a specified temperature for a specified time—holds promise for killing bacteria without cooking the oyster or altering its texture or flavor.

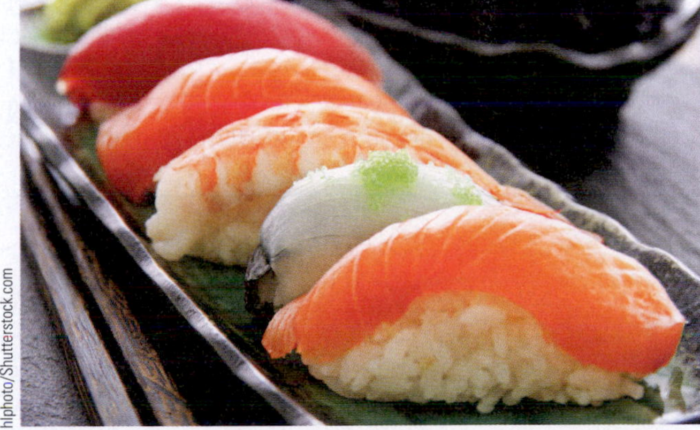

hlphoto/Shutterstock.com

> PHOTO 19-6 Eating raw seafood is a risky proposition.

As population density increases along the shores of seafood-harvesting waters, pollution inevitably invades the sea life there. Preventing seafood-borne illness is in large part a task of controlling water pollution. To help ensure a safe seafood market, the FDA requires processors to adopt food safety practices based on the HACCP system mentioned earlier.

Chemical pollution and microbial contamination lurk not only in the water, but also in the boats and warehouses where seafood is cleaned, prepared,

sushi: vinegar-flavored rice and seafood, typically wrapped in seaweed and stuffed with colorful vegetables. Some sushi is stuffed with raw fish; other varieties contain cooked seafood.

> How To 19-1 Prevent Foodborne Illnesses

Most foodborne illnesses can be prevented by following four simple rules: clean, separate, cook, and chill.

Clean

- Wash fruits and vegetables in a clean sink with a scrub brush and warm water; store washed and unwashed produce separately. Do not rinse raw seafood, meat, or poultry.
- Use hot, soapy water to wash hands, utensils, dishes, nonporous cutting boards, and countertops before handling food and between tasks when working with different foods. Use a bleach solution to sanitize surfaces, including cutting boards (one capful per gallon of water).
- Cover cuts with clean bandages before food preparation; dirty bandages carry harmful microorganisms.
- Mix foods with utensils, not hands; keep hands and utensils away from mouth, nose, and hair.
- Anyone may be a carrier of bacteria and should avoid coughing or sneezing over food. A person with a skin infection or infectious disease should not prepare food.
- Clean sponges every day by microwaving wet sponges at full power for one minute or running them through the dishwasher. Wash dish cloths and dish towels regularly and use fresh, clean ones every day.
- Clean up food spills and crumb-filled crevices.

Separate

- Separate raw seafood, meat, and poultry from other foods in the grocery cart and in shopping bags; clean reusable shopping bags regularly.
- Wash all surfaces that have been in contact with raw meats, poultry, eggs, fish, and shellfish before reusing.
- Serve cooked foods on a clean plate with a clean utensil. Separate raw foods from those that have been cooked.
- Don't use marinade that was in contact with raw meat for basting or sauces.

Cook

- When cooking meats or poultry, use a thermometer to test the internal temperature. Insert the thermometer between the thigh and the body of a turkey or into the thickest part of other meats, making sure the tip of the thermometer is not in contact with bone or the pan. Cook to the temperature indicated for that particular meat (see Figure 19-3, p. 614); cook hamburgers to at least medium well done. If you have safety questions, call the USDA Meat and Poultry Hotline: (800) 535-4555.
- Cook stuffing separately, or stuff poultry just prior to cooking.
- Do not cook large cuts of meat or turkey in a microwave oven; it leaves some parts undercooked while overcooking others.
- Cook eggs before eating them (soft-boiled for at least 3½ minutes; scrambled until set, not runny; fried for at least 3 minutes on one side and 1 minute on the other).
- Cook seafood thoroughly. If you have safety questions about seafood, call the FDA hotline: (800) FDA-4010.
- When serving foods, maintain temperatures at 140°F or higher.
- Heat leftovers thoroughly to at least 165°F. Do not reheat leftovers in crock pots, slow cookers, or chafing dishes.
- Bring sauces, soups, and gravies to a boil.

Chill

- When running errands, stop at the grocery store last. When you get home, refrigerate the perishable groceries (such as meats and dairy products) immediately. Do not leave perishables in the car any longer than it takes for ice cream to melt.
- Put packages of raw meat, fish, or poultry on a plate before refrigerating to prevent juices from dripping on food stored below.
- Buy only foods that are solidly frozen in store freezers.
- Keep cold foods at 40°F or less; keep frozen foods at 0°F or less (keep a thermometer in the refrigerator).
- Marinate meats in the refrigerator, not on the counter.
- Look for "Keep Refrigerated" or "Refrigerate After Opening" on food labels.
- Refrigerate leftovers promptly; use shallow containers to cool foods faster; use leftovers within 3 to 4 days.

and refrigerated. Because seafood is one of the most perishable foods, time and temperature are critical to its freshness, flavor, and safety. To keep seafood as fresh as possible, people in the industry must "keep it cold, keep it clean, and keep it moving." Wise consumers eat it cooked.

Other Precautions and Procedures Fresh food generally smells fresh. Not all types of food poisoning are detectable by odor, but some bacterial wastes produce "off" odors—and food with an abnormal odor is spoiled. Throw it out or, if it was recently purchased, return it to the grocery store. Do not taste it. Table 19-2 (p. 618) lists safe refrigerator storage times for selected foods.

Local health departments and the USDA and FDA websites can provide additional information about food safety. If precautions fail and a mild foodborne illness develops, drink clear liquids to replace fluids lost through vomiting and diarrhea. If serious foodborne illness is suspected, first call a physician. Then wrap the remainder of the suspected food and label the container so that the food cannot be

- Thaw meats or poultry in the refrigerator, not at room temperature. If you must hasten thawing, use cool water (changed every 30 minutes) or a microwave oven.
- Freeze meat, fish, or poultry immediately if not planning to use within a few days.
- Wipe up spills immediately; clean the refrigerator interior regularly and the handles daily.
- At least once a week, review the contents of the refrigerator and throw out foods that should no longer be eaten.

In General

- Do not reuse disposable containers; use nondisposable containers or recycle instead.
- Do not taste food that is suspect. "If in doubt, throw it out."
- Throw out foods with danger-signaling odors. Be aware, though, that most food-poisoning bacteria are odorless, colorless, and tasteless.
- Do not buy or use items that have broken seals or mangled packaging; such containers cannot protect against microbes, insects, spoilage, or even vandalism. Check safety seals, buttons, and expiration dates.
- Follow label instructions for storing and preparing packaged and frozen foods; throw out foods that have been thawed or refrozen.
- Discard foods that are discolored, moldy, or decayed or that have been contaminated by insects or rodents.

For Specific Food Items

- *Canned goods.* Carefully discard food from cans that leak or bulge so that other people and animals will not accidentally ingest it; before canning, seek professional advice from the USDA Extension Service (find information and local offices at the USDA website).
- *Milk and cheeses.* Use only pasteurized milk and milk products. Aged cheeses, such as cheddar and Swiss, do well for an hour or two without refrigeration, but they should be refrigerated or stored in an ice chest for longer periods.
- *Eggs.* Use clean eggs with intact shells. Do not eat eggs, even pasteurized eggs, raw; raw eggs are commonly found in Caesar salad dressing, eggnog, cookie dough, hollandaise sauce, and key lime pie. Cook eggs until whites are firmly set and yolks begin to thicken.
- *Honey.* Honey may contain dormant bacterial spores, which can awaken in the human body to produce botulism. In adults, this poses little hazard, but infants younger than 1 year of age should never be fed honey. Honey can accumulate enough toxin to kill an infant; it has been implicated in several cases of sudden infant death. (Honey can also be contaminated with environmental pollutants picked up by the bees.)
- *Mayonnaise.* Commercial mayonnaise may actually help a food to resist spoilage because of the acid content. Still, keep it refrigerated after opening.
- *Mixed salads.* Mixed salads of chopped ingredients spoil easily because they have extensive surface area for bacteria to invade, and they have been in contact with cutting boards, hands, and kitchen utensils that easily transmit bacteria to food (regardless of their mayonnaise content). Chill them well before, during, and after serving.
- *Picnic foods.* Choose foods that last without refrigeration, such as fresh fruits and vegetables, breads and crackers, and canned spreads and cheeses that can be opened and used immediately. Pack foods cold, layer ice between foods, and keep foods out of water.
- *Seafood.* Buy only fresh seafood that has been properly refrigerated or iced. Cooked seafood should be stored separately from raw seafood to avoid cross-contamination.

NOTE: Learn more about food safety at www.HomeFoodSafety.org or by downloading *Is My Food Safe?,* a free phone app sponsored by the Academy of Nutrition and Dietetics.

› TRY IT After cutting the fat from a pork loin, you rinse the wooden cutting board under warm water before using it to chop vegetables. Discuss whether this precaution is adequate to protect against cross-contamination.

mistakenly eaten, place it in the refrigerator, and hold it for possible inspection by health authorities.

Food Safety while Traveling People who travel to other countries have a 50–50 chance of contracting a foodborne illness, commonly described as **travelers' diarrhea.** Like many other foodborne illnesses, travelers' diarrhea is a sometimes serious, always annoying bacterial infection of the digestive tract. The risk is high because, for one thing, some countries' cleanliness standards for food and water are lower than those in the United States. For another, every region's microbes are different, and although people are immune to the microbes in their own neighborhoods, they have had no chance to develop immunity to the pathogens in places they are visiting for the first time. In addition to the food safety tips outlined in How To 19-1, precautions while traveling include:

- Wash hands frequently with soap and hot water, especially before handling food or eating. Use sanitizing gel or hand wipes regularly.

travelers' diarrhea: nausea, vomiting, and diarrhea caused by consuming food or water contaminated by any of several organisms, most commonly, *E. coli, Shigella, Campylobacter jejuni,* and *Salmonella.*

TABLE 19-2 Refrigerator Home Storage (at 40°F or below)

If product has a "use-by" date, follow that date. If product has a "sell-by" date or no date, cook or freeze the product by the time on the following chart.

Fresh or Uncooked Products	
Product	**Storage Times after Purchase**
Poultry	1 or 2 days
Beef, veal, pork, and lamb	3 to 5 days
Ground meat and ground poultry	1 or 2 days
Fresh variety meats (liver, tongue, brain, kidneys, heart, chitterlings)	1 or 2 days
Cured ham, cook-before-eating	5 to 7 days
Sausage from pork, beef, or turkey (uncooked)	1 or 2 days
Eggs	3 to 5 weeks

Sealed Processed Products		
Processed Product	**Unopened, after Purchase**	**After Opening**
Cooked poultry	3 to 4 days	3 to 4 days
Cooked sausage	3 to 4 days	3 to 4 days
Sausage, hard/dry, shelf-stable	6 weeks/pantry	3 weeks
Corned beef, uncooked, in pouch with pickling juices	5 to 7 days	3 to 4 days
Vacuum-packed dinners, commercial brand with USDA seal	2 weeks	3 to 4 days
Bacon	2 weeks	7 days
Hot dogs	2 weeks	1 week
Luncheon meat	2 weeks	3 to 5 days
Ham, fully cooked	7 days	slices, 3 days; whole, 7 days
Ham, canned, labeled "keep refrigerated"	9 months	3 to 4 days
Ham, canned, shelf-stable	2 years/pantry	3 to 5 days
Canned meat and poultry, shelf-stable	2 to 5 years/pantry	3 to 4 days

- Eat only foods that have been recently prepared and are served hot. Eat raw fruits or vegetables only if washed in purified water or peeled with clean hands.
- Use purified water for drinking, making ice cubes, and brushing teeth. Alternatively, use disinfecting tablets or boil water. Drink beverages made with boiling water (such as hot tea or coffee) or from factory sealed containers (such as bottled water or canned sodas).
- Refuse dairy products that have not been pasteurized and refrigerated properly.
- Travel with antibacterial and antidiarrheal medication in case efforts to avoid illness fail.[7]

To sum up these recommendations, "Boil it, cook it, peel it, or forget it."

Advances in Food Safety Advances in technology have dramatically improved the quality and safety of foods available on the market. From pasteurization in the early 1900s to irradiation in the early 2000s, these advances offer numerous benefits, but they also raise consumer concerns.*

*During the past century, pasteurization of milk helped control typhoid fever, tuberculosis, scarlet fever, diphtheria, and other infectious diseases.

Irradiation The use of low-dose **irradiation** protects consumers from foodborne illnesses by:

- Sterilizing some foods, such as spices and teas, for storage at room temperature
- Controlling insects and extending shelf life in fresh fruits and vegetables
- Delaying the growth of sprouts on potatoes and onions and delaying the ripening in some fruits such as strawberries and mangoes
- Preventing foodborne illness by destroying harmful bacteria in fresh and frozen beef, poultry, lamb, and pork
- Extending the shelf life of foods by destroying organisms that cause spoilage

Some foods, however, are not candidates for irradiation. For example, when irradiated, high-fat meats develop off-odors, egg whites turn milky, grapefruits become mushy, and milk products change flavor. Incidentally, the milk in those boxes kept at room temperature on grocery-store shelves is *not* irradiated; it is sterilized with an **ultrahigh temperature (UHT) treatment.**

The use of food irradiation has been extensively evaluated over the past 50 years; approved for use in more than 40 countries; and supported by numerous health agencies, including the **FAO**, **WHO**, and the American Medical Association. Irradiation does not make foods radioactive, nor does it noticeably change the taste, texture, or appearance of approved foods. Vitamin loss is minimal and comparable to amounts lost in other food-processing methods such as canning. Because irradiation kills bacteria without the use of heat, it is sometimes called "cold pasteurization."

Consumer Concerns about Irradiation Many consumers associate the term *radiation* with cancer, birth defects, and mutations, and consequently have strong negative emotions about using irradiation on foods. Some may mistakenly fear that irradiated food has been contaminated by radioactive particles, such as occurs in the aftermath of a nuclear accident. Some balk at the idea of irradiating, and thus sterilizing, contaminated foods and prefer instead the elimination of unsanitary slaughtering and food preparation conditions. Food producers, on the other hand, are eager to use irradiation, but they hesitate to do so until consumers are ready to accept it and willing to pay for it. Once consumers understand the benefits of irradiation, about half are willing to use irradiated foods, but most are not willing to pay more.

Regulation of Irradiation The FDA has established regulations governing the specific uses of irradiation and allowed doses. Each food that has been treated with irradiation must say so on its label (see Figure 19-5). Labels can be misleading, however. Products that use irradiated foods as ingredients are not required to say so on the label. Furthermore, consumers may interpret the *absence* of the irradiation symbol to mean that the food was produced without any kind of treatment. This is not true; it is just that the FDA does not require label statements for other treatments used for the same purpose, such as postharvest fumigation with pesticides.

Other Pasteurizing Systems Other technologies using high-intensity pulsed light or electron beams have also been approved by the FDA. Like irradiation, these technologies kill microorganisms and extend the shelf life of foods without diminishing their nutrient content.

REVIEW IT Describe how foodborne illnesses can be prevented.
Millions of people suffer mild to life-threatening symptoms caused by foodborne illnesses (review Table 19-1, p. 611). As How To 19-1 (pp. 616–617) describes, most of these illnesses can be prevented by storing and cooking foods at their proper temperatures and by preparing them in sanitary conditions. Irradiation of certain foods protects consumers from foodborne illnesses, but it also raises some concerns.

> **FIGURE 19-5 Irradiation symbol**

This international symbol, called the radura, identifies retail foods that have been irradiated. The phrases "Treated by irradiation" or "Treated with radiation" must accompany the symbol. The irradiation label is not required on commercially prepared foods that contain irradiated ingredients, such as spices. Foods approved for irradiation include eggs; fresh fruit (strawberries, citrus, papaya); oysters, clams, mussels, scallops, crabs, lobsters, shrimp; raw beef, lamb, poultry, pork; spices, tea; vegetables (iceberg lettuce, fresh spinach, potatoes, tomatoes, onions); and wheat.

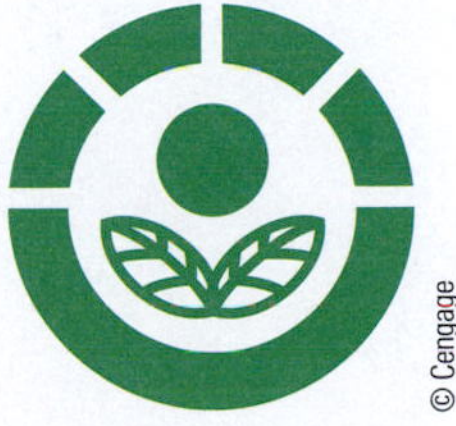

irradiation: sterilizing a food by exposure to energy waves, similar to ultraviolet light and microwaves; sometimes called *ionizing radiation.*

ultrahigh temperature (UHT) treatment: sterilizing a food by brief exposure to temperatures above those normally used.

19.2 Nutritional Adequacy of Foods and Diets

LEARN IT Explain how to minimize nutrient losses in the kitchen.

In years past, when most foods were whole and farm fresh, the task of meeting nutrient needs primarily involved balancing servings from the various food groups. Today, however, foods have changed. Advances in food production over the past century have set the stage for the widespread dissemination of ultraprocessed products—new creations that have little to do with natural foods and contain highly processed ingredients. Many of these foods appeal to consumers' demands for convenience and flavor, but do not necessarily deliver a balanced assortment of needed nutrients. In fact, most lack fiber, vitamins, minerals, and phytochemicals, but deliver excessive amounts of sugar, salt, and *trans* and saturated fats—the perfect combination of dietary factors to promote obesity and chronic diseases.[8] Advertisers spend much effort and money encouraging consumers to buy their products quickly, frequently, and abundantly, not on promoting healthy eating habits—unless that would increase sales too. For health's sake, consumers will want to buy fewer processed foods, prepare more meals at home using whole fresh foods, and dine at restaurants that prepare meals from scratch.

Obtaining Nutrient Information To help consumers find their way among the abundance of available foods, the FDA has developed extensive nutrition labeling regulations, as Chapter 2 described. In addition, the USDA's *Dietary Guidelines for Americans* help consumers combine foods into healthful eating patterns, and MyPlate helps them put those guidelines into practice (see Chapter 2).

Minimizing Nutrient Losses In addition to selecting nutritious foods and preparing them safely, consumers can improve their nutrition health by learning to store and cook foods in ways that minimize nutrient losses. Water-soluble vitamins are the most vulnerable of the nutrients, but both vitamins and minerals can be lost when they dissolve in water that is then discarded.

Fruits and vegetables contain enzymes that both synthesize and degrade vitamins. After a fruit or vegetable has been harvested, vitamin synthesis stops, but degradation continues. To slow the degradation of vitamins, most fruits and vegetables should be immediately frozen or kept refrigerated until used. In general, the nutrient content of frozen fruits and vegetables is comparable to their fresh counterparts.[9] Because many vitamins are easily destroyed by oxygen, fruits and vegetables that have been cut and juice that has been opened should be stored in airtight containers and refrigerated. (Degradative enzymes are most active at warmer temperatures.)

Water-soluble vitamins readily dissolve in water. To prevent losses during washing, rinse fresh fruits and vegetables before cutting. To minimize losses during cooking, steam, griddle, or microwave vegetables; pressure cooking and boiling cause the greatest nutrient losses. Alternatively, use the cooking water when preparing meals such as casseroles and soups.

Finally, keep in mind that most vitamin losses are not catastrophic and that a law of diminishing returns operates. Do not fret over small losses or waste time that may be valuable in improving your health in other ways. Be assured that if you start with plenty of fruits and vegetables and are reasonably careful in their storage and preparation, you will receive a sufficient supply of all the nutrients they provide.

REVIEW IT Explain how to minimize nutrient losses in the kitchen.
In the marketplace, food labels, the *Dietary Guidelines for Americans,* and MyPlate all help consumers learn about nutrition and how to plan healthy diets. At home, consumers can minimize nutrient losses from fruits and vegetables by refrigerating them, washing them before cutting them, storing them in airtight containers, and cooking them for short times in minimal water.

19.3 Environmental Contaminants

LEARN IT Explain how environmental contaminants get into foods and how people can protect themselves against contamination.

Concern about environmental contamination of foods is growing as the world becomes more populated and more industrialized. Industrial processes pollute the air, water, and soil. Plants absorb the **contaminants,** and people consume the plants (grains, vegetables, legumes, and fruits) or the meat and milk products from livestock that have eaten the plants. Similarly, polluted water contaminates the fish and other seafood that people eat. Environmental contaminants in air, water, and foods find their way into our bodies and have the potential to cause numerous health problems.

Harmfulness of Environmental Contaminants The potential harmfulness of a contaminant depends in part on its **persistence**—the extent to which it lingers in the environment or in the body. Some contaminants in the environment are short-lived because microorganisms or agents such as sunlight or oxygen break them down. Some contaminants in the body may linger for only a short time because the body rapidly excretes them or metabolizes them to harmless compounds. These contaminants present little cause for concern. Some contaminants, however, resist breakdown and can accumulate. Each level of the **food chain,** then, has a greater concentration than the one below—a process known as **bioaccumulation.** Figure 19-6 shows how bioaccumulation leads to high concentrations of toxins in animals and in people at the top of the food chain.

contaminants: substances that make a food impure and unsuitable for ingestion.

persistence: stubborn or enduring continuance; with respect to food contaminants, the quality of persisting, rather than breaking down, in the bodies of animals and human beings.

food chain: the sequence in which living things depend on other living things for food.

bioaccumulation: the accumulation of contaminants in the flesh of animals high on the food chain.

> **FIGURE 19-6 Bioaccumulation of Toxins in the Food Chain**

This example features fish as the food for human consumption, but bioaccumulation of toxins occurs on land as well when cows, pigs, and chickens eat or drink contaminated foods or water.

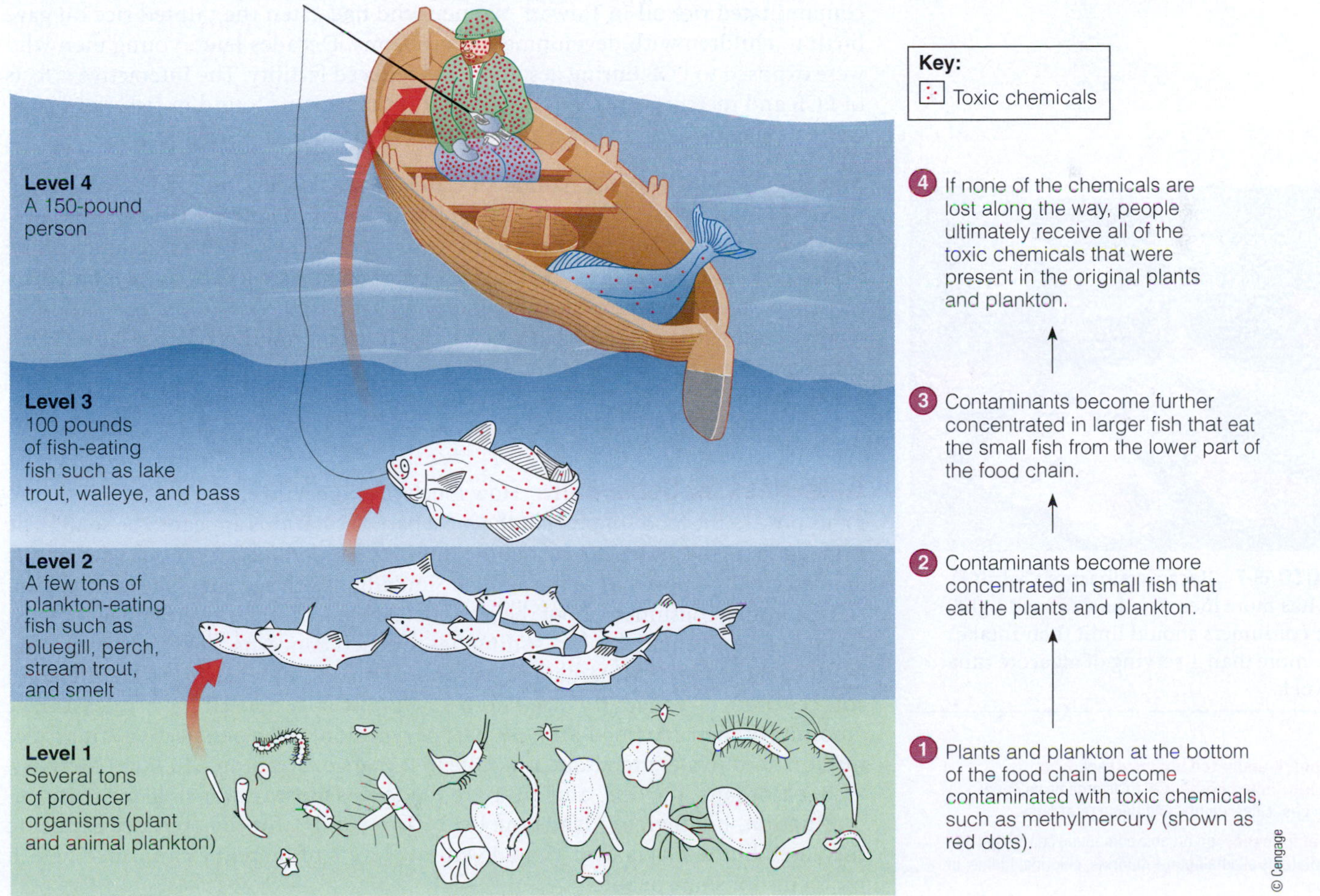
Key:
Toxic chemicals
Level 4
A 150-pound person
4 If none of the chemicals are lost along the way, people ultimately receive all of the toxic chemicals that were present in the original plants and plankton.
Level 3
100 pounds of fish-eating fish such as lake trout, walleye, and bass
3 Contaminants become further concentrated in larger fish that eat the small fish from the lower part of the food chain.
Level 2
A few tons of plankton-eating fish such as bluegill, perch, stream trout, and smelt
2 Contaminants become more concentrated in small fish that eat the plants and plankton.
Level 1
Several tons of producer organisms (plant and animal plankton)
1 Plants and plankton at the bottom of the food chain become contaminated with toxic chemicals, such as methylmercury (shown as red dots).
© Cengage

Contaminants enter the environment in various ways. Accidental spills are rare but can have devastating effects. More commonly, small amounts are released into the environment from industrial wastes over long periods.[10] The following paragraphs describe how contaminants can enter the food supply.

Methylmercury A classic example of acute contamination occurred in 1953 when a number of people in Minamata, Japan, became ill with a disease no one had seen before. By 1960, 121 cases had been reported, including 23 in infants. Mortality was high; 46 died, and the survivors suffered blindness, deafness, lack of coordination, and intellectual deterioration. The cause was ultimately revealed to be methylmercury contamination of fish from the bay where these people lived. The infants who contracted the disease had not eaten any fish, but their mothers had, and even though the mothers exhibited no symptoms during their pregnancies, the poison affected their unborn babies. Manufacturing plants in the region were discharging mercury-containing waste into the waters of the bay, the mercury was turning into methylmercury, and the fish in the bay were accumulating this poison in their bodies. Some of the affected families had been eating fish from the bay every day.

PBB and PCB In 1973, half a ton of **PBB (polybrominated biphenyls),** toxic **organic halogens**, were accidentally mixed into some livestock feed that was distributed throughout the state of Michigan. The PBB found its way into millions of animals and then into the people who ate the meat. The seriousness of the accident came to light when dairy farmers reported that their cows were going dry, aborting their calves, and developing abnormal growths on their hooves. Although more than 30,000 cattle, sheep, and swine and more than a million chickens were destroyed, an estimated 97 percent of Michigan's residents had been exposed to PBB. Some of the exposed farm residents suffered nervous system aberrations and liver disorders.

A similar accident occurred in 1979 when **PCB (polychlorinated biphenyls)** contaminated rice oil in Taiwan. Women who had eaten the tainted rice oil gave birth to children with developmental problems. Decades later, young men who were exposed to PCB during gestation had reduced fertility. The interactive effects of PCB and mercury—two environmental contaminants found in fish—are especially damaging to brain functions such as balance and coordination.

Arsenic Arsenic—whether naturally occurring or a result of industrial contamination—is found in the water, air, food, and soil. Arsenic-based pesticides were commonly used in the United States until 1970, and so low levels of arsenic can be detected in agricultural fields. For this reason, even organic foods may contain arsenic. The FDA routinely tests rice and juices and has found trace amounts of arsenic.[11] After assessing the quantities of arsenic children commonly consume, the FDA is confident about the overall safety of rice products and apple juice. The FDA will take action when the arsenic level is at 10 parts per billion, or greater. (For perspective, 1 part per billion is equivalent to about 1 second in 32 years or 1 cent in $10 million.)

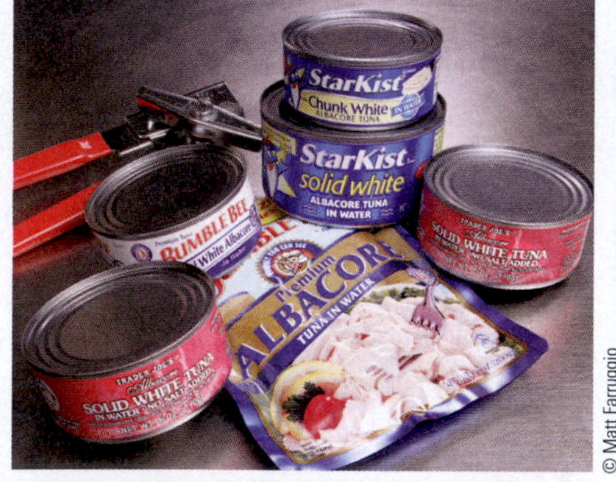
StarKist
Chunk White
StarKist
solid white
ALBACORE TUNA
BUMBLE BEE
SOLID WHITE TUNA
ALBACORE
SOLID WHITE TUNA

© Matt Farruggio

> **PHOTO 19-7** Because albacore ("white") tuna has more mercury than canned light tuna, consumers should limit their intake to no more than 1 serving of albacore tuna per week.

PBB (polybrominated biphenyl) and **PCB (polychlorinated biphenyl):** toxic organic halogens used in pesticides, paints, and flame retardants.

organic halogens: an organic compound containing one or more atoms of a halogen—fluorine, chlorine, iodine, or bromine.

Guidelines for Consumers

How much of a threat do environmental contaminants pose to the food supply? For the most part, the hazards appear to be small. The FDA regulates the presence of contaminants in foods and requires foods with unsafe amounts to be removed from the market. Similarly, health agencies may issue advisories informing consumers about the potential dangers of eating contaminated foods.

Most recently, mercury poisoning has aroused concerns—even at levels one-tenth of those in the Minamata catastrophe. Fish and other seafood are the main sources of dietary mercury (see Photo 19-7). Virtually all fish have at least trace amounts of mercury (median, 0.17 part per million). (For perspective, 1 part per million is equivalent to about 1 minute in 2 years or 1 cent in $10,000.) Mercury, PCB, chlordane, dioxins, and DDT are the toxins most responsible for fish contamination, but mercury leads the list by threefold. Chronic mercury exposure increases blood levels over time. Even low levels of mercury can cause health problems for some people.[12]

Review Figure 19-6 (p. 621) and notice how toxins such as mercury become more concentrated in animals and in people high in the food chain. Because of bioaccumulation, large game fish at the top of the aquatic food chain (such as tilefish, swordfish, king mackerel, and shark) generally have the highest concentrations of mercury (10 times the average). Consumers who enjoy eating these fish should select the smaller, younger ones (within legal limits). Also because of bioaccumulation, the concentrations in fish may be a million times higher than the concentrations in the water itself.

The **Environmental Protection Agency (EPA)** regulates commercial fishing to help ensure that fish destined for consumption in the United States meet safety standards for mercury and other contaminants. Farm-raised fish usually have lower concentrations of mercury than fish caught in the wild. Consequently, most consumers in the United States are not in danger of receiving harmful levels of mercury from fish.

The potential harm from contaminants must be balanced against the potential benefits from nutrients. Pregnant and lactating women and young children are most vulnerable because mercury toxicity damages the developing brain. Yet they are also likely to benefit from consuming seafood rich in omega-3 fatty acids. Table 15-8 (p. 480) presented the best choices—and those to avoid—to receive the benefits and minimize the risks of eating seafood.

What about the noncommercial fish a person catches from a local lake, river, or ocean? After all, it's almost impossible to tell whether water is contaminated without sophisticated equipment. Each state monitors its waters and issues advisories to inform the public if chemical contaminants have been found in the local fish. To find out whether a fish advisory has been posted in your region, call the local or state environmental health department.

REVIEW IT Explain how environmental contaminants get into foods and how people can protect themselves against contamination.

Foods may become contaminated as pollutants enter the air, land, and sea. So far, the hazards appear relatively small. In all cases, two principles apply. First, remain alert to the possibility of contamination of foods and keep an ear open for public health announcements and advice. Second, eat a variety of foods. Varying food choices is an effective defensive strategy against the accumulation of toxins in the body. Each food eaten dilutes contaminants that may be present in other components of the diet.

19.4 Natural Toxicants in Foods

LEARN IT Identify natural toxicants and determine whether they are hazardous.

Consumers concerned about food contamination may think that they can eliminate all poisons from their diets by eating only "natural" foods. On the contrary, nature has provided plants with an abundant array of toxicants. A few examples will show how even "natural" foods may contain potentially harmful substances. They also show that although the *potential* for harm exists, *actual* harm rarely occurs.

Poisonous mushrooms are a familiar example of plants that can be harmful when eaten. Few people know, though, that other commonly eaten foods contain substances that can cause illnesses. Cabbage, bok choy, turnips, mustard greens, kale, brussels sprouts, cauliflower, broccoli, kohlrabi, and radishes contain small quantities of goitrogens—compounds that can enlarge the thyroid gland. Eating exceptionally large amounts of goitrogen-containing vegetables can aggravate a preexisting thyroid problem, but it usually does not initiate one. Problems may develop when exceptionally large amounts (2 to 3 pounds a day) of these vegetables are eaten raw; cooking deactivates the enzyme that normally inhibits the uptake of iodine in the thyroid.

Lima beans and fruit seeds such as apricot pits contain cyanogens—inactive compounds that produce the deadly poison cyanide upon activation by a specific plant enzyme. For this reason, many countries restrict commercially grown lima beans to those varieties with the lowest cyanogen contents. As for fruit seeds, they are seldom deliberately eaten. An occasional swallowed seed or two presents no danger, but a couple of dozen seeds can be fatal to a small child. Perhaps the most infamous cyanogen in seeds is laetrile—a compound erroneously represented as a cancer cure. True, laetrile kills cancer, but only at doses that kill the person too. The combination of cyanide poisoning and lack of medical attention is life-threatening.

The humble potato contains many natural poisons, including **solanine**, a powerful narcotic-like substance. Most of a potato's solanine is found in the sprouts and in the green layer that develops just beneath the skin. Solanine poisoning is extremely rare, however, because the small amounts of solanine (8 milligrams per 100 grams of potato) normally found in potatoes are harmless—even when the potato skin is eaten. Solanine can be toxic, however, and presents a hazard when consumed in large quantities (20 to 25 milligrams per 100 grams of potato). Solanine is not destroyed by cooking, but it can be removed by peeling the potato. Symptoms of solanine poisoning include gastrointestinal disturbances and neurological disorders.

REVIEW IT Identify natural toxicants and determine whether they are hazardous.
Natural toxicants include the goitrogens in cabbage, cyanogens in lima beans, and solanine in potatoes. These examples of naturally occurring toxicants illustrate two familiar principles. First, any substance can be toxic when consumed in excess. Second, poisons are poisons, whether made by people or by nature. Remember, it is not the source of a chemical that makes it hazardous, but its chemical structure and the quantity consumed.

19.5 Pesticides

LEARN IT Debate the risks and benefits of using pesticides.

The use of **pesticides** in agriculture is controversial. They help ensure the survival of crops, but they leave **residues** in the environment and on some of the foods we eat. Balancing the benefits of pesticides to agriculture and food production against the risks to the environment and human health is an ongoing challenge.

Hazards and Regulation of Pesticides

Ideally, a pesticide destroys the pest and quickly degenerates to nontoxic products without accumulating in the food chain. Then, by the time consumers eat the food, no harmful residues remain. Unfortunately, no such perfect pesticide exists. As new pesticides are developed, government agencies assess their risks and benefits and monitor their use.

Hazards of Pesticides Pesticides applied in the field may linger on foods. Health risks from pesticide exposure are probably small for healthy adults, but children, the elderly, and people with weakened immune systems may be vulnerable to pesticide toxicity.

Regulation of Pesticides Consumers depend on the EPA and the FDA to keep pesticide use within safe limits. These agencies evaluate the risks and benefits of a pesticide's use by asking such questions as: How dangerous is it? How much residue is left on the crop? How much harm does the pesticide do to the environment? How necessary is it? What are the alternatives to its use?

If the pesticide is approved, the EPA establishes a **tolerance level** for its presence in foods, well below the level at which it could cause any conceivable harm. Tolerance regulations also state the specific crops to which each pesticide can be applied. If a pesticide is misused, growers risk fines, lawsuits, and destruction of their crops.

Once tolerances are set, the FDA enforces them by monitoring foods and livestock feeds for the presence of pesticides. Over the past several decades of testing, the FDA has seldom found residues above tolerance levels (less than 3 percent of domestic foods tested), so it appears that pesticides are generally used according to regulations.[13] Minimal pesticide use means lower costs for growers. In addition to costs, many farmers are also concerned about the environment, the quality of their

solanine (SOH-lah-neen): a poisonous narcotic-like substance present in potato skins and sprouts.

pesticides: chemicals used to control insects and other organisms on plants, vegetables, fruits, and animals. Used broadly, the term includes herbicides (to kill weeds), insecticides (to kill insects), and fungicides (to kill fungi).

residues: whatever remains. In the case of pesticides, those amounts that remain on or in foods when people buy and use them.

tolerance level: the maximum amount of a residue permitted in a food when a pesticide is used according to label directions.

farmland, and a safe food supply. Where violations are found, they are usually due to unusual weather conditions, use of unapproved pesticides, or misuse—for example, application of a particular pesticide to a crop for which it has not been approved.

Pesticides from Other Countries A substantial and increasing amount of the fruits and vegetables consumed in the United States are imported from other countries (see Photo 19-8). These countries have their own pesticide regulations—some more, and others less, stringent than those in the United States. To export into the United States, countries are required to comply with US pesticide tolerance limits and, for the most part, they do. The FDA finds violations of residue limits in about 13 percent of imported foods tested. Close to 200 member nations work together to develop international food standards through the Food and Agriculture Organization (FAO) and the World Health Organization (WHO) to help protect consumer health and promote fair practices in food trade, but compliance is voluntary.[14]

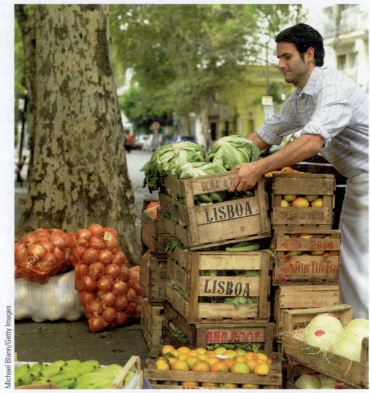
LISBOA
LISBOA
2006
Michael Blann/Getty Images

> **PHOTO 19-8** As many as 400 varieties of fruits and vegetables are imported from other countries.

Monitoring Pesticides

The FDA collects and analyzes samples of both domestic and imported foods. If the agency finds samples in violation of regulations, it can seize the products or order them destroyed. Individual states also scan for pesticides (as well as for industrial chemicals) and provide information to the FDA.

Food in the Fields In addition to its ongoing surveillance, the FDA conducts focused sampling to determine the presence of particular pesticides in specific crops. For example, the agency might search for aldicarb in potatoes, captan in cherries, and diaminozide (the chemical name for Alar) in apples, among others.

Food on the Plate In addition to monitoring crops in the field for pesticides, the FDA also monitors people's actual intakes. The agency conducts the Total Diet Study (sometimes called the "Market Basket Survey") to estimate the dietary intakes of pesticide residues by eight age and gender groups from infants to senior citizens. Four times a year, FDA surveyors buy almost 300 foods from US grocery stores, each time in several cities. They prepare the foods table ready and then analyze them not only for pesticides, but also for essential minerals, industrial chemicals, **heavy metals**, and radioactive materials. In all, the survey reports on more than 6000 samples a year, including samples imported from 100 countries. Most heavily sampled are fresh vegetables, fruits, and dairy products.

The Total Diet Study provides a direct estimate of the amounts of pesticide residues that remain in foods as they are usually eaten—after they have been washed, peeled, and cooked. Analyses reveal that almost all samples fall well below the amounts considered acceptable. The amount considered acceptable is "the daily intake of a chemical, which, if ingested over a lifetime, appears to be without appreciable risk." *Without appreciable risk* means "practical certainty that injury will not result even after a lifetime of exposure." All in all, these findings confirm the safety of the US food supply.

Consumer Concerns

Despite these reassuring reports, consumers still worry that food monitoring may not be adequate. For one thing, manufacturers develop new pesticides all the time. For another, as described earlier, other countries may use different pesticides and follow less stringent guidelines. For still another, although US regulations may protect crops adequately, they may not necessarily protect the environment or the people who work in the fields. Concerns over poisoning of soil, waterways, wildlife, and workers and their families may well be valid.

heavy metals: mineral ions such as mercury or lead, so called because of their relatively high atomic weight. Many heavy metals are poisonous.

TABLE 19-3 Tips to Minimize Pesticide Residues and Bacteria Contamination

When Shopping for Foods
• Select fruits and vegetables that do not have holes. • Select a variety of foods to minimize exposure to any one pesticide. • Consider buying certified organic foods when shopping for produce most likely to be contaminated (see Table 19-4, p. 628).
When Preparing Foods
• Wash your hands for 20 seconds with warm water and soap before and after preparing foods. • Trim the fat from meat, and remove the skin from poultry and fish; discard fats and oils in broths and pan drippings (pesticide residues concentrate in the animal's fat). • Wash fresh produce in warm running water, gently rub soft produce or use a scrub brush on firm produce, and rinse thoroughly. • Use a knife to peel an orange and grapefruit; do not bite into the peel. • Discard the outer leaves of leafy vegetables such as cabbage and lettuce. • Cut away damaged or bruised areas. • Wash fruits and vegetables before peeling to avoid transferring dirt and bacteria from the knife onto the produce. Peel waxed fruits and vegetables; waxes don't wash off and can seal in pesticide residues. • Peel vegetables such as carrots and fruits such as apples when possible (peeling removes dirt, bacteria, and pesticides that remain in or on the peel, but also removes fibers, vitamins, and minerals).

The FDA does not sample *all* food shipments or test for *all* pesticides in each sample. The FDA is a *monitoring* agency, and as such, it cannot, nor can it be expected to, guarantee 100 percent safety in the food supply. Instead, it sets standards so that substances do not become a hazard, checks enough samples to adequately assess average food safety, and acts promptly when problems or suspicions arise.

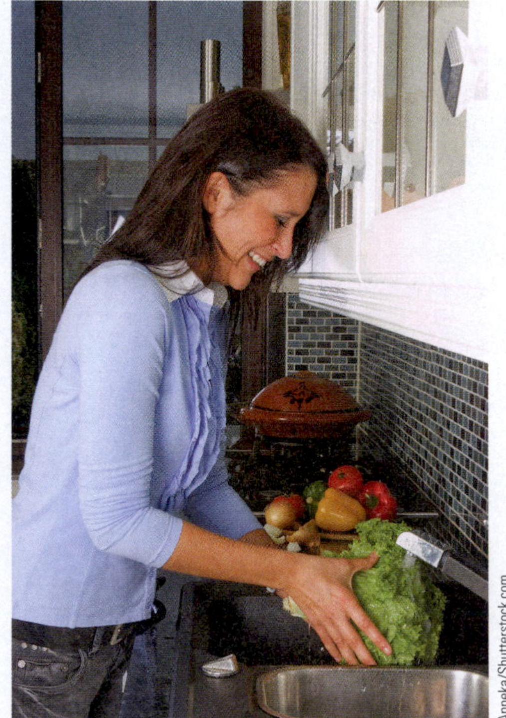

Anneka/Shutterstock.com

> **PHOTO 19-9** Washing fresh fruits and vegetables removes most, if not all, of the pesticide residues that might have been present.

Minimizing Risks Whether consumers ingest pesticide residues depends on a number of factors. How much of a given food does the consumer eat? What pesticide was used on it? How much was used? How long ago was the food last sprayed? Did environmental conditions promote pest growth or pesticide breakdown? How well was the produce washed? Was it peeled or cooked? With so many factors, consumers cannot know for sure whether pesticide residues remain on foods, but they can minimize their risks by following the guidelines offered in Table 19-3; washing, peeling, and cooking fruits and vegetables reduces pesticide residue levels (see Photo 19-9). The food supply is protected well enough that consumers who take these precautions can feel secure that the foods they eat are safe.

Alternatives to Pesticides The use of pesticides has helped generate higher crop yields that feed the world and protect against diseases transmitted by insects. Still, many consumers are concerned. To feed a nation while using fewer pesticides requires creative farming methods. Highlight 19 describes how scientists can genetically alter plants to enhance their production of natural pesticides, and Chapter 20 presents alternative, or sustainable, agriculture methods. These methods include such practices as rotating crops, releasing organisms into fields to destroy pests, and planting nonfood crops nearby to kill pests or attract them away from the food crops. For example, releasing beetles into orange groves helps reduce the population of aphids; some flowers, such as marigolds, release natural insecticides that protect crops such as tomatoes. Sometimes alternative farming methods are more labor-intensive and may produce smaller yields than conventional methods, at least initially. Over time, though, by eliminating expensive pesticides, fertilizers, and fuels, these alternatives may actually cut costs more than they cut yields.

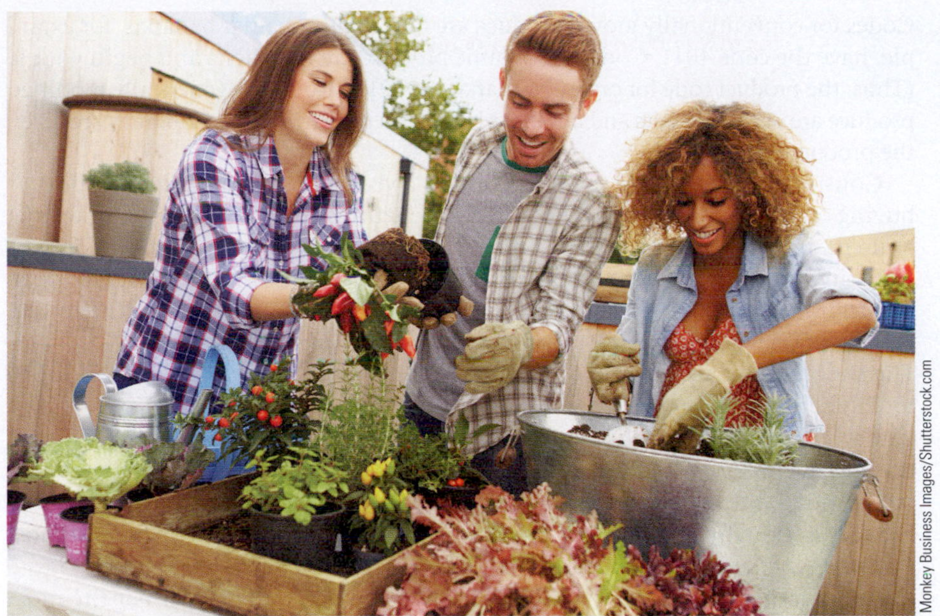

Monkey Business Images/Shutterstock.com

> **PHOTO 19-10** People can grow organic vegetables when their gardens or farms are relatively small. Even when land isn't readily available, vegetables can be grown in pots on windowsills, balconies, or rooftops.

Organically Grown Crops Alternative methods are especially useful for gardeners and farmers who want to produce and market **organic** crops that are grown and processed according to USDA regulations defining the use of synthetic fertilizers, herbicides, insecticides, fungicides, preservatives, and other chemical ingredients (see Photo 19-10). Similarly, meat, poultry, eggs, and dairy products may be called organic if the livestock has been raised according to USDA regulations defining the grazing conditions and the use of organic feed, hormones, and antibiotics. In addition, producers may *not* claim products are organic if they have been irradiated, genetically engineered, or grown with fertilizer made from sewer sludge. Figure 19-7 shows examples of food labels for products using organic ingredients.

organic: in agriculture, crops grown and processed according to USDA regulations defining the use of fertilizers, herbicides, insecticides, fungicides, preservatives, and other chemical ingredients.

Most organic foods are marked as such, but consumers can also determine whether fruits and vegetables are organic by reading the product code on produce stickers.

> **FIGURE 19-7 Food Labels for Organic Products**

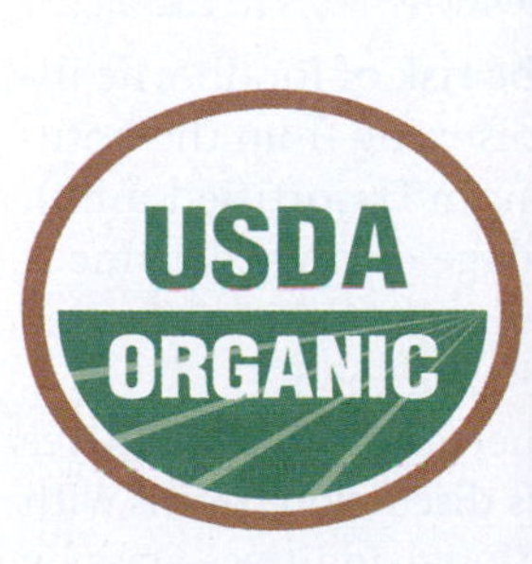
USDA
ORGANIC

Organic foods that have met USDA standards may use this seal on their labels.

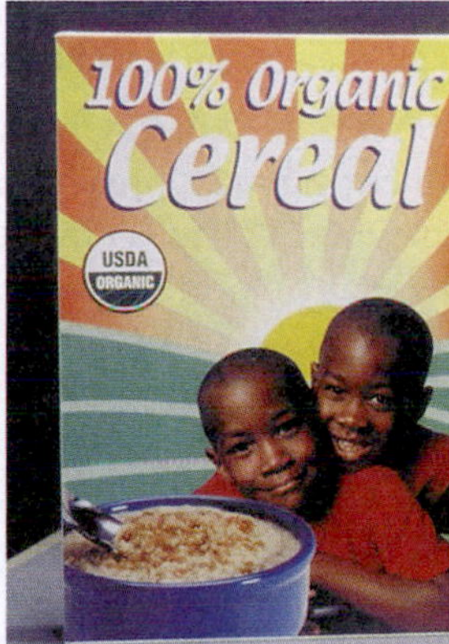
100% Organic
Cereal
USDA
ORGANIC

Foods made with 100 percent organic ingredients may claim "100% organic" and use the seal.

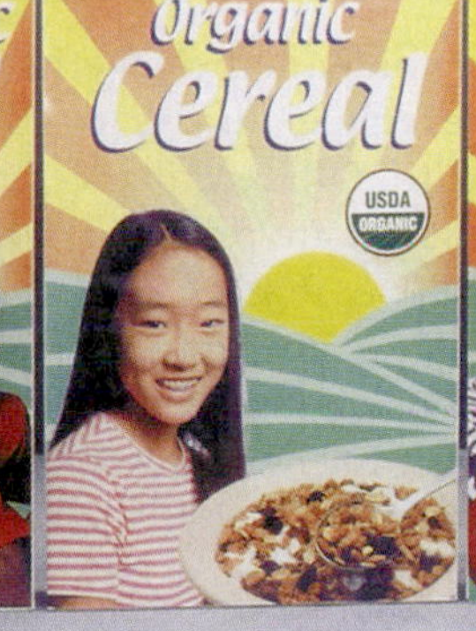
Organic
Cereal
USDA
ORGANIC

Foods made with at least 95 percent organic ingredients may claim "organic" and use the seal.

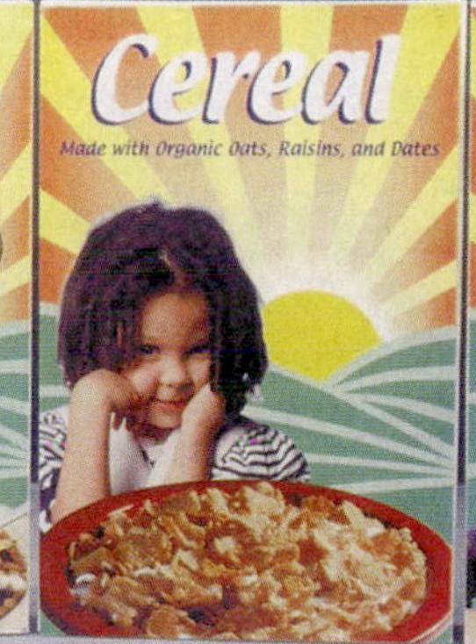
Cereal
Made with Organic Oats, Raisins, and Dates

Foods made with at least 70 percent organic ingredients may list up to three of those ingredients on the front panel.

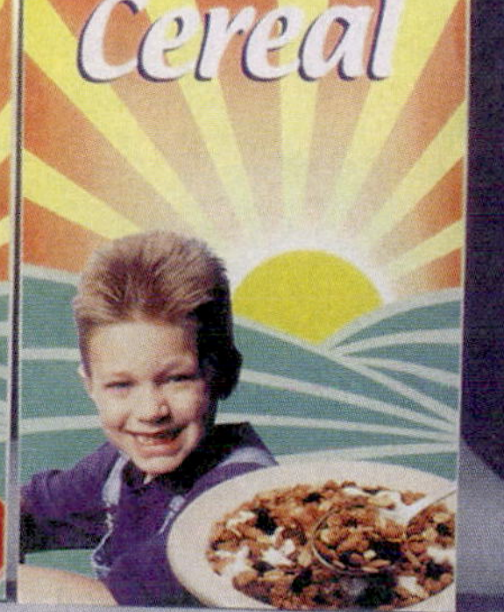
Cereal

Foods made with less than 70 percent organic ingredients may list them on the side panel, but cannot make any claims on the front.

United States Department of Agriculture

TABLE 19-4 Most and Least Pesticide-Contaminated Fruits and Vegetables

Most Contaminated	Least Contaminated
Strawberries	Avocados
Apples	Corn
Nectarines	Pineapples
Peaches	Cabbage
Celery	Peas (frozen)
Grapes	Onions
Cherries	Asparagus
Spinach	Mangoes
Tomatoes	Papayas
Bell peppers	Kiwi
Cherry tomatoes	Eggplant
Cucumbers	Honeydew melon
Snap peas (imported)	Grapefruit
Blueberries	Cantaloupe
Potatoes	Cauliflower

NOTE: These fruits and vegetables are ranked in order of their pesticide load. The top 12 most contaminated are commonly referred to as "the dirty dozen" and the top 15 least contaminated, as "the clean fifteen."

Codes for conventionally grown produce are four digits. Regular bananas, for example, have the code 4011. Codes for organic produce are five digits and begin with 9. (Thus, the product code for organic bananas is 94011.) Codes for genetically modified produce are also five digits and begin with 8. (Genetically modified bananas are given the product code 84011.)

Consumers spend more than $40 billion a year on organic foods. Reasons for buying organic include avoiding pesticides, benefiting the environment, protecting animals, improving worker safety, and obtaining safer and more nutritious foods.

Eating organic foods does reduce exposure to pesticide residues.[15] Each year, an environmental advocacy group publishes a list of the most popular fruits and vegetables that are most and least likely to have pesticide residues (see Table 19-4).[16] The suggestion is that because pesticide residues in conventionally grown foods are higher than in organic foods, consumers may want to pay attention to these lists when considering whether to make organic purchases. Some research contradicts such advice and indicates that the pesticide residues on even the most contaminated fruits and vegetables pose negligible health risks.[17] Whether buying conventionally grown or organically grown produce, consumers benefit most from eating at least five servings of fruits and vegetables daily.

Are organic foods nutritionally superior to conventional foods? For the most part, nutrient differences are relatively small and within the range that normally occurs in crops.[18]

Interestingly, organic has intense meanings for many consumers (see Photo 19-11). In one study, participants tasting foods, such as two yogurts, rated the one labeled "organic" as more nutritious, lower in fat, and worth more money and the one labeled "regular" as more flavorful—even though both yogurts were organic and identical (only their labels differed).[19]

REVIEW IT Debate the risks and benefits of using pesticides.

Pesticides can safely improve crop yields when used according to regulations, but they can also be hazardous when used inappropriately. The FDA tests both domestic and imported foods for pesticide residues in the fields and in market basket surveys of foods prepared table ready. Consumers can minimize their ingestion of pesticide residues on foods by following the suggestions in Table 19-3 (p. 626). Alternative farming methods may allow farmers to grow crops with few or no pesticides.

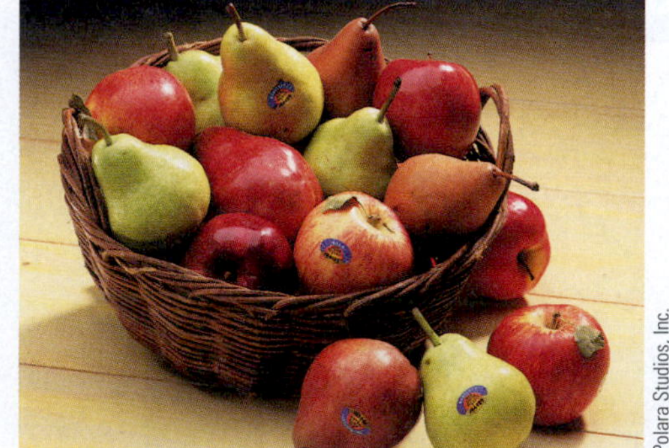

> **PHOTO 19-11** Many consumers are willing to pay a little more for organic produce.

19.6 Food Additives

LEARN IT List common food additives, their purposes, and examples.

Additives confer many benefits on foods. Some reduce the risk of foodborne illness (for example, nitrites used in curing meat prevent poisoning from the botulinum toxin). Others enhance nutrient quality (as in vitamin D–fortified milk). Most additives are **preservatives** that help prevent spoilage during the time it takes to deliver foods long distances to grocery stores and then to kitchens (see Photo 19-12). Some additives simply make foods look and taste good.

Intentional additives are put into foods on purpose, whereas indirect additives may get in unintentionally before or during processing. This discussion begins with the regulations that govern additives, then presents intentional additives class by class, and finally says a word about indirect additives.

Regulations Governing Additives The FDA's regulation of additives focuses primarily on safety. To receive permission to use a new additive in food products, a manufacturer must satisfy the FDA that the additive is:

- Effective (it does what it is supposed to do)
- Detectable and measurable in the final food product

additives: substances not normally consumed as foods but added to food either intentionally or by accident.

preservatives: antimicrobial agents, antioxidants, and other additives that retard spoilage or maintain desired qualities, such as softness in baked goods.

- Safe (when fed in large doses to animals under strictly controlled conditions, it causes no cancer, birth defects, or other injury)

On approving an additive's use, the FDA writes a regulation stating in what amounts and in what foods the additive may be used. No additive receives permanent approval, and all must undergo periodic review.

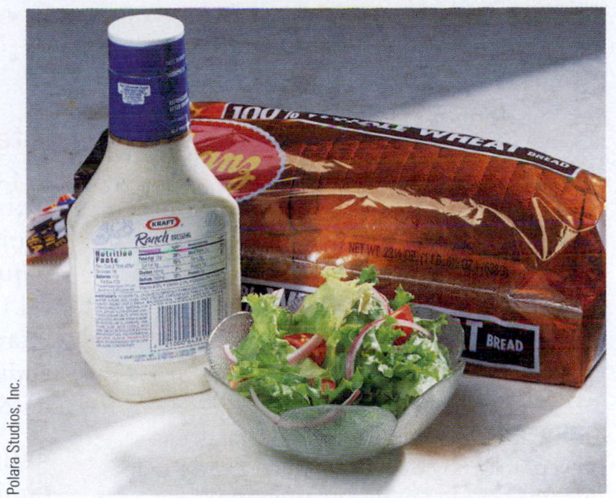
KRAFT
Ranch
BREAD

Polara Studios, Inc.

> **PHOTO 19-12** Without additives, bread would quickly get moldy, and salad dressing would go rancid.

The GRAS List Many familiar substances are exempted from complying with the FDA's approval process because they are **generally recognized as safe (GRAS),** based either on their extensive, long-term use in foods or on current scientific evidence. Several hundred substances are on the GRAS list, including such items as salt, sugar, caffeine, and many spices. Whenever substantial scientific evidence or public outcry has questioned the safety of any substance on the GRAS list, it has been reevaluated. If a legitimate question has been raised about a substance, it has been removed or reclassified. Meanwhile, the entire GRAS list is subjected to ongoing review.

The Delaney Clause One risk that the US law on additives refuses to tolerate at any level is the risk of cancer. To remain on the GRAS list, an additive must not have been found to be a **carcinogen** in any test on animals or human beings. The **Delaney Clause** (the part of the law that states this criterion) is uncompromising in addressing carcinogens in foods and drugs; in fact, its limitations have been intensely debated over the years.

The Delaney Clause is best understood as a product of a different historical era. It was adopted decades ago, at a time when scientists knew less about the relationships between carcinogens and cancer development. At that time, most substances were detectable in foods only in relatively large amounts, such as parts per thousand. Today, scientific understanding of cancer has progressed, and technology has advanced so that carcinogens in foods can be detected even when they are present only in parts per billion or even per trillion. (For perspective, one part per trillion is equivalent to about 1 inch in 16 million miles; or 1 second in 32,000 years.) Earlier, "zero risk" may have seemed attainable, but today we know it is not: all substances, no matter how pure, can be shown to be contaminated at some level with one carcinogen or another. For these reasons, the FDA prefers to deem additives (and pesticides and other contaminants) safe if lifetime use presents no more than a one-in-a-million risk of cancer to human beings. Thus, instead of the "zero-risk" policy of the Delaney Clause, the FDA uses a "negligible-risk" standard, sometimes referred to as the ***de minimis* rule.**

Margin of Safety Whatever risk level is permitted, actual risks must be determined by research. To determine risks posed by an additive, researchers feed test animals the additive at several concentrations throughout their lives. The additive is then permitted in foods in amounts 100 times *below* the lowest level that is found to cause any harmful effect—that is, at a 1/100 **margin of safety.** In many foods, *naturally* occurring substances occur with narrower margins of safety. Even nutrients pose risks at dose levels above those recommended and normally consumed: for older adults, the RDA for vitamin D is only 1/5 of the Upper Level.

Risks versus Benefits Of course, additives would not be added to foods if they only presented risks. In general, additives are used in foods when they offer benefits that outweigh the risks or make the risks worth taking. No amount of risk may be worth taking in the case of color additives that only enhance appearance but do not improve health or safety. In contrast, the FDA finds it worth taking the small risks associated with the use of nitrites on meat products, for example, because nitrites inhibit the formation of the deadly botulinum toxin. The choice involves a compromise between the risks of using additives and the risks of doing without them.

It is the manufacturers' responsibility to use only the amounts of additives that are necessary to achieve the needed effect, and no more. The FDA also requires that additives *not* be used:

- To disguise faulty or inferior products
- To deceive the consumer

generally recognized as safe (GRAS): food additives that have long been in use and are believed to be safe. First established by the FDA in 1958, the GRAS list is subject to revision as new facts become known.

carcinogen: a substance that can cause cancer; the adjective is *carcinogenic.*

Delaney Clause: a 1958 amendment to the Food, Drug, and Cosmetic Act of 1938, named after Congressman James Delaney of New York that states that no substance known to cause cancer in animals or human beings at any dose level shall be added to foods.

***de minimis* rule:** a guideline that defines risk as a cancer rate of less than one cancer per million people exposed to a contaminant over a 70-year lifetime.

margin of safety: when speaking of food additives, a zone between the concentration normally used and that at which a hazard exists. For common table salt, for example, the margin of safety is 1/5 (five times the amount normally used would be hazardous).

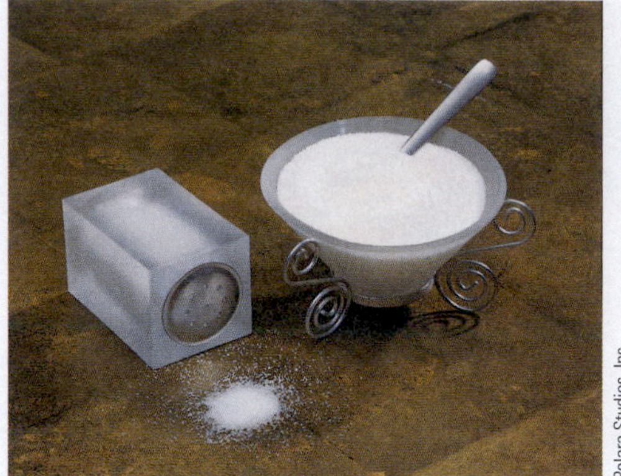
Polara Studios, Inc.

> **PHOTO 19-13** Both salt and sugar act as preservatives by extracting water from food; microbes cannot grow without water.

- If use would significantly destroy nutrients
- If effects can be achieved by economical, sound manufacturing processes instead

Intentional Food Additives **Intentional food additives** are added to foods to give them some desirable characteristic: resistance to spoilage, color, flavor, texture, stability, or nutritional value. Some food additives derive from natural sources (for example, beets may provide food coloring); others are not found in nature, but can be synthesized as artificial ingredients. In addition, some natural ingredients can also be synthesized as artificial ingredients (for example, vitamin C may be derived from an orange or manufactured in a laboratory). All additives—whether natural or artificial—are subject to the same FDA safety standards. This section describes additives people most often ask about.

Antimicrobials Foods can go bad in many ways. One way is by becoming contaminated with microbes that cause foodborne illnesses, a hazard that justifies the use of antimicrobial agents. The most widely used antimicrobial agents are ordinary salt and sugar. Salt has been used throughout history to preserve meat and fish; sugar serves the same purpose in canned and frozen fruits and in jams and jellies (see Photo 19-13). Both exert their protective effect primarily by capturing water and making it unavailable to microbes.

Other antimicrobial agents, the **nitrites,** are added to foods for three main purposes: to preserve color, especially the pink color of hot dogs and other cured meats; to enhance flavor by inhibiting rancidity, especially in cured meats and poultry; and to protect against bacterial growth. In amounts smaller than those needed to confer color, nitrites prevent the growth of the bacteria that produce the deadly botulinum toxin.

Nitrites clearly prevent food spoilage and bacterial contamination, but their use has been controversial. During the curing process and in the human body, nitrites can be converted to **nitrosamines.** Some nitrosamines are known to cause cancer in animals, but evidence is inconclusive in humans.[20] In fact, limited evidence suggests that nitrites may actually be beneficial to human health.[21] The USDA and FDA regulate and monitor the use of nitrites in foods and beverages.

Another food additive used in processed meat and poultry products—such as sausages, hot dogs, and bologna—is a mixture of viruses known as **bacteriophages.** Bacteriophages destroy the bacterium *Listeria monocytogenes,* thus protecting consumers from the potentially life-threatening foodborne illness listeriosis. These additives are included in the ingredients list on food labels as a "bacteriophage preparation."

Antioxidants Another way food can go bad is by exposure to oxygen (oxidation). Often, these changes involve no hazard to health, but they damage the food's appearance, flavor, and nutritional quality. Oxidation is easy to detect when sliced apples or potatoes turn brown or when oil goes rancid. Antioxidants prevent these reactions. Among the antioxidants approved for use in foods are vitamin C (ascorbate) and vitamin E (tocopherol).

Another group of antioxidants, the **sulfites,** cost less than the vitamins. Sulfites prevent oxidation in many processed foods and alcoholic beverages (especially wine). Because some people experience adverse reactions, the FDA prohibits sulfite use on foods intended to be consumed raw, with the exception of grapes, and requires foods and drugs that contain sulfite additives to declare it on their labels. For most people, sulfites pose no hazard in the amounts used in products, but there is one more consideration—sulfites destroy the B vitamin thiamin. For this reason, the FDA prohibits their use in foods that are important sources of the vitamin, such as enriched grain products.

Two other antioxidants in wide use are **BHA and BHT,** which prevent rancidity in baked goods and snack foods. Several tests have shown that animals fed large amounts

intentional food additives: additives intentionally added to foods, such as nutrients, colors, and preservatives.

nitrites (NYE-trites): salts added to food to prevent botulism. One example is sodium nitrite, which is used to preserve meats.

nitrosamines (nye-TROHS-uh-meens): derivatives of nitrites that may be formed in the stomach when nitrites combine with amines. Nitrosamines are carcinogenic in animals.

bacteriophages (bak-TIR-ee-oh-fayjz): viruses that infect bacteria.

- **bacterio** = bacteria
- **phage** = eat

sulfites: salts containing sulfur that are added to foods to prevent spoilage.

BHA and **BHT:** preservatives commonly used to slow the development of off-flavors, odors, and color changes caused by oxidation. BHA is butylated hydroxyanisole, and BHT is butylated hydroxytoluene.

of BHT develop *less* cancer when exposed to carcinogens and live *longer* than controls. Apparently, BHT protects against cancer through its antioxidant effect, which is similar to that of the antioxidant nutrients. The amount of BHT ingested daily from the US diet, however, contributes little to the body's antioxidant defense system. A caution: at intakes higher than those that protect against cancer, BHT *causes* cancer. Vitamins E and C remain the most important dietary antioxidants to strengthen defenses against cancer. (See Highlight 11 for a full discussion.)

Colors Only a few artificial colors remain on the FDA's list of additives approved for use in foods—a highly select group that has survived considerable testing (see Photo 19-14). Colors derived from the natural pigments of plants must meet standards of purity and safety, just as artificial colors do. Examples of natural pigments commonly used by the food industry are the caramel that tints cola beverages and baked goods and the carotenoids that color margarine, cheeses, and pastas. Carotenoids are also added to the feed for farm-raised salmon, which deepens the pink flesh color.

Flavors Myriad natural flavors, artificial flavors, and flavor enhancers are among the most often used food additives. Many foods taste delicious because manufacturers have added the natural flavors of spices, herbs, essential oils, fruits, and fruit juices. Some spices provide antioxidant protection as well as flavors. Often, natural flavors are used in combination with artificial flavors.

One of the best-known flavor enhancers is **monosodium glutamate**, or **MSG**—a sodium salt of the amino acid glutamic acid. MSG is used widely in a number of foods, especially Asian foods, canned vegetables, soups, and processed meats. Besides enhancing the well-known sweet, salty, bitter, and sour tastes, MSG itself may possess a unique flavor (known as umami). Adverse reactions to MSG—known as the **MSG symptom complex**—may occur in people with asthma and in sensitive individuals who consume large amounts of MSG, especially on an empty stomach. Otherwise, MSG is considered safe for adults. It is not allowed in foods designed for infants, however. Food labels require ingredient lists to itemize all additives, including MSG.

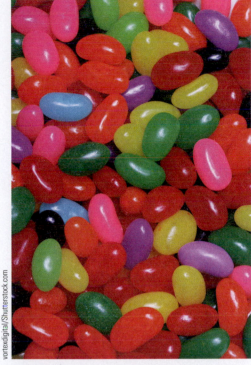

vortexdigital/Shutterstock.com

> **PHOTO 19-14** Color additives not only make foods attractive, but they identify flavors as well. Everyone agrees that yellow jellybeans should taste lemony and black ones should taste like licorice.

Sugar Alternatives The sugar alternatives, introduced in Chapter 4, are among the most widely used artificial flavor additives. Table 4-8 (p. 114) provides a summary of alternative sweeteners. This section presents safety issues surrounding a few of the most controversial ones.

Questions about the safety of the artificial sweetener saccharin surfaced in 1977, when experiments suggested that large doses of saccharin (equivalent to hundreds of cans of diet soda daily for a lifetime) increased the risk of bladder cancer in rats. As a result, the FDA proposed banning saccharin. Public outcry in favor of saccharin was so loud, however, that Congress imposed a moratorium on the ban while additional safety studies were conducted. Products containing saccharin were required to carry a warning label until 2001, when studies concluded that saccharin did not cause cancer in humans. Common sense dictates that consuming large amounts of any substance is probably not wise, but at current, moderate intake levels, saccharin appears to be safe for most people.

Aspartame—a simple chemical compound made of two amino acids (phenylalanine and aspartic acid) and a methyl group (CH_3)—must bear a warning label for people with the inherited disease phenylketonuria (PKU). People with PKU are unable to dispose of any excess phenylalanine. The accumulation of phenylalanine and its by-products is toxic to the developing nervous system, causing irreversible brain damage. The little extra phenylalanine from aspartame poses only a small risk, even in heavy aspartame users, but people with PKU need to get all their required phenylalanine from protein- and nutrient-rich foods instead of from an artificial sweetener.

During metabolism in the body, the methyl group of aspartame temporarily becomes methyl alcohol (methanol)—a potentially toxic compound. This breakdown also occurs in aspartame-sweetened beverages when they are stored at warm temperatures over time. The amount of methanol produced may be safe to consume, but a person may not want to, considering that the beverage has lost its sweetness. In the body,

monosodium glutamate (MSG): a sodium salt of the amino acid glutamic acid commonly used as a flavor enhancer. The FDA classifies MSG as a "generally recognized as safe" ingredient.

MSG symptom complex: an acute, temporary intolerance reaction that may occur after the ingestion of the additive MSG (monosodium glutamate). Symptoms include burning sensations, chest and facial flushing and pain, and throbbing headaches.

enzymes convert methanol to formaldehyde, another toxic compound. Finally, formaldehyde is broken down to carbon dioxide. Before aspartame could be approved, the quantities of these products generated during metabolism had to be determined, and they were found to fall below the threshold at which they would cause harm. In fact, ounce for ounce, tomato juice yields six times as much methanol as a diet soda.

The amount of artificial sweetener considered safe is called the **Acceptable Daily Intake (ADI)** and represents the amount of consumption that, if maintained every day throughout a person's life, would still be considered safe by a wide margin. It usually reflects an amount 100 times less than the level at which no observed effects occur in animal research studies. The ADI for aspartame, for example, is 50 milligrams per kilogram of body weight. For a 150-pound adult, the ADI is equivalent to almost 20 cans of soft drinks sweetened only with aspartame every day for a lifetime. Most people who use aspartame consume less than 5 milligrams per kilogram of body weight per day. Table 4-8 (p. 114) included the ADI for approved sweeteners.

Texture and Stability Some additives help maintain a desirable consistency in foods. Emulsifiers keep mayonnaise stable, control crystallization in syrups, disperse spices in salad dressings, and allow powdered coffee creamer to dissolve easily. Gums are added to thicken foods and help form gels. Yeast may be added to provide leavening, and bicarbonates and acids may be used to control acidity.

Nutrients As mentioned earlier, nutrients are sometimes added as antioxidants (vitamins C and E) or for color (beta-carotene and other carotenoids). In addition, manufacturers sometimes add nutrients to fortify or maintain the nutritional quality of foods. Included among nutrient additives are the five nutrients added to grains (thiamin, riboflavin, niacin, folate, and iron), the iodine added to salt, the vitamins A and D added to milk, and the nutrients added to fortified breakfast cereals. Appropriate uses of nutrient additives are to:

- Correct dietary deficiencies known to result in diseases
- Restore nutrients to levels found in the food before storage, handling, and processing
- Balance the vitamin, mineral, and protein contents of a food in proportion to the energy content
- Correct nutritional inferiority in a food that replaces a more nutritious traditional food

A nutrient-poor food with nutrients added may appear to be nutrient-rich, but it is rich only in those nutrients chosen for addition. Table 19-5 summarizes intentional food additives.

Acceptable Daily Intake (ADI): the estimated amount of a sweetener that individuals can safely consume each day over the course of a lifetime without adverse effect.

TABLE 19-5 Intentional Food Additives

Food Additive	Purpose	Common Examples
Antimicrobials	Prevent food spoilage from microorganisms	Salt, sugar, nitrites and nitrates (such as sodium nitrate), bacteriophages
Antioxidants	Prevent oxidative changes in color, flavor, or texture and delay rancidity and other damage to foods caused by oxygen	Vitamin C (erythorbic acid, sodium ascorbate), vitamin E (tocopherol), sulfites (sulfur dioxide, sodium sulfite, sodium bisulfite, potassium bisulfite, sodium metabisulfite, potassium metabisulfite), BHA and BHT
Colors	Enhance appearance	Artificial: indigotine, erythrosine, tartrazine Natural: annatto (yellow), caramel (yellowish brown), carotenoids (yellowish orange), dehydrated beets (reddish brown), grape skins (red, green)
Flavors	Enhance taste	Salt, sugar, spices, artificial sweeteners, MSG
Emulsifiers and gums	Thicken, stabilize, or otherwise improve consistency and texture	Emulsifiers: lecithin, alginates, mono- and diglycerides Gums: agar, alginates, carrageenan, guar, locust bean, psyllium, pectin, xanthan gum, gum arabic, cellulose derivatives
Nutrients (vitamins and minerals)	Improve the nutritive value by replacing vitamins and minerals lost in processing (enrichment) or adding vitamins or minerals that may be lacking in the diet (fortification)	Thiamin, niacin, riboflavin, folate, iron (in grain products); iodine (in salt); vitamins A and D (in milk); vitamin C and calcium (in fruit drinks); vitamin B_{12} (in vegetarian foods)

Indirect Food Additives **Indirect** or **incidental additives** find their way into foods during harvesting, production, processing, storage, or packaging. Incidental additives may include tiny bits of plastic, glass, paper, tin, and other substances from packages as well as chemicals from processing, such as the solvent used to decaffeinate coffee. The following paragraphs discuss a few different types of indirect additives that sometimes make headline news.

Acrylamide Raw potatoes don't have it, but french fries do—acrylamide, a compound that forms when carbohydrate-rich foods containing sugars and the amino acid asparagine are cooked at high temperatures. Apparently, acrylamide has been in foods ever since we started baking, frying, and roasting, but only recently has its presence been analyzed. At high doses, acrylamide causes cancer in animals and nerve damage in people. As such, scientists classify it as a probable carcinogen. Quantities commonly found in foods such as french fries, potato chips, breakfast cereals, and cookies, however, appear to be well below the amounts that cause such damage. The FDA is investigating how acrylamide is formed in foods, how its formation can be limited, and whether its presence is harmful.

Food Packaging The FDA ensures the safety of food packaging and assesses whether packaging materials might migrate into foods. These materials include coatings on can interiors, plastics, papers, and sealants.

Some microwave products are sold in "active packaging" that helps cook the food; for example, pizzas are often heated on a metalized film laminated to paperboard. This film absorbs the microwave energy in the oven and reaches temperatures as high as 500°F. At such temperatures, packaging components migrate into the food. For this reason, manufacturers must perform specific tests to determine whether materials are migrating into foods. If they are, their safety must be confirmed by strict procedures similar to those governing intentional additives.

Most microwave products are sold in "passive packaging" that is transparent to microwaves and simply holds the food as it cooks. These containers don't get much hotter than the foods, but materials still migrate at high temperatures. Consumers should not reuse these containers in the microwave oven. Instead they should use only glass or ceramic containers labeled as microwave safe; tiny air bubbles in some glass may expand when microwaved, causing the glass to break and glazes on some ceramics to leach, contaminating the food. In the United States, these ceramic containers cannot be sold without a permanent marking stating "Not for food use." Similarly, use only plastic wraps labeled as microwave-safe. Avoid using disposable styrofoam or plastic containers such as those used for carryout or margarine.

Similarly, a chemical known as bisphenol A (BPA) can leach from hard-plastic bottles and coatings of some food cans into food and beverages. The FDA has some concern about the potential health effects of BPA and is taking steps to reduce exposure in the food supply, including banning its use in baby bottles and sippy cups. Bisphenol S (BPS), a chemically related compound, has been used as a replacement in BPA-free products and has the same toxic effects.[22] Consumers who want to limit their exposure to toxic plastics should know that containers marked with recycle codes 3 or 7 may be made with BPA; those marked 6 contain polystyrene. The safest choices for food use are numbers 1, 2, 4, and 5. In addition, consumers should not use any plastic containers for hot foods or liquids.

To limit contamination and waste from packaging, some manufacturers are creating food wrappers and containers that are edible and soluble. For example, coatings similar to those used to cover pills might encase powdered cocoa; when dropped into hot water, the casing dissolves.

Decaffeinated Coffee In an effort to eliminate caffeine from their diets, some consumers select decaffeinated coffee. To remove caffeine from coffee beans, manufacturers often use methylene chloride in a process that leaves traces of the

indirect or **incidental additives:** substances that can get into food as a result of contact during growing, processing, packaging, storing, cooking, or some other stage before the foods are consumed; sometimes called *accidental additives.*

chemical in the final product. The FDA estimates that the average cup of coffee decaffeinated this way contains about 0.1 part per million of methylene chloride, which seems to pose no significant threat. A person drinking decaffeinated coffee containing 100 times as much methylene chloride every day for a lifetime has a one-in-a-million chance of developing cancer from it. People are exposed to much more methylene chloride from other sources such as hair sprays and paint-stripping solutions. Still, some consumers prefer either to return to caffeine or to select coffee decaffeinated in another way, perhaps by steam. Unfortunately, manufacturers are not required to state on their labels the type of decaffeination process used in their products. Many labels provide consumer-information telephone numbers for those who have such questions.

Hormones Hormones are a unique type of incidental additive in that their use is intentional, but their presence in the final food product is not. The FDA has approved about a dozen hormones for use in food-producing animals, and the USDA has established limits for residues allowed in meat products.

Some ranchers in the United States treat cattle with **bovine growth hormone (BGH).** All cows make BGH naturally, but when given higher doses, animals produce leaner meats, and dairy cows produce more milk.

Indeed, traces of BGH do remain in the meat and milk of both hormone-treated and untreated cows. BGH residues have not been tested for safety in human beings because residues of the natural hormone have always been present in milk and meat, and the amount found in treated cows is within the range that can occur naturally. Furthermore, BGH, being a peptide hormone, is denatured by the heat used in processing milk and cooking meat, and it is also digested by enzymes in the GI tract. The FDA has determined that BGH absorption does not occur in humans and that BGH is biologically inactive in humans even if injected. According to the National Institutes of Health, "As currently used in the United States, meat and milk from [hormone] treated cows are as safe as those from untreated cows." Whether hormones that have passed through the animals into feces and then contaminated the soil and water interfere with plants or animals in the environment remains controversial.

Antibiotics Like hormones, antibiotics are also intentionally given to livestock, and residues may remain in the meats and milks. Consequently, people consuming these foods receive tiny doses of antibiotics regularly, and those with sensitivity to antibiotics may suffer allergic reactions. To minimize drug residues in foods, the FDA requires a specified time between the time of medication and the time of slaughter to allow for drug metabolism and excretion.

Of greater concern to the public's health is the widespread use of antibiotics in food animal production and the consequent development of antibiotic resistance. Ranchers and farmers add an estimated 30 million pounds of antibiotics to livestock feed every year in an effort to defend against infections common in animals living in crowded conditions. These drugs also allow animals to gain weight faster, thus saving on feed costs. Because bacteria continuously exposed to antibiotics begin to adapt, they eventually lose their sensitivity to the drugs. The resulting antibiotic-resistant bacteria can cause severe infections that do not respond to standard antibiotic therapy, which is catastrophic in the treatment of disease in human beings.[23] The FDA continues to monitor the use of antibiotics in the food industry with the goal of ensuring that antibiotics remain effective in treating human disease.

bovine growth hormone (BGH): a hormone produced naturally in the pituitary gland of a cow that promotes growth and milk production; now produced for agricultural use by bacteria.

- **bovine** = of cattle

REVIEW IT List common food additives, their purposes, and examples.

On the whole, the benefits of food additives seem to justify the risks associated with their use. The FDA regulates the use of the intentional additives (summarized in Table 19-5, p. 632). Incidental additives sometimes get into foods during processing, but rarely present a hazard, although some processes such as treating livestock with hormones and antibiotics raise consumer concerns.

19.7 Consumer Concerns about Water

LEARN IT Discuss consumer concerns about water.

Foods are not alone in transmitting diseases; water is guilty too. In fact, *Cryptosporidium* and *Cyclospora*, commonly found in fresh fruits and vegetables, and *Vibrio vulnificus*, found in raw oysters, are commonly transmitted through contaminated water. In addition to microorganisms, water may contain many of the same impurities that foods do: environmental contaminants, pesticides, and additives such as chlorine used to kill pathogenic microorganisms and fluoride used to protect against dental caries. A glass of "water" is more than just H_2O. This discussion examines the sources of drinking water, harmful contaminants, and ways to ensure water safety.

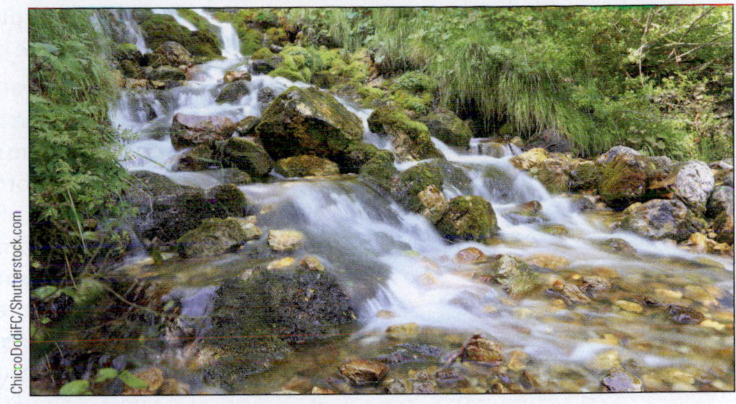

ChiccoDodiFC/Shutterstock.com

> **PHOTO 19-15** Clean rivers represent irreplaceable water resources.

Sources of Drinking Water

Water that is suitable for drinking is called **potable.** Only 1 percent of all the earth's water is potable (see Photo 19-15). Drinking water comes from two sources—surface water and groundwater. In the United States, each source supplies water for about half of the population.

Most major cities obtain their drinking water from surface water—the water in lakes, rivers, and reservoirs. Surface water is readily contaminated because it is directly exposed to acid rain, runoff from highways and urban areas, pesticide runoff from agricultural areas, and industrial wastes that are dumped directly into it. Surface water contamination is reversible, however, because fresh rain constantly replaces the water. It is also cleansed to some degree by aeration, sunlight, and plants and microorganisms that live in it.

Groundwater is the water in underground aquifers—rock formations that are saturated with and yield usable water. People who live in rural areas rely mostly on groundwater pumped up from private wells. Groundwater is contaminated more slowly than surface water, but also more permanently. Contaminants deposited on the ground migrate slowly through the soil before reaching groundwater. Once there, the contaminants break down less rapidly than in surface water because of the lack of aeration, sunlight, and aerobic microorganisms. The slow replacement of groundwater also allows contaminants to remain for a long time. Groundwater is especially susceptible to contamination from hazardous waste sites, dumps and landfills, underground tanks storing gasoline and other chemicals, and improperly discarded household chemicals and solvents.

Water Systems and Regulations

Public water systems treat water to remove contaminants that have been detected above acceptable levels. During treatment, a disinfectant (usually, chlorine) is added to kill bacteria. The addition of chlorine to public water is an important public health measure that appears to offer great benefits and small risks. On the one hand, chlorinated water has eliminated such waterborne diseases as typhoid fever, which once ravaged communities, killing thousands of people. On the other hand, it has been associated with an increase in bladder cancer and dioxin contamination of the environment. The EPA is responsible for ensuring that public water systems meet minimum standards for protecting public health.*

Even safe water may have characteristics that some consumers find unpleasant. Most of these problems reflect the mineral content of the water. For example, manganese and copper give water a metallic taste, and sulfur produces a "rotten egg" odor. Iron leaves a rusty brown stain on plumbing fixtures and laundry. Calcium and magnesium (commonly found in "hard water") build up in coffeemakers and hot water heaters. Similarly, soap is not easily rinsed away in hard water, leaving bathtubs and

*The EPA's safe drinking water hotline: (800) 426–4791.

potable (POH-tah-bul): suitable for drinking.

laundry looking dingy. For these and other reasons, some consumers have adopted alternatives to the public water system.

Home Water Treatments To ease concerns about the quality of drinking water, some people purchase home water-treatment systems. Because the EPA does not certify or endorse these water-treatment systems, consumers must shop carefully. Manufacturers offer a variety of units for removing contaminants from drinking water. None of them removes all contaminants, and each has its own advantages and disadvantages. Choosing the right treatment unit depends on the kinds of contaminants in the water. For example, activated carbon filters are particularly effective in removing chlorine, heavy metals such as mercury, and organic contaminants from sediment. Reverse osmosis forces pressurized water through a membrane, flushing out minerals such as sodium and some microorganisms such as *Giardia.* Ozonation uses ozone gas to disinfect water. And distillation systems, which boil water and condense the steam to water, kill microorganisms but leave behind minerals such as lead. Therefore, before purchasing a home water-treatment unit, a consumer must first determine the quality of the water. In some cases, a state or county health department will test water samples or can refer the consumer to a certified laboratory. Consumers need to be aware that unscrupulous vendors may use scare tactics during home inspections to prompt sales.

Bottled Water Despite the higher cost, many people turn to bottled water as an alternative to tap water. Almost 12 billion gallons of bottled water are sold in the United States annually—an average of more than 35 gallons per person. The FDA regulates bottled drinking water and has established quality and safety standards compatible with those set by the EPA for public water systems. In fact, some bottled waters come from the same municipal water sources as that for consumers' home taps. In addition, all bottled waters must be processed, packaged, and labeled in accordance with FDA regulations. Water quality may vary among brands because of variations in the source water used and company practices, but bottled water is neither safer nor healthier than tap water.

As Chapter 14 discussed, some bottled waters are marketed as "enhanced water"—water that has been enhanced with sweeteners, juices, coloring, flavors, vitamins, minerals, protein, or extra oxygen. Consumers perceive these bottled waters as healthful and sales have skyrocketed.

Labels on bottled water must identify the water's source. Approximately 75 percent of bottled waters derive from protected groundwater (from springs or wells)—the same as tap water. This water is usually treated before being bottled. For example, it may be disinfected with ozone gas rather than chlorine. Ozone kills microorganisms, then disintegrates spontaneously into water and oxygen, leaving behind no toxic by-products. Other bottled waters may be treated by filtration to remove pathogens and other particles. Bottled waters may also be treated by reverse osmosis or ion exchange to remove minerals. Alternatively, the water may be distilled into a vapor and then condensed again into water, thus removing any dissolved solids. These processes allow the bottle to be labeled "purified water." Most bottled waters do not contain fluoride; consequently, they do not provide the tooth protection of fluoridated water from community public water systems.

Consumers should be aware that bottled water is not necessarily purer than the water from their taps (see Photo 19-16). In fact, some bottled waters were recently recalled when *E. coli* contamination was discovered. As a safeguard, the FDA recommends that bottled water be handled like other foods and be refrigerated after opening.

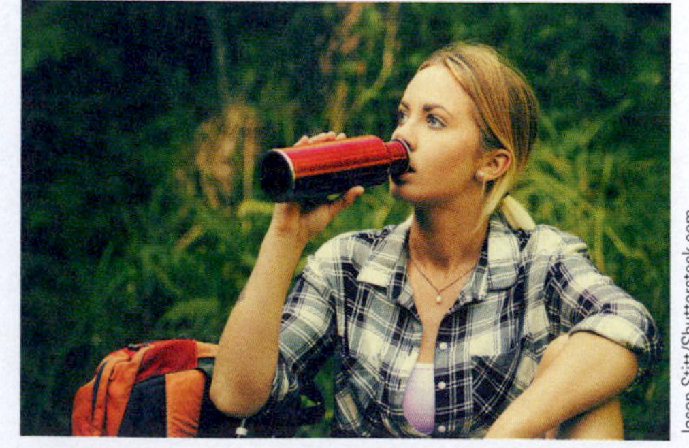

Jason Stitt/Shutterstock.com

> **PHOTO 19-16** Realizing that fossil fuels and many gallons of water are used to create and transport plastic water bottles, concerned consumers use refillable bottles to save money and the environment.

Protection of drinking water is a subject of ongoing concern and controversy. It may soon become a source of conflict between the world's nations as the population continues to grow and the renewable water supply remains constant. Estimates are that by 2030, half of the world's people will not have enough clean water to meet their needs.[24] To avert this potential calamity, we must take active steps to conserve water, clean polluted water, desalinate seawater, and curb population growth.

REVIEW IT Discuss consumer concerns about water.

Like foods, water may contain infectious microorganisms, environmental contaminants, pesticide residues, and additives. The EPA monitors the safety of the public water system, but many consumers choose home water-treatment systems or bottled water instead of tap water.

As this chapter said at the start, supplying safe food and clean water to hundreds of millions of people in the United States is an incredible challenge—one that is met, for the most part, with incredible efficiency.[25] The following chapter describes a contrasting situation—that of the food supply not reaching the people.

What's Online

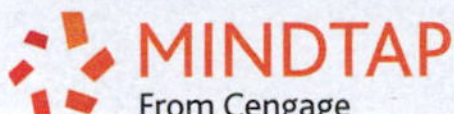
MINDTAP
From Cengage

Visit **www.cengagebrain.com** to access MindTap, a complete digital course that includes Diet & Wellness Plus, interactive quizzes, videos, and more.

REFERENCES

1. Centers for Disease Control and Prevention, *Estimates of foodborne illness in the United States*, www.cdc.gov/foodborneburden, August 19, 2016.
2. S. J. Crowe and coauthors, Vital signs: Multistate foodborne outbreaks—United States, 2010-2014, *Morbidity and Mortality Weekly Report* 64 (2015): 1221–1225.
3. L. H. Gould and coauthors, Outbreaks of disease associated with food imported into the United States, 1996-2014, *Emerging Infectious Diseases* 23 (2017): 525–528; *FDA Globalization*, www.fda.gov, June 24, 2016.
4. Centers for Disease Control and Prevention, Handwashing: Clean hands save lives, www.cdc.gov/handwashing, January 27, 2016.
5. K. Stein, The results of an international germ study: Should registered dietitians be surprised by the surprise? *Journal of the Academy of Nutrition and Dietetics* 113 (2013): 1288–1294.
6. R. C. Miranda and D. W. Schaffner, Longer contact times increase cross-contamination of *Enterobacter aerogenes* from surfaces to food, *Applied and Environmental Microbiology* 82 (2016): 6490–6496.
7. R. Steffen, D. R. Hill, and H. L. DuPont, Traveler's diarrhea—A clinical review, *Journal of the American Medical Association* 313 (2015): 71–80.
8. K. R. Siegel and coauthors, Association of higher consumption of foods derived from subsidized commodities with adverse cardiometabolic risk among US adults, *JAMA Internal Medicine* 176 (2016): 1124–1132.
9. A. Bouzari, D. Holstege, and D. M. Barrett, Vitamin retention in eight fruits and vegetables: A comparison of refrigerated and frozen storage, *Journal of Agricultural and Food Chemistry* 63 (2015): 957–62.
10. P. E. Drevnick, C. H. Lamborg, and M. J. Horgan, Increase in mercury in Pacific yellowfin tuna, *Environmental Toxicology and Chemistry* 34 (2015): 931–934.
11. US Food and Drug Administration, Arsenic, https://www.fda.gov/food/foodborneillnesscontaminants/metals/ucm280202.htm, April 1, 2016.
12. E. C. Somers and coauthors, Mercury exposure and antinuclear antibodies among females of reproductive age in the United States: NHANES, *Environmental Health Perspectives* 123 (2015): 792–798.
13. US Food and Drug Administration, *Pesticide Monitoring Program Fiscal Year 2013 Pesticide Report*, July 2016.
14. A. Ambrus and Y. Z. Yang, Global harmonization of maximum residue limits for pesticides, *Journal of Agricultural and Food Chemistry* 64 (2015): 30–35.
15. A. Zalecka and coauthors, The influence of organic production on food quality: Research findings, gaps and future challenges, *Journal of Science and Food Agriculture* 94 (2014): 2600–2604.
16. Environmental Working Group, *EWG's 2016 Shopper's Guide to Pesticides in Produce*, www.ewg.org/foodnews, 2016.
17. C. K. Winter, Pesticide residues in imported, organic, and "suspect" fruits and vegetables, *Journal of Agricultural and Food Chemistry* 60 (2012): 4425–4429.
18. M. R. Freedman and M. Mirabrishami, Vitamin C content of refrigerated, commercially available orange juice from organically grown and conventionally grown oranges is not different, *Nutrition Today* 50 (2015): 306–309; E. Johansson and coauthors, Contribution of organically grown crops to human health, *International Journal of Environmental Research and Public Health* 11 (2014): 3870–3893.
19. J. L. Wan-chen and coauthors, You taste what you see: Do organic labels bias taste perceptions? *Food Quality and Preference* 29 (2013): 33–39.
20. P. Song, L. Wu, and W. Guan, Dietary nitrates, nitrites, and nitrosamines intake and the risk of gastric cancer: A meta-analysis, *Nutrients* 7 (2015): 9872–9895.
21. A. Butler, Nitrites and nitrates in the human diet: Carcinogens or beneficial hypotensive agents? *Journal of Ethnopharmacology* 167 (2015): 105–107.
22. B. Mole, Doubts grow over BPA replacement, *Science News*, April 4, 2015, p. 10; C. D. Kinch and coauthors, Low-dose exposure to bisphenol A and replacement bisphenol S induces precocious hypothalamic neurogenesis in embryonic zebrafish, *Proceedings of the National Academy of Sciences of the United States of America* 112 (2015): 1475–1480.
23. A. Knoblock-Hahn, K. Brown, and L. Medrow, A balanced approach to understanding the science of antibiotics in animal agriculture, *Journal of the Academy of Nutrition and Dietetics* 116 (2016): 1332–1335.
24. United Nations, International decade for action 'Water For Life' 2005–2015, www.un.org/waterforlifedecade/scarcity.shtml.
25. Position of the Academy of Nutrition and Dietetics: Food and Water Safety, *Journal of the Academy of Nutrition and Dietetics* 114 (2014): 1819–1829.

LEARN IT Debate the pros and cons surrounding genetically engineered foods.

Food Biotechnology

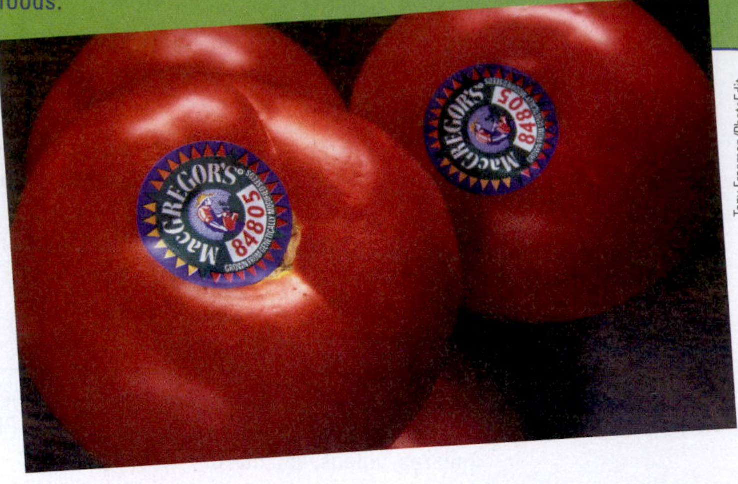
MacGREGOR'S
84805

Tony Freeman/PhotoEdit

Advances in food **biotechnology** promise just about everything from the frivolous (a tear-free onion) to the profound (a hunger-free world). Already biotechnology has produced leaner meats, longer shelf lives, better nutrient composition, and greater crop yields grown with fewer pesticides. Overall, biotechnology offers numerous opportunities to overcome food shortages, improve the environment, and eliminate disease. But it also raises concerns about possible risks to the environment and human health. Critics assert that biotechnology will exacerbate world hunger, destroy the environment, and endanger health. Foods and ingredients produced through biotechnology have been on the market for more than 25 years, yet the controversies and debates continue. This highlight presents some of the many issues surrounding genetically engineered foods, and Glossary H19-1 defines key terms.

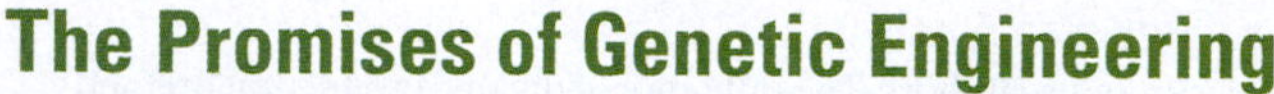

The Promises of Genetic Engineering

For centuries, farmers have been selectively breeding plants and animals to shape the characteristics of their crops and livestock. They have created prettier flowers, hardier vegetables, and leaner animals. Consider the success of selectively breeding corn (see Photo H19-1). Early farmers in Mexico began with a wild, native plant called teosinte (tay-oh-SEEN-tay) that bears only five or six kernels on each small spike. Many years of patient selective breeding have produced large ears filled with hundreds of plump kernels aligned in perfect formation, row after row.

Such genetic improvements, together with the use of irrigation, fertilizers, and pesticides, were responsible for more than half of the increases in US crop yields in the 20th century. Farmers still use selective breeding, but now, in the 21st century, **genetic engineering** allows scientists to insert or modify the genes in an organism to express a new trait or change the expression of an existing trait.[1] These advances have brought rapid and dramatic changes to agriculture and food production.

Selective breeding works, but it is slow and imprecise. With genetic engineering, scientists can improve crops (or livestock) by introducing a copy of the specific gene needed to produce the desired trait. Figure H19-1 illustrates the difference. Once introduced, the selected gene acts like any other gene—it provides instructions for making a protein. The protein then determines a characteristic in the genetically modified plant or animal. In short, the process is now faster and more refined. Farmers no longer need to wait patiently for breeding to yield improved crops and animals, nor must they even respect natural lines of reproduction among species. Laboratory scientists can copy genes from one organism and insert them into almost any other organism—plant, animal, or microbe. Alternatively, instead of genetically modifying crops, they might genetically edit crops by snipping and tweaking DNA at precise locations. Their work is changing not only the way farmers plant, fertilize, and harvest their crops, but also the ways the food industry processes food and consumers receive nutrients, phytochemicals, and drugs.

Extended Shelf Life

Among the first products of genetic engineering were tomatoes that stay firm and ripe longer than regular tomatoes that are typically harvested green and ripened in the stores. These genetically modified tomatoes promise less waste and higher profits. Normally, tomatoes

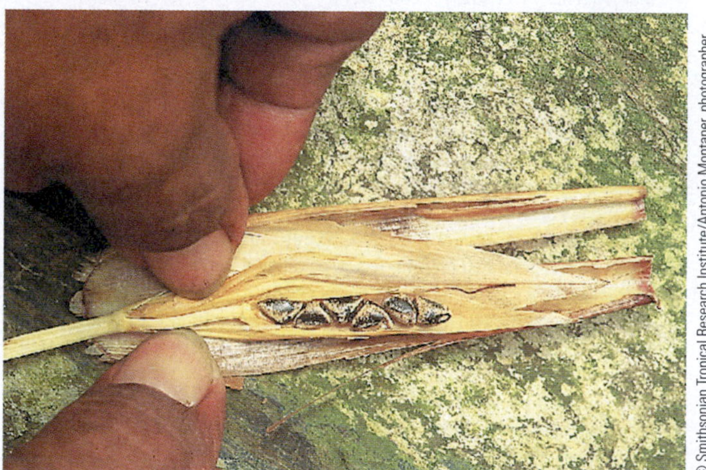

© Smithsonian Tropical Research Institute/Antonio Montaner, photographer

> **PHOTO H19-1** This wild predecessor of corn, with its sparse five or six kernels, bears little resemblance to today's large, full, sweet ears.

GLOSSARY H19-1

biotechnology: the science of manipulating biological systems or organisms to create or modify their products.

clone: an organism created without sexual reproduction and genetically identical to one ancestor.

genetic engineering: the intentional manipulation of the genetic material of living cells in order to produce some desirable trait not present in the original. Foods produced via this technology are called *genetically modified (GM)* or *genetically engineered (GE) foods.*

> **FIGURE H19-1 Selective Breeding and Genetic Engineering Compared**

Traditional Selective Breeding

Traditional selective breeding combines many genes from two varieties of the same species to produce one with the desired characteristics.

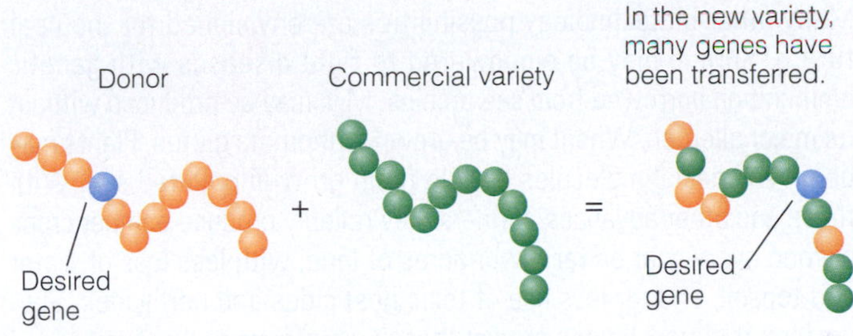
Donor
Commercial variety
In the new variety, many genes have been transferred.
Desired gene
Desired gene

Genetic Engineering

Through genetic engineering, a single gene is (or several are) transferred from the same or different species to produce one with the desired characteristics.

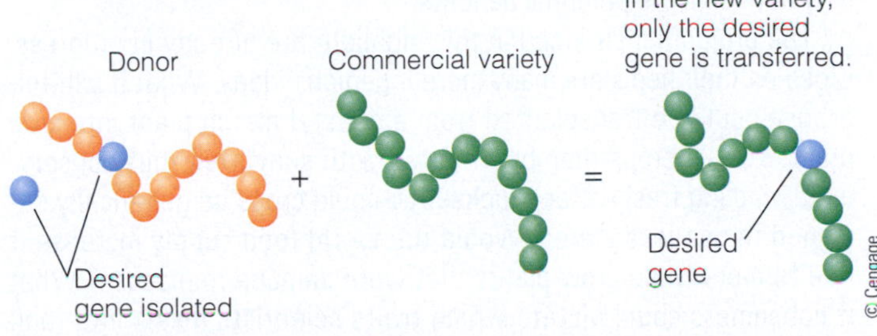
Donor
Commercial variety
In the new variety, only the desired gene is transferred.
Desired gene isolated
Desired gene
© Cengage

produce an enzyme (remember that enzymes are proteins) that softens them after they have been picked. Scientists can now introduce into a tomato plant a gene that is a mirror image of the one that codes for the "softening" enzyme. This gene blocks synthesis of the softening enzyme. Without this enzyme, the genetically altered tomato softens more slowly than a regular tomato, allowing growers to harvest it at its most flavorful and nutritious vine-ripe stage.

Similarly, apples have been genetically engineered not to turn brown when cut. Scientists accomplished this feat by turning off a gene that produces the enzyme that causes browning when apples are cut and exposed to oxygen. Minor damage won't create brown spots either, thus reducing food waste.

Improved Food Safety

Some genetic changes alter a food in ways that improve its safety. Potatoes, for example, have been genetically engineered to produce less acrylamide—the potentially cancer-causing chemical that forms in high-carbohydrate foods during high-temperature cooking. The FDA has concluded that these potatoes are as safe and nutritious as any other potato; those concerned about acrylamide may suggest they are safer.[2]

Improved Nutrient Composition

Genetic engineering can also improve the nutrient composition of foods. Instead of manufacturers adding nutrients to foods during processing, plants can be genetically altered to do the fortification work—a strategy called *biofortification*. Biofortification of crops with key vitamins and minerals can effectively combat the nutrient deficiency diseases that claim so many lives worldwide.[3] Soybeans may be implanted with a gene that upgrades soy protein to a quality approaching that of milk. Corn has been modified to contain twice the amount of lysine and tryptophan, its two limiting amino acids. Soybean and canola plants can be genetically modified to alter the composition of their oils, making them richer in the heart-healthy monounsaturated fatty acids.

"Golden rice," which has received genes from a daffodil and a bacterium that enable it to make beta-carotene, offers promise in treating vitamin A deficiency worldwide (see Photo H19-2). (Chapter 11 described how vitamin A deficiency contributes to the deaths of 2 million children and the blindness of a half million each year.) Of course, increasing nutrients in crops may have unintended consequences as well. For example, when broccoli is manipulated to increase its selenium content, production of the cancer-fighting phytochemical sulforaphane declines.

In addition to enhancing the nutrient composition, genetically modified crops can also produce more of the phytochemicals that help maintain health and reduce the risks of chronic diseases (see Highlight 13, p. 417). For example, pineapples can be genetically engineered to silence the gene that uses up the natural levels of pink lycopene to make yellow carotene.[4] The pink pineapples, with their abundant lycopene, are similar to red tomatoes in providing this powerful disease-fighting antioxidant. The possibilities seem endless.

Efficient Food Production

Genetic engineering also helps process foods more efficiently, which saves money.[5] For example, the protein chymosin, which prompts the ripening of cheese, has traditionally been harvested from the stomachs

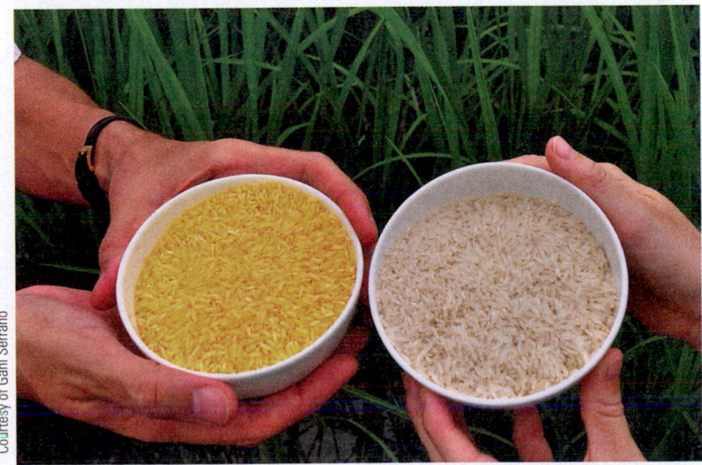
Courtesy of Gani Serrano

> **PHOTO H19-2** The vitamin A precursor beta-carotene gives golden rice its yellow color.

of nursing calves, a costly process. Now scientists have genetically engineered the bacterium *E. coli* to mass-produce chymosin—saving time, money, space, and animals.

Genetic engineering can also help bypass costly food-processing steps. At present, people who are lactose intolerant can buy milk that has been processed to include the lactase enzyme. Wouldn't it be more convenient, and less expensive, if scientists could genetically modify cows to make lactose-free milk directly? They've done it. Decaffeinated coffee beans are another real possibility.

Much of the research on genetic engineering of foods has focused on fruits and vegetables, but genetically engineered animals are also being grown for food. Scientists have inserted a gene into a salmon that enables the fish to reach adult size in a year and a half instead of three. The FDA confirms that the salmon is as safe and nutritious as other salmon and that the inserted genes remain stable over several generations of fish.[6]

Genetic research today has progressed well beyond tweaking a gene here and there to produce a desired trait. Scientists can now **clone** animals. By cloning animals, scientists have the ability to produce prized breeding stock. The FDA has declared that food from cloned livestock is safe to eat, but the USDA has asked farmers to keep cloned animals off the market. Because cloning an animal costs tens of thousands of dollars, it is incredibly unprofitable to slaughter it for meat. For this reason, cloned animals are used primarily for breeding and their natural-born offspring are used primarily for food. Because the FDA does not distinguish between foods from cloned animals or their offspring and foods from conventional animals, food labels are not required to provide this information.

Efficient Drug Delivery

Using cloned animals and other organisms in the development of pharmaceuticals is whimsically called "biopharming." For example, a goat that has been genetically modified to produce a malaria vaccine in its milk could provide both nourishment and immunization to a whole village of people now left unprotected because they lack food and medical help. Similarly, researchers have figured out how to induce hens to produce eggs with a drug to treat multiple sclerosis. Bananas and potatoes have been designed to make hepatitis vaccines, and tobacco leaves to make AIDS drugs. Researchers can also harvest vaccines by genetically altering hydroponically grown tomato plants to secrete a protein through their root systems into the water. Using foods to deliver drugs is only a small part of the promise and potential that biotechnology offers the field of medicine.

Genetically Assisted Agriculture

Currently eight genetically modified crops are grown in the United States. Only sweet corn, summer squash, and papayas are available directly to consumers in markets. Soybeans, cotton, canola, alfalfa, and sugar beets are used for animal feed and as ingredients in processed foods such as sugar or vegetable oil. The sugar and oil may derive from genetically modified crops but they are chemically identical to other sugars and oils.

Genetic engineering has helped farmers increase yields, extend growing seasons, and grow crops more efficiently. Crops that have been engineered to tolerate herbicides allow farmers to farm without tilling, which improves soil health and water retention. Similarly, farmers can grow crops that produce their own pesticides, thus allowing farmers to save time, increase yields, and use fewer, or less harmful, pesticides. Genetically modified crops have decreased the environmental impact associated with herbicide, pesticide, and fertilizer use.

Other Possibilities

Many other biotechnology possibilities are envisioned for the near future. Shrimp may be empowered to fight diseases with genetic ammunition borrowed from sea urchins. Milk may be produced without its major allergen. Wheat may be grown without its gluten. Plants may be given special molecules to help them grow in polluted soil. With these and other advances, farmers may reliably produce bumper crops of food every year on far fewer acres of land, with less loss of water and topsoil, and far less use of toxic pesticides and herbicides. Supporters of biotechnology predict that these efforts will enhance food production and help meet the challenge of feeding an ever-increasing world population. They contend that genetically modified crops have the potential to eliminate hunger and starvation. Others suggest that the problems of world hunger are more complex than biotechnology alone can resolve and that the potential risks of genetic engineering may outweigh the potential benefits.

The projects mentioned in this highlight are already in progress. Close on their heels are many more ingenious ideas. What if salt tolerance could be transplanted from a coastal marsh plant into crop plants? Could crops then be irrigated with seawater, thus conserving dwindling freshwater supplies? Or could crops be genetically designed to use less water? Would the world food supply increase if rice farmers could grow plants that were immune to disease? What if consumers could dictate which traits scientists insert into food plants? Would they choose to add phytochemicals to fight cancer or reduce the risk of heart disease? These and other possibilities seem unlimited, and though they may sound incredible, many such products have already been developed and are awaiting approval from the FDA, EPA, and USDA.

The Potential Problems and Concerns

Even as scientific evidence supports the value of genetically modified foods, public opposition remains strong.[7] Consumers accept or reject foods and technology depending on their perceptions of the associated benefits and risks. For the most part, when something is perceived as being beneficial, it is also perceived as having low risk. Perceptions of risk and rejection increase when conditions are unfamiliar, uncertain, unknown, or uncontrollable or consequences are severe, whereas perceptions of benefits and acceptance increase when conditions are traditional, well known, and familiar. In the case of genetically modified foods, many consumers are understandably suspicious of an unfamiliar and complicated processing technique; they haven't accepted that the benefits might outweigh the risks. Those with higher scientific knowledge tend to have less negative attitudes toward genetically modified foods.[8]

Most scientists hail biotechnology with confidence, but many consumers have reservations. Those who oppose biotechnology fear for the safety of a world where genetic tampering produces effects that are not yet fully understood. They suspect that the food industry may be driven by potential profits, without ethical considerations or laws to harness the effects. They point out that even the scientists who developed the techniques cannot predict the ultimate outcomes of their discoveries. These consumers don't want to eat a scientific experiment or interfere with natural systems. Genetic decisions, they say, are best left to the powers of nature.

If science and the marketplace are allowed to drive biotechnology without restraint, critics fear that the following problems may result:

- *Disruption of natural ecosystems.* New, genetically unique organisms that have no natural place in the food chain or evolutionary biological systems could escape into the environment and reproduce.
- *Introduction of diseases.* Newly created viruses may mutate to cause deadly diseases that may attack plants, animals, or human beings. Genetically modified bacteria may develop resistance to antibiotics, making the drugs useless in fighting infections.
- *Introduction of allergens and toxins.* Genetically modified crops may contain new substances that have consequences, such as causing allergies.
- *Creation of biological weapons.* Fatal bacterial and viral diseases may be developed for use as weapons.
- *Ethical dilemmas.* Critics pose the question "How many human genes does an organism have to contain before it is considered human? For instance, how many human genes would a green pepper have to contain before one would have qualms about eating it?"

Proponents of biotechnology respond that evidence to date does not justify these concerns. Opponents counter that the lack of evidence showing harm does not provide evidence showing safety. These opposing views illustrate the tension between the forward thrust of science and the hesitation of consumers. Some would argue for more research on the safety of genetically modified food, while others assert that more research is a waste of resources and that it is time to embrace biotechnology. In addition to evaluating the potential risks and benefits, genetically modified crops need international oversight. Table H19-1 (p. 642) summarizes some of the issues.

From another perspective, some argue that the concerns expressed by those protesting genetically engineered foods reflect prejudices acquired in an elitist world of fertile land and abundant food. Those living in poverty-stricken areas of the world do not have the luxury of determining how to grow crops and process foods. They cannot afford the delays created when protesters destroy test crops and disrupt scientific meetings. They need solutions now. People are starving, and genetic engineering holds great promise for increasing crop yields and providing those people with food.

More than 100 Nobel Peace Prize Laureates have spoken up in defense of genetically modified foods.[9] The work of one of them, Dr. Norman Borlaug, and his team over the past four decades attests to the benefits of using technology to defend against hunger. By developing grains that resist pests and diseases, they have been able to increase yields and provide real solutions to global hunger problems. When Mexico used Borlaug's special breed of dwarf wheat, yields increased threefold compared with traditional varieties. India increased wheat production tenfold and became self-sufficient in its grain production. Pakistan increased its wheat production fivefold and sub-Saharan Africa more than tripled crop yields by changing farming practices. The combination of improved conventional systems and biotechnology produces more food to meet the nutritional needs of more people.

The products of biotechnology must undergo rigorous safety testing. When a new gene has been introduced into a food, tests need to ensure that other, unwanted genes have not accompanied it. If a disease-producing microorganism has donated genetic material, scientists must prove that no dangerous characteristic from the microorganism has also entered the food. If the inserted genetic material comes from a source to which some people develop allergies, such as nuts, then the new product must be labeled to alert them. Furthermore, if the newly altered genetic material creates proteins that have never before been encountered by the human body, their effects are rigorously studied to ensure that people can eat them safely.

FDA Regulations

The FDA has taken the position that foods produced through biotechnology and cloning are not substantially different from others and require no special testing, regulations, or labeling (see Photo H19-3). After all, most foods available today have been genetically altered by years of selective breeding. The new vegetable broccoflower, a product of sophisticated cross-breeding of broccoli with cauliflower, met no testing or approval barriers on its way to the dinner plate. When the

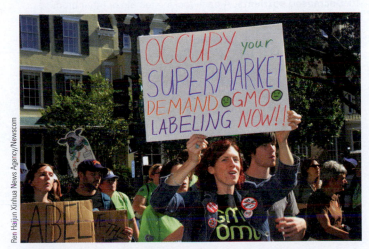
OCCUPY your
SUPERMARKET
DEMAND GMO
LABELING NOW!!

Ren Haijun Xinhua News Agency/Newscom

> **PHOTO H19-3** Many consumers believe that genetically modified foods should be labeled as such.

TABLE H19-1 **Food Biotechnology: Point, Counterpoint**

Arguments in Opposition to Genetic Engineering	Arguments in Support of Genetic Engineering
1. **Ethical and moral issues.** It's immoral to "play God" by mixing genes from organisms unable to do so naturally. Religious and vegetarian groups object to genes from prohibited species occurring in their allowable foods.	1. **Ethical and moral issues.** Scientists throughout history have been persecuted and even put to death by fearful people who accuse them of playing God. Yet, today many of the world's citizens enjoy a long and healthy life of comfort and convenience because of once-feared scientific advances put to practical use.
2. **Imperfect technology.** The technology is young and imperfect—genes rarely function in just one way, their placement is imprecise ("shotgun"), and all of their potential effects are impossible to predict. Toxins are as likely to be produced as the desired trait. More than 95 percent of DNA is called "junk" because scientists have not yet determined its function.	2. **Advanced technology.** Recombinant DNA technology is precise and reliable. Many of the most exciting recent advances in medicine, agriculture, and technology were made possible by the application of this technology.
3. **Environmental concerns.** Environmental side effects are unknown. The power of a genetically modified organism to change the world's environments is unknown until such changes actually occur—then the "genie is out of the bottle." Once out, insects, birds, and the wind distribute genetically altered seed and pollen to points unknown.	3. **Environmental protection.** Genetic engineering may be the only hope of saving rain forest and other habitats from destruction. Through genetic engineering, farmers can make use of previously unproductive lands such as salt-rich soils and arid areas.
4. **"Genetic pollution."** Other kinds of pollution can often be cleaned up with money, time, and effort. Once genes are spliced into living things, those genes forever bear the imprint of human tampering.	4. **Genetic improvements.** Genetic side effects are more likely to benefit the environment than to harm it.
5. **Crop vulnerability.** Pests and diseases can quickly adapt to overtake genetically identical plants or animals around the world. Diversity is key to defense.	5. **Improved crop resistance.** Pests and diseases can be specifically fought on a case-by-case basis. Biotechnology is the key to defense.
6. **Loss of gene pool.** Loss of genetic diversity threatens to deplete valuable gene banks from which scientists can develop new agricultural crops.	6. **Gene pool preserved.** Thanks to advances in genetics, laboratories around the world are able to stockpile the genetic material of millions of species that, without such advances, would have been lost forever.
7. **Profit motive.** Genetic engineering will profit industry more than the world's poor and hungry.	7. **Everyone profits.** Industries benefit from genetic engineering, and a thriving food industry benefits the nation and its people, as witnessed by countries lacking such industries. Genetic engineering promises to provide adequate nutritious food for millions who lack such food today. Developed nations gain cheaper, more attractive, more delicious foods with greater variety and availability year round.
8. **Unproven safety for people.** Human safety testing of genetically altered products is generally lacking. The population is an unwitting experimental group in a nationwide laboratory study for the benefit of industry.	8. **Safe for people.** Human safety testing of genetically altered products is unneeded because the products are essentially the same as the original foodstuffs.
9. **Increased allergens.** Allergens can be unwittingly transferred into foods.	9. **Control of allergens.** A few allergens can be transferred into foods, but these are known. Also, foods likely to contain them are clearly labeled to warn consumers. Some foods are being designed to eliminate the allergen.
10. **Decreased nutrients.** A fresh-looking tomato or other produce held for several weeks may have lost substantial nutrients.	10. **Increased nutrients.** Genetic modifications can easily enhance the nutrients in foods.
11. **No product tracking.** Without labeling, the food industry cannot track problems to the source.	11. **Excellent product tracking.** The identity and location of genetically altered foodstuffs are known, and they can be tracked should problems arise.
12. **Overuse of herbicides.** Farmers, knowing that their crops resist herbicide effects, will use them liberally.	12. **Conservative use of herbicides.** Farmers will not waste expensive herbicides in second or third applications when the prescribed amount gets the job done the first time.
13. **Increased consumption of pesticides.** When a pesticide is produced by the flesh of produce, consumers cannot wash it off the skin of the produce with running water as they can with ordinary sprays.	13. **Reduced pesticides on foods.** Pesticides produced by plants in tiny amounts known to be safe for consumption are more predictable than applications by agricultural workers who make mistakes. Because other genetic manipulations will eliminate the need for postharvest spraying, fewer pesticides will reach the dinner table.
14. **Lack of oversight.** Government oversight is run by industry people for the benefit of industry—no one is watching out for the consumer.	14. **Sufficient regulation and rapid response.** Government agencies are efficient in identifying and correcting problems as they occur in the industry.

vegetable became available on the market, scientists studied its nutrient contents, but they did not question its safety.

In most cases, a new genetically modified food differs from the old conventional one only by a gene or two. The chymosin produced by bacteria is structurally and functionally the same as the chymosin produced by calves, for example. For that reason, the FDA considers it and other genetically engineered foods "generally recognized as safe (GRAS)."

A product such as the tomato described earlier need not be tested because its new gene *prevents* synthesis of a protein and adds nothing but a tiny fragment of genetic material. Nor does this tomato require special labeling because it is not significantly different from the many other varieties of tomatoes on the market. On the other hand, any substance introduced into a food (such as a hormone or protein) by way of bioengineering must meet the same safety standards applied to all additives. A tomato plant with a gene that, for example, produces a pesticide cannot be marketed until tests prove it safe for consumption. The FDA assures consumers that all bioengineered foods on the market today are as safe as their traditional counterparts.

All foods, including those produced through biotechnology, that present a safety risk to anyone must be labeled. For example, if an allergy-causing protein has been introduced to a nonallergenic food, then labeling must warn consumers.

Proponents of mandatory labeling for genetically modified foods say that consumers have the right to know, especially if the foods carry risks without benefits. Opponents say labeling a food as genetically modified sends an erroneous message that the food is less safe than its conventional counterpart. Currently, labeling is voluntary in the United States.[10] Manufacturers may state that a product has been "genetically engineered." Those who do would be wise to explain its purpose and benefit. When consumers recognize a personal health benefit, most tend to accept genetically engineered foods. To help consumers who prefer foods that are free of genetically modified ingredients, the USDA is developing a voluntary certification and labeling system (see Photo H19-4). Certified manufacturers may label their food as "not genetically engineered" or "not bioengineered."

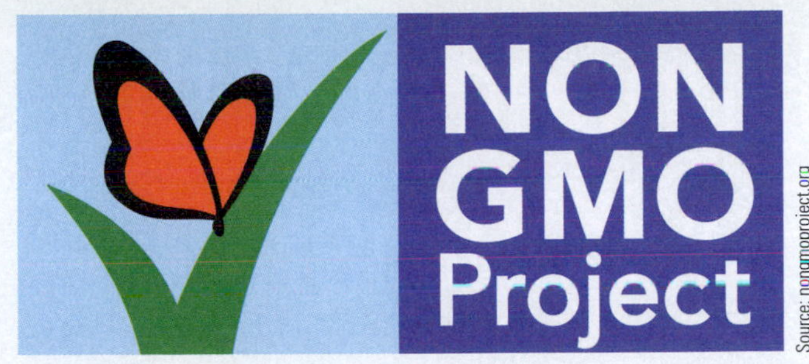
NON
GMO
Project
Source: nongmoproject.org

> **PHOTO H19-4** Until the USDA creates a label to certify a food as GMO-free, many companies use this label, which was developed by the Non-GMO Project, a nonprofit agency.

Will these new technologies provide foods to meet the needs of the future? Some would say yes. Biotechnology holds a world of promise, and with proper safeguards and controls, it may yield products that meet the needs of consumers almost perfectly.

CRITICAL THINKING QUESTIONS

A. How might people from different countries view the risks and benefits of biotechnology?

B. Controversy surrounds the safety and use of food biotechnology. Genetically modified foods raise concerns about long-term health and environmental consequences. Even though most scientists agree that these foods are safe and perhaps even beneficial to consumers, many consumers still express uncertainty. What is your position on food biotechnology and genetically modified foods? What could be done to minimize any associated risks and alleviate fears?

REFERENCES

1. National Academies of Sciences, Engineering, and Medicine, *Genetically engineered crops: Experiences and prospects,* (Washington, DC: National Academies Press, 2016), www.nap.edu/23395.
2. Food and Drug Administration, FDA concludes Arctic Apples and Innate Potatoes are safe for consumption, https://www.fda.gov/NewsEvents/Newsroom/PressAnnouncements/ucm439121.htm, March 20, 2015.
3. C. Shekhar, Hidden hunger: Addressing micronutrient deficiencies using improved crop varieties, *Chemistry and Biology* 20 (2013): 1305–1306.
4. Food and Drug Administration, FDA concludes consultation on pink flesh pineapple, https://www.fda.gov/Food/NewsEvents/ConstituentUpdates/ucm533075.htm, December 14, 2016.
5. R. Ehrenberg, GMOs under scrutiny, *Science News*, February 6, 2016, pp. 22–27.
6. FDA has determined that the AquAdvantage salmon is as safe to eat as non-GE salmon, *FDA Consumer Health Information,* November 2015.
7. S. Blancke and coauthors, Fatal attraction: The intuitive appeal of GMO opposition, *Trends in Plant Science* 20 (2015): 414–418; D. A. Goldstein, Tempest in a tea pot: How did the public conversation on genetically modified crops drift so far from the facts? *Journal of Medical Toxicology* 10 (2014): 194–201.
8. S. Wunderlich and K. A. Gatto, Consumer perception of genetically modified organisms and sources of information, *Advances in Nutrition* 6 (2015): 842–851.
9. J. Lyon, Nobel laureates pick food fight with GMO foes, *Journal of the American Medical Association* 316 (2016): 1752–1753.
10. Food and Drug Administration, Labeling of foods derived from genetically engineered plants, https://www.fda.gov/Food/IngredientsPackagingLabeling/GEPlants/ucm346858.htm, January 18, 2017.

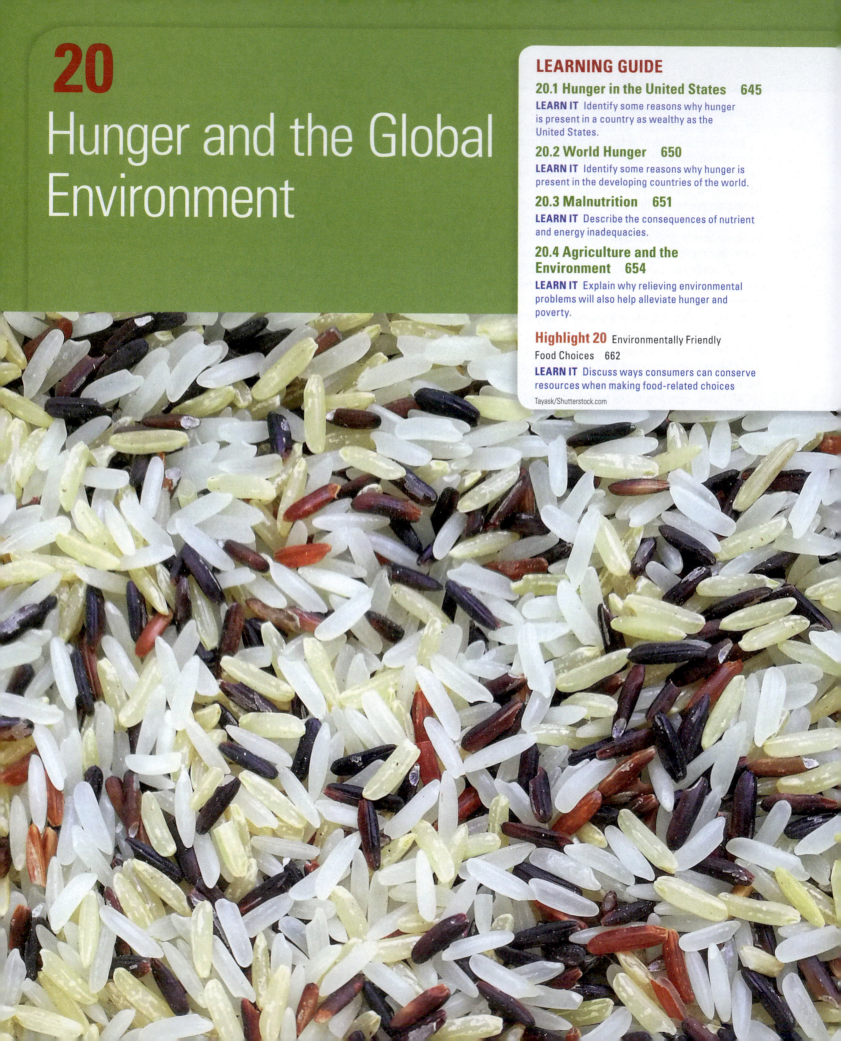

20 Hunger and the Global Environment

LEARNING GUIDE

Tayask/Shutterstock.com

Nutrition in Your Life

Imagine living with hunger from the moment you wake up until the time you thankfully fall asleep—and all through your dreams as well. Meal after meal, day after day, you have little or no food to eat. You need food, but you have no money. Would you beg on the street corner or go "dumpster diving" at a fast-food restaurant? And then where would you find your next meal? How will you ever get enough to eat as long as you live in poverty? Resolving the hunger problem—whether in your community or on the other side of the world—depends on alleviating poverty and using resources wisely. As you read this chapter, consider ways to get involved in hunger relief.

Worldwide, one person in every nine experiences persistent hunger—not the healthy appetite triggered by anticipation of a meal, but the painful sensation caused by a lack of food.[1] In this chapter, **hunger** takes on the greater meaning—hunger that develops from prolonged, recurrent, and involuntary lack of food and results in illness, weakness, or pain that exceeds the usual uneasy sensation. Such hunger deprives a person of the physical and mental energy needed to enjoy a full life and often leads to severe malnutrition and death. Millions of people die of hunger-related causes every year—one child every 10 seconds.[2]

The enormity of the world hunger problem is reflected not only by huge numbers, but also by major challenges. How do we provide enough food to meet the needs of the world's growing population without destroying the natural resources needed to continue producing food? How can we ensure that all people have access to enough nutritious food to live active, healthy lives? The solutions depend on finding the balance among the production and distribution of food, the numbers of people, and the care of the environment.

20.1 Hunger in the United States

LEARN IT Identify some reasons why hunger is present in a country as wealthy as the United States.

Ideally, all people at all times would have access to enough food to support an active, healthy life. In other words, they would experience **food security.** Unfortunately, an estimated 42 million people in the United States, including more than 6 million children, live in poverty and cannot afford to buy enough food to maintain good health.[3] Said another way, one out of eight households experiences hunger or the threat of hunger. Given the agricultural bounty and enormous wealth in this country, do these numbers surprise you? The limited or uncertain availability of nutritionally adequate and safe foods is known as **food insecurity** and is a major social problem in our nation today. Inadequate diets lead to poor health in adults and impaired physical, psychological, and cognitive development in children.

Table 20-1 (p. 646) presents the questions used in national surveys to identify food insecurity in the United States, and Figure 20-1 (p. 646) shows the most recent findings.Responses to these questions provide crude, but necessary, data to estimate the degree of hunger in this country. Specific questions focus on food insecurity in children. Even short-term food insecurity in a household can interfere with a young child's development.

Defining Hunger in the United States

At its most extreme, people experience hunger because they have absolutely no food. More often, they have too little food (**food insufficiency**) and try to stretch their limited resources by eating small meals or skipping meals—often for days at a time. Sometimes hungry people

hunger: the painful sensation caused by a lack of food that initiates food-seeking behavior; a consequence of food insecurity that, because of prolonged, involuntary lack of food, results in discomfort, illness, weakness, or pain that goes beyond the usual uneasy sensation.

food security: access to enough food to sustain a healthy and active life. Food security categories include:

- *High food security:* no indications of food-access problems or limitations
- *Marginal food security:* one or two indications of food-access problems but with little or no change in food intake

food insecurity: limited or uncertain access to foods of sufficient quality or quantity to sustain a healthy and active life. Food insecurity categories include:

- *Low food security:* reduced quality of life with little or no indication of reduced food intake; formerly known as *food insecurity without hunger*
- *Very low food security:* multiple indications of disrupted eating patterns and reduced food intake; formerly known as *food insecurity with hunger*

food insufficiency: an inadequate amount of food due to a lack of resources.

TABLE 20-1 Questions to Identify Food Insecurity in a US Household

To determine the extent of food insecurity in a household, surveys ask questions about behaviors and conditions known to characterize households having difficulty meeting basic food needs during the past 12 months. Most often, adults tend to protect their children from hunger. In the most severe cases, children also suffer from hunger and eat less.

1. Did you worry whether food would run out before you got money to buy more?
2. Did you find that the food you bought just didn't last and you didn't have money to buy more?
3. Were you unable to afford to eat balanced meals?
4. Did you or other adults in your household ever cut the size of your meals or skip meals because there wasn't enough money for food?
5. If so, how often did this happen?
6. Did you ever eat less than you felt you should because there wasn't enough money for food?
7. Were you ever hungry but didn't eat because there wasn't enough money for food?
8. Did you lose weight because there wasn't enough money for food?
9. Did you or other adults in your household ever not eat for a whole day because there wasn't enough money for food?
10. If so, how often did this happen?
11. Did you rely on only a few kinds of low-cost food to feed your children because you were running out of money to buy food?
12. Were you unable to feed your children a balanced meal because you couldn't afford it?
13. Were your children not eating enough because you just couldn't afford enough food?
14. Did you ever cut the size of your children's meals because there wasn't enough money for food?
15. Were your children ever hungry but you just couldn't afford more food?
16. Did your children ever skip a meal because there wasn't enough money for food?
17. If so, how often did this happen?
18. Did your children ever not eat for a whole day because there wasn't enough money for food?

The more positive responses, the greater the food insecurity. Households with children answer all of the questions and are categorized as follows:

- ≤2 positive responses = food secure
- 3–7 positive responses = low food security
- ≥8 positive responses = very low food security

Households without children answer the first 10 questions and are categorized as follows:

- ≤2 positive responses = food secure
- 3–5 positive responses = low food security
- ≥6 positive responses = very low food security

Figure 20-1 shows the results of the 2014 surveys.

SOURCE: A. Coleman-Jensen and coauthors, *Household Food Security in the United States in 2014*, US Department of Agriculture, *Economic Research Report 194, September 2015*.

> FIGURE 20-1 Prevalence of Food Security in US Households

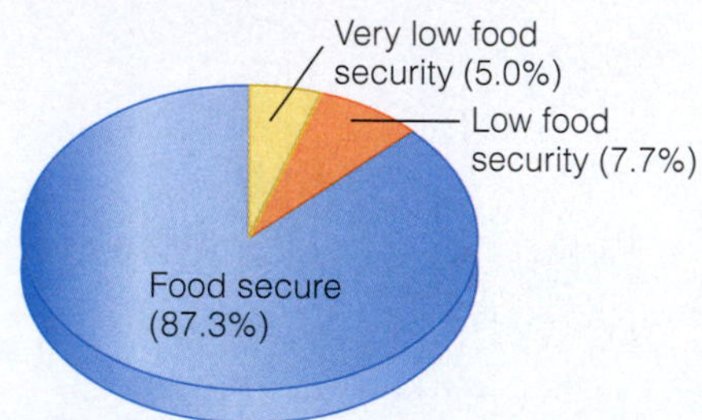

Very low food security (5.0%)
Low food security (7.7%)
Food secure (87.3%)

SOURCE: Economic Research Service, US Department of Agriculture, www.ers.usda.gov, October 2016.

obtain enough food to satisfy their hunger, perhaps by seeking food assistance or finding food through socially unacceptable ways—begging from strangers, stealing from markets, or scavenging through garbage cans, for example. Sometimes obtaining food raises concerns for food safety—for example, when rot, mold, or insects have damaged foods or when people eat outdated foods or meat from roadkill.

Food Poverty Hunger has many causes, but in developed countries, the primary cause is **food poverty**. People are hungry not because there is no food nearby to purchase, but because they lack money. The rate and severity of US poverty increased over the past decade. An estimated 15 percent of the people in the United States lives in poverty.[4] Even those above the poverty line (about $11,770 per year for an individual) may not have food security. Physical and mental illnesses and disabilities, unemployment, low-paying jobs, unexpected or ongoing medical expenses, and high living expenses threaten financial stability. When money is tight, people must choose between food and life's other necessities—utilities, housing, and medical care. Food costs are more variable and flexible; people can purchase fewer groceries to lower the monthly food bill, but they usually can't pay only a portion of the bills for electricity, rent, or medication. Other problems further contribute to food poverty, such as abuse of alcohol and other drugs; lack of awareness of available food assistance programs; and the reluctance of people, particularly the elderly, to accept what they perceive as "welfare" or "charity."

In the United States, poverty and hunger reach across various segments of society, touching some more than others—notably, single parents living in households with their children, Hispanics and African Americans, and those living in the inner cities. People living in poverty are simply unable to buy sufficient amounts of nourishing foods, even if they are wise shoppers. Consequently, their diets tend to be inadequate. For many of the children in these families, school lunch (and breakfast, where available) may be the only nourishment for the day. Otherwise they go hungry, waiting for an adult to find money for food. Not surprisingly, these children are more likely to have chronic health problems than those who eat regularly.[5] They also tend to perform poorly in school and in social situations. For adults, the risk of developing chronic diseases increases.

food poverty: hunger resulting from inadequate access to available food for various reasons, including inadequate resources, political obstacles, social disruptions, poor weather conditions, and lack of transportation.

Obesity Paradox Ironically, hunger and obesity often exist side by side—sometimes within the same household or even the same person. That hunger reflects an inadequate food intake and obesity implies an excessive intake seems paradoxical, but research studies have confirmed the association.[6] The highest rates of obesity occur among those living in the greatest poverty—the same people who live with food insecurity.

Unfortunately, many healthful food choices, such as fruits and vegetables, are not readily available in low-income or rural neighborhoods. Instead of supermarkets, these neighborhoods typically have corner stores that stock canned foods, sodas, and chips, but not fresh produce. Neighborhoods and communities characterized by limited access to nutritious and affordable foods are known as **food deserts.** Food deserts are more prevalent in low-income and African American communities. With limited access to grocery stores carrying varieties of fruits and vegetables, residents in these neighborhoods fall short of meeting dietary guidelines.[7] Furthermore, fruits and vegetables tend to cost more than the energy-dense foods that foster weight gain. Foods such as doughnuts, pizzas, and hamburgers provide the most energy and satiety for the least cost. Quite simply, poor-quality diets deliver more kcalories, but fewer nutrients, for less money; high-quality diets deliver fewer kcalories, but more nutrients, for more money. The challenge, of course, is finding the foods that deliver the most nutrients for the least cost.[8] Lowering the price of fruits and vegetables is one easy and effective way to improve diet quality.[9] Increasing accessibility of low-fat milk in low-income neighborhoods is another.[10]

Economic uncertainty and stress greatly influence the prevalence of obesity. People who are unsure about their next meal may overeat when food or money is available. Interestingly, food insecure people who do *not* participate in food assistance programs have a *greater* risk of obesity than those who do participate—illustrating that providing food actually helps prevent obesity. Figure 20-2 shows how poverty and food insecurity can lead to both malnutrition and obesity.

> **FIGURE 20-2 The Poverty-Obesity Paradox**

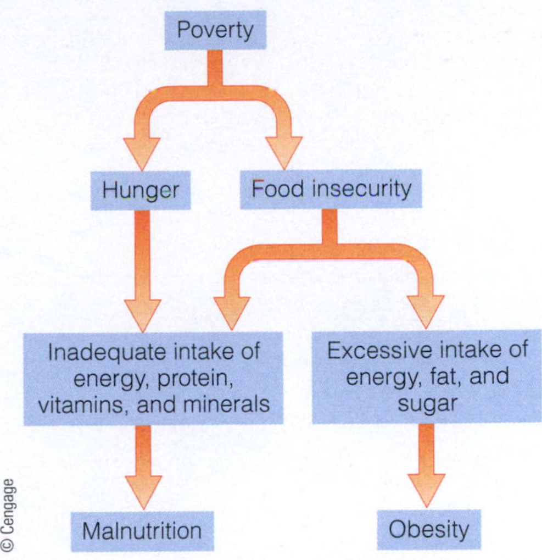
Poverty
Hunger
Food insecurity
Inadequate intake of energy, protein, vitamins, and minerals
Excessive intake of energy, fat, and sugar
Malnutrition
Obesity
© Cengage

Relieving Hunger in the United States

The Academy of Nutrition and Dietetics calls for aggressive action to bring an end to domestic food insecurity and hunger and to achieve food and nutrition security for everybody living in the United States.[11] Many federal and local programs aim to prevent or relieve malnutrition and hunger in the United States (see Photo 20-1).

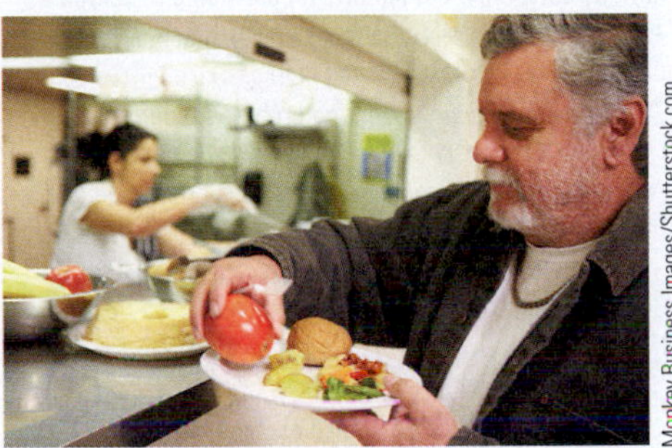
Monkey Business Images/Shutterstock.com

> **PHOTO 20-1** Feeding the hungry—in the United States.

Federal Food Assistance Programs Adequate nutrition and food security are essential to supporting good health and achieving the public health goals of the United States. To that end, an extensive network of federal assistance programs provides life-sustaining food to millions of US citizens daily. Programs described in earlier chapters include the WIC program for low-income pregnant women, breastfeeding mothers, and their young children (Chapter 15); the school lunch, breakfast, and child-care food programs for children (Chapter 16); and the food assistance programs for older adults such as congregate meals and Meals on Wheels (Chapter 17).

The Supplemental Nutrition Assistance Program (SNAP), administered by the US Department of Agriculture (USDA), is the largest of the federal food assistance programs, both in amount of money spent and in number of people served. Participation in SNAP significantly decreases food insecurity.[12] It provides assistance to more than 44 million people at a cost of $70 billion per year; about half of the recipients are children. The USDA issues debit cards through state agencies to households—people who buy and prepare food together. The amount a household receives depends on its size, resources, and income. The average monthly benefit is about $125 per person. Recipients may use the cards to purchase food and food-bearing plants and seeds, but not to buy tobacco, cleaning items, alcohol, or other nonfood items.

Controversy surrounds the question of whether SNAP participants should be allowed to purchase soft drinks and other nonnutritious foods and beverages. Some argue that government programs should not support poor-quality foods that promote obesity and other diseases; others argue that government programs should not tell consumers what they cannot eat and drink and to do so is discriminatory and

food deserts: neighborhoods and communities characterized by limited access to nutritious and affordable foods.

unfair. This lack of quality control on food purchases may not only promote obesity and disease, but it may also exacerbate hunger; consider that, given the same number of kcalories, a child will become hungrier sooner after drinking a 20-ounce soft drink than after eating a large apple with a heaping spoonful of peanut butter. In general, SNAP participants have low-quality diets and poor health. Providing sufficient benefits and aligning SNAP policy with the *Dietary Guidelines for Americans* would help improve the nutritional quality of diets and health of participants.[13] How To 20-1 offers healthy shopping tips for those on a limited budget.

Food assistance programs improve nutrient intakes significantly, but hunger remains a problem in the United States. Homeless people are eligible, but relatively few receive food assistance. For some, reading, understanding, and completing the application can be difficult. For others, having to verify identity and homelessness can be frustrating. For many, accepting hunger is simply easier than meeting these challenges.

National Food Recovery Programs Efforts to resolve the problem of hunger in the United States do not depend solely on federal assistance programs. National **food recovery** programs have made a dramatic difference. The largest hunger relief program, Feeding America, coordinates the efforts of 200 **food banks** and 60,000 food pantries and meal programs across the country that feed an estimated 46 million people a year.

food recovery: collecting wholesome food for distribution to low-income people who are hungry. Four common methods of food recovery include:

- *Field gleaning:* collecting crops from fields that either have already been harvested or are not profitable to harvest
- *Perishable food rescue or salvage:* collecting perishable produce from wholesalers and markets
- *Prepared food rescue:* collecting prepared foods from commercial kitchens
- *Nonperishable food collection:* collecting processed foods from wholesalers and markets

food banks: facilities that collect and distribute food donations to authorized organizations feeding the hungry.

Each year, an estimated 40 percent of the US food supply is wasted along the way from farm to final consumption—that's an estimated 90 billion pounds of food. The uneaten foods represent 1250 kcalories per person per day—enough to feed a hungry child.[14]

Reducing that food waste and alleviating food insecurity is a national goal, and every step from farm to fork has a role to play.[15] Federal legislation has been introduced to reduce food waste on the farm, in stores, and at home; to redirect food from manufacturers, retailers, and restaurants to hunger-relief organizations; and to use food waste and crop waste to produce energy. In addition, manufacturers have been urged to make food date labels more consistent and less confusing, so less food is needlessly thrown out. The EPA's Food Recovery Hierarchy (see Figure 20-3) prioritizes actions

> **FIGURE 20-3 Food Recovery Hierarchy**

Each tier of the hierarchy focuses on different strategies to prevent or divert wasted food. The top tiers are most preferred because they provide benefits for the environment, society, and the economy.

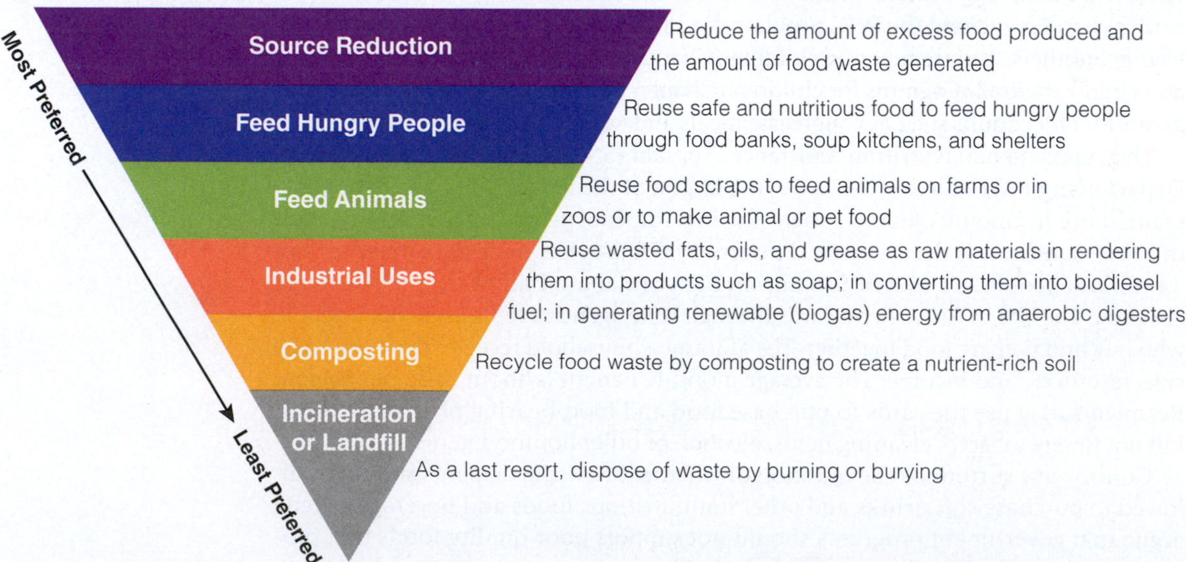
Most Preferred
Source Reduction
Reduce the amount of excess food produced and the amount of food waste generated
Feed Hungry People
Reuse safe and nutritious food to feed hungry people through food banks, soup kitchens, and shelters
Feed Animals
Reuse food scraps to feed animals on farms or in zoos or to make animal or pet food
Industrial Uses
Reuse wasted fats, oils, and grease as raw materials in rendering them into products such as soap; in converting them into biodiesel fuel; in generating renewable (biogas) energy from anaerobic digesters
Composting
Recycle food waste by composting to create a nutrient-rich soil
Incineration or Landfill
As a last resort, dispose of waste by burning or burying
Least Preferred

SOURCE: US Environmental Protection Agency, Sustainable management of food, www.epa.gov/sustainable-management-food/food-recovery-hierarchy.

> How To 20-1 Stretch Food Dollars and Reduce Waste

Chapter 2 introduced the principles for planning a healthy diet. Meeting that goal on a limited budget adds to the challenge. To save money and spend wisely, plan and shop for healthy meals with the following tips in mind.

Plan Ahead

- Plan menus and make a grocery list before going to the store to avoid expensive "impulse" items.
- Center meals on whole grains, legumes, and vegetables.
- Use small quantities of meat, poultry, fish, or eggs.
- Use cooked cereals such as oatmeal instead of ready-to-eat breakfast cereals.
- Cook large quantities when time and money allow; freeze portions for convenient meals another time.
- Check for sales and use coupons for products you need; plan meals to take advantage of sale items.

Shop Smart

- Do not shop when hungry.
- Look for bargains on day-old bread and other bakery products.
- Select whole foods instead of convenience foods (potatoes instead of instant mashed potatoes, for example).
- Try store brands.
- Buy fresh produce that is in season; buy canned or frozen items at other times.
- Buy large bags of frozen items or dry goods; when cooking, take out the amount needed and store the remainder.
- Buy fat-free dry milk; mix and refrigerate quantities needed for a day or two. Buy fresh milk by the gallon or half-gallon if you can use it before it spoils.
- Buy less expensive cuts of meat, such as beef chuck and pork shoulder roasts; cover during cooking and cook with liquid long enough to make meat tender.
- Buy whole chickens instead of pieces; ask the butcher to show you how to cut them up.
- Compare the unit price (cost per ounce, for example) of similar foods so that you can select the least expensive brand or size.
- Buy only what you need and are able to eat before it spoils.
- Buy nonfood items such as toilet paper and laundry detergent at discount stores instead of grocery stores.

Reduce Waste

- Be creative with the foods you have available. Consumers can search websites for recipes using ingredients they have on hand.
- Use leftovers to save time and money as well as to reduce waste.
- Store foods properly and use older foods first.
- Freeze extra food.
- Donate nonperishable foods that you are not going to use.
- Use every little bit. The ends of a loaf of bread can become croutons, excess rice can become the start of a casserole, leftover fruit can be a yogurt topping, and vegetable trimmings can form a base for soups, sauces, and stocks.
- Compost fruit and vegetable scraps to use in the garden or other outdoor plants.

For daily menus and recipes to help you eat better on a budget, visit the Healthy Eating on a Budget section of the MyPlate website: www.choosemyplate.gov/budget. For information on food waste, visit the Let's Talk Trash section: www.choosemyplate.gov/lets-talk-trash.

> TRY IT Review the sample meals at the Healthy Eating on a Budget section of the MyPlate website (www.choosemyplate.gov/budget) and select a day's meals to analyze using your personal profile in a diet analysis program.

to prevent and divert wasted food.[16] The hierarchy aims to reduce, reuse, and recycle food waste. How To 20-1 includes tips for reducing waste in the home.

Food recovery programs collect and distribute good food that would otherwise go to waste. Volunteers might pick corn left in an already harvested field, a grocer might deliver ripe bananas to a local food bank, and a caterer might take leftover chicken salad to a community shelter, for example. All of these efforts help feed the hungry in the United States.

Community Efforts Food recovery programs depend on volunteers (see Photo 20-2). Concerned citizens work through local agencies and churches to feed the hungry. Community-based food pantries provide groceries, and soup kitchens serve prepared meals. A combination of various strategies helps build food security in a community.

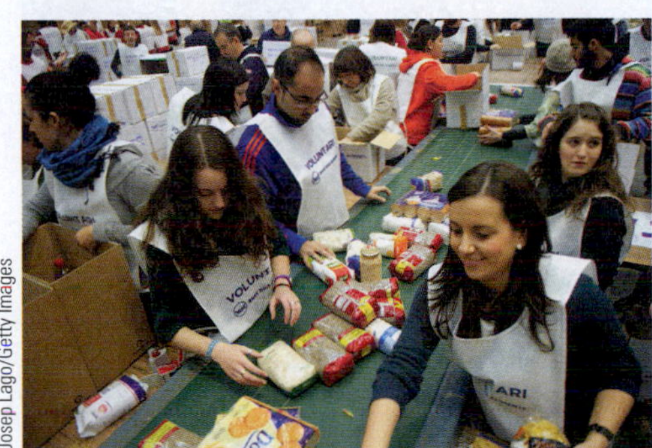

Josep Lago/Getty Images

> PHOTO 20-2 The fight against hunger depends on the helping hands of caring volunteers.

REVIEW IT Identify some reasons why hunger is present in a country as wealthy as the United States.

Food insecurity and hunger are widespread in the United States among those living in poverty. Ironically, hunger and poverty coexist with obesity. Government assistance programs help relieve poverty and hunger. Food recovery programs and other community efforts also provide some hunger relief.

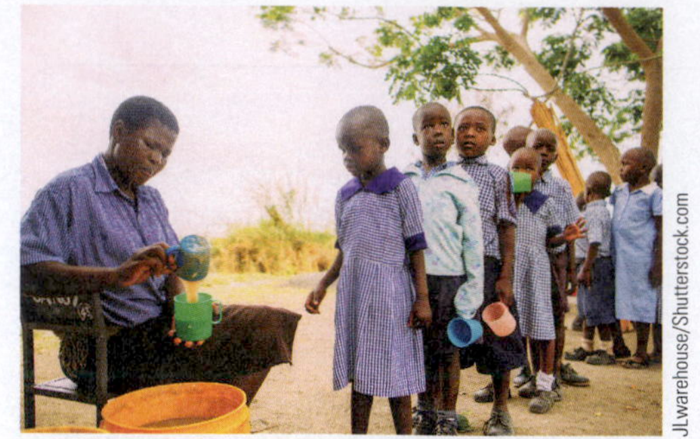

> **PHOTO 20-3** Feeding the hungry—in Kenya.

JLwarehouse/Shutterstock.com

20.2 World Hunger

LEARN IT Identify some reasons why hunger is present in the developing countries of the world.

As distressing as hunger is in the United States, the prevalence is far greater and the consequences more severe in developing countries, where an estimated 795 million people do not have enough to eat (see Photo 20-3).[17] Although hunger in developing countries has diverse causes, once again, the primary cause is poverty, and the poverty is far more extreme than in the United States. Most people cannot grasp the severity of poverty in the developing world. Of the more than 7 billion people in the world, 25 percent have no land and no possessions *at all.* They are the "poorest poor." They survive on little more than $1 a day each, and they lack safe housing, clean water, and health care. They cannot read or write. The average US housecat receives twice as much protein every day as one of these people, and the cost of keeping a pet cat is greater than such a person's annual income.

The "poorest poor" are usually female. Many societies around the world undervalue females, providing girls with poorer diets, less education, and fewer opportunities than boys. Malnourished girls become malnourished mothers who give birth to low-birthweight infants—and the cycle of hunger, malnutrition, and poverty continues. The consequences of stunted growth in early childhood are evident throughout life.

Not only does poverty cause hunger, but tragically, hunger worsens poverty by robbing a person of the good health and the physical and mental energy needed to be active and productive. Hungry people simply cannot work hard enough to get themselves out of poverty. Providing nourishment is a necessary investment in the well-being of both individuals and nations. Economists calculate that every $1 spent ending hunger and malnutrition by 2030 would generate a value of $16 in longer, healthier, and more productive lives.[18]

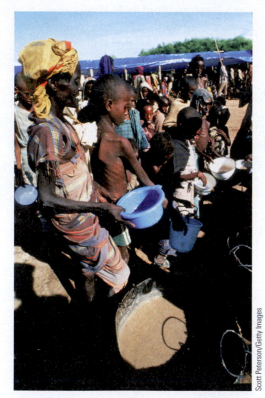

> **PHOTO 20-4** International efforts cannot fully relieve the hunger and poverty in Somalia and other parts of the world.

Scott Peterson/Getty Images

Food Shortages

World hunger brings to mind victims of **famine,** a severe food shortage in an area that causes widespread starvation and death. In recent years, the natural causes of famine—drought, flood, and pests—have become less important than the political and economic crises created by people. Figure 20-4 shows the hunger hotspots in the world.

Economic and Political Turbulence A sudden increase in food prices, a drop in workers' wages, or a change in government policy can quickly leave millions hungry. An estimated 30 million people died during the Chinese famine of 1959 through 1961, the worst famine of the 20th century. The main cause was government policies associated with the Great Leap Forward, a government initiative that was intended to transform China's economy. The poorly planned communal farm system and the widespread waste of resources, however, devastated the Chinese agricultural system.

Armed Conflicts Armed conflict is a major cause of famine worldwide. Years of civil war have left more than 6 million people in Syria hungry and dying as the Syrian government and opposing armed groups use starvation as a weapon of war. Intentionally starving civilians is considered a war crime, but no one ever faces charges. International relief agencies try to deliver food to the people, but aid workers face numerous obstacles as they try to navigate through war-torn cities.

Natural Disasters Natural disasters and other poor weather conditions create food shortages. The current drought in Ethiopia has left 15 million people without access to adequate food for survival. During such natural disasters, emergency food relief from countries around the world provides a safety net for countries in need. International food relief programs also provide ongoing food assistance to countries such as Sudan that are chronically short of food because of ongoing drought and poverty (see Photo 20-4).

famine: widespread and extreme scarcity of food in an area that causes starvation and death in a large portion of the population.

> **FIGURE 20-4 Hunger Hot Spots**

Hunger is prevalent in the developing world, with some countries reporting hunger and malnutrition in more than half of their population. Most of the world's undernourished people live in Sub-Saharan Africa.

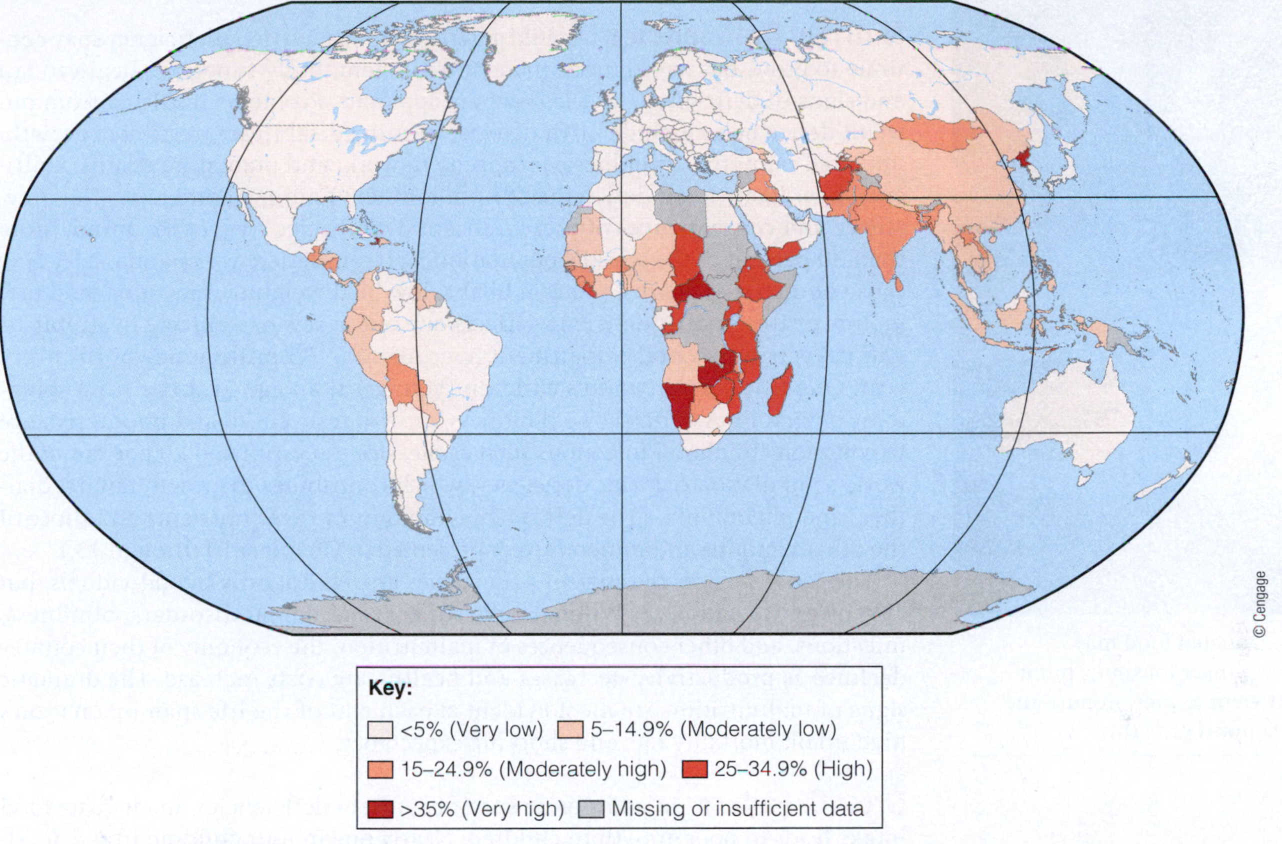
© Cengage
Key:
<5% (Very low)
5–14.9% (Moderately low)
15–24.9% (Moderately high)
25–34.9% (High)
>35% (Very high)
Missing or insufficient data

Population Needs The world's population continues to increase even as the rate slows (see Figure 20-5). Ever-increasing numbers threaten earth's **carrying capacity** to provide safe water and adequate food for its inhabitants. Contaminated water and food shortages are responsible for much of the world's disease and death.

As the world's population continues to grow, much of the increase is occurring in developing countries where hunger and malnutrition are already widespread. With more mouths to feed, hunger and poverty worsen.

REVIEW IT Identify some reasons why hunger is present in the developing countries of the world.

Natural causes such as drought, flood, and pests and political causes such as armed conflicts and government policies all contribute to the extreme hunger and poverty seen in the developing countries. In addition, overpopulation means more mouths to feed, which worsens the problems of poverty and hunger.

> **FIGURE 20-5 World Population**

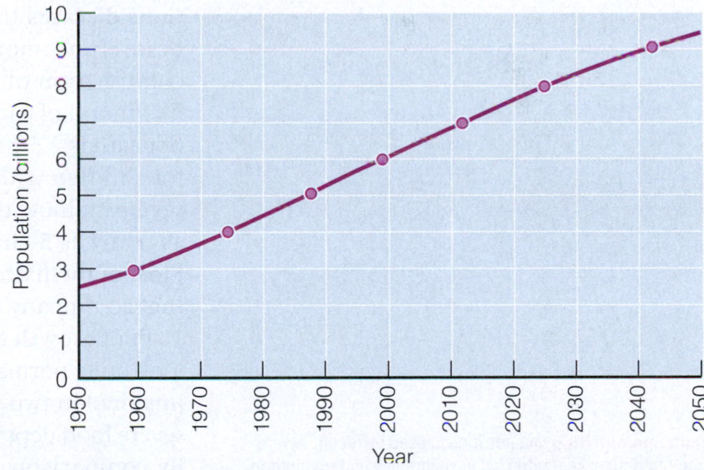
Population (billions)
0
1
2
3
4
5
6
7
8
9
10
1950
1960
1970
1980
1990
2000
2010
2020
2030
2040
2050
Year

SOURCE: US Census Bureau, International Data Base, updated June 2011.

20.3 Malnutrition

LEARN IT Describe the consequences of nutrient and energy inadequacies.

Persistent hunger inevitably leads to malnutrition. Although malnutrition touches many adult lives, it most often strikes early in childhood and results in specific nutrient deficiencies or overall growth failure. Providing optimal nutrition during the critical time of gestation and the first 2 years of life—commonly called the

carrying capacity: the number of people, other living organisms, or crops that a region can support without environmental degradation.

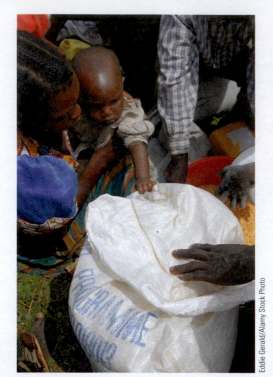
Eddie Gerald/Alamy Stock Photo

> **PHOTO 20-5** Donated food may temporarily ease hunger for some, but it is usually insufficient to prevent nutrient deficiencies or support growth.

first 1000 days—best supports an infant's growth and development, but dietary interventions whenever possible throughout childhood and adolescence, is also helpful (see Photo 20-5).[19]

Nutrient Deficiencies A child suffering from a nutrient deficiency may continue to grow, but without adequate nourishment, body functions begin to fail and signs of deficiency diseases become apparent. Problems resulting from nutrient deficiencies include birth defects, learning disabilities, restricted growth, impaired immunity, blindness, incapacity to work, and premature deaths. Nutrients most likely to be deficient are iron, iodine, vitamin A, and zinc. The prevalence and consequences of these nutrient deficiencies stagger the mind. More than 30 percent of the world's population has iron-deficiency anemia, a leading cause of maternal deaths, preterm births, low birthweights, infections, and premature deaths. Iodine deficiency affects one out of seven, resulting in stillbirths and irreversible mental impairment (cretinism) in 35 million newborns every year. One-third of the world's children (younger than age 5) suffer from symptoms of vitamin A deficiency—blindness, growth restriction, and poor resistance to common childhood infections such as measles. An estimated 20 percent of the world's population risk zinc deficiency, which contributes to growth failure, diarrhea, and pneumonia. (The deficiency symptoms of these nutrients and those of the other vitamins and minerals were presented in Chapters 10 through 13.)

The consequences of nutrient deficiencies are felt not only by individuals, but also by entire nations.[20] When people suffer from mental disorders, blindness, infections, and other consequences of malnutrition, the economy of their country declines as productivity decreases and health-care costs increase. The dramatic signs of malnutrition are most evident at each end of the life span in a nation's high infant mortality rate and short life expectancy.

Growth Failure In addition to specific nutrient deficiencies, inadequate food intake leads to poor growth in children. Nearly one in four children in the developing world is severely underweight by the age of 5. These underweight children are malnourished and readily develop the diseases of poverty: parasitic and infectious diseases that cause diarrhea (dysentery and cholera), acute respiratory illnesses (pneumonia and whooping cough), measles, and malaria.[21] The synergistic combination of infectious disease and malnutrition dramatically increases the likelihood of early death. Compared with adequately nourished children, the risk of death is 2.5 times greater for children with mild malnutrition, 4.6 times greater for children with moderate malnutrition, and 8.4 times greater for children with severe malnutrition. Each year, 5.9 million children younger than the age of 5 die; as many as 5 children *every minute* die as a result of hunger and malnutrition.[22] Most of them do not starve to death—they die from the diarrhea and dehydration that accompany infections.

Poor growth due to malnutrition is easy to overlook because a small child may look quite normal, but it is the most common sign of malnutrition. Growth may be impaired in two ways. Children who are suffering from **acute malnutrition** (recent severe food deprivation) may be underweight for their height (described as *wasting*). By comparison, children who have experienced **chronic malnutrition** (long-term food deprivation) are short for their age (described as *stunting*). An estimated 25 percent of the world's children younger than the age of 5 are stunted and about 10 percent are wasted. Children with both stunting and wasting have an exceptionally high risk of mortality.[23] Table 20-2 compares key features of acute malnutrition with those of chronic malnutrition.

Acute malnutrition presents itself in three clinical forms: marasmus, kwashiorkor, and marasmus-kwashiorkor mix.[24] Historically, **kwashiorkor** was attributed to protein deficiency and **marasmus** was attributed to energy deficiency. Together, they were named *protein-energy malnutrition*. Traditional thinking about protein-energy malnutrition was challenged by findings that the

acute malnutrition: malnutrition caused by recent severe food restriction; characterized in children by underweight for height (*wasting*).

chronic malnutrition: malnutrition caused by long-term food deprivation; characterized in children by short height for age (*stunting*).

kwashiorkor (kwash-ee-OR-core or kwash-ee-or-CORE): severe malnutrition characterized by failure to grow and develop, edema, changes in the pigmentation of hair and skin, fatty liver, anemia, and apathy.

marasmus (ma-RAZ-mus): severe malnutrition characterized by poor growth, dramatic weight loss, loss of body fat and muscle, and apathy.

diets of children with marasmus or kwashiorkor do not differ. Furthermore, treatment based on the concepts of protein-energy malnutrition failed to restore physiological homeostasis or healthy body composition. Most cases are a mix of the two diseases.

Current understanding of kwashiorkor and marasmus recognizes that the primary cause of malnutrition is a deficiency of *many* nutrients, including amino acids, potassium, magnesium, zinc, and phosphorus. Such poor-quality diets result in loss of appetite, diminished growth, and inability to resist infection or respond to environmental stresses. The following paragraphs present descriptions of kwashiorkor and marasmus.

TABLE 20-2 Acute and Chronic Malnutrition Compared

	Acute malnutrition	Chronic malnutrition
Food deprivation	Severe and recent	Long-term
Physical features	Rapid weight loss Wasting (underweight for height)	Minimal height gains Stunting (short for age)
World prevalence of children younger than age 5	5 to 15%	20 to 50%
Clinical forms	Marasmus (wasting) Kwashiorkor (edema) Marasmic-kwashiorkor mix	

Kwashiorkor *Kwashiorkor* is a Ghanaian word that refers to the birth position of a child and is used to describe the illness a child develops when the next child is born. When a mother who has been nursing her first child bears a second child, she weans the first child and puts the second one on the breast. The first child, suddenly switched from nutrient-dense, protein-rich breast milk to a starchy, nutrient-poor cereal, soon begins to sicken and die. The child appears withdrawn or irritable and obviously ill. Loss of appetite interferes with any attempts to provide nourishment.

In kwashiorkor, some muscle wasting may occur, but it may not be apparent because the child's face, limbs, and abdomen become swollen with edema—a distinguishing feature of kwashiorkor (see Photo 20-6). Fluid balance shifts in response to decreased concentrations of the blood protein albumin. A fatty liver develops because of a lack of the protein carriers to transport lipids out of the liver. The fatty liver lacks enzymes to clear metabolic toxins from the body, so their harmful effects are prolonged. Inflammation in response to these toxins and to infections further contributes to the edema that accompanies kwashiorkor. Without sufficient tyrosine to make melanin, hair loses its color, and inadequate protein synthesis leaves the skin patchy and scaly, often with sores that fail to heal. The lack of proteins to carry or store iron leaves iron free. Free iron is common in kwashiorkor and may contribute to edema by increasing the secretion of ADH—the antidiuretic hormone responsible for water retention. In addition, iron may contribute to illness and death by promoting bacterial growth and free-radical damage. (Free-radical damage was discussed fully in Highlight 11, p. 353.)

Marasmus Appropriately named from the Greek word meaning "dying away," marasmus occurs most commonly in children in all the overpopulated and impoverished areas of the world. Children living in poverty simply do not have enough to eat. They subsist on diluted cereal drinks that supply scant energy and protein of low quality; such food can barely sustain life, much less support growth. The loose skin on the buttocks and thighs sags down and looks as if the child is wearing baggy pants. Sadly, children with marasmus are often described as just "skin and bones" (see Photo 20-7, p. 654).

Because the brain normally grows to almost its full adult size within the first 2 years of life, marasmus impairs brain development and learning ability. Reduced synthesis of key hormones slows metabolism and lowers body temperature. There is little or no fat under the skin to insulate against cold. Hospital workers find that children with marasmus need to be clothed, covered, and kept warm. Because these children often suffer delays in their mental and behavioral development, they also need loving care, a stimulating environment, and parental attention.

The starving child faces this threat to life by engaging in as little activity as possible—not even crying for food. The body musters all its forces to meet the

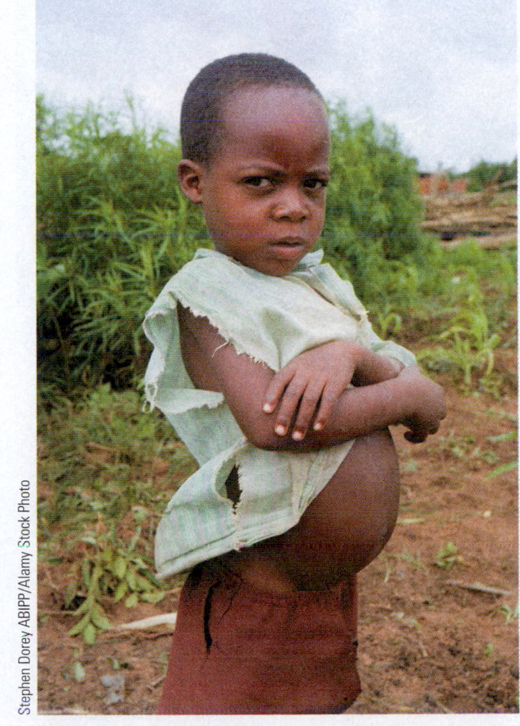

> **PHOTO 20-6** The edema characteristic of kwashiorkor is apparent in this child's swollen belly. Malnourished children commonly have an enlarged abdomen from parasites as well.

crisis, so it cuts down on any expenditure of energy not needed for the functioning of the heart, lungs, and brain. Growth ceases; the child is no larger at age 4 than at age 2. Enzymes are in short supply, and the GI tract lining deteriorates. Consequently, what little food is eaten can't be digested and absorbed.

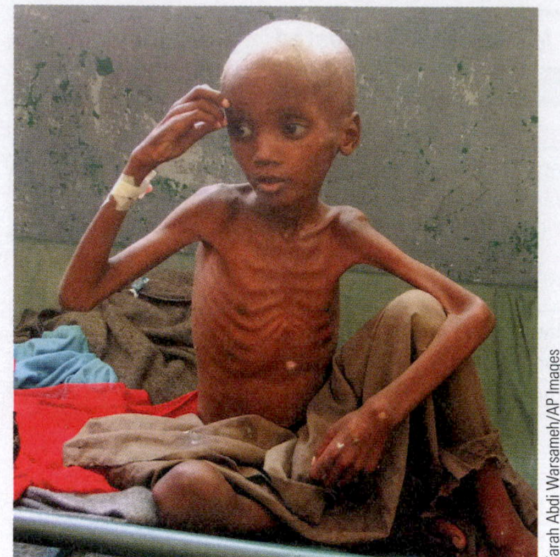
Farah Abdi Warsameh/AP Images

> **PHOTO 20-7** The severe wasting characteristic of marasmus is apparent in this child's "matchstick" arms.

Rehabilitation Ideally, optimal breastfeeding and improved complementary feedings would prevent malnutrition and save the lives of children. When mild to moderate malnutrition did occur, it might be quickly remedied with supplemental foods in the community. Severe acute malnutrition, on the other hand, may require hospitalization, which demands intensive nursing care, a therapeutic diet, and medication. Maintaining supplementary feedings for an extended period of time helps prevent relapse.[25]

Because the causes of malnutrition extend beyond insufficient food to include an individual's genetics, environmental stresses, and gastrointestinal bacteria, treatment must be individualized. Providing foods fortified with multiple vitamins and minerals protects against some deficiency diseases; whether it improves illnesses, growth, or cognition is less clear. To support physical growth, mental development, metabolic balance, and recovery from illnesses, malnourished children need specially formulated diets. They also need antibiotics to alter the GI bacteria, improve recovery rates, and decrease mortality; the GI bacteria of children with kwashiorkor impair energy metabolism and contribute to weight loss.[26]

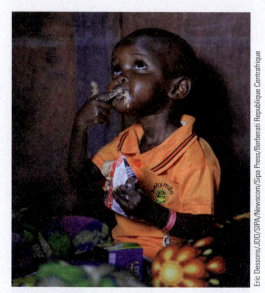
Eric Dessons/JDD/SIPA/Newscom/Sipa Press/Berberati Republique Centrafrique

> **PHOTO 20-8** Ready-to-use therapeutic food (RUTF)—made of peanut butter and powdered milk fortified with vitamins and minerals—nourishes hundreds of thousands of malnourished children each year.

To ensure rapid weight gain and correct nutrient deficiencies, children suffering from uncomplicated, but severe acute malnutrition may be given ready-to-use therapeutic food (RUTF)—a paste made of local commodities such as peanut butter and powdered milk and fortified with vitamins and minerals (see Photo 20-8).[27] Because it does not need to be mixed with water, the risk of bacterial contamination is greatly minimized. Another benefit is that it can be stored for 3 to 4 months without refrigeration. Whether these therapeutic foods should be used for the *prevention* of childhood malnutrition is currently being studied.

In addition to nutrition intervention, children suffering from diarrhea commonly need rehydration. In severe cases, diarrhea will have incurred dramatic fluid and mineral losses that need to be replaced immediately to help raise the blood pressure and strengthen the heartbeat. Health-care workers around the world save millions of lives each year by effectively reversing dehydration and correcting the diarrhea with **oral rehydration therapy (ORT).** ORT is a simple, inexpensive, and effective treatment that consists of giving a sugar and salt solution orally. In addition to ORT, adequate sanitation and clean water are essential to prevent death from diarrheal disease.

oral rehydration therapy (ORT): the administration of a simple solution of sugar, salt, and water, taken by mouth, to treat dehydration caused by diarrhea. A simple ORT recipe:

- ½ L boiling water
- 4 tsp sugar
- ½ tsp salt

REVIEW IT **Describe the consequences of nutrient and energy inadequacies.**
Hunger leads to malnutrition, which appears most evident in nutrient deficiencies and growth failure. Children suffering from acute malnutrition (recent severe food deprivation) may be underweight for their height, while those experiencing chronic malnutrition (long-term food deprivation) are short for their age. Problems resulting from nutrient deficiencies include preterm births and low birth weights (iron), stillbirths and cretinism (iodine), blindness (vitamin A), and growth failure (zinc). Treatment should be individualized to ensure rapid weight gain and correct nutrient deficiencies.

20.4 Agriculture and the Environment

LEARN IT **Explain why relieving environmental problems will also help alleviate hunger and poverty.**

Much progress has been made in recent years to alleviate hunger, improve agriculture, and protect the environment. Such progress gives hope that enough quality food can be grown in a sustainable way with minimal environment impact to feed all the world's people people adequately.[28] The challenges are enormous as the food demand is expected to double by 2050. The remainder of this chapter first examines the problems agriculture imposes on the environment and then explores possible solutions (see Photo 20-9).[29]

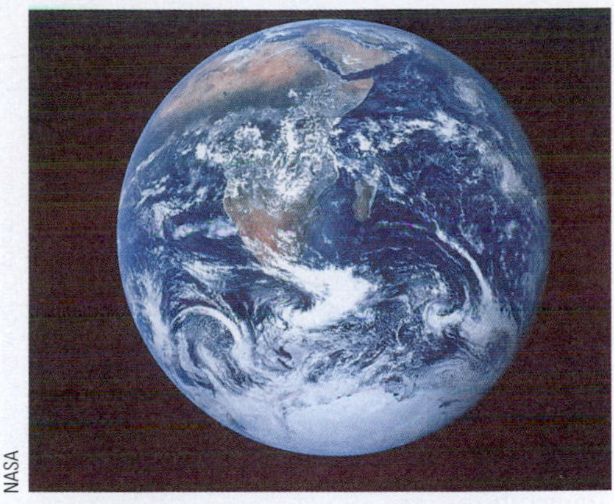

NASA

> **PHOTO 20-9** A reminder that caring for our planet will serve us well for future generations: "We do not inherit the earth from our ancestors, we borrow it from our children." —ascribed to Chief Seattle, a 19th-century Native American leader

Agricultural Consequences

Food production to feed billions of people around the world damages the environment. Because a damaged environment cannot support food production, concerted efforts are needed to improve food production in ways that will protect the environment. Only then will the vicious cycle of hunger and environmental degradation end.

Planting Crops Growing crops has major environmental consequences. The soil loses nutrients as each crop is harvested, so fertilizer is applied. Some nitrogen in the fertilizer is released as a gas that contributes to greenhouse gas emissions. With rain or irrigation, fertilizer leaches into ground water or runs off into the waterways where it stimulates algae growth, which depletes oxygen and kills aquatic plants and animals.

To protect crops against weeds and pests, farmers apply herbicides and pesticides, which pollute the water and kill native plants, native insects, and animals that eat those plants and insects. Ironically, with continued widespread use of pesticides and herbicides, pests and weeds become more resistant. Consequently, farmers must use more pesticides and herbicides. These chemicals pose hazards for farm workers who handle them, and the residues can create health problems for consumers as well (as Chapter 19 discussed).

Finally, when fields are irrigated, the water evaporates, but the salts do not. As salts accumulate on the soil surface, plant growth fails. Irrigation can also deplete the water supply over time as much of the water taken from surface waters or from underground evaporates or runs off. Excessive irrigation can dry up rivers and lakes and lower the water table of entire regions. A vicious cycle develops. The drier the region becomes, the more farmers must irrigate, and the more they irrigate, the drier the region becomes.

> **FIGURE 20-6 Pounds of Grain Needed to Produce 1 Pound of Bread and 1 Pound of Animal Weight Gain**

To gain 1 pound, animals raised for food have to eat many more pounds of grain than it takes to make a pound of bread.

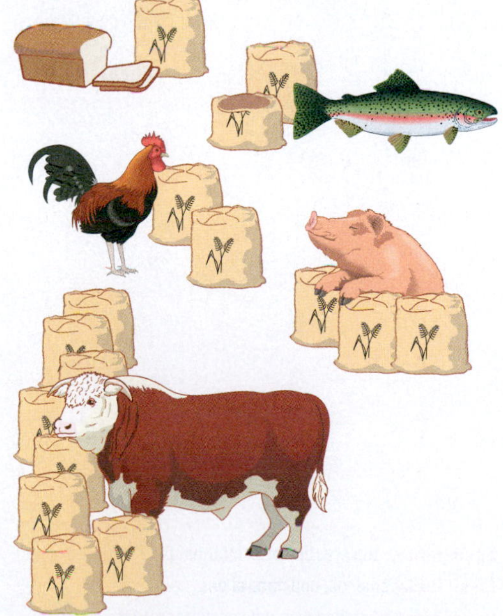

SOURCE: Idea and data from T. R. Reid, Feeding the planet, National Geographic, October 1998, pp. 58–74.

Raising Livestock Consumers are not typically aware of the environmental impact of eating meat, but raising livestock takes an enormous toll on land and energy resources.[30] Animals raised in large concentrated areas such as cattle feedlots or hog farms create environmental problems when huge masses of animal wastes are produced. The ammonia from their wastes pollutes the air and is a major cause of acid rain, which damages plants, acidifies soils, and pollutes waterways. In addition to urine and manure, animals produce large quantities of methane—a greenhouse gas that contributes to climate change. In an effort to prevent contamination of air, soil, and water, the US Environmental Protection Agency offers incentives to livestock farmers who clean up their wastes and allow inspections.

In addition to the waste problems, animals in feedlots must be fed, and grain is grown for them on other land. That grain may require fertilizers, herbicides, pesticides, and irrigation, too. In the United States, more cropland is used to produce grains for livestock than to produce grains for people. Figure 20-6 compares the grain required to produce various foods.

Fishing Fishing also incurs environmental costs. On the sea, we harvest fish, often with little thought to the dwindling supplies or the environmental damage incurred. Excessive fishing—catching fish at a faster rate than they can reproduce—diminishes the availability of seafood for people to eat, upsets the balance of marine life, and reduces water quality. Some fishing methods, such as nets and filament line, kill nonfood species and deplete large populations of aquatic animals such as turtles. Some fishing methods damage the ocean floor.

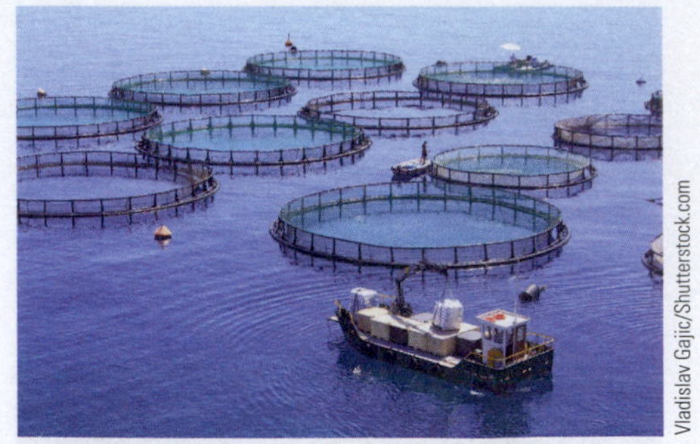
Vladislav Gajic/Shutterstock.com

> **PHOTO 20-10** About half of the seafood consumed in the United States comes from aquaculture.

Catching wild fish cannot keep pace with consumer consumption. The shortfall has spurred the rapid growth of **aquaculture**, which now provides roughly half of the world's food fish and shellfish (see Photo 20-10). Aquaculture continues to grow more rapidly than any other kind of food animal production.

Some aquaculture farms consist of vast net cages that enclose fish in ocean water or freshwater lakes, where natural water flow refreshes the cages. Other types of farms house fish in artificial ponds positioned close to natural water or farther inland. On the coast, natural water is diverted through the ponds, bringing fresh water in and carrying out wastes. Farther inland, pond water is continuously filtered and cleansed, recycling through the ponds. All farmed fish must be fed, and fish chow consists of grains and fish harvested from wild species, diminishing their stocks for human consumption. Adequate environmental safeguards are a must to prevent environmental degradation from aquaculture. Aquaculture can be sustainable, however, with the appropriate technologies and practices.

Fishing is also energy-intensive, requiring fuel for boats, refrigeration, processing, packing, and transport. Water pollution incurs health risks when people eat contaminated fish. Bioaccumulation of toxins in fish may rule out fish consumption altogether in some areas (review Figure 19-6, p. 621).

Energy Overuse The entire food industry, whether based on growing crops, raising livestock, or fishing, requires energy, which primarily entails burning **fossil fuels.** Massive fossil fuel use threatens the environment by causing air and water pollution, changing climate patterns, depleting the ozone layer, and more. In the United States, the food industry consumes about 20 percent of all the energy the nation uses. Most of this energy is used to run farm machinery and to produce fertilizers and pesticides. Energy is also used to process, package, transport, refrigerate, store, and prepare foods.

Water Misuse Food production also uses an enormous amount of water—approximately 80 percent of the total amount used in the United States. It takes an estimated 1.5 million gallons of water to produce the food for one US consumer for 1 year. According to the Environmental Protection Agency, current farming practices are responsible for much most of the pollution in US rivers and streams. Growing crops adds sediment, nutrients, and pesticides to the water. Irrigating crops depletes groundwater supplies, causing the land to become desert, which ironically can lead to flooding.

As human populations grow, so does the demand for clean potable water. In areas of high **water stress,** natural and manmade influences converge to limit access to safe drinking water (see Figure 20-7). Poor water management causes many of the world's water problems as wastewater is dumped into the world's rivers, lakes, and streams without treatment. Nearly 4 million children die each year because of unclean water and poor sanitation. By 2025, if present patterns continue, half of the world's population will live in water-stressed regions.

Biodiversity Biodiversity is declining and plant species are becoming extinct. Agricultural practices and the increasing uniformity of global food habits have contributed to the loss of species. Wheat, rice, soybeans, and maize provide 75 percent of the food energy around the world. Only two dozen other crops provide the remainder. As people everywhere eat the same limited array of foods, demand for a local regions' native, genetically diverse plants is no longer financially worth preserving. Yet, in the future, as the climate and environment change, those very plants may be needed for food. A wild species of corn that grows in a dry climate, for example, might contain the genetic information necessary to help make domestic corn resistant to drought.

Pollinators are also disappearing and becoming extinct. The disappearance of birds, bugs, bees, and other creatures that pollinate food crops could dramatically diminish the food supply and increase malnutrition (and related diseases

aquaculture: the practice of fish farming.

fossil fuels: coal, oil, and natural gas.

water stress: intense demands on water resources by human activities such as municipal water supplies, industries, power plants, and agriculture.

> **FIGURE 20-7 Water-Scarcity Hot Spots**

Water scarcity is the lack of sufficient available water to fully meet the demands of a region. Water stress occurs when the demand for water exceeds the amount available or when poor quality limits its use.

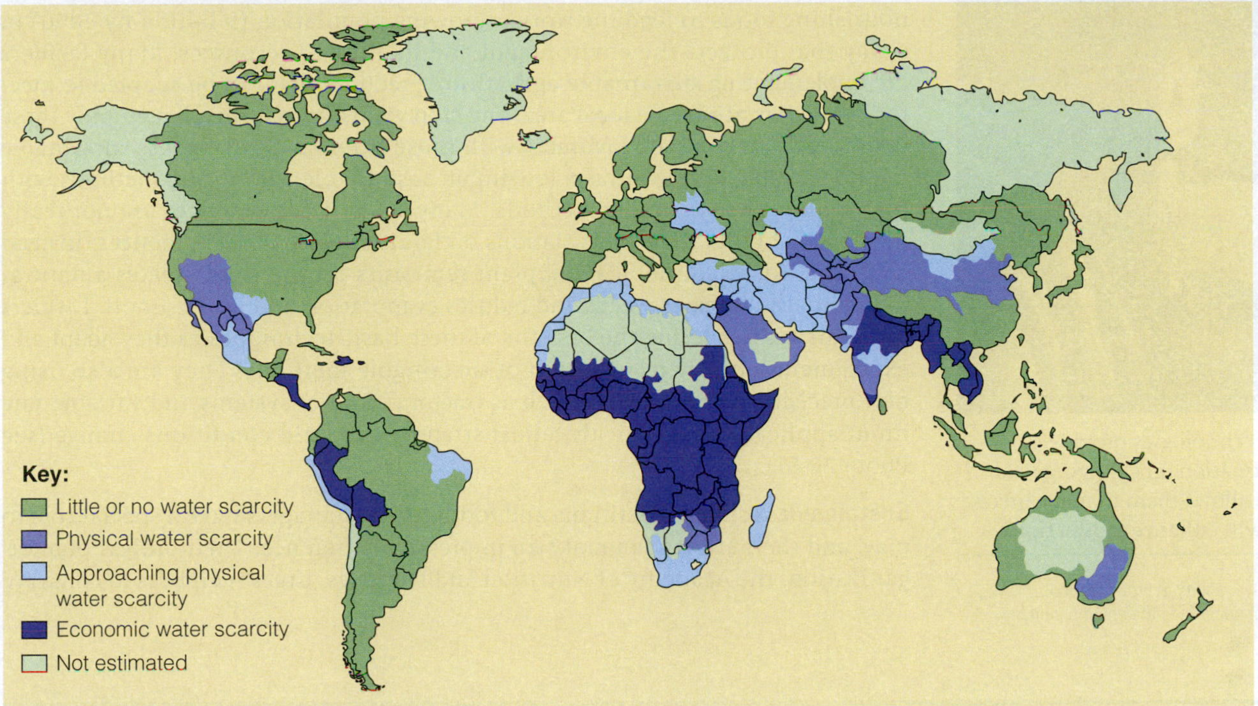

Key:
Little or no water scarcity
Physical water scarcity
Approaching physical water scarcity
Economic water scarcity
Not estimated

SOURCE: *World Water Assessment Programme,* The United Nations World Water Development Report 3: Water in a Changing World (*Paris: UNESCO, and London: Earthscan, 2009*). p. 92.

and death) in many parts of the world. The nutrient most likely to be lacking is vitamin A and its deficiency already claims the lives of hundreds of thousands of women and children each year.[31] Taken to the extreme of total pollinator extinction, researchers calculate a reduction in global supplies of fruit by 23 percent, vegetables by 16 percent, and nuts and seeds by 22 percent.[32]

Food Waste Each year, an estimated one-third of the world's food supply is wasted along the way from farm to final consumption. Consumers in wealthy nations such as the United States waste an estimated 200 to 250 pounds of food per person per year. By comparison, consumers in the developing regions of Southern Asia, Sub-Saharan Africa, and Eastern Asia waste only 10 to 25 pounds per person per year. Saving even 25 percent of food wasted globally would be enough to feed 870 million hungry people.

Food waste has a major environmental impact as well—both by squandering resources and by contributing to greenhouse gases. Each year, food waste accounts for more than 25 percent of the water used and about 300 million barrels of oil. In addition, the methane and carbon dioxide from decomposing food contributes to greenhouse gases and climate change.

In short, food production takes a tremendous toll on the environment. And environmental problems can limit the world's ability to feed its people and keep them healthy. For the most part, our current food production systems are not **sustainable**.

Sustainable Solutions

Historically, agricultural yields improved with advances in irrigation systems, fertilizers, and genetic strains. Today, however, the contributions these measures can make are reaching their limits, in part because they have also created environmental problems. The time has come for

sustainable: able to continue indefinitely; using resources at such a rate that the earth can keep on replacing them and producing pollutants at a rate with which the environment and human cleanup efforts can keep pace, so that no net accumulation of pollution occurs.

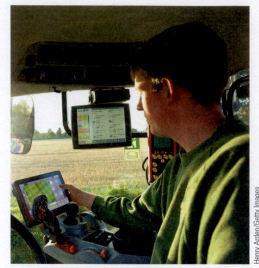

Henry Arden/Getty Images

> **PHOTO 20-11** Technologies provide farmers with information on changing field conditions, which allows them to make precise adjustments that will enhance production.

sustainable agriculture: ability to produce food indefinitely, with little or no harm to the environment.

agricultural practices to shift from damaging the environment to supporting a sustainable world that is capable of eradicating poverty and hunger.[33]

Sustainable Agriculture The challenge we face is figuring out how to grow enough nourishing foods to feed the world's growing population (9 billion by 2050) in a way that protects the environment and its limited resources. Many farmers are implementing **sustainable agriculture** practices that can be adapted to meet the particular needs of a local area. The crop yields from farms that employ these practices often compare favorably with those from farms using less sustainable methods. Table 20-3 contrasts low-input, sustainable agriculture methods with high-input, unsustainable methods. Many sustainable practices are not really new, incidentally; they are variations on familiar agricultural practices. Instead of tilling, for example, leaving plant remnants on the field creates a natural mulch that suppresses weeds and reduces evaporation and water runoff. Farmers today are rediscovering the benefits of these basic techniques as they adapt and experiment with them in search of sustainable methods. They are also using new precision technologies—such as tractor guidance systems and variable-rate input applications to quickly adjust strategies as field conditions change (see Photo 20-11).

Sustainable Actions Dietitians and foodservice managers have a special role to play, and their efforts can make an impressive difference. Their professional organization, the Academy of Nutrition and Dietetics, urges members to conserve

TABLE 20-3 Acute and Chronic Malnutrition Compared

Environmental issues	Unsustainable methods	Sustainable methods
Soil	Growing the same crop repeatedly on the same land takes nutrients out of the soil, making fertilizer use necessary; favors soil erosion; and invites weeds and pests to become established, making pesticide use necessary. Plowing the same way everywhere, allows water runoff and erosion.	Rotating crops increases nitrogen in the soil so there is less need to use fertilizers. Using appropriate plowing methods reduces soil erosion and problems caused by weeds and pests. Using cover crops, crop rotation, no-till planting, contour planting, ridge till, mulch, terraces, and grass strips conserves both soil and water.
Fertilizer	Using fertilizers pollutes ground and surface water and increases costs.	Reducing the use of fertilizers and using livestock manure more effectively lowers costs. Planting cover crops, such as legumes, after harvest restores nutrients and reduces erosion. Composting all plant residues not harvested into the soil improves its nutrient content and water-holding capacity.
Livestock	Feeding livestock in feedlots concentrates manure that pollutes water and releases methane, a global warming gas. Injecting animals with antibiotics prevents diseases.	Feeding livestock or buffalo on the open range allows their manure to fertilize the ground. Collecting feedlot animals' manure enables it to be used as fertilizer or treated before it is released. Maintaining animals' health can prevent disease.
Herbicide/ pesticide	Spraying herbicides and pesticides over large areas wipes out weeds, pests, and other plants and insects.	Using crop rotations, cover crops, and mechanical cultivation can control weeds. Using resistant crops and rotating crops foils pests that lay their eggs in the soil where last year's crop was grown. Using biological controls such as predators can destroy pests.
Water	Irrigating on a large scale depletes water supplies and concentrates salts in the soil.	Irrigating only during dry spells and applying only spot irrigation conserves water.
Energy	Using only fossil fuels depletes resources.	Using renewable energy technologies such as hydroelectric, biomass, photovoltaics, wind power, solar thermal, geothermal, biogas, and methanol conserves resources. Using machinery scaled to the job at hand, and operating it at efficient speeds conserves energy. Combining operations such as harrowing, planting, and fertilizing in the same operation conserves energy.

resources and minimize waste in both their professional and their personal lives. In addition, members can educate themselves and others on hunger, its consequences, and programs to fight it; conduct research on the effectiveness and benefits of programs; and serve as advocates on the local, state, and national levels to help end hunger in the United States. Globally, these professionals support programs that combat malnutrition, provide food security, promote sustainable diets, respect local cultures, protect the environment, and sustain the economy.[34]

Sustainable Diets The foods and beverages people consume influence both personal well-being and that of the environment. The goal, then, is to select a meal pattern that is both healthy and sustainable. Fortunately, that is relatively easy. **Sustainable diets:**

- Minimize the consumption of energy-dense, ultraprocessed, and packaged foods
- Include more plant-based foods and fewer animal-derived foods, especially beef
- Meet daily energy needs without excess

These shifts in eating patterns reduce overconsumption of foods, especially resource-intensive foods, and contribute to a sustainable future.[35] The benefits are threefold—improving food security, minimizing environmental impacts, and promoting good health.[36]

Diet composition dramatically influences the environmental footprint. Changing eating patterns toward plant-based diets reduces the environmental costs and increases the carrying capacity of US agricultural resources. Reducing kcalorie intake helps as well; overconsumption of kcalories places unnecessary demands on the environment. A study that calculated the carrying capacity of ten different eating patterns concluded that the best options were vegetarian (not vegan) diets and those that included only small amounts of meat and dairy products.[37] Such findings confirm that dietary sustainability can be achieved without drastic changes.[38]

Can one person's choice to reduce food waste or to recycle a bottle or to volunteer at a food recovery program make a difference? In truth, such choices produce several benefits (see Photo 20-12). For one, a person's action may influence many other people over time. For another, a repeated action becomes a habit, with compounded benefits. For still another, making choices with an awareness of the consequences improves behaviors and gives a person a sense of personal control, hope, and effectiveness. The daily actions of many concerned people can help solve the problems of hunger in their own communities or on the other side of the world. As Margaret Mead said, "Never doubt that a small group of thoughtful, committed people can change the world. Indeed, it is the only thing that ever has."

Individuals can assist the global community in solving its poverty and hunger problems by joining and working for hunger-relief organizations (see Table 20-4, p. 660). They can also support the needed changes in economic policies that influence food availability and price volatility both at home and in developing countries.

Most importantly, all individuals can try to make lifestyle choices that consider the environmental consequences. Many small decisions each day have major consequences for the environment. Highlight 20 (p. 662) describes how consumers can conserve resources and minimize waste when making food-related choices.

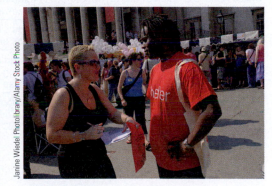

Janine Wiedel Photolibrary/Alamy Stock Photo

> **PHOTO 20-12** Each person's choice to get involved and be heard can help lead to needed change.

sustainable diets: patterns of eating that promote health and provide food security for the present population while sustaining environmental resources for future generations.

TABLE 20-4 Hunger-Relief Organizations

Organization	Mission Statement
Bread for the World **www.bread.org**	Nonpartisan, Christian citizens' movement seeking to influence reform in policies, programs, and conditions that allow hunger and poverty to persist globally.
Catholic Relief Services **www.crs.org**	Humanitarian service agency assisting the impoverished and disadvantaged through community-based, sustainable development initiatives.
Feed the Future **www.feedthefuture.gov**	US government global initiative helping countries transform their own agricultural sectors to grow enough food to sustainably feed their people.
Food First **www.foodfirst.org**	North American organization dedicated to building strong, sustainable, local and regional food systems that ensure access to affordable, nutritious, and culturally appropriate food for all people at all times.
Congressional Hunger Center **www.hungercenter.org**	Bipartisan organization training and inspiring leaders with the intent to end hunger, and advocating public policies to create a food-secure world.
Feeding America **www.feedingamerica.org**	Domestic organization providing food assistance through a nationwide network of member food banks and facilitating education to end hunger nationally. The Healthy Food Bank Hub is an interactive section of Feeding America that provides tools and resources for both public health professionals looking to learn more about hunger, and food banking professionals looking to further promote a healthful lifestyle to their clients.
Food and Agriculture Organization (FAO) of the United Nations **www.fao.org**	International organization leading efforts to help eliminate hunger, food insecurity, and malnutrition; make agriculture, forestry, and fisheries more productive and sustainable; reduce rural poverty; and enable inclusive and efficient agricultural and food systems.
Idealist **www.idealist.org**	International organization seeking to connect people, organizations, and resources to help build a world where all people can live free and dignified lives.
Oxfam America **www.oxfamamerica.org**	International relief and development organization aiming to create lasting solutions to poverty, hunger, and injustice.
Pan American Health Organization **www.paho.org**	International public health agency aiming to strengthen national and local health systems with the purpose of improving the quality of, and lengthening, the lives of peoples in the Americas.
Society of St. Andrew **www.endhunger.org**	Ecumenical Christian ministry salvaging and redirecting large amounts of fresh produce to hunger agencies for distribution to the poor.
The Hunger Project **www.thp.org**	International organization committed to ending world hunger by empowering people to lead lives of self-reliance, meet their own basic needs, and build better futures for their children.
United Nations Children's Fund (UNICEF) **www.unicef.org**	International organization advocating for the protection of children's rights, to help meet their basic needs and to expand their opportunities to reach their full potentials.
World Food Programme **www.wfp.org**	Food aid branch of the United Nations aiming to prepare for, protect during, and provide assistance after, emergencies, as well as to reduce hunger and undernutrition.
World Health Organization (WHO) **www.who.int**	United Nations agency acting as the authority on international public health by influencing policy, setting research agendas, establishing standards, and providing technical support to monitor and assess health trends.
WhyHunger **www.whyhunger.org**	Domestic organization supporting and funding community-based organizations intent on empowering individuals and building self-reliance to provide long-term solutions to hunger and poverty.

REVIEW IT Explain why relieving environmental problems will also help alleviate hunger and poverty.

Environmental degradation reduces our ability to produce enough food to feed the world's people. Governments, businesses, and all individuals have many opportunities to make environmentally conscious choices, which may help solve the hunger problem and improve quality of life. Personal choices, made by many people, can have a great impact.

What's Online

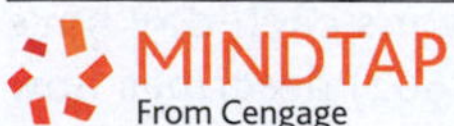
MINDTAP
From Cengage

Visit **www.cengagebrain.com** to access MindTap, a complete digital course that includes Diet & Wellness Plus, interactive quizzes, videos, and more.

REFERENCES

1. Food and Agriculture Organization of the United Nations, *The state of food insecurity in the world, 2015,* http://www.fao.org/3/a-i4646e.pdf.
2. UNICEF, Undernutrition contributes to nearly half of all deaths in children under 5 and is widespread in Asia and Africa, http://data.unicef.org/topic/nutrition/malnutrition/#sthash.cge75ymc.dpuf, February 2017.
3. *Food Security in the United States in 2015,* US Department of Agriculture, October 11, 2016.
4. C. DeNavas-Walt and B. D. Proctor, US Census Bureau, *Income and poverty in the United States: 2014,* https://www.census.gov/library/publications/2015/demo/p60-252.html, September 2015.
5. Council on Community Pediatrics, Poverty and child health in the United States, *Pediatrics* 137 (2016): 59–72.
6. J. Kaur, M. M. Lamb, and C. L. Ogden, The association between food insecurity and obesity in children: The National Health and Nutrition Examination Survey, *Journal of the Academy of Nutrition and Dietetics* 115 (2015): 751–58.
7. N. M. Widick and coauthors, Access to healthy food stores modifies effect of a dietary intervention, *American Journal of Preventive Medicine* 48 (2015): 309–317.
8. A. Drewnowski, New metrics of affordable nutrition: Which vegetables provide most nutrients for least cost? *Journal of the Academy of Nutrition and Dietetics* 113 (2013): 1182–1187.
9. W. E. Waterlander and coauthors, Price discounts significantly enhance fruit and vegetable purchases when combined with nutrition education: A randomized controlled supermarket trial, *American Journal of Clinical Nutrition* 97 (2013): 886–895.
10. L. Rimkus and coauthors, Disparities in the availability and price of low-fat and higher-fat milk in US food stores by community characteristics, *Journal of the Academy of Nutrition and Dietetics* 115 (2015): 1975–1985.
11. Position of the American Dietetic Association: Food insecurity in the United States, *Journal of the American Dietetic Association* 110 (2010): 1368–1377.
12. J. Mabli and coauthors, Measuring the effect of Supplemental Nutrition Assistance Program (SNAP) participation on food security, www.fns.usda.gov/research-and-analysis, August 2013.
13. L. Harnack and coauthors, Effects of subsidies and prohibitions on nutrition in a food benefit program: A randomized clinical trial, *JAMA Internal Medicine* 176 (2016): 1610–1618.
14. 1. J. C. Buzby, H. F. Wells, and J. Hyman, The estimated amount, value, and calories of postharvest food losses at the retail and consumer levels in the United States, US Department of Agriculture, *Economic Information Bulletin Number 121,* February 2014.
15. C. Vogliano and K. Brown, The state of America's wasted food and opportunities to make a difference, *Journal of the Academy of Nutrition and Dietetics* 116 (2016): 1199–1207; A. Tagtow and coauthors, Food waste reduction efforts at the USDA, *Journal of the Academy of Nutrition and Dietetics* 115 (2015): 1914-1918.
16. US Environmental Protection Agency, 3. Sustainable Management of Food: Food Recovery Hierarchy, www.epa.gov/sustainable-management-food/food-recovery-hierarchy.
17. World Hunger Education Service, 2016 World hunger and poverty facts and statistics, http://www.worldhunger.org/2015-world-hunger-and-poverty-facts-and-statistics, December 28, 2016.
18. *The Global Nutrition Report,* 2016, www.globalnutritionreport.org.
19. A. M. Prentice and coauthors, Critical windows for nutritional interventions against stunting, *American Journal of Clinical Nutrition* 97 (2013): 911–918.
20. G. Fink and coauthors, Schooling and wage income losses due to early-childhood growth faltering in developing countries: National, regional, and global estimates, *American Journal of Clinical Nutrition* 104 (2016): 104–112.
21. Z. A. Bhutta and J. K. Das, Global burden of childhood diarrhea and pneumonia: What can and should be done? *Pediatrics* 131 (2013): 634–636.
22. World Health Organization, Children: Reducing mortality, www.who.int/mediacentre/factsheets/fs178/en, September 2016.
23. C. M. McDonald and coauthors, The effect of multiple anthropometric deficits on child mortality: Meta-analysis of individual data in 10 prospective studies from developing countries, *American Journal of Clinical Nutrition* 97 (2013): 896–901.
24. I. Trehan and M. J. Manary, Management of severe acute malnutrition in low-income and middle-income countries, *Archives of Disease in Childhood* 100 (2015): 283–287; S. Frison, F. Checchi, and M. Kerac, Omitting edema measurement: How much acute malnutrition are we missing? *American Journal of Clinical Nutrition* 102 (2015): 1176–1181.
25. I. Trehan and coauthors, Extending supplementary feeding for children younger than 5 years with moderate acute malnutrition leads to lower relapse rates, *Journal of Pediatric Gastroenterology and Nutrition* 60 (2015): 544–549.
26. I. Trehan and coauthors, Antibiotics as part of the management of severe acute malnutrition, *New England Journal of Medicine* 368 (2013): 425–435; W. S. Garrett, Kwashiorkor and the gut microbiota, *New England Journal of Medicine* 368 (2013): 1746–1747; H. Tilg and A. R. Moschen, Malnutrition and microbiota—A new relationship? *Nature Reviews: Gastroenterology and Hepatology* 10 (2013): 261–262.
27. P. Bahwere and coauthors, Cereals and pulse-based ready-to-use therapeutic food as an alternative to the standard milk- and peanut paste-based formulation for treating severe acute malnutrition: A noninferiority, individually randomized controlled efficacy clinical trial, *American Journal of Clinical Nutrition* 103 (2016): 1145–1161; A. Santini and coauthors, State of the art of Ready-to-Use Therapeutic Food: A tool for nutraceuticals addition to foodstuff, *Food Chemistry* 140 (2013): 843–849.
28. B. M. Popkin, Relationship between shifts in food system dynamics and acceleration of the global nutrition transition, *Nutrition Reviews* 75 (2017): 73–82.
29. FAO Economic and Social Development Department, *World Agriculture: Towards 2015/2030 Executive Summary,* http://www.fao.org/docrep/004/y3557e/y3557e00.htm.
30. A. Clonan and coauthors, Red and processed meat consumption and purchasing behaviours and attitudes: Impacts for human health, animal welfare and environmental sustainability, *Public Health Nutrition* 18 (2015): 2446–2456.
31. A. M. Ellis, S. S. Myers, and T. H. Rickets, Do pollinators contribute to nutritional health? *PLoS One* 10 (2015): e114805.
32. M. R. Smith and coauthors, Effects of decreases of animal pollinators on human nutrition and global health: A modeling analysis, *Lancet* 386 (2015): 1964–1972.
33. J. Rockström and coauthors, Sustainable intensification of agriculture for human prosperity and global sustainability, *Ambio* 46 (2017): 4–17.
34. C. Vogliano and coauthors, Plentiful, nutrient-dense food for the world: A guide for registered dietitian nutritionists, *Journal of the Academy of Nutrition and Dietetics* 115 (2015): 2014–2018; Position of the Academy of Nutrition and Dietetics: Nutrition security in developing nations: Sustainable food, water, and health, *Journal of the Academy of Nutrition and Dietetics* 113 (2013): 581–595.
35. J. Ranganathan and coauthors, Shifting diets for a sustainable food future, Washington, DC: World Resources Institute, April 2016.
36. A. A. Alsaffar, Sustainable diets: The interaction between food industry, nutrition, health, and the environment, *Food Science and Technology International* 22 (2016): 102–111.
37. C. J. Peters and coauthors, Carrying capacity of US agricultural land: Ten diet scenarios, *Elementa Science of the Anthropocene* (2016): doi.org/10.12952/journal.elementa.000116.
38. M. Perignon and coauthors, Improving diet sustainability through evolution of food choices: Review of epidemiological studies on the environmental impact of diets, *Nutrition Reviews* 75 (2017): 2–17.

LEARN IT Discuss ways consumers can conserve resources when making food-related choices.

Environmentally Friendly Food Choices

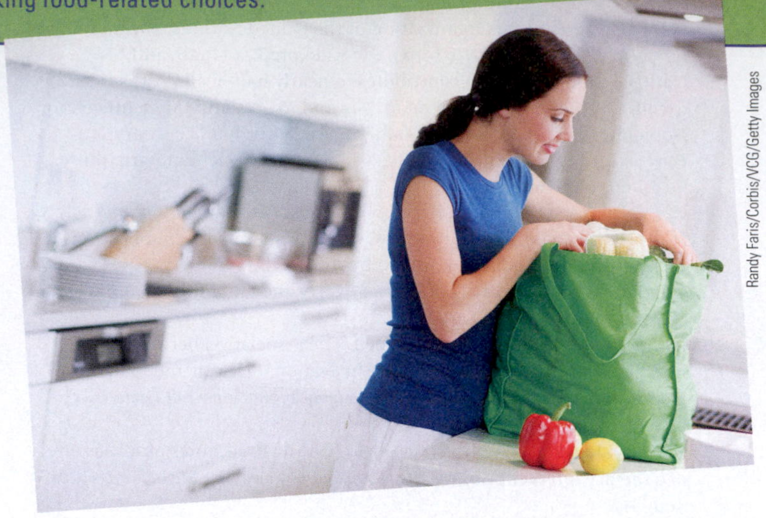

Randy Faris/Corbis/VCG/Getty Images

Chapter 20 concludes its examination of US and world hunger by focusing on the environment. It explains how producing enough food to feed billions of people around the world damages the environment—and how a damaged environment cannot adequately feed billions of people around the world. Efforts to resolve hunger and protect the environment demand improvements in our ways of producing, processing, packaging, transporting, storing, and preparing foods. Because sustainable food strategies have social, economic, and environmental impacts, their success depends on pleasing the people, providing reasonably priced products, and protecting the planet. Consumers' preferences for sustainable practices seems to be a growing trend.[1]

The United Nations describes a nation's impact on the environment as its "ecological footprint"—a measure of the resources used to support a nation's consumption of food, materials, and energy. This measure takes into account the two most challenging aspects of sustainability—per capita resource consumption and population growth. As Figure H20-1 shows, the people of North America are the world's greatest consumers on a per capita basis. Some have estimated that it would take four more planet earths to accommodate every person in the world using resources at the level currently used in the United States. This highlight explores ways that consumers can conserve resources when making food-related choices. Such conscientious food choices can reduce pollution production and resource use.

Choice: Animal or Vegetable?

Some foods require more water, more fertilizer, more pesticides, and more energy for their production than others. One way to reduce these costs of food production is for consumers to eat low on the food chain. For the most part, that means eating more foods derived from plants and fewer foods derived from animals. Plant-based diets use fewer natural resources and are less environmentally damaging than meat-based diets.[2] Compared with vegetarian diets, meat-based diets use 2.9 times more water, 2.5 times more energy, 13 times more fertilizer, and 1.4 times more pesticides.

Consider that relatively little energy is needed to produce grains: it takes less than 1 kcalorie of fuel to produce each kcalorie of grain, whereas most animal-derived foods require from 10 to 90 kcalories of fuel per kcalorie of edible food; kcalories to produce fruits and vegetables are generally greater than grains, but less than animal-derived foods. In general, meat-based diets require much more energy, as well as more land and water, than do plant-based diets. An exception is livestock raised on the open range; these animals require about as much energy as most plant foods. Because we raise so much more grain-fed, than range-fed, livestock, however, the average energy requirement for meat production is high.

To support our meat intake, we maintain several billion livestock, about four times our own weight in animals. Livestock consume 10 times as much grain each day as we do. We could use much of that grain to make grain products for ourselves and for others around the world. Making this shift could free up enough grain to feed 400 million people while using less fuel, water, and land.

> **FIGURE H20-1 Ecological Footprints**

The width of a bar represents the region's population, and the height represents per capita consumption (in terms of area of productive land or sea required to produce the natural resources consumed). Thus, the footprint of the bar represents the region's total consumption. For example, Asia's population is more than 10 times as great as North America's, but because its consumption is only one-sixth as large, their footprints are similar in size.

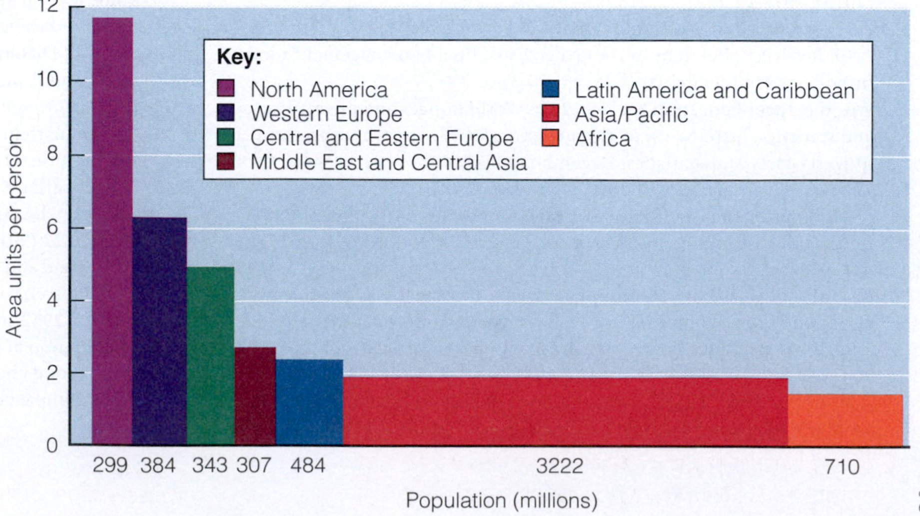
Key:
North America
Western Europe
Central and Eastern Europe
Middle East and Central Asia
Latin America and Caribbean
Asia/Pacific
Africa
Area units per person
0
2
4
6
8
10
12
299
384
343
307
484
3222
710
Population (millions)
© Cengage

Part of the solution to the livestock problem may be to cease feeding grain to animals and return to grazing them on the open range, which can be a sustainable practice. Ranchers have to manage the grazing carefully to hold the cattle's numbers to what the land can support without environmental degradation. To accomplish this, the economic benefits of traditional livestock and feed-growing operations would have to end. If producers were to pay the true costs of the environmental damage incurred by irrigation water, fertilizers, pesticides, and fuels, the price of meats might double or triple. According to classic economic theory, people would then buy less meat (reducing demand), and producers would respond by producing less meat (reducing supply). Meat production would then fall to a sustainable level.

Because meat production demands such a large and disproportionate share of natural resources, it provides a great opportunity to make significant improvements in sustainability.[3] Modest reductions in meat consumption can have a significant impact. Completely eliminating meat from the diet is not necessary to design a sustainable diet that meets dietary requirements and lowers greenhouse gas emissions.[4] In fact, a study mentioned earlier in the chapter concluded that vegetarian diets or diets that included only small amounts of meat and dairy products were better than vegan diets with respect to the earth's carrying capacity.[5] Consumers can choose smaller portions of meat or select range-fed beef or buffalo. Livestock on the range eat grass, which people cannot eat. "Rangeburger" buffalo also offers nutrient advantages over grain-fed beef because it is lower in fat and because the fat has more polyunsaturated fatty acids, including the omega-3 fatty acids.

Some consumers are opting for vegetarian diets—at least occasionally. Choosing fish instead of meat may be a practical alternative if seafood is selected with an awareness of the environmental consequences. To learn more about how to select seafood that's fished or farmed in environmentally responsible ways, visit Seafood Watch at www.seafoodwatch.org.

Choice: Global or Local?

Plant-based diets have an environmental advantage over meat-based diets, but some would argue that they don't go far enough. A more ecologically responsible diet is also based on locally grown products (see Photo H20-1). On average, an item of food is transported 1500 miles before it is eaten— even when the crops are grown and the final destination are both in the United States. That our foods now travel more than we do has several costly ramifications:

- *Energetically costly.* Foods must be refrigerated and transported thousands of miles to provide a full array of all produce all year round.
- *Socially unjust.* Farmers in impoverished countries, where the people are malnourished, are paid meager wages to grow food for wealthy nations.
- *Economically unwise.* It supports agribusinesses that buy land and labor cheaply in foreign countries instead of supporting local farmers raising crops in our communities.

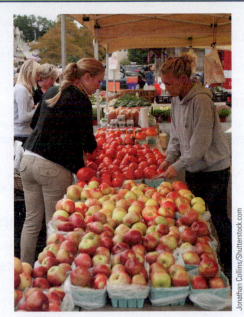

Jonathan Collins/Shutterstock.com

> **PHOTO H20-1** Locally grown foods offer benefits to both the local economy and the global environment.

- *Biologically risky.* Highly perishable foods are shipped from countries with unsafe drinking water and sanitation practices.

For all these reasons, consumers may want to support the global environment by buying locally.

Buying locally offers other benefits as well. Families buying home-grown produce tend to eat a greater quantity and selection of fruits and vegetables.

Adopting a local diet presents a bit of a challenge at first, especially when local fruits and vegetables are "out of season." But a nutritionally balanced diet of delicious foods is quite possible with a little creative planning.

Defining *Local*

Consumers shopping for "locally grown" produce are often trying to find fresh foods that will both help support small farms and protect the environment. Grocers tapping into this "local" marketing concept have seen significant increases in sales. But what exactly does *local* mean? How far is "locally grown" from the farm to the market? Given that *local* is not defined by the FDA, consumers and grocers do not always share the same understanding of the term. Some would say *local* means reasonably nearby—say, within 10 to 50 miles, or up to 100 miles. Others say it means within a day's drive, or within the state or a geographic region. Without agreement, consumers are left to identify which goods meet their limited definition, and grocers are free to market their goods with a broad definition.

Consumers who think of *local* as "fresh from a small farm" may be surprised to learn that is not always the case. "Local" may be a corporate-managed 1000-acre tomato farm or a family-run 3-acre blueberry farm. Because large retail stores need large volumes, they tend to deal with a few large producers. Shipments typically go through a distribution center, which can delay deliveries for several hours or even days. In contrast, small producers tend to sell to farmers' markets and small stores. Deliveries often arrive within hours of harvest.

Eco-Friendly Miles

Consumers who support the concept of purchasing local foods may believe that the fewer miles a food travels, the better for the environment—but this is not always the case. The type of transportation also contributes to environmental costs. In general, transporting by ship is cleaner than by airplane; by train is cleaner than by truck. It may be obvious that the eco-friendly choice for a person living in San Francisco is a California wine, but what about a person living in Atlanta? Is it "greener" to buy wine trucked across the country from California or shipped across the ocean from France?

Eco-Friendly Products and Packaging

Some consumers are attracted to products and packaging that claim to be "eco-friendly," expecting far-reaching environmental benefits, even though such claims may be unsubstantiated. The Federal Trade Commission, which is responsible for enforcing truth-in-advertising

> How To H20-1 Make Environmentally Friendly Food-Related Choices

Food production taxes environmental resources and causes pollution. Consumers can make environmentally friendly choices at every step from food shopping to cooking and use of kitchen appliances to serving, cleanup, and waste disposal.

Food Shopping

Transportation

- Whenever possible, walk or ride a bicycle; use carpools and mass transit.
- Shop only once a week, share trips, or take turns shopping with others.
- When buying a car, choose an energy-efficient one.

Food Choices

- Choose foods low on the food chain; that is, eat more plants and fewer animals that eat plants (this suggestion also complements the *Dietary Guidelines for Americans* for eating for good health).
- Eat small portions of meat; select range-fed beef, buffalo, and poultry.
- Shop at farmers' markets and roadside stands for local foods; they require less transportation, packaging, and refrigeration.
- Limit use of imported canned beef products such as stews, chili, and corned beef that frequently come from cleared rain forest land.
- Choose seafood that has been farmed or fished in environmentally responsible ways.
- Choose chickens from local farms.
- Plan wisely and buy smart to reduce the amount of food wasted.
- Donate excess food to food banks or shelters.
- Give food scraps to farmers for animal feed.

Food Packages

- Whenever possible, select foods with no packages; next best are minimal, reusable, or recyclable ones.
- Buy juices and sodas in large glass or recyclable plastic bottles (not small individual cans or cartons); grains, legumes, and nuts in bulk (not separate little packages); and eggs in pressed fiber cartons (not foam, unless it is recycled locally).
- Carry reusable string or cloth shopping bags; alternatively, reuse plastic bags.

Gardening

- Grow some of your own food, even if it is only herbs planted in pots on your kitchen windowsill.
- Compost all vegetable scraps, fruit peelings, and leftover plant foods.

Cooking Food

- Cook foods quickly in a stir-fry, pressure cooker, or microwave oven.
- When using the oven, bake a lot of food at one time and keep the door closed tightly.
- Use nondisposable utensils, dishes, and pans.
- Use pumps instead of spray products.
- Prepare smaller recipes to minimize waste.
- Eat leftovers.

Kitchen Appliances

- Use fewer small electrical appliances; open cans, mix batters, sharpen knives, and chop vegetables by hand.
- When buying a large appliance, choose an energy-efficient one.
- Consider solar power to meet home electrical needs.
- Set the water heater at <130°F (54°C), no hotter; put it on a timer; wrap it and the hot-water pipes in insulation; install water-saving faucets.
- Set the refrigerator at 37°F to 40°F and the freezer to 0°F.
- Keep all appliances clean and in good repair.

Food Serving, Dish Washing, and Waste Disposal

- Use "real" plates, cups, and glasses instead of disposable ones.
- Use cloth towels and napkins, reusable storage containers with lids, reusable pans, and dishcloths instead of paper towels, plastic wrap, plastic storage bags, aluminum foil, and sponges.
- Run the dishwasher only when it is full.
- Recycle all paper, glass, plastic, and aluminum.

These suggested lifestyle changes can easily be extended from food to other areas.

> TRY IT Find out if you are living a sustainable life by exploring the Sustainable Table website at www.sustainabletable.org.

laws, has created "green guidelines." To claim that a product is "biodegradable," it must completely break down and return to nature within one year. Claims of "being green" cannot be used if the environmental costs of creating and delivering the product exceed the benefits of using it. For example, it is deceptive to claim a product is eco-friendly when the environmental damage of long-distance shipping outweighs the benefits of using recycled packaging.

Other Food-Related Choices

Eating more foods derived from plants and produced locally are two major trends that can influence the food industry. Consumers can also make dozens of other smaller decisions every day to help conserve resources and protect the environment. How To H20-1 lists some of the ways consumers can "tread lightly on the earth" through their daily food choices. Among those strategies is a message to reduce food waste. In addition to the tips to reduce food waste listed here and in How To 20-1 (p. 649), consumers may need to eat closer to their nutrient requirements. Overeating contributes to food losses as much as any other food waste does.[6] Individual consumer behaviors can have a substantial influence on providing food security for the growing world population.

Chapter 20 and this highlight have presented many problems and have suggested that, although many of the problems are global in scope, the solutions depend on the actions of individual people at the local level. On learning of this, concerned people may take a perfectionist attitude, believing that they should be doing more than they realistically can, and so feel defeated. Keep in mind that striving for perfection even while falling short is progress. A positive attitude can bring about improvement, and sometimes improvement is enough. Celebrate the changes that are possible today by making them a permanent part of your life; do the same with changes that become possible tomorrow and every day thereafter. The results may surprise you.

CRITICAL THINKING QUESTIONS

A. What do choices about food shopping, cooking, storage, and disposal say about a person's values?

B. At first glance, labeling appears to be a helpful way for consumers to make informed choices about the products they are buying. But given the lack of consensus on criteria to qualify as "green," manufacturers have taken advantage of this marketing scheme and slapped "eco-labels" on a variety of products with little, or no, thought given to the environment. If you served on a labeling-regulation committee, what criteria would you propose in determining which, if any, food products and packages could claim to be environmentally friendly? How important is it for consumers to adopt environmentally friendly food behaviors?

REFERENCES

1. B. Boyce, Trends in farm-to-table from a sociological perspective, *Journal of the Academy of Nutrition and Dietetics* 113 (2013): 892–898.
2. J. Sabaté and S. Soret, Sustainability of plant-based diets: Back to the future, *American Journal of Clinical Nutrition* 100 (2014): 476S–482S.
3. H. Aiking, Protein production: Planet, profit, plus people? *American Journal of Clinical Nutrition* 100 (2014): 483S–489S.
4. J. I. Macdiarmid and coauthors, Sustainable diets for the future: Can we contribute to reducing greenhouse gas emissions by eating a healthy diet? *American Journal of Clinical Nutrition* 96 (2012): 632–639.
5. C. J. Peters and coauthors, Carrying capacity of US agricultural land: Ten diet scenarios, *Elementa Science of the Anthropocene* (2016): doi.org/10.12952/journal.elementa.000116.
6. P. Alexander and coauthors, Losses, inefficiencies and waste in the global food system, *Agricultural Systems* 153 (2017): 190–200.

Appendixes

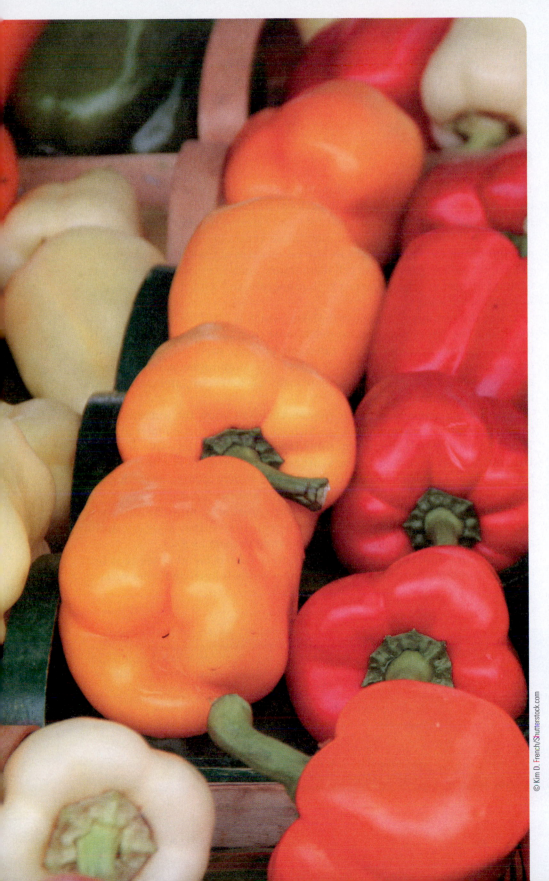

© Kim D. French/Shutterstock.com

Appendix A Cells, Hormones, and Nerves

CONTENTS

This appendix offers an understanding of how the body coordinates its activities. It presents a brief summary of the structure and function of the body's basic working unit (the cell) and of the body's two major regulatory systems (the hormonal system and the nervous system).

Cells

The body's organs are made up of millions of cells and of materials produced by them. Each **cell** is specialized to perform its organ's functions, but all cells have common structures (see Glossary A-1 and Figure A-l). Every cell is contained within a **cell membrane.** The cell membrane assists in moving materials into and out of the cell, and some of its special proteins act as "pumps" (described in Chapter 6). Some features of cell membranes, such as microvilli (described in Chapter 3), permit cells to interact with other cells and with their environments in highly specific ways.

Inside the membrane lies the **cytoplasm,** which is filled with **cytosol,** a jelly-like fluid. The cytoplasm contains much more than just cytosol, though. It is a highly organized system of fibers, tubes, membranes, particles, and subcellular **organelles** as complex as a city. These parts intercommunicate, manufacture and exchange materials, package and prepare materials for export, and maintain and repair themselves.

Within each cell is another membrane-enclosed body, the **nucleus.** Inside the nucleus are the **chromosomes,** which contain the genetic material, DNA. The DNA encodes all the instructions for carrying out the cell's activities. The role of DNA in coding for the synthesis of cell proteins is summarized in Figure 6-7 (p. 175). Chapter 6 also describes the variety of proteins produced by cells and some of the ways they perform the body's work.

Among the organelles within a cell are ribosomes, mitochondria, and lysosomes. Figure 6-7 briefly referred to the **ribosomes;** they assemble amino acids into proteins, following directions conveyed to them by RNA.

The **mitochondria** are made of intricately folded membranes that bear thousands of highly organized sets of enzymes on their inner and outer surfaces.

GLOSSARY A-1 CELL STRUCTURE TERMS

cell: the basic structural unit of all living things.

cell membrane: the thin layer of tissue that surrounds the cell and encloses its contents, made primarily of lipid and protein.

chromosomes: structures within the nucleus of a cell made of DNA and associated proteins. Human beings have 46 chromosomes in 23 pairs. Each chromosome has many genes.

cytoplasm (SIGH-toh-plazm): the cell contents, except for the nucleus.

cytosol: the fluid of cytoplasm that contains water, ions, nutrients, and enzymes.

endoplasmic reticulum (en-doh-PLAZ-mic reh-TIC-you-lum): a complex network of intracellular membranes. The *rough endoplasmic reticulum* is dotted with ribosomes, where protein synthesis takes place. The *smooth endoplasmic reticulum* bears no ribosomes.

Golgi (GOAL-gee) **apparatus:** a set of membranes within the cell where secretory materials are packaged for export.

lysosomes (LYE-so-zomes): cellular organelles; membrane-enclosed sacs of degradative enzymes.

mitochondria (my-toh-KON-dree-uh): the cellular organelles responsible for producing ATP aerobically; made of membranes with enzymes mounted on them. (The singular is *mitochondrion.*)

nucleus: a major membrane-enclosed body within cells, which contains the cell's genetic material (DNA) embedded in chromosomes.

organelles: subcellular structures such as ribosomes, mitochondria, and lysosomes.

ribosomes (RYE-boh-zomes): protein-making organelles in cells that are composed of RNA and protein.

> FIGURE A-1 The Structure of a Typical Cell

The cell shown might be one in a gland (such as the pancreas) that produces secretory products (enzymes) for export (to the intestine). The rough endoplasmic reticulum with its ribosomes produces the enzymes; the smooth reticulum conducts them to the Golgi region; the Golgi membranes merge with the cell membrane, where the enzymes can be released into the extracellular fluid.

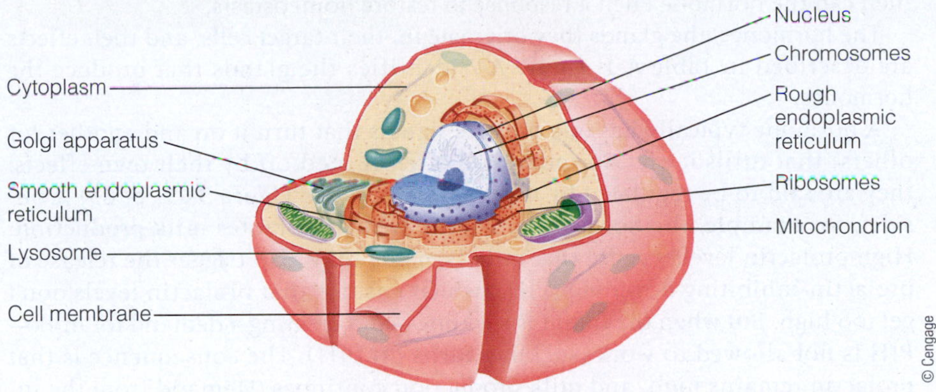

Nucleus
Chromosomes
Rough endoplasmic reticulum
Ribosomes
Mitochondrion
Cytoplasm
Golgi apparatus
Smooth endoplasmic reticulum
Lysosome
Cell membrane
© Cengage

Mitochondria are crucial to energy metabolism (described in Chapter 7) and muscles conditioned to work aerobically are packed with them. Their presence is implied whenever the TCA cycle and electron transport chain are mentioned because the mitochondria house the needed enzymes.*

The **lysosomes** are membrane-enclosed sacs of degradative enzymes. When a cell needs to self-destruct or to digest materials in its surroundings, its lysosomes release their enzymes. Lysosomes are active when tissue repair or remodeling is taking place—for example, in cleaning up infections, healing wounds, shaping embryonic organs, and remodeling bones.

In addition to these and other cellular organelles, the cell's cytoplasm contains a highly organized system of membranes, the **endoplasmic reticulum.** The ribosomes, mentioned earlier, may either float freely in the cytoplasm or be mounted on the endoplasmic reticulum. A surface dotted with ribosomes looks speckled under the microscope and is called "rough" endoplasmic reticulum; such a surface without ribosomes is called "smooth." Some intracellular membranes are organized into tubules that collect cellular materials, merge with the cell membrane, and discharge their contents to the outside of the cell; these membrane systems are named the **Golgi apparatus,** after the scientist who first described them. The rough and smooth endoplasmic reticula and the Golgi apparatus are continuous with one another, so secretions produced deep in the interior of the cell can be efficiently transported and released to the outside. These and other cell structures enable cells to perform a multitude of specialized functions.

The actions of cells are coordinated by both hormones and nerves. Among the types of cellular organelles are receptors for the hormones delivering instructions that originate elsewhere in the body. Some hormones penetrate the cell and its nucleus and attach to receptors on chromosomes, where they activate certain genes to initiate, stop, speed up, or slow down synthesis of certain proteins as needed. Other hormones attach to receptors on the cell surface and transmit their messages from there. The hormones are described in the next section; the nerves, in the one following.

*For the reactions of glycolysis, the TCA cycle, and the electron transport chain, see Chapter 7 and Appendix C. The reactions of glycolysis take place in the cytoplasm; the conversion of pyruvate to acetyl CoA takes place in the mitochondria, as do the TCA cycle and electron transport chain reactions. The mitochondria then release carbon dioxide, water, and ATP as their end products.

APPENDIX A

Hormones

Hormones are chemical messengers secreted by a variety of glands in response to altered conditions in the body. Each hormone travels in the blood to all parts of the body, but only its specific target cells possess receptors to accept it. Only then can the hormone elicit a response to restore homeostasis.

The hormones, the glands they originate in, their target cells, and their effects are described in Table A-1. Figure A-2 identifies the glands that produce the hormones.

A hormone typically has one or more signals that turn it on and another (or others) that turns it off. Hormones are often turned off by their own effects; they are said to be regulated by *negative feedback* (see Figure 3-12, p. 83). Consider, for example, the hormone prolactin, which promotes milk production. High prolactin levels ensure that milk is made; they also trigger the release of prolactin-inhibiting hormone (PIH), which ensures that prolactin levels don't get too high. But when the infant is suckling—and creating a demand for milk—PIH is not allowed to work (suckling turns off PIH). The consequence is that prolactin remains high, and milk production continues. Demand from the infant thus directly adjusts the supply of milk. The need is met through the interaction of the nerves and hormones.

Every body part is affected by hormones. Each different hormone has unique effects, and hormones that oppose each other are produced in carefully regulated amounts, so each can respond to the exact degree that is appropriate to the condition.

As Table A-1 summarizes, hormones have an enormous impact on body processes. The body's other overall regulating agency is the nervous system.

> FIGURE A-2 The Endocrine System

These organs and glands release hormones that regulate body processes. An *endocrine gland* secretes its product directly into *(endo)* the blood; for example, the pancreas cells that secrete insulin into the blood. An *exocrine gland* secretes its product(s) out *(exo)* to an epithelial surface either directly or through a duct; the sweat glands of the skin and the pancreas cells that secrete digestive enzymes into the gastrointestinal tract are both examples. The pancreas is therefore both an endocrine and an exocrine gland.

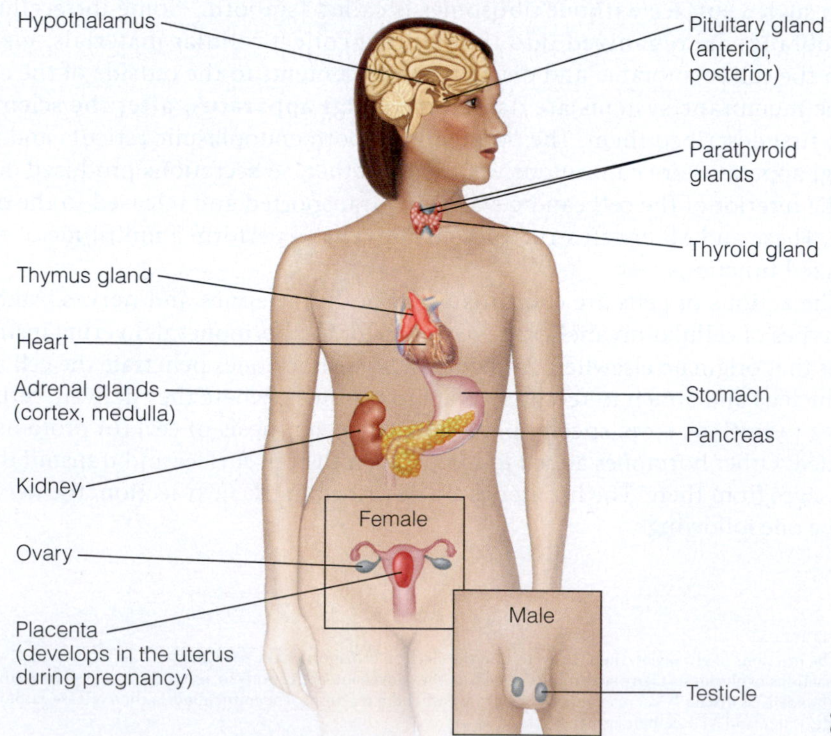
Hypothalamus
Pituitary gland (anterior, posterior)
Parathyroid glands
Thyroid gland
Thymus gland
Heart
Adrenal glands (cortex, medulla)
Stomach
Pancreas
Kidney
Female
Ovary
Placenta (develops in the uterus during pregnancy)
Male
Testicle
© Cengage

hormones: chemical messengers. Hormones are secreted by a variety of endocrine glands in response to altered conditions in the body. Each hormone travels to one or more specific target tissues or organs, where it elicits a specific response to maintain homeostasis. The study of hormones and their actions is called *endocrinology*.

TABLE A-1 Summary of Major Hormones

Gland	Hormone	Target Cells	Action
Anterior pituitary	Adrenocorticotropin (ACTH)	Adrenal cortex	Stimulates secretion of glucocorticoids and androgens
Adrenal cortex	Aldosterone	Kidneys	Stimulates sodium reabsorption, thereby regulating acid-base balance, blood volume, and blood pressure
Posterior pituitary	Antidiuretic hormone (ADH); also called vasopressin	Arteries	Causes vasoconstriction
		Kidneys	Promotes water retention
Thyroid gland	Calcitonin	Bones	Lowers blood calcium by moving calcium from the bloodstream into the bones whenever blood calcium rises above normal
		Kidneys	Increases excretion of calcium and phosphorus
Duodenum	Cholecystokinin	Gallbladder	Releases bile into the intestine
		Pancreas	Releases pancreatic juices into the intestine
Hypothalamus	Corticotropin-releasing hormone (CRH)	Anterior pituitary	Controls release of adrenocorticotropin (ACTH)
Kidneys	Erythropoietin	Bone marrow	Stimulates red blood cell production
Ovaries	Estrogens	Female sexual tissues	Promotes growth, development, and health of all tissues involved in female sexuality
Anterior pituitary	Follicle-stimulating hormone (FSH)	Ovaries (female)	Stimulates follicular development and ovulation
		Testicles (male)	Stimulates sperm production
Stomach, duodenum	Gastrin	Stomach	Stimulates gastric acid secretion; slows motility
Hypothalamus	Growth hormone releasing hormone (GHRH) and growth hormone inhibiting hormone (GHIH or somatostatin)	Anterior pituitary	Controls release of growth hormone (GH)
Pancreas (alpha cells)	Glucagon	Liver	Promotes the breakdown of glycogen to glucose
		Most cells	Increases use of fat and amino acids for energy
Adrenal cortex	Glucocorticoids	Most cells	Protects against stress; raises blood glucose
Hypothalamus	Gonadotropin-releasing hormone (GnRH)	Anterior pituitary	Controls release of follicle-stimulating hormone (FSH) and luteinizing hormone (LH)
Anterior pituitary	Growth hormone (GH); also called somatotropin	All tissues	Stimulates growth; regulates metabolism
Pancreas (beta cells)	Insulin	Most cells	Stimulates nutrient uptake into cells
Anterior pituitary	Luteinizing hormone (LH)	Ovaries (female)	Stimulates follicular development and ovulation
		Testicles (male)	Stimulates testosterone production
Adrenal medulla	Norepinephrine and epinephrine; formerly called noradrenaline and adrenaline, respectively	Many cells	Facilitates the body's readiness for fight or flight: maintains blood pressure, increases cardiac output, constricts blood vessels, keeps airways open, raises blood glucose levels
Posterior pituitary	Oxytocin	Uterus (female in late pregnancy)	Induces muscle contractions during childbirth
		Mammary glands (female in lactation)	Causes milk ejection during lactation
Parathyroid gland	Parathyroid hormone (PTH); also called parathormone	Bones	Releases stored calcium into the blood
		Kidneys	Slows calcium excretion
		Intestines	Increases calcium absorption
Corpus luteum, placenta	Progesterone	Uterus	Facilitates implantation at the start of pregnancy
		Mammary glands	Stimulates mammary gland development for lactation
Anterior pituitary	Prolactin	Mammary glands (female in lactation)	Stimulates milk production
Hypothalamus	Prolactin-inhibiting hormone (PIH)	Anterior pituitary	Controls release of prolactin
Duodenum	Secretin	Pancreas	Stimulates bicarbonate secretion into the intestine; slows stomach motility
Testicles	Testosterone	Male sexual tissues	Promotes growth, development, and health of all tissues involved in male sexuality
Anterior pituitary	Thyroid-stimulating hormone (TSH)	Thyroid gland	Stimulates synthesis and release of thyroid hormones (thyroxine and triiodothyronine)
Thyroid gland	Thyroxine	Many cells	Regulates metabolic rate, growth, and heat production
Hypothalamus	TSH-releasing hormone (TRH)	Anterior pituitary	Controls release of thyroid-stimulating hormone (TSH)
Skin	Vitamin D	Intestines	Increases calcium absorption

APPENDIX A

Nerves

The nervous system has a central control system that can evaluate information about conditions within and outside the body, and an expansive communication system that receives information and sends instructions. The control system is the brain and spinal cord, called the **central nervous system;** and the communication system between the center and the parts is the **peripheral nervous system.** (Glossary A-2 defines these and other related terms.) The smooth functioning that results from the systems' adjustments to changing conditions is homeostasis.

The nervous system is best understood as two systems that use the same or similar pathways to receive and transmit their messages. The **somatic nervous system** controls the voluntary muscles; the **autonomic nervous system** controls the involuntary, internal muscles and organs.

When scientists were first studying the autonomic nervous system, they noticed that when something hurt one organ of the body, some of the other organs reacted as if in sympathy for the afflicted one. They, therefore, named the nerve network they were studying the **sympathetic nervous system.** The term is still used today to refer to the branch of the autonomic nervous system that responds to stressful conditions. The other branch that supports normal conditions is called the **parasympathetic nervous system.** (Think of the sympathetic branch as the emergency responder when homeostasis needs prompt restoring and the parasympathetic branch as the steady commander during normal times.) Both systems transmit their messages through the brain and spinal cord. Nerves of the two branches travel side by side along the same pathways to transmit their messages, but they oppose each other's actions (see Figure A-3).

An example will show how the sympathetic and parasympathetic nervous systems work to maintain homeostasis. When you go outside in cold weather, your skin's temperature receptors send "cold" messages to the spinal cord and brain. Your conscious mind may intervene at this point to tell you to zip your jacket, but let's say you have no jacket. Your sympathetic nervous system reacts to the external stressor, the cold. It signals your skin-surface capillaries to shut down so that your blood will circulate deeper in your tissues, where it will conserve heat. Your sympathetic nervous system also signals involuntary contractions of the small muscles just under the skin surface. The product of these muscle contractions is heat, and the visible result is goose bumps. If these measures do not raise your body temperature enough, then the sympathetic nerves signal your large muscle groups to shiver; the contractions of these large muscles produce still more heat. All of this activity helps maintain your homeostasis (with respect to temperature) under conditions of external extremes (cold) that would throw it off balance. The cold was a stressor; the body's response was resistance.

Now let's say you come in and sit by a fire and drink hot cocoa. You are warm and no longer need all that sympathetic activity. At this point, your parasympathetic nerves take over; they signal your skin-surface capillaries to dilate again, your goose bumps to subside, and your muscles to relax. Your body is back to normal. This is recovery.

GLOSSARY A-2 NERVOUS SYSTEM TERMS

autonomic nervous system: the division of the nervous system that controls the body's automatic responses. Its two branches are the *sympathetic* branch, which helps the body respond to stressors from the outside environment, and the *parasympathetic* branch, which regulates normal body activities between stressful times.

central nervous system: the central part of the nervous system; the brain and spinal cord.

parasympathetic nervous system: the part of the autonomic nervous system that dominates during nonstressful conditions and includes such effects as normal heart rate, pupil dilation, and peristalsis.

peripheral (puh-RIFF-er-ul) **nervous system:** the peripheral (outermost) part of the nervous system; the vast complex of wiring that extends from the central nervous system to the body's outermost areas. It contains both *somatic* and *autonomic* components.

somatic (so-MAT-ick) **nervous system:** the division of the nervous system that controls the voluntary muscles, as distinguished from the autonomic nervous system, which controls involuntary functions.

sympathetic nervous system: the part of the autonomic nervous system that dominates during stressful conditions and includes such effects as increased heart rate, dilated pupils, slowed peristalsis, and secretion of epinephrine and norepinephrine.

> **FIGURE A-3 The Organization of the Nervous System**

The brain and spinal cord evaluate information about conditions within and outside the body, and the peripheral nerves receive information and send instructions.

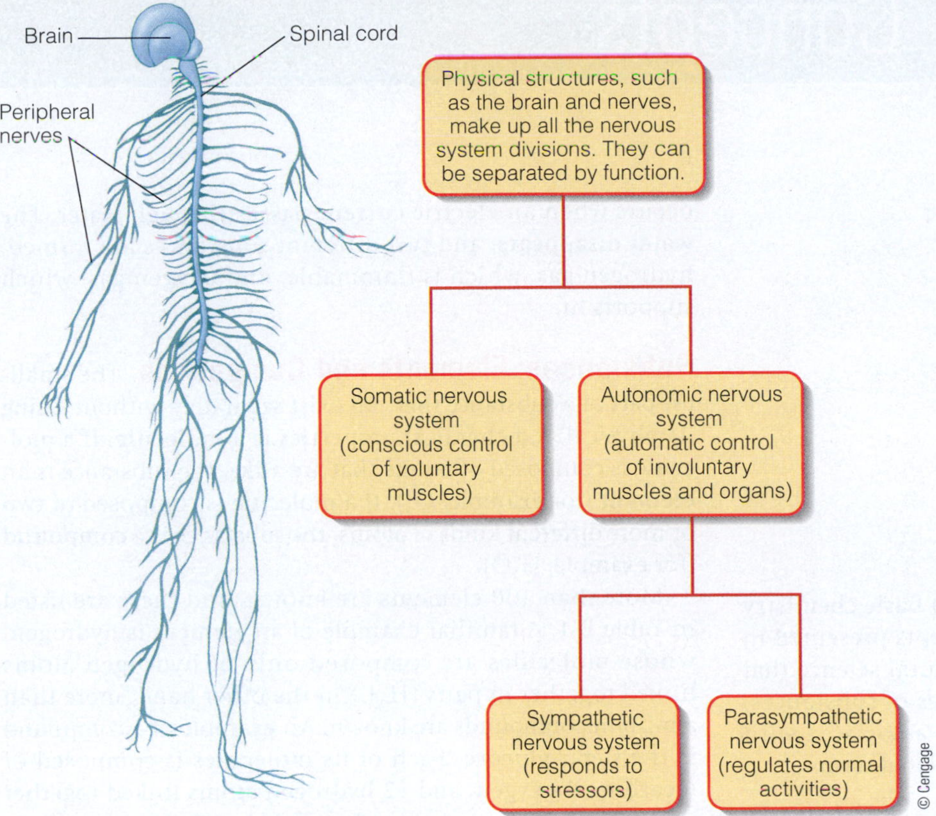

Brain
Spinal cord
Peripheral nerves
Physical structures, such as the brain and nerves, make up all the nervous system divisions. They can be separated by function.
Somatic nervous system (conscious control of voluntary muscles)
Autonomic nervous system (automatic control of involuntary muscles and organs)
Sympathetic nervous system (responds to stressors)
Parasympathetic nervous system (regulates normal activities)
© Cengage

Putting It Together

The hormonal and nervous systems coordinate body functions by transmitting and receiving messages. The point-to-point messages of the nervous system travel through the spinal cord and brain, whereas the messages of the hormonal system are sent through the bloodstream, and any organ with the appropriate receptors can pick them up. Nerve impulses travel faster than hormonal messages do—although both are remarkably swift. Whereas your brain's command to wiggle your toes reaches the toes within a fraction of a second and stops as quickly, a gland's message to alter a body condition may take several seconds or minutes to get started and may fade away equally slowly.

Together, the two systems possess every characteristic a superb communication network needs: varied speeds of transmission, along with private communication lines or public broadcasting systems, depending on the needs of the moment. The hormonal system, together with the nervous system, integrates the whole body's functioning so that all parts act smoothly together.

Appendix B Basic Chemistry Concepts

APPENDIX B

CONTENTS

This appendix provides the background in basic chemistry needed to understand the nutrition concepts presented in this book. Chemistry is the branch of natural science that deals with the composition and properties of substances, how substances interact, and the **energy** associated with these interactions. Glossary B-1 defines related terms.

The Properties of Atoms

Every substance has physical and chemical properties that distinguish it from all other substances and thus give it a unique identity. The physical properties include such characteristics as color, taste, texture, and odor, as well as the temperatures at which a substance changes its state (from a solid to a liquid or from a liquid to a gas) and the weight of a unit volume (its density). The chemical properties of a substance have to do with how it reacts with other substances or responds to a change in its environment.

A physical change does not change a substance's chemical composition. The three physical states—ice, water, and steam—all consist of two hydrogen atoms and one oxygen atom bound together. In contrast, a chemical change occurs when an electric current passes through water. The water disappears, and two different substances are formed: hydrogen gas, which is flammable, and oxygen gas, which supports life.

Substances: Elements and Compounds

The smallest part of a substance that can exist separately without losing its physical and chemical properties is a **molecule**. If a molecule is composed of **atoms** that are alike, the substance is an **element** (for example, O_2). If a molecule is composed of two or more different kinds of atoms, the substance is a **compound** (for example, H_2O).

More than 100 elements are known, and these are listed in Table B-1. A familiar example of an element is hydrogen, whose molecules are composed only of hydrogen atoms linked together in pairs (H_2). On the other hand, more than a million compounds are known. An example of a compound is the sugar glucose. Each of its molecules is composed of 6 carbon, 6 oxygen, and 12 hydrogen atoms linked together in a specific arrangement (as described in Chapter 4).

The Nature of Atoms

Atoms themselves are made of smaller particles. Within an atom's nucleus are protons (positively charged particles), and surrounding the nucleus are an equal number of electrons (negatively charged particles). The number of protons in the nucleus of an atom determines the atomic number. The positive charge on a proton is equal to the negative charge on an electron, so the charges cancel each other out and leave the atom neutral to its surroundings.

The nucleus may also include neutrons, subatomic particles that have no charge. Protons and neutrons are of equal mass, and together they give an atom its atomic mass. Electrons bond atoms together to make molecules, and they are involved in chemical reactions.

Each element has a characteristic number of protons in its atom's nucleus. For example, the hydrogen atom (the simplest

GLOSSARY B-1
CHEMISTRY TERMS

anions (AN-eye-uns): negatively changed ions.

atoms: the smallest components of an element that have all of the properties of the element.

cations (CAT-eye-uns): positively changed ions.

compound: a substance composed of two or more different atoms—for example, water (H_2O).

covalent bonds: strong chemical bonds formed between atoms by sharing electrons.

element: a substance composed of atoms that are alike—for example, iron (Fe).

energy: the capacity to do work. The energy in food is chemical energy. The body can convert this chemical energy to mechanical, electrical, or heat energy.

ions (EYE-uns): atoms or molecules that have gained or lost one or more electrons and therefore have electrical charges. Examples include the positively charged sodium ion (Na^+) and the negatively charged chloride ion (Cl^-).

molecule: two or more atoms of the same or different elements joined by chemical bonds. Examples are molecules of the element oxygen, composed of two oxygen atoms (O_2), and molecules of the compound water, composed of two hydrogen atoms and one oxygen atom (H_2O).

polar: characteristic of a neutral molecule, such as water, that has opposite charges spatially separated within the molecule.

TABLE B-1 The Elements

Number of Protons (Atomic Number)	Element	Number of Electrons in Outer Shell
1	Hydrogen (H)	1
2	Helium (He)	2
3	Lithium (Li)	1
4	Beryllium (Be)	2
5	Boron (B)	3
6	Carbon (C)	4
7	Nitrogen (N)	5
8	Oxygen (O)	6
9	Fluorine (F)	7
10	Neon (Ne)	8
11	Sodium (Na)	1
12	Magnesium (Mg)	2
13	Aluminum (Al)	3
14	Silicon (Si)	4
15	Phosphorus (P)	5
16	Sulfur (S)	6
17	Chlorine (Cl)	7
18	Argon (Ar)	8
19	Potassium (K)	1
20	Calcium (Ca)	2
21	Scandium (Sc)	2
22	Titanium (Ti)	2
23	Vanadium (V)	2
24	Chromium (Cr)	1
25	Manganese (Mn)	2
26	Iron (Fe)	2
27	Cobalt (Co)	2
28	Nickel (Ni)	2
29	Copper (Cu)	1
30	Zinc (Zn)	2
31	Gallium (Ga)	3
32	Germanium (Ge)	4
33	Arsenic (As)	5
34	Selenium (Se)	6
35	Bromine (Br)	7
36	Krypton (Kr)	8
37	Rubidium (Rb)	1
38	Strontium (Sr)	2
39	Yttrium (Y)	2
40	Zirconium (Zr)	2
41	Niobium (Nb)	1
42	Molybdenum (Mo)	1
43	Technetium (Tc)	1
44	Ruthenium (Ru)	1
45	Rhodium (Rh)	1
46	Palladium (Pd)	—
47	Silver (Ag)	1
48	Cadmium (Cd)	2
49	Indium (In)	3
50	Tin (Sn)	4
51	Antimony (Sb)	5
52	Tellurium (Te)	6
53	Iodine (I)	7
54	Xenon (Xe)	8
55	Cesium (Cs)	1
56	Barium (Ba)	2
57	Lanthanum (La)	2
58	Cerium (Ce)	2
59	Praseodymium (Pr)	2
60	Neodymium (Nd)	2
61	Promethium (Pm)	2
62	Samarium (Sm)	2
63	Europium (Eu)	2
64	Gadolinium (Gd)	2
65	Terbium (Tb)	2
66	Dysprosium (Dy)	2
67	Holmium (Ho)	2
68	Erbium (Er)	2
69	Thulium (Tm)	2
70	Ytterbium (Yb)	2
71	Lutetium (Lu)	2
72	Hafnium (Hf)	2
73	Tantalum (Ta)	2
74	Tungsten (W)	2
75	Rhenium (Re)	2
76	Osmium (Os)	2
77	Iridium (Ir)	2
78	Platinum (Pt)	1
79	Gold (Au)	1
80	Mercury (Hg)	2
81	Thallium (Tl)	3
82	Lead (Pb)	4
83	Bismuth (Bi)	5
84	Polonium (Po)	6
85	Astatine (At)	7
86	Radon (Rn)	8
87	Francium (Fr)	1
88	Radium (Ra)	2
89	Actinium (Ac)	2
90	Thorium (Th)	2
91	Protactinium (Pa)	2
92	Uranium (U)	2
93	Neptunium (Np)	2
94	Plutonium (Pu)	2
95	Americium (Am)	2
96	Curium (Cm)	2
97	Berkelium (Bk)	2
98	Californium (Cf)	2
99	Einsteinium (Es)	2
100	Fermium (Fm)	2
101	Mendelevium (Md)	2
102	Nobelium (No)	2
103	Lawrencium (Lr)	2
104	Rutherfordium (Rf)	2
105	Dubnium (Db)	2
106	Seaborgium (Sg)	2
107	Bohrium (Bh)	2
108	Hassium (Hs)	2
109	Meitnerium (Mt)	2
110	Darmstadtium (Ds)	2

Key
- Elements found in energy-yielding nutrients, vitamins, and water
- Major minerals
- Trace minerals

of all) possesses a single proton, with a single electron associated with it:

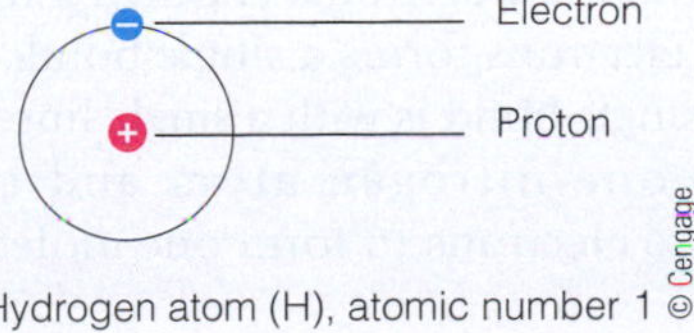
Electron
Proton
© Cengage

Hydrogen atom (H), atomic number 1

Just as hydrogen always has one proton, helium always has two, lithium three, and so on. The atomic number of each element is the number of protons in the nucleus of that atom, and this never changes in a chemical reaction; it gives the atom its identity. The atomic numbers for the known elements are listed in Table B-1.

In addition to hydrogen, the atoms most common in living things are carbon (C), nitrogen (N), and oxygen (O), whose atomic numbers are 6, 7, and 8, respectively. Their structures are more complicated than that of hydrogen, but each of them possesses the same number of electrons as there are protons in the nucleus. These electrons are found in orbits, or shells (shown below).

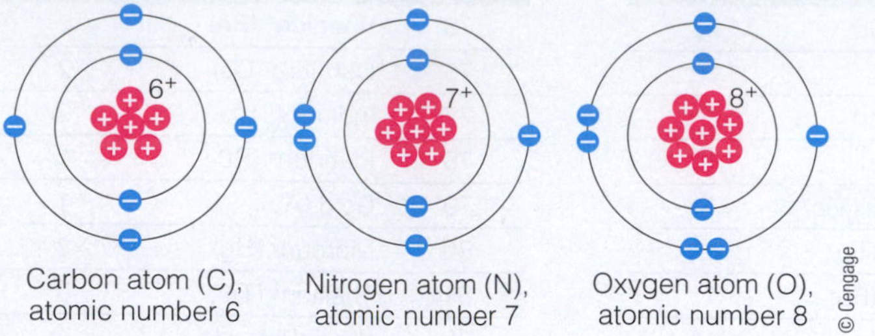
6+
7+
8+
Carbon atom (C), atomic number 6
Nitrogen atom (N), atomic number 7
Oxygen atom (O), atomic number 8
© Cengage

In these and all diagrams of atoms that follow, only the protons and electrons are shown. The neutrons, which contribute only to atomic weight, not to charge, are omitted.

The most important structural feature of an atom for determining its chemical behavior is the number of electrons in its outermost shell. The first, or innermost, shell is full when it is occupied by two electrons; so an atom with two or more electrons has a filled first shell. When the first shell is full, electrons begin to fill the second shell.

The second shell is completely full when it has eight electrons. A substance that has a full outer shell tends not to enter into chemical reactions. Atomic number 10, neon, is a chemically inert substance because its outer shell is complete. Fluorine, atomic number 9, has a great tendency to attract an electron from other substances to complete its outer shell, and thus it is highly reactive. Carbon has a half-full outer shell, which helps explain its great versatility; it can combine with many other elements in a variety of ways to form a large number of compounds.

Atoms seek to reach a state of maximum stability or of lowest energy in the same way that a ball will roll down a hill until it reaches the lowest place. An atom achieves a state of maximum stability:

- By gaining or losing electrons to either fill or empty its outer shell.
- By sharing its electrons with other atoms and thereby completing its outer shell.

The number of electrons determines how the atom will chemically react with other atoms.

hydrogen effectively has the required 2 electrons in its first (outer) shell, and carbon has 8 electrons in its second (outer) shell; and the molecule is electrically neutral, with a total of 10 protons and 10 electrons.

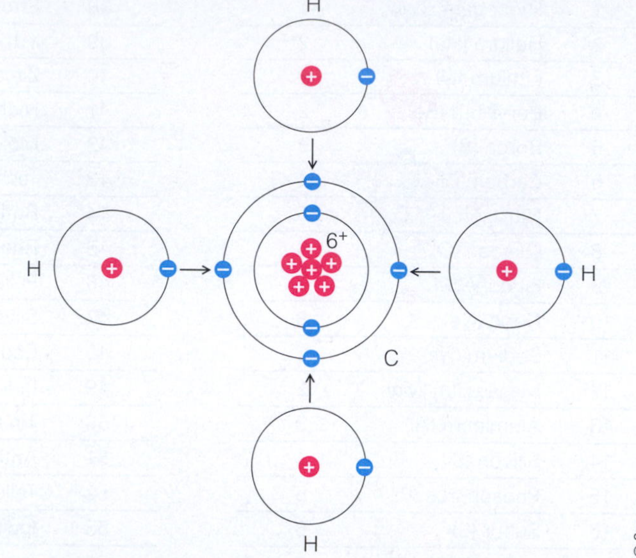
H
H
6+
H
C
H
© Cengage

When a carbon atom shares electrons with four hydrogen atoms, a methane molecule is made.

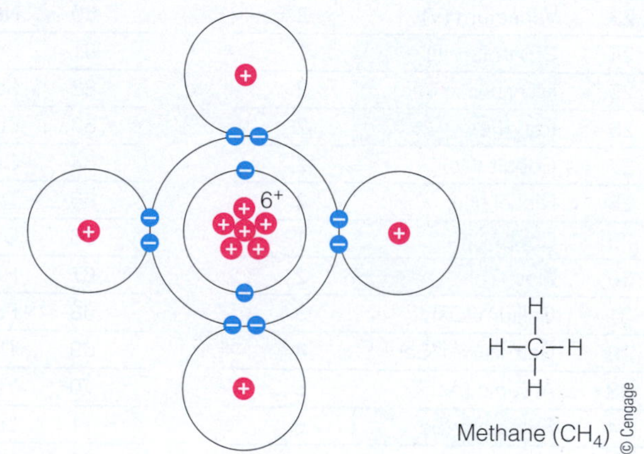
6+
H
H—C—H
H
Methane (CH_4)
© Cengage

The chemical formula for methane is CH_4. Note that by sharing electrons, every atom achieves a filled outer shell.

Chemical Bonding

Atoms often complete their outer shells by sharing electrons with other atoms. In order to complete its outer shell, a carbon atom requires four electrons. A hydrogen atom requires one. Thus, when a carbon atom shares electrons with four hydrogen atoms, each completes its outer shell (as shown in the next drawing). Electron sharing binds the atoms together and satisfies the conditions of maximum stability for the molecule. The outer shell of each atom is complete because

Bonds that involve the sharing of electrons, like the bonds in methane between the one carbon and the four hydrogens, are the most stable kind of association that atoms can form with one another. These bonds are called **covalent bonds,** and the resulting combination of atoms is called a molecule. A single pair of shared electrons forms a single bond. A simplified way to represent a single bond is with a single line.

Similarly, one nitrogen atom and three hydrogen atoms can share electrons to form one molecule of ammonia (NH_3):

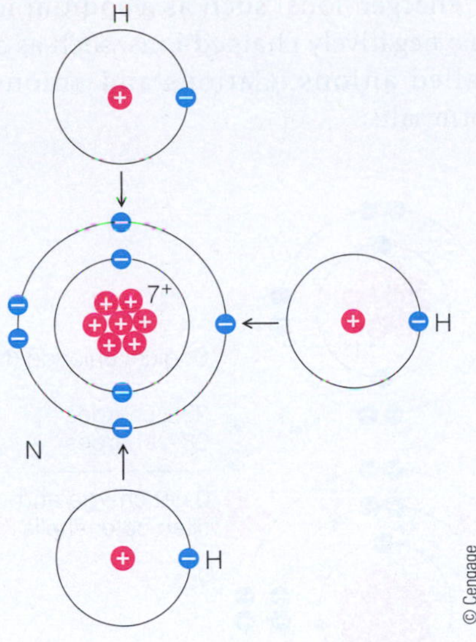
H
7+
H
N
H
© Cengage

When a nitrogen atom shares electrons with three hydrogen atoms, an ammonia molecule is made.

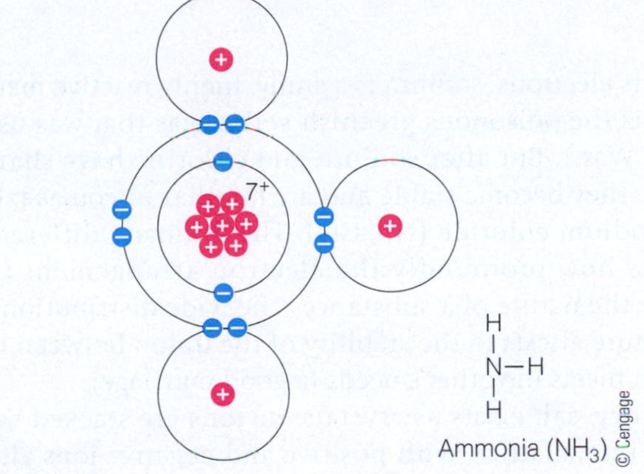
7+
H
N—H
H
Ammonia (NH_3)
© Cengage

The chemical formula for ammonia is NH_3. Count the electrons in each atom's outer shell to confirm that it is filled.

One oxygen atom may be bonded to two hydrogen atoms to form one molecule of water (H_2O):

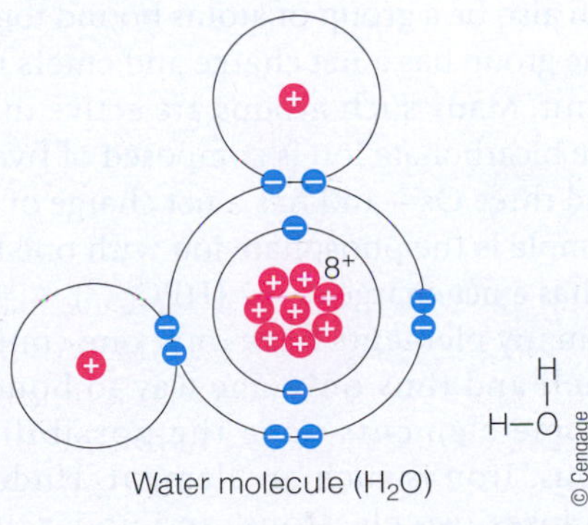
8+
H
H—O
Water molecule (H_2O)
© Cengage

When two oxygen atoms form a molecule of oxygen, they must share two pairs of electrons. This double bond may be represented as two lines:

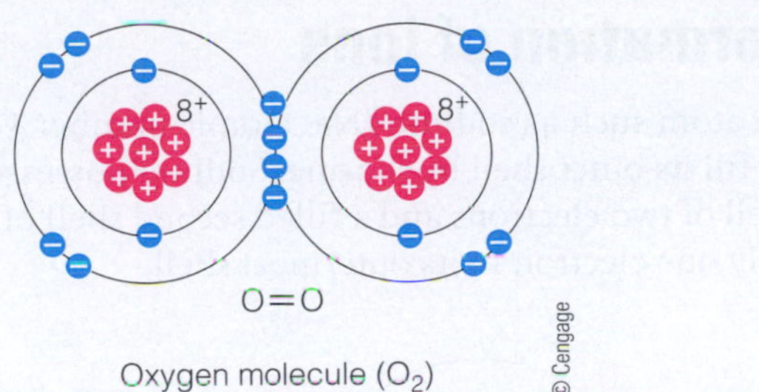
8+
8+
O=O
Oxygen molecule (O_2)
© Cengage

Small atoms form the tightest, most stable bonds. H, O, N, and C are the smallest atoms capable of forming one, two, three, and four electron-pair bonds, respectively. This is the basis for the statement in Chapter 4 that in drawings of compounds containing these atoms, hydrogen must always have one, oxygen two, nitrogen three, and carbon four bonds radiating to other atoms:

H— —O— —N— —C—

© Cengage

The stability of the associations between these small atoms (hydrogen, carbon, nitrogen, and oxygen) and the versatility with which they can combine make them very common in living things. Interestingly all cells—whether they come from animals, plants, or bacteria—contain the same elements in very nearly the same proportions. The elements commonly found in living things are shown in Table B-2.

TABLE B-2 Elemental Composition of the Human Body

Element	Chemical Symbol	By Weight (%)
Oxygen	O	65.0
Carbon	C	18.0
Hydrogen	H	10.0
Nitrogen	N	3.0
Calcium	Ca	1.5
Phosphorus	P	1.0
Potassium	K	0.4
Sulfur	S	0.3
Sodium	Na	0.2
Chloride	Cl	0.1
Magnesium	Mg	0.1
Total		99.6[a]

[a]The remaining 0.4 percent by weight is contributed by the trace elements: chromium (Cr), copper (Cu), zinc (Zn), selenium (Se), molybdenum (Mo), fluorine (F), iodine (I), manganese (Mn), and iron (Fe). Cells may also contain variable traces of some of the following: boron (B), cobalt (Co), Lithium (Li), strontium (Sr), aluminum (Al), silicon (Si), Lead (Pb), vanadium (V), arsenic (As), bromine (Br), and others.

© Cengage

Formation of Ions

An atom such as sodium (Na, atomic number 11) cannot easily fill its outer shell by sharing. Sodium possesses a filled first shell of two electrons and a filled second shell of eight; there is only one electron in its outermost shell:

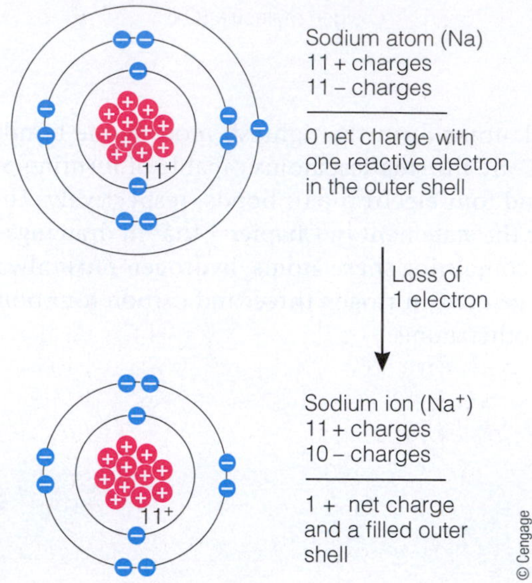

Sodium atom (Na)
11 + charges
11 – charges
0 net charge with one reactive electron in the outer shell
11+
Loss of 1 electron
Sodium ion (Na+)
11 + charges
10 – charges
1 + net charge and a filled outer shell
11+
© Cengage

If sodium loses this electron, it satisfies one condition for stability: a filled outer shell (now its second shell counts as the outer shell). However, it is not electrically neutral. It has 11 protons (positive) and only 10 electrons (negative). It therefore has a net positive charge. An atom or molecule that has lost or gained one or more electrons and so is electrically charged is called an **ion**.

An atom such as chlorine (Cl, atomic number 17), with seven electrons in its outermost shell, can share electrons to fill its outer shell, or it can gain one electron to complete its outer shell and thus give it a negative charge:

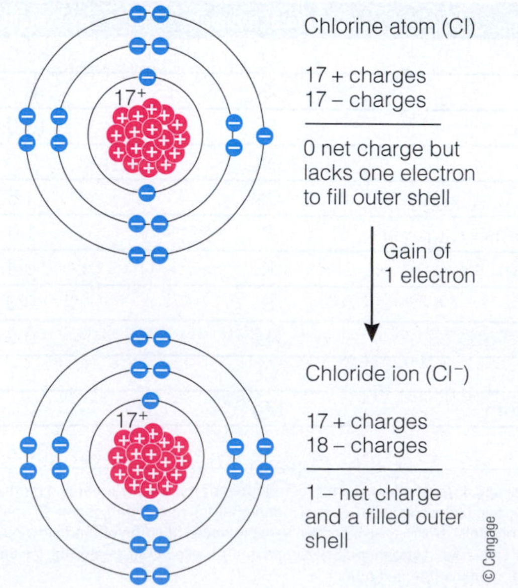

Chlorine atom (Cl)
17 + charges
17 – charges
0 net charge but lacks one electron to fill outer shell
17+
Gain of 1 electron
Chloride ion (Cl−)
17 + charges
18 – charges
1 – net charge and a filled outer shell
17+
© Cengage

Positively charged ions, such as a sodium ion (Na^+), are called **cations**; negatively charged ions, such as a chloride ion (Cl^-), are called **anions**. Cations and anions attract one another to form salts:

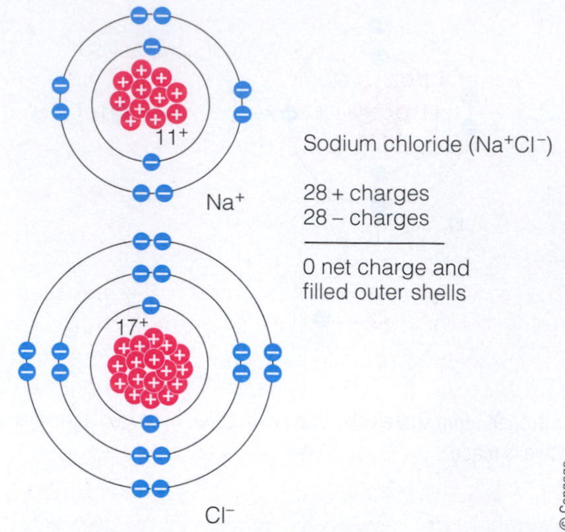

11+
Na+
Sodium chloride (Na+Cl−)
28 + charges
28 – charges
0 net charge and filled outer shells
17+
Cl−
© Cengage

With all its electrons, sodium is a shiny, highly reactive metal; chlorine is the poisonous greenish yellow gas that was used in World War I. But after sodium and chlorine have shared electrons, they become stable and are familiar to you as table salt, or sodium chloride (Na^+Cl^-). The dramatic difference illustrates how profoundly the electron arrangement can influence the nature of a substance. The wide distribution of salt in nature attests to the stability of the union between the ions. Each meets the other's needs (a good marriage).

When dry, salt exists as crystals; its ions are stacked very regularly into a lattice, with positive and negative ions alternating in a three-dimensional checkerboard structure. In water, however, the salt quickly dissolves, and its ions separate from one another, forming an electrolyte solution in which they move about freely. Covalently bonded molecules rarely dissociate like this in a water solution. The most common exception is when they behave like acids and release H^+ ions, as discussed in the next section.

An ion can also be a group of atoms bound together in such a way that the group has a net charge and enters into reactions as a single unit. Many such groups are active in the fluids of the body. The bicarbonate ion is composed of five atoms—one H, one C, and three Os—and has a net charge of −1 (HCO_3^-). Another example is the phosphate ion with one H, one P, and four O, that has a net charge of −2 (HPO_4^{-2}).

Whereas many elements have only one configuration in the outer shell and thus only one way to bond with other elements, some elements have the possibility of varied configurations. Iron is such an element. Under some conditions iron loses two electrons, and under other circumstances it loses three. If iron loses two electrons, it then has a net charge of +2 and is called ferrous iron (Fe^{++}). If it loses three electrons, it becomes the +3 ion called ferric iron (Fe^{+++}).

Ferrous iron (Fe^{++}) (lost 2 outer-shell electrons)	Ferric iron (Fe^{+++}) (lost 3 outer-shell electrons)
26 + charges	26 + charges
24 − charges	23 − charges
2 + net charge	3 + net charge

Remember that a positive charge on an ion means that negative charges—electrons—have been lost and not that positive charges have been added to the nucleus.

Water, Acids, and Bases

Water The water molecule is electrically neutral, having equal numbers of protons and electrons. When a hydrogen atom shares its electron with oxygen, however, that electron will spend most of its time closer to the positively charged oxygen nucleus. This leaves the positive proton (nucleus of the hydrogen atom) exposed on the outer part of the water molecule. We know, too, that the two hydrogens both bond toward the same side of the oxygen. These two facts explain why water molecules are **polar**: they have regions that are more positively and more negatively charged.

Polar molecules like water are attracted to one another by the forces between the positive areas of one and the negative areas of another. These attractive forces, sometimes known as polar bonds or hydrogen bonds, occur among many molecules and also within different parts of the same molecule. Although very weak in comparison with covalent bonds, polar bonds may occur in such abundance that they become exceedingly important in determining the structure of large molecules such as proteins and DNA.

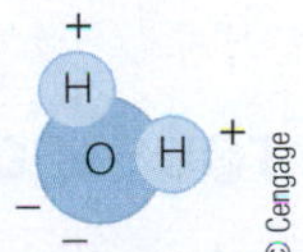
H
O
H
+
+
−
−

This diagram of a polar water molecule shows the negative area near the O and the positive area near the H atoms.

Water molecules have a slight tendency to ionize, separating into positive (H^+) and negative (OH^-) ions. In pure water, a small but constant number of these ions is present, and the number of positive ions exactly equals the number of negative ions.

Acids An acid is a substance that releases H^+ ions (protons) in a water solution. Hydrochloric acid (HCl^-) is such a substance because it dissociates in a water solution into H^+ and Cl^- ions. Acetic acid is also an acid because it dissociates in water to acetate ions and free H^+:

Acetic acid dissociates into an acetate ion and a hydrogen ion.

The more H^+ ions released, the stronger the acid. Chemists define degrees of acidity by means of the pH scale, which runs from 0 to 14. The pH expresses the concentration of H^+ ions: a pH of 1 is extremely acidic, 7 is neutral, and 13 is very basic. There is a tenfold difference in the concentration of H^+ ions between points on this scale. A solution with pH 3, for example, has 10 times as many H^+ ions as a solution with pH 4. Figure 3-6 (p. 75) presented the pH of common substances.

Bases A base is a substance that can combine with H^+ ions, thus reducing the acidity of a solution. The compound ammonia is such a substance. The ammonia molecule has two electrons that are not shared with any other atom; a hydrogen ion (H^+) is a proton without an outer shell of electrons. The proton readily combines with the ammonia molecule to form an ion; thus a free H^+ is withdrawn from the solution and no longer contributes to its acidity. Many nitrogen-containing compounds are important bases in living systems. Acids and bases neutralize each other to produce substances that are neither acid nor base.

Chemical Reactions

A chemical reaction results in the breakdown or formation of substances. Almost all such reactions involve a change in the bonding of atoms. Old bonds are broken, and new ones are formed. The nuclei of atoms are never involved in chemical reactions—only the outer-shell electrons participate. At the end of a chemical reaction, the number of atoms of each type is always the same as at the beginning. For example, two hydrogen molecules ($2H_2$) can react with one oxygen molecule (O_2) to form two water molecules ($2H_2O$). In this reaction, two substances (hydrogen and oxygen) disappear, and a new one (water) is formed, but at the end of the reaction there are still four H atoms and two O atoms, just as there were at the beginning. Because the atoms are now linked in a different way, their characteristics and properties have changed.

In many instances chemical reactions involve the exchange of electrons or protons between molecules. In such reactions the molecule that gains one or more electrons (or loses one or more protons) is said to be reduced; the molecule that loses electrons (or gains protons) is oxidized. A hydrogen ion is equivalent to a proton.

Oxidation and reduction reactions take place simultaneously because an electron or proton that is lost by one molecule is accepted by another. The addition of an atom of oxygen is also oxidation because oxygen (with six electrons in the outer shell) accepts two electrons in becoming bonded. Oxidation occurs, then, with the loss of electrons, the gain of protons, or the addition of oxygen (with six electrons); reduction occurs with the opposite—a gain of electrons, a loss of protons, or a loss of oxygen. The addition of hydrogen atoms to oxygen to form water can thus be described as the reduction of oxygen *or* the oxidation of hydrogen.

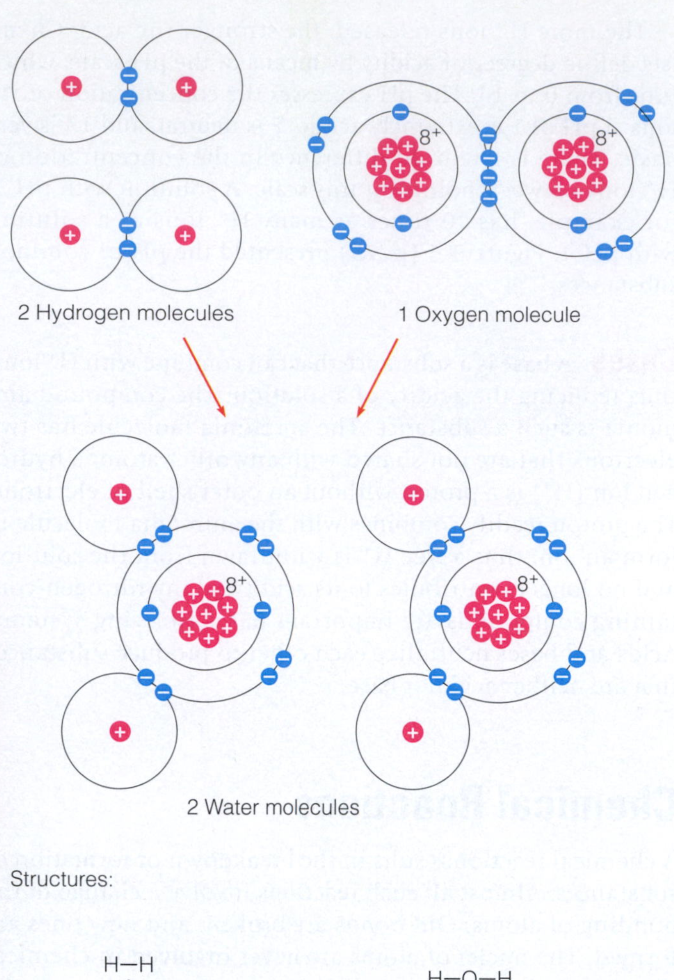
2 Hydrogen molecules
1 Oxygen molecule
8+
8+
8+
8+
2 Water molecules

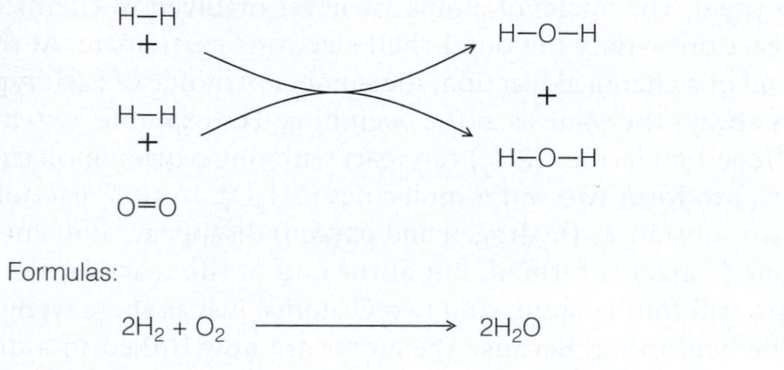
Structures:
H—H
+
H—H
+
O=O
H—O—H
+
H—O—H
Formulas:
2H2 + O2
2H2O
© Cengage

Hydrogen and oxygen react to form water.

Reactions in which the end products contain more energy than the reacting compounds started with are called endergonic, or "uphill," reactions and do not occur until an energy source is provided. An example of such an energy source is the sunlight used in photosynthesis reactions that combine carbon dioxide and water (low-energy compounds) to form glucose (a higher-energy compound). Conversely, the oxidation of glucose to carbon dioxide and water is an exergonic, or "downhill," reaction because the end products have less energy than the starting product. Oftentimes, but not always, reduction reactions are endergonic, resulting in an increase in the energy of the end products. Oxidation reactions often, but not always, are exergonic.

Chemical reactions tend to occur spontaneously if the end products are in a lower energy state and therefore are more stable than the reacting compounds. These reactions often give off energy in the form of heat as they occur. The generation of heat by wood burning in a fireplace and the maintenance of warmth in the human body both depend on energy-yielding chemical reactions. These downhill reactions occur easily although they may require some activation energy to get them started, just as a ball requires a push to start rolling.

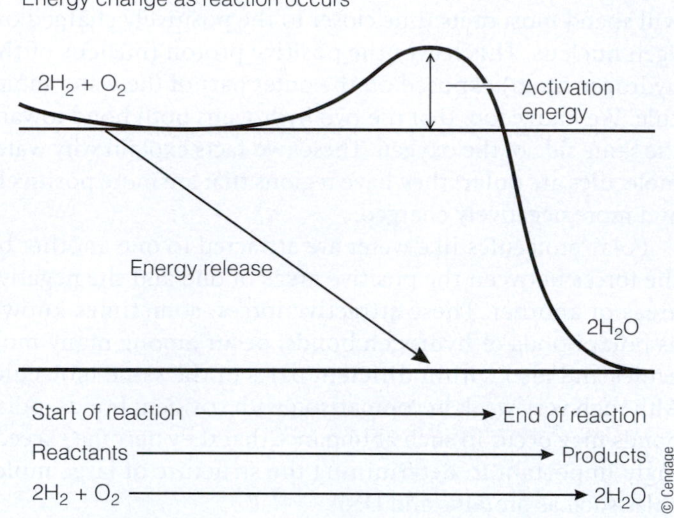
Energy change as reaction occurs
2H2 + O2
Activation
energy
Energy release
2H2O
Start of reaction
End of reaction
Reactants
Products
2H2 + O2
2H2O
© Cengage

Formation of Free Radicals

Normally, when a chemical reaction takes place, bonds break and re-form to create new, stable compounds. Occasionally, bonds break in such a way as to create a free radical—a molecule with one or more unpaired electrons. When they do, free radicals are formed. Free radicals are highly unstable and quickly react with other compounds, forming more free radicals in a chain reaction. A cascade may ensue in which many highly reactive radicals are generated, resulting in damage that contributes to the development of many chronic diseases (see Highlight 11, p. 353, for more details). Free radicals are of special interest in nutrition because the antioxidant properties of vitamins C and E as well as those of beta-carotene and the mineral selenium protect against the destructive effects of these free radicals.

Appendix C Biochemical Structures and Pathways

This appendix describes the biochemical structures and pathways most important to the study of nutrition. It begins by presenting diagrams of nutrients commonly found in the human diet. Following the diagrams of nutrients are sections on the major metabolic pathways mentioned in Chapter 7—glycolysis, fatty acid oxidation, amino acid degradation, the TCA cycle, and the electron transport chain—and a description of how alcohol interferes with these pathways. Discussions of the urea cycle and the formation of ketone bodies complete the appendix.

CONTENTS

Carbohydrates

Monosaccharides

Glucose (alpha form). The ring would be at right angles to the plane of the paper. The bonds directed upward are above the plane; those directed downward are below the plane. This molecule is considered an alpha form because the OH on carbon 1 points downward.

Glucose (beta form). The OH on carbon 1 points upward.
Fructose, galactose: see Chapter 4.

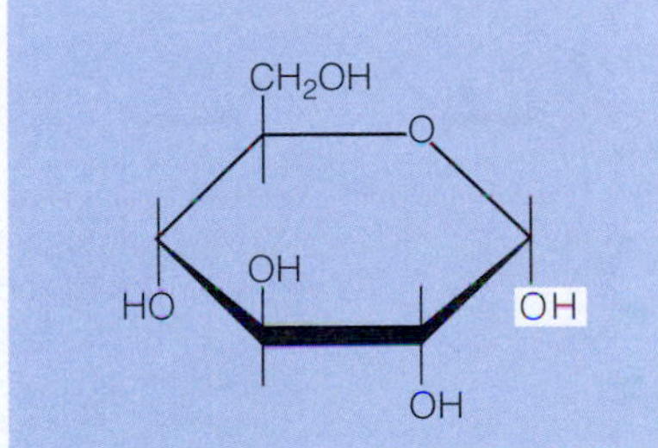

CH_2OH
O
HO
OH
OH
OH

Glucose (alpha form) shorthand notation. This notation, in which the carbons in the ring and single hydrogens have been eliminated, will be used throughout this appendix.

Disaccharides

Maltose.

Lactose (alpha form).

Sucrose.

Polysaccharides: Starches

As described in Chapter 4, starch, glycogen, and cellulose are all long chains of glucose molecules covalently linked together. (Appendix B discussed covalent bonding.)

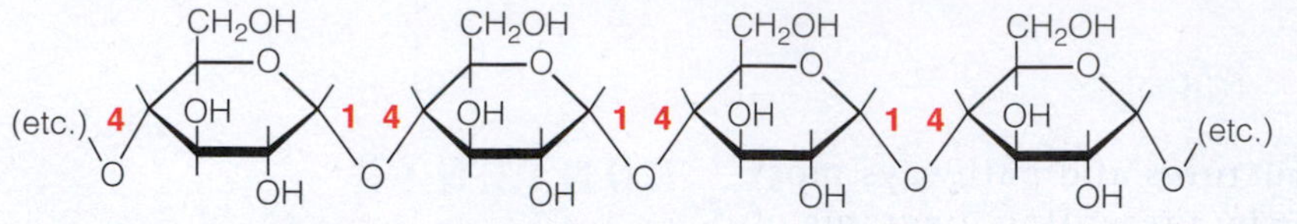

Amylose (unbranched starch)

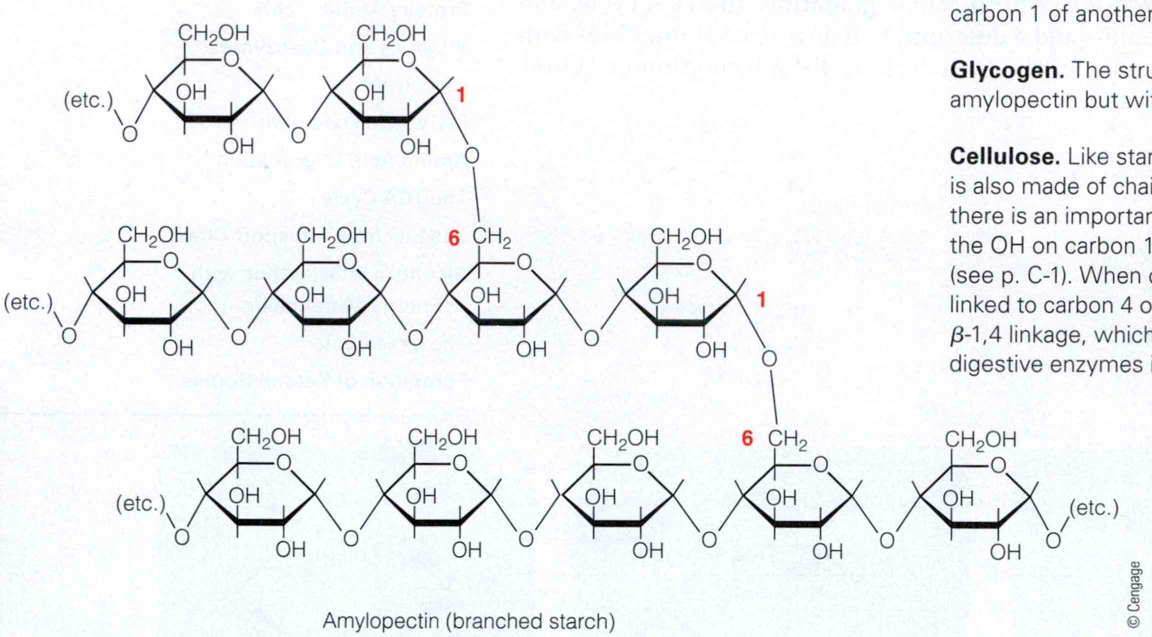

Amylopectin (branched starch)

Starch. Two kinds of covalent bonds link the glucose molecules in starch, giving rise to two kinds of chains. Amylose is composed of straight chains, with carbon 1 of one glucose linked to carbon 4 of the next (α-1,4 linkage). Amylopectin is made up of straight chains like amylose, but has occasional branches where the carbon 6 of a glucose is also linked to the carbon 1 of another glucose (α-1,6 linkage).

Glycogen. The structure of glycogen is like amylopectin but with many more branches.

Cellulose. Like starch and glycogen, cellulose is also made of chains of glucose units, but there is an important difference: in cellulose, the OH on carbon 1 is in the beta position (see p. C-1). When carbon 1 of one glucose is linked to carbon 4 of the next, it forms a β-1,4 linkage, which cannot be broken by digestive enzymes in the human GI tract.

Polysaccharides: Fibers

Fibers, such as hemicelluloses, consist of long chains of various monosaccharides.

The following structures illustrate the monosaccharides common in the backbone chain of hemicelluloses.*

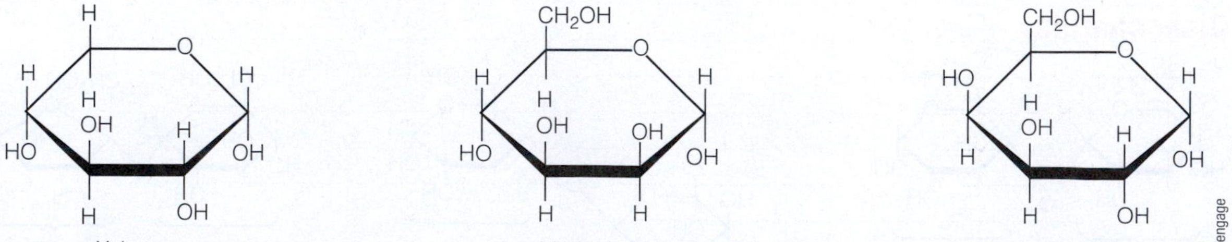

Xylose

Mannose

Galactose

*These structures are shown in the alpha form with the H on the carbon pointing upward and the OH pointing downward, but they may also appear in the beta form with the H pointing downward and the OH upward.

Monosaccharides common in the side chains of hemicelluloses:

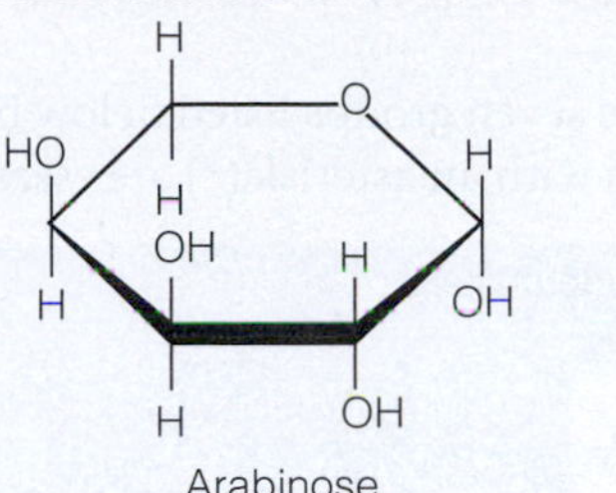
H
HO
O
H
H
OH
H
H
OH
H
OH
Arabinose

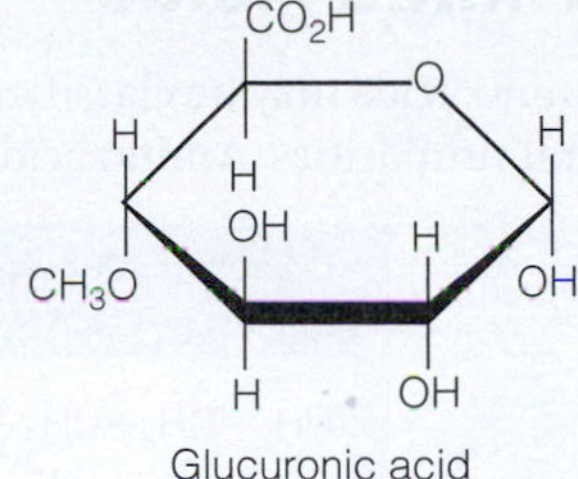
CO_2H
O
H
H
H
OH
H
CH_3O
OH
H
OH
Glucuronic acid

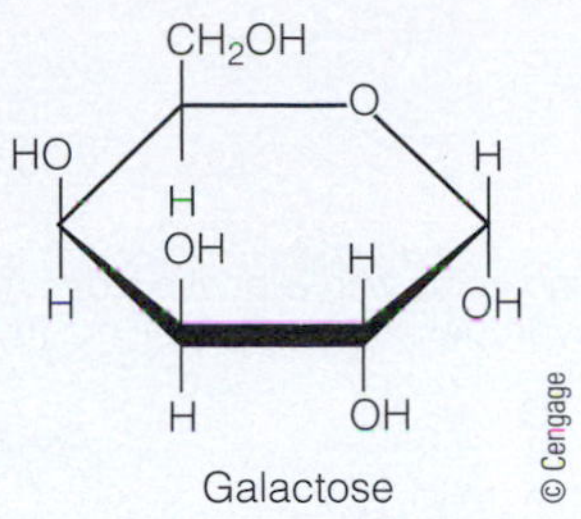
CH_2OH
HO
O
H
H
OH
H
H
OH
H
OH
Galactose

Hemicelluloses. The most common hemicelluloses are composed of a backbone chain of xylose, mannose, and galactose, with branching side chains of arabinose, glucuronic acid, and galactose.

Lipids

TABLE C-1 Saturated Fatty Acids Found in Natural Fats

Saturated Fatty Acids	Chemical Formulas	Number of Carbons	Major Food Sources
Butyric	C_3H_7COOH	4	Butterfat
Caproic	$C_5H_{11}COOH$	6	Butterfat
Caprylic	$C_7H_{15}COOH$	8	Coconut oil
Capric	$C_9H_{19}COOH$	10	Palm oil
Lauric	$C_{11}H_{23}COOH$	12	Coconut oil, palm oil
Myristic	$C_{13}H_{27}COOH$	14	Coconut oil, palm oil
Palmitic	$C_{15}H_{31}COOH$	16	Palm oil
Stearic	$C_{17}H_{35}COOH$	18	Most animal fats
Arachidic	$C_{19}H_{39}COOH$	20	Peanut oil
Behenic	$C_{21}H_{43}COOH$	22	Seeds
Lignoceric	$C_{23}H_{47}COOH$	24	Peanut oil

NOTE: The most common fatty acids are myristic, palmitic, and stearic.

TABLE C-2 Unsaturated Fatty Acids Found in Natural Fats

Unsaturated Fatty Acids	Chemical Formulas	Number of Carbons	Number of Double Bonds	Standard Notation[a]	Omega Notation[b]	Major Food Sources
Palmitoleic	$C_{15}H_{29}COOH$	16	1	16:1;9	16:1ω7	Seafood, beef
Oleic	$C_{17}H_{33}COOH$	18	1	18:1;9	18:1ω9	Olive oil, canola oil
Linoleic	$C_{17}H_{31}COOH$	18	2	18:2;9,12	18:2ω6	Sunflower oil, safflower oil
Linolenic	$C_{17}H_{29}COOH$	18	3	18:3;9,12,15	18:3ω3	Soybean oil, canola oil
Arachidonic	$C_{19}H_{31}COOH$	20	4	20:4;5,8,11,14	20:4ω6	Eggs, most animal fats
Eicosapentaenoic	$C_{19}H_{29}COOH$	20	5	20:5;5,8,11,14,17	20:5ω3	Seafood
Docosahexaenoic	$C_{21}H_{31}COOH$	20	6	22:6;4,7,10,13,16,19	22:6ω3	Seafood

NOTE: A fatty acid has two ends; designated the methyl (CH_3) end and the carboxyl, or acid (COOH), end.

[a]Standard chemistry notation begins counting carbons at the acid end. The number of carbons the fatty acid contains comes first, followed by a colon and another number that indicates the number of double bonds; next comes a semicolon followed by a number or numbers indicating the positions of the double bonds. Thus the notation for linoleic acid, an 18-carbon fatty acid with two double bonds between carbons 9 and 10 and between carbons 12 and 13, is 18:2;9,12.

[b]Because fatty acid chains are lengthened by adding carbons at the acid end of the chain, chemists use the omega system of notation to ease the task of identifying them. The omega system begins counting carbons at the methyl end. The number of carbons the fatty acid contains comes first, followed by a colon and the number of double bonds; next come the omega symbol (ω) and a number indicating the position of the double bond nearest the methyl end. Thus linoleic acid with its first double bond at the sixth carbon from the methyl end would be noted 18:2ω6 in the omega system.

Protein: Amino Acids

The common amino acids may be classified into the seven groups listed below based on their structural similarities. Amino acids marked with an asterisk (*) are essential.

1. Amino acids with aliphatic side chains, which consist of hydrogen and carbon atoms (hydrocarbons):

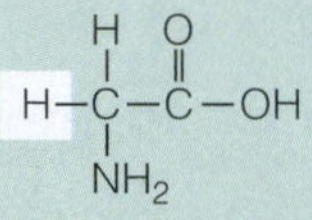

$H-C-C-OH$ **Glycine (Gly)**

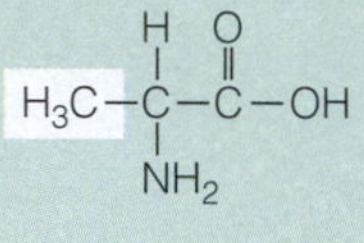

$H_3C-C-C-OH$ **Alanine (Ala)**

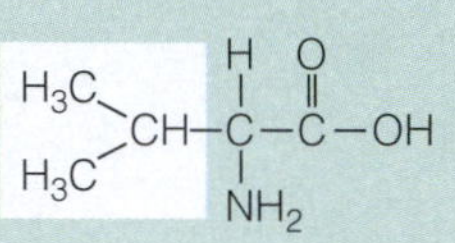

$(H_3C)_2CH-C-C-OH$ **Valine* (Val)**

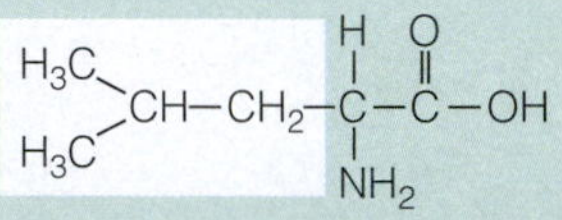

$(H_3C)_2CH-CH_2-C-C-OH$ **Leucine* (Leu)**

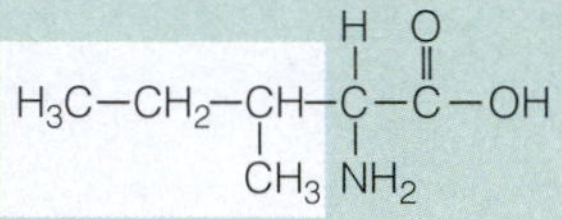

$H_3C-CH_2-CH(CH_3)-C-C-OH$ **Isoleucine* (Ile)**

2. Amino acids with hydroxyl (OH) side chains:

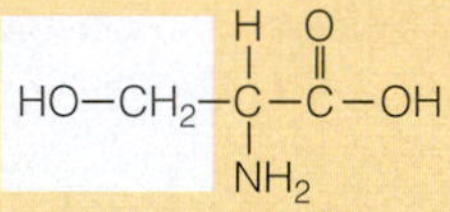

$HO-CH_2-C-C-OH$ **Serine (Ser)**

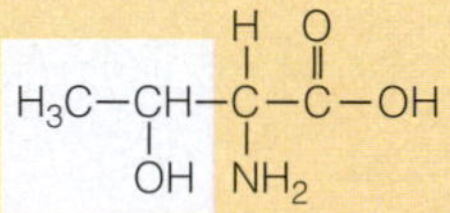

$H_3C-CH(OH)-C-C-OH$ **Threonine* (Thr)**

3. Amino acids with side chains containing acidic groups or their amides, which contain the group NH_2:

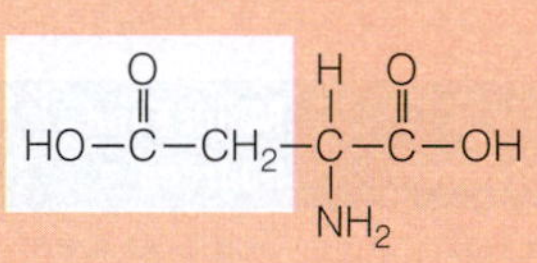

$HO-C-CH_2-C-C-OH$ **Aspartic acid (Asp)**

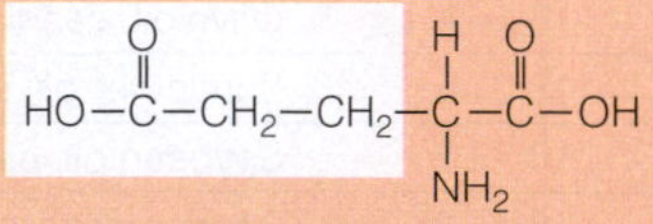

$HO-C-CH_2-CH_2-C-C-OH$ **Glutamic acid (Glu)**

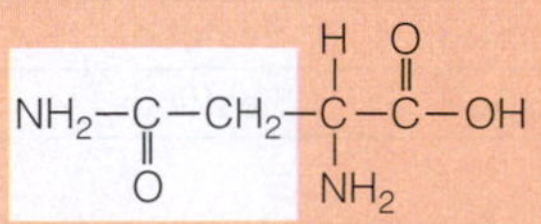

$NH_2-C-CH_2-C-C-OH$ **Asparagine (Asn)**

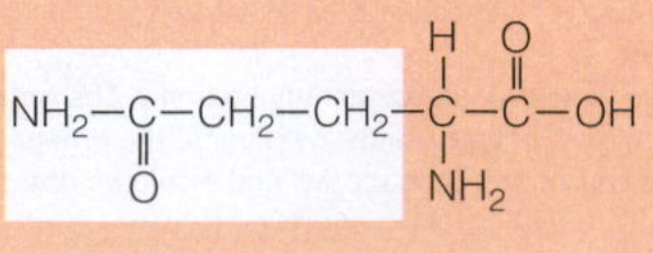

$NH_2-C-CH_2-CH_2-C-C-OH$ **Glutamine (Gln)**

4. Amino acids with basic side chains:

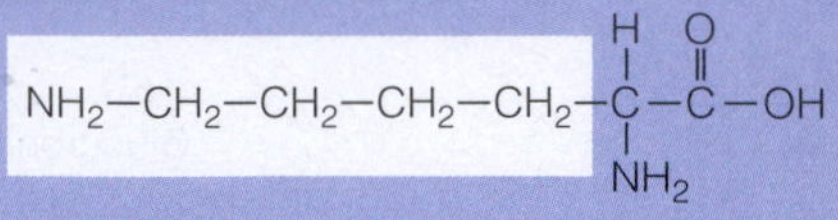

$NH_2-CH_2-CH_2-CH_2-CH_2-C-C-OH$ **Lysine* (Lys)**

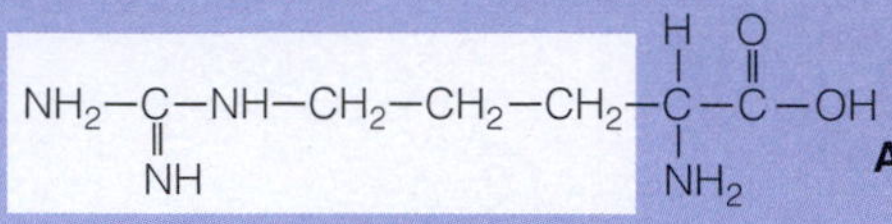

$NH_2-C(=NH)-NH-CH_2-CH_2-CH_2-C-C-OH$ **Arginine (Arg)**

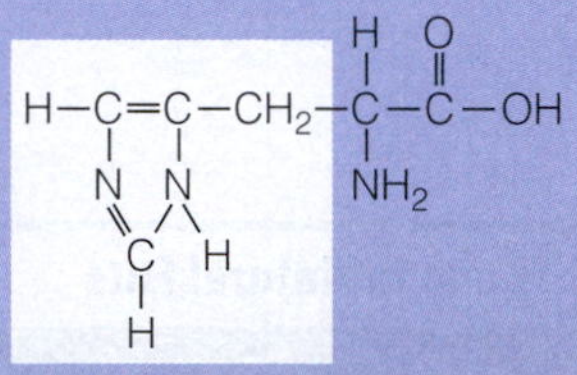

Histidine* (His)

5. Amino acids with aromatic side chains, which are characterized by the presence of at least one ring structure:

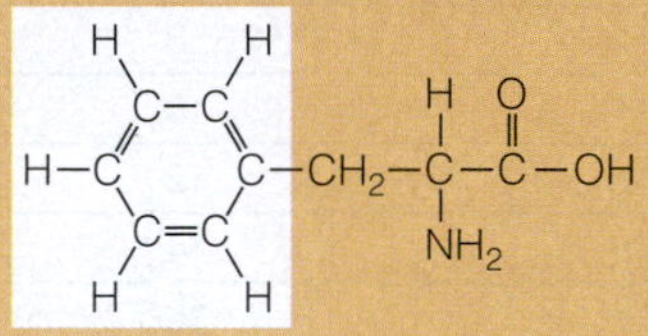

Phenylalanine* (Phe)

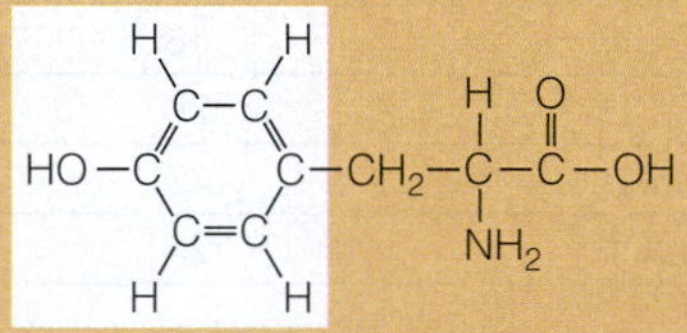

Tyrosine (Tyr)

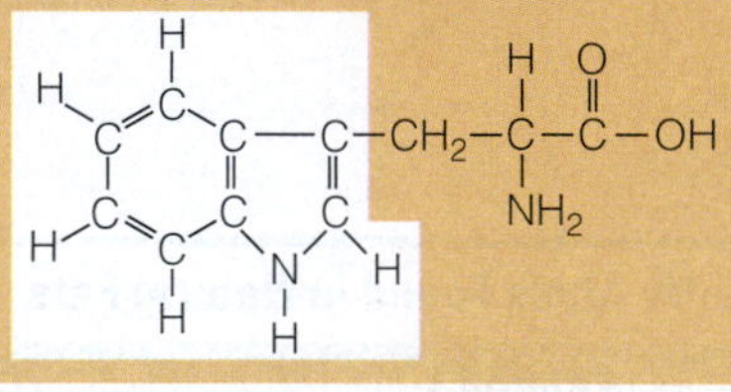

Tryptophan* (Trp)

6. Amino acids with side chains containing sulfur atoms:

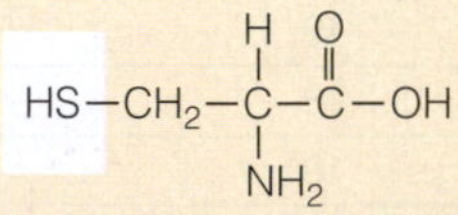

$HS-CH_2-C-C-OH$ **Cysteine (Cys)**

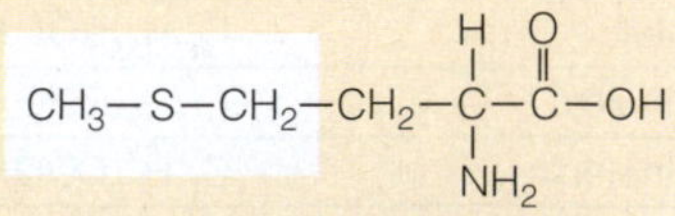

$CH_3-S-CH_2-CH_2-C-C-OH$ **Methionine* (Met)**

7. Imino acid:

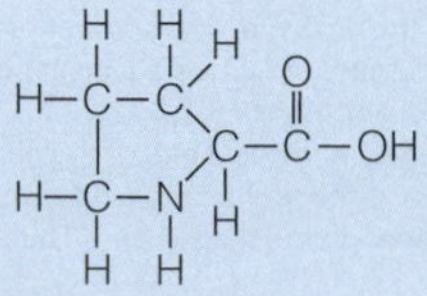

Proline (Pro)

Proline has the same chemical structure as the other amino acids, but its amino group has given up a hydrogen to form a ring.

Vitamins and Coenzymes

Vitamin A: retinol. Retinol is the alcohol form of vitamin A.

Vitamin A: retinal. Retinal is the aldehyde form of vitamin A.

Vitamin A: retinoic acid. Retinoic acid is the acid form of vitamin A.

Vitamin A precursor: beta-carotene. Beta-carotene is the carotenoid with the most vitamin A activity.

Thiamin. Thiamin is part of the coenzyme thiamin pyrophosphate (TPP).

Thiamin pyrophosphate (TPP). TPP is a coenzyme that includes the thiamin molecule as part of its structure.

Riboflavin. Riboflavin is a part of two coenzymes—flavin mononucleotide (FMN) and flavin adenine dinucleotide (FAD).

Flavin mononucleotide (FMN). FMN is a coenzyme that includes the riboflavin molecule as part of its structure.

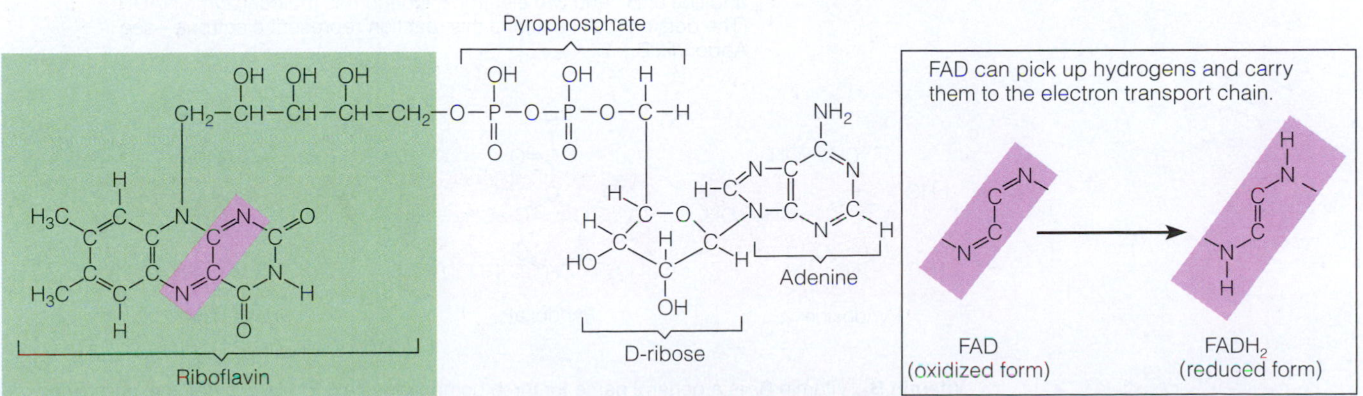

Pyrophosphate
Riboflavin
D-ribose
Adenine
FAD can pick up hydrogens and carry them to the electron transport chain.
FAD
(oxidized form)
$FADH_2$
(reduced form)

Flavin adenine dinucleotide (FAD). FAD is a coenzyme that includes the riboflavin molecule as part of its structure.

APPENDIX C

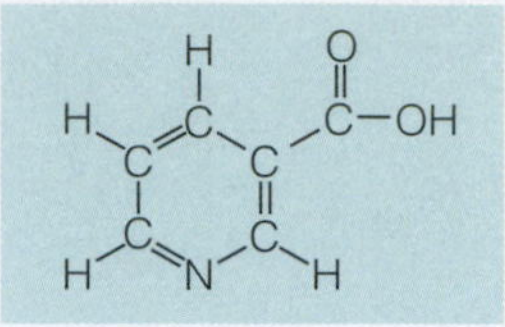

Nicotinic acid

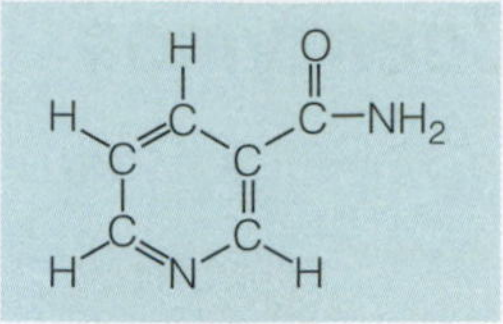

Nicotinamide

Niacin (nicotinic acid and nicotinamide). Niacin is a part of two coenzymes—nicotinamide adenine dinucleotide (NAD^+) and nicotinamide adenine dinucleotide phosphate ($NADP^+$).

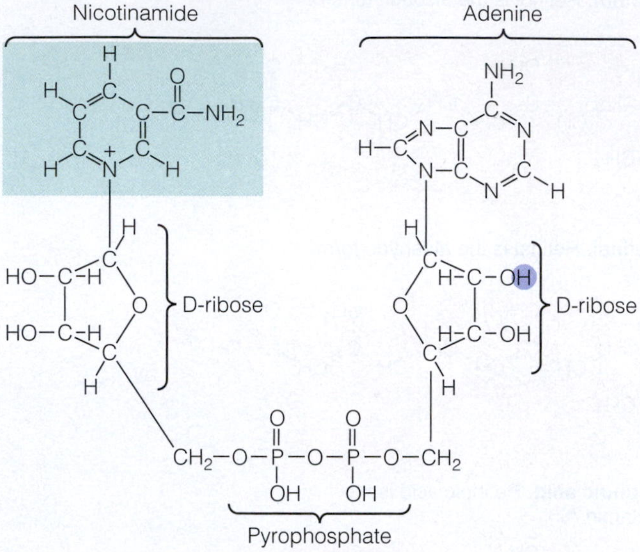

Nicotinamide

Adenine

D-ribose

D-ribose

Pyrophosphate

Nicotinamide adenine dinucleotide (NAD^+). NAD is a coenzyme that includes niacin as part of its structure. NADP has the same structure as NAD but with a phosphate group attached to the O instead of the H.

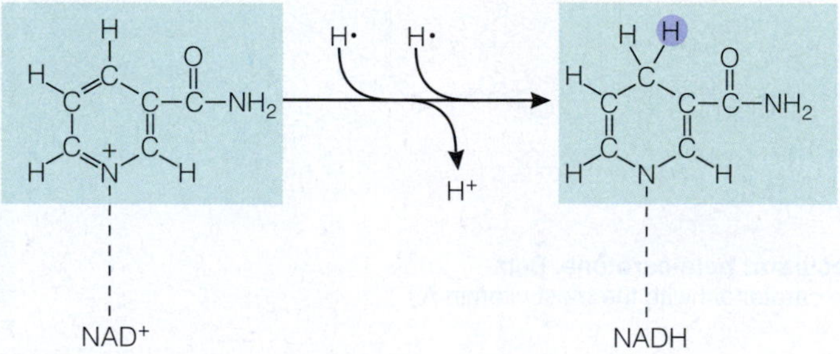

NAD^+

NADH

Reduced NAD^+ (NADH). When NAD^+ is reduced by the addition of H^+ and two electrons, it becomes the coenzyme NADH. (The dots on the H entering this reaction represent electrons—see Appendix B.)

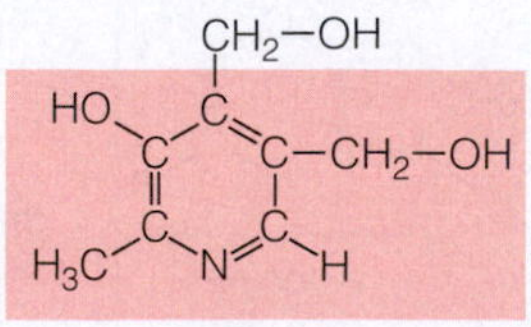

Pyridoxine

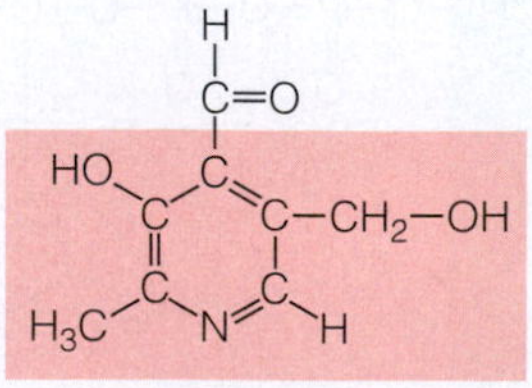

Pyridoxal

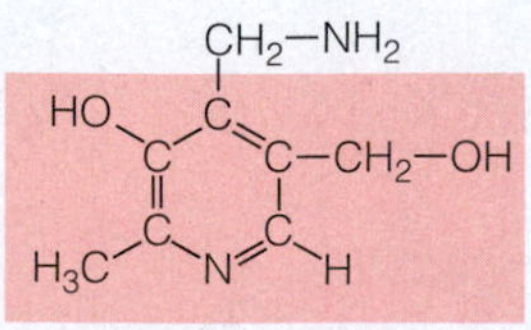

Pyridoxamine

Vitamin B_6. Vitamin B_6 is a general name for three compounds—pyridoxine, pyridoxal, and pyridoxamine, which become a part of two coenzymes—pyridoxal phosphate and pyridoxamine phosphate.

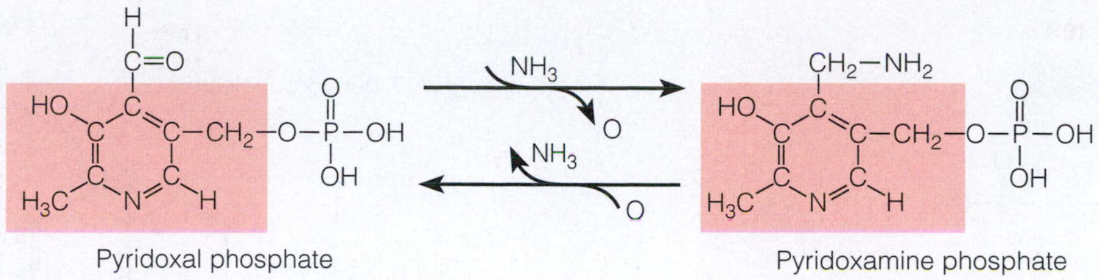

Pyridoxal phosphate

Pyridoxamine phosphate

Pyridoxal phosphate (PLP) and pyridoxamine phosphate. These coenzymes include vitamin B_6 as part of their structures.

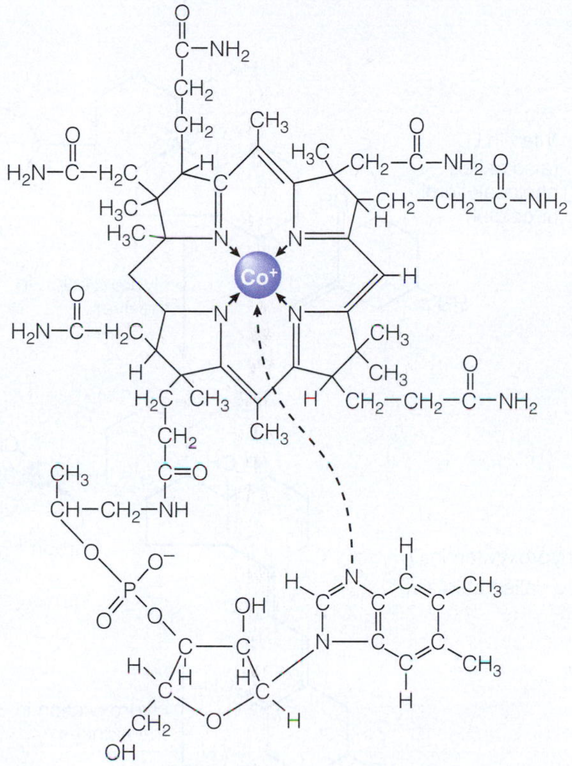

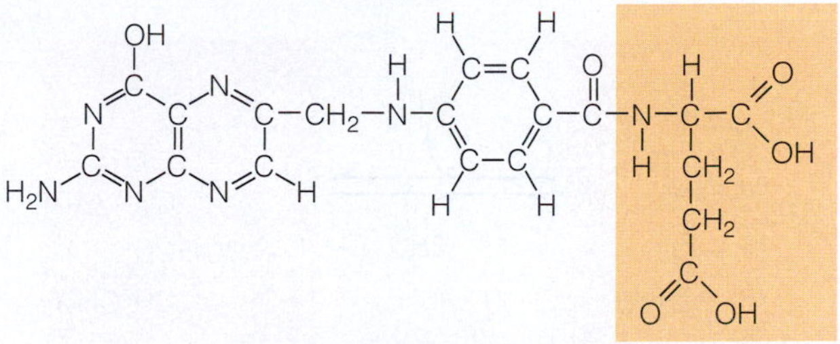

Folate (folacin or folic acid). Folate consists of a double ring combined with a single ring and at least one glutamate (a nonessential amino acid highlighted in color). Folate is a part of the coenzyme tetrahydrofolate (THF).

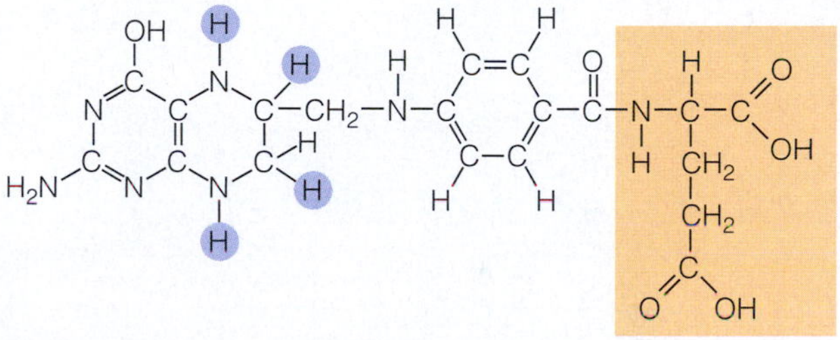

Vitamin B_{12} (cyanocobalamin). The arrows in this diagram indicate that the spare electron pairs on the nitrogens attract them to the cobalt.

Tetrahydrofolate (THF). THF is the active coenzyme form of folate and has four added hydrogens. An intermediate form, dihydrofolate, has two added hydrogens.

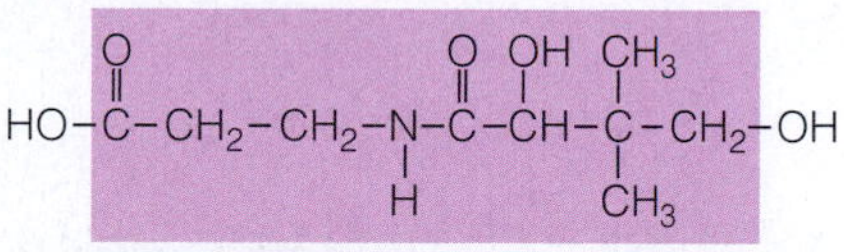

Pantothenic acid. Pantothenic acid is part of coenzyme A (CoA).

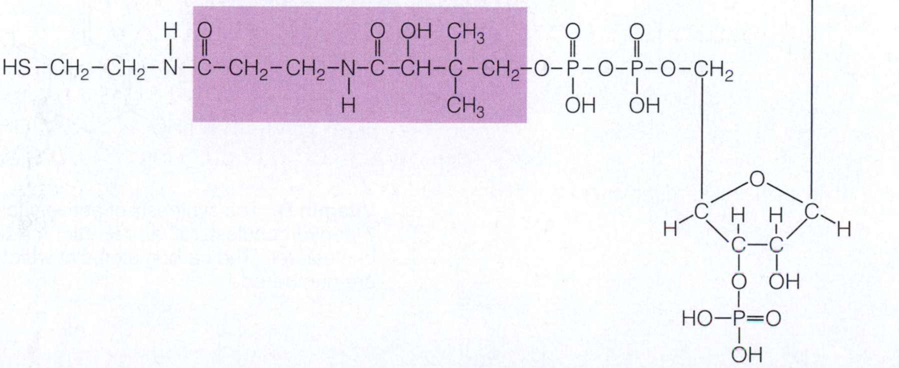

Coenzyme A (CoA). Coenzyme A is a coenzyme that includes pantothenic acid as part of its structure.

Biotin.

Ascorbic acid (reduced form)

Dehydroascorbic acid (oxidized form)

Vitamin C. Two hydrogen atoms with their electrons are lost when ascorbic acid is oxidized and gained when it is reduced again.

7-dehydrocholesterol

Carbon #7

Ultraviolet light on the skin

Vitamin D_3 (also called cholecalciferol or calciol)

Hydroxylation in the liver

25-hydroxyvitamin D_3 (also called calcidiol)

Carbon #25

Hydroxylation in the kidneys

1,25-dihydroxyvitamin D_3 (also called calcitriol)

Carbon #1

Vitamin D. The synthesis of active vitamin D begins with 7-dehydrocholesterol, a precursor made in the liver from cholesterol. (The carbon atoms at which changes occur are numbered.)

Tocotrienols contain double bonds here.

Vitamin E (alpha-tocopherol). Vitamin E consists of two subgroups—the tocopherols and the tocotrienols. All are made up of a complex ring structure with a long saturated (in tocopherols) or unsaturated (in tocotrienols) side chain. The number and positions of methyl groups (CH_3) distinguish the members within each subgroup.

Vitamin K (phylloquinone). Naturally occurring compounds with vitamin K activity include phylloquinones (from plants) and menaquinones (from bacteria). The chemical structure of menaquinones differs only slightly from that of phylloquinones.

Vitamin K (menadione). Menadione is a synthetic compound that has the same activity as natural vitamin K.

Triphosphate

Cleavage

Adenine

Ribose

Adenosine triphosphate (ATP). The high-energy compound ATP releases energy when one or two phosphate groups split off. The cleavage point marks the bond that is broken when ATP splits to become ADP + P.

Cleavage

+ H—O—H (Water)

Phosphate + ADP

Adenosine diphosphate (ADP).

APPENDIX C

Glycolysis

Figure C-1 depicts glycolysis. The following text describes key steps as numbered on the figure.

> **FIGURE C-1 Glycolysis**

Notice that galactose and fructose enter at different places but continue on the same pathway.

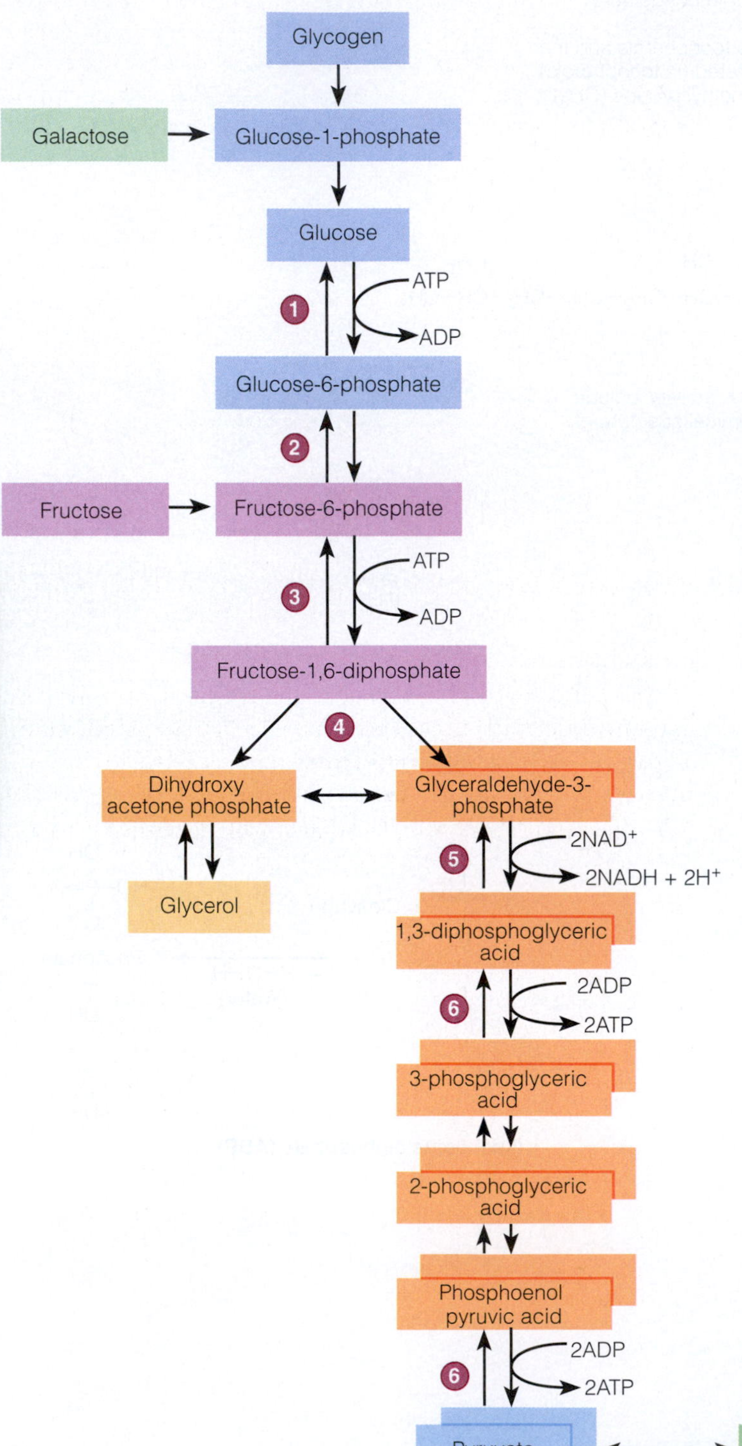

Glycogen
Galactose
Glucose-1-phosphate
Glucose
ATP
ADP
1
Glucose-6-phosphate
2
Fructose
Fructose-6-phosphate
ATP
ADP
3
Fructose-1,6-diphosphate
4
Dihydroxy acetone phosphate
Glyceraldehyde-3-phosphate
Glycerol
5
2NAD+
2NADH + 2H+
1,3-diphosphoglyceric acid
6
2ADP
2ATP
3-phosphoglyceric acid
2-phosphoglyceric acid
Phosphoenol pyruvic acid
6
2ADP
2ATP
Pyruvate
Lactate
2NADH + 2H+
2NAD+

1. A phosphate is attached to glucose at the carbon that chemists call number 6 (review the first diagram of glucose, p. C-1, to see how chemists number the carbons in a glucose molecule). The product is called, logically enough, glucose-6-phosphate. One ATP molecule is used to accomplish this.
2. Glucose-6-phosphate is rearranged by an enzyme.
3. A phosphate is added in another reaction that uses another molecule of ATP. The resulting product is fructose-1,6-diphosphate. At this point the 6-carbon sugar has a phosphate group on its first and sixth carbons and is ready to break apart.
4. When fructose-1,6-diphosphate breaks in half, the two 3-carbon compounds are not identical. Each has a phosphate group attached, but only glyceraldehyde-3-phosphate converts directly to pyruvate. The other compound, however, converts easily to glyceraldehyde-3-phosphate.
5. In the next step, NAD^+ is reduced to $NADH + H^+$.
6. In two of the following steps ATP is regenerated.

Remember that in effect two molecules of glyceraldehyde-3-phosphate are produced from glucose; therefore, four ATP molecules are generated from each glucose molecule. Two ATP were needed to get the sequence started, so the net gain at this point is two ATP and two molecules of $NADH + H^+$. As you will see later, each $NADH + H^+$ moves to the electron transport chain to unload its hydrogens, producing more ATP.

Fatty Acid Oxidation

Figure C-2 presents fatty acid oxidation. The sequence is as follows.

1. The fatty acid is activated by combining with coenzyme A (CoA). In this reaction, ATP loses two phosphorus atoms and becomes AMP (adenosine monophosphate)—the equivalent of a loss of two ATP.
2. In the next reaction, two H with their electrons are removed and transferred to FAD, forming $FADH_2$.
3. In a later reaction, two H are removed and go to NAD^+ (forming $NADH + H^+$).
4. The fatty acid is cleaved at the "beta" carbon, the second carbon from the carboxyl (COOH) end. This break results in a fatty acid that is two carbons shorter than the previous one and a 2-carbon molecule of acetyl CoA. At the same time, another CoA is attached

> FIGURE C-2 Fatty Acid Oxidation

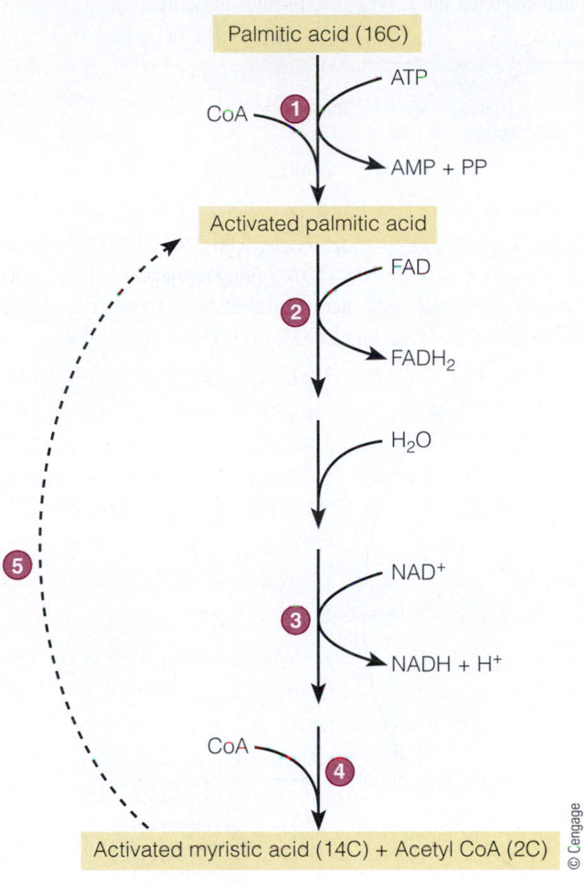

Palmitic acid (16C)
ATP
CoA
1
AMP + PP
Activated palmitic acid
FAD
2
$FADH_2$
H_2O
5
NAD^+
3
$NADH + H^+$
CoA
4
Activated myristic acid (14C) + Acetyl CoA (2C)
© Cengage

to the fatty acid, thus activating it for its turn through the series of reactions.

5. The sequence is repeated with each cycle producing an acetyl CoA and a shorter fatty acid until only a 2-carbon fatty acid remains—acetyl CoA.

In the example shown in Figure C-2, palmitic acid (a 16-carbon fatty acid) will go through this series of reactions seven times, using the equivalent of two ATP for the initial activation and generating seven $FADH_2$, seven $NADH + H^+$, and eight acetyl CoA. As you will see later, each of the seven $FADH_2$ will enter the electron transport chain, yielding two ATP (for a total of 14). Similarly, each $NADH + H^+$ will enter the electron transport chain, yielding three ATP (for a total of 21). Thus the oxidation of a 16-carbon fatty acid uses 2 ATP and generates 35 ATP. When the eight acetyl CoA enter the TCA cycle, even more ATP will be generated, as a later section describes.

Amino Acid Degradation

The first step in amino acid degradation is the removal of the nitrogen-containing amino group through either transamination (see Figure 6-11, p. 181) or deamination (see Figure 6-12, p. 181) reactions. Then the remaining carbon skeletons may enter the metabolic pathways at different places, as shown in Figure C-3 (p. C-12).

The TCA Cycle

The tricarboxylic acid, or TCA, cycle is the set of reactions that break down acetyl CoA to carbon dioxide and hydrogen atoms. Pyruvate derived from glycolysis does not enter the TCA cycle directly; instead pyruvate enters the mitochondrion, loses a carbon group, and bonds with a molecule of CoA to become acetyl CoA. The TCA cycle uses any substance that can be converted to acetyl CoA directly or indirectly through pyruvate.

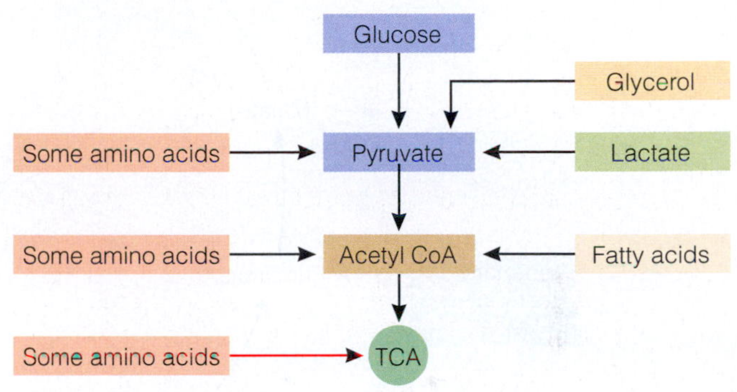

Glucose
Glycerol
Some amino acids
Pyruvate
Lactate
Some amino acids
Acetyl CoA
Fatty acids
Some amino acids
TCA
© Cengage

Any substance that can be converted to acetyl CoA directly, or indirectly through pyruvate, may enter the TCA cycle.

The pathway from pyruvate to acetyl CoA is complex. We have included only those steps that will help you understand the transfer of energy from the nutrients. Pyruvate loses a carbon to carbon dioxide and is attached to a molecule of CoA. In the process, NAD^+ picks up two hydrogens with their associated electrons, becoming $NADH + H^+$.

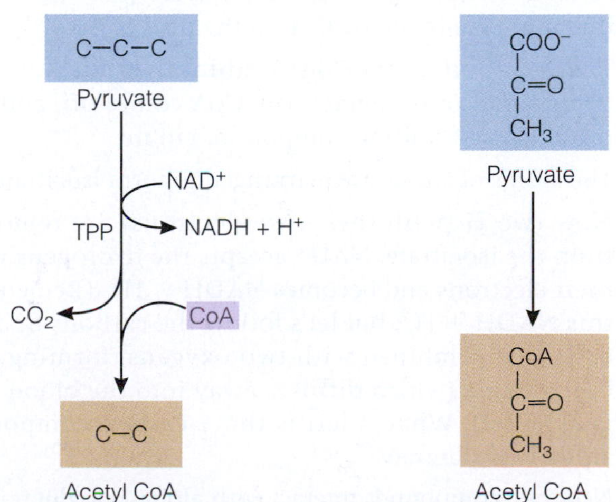

C–C–C
Pyruvate
NAD^+
TPP
$NADH + H^+$
CO_2
CoA
C–C
Acetyl CoA
COO^-
C=O
CH_3
Pyruvate
CoA
C=O
CH_3
Acetyl CoA
© Cengage

The step from pyruvate to acetyl CoA. (TPP and NAD are coenzymes containing the B vitamins thiamin and niacin, respectively.)

APPENDIX C

> FIGURE C-3 Amino Acids Enter the Metabolic Pathways

After losing their amino groups, carbon skeletons can be converted to one of seven molecules that can enter the TCA cycle (presented in Figure C-4).

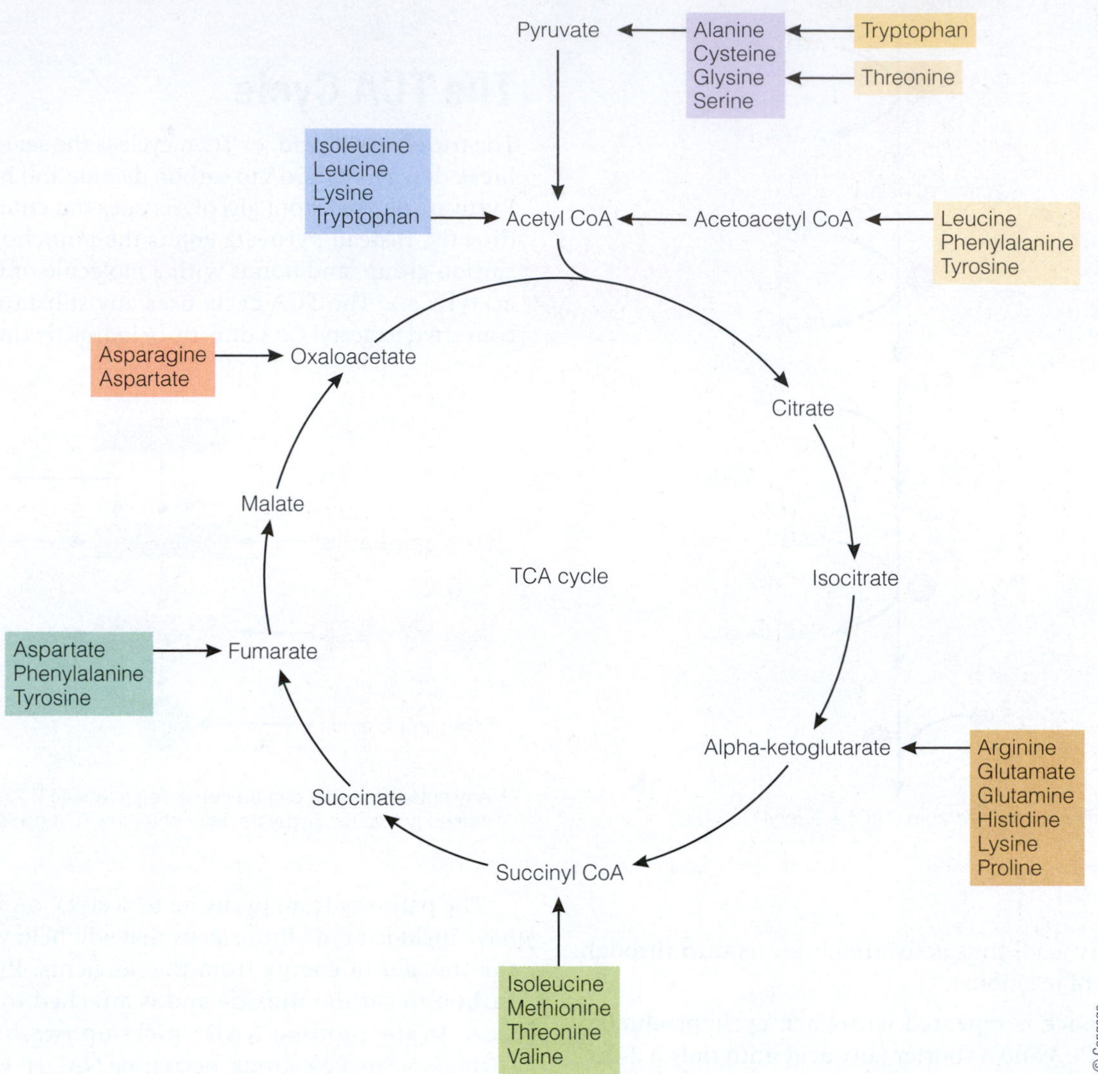

Pyruvate
Alanine
Cysteine
Glysine
Serine
Tryptophan
Threonine
Isoleucine
Leucine
Lysine
Tryptophan
Acetyl CoA
Acetoacetyl CoA
Leucine
Phenylalanine
Tyrosine
Asparagine
Aspartate
Oxaloacetate
Citrate
Malate
TCA cycle
Isocitrate
Aspartate
Phenylalanine
Tyrosine
Fumarate
Alpha-ketoglutarate
Arginine
Glutamate
Glutamine
Histidine
Lysine
Proline
Succinate
Succinyl CoA
Isoleucine
Methionine
Threonine
Valine

Let's follow the steps of the TCA cycle (see the corresponding numbers in Figure C-4 on the next page).

1. The 2-carbon acetyl CoA combines with a 4-carbon compound, oxaloacetate. The CoA comes off, and the product is a 6-carbon compound, citrate.
2. The atoms of citrate are rearranged to form isocitrate.
3. Now two H (with their two electrons) are removed from the isocitrate. NAD^+ accepts the hydrogens with their electrons and becomes $NADH + H^+$. (Remember this $NADH + H^+$, but let's follow the carbons first.) A carbon is combined with two oxygens, forming carbon dioxide (which diffuses away into the blood and is exhaled). What is left is the 5-carbon compound alpha-ketoglutarate.
4. Now two compounds interact with alpha-ketoglutarate—a molecule of CoA and a molecule of NAD^+. In this complex reaction, a carbon and two oxygens are removed (forming carbon dioxide); two hydrogens are removed and go to NAD^+ (forming $NADH + H^+$); and the remaining 4-carbon compound is attached to the CoA, forming succinyl CoA. (Remember this $NADH + H^+$ also. You will see later what happens to it.)
5. Now two molecules react with succinyl CoA—a molecule called GDP and one of phosphate (P). The CoA comes off, the GDP and P combine to form the high-energy compound GTP (similar to ATP), and succinate remains. (Remember this GTP.)
6. In the next reaction, two H with their electrons are removed from succinate and are transferred to a molecule of FAD (a coenzyme like NAD^+) to form $FADH_2$. The product that remains is fumarate. (Remember this $FADH_2$.)
7. Next a molecule of water is added to fumarate, forming malate.

> **FIGURE C-4** The TCA Cycle

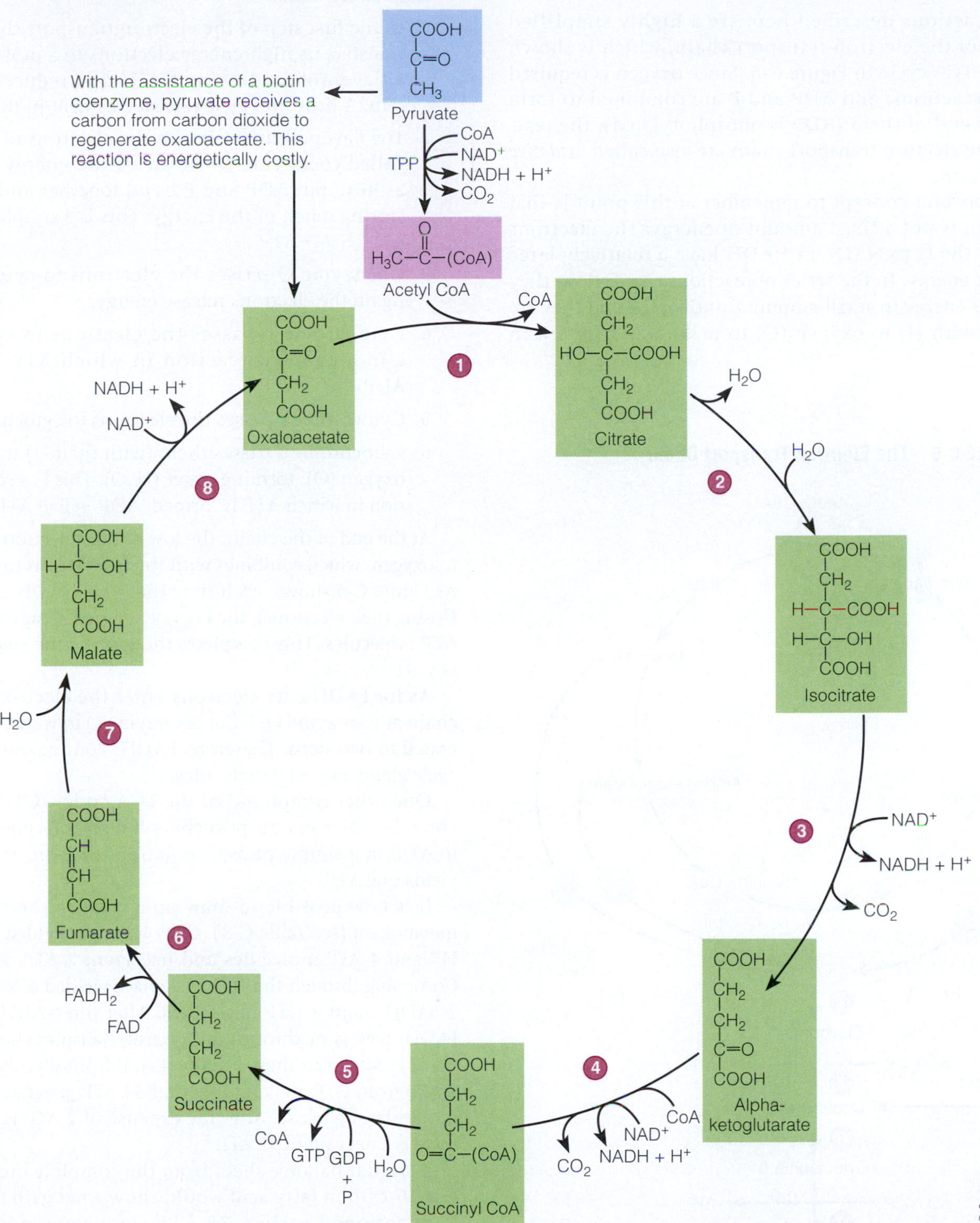

COOH
C=O
CH3
Pyruvate
With the assistance of a biotin coenzyme, pyruvate receives a carbon from carbon dioxide to regenerate oxaloacetate. This reaction is energetically costly.
TPP
CoA
NAD+
NADH + H+
CO2
H3C–C–(CoA)
Acetyl CoA
CoA
1
Oxaloacetate
Citrate
HO–C–COOH
H2O
2
Isocitrate
H–C–COOH
H–C–OH
3
NAD+
NADH + H+
CO2
Alpha-ketoglutarate
4
CoA
NAD+
NADH + H+
CO2
Succinyl CoA
O=C–(CoA)
5
H2O
GDP + P
GTP
CoA
Succinate
6
FAD
FADH2
Fumarate
7
H2O
Malate
H–C–OH
8
NAD+
NADH + H+
© Cengage

8. A molecule of NAD^+ accepts two H with their associated electrons and forms $NADH + H^+$. The product that remains is the 4-carbon compound oxaloacetate. (Remember this $NADH + H^+$.)

The cycle is complete and we are back where we started. The oxaloacetate can combine with another molecule of acetyl CoA (step 1), and the cycle can begin again.

So far, we have seen two carbons brought in with acetyl CoA and two carbons ending up in carbon dioxide. But where are the energy and the ATP that were promised?

A review of the eight steps of the TCA cycle shows that the compounds $NADH + H^+$ (three molecules), $FADH_2$, and GTP captured energy along the way. To see how this energy ends up in ATP, we must follow the electrons further—into the electron transport chain.

The Electron Transport Chain

The six reactions described here are a highly simplified overview of the electron transport chain, which is shown below the TCA cycle in Figure C-5. Since oxygen is required for these reactions, and ADP and P are combined to form ATP in several of them (ADP is phosphorylated), the reactions of the electron transport chain are also called *oxidative phosphorylation*.

An important concept to remember at this point is that an electron is not a fixed amount of energy. The electrons that bond the H to NAD^+ in NADH have a relatively large amount of energy. In the series of reactions that follow, they release this energy in small amounts, until at the end they are attached (with H) to oxygen (O) to make water (H_2O). In some of the steps, the energy they release is captured into ATP in coupled reactions.

1. In the first step of the electron transport chain, NADH transfers its high-energy electrons to a molecule called a flavoprotein, leaving NAD^+ and reduced flavoprotein. A little energy is released as heat in this reaction.
2. The flavoprotein passes on the electrons to a molecule called coenzyme Q. Again a little energy is released as heat, but ADP and P bond together and form ATP, storing much of the energy. This is a coupled reaction: ADP + P → ATP.
3. Coenzyme Q passes the electrons to cytochrome *b*. Again the electrons release energy.
4. Cytochrome *b* passes the electrons to cytochrome *c* in a coupled reaction in which ATP is formed: ADP + P → ATP.
5. Cytochrome *c* passes the electrons to cytochrome *a*.
6. Cytochrome *a* passes them (with their H) to an atom of oxygen (O), forming water (H_2O). This is a coupled reaction in which ATP is formed: ADP + P → ATP.

> **FIGURE C-5 The Electron Transport Chain**

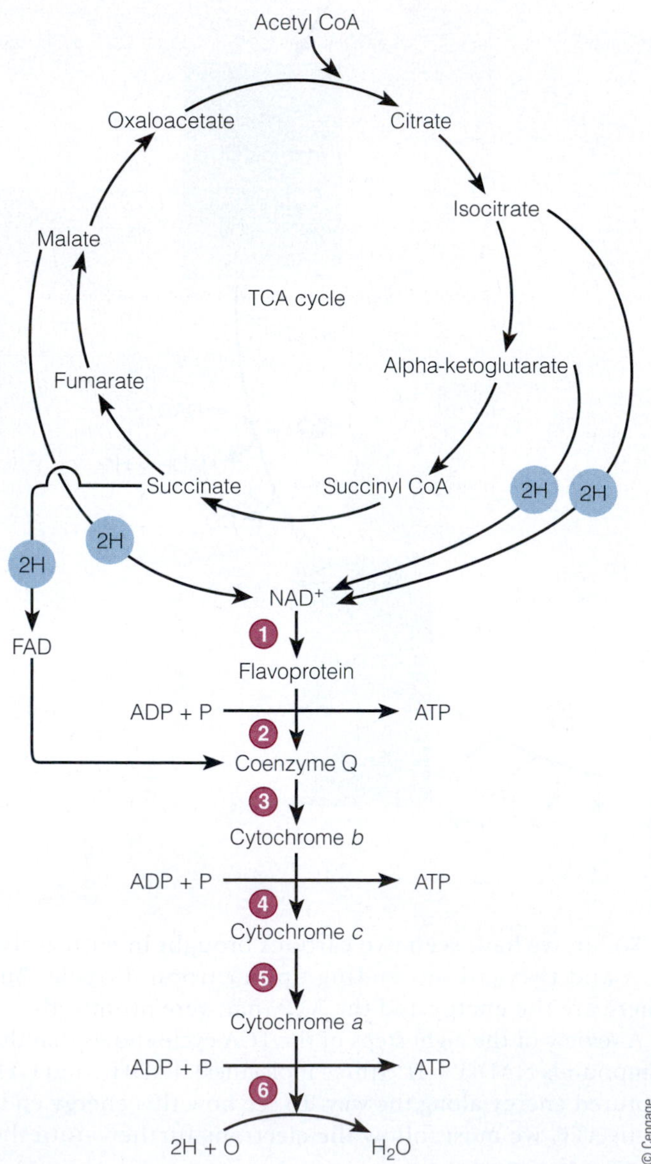
Acetyl CoA
Citrate
Isocitrate
Alpha-ketoglutarate
Succinyl CoA
Succinate
Fumarate
Malate
Oxaloacetate
TCA cycle
2H
2H
2H
2H
NAD+
FAD
1
Flavoprotein
ADP + P
ATP
2
Coenzyme Q
3
Cytochrome b
ADP + P
ATP
4
Cytochrome c
5
Cytochrome a
ADP + P
ATP
6
2H + O
H2O
© Cengage

At the end of the chain, the low-energy electrons are passed to oxygen, which combines with the free H^+ ions to form water. As Figure C-5 shows, each time the three NADH are oxidized (losing their electrons), the energy released is captured in three ATP molecules. This completes the story of the electrons from NADH.

As for $FADH_2$, its electrons enter the electron transport chain at coenzyme Q. From coenzyme Q to water, ATP is generated in two steps. Therefore, $FADH_2$ coming out of the TCA cycle yields two ATP molecules.

One other compound of the TCA cycle—GTP—does not enter the electron transport chain but gives its energy directly to ADP in a simple phosphorylation reaction. This reaction yields one ATP.

It is now possible to draw up a balance sheet of glucose metabolism (see Table C-3). Glycolysis has yielded 4 NADH + H^+ and 4 ATP molecules and has spent 2 ATP. The 2 acetyl CoA going through the TCA cycle have yielded 6 NADH + H^+, 2 $FADH_2$, and 2 GTP molecules. After the NADH + H^+ and $FADH_2$ have gone through the electron transport chain, there are 28 ATP. Added to these are the 4 ATP from glycolysis and the 2 ATP from GTP, making the total 34 ATP generated from one molecule of glucose. After the expense of 2 ATP is subtracted, there is a net gain of 32 ATP.*

A similar balance sheet from the complete breakdown of one 16-carbon fatty acid would show a net gain of 129 ATP. As mentioned earlier, 35 ATP were generated from the 7 $FADH_2$ and 7 NADH + H^+ produced during fatty acid

*The total may sometimes be 30 ATP. The NADH + H^+ generated in the cytoplasm during glycolysis pass their electrons on to shuttle molecules, which move them into the mitochondria. One shuttle, malate, contributes its electrons to the electron transport chain before the first site of ATP synthesis, yielding 5 ATP. Another, glycerol phosphate, adds its electrons into the chain beyond that first site, yielding 3 ATP. Thus sometimes 5, and sometimes 3, ATP result from the NADH + H^+ that arise from glycolysis. The amount depends on the cell.

TABLE C-3 Balance Sheet for Glucose Metabolism

		ATP
Glycolysis:	4 ATP − 2 ATP	2
1 glucose to 2 pyruvate	2 NADH + H^+	3–5[a]
2 pyruvate to 2 acetyl CoA	2 NADH + H^+	5
TCA cycle and electron transport chain:		
2 isocitrate	2 NADH + H^+	5
2 alpha-ketoglutarate	2 NADH + H^+	5
2 succinyl CoA	2 GTP	2
2 succinate	2 $FADH_2$	3
2 malate	2 NADH + H^+	5
Total ATP collected from one molecule glucose:		30–32

[a]Each NADH + H^+ from glycolysis can yield 1.5 or 2.5 ATP. See the accompanying text.

oxidation. The 8 acetyl CoA produced will each generate 12 ATP as they go through the TCA cycle and the electron transport chain, for a total of 96 more ATP. After subtracting the 2 ATP needed to activate the fatty acid initially, the net yield from one 16-carbon fatty acid: 35 + 96 − 2 = 129 ATP.

These calculations help explain why fat yields more energy (measured as kcalories) per gram than carbohydrate or protein. The more hydrogen atoms a fuel contains, the more ATP will be generated during oxidation. The 16-carbon fatty acid molecule, with its 32 hydrogen atoms, generates 129 ATP, whereas glucose, with its 12 hydrogen atoms, yields only 32 ATP.

The TCA cycle and the electron transport chain are the body's major means of capturing the energy from nutrients in ATP molecules. Other means, such as anaerobic glycolysis, contribute energy quickly, but the aerobic processes are the most efficient.

Alcohol's Interference with Energy Metabolism

Highlight 7 (p. 219) provided an overview of how alcohol interferes with energy metabolism. With an understanding of the TCA cycle, a few more details may be appreciated. During alcohol metabolism, the enzyme alcohol dehydrogenase oxidizes alcohol to acetaldehyde while it simultaneously reduces a molecule of NAD^+ to NADH + H^+. The related enzyme acetaldehyde dehydrogenase reduces another NAD^+ to NADH + H^+ while it oxidizes acetaldehyde to acetyl CoA, the compound that enters the TCA cycle to generate energy. Thus, whenever alcohol is being metabolized in the body, NAD^+ diminishes, and NADH + H^+ accumulates, thus altering the body's "redox state." NAD^+ can oxidize, and NADH + H^+ can reduce, many other compounds as well. During alcohol metabolism, however, NAD^+ becomes unavailable for the multitude of reactions for which it is required.

As the previous sections just explained, for glucose to be completely metabolized, the TCA cycle must be operating, and NAD^+ must be present. If these conditions are not met (and when alcohol is present, they may not be), the pathway will be blocked, and traffic will back up—or an alternate route will be taken. Think about this as you follow the pathway shown in Figure C-6.

In each step of alcohol metabolism in which NAD^+ is converted to NADH + H^+, hydrogen ions accumulate, resulting in a dangerous shift of the acid–base balance toward acid (Chapter 12 explained acid-base balance). The accumulation of NADH + H^+ slows TCA cycle activity, so pyruvate and acetyl CoA build up. This condition favors the conversion of pyruvate to lactate, which serves as a temporary storage place

> FIGURE C-6 Ethanol Enters the Metabolic Pathways

This is a simplified version of the glucose-to-energy pathway showing the entry of ethanol. The coenzyme NAD (which is the active form of the B vitamin niacin) is the only one shown here; however, many others are involved.

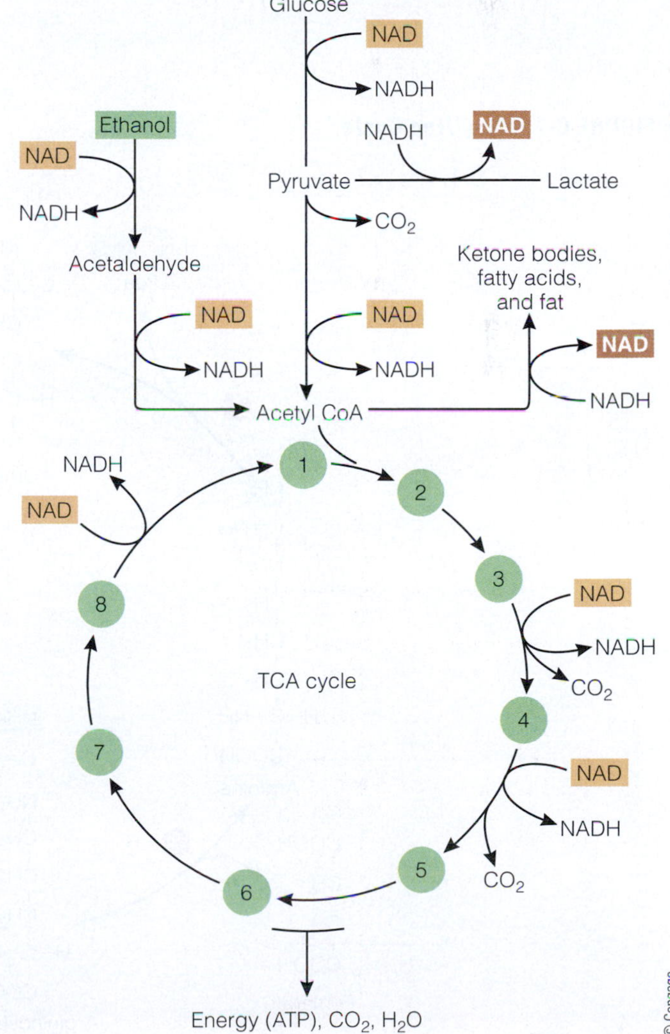

Glucose
NAD
NADH
Ethanol
NAD
NADH
NADH
NAD
Pyruvate
Lactate
CO_2
Acetaldehyde
Ketone bodies, fatty acids, and fat
NAD
NADH
NAD
NADH
NAD
NADH
Acetyl CoA
NADH
NAD
1
2
3
4
5
6
7
8
TCA cycle
NAD
NADH
CO_2
NAD
NADH
CO_2
Energy (ATP), CO_2, H_2O

for hydrogens from NADH + H^+. The conversion of pyruvate to lactate restores some NAD^+, but a lactate buildup has serious consequences of its own. It adds to the body's acid burden and interferes with the excretion of uric acid, causing goutlike symptoms. Molecules of acetyl CoA become building blocks for fatty acids or ketone bodies. The making of ketone bodies consumes acetyl CoA and generates NAD^+; but some ketone bodies are acids, so they push the acid-base balance further toward acid.

Thus alcohol cascades through the metabolic pathways, wreaking havoc along the way. These consequences have physical effects, as Highlight 7 described.

The Urea Cycle

Chapter 6 summed up the process by which waste nitrogen is eliminated from the body by stating that ammonia molecules combine with carbon dioxide to produce urea. This is true, but it is not the whole story. Urea is produced in a multistep process within the cells of the liver.

Ammonia, freed from an amino acid or other compound during metabolism anywhere in the body, arrives at the liver by way of the bloodstream and is taken into a liver cell. There, it is first combined with carbon dioxide and a phosphate group from ATP to form carbamyl phosphate:

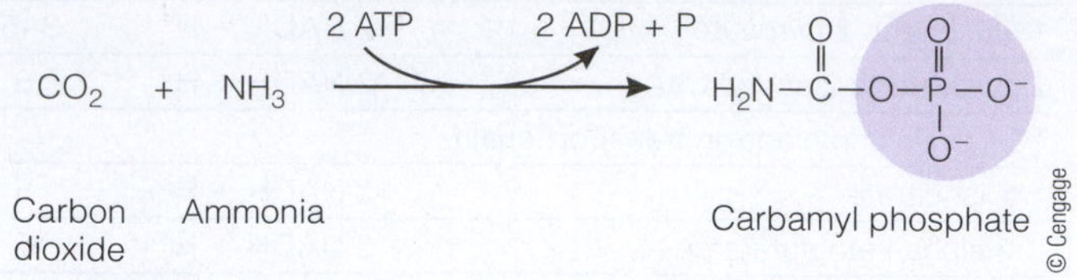

$$\underset{\text{Carbon dioxide}}{CO_2} + \underset{\text{Ammonia}}{NH_3} \xrightarrow[]{\text{2 ATP} \rightarrow \text{2 ADP + P}} \underset{\text{Carbamyl phosphate}}{H_2N{-}C({=}O){-}O{-}P({=}O)(O^-){-}O^-}$$

© Cengage

Figure C-7 shows the cycle of four reactions that follow.

1. Carbamyl phosphate combines with the amino acid ornithine, losing its phosphate group. The compound formed is citrulline.
2. Citrulline combines with the amino acid aspartic acid, to form argininosuccinate. The reaction requires energy from ATP. (In this reaction, ATP loses two phosphorus atoms, and becomes adenosine monophosphate, AMP.)
3. Argininosuccinate is split, forming another acid, fumarate, and the amino acid arginine.
4. Arginine loses its terminal carbon with two attached amino groups and picks up an oxygen from water.

> **FIGURE C-7** **The Urea Cycle**

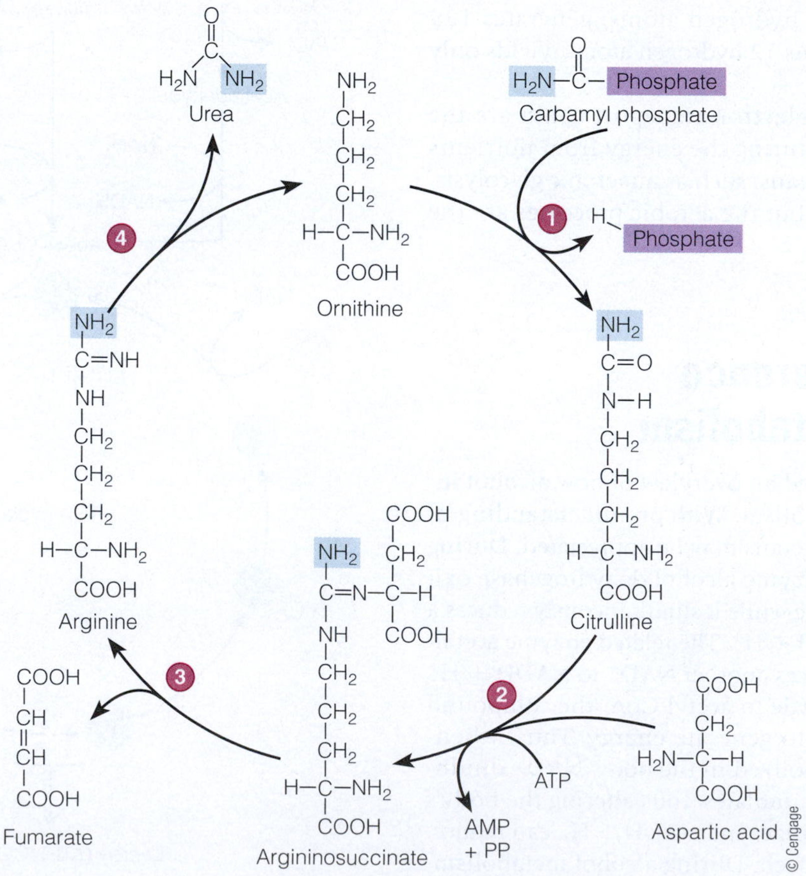

© Cengage

The end product is urea, which the kidneys excrete in the urine. The compound that remains is ornithine, identical to the ornithine with which this series of reactions began, ready to react with another molecule of carbamyl phosphate and turn the cycle again.

Formation of Ketone Bodies

Normally, fatty acid oxidation proceeds all the way to carbon dioxide and water. In ketosis, however, an intermediate is formed from the condensation of two molecules of acetyl CoA: acetoacetyl CoA. Figure C-8 shows the formation of ketone bodies from that intermediate.

1. Acetoacetyl CoA condenses with acetyl CoA to form a 6-carbon intermediate, beta-hydroxy-beta-methylglutaryl CoA.
2. This intermediate is cleaved to acetyl CoA and acetoacetate.
3. Acetoactate can be metabolized either to beta-hydroxybutyrate acid (step 3a) or to acetone (3b).

Acetoacetate, beta-hydroxybutyrate, and acetone are the ketone bodies of ketosis. Two are real ketones (they have a C=O group between two carbons); the other is an alcohol that has been produced during ketone formation—hence the term *ketone bodies,* rather than ketones, to describe the three of them. There are many other ketones in nature; these three are characteristic of ketosis in the body.

> **FIGURE C-8 The Formation of Ketone Bodies**

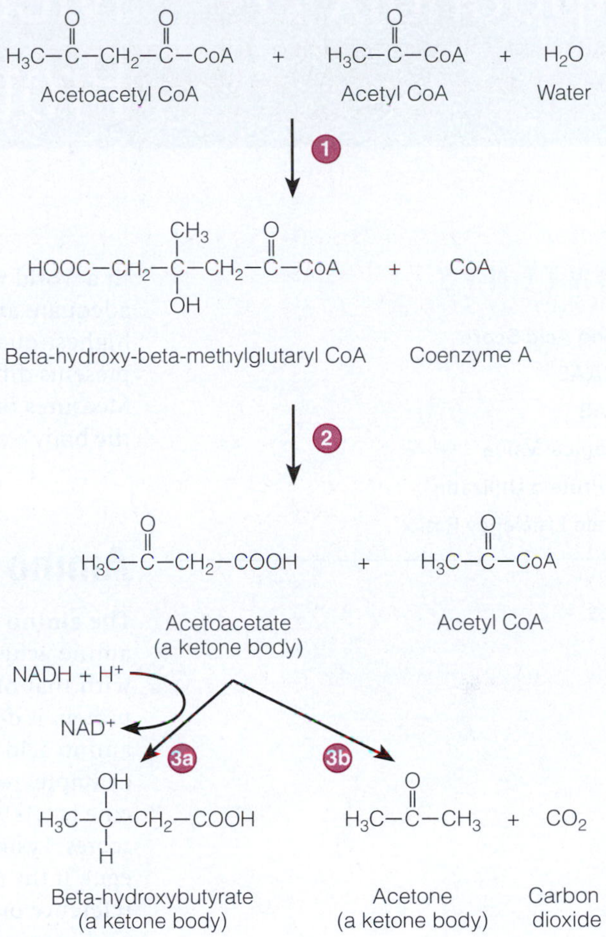

$H_3C{-}C({=}O){-}CH_2{-}C({=}O){-}CoA$ (Acetoacetyl CoA) + $H_3C{-}C({=}O){-}CoA$ (Acetyl CoA) + H_2O (Water)

↓ 1

$HOOC{-}CH_2{-}C(CH_3)(OH){-}CH_2{-}C({=}O){-}CoA$ (Beta-hydroxy-beta-methylglutaryl CoA) + CoA (Coenzyme A)

↓ 2

$H_3C{-}C({=}O){-}CH_2{-}COOH$ (Acetoacetate (a ketone body)) + $H_3C{-}C({=}O){-}CoA$ (Acetyl CoA)

3a (NADH + H^+ → NAD^+): $H_3C{-}CH(OH){-}CH_2{-}COOH$ (Beta-hydroxybutyrate (a ketone body))

3b: $H_3C{-}C({=}O){-}CH_3$ (Acetone (a ketone body)) + CO_2 (Carbon dioxide)

Appendix D Measures of Protein Quality

CONTENTS

In a world where food is scarce and many people's diets contain marginal or inadequate amounts of protein, it is important to know which foods contain the highest-quality protein. Chapter 6 described protein quality, and this appendix presents different measures researchers use to assess the quality of a food protein. Measures of protein quality aim to determine how well a food protein supports the body's normal metabolism and growth. Glossary D-1 defines related terms.

Amino Acid Score

The **amino acid score** predicts protein quality based on the pattern of essential amino acids. It compares the essential amino acid composition of a food protein with that of a reference protein (egg). The score of each amino acid in the food protein is described as a percentage of the amino acid in the reference protein. The amino acid with the lowest percentage score is the most limiting amino acid. For example, results might find that compared with the reference amino acids, leucine gets a 93, lysine gets an 80, and all the other essential amino acids get higher scores. Lysine is the limiting amino acid (the one that falls shortest compared with egg). If the protein's limiting amino acid is 80 percent of the amount found in the reference protein, it receives an amino acid score of 80. The advantages of amino acid scoring are that it is simple and inexpensive, it easily identifies the limiting amino acid, and it can be used to score mixtures of different proportions of multiple proteins mathematically without having to create a mixture to test. Its chief weakness is that it fails to estimate the digestibility of a protein, which may strongly affect the protein's quality.

PDCAAS

The **protein digestibility-corrected amino acid score,** or **PDCAAS,** is a widely used measurement of protein quality.[1] The PDCAAS compares the amino acid composition of a food protein with human amino acid requirements and corrects for digestibility. First the protein's essential amino acid composition is determined, and then it is compared against the amino acid requirements of

GLOSSARY D-1 PROTEIN QUALITY TERMS

amino acid score: a measure of protein quality assessed by comparing a protein's amino acid pattern with that of a reference protein; also called the *chemical score.*

biological value (BV): a measure of protein quality assessed by measuring the amount of protein nitrogen that is retained from a given amount of protein nitrogen absorbed.

DIAAS (digestible indispensable amino acid score): a measure of protein quality similar to PDCAAS, except it determines protein digestibility at the end of the small intestine, which more accurately reflects the extent of amino acid absorption.

net protein utilization (NPU): a measure of protein quality assessed by measuring the amount of protein nitrogen that is retained from a given amount of protein nitrogen eaten.

PDCAAS (protein digestibility-corrected amino acid score): a measure of protein quality assessed by comparing the amino acid score of a food protein with the amino acid requirements of preschool-aged children and then correcting for the true digestibility of the protein.

protein efficiency ratio (PER): a measure of protein quality assessed by determining how well a given protein supports weight gain in growing rats; used to establish the protein quality for infant formulas and baby foods.

preschool-aged children.[2] This comparison reveals the most limiting amino acid—the one that falls shortest compared with the reference. If a food protein's limiting amino acid is 70 percent of the amount found in the reference protein, it receives a score of 70. The amino acid score is multiplied by the food's protein digestibility percentage to determine the PDCAAS. How To D-1 provides an example of how to calculate the PDCAAS, and Table D-1 lists the PDCAAS values of selected foods.

TABLE D-1 PDCAAS Values of Selected Foods

Food	PDCAAS
Casein (milk protein)	1.00
Egg white	1.00
Soybean (isolate)	.99
Beef	.92
Pea flour	.69
Kidney beans (canned)	.68
Chickpeas (canned)	.66
Pinto beans (canned)	.66
Rolled oats	.57
Lentils (canned)	.52
Peanut meal	.52
Whole wheat	.40

NOTE: 1.0 is the maximum PDCAAS a food protein can receive.

DIAAS

The Food and Agriculture Organization (FAO) of the United Nations recommends another method, known as the Digestible Indispensable Amino Acid Score (DIAAS), to replace PDCAAS as the preferred method to determine protein quality.[3] The DIAAS overcomes some of the weaknesses of the current PDCAAS method. Whereas PDCAAS estimates protein digestibility over the entire intestine and uses a single digestibility score, the DIAAS determines amino acid digestibility at the end of the small intestine, which more accurately reflects the extent of amino acids absorption, and considers the digestibility of individual amino acids, as opposed to the protein as a whole.

Biological Value

The **biological value (BV)** of a food protein measures its efficiency in supporting the body's growth and maintenance. In a test of biological value, two nitrogen balance studies are done. In the first, no protein is fed, and nitrogen (N) excretions

> How To D-1 Measure Protein Quality Using PDCAAS

To calculate the PDCAAS (protein digestibility-corrected amino acid score), researchers first determine the amino acid profile of the test protein (in this example, pinto beans). The second column of the table below presents the essential amino acid profile of pinto beans. The third column presents the amino acid reference pattern.

To determine how well the food protein meets human needs, researchers calculate the ratio by dividing the second column by the third column (for example, 30 ÷ 18 = 1.67). The amino acid with the lowest percentage is the most limiting amino acid—in this case, methionine. Its percentage is the amino acid score for the protein—in this case, 0.84.

The amino acid score alone, however, does not account for digestibility. Protein digestibility, as determined by animal studies, yields a value of 79 percent for pinto beans. Together, the amino acid score and the digestibility value determine the PDCAAS:

$$\text{PDCAAS} = \text{protein digestibility} \times \text{amino acid score}$$

$$\text{PDCAAS for pinto beans} = 0.79 \times 0.84 = 0.66$$

Thus the PDCAAS for pinto beans is 0.66 as Table D-1 shows.

Essential Amino Acids	Amino Acid Profile of Pinto Beans (mg/g protein)	Amino Acid Reference Pattern (mg/g protein)	Amino Acid Score
Histidine	30.0	18	1.67
Isoleucine	42.5	25	1.70
Leucine	80.4	55	1.46
Lysine	69.0	51	1.35
Methionine (+ cystine)	21.1	25	0.84
Phenylalanine (+ tyrosine)	90.5	47	1.93
Threonine	43.7	27	1.62
Tryptophan	8.8	7	1.26
Valine	50.1	32	1.57

in the urine and feces are measured. It is assumed that under these conditions, N lost in the urine is the amount the body loses each day, regardless of food protein; this endogenous N is "urinary N on a zero-protein diet." The N lost in the feces is the amount the body loses each day, regardless of food protein; this metabolic N is "fecal N on a zero-protein diet."

In the second study, a diet containing the test protein in an amount equal to the requirement is fed. Intakes and losses are measured; then the BV is derived using this formula:

$$BV = \frac{\text{N retained}}{\text{N absorbed}} \times 100$$

The more nitrogen retained, the higher the protein quality. (Recall that when an essential amino acid is missing, protein synthesis stops, and the remaining amino acids are deaminated and the nitrogen excreted.)

Egg protein has a BV of 100, indicating that 100 percent of the nitrogen absorbed is retained. Supplied in adequate quantity, a protein with a BV of 70 or greater can support human growth as long as energy intake is adequate. Table D-2 presents the BV for selected foods.

TABLE D-2 Biological Values (BV) of Selected Foods

Food	BV
Egg	100
Milk	93
Beef	75
Fish	75
Corn	72

NOTE: 100 is the maximum BV a food protein can receive.

Net Protein Utilization

Like BV, **net protein utilization (NPU)** measures how efficiently a protein is used by the body and involves two balance studies. The difference is that NPU measures retention of food nitrogen consumed rather than food nitrogen absorbed (as in BV). The formula for NPU is:

$$NPU = \frac{\text{N retained}}{\text{N intake}} \times 100$$

The numerator is the same as for BV, but the denominator represents food N intake only—not N absorbed.

Protein Efficiency Ratio

The **protein efficiency ratio (PER)** measures the weight gain of a growing animal and compares it to the animal's protein intake. To determine the PER of a food protein, young, growing animals are given a standard diet containing about 10 percent (by weight) of the test protein. After a specified period of time, weight gain is measured and compared to the amount of test protein consumed. The PER is expressed as:

$$PER = \frac{\text{weight gain (g)}}{\text{protein intake (g)}}$$

Table D-3 presents PER values for selected foods.

TABLE D-3 Protein Efficiency Ratio (PER) Values of Selected Proteins

Protein	PER
Casein (milk)	2.8
Soy	2.4
Glutein (wheat)	0.4

APPENDIX D

REFERENCES

1. G. Schaafsma, Advantages and limitations of the protein digestibility-corrected amino acid score (PDCAAS) as a method for evaluating protein quality in human diets, *British Journal of Nutrition* 108 (2012): S333–S336.
2. D. J. Millward, Amino acid scoring patterns for protein quality assessment, *British Journal of Nutrition* 108 (2012): S31–S43.
3. R. R. Wolfe and coauthors, Protein quality as determined by the Digestible Indispensable Amino Acid Score: Evaluation of factors underlying the calculation, *Nutrition Reviews* 74 (2016): 584–599; S. Leser, The 2013 FAO report on dietary protein quality evaluation in human nutrition: Recommendations and implications, *Nutrition Bulletin* 38 (2013): 421–428.

Appendix E Nutrition Assessment

CONTENTS

Nutrition assessment evaluates a person's health from a nutrition perspective. Many factors influence or reflect nutrition status. Consequently, the assessor, usually a registered dietitian nutritionist (RDN) assisted by other qualified health-care professionals, gathers information from many sources, including:

- Historical information.
- Anthropometric measurements.
- Physical examinations.
- Biochemical analyses (laboratory tests).

Each of these methods involves collecting data in a variety of ways and interpreting each finding in relation to the others to create a total picture.

The accurate gathering of this information and its careful interpretation are the basis for a meaningful evaluation. The more information gathered about a person, the more accurate the assessment will be. Gathering information is a time-consuming process, however, and time is often a rare commodity in the health care setting. Nutrition care is only one part of total care. It may not be practical or essential to collect detailed information on each person.

A strategic compromise is to screen patients by collecting preliminary data. Data such as height-weight and hematocrit are easy to obtain and can alert health-care workers to potential problems. **Nutrition screening** identifies patients who will require additional nutrition assessment. This appendix provides a sample of the procedures, standards, and charts commonly used in nutrition assessment.

Historical Information

Historical information provides valuable clues about a person's nutrition status and nutrient requirements; it also reveals personal preferences that need consideration when developing a nutrition care plan. Table E-1 summarizes the different

TABLE E-1 Historical Information Used in Nutrition Assessments

Type of History	What It Identifies
Medical history	Current and previous mental, emotional, and physical health problems, treatments, and surgeries; chronic disease risks; and family medical history that affect nutrient needs, nutrition status, or the need for intervention to prevent or alleviate health problems
Personal and social history	Cognitive, educational, family, religious, cultural, financial, and environmental influences on food intake, nutrient needs, and diet therapy options
Medication and supplement history	Medications (prescription and over-the-counter), illicit drugs, dietary supplements, and alternative therapies that affect nutrition status
Food and nutrition history	Food intake and availability, recent weight changes, dietary restrictions, food allergies or intolerances, physical activity habits, nutrition and health knowledge

nutrition screening: a brief assessment of health-related variables to identify people who are malnourished or are at risk for malnutrition.

APPENDIX E

TABLE E-2 Medical Conditions Associated with Malnutrition

- Acquired immune deficiency syndrome (AIDS)
- Alcoholism
- Anorexia (lack of appetite)
- Anorexia nervosa
- Bulimia nervosa
- Burns (extensive or severe)
- Cancer
- Celiac disease
- Chewing or swallowing difficulties (including poorly fitted dentures, dental caries, missing teeth, and mouth ulcers)
- Chronic obstructive pulmonary disease
- Circulatory problems
- Constipation
- Crohn's disease
- Cystic fibrosis
- Decubitus ulcers (pressure sores)
- Dementia
- Depleted blood proteins
- Depression
- Diabetes mellitus
- Diarrhea, prolonged or severe
- Drug addiction
- Dysphagia
- Failure to thrive
- Feeding disabilities
- Fever
- GI tract disorders or surgery
- Heart disease
- HIV infection
- Hormonal imbalance
- Hyperlipidemia
- Hypertension
- Infections
- Inflammatory bowel diseases
- Kidney disease
- Liver disease
- Lung disease
- Malabsorption
- Mental illness
- Mental retardation
- Multiple pregnancies
- Nausea
- Neurologic disorders
- Organ failure
- Overweight
- Pancreatic insufficiency
- Paralysis
- Physical disability
- Pneumonia
- Pregnancy
- Radiation therapy
- Surgery (recent or major)
- Tobacco use
- Trauma
- Ulcerative colitis
- Ulcers
- Underweight
- Vomiting (prolonged or severe)

types of historical data that contribute to a nutrition assessment; this information is obtained from the medical record and interviews with the patient or caregiver.

An adept history taker uses the interview both to gather facts and to establish a rapport with the patient. This section briefly reviews the major areas of nutrition concern in a person's history.

Medical History

The assessor can obtain a **medical history** from records completed by the attending physician, nurse, or other health-care professional. In addition, conversations with the patient can uncover valuable information previously overlooked because no one thought to ask or because the patient was not thinking clearly when asked.

An accurate, complete medical history includes the person's current and ongoing medical issues; this information helps identify conditions and treatments that might lead to malnutrition (see Table E-2). A medical history includes the family medical history as well, which may reveal genetic susceptibilities for diseases that might be prevented with dietary and other lifestyle changes.

Personal and Social History

A **personal and social history** reveals factors that influence food choices and a person's ability to manage health and nutrition problems. The ethnic background and religious beliefs of both the patient and the other members of the household influence food choices. Financial concerns might restrict access to nutritious food and health care. In general, the quality of the diet declines as income falls. At some point, the ability to purchase the foods required to meet nutrient needs is lost; an inadequate income puts an adequate diet out of reach. Agencies use poverty indexes to identify people at risk for poor nutrition and to qualify people for government food assistance programs.

Low income affects not only the power to purchase foods but also the ability to shop for, store, and cook them; some individuals depend on others to procure and prepare meals. A person who lives alone or is depressed may eat poorly or be unable to follow complex dietary instructions. Use of alcohol, tobacco, or illicit drugs interferes with good health and nutrition status. A skilled assessor will note such concerns in the history.

medical history: an account of a patient's current and past health status and disease risks.

personal and social history: a record of a person's social and economic background, including such factors as education, income, and ethnic identity.

Medication and Supplement History

The many interactions of foods and drugs require that healthcare professionals take a **medication and supplement history** and pay special attention to any patient who takes drugs routinely. If a person is taking any drug, the assessor records the name of the drug; the dose, frequency, and duration of intake; the reason for taking the drug; and signs of any adverse effects. Highlight 17 (p. 560) discussed nutrient-drug interactions in more detail, and Table H17-1 (p. 561) summarizes the mechanisms by which these interactions occur and provides specific examples.

Food and Nutrition History

A **food and nutrition history** (often called a *diet history*) provides a record of a person's dietary practices. It includes information about food intake, lifestyle habits, and other factors that affect food choices, such as food allergies or beliefs about nutrition and health. The assessment often examines recent food intake as well as usual food choices.

Besides identifying possible nutrient imbalances, food and nutrition histories provide valuable clues about how a person will accept diet changes should they be necessary. Information about what and how a person eats provides the background for realistic and attainable nutrition goals. The following section describes the most common methods of gathering food intake information.

Food Intake Data

Assessors evaluate food intake using various tools such as the 24-hour recall, the food record, the food frequency questionnaire, and direct observation. Food models or photos and measuring devices can help patients identify the types of foods and quantities consumed. The assessor also needs to know how the foods are prepared and when they are eaten. In addition to asking about foods, assessors will ask about beverage consumption, including beverages containing alcohol or caffeine.

24-Hour Dietary Recall

The **24-hour dietary recall** provides data for one day only and is commonly used in nutrition surveys to obtain estimates of the typical food intakes for a population. The assessor asks an individual to recount all the foods and beverages consumed in the past 24 hours or for the previous day. The interview includes questions about the times of meals and snacks, amounts consumed, and methods of food preparation.

The multiple-pass method is the most effective approach for obtaining an accurate 24-hour recall. In this procedure, the interview includes four or five separate passes through the 24-hour period of interest. In the first pass, the person provides a "quick list" of foods consumed without prompts from the interviewer. The second pass helps the person remember foods that are often forgotten, such as beverages, bread, additions to foods (such as butter on toast), savory snacks, and sweets. Third and fourth passes elicit additional details about the foods consumed, such as the amounts eaten, preparation methods, and places where foods were obtained or consumed. A final pass provides an opportunity to recall foods and to probe for additional details. The entire multiple-pass interview can be conducted in about 30 to 45 minutes.

An advantage of the 24-hour recall is that it is relatively easy to obtain. It does not, however, provide enough information to allow accurate generalizations about an individual's usual food intake. The previous day's intake may not be typical, for example, or the person may be unable to report portion sizes accurately or may conceal or forget information about foods eaten. This limitation is partially overcome when 24-hour dietary recalls are collected on several nonconsecutive days.

Food Record

Another tool for history taking is the **food record**, in which the person records food and beverages consumed, including the quantity and method of preparation. Figure E-1 (p. E-4) provides an example. A food record can help both the assessor and the patient to determine factors associated with eating that may affect dietary balance and adequacy.

medication and supplement history: a record of all the drugs, over-the-counter and prescribed, as well as dietary and herbal supplements that a person takes routinely.

food and nutrition history: a record of eating behaviors and the foods a person eats.

24-hour dietary recall: a record of foods consumed during the previous day or in the past 24 hours; sometimes modified to include foods consumed in a typical day.

food record: a detailed log of all foods eaten during a specified time period, usually several days; also called a *food diary*. A food record may also include associated information such as when, where, and with whom each food as well as details about physical activity, medications, and disease symptoms.

> **FIGURE E-1 Food Record**

The entries in a food record should include the times and places of meals and snacks, the types and amounts of foods eaten, and a description of the individual's feelings when eating. The diary should also record physical activities: the kind, the intensity level, the duration, and the person's feelings about them.

Time	Place	Activity or food eaten	People present	Mood
10:30–10:40	School vending machine	6 peanut butter crackers and 12 oz. cola	by myself	starved
12:15–12:30	Restaurant	Sub sandwich and 12 oz. cola	friends	relaxed & friendly
3:00–3:45	Gym	Weight training	work out partner	tired
4:00–4:10	Snack bar	Small frozen yogurt	by myself	OK

© Cengage

Food records work especially well with cooperative people but require considerable time and effort on their part. A prime advantage is that the record keeper assumes an active role and may for the first time become aware of personal food habits and assume responsibility for them. It also provides the assessor with an accurate picture of the person's lifestyle and factors that affect food intake. For these reasons, a food record can be particularly useful in outpatient counseling for such nutrition problems as overweight, underweight, or food allergy. The major disadvantages stem from poor compliance in recording the data and conscious or unconscious changes in eating habits that may occur while the person is keeping the record.

Food Frequency Questionnaire An assessor uses a **food frequency questionnaire** to survey the foods and beverages regularly consumed during a specific time period. Some questionnaires are qualitative only: food lists contain common foods, organized by food group, with check boxes to indicate frequency of consumption (see Figure E-2). Other types of questionnaires can collect semiquantitative information by including portion sizes as well. This information helps pinpoint foods and food groups, and therefore nutrients, that may be excessive or deficient in the diet. That a person ate no vegetables yesterday may not seem particularly significant, but never eating vegetables is a warning of possible nutrient deficiencies. When used with the usual intake or 24-hour recall approach, the food frequency questionnaire enables the assessor to double-check the accuracy of the information obtained.

food frequency questionnaire: a checklist of foods routinely consumed. Some questionnaires ask only about the types of food eaten and yield qualitative information; others include questions about portions as well and yield semiquantitative data.

> **FIGURE E-2 Sample Section of a Food Frequency Questionnaire**

FRUIT	HOW OFTEN								HOW MUCH			
	Never or less than once per month	1 per mon.	2–3 per mon.	1 per week	2 per week	3–4 per week	5–6 per week	Every day	MEDIUM SERVING	YOUR SERVING SIZE S	M	L
EXAMPLE: Bananas	○	○	○	●	○	○	○	○	1 medium	○ 1/2	● 1	○ 2
Bananas	○	○	○	○	○	○	○	○	1 medium	○ 1/2	○ 1	○ 2
Apples, applesauce	○	○	○	○	○	○	○	○	1 medium or 1/2 cup	○ 1/2	○ 1	○ 2
Oranges (not including juice)	○	○	○	○	○	○	○	○	1 medium	○ 1/2	○ 1	○ 2
Grapefruit (not including juice)	○	○	○	○	○	○	○	○	1/2 medium	○ 1/4	○ 1/2	○ 1
Cantaloupe	○	○	○	○	○	○	○	○	1/4 medium	○ 1/8	○ 1/4	○ 1/2
Peaches, apricots (fresh, in season)	○	○	○	○	○	○	○	○	1 medium	○ 1/2	○ 1	○ 2
Peaches, apricots (canned or dried)	○	○	○	○	○	○	○	○	1 medium or 1/2 cup	○ 1/2	○ 1	○ 2
Prunes, or prune juice	○	○	○	○	○	○	○	○	1/2 cup	○ 1/4	○ 1/2	○ 1
Watermelon (in season)	○	○	○	○	○	○	○	○	1 slice	○ 1/2	○ 1	○ 2
Strawberries, other berries (in season)	○	○	○	○	○	○	○	○	1/2 cup	○ 1/4	○ 1/2	○ 1
Any other fruit, including kiwi, fruit cocktail, grapes, raisins, mangoes	○	○	○	○	○	○	○	○	1/2 cup	○ 1/4	○ 1/2	○ 1

© Cengage

Direct Observation In facilities that serve meals, food intakes can be directly observed and analyzed. This method can also reveal a person's food preferences, changes in appetite, and any problems with a prescribed diet. Health practitioners use direct observation to estimate a patient's intake of food energy (and often, protein) during a single day or on several consecutive days. To estimate food and nutrient intakes, the clinician records the dietary items that a patient is given at meals and subtracts the amounts remaining after meals are completed; this procedure allows an estimate of the amounts of foods and beverages actually consumed. Although a useful means of discerning patients' intakes, direct observation requires regular and careful documentation and can be labor-intensive and costly.

Analysis of Food Intake Data After collecting food intake data, the assessor estimates nutrient intakes, either informally by using food guides or formally by using diet analysis programs. The assessor compares intakes with standards, usually standards such as the RDA or dietary guidelines, to determine how closely the person's diet comes to meeting the standards. Are the types and amounts of proteins, carbohydrates (including fiber), and fats (including saturated fats and omega-3 fatty acids) appropriate? Are all food groups included in appropriate amounts? Is caffeine or alcohol consumption excessive? Are intakes of any vitamins or minerals (including sodium and iron) excessive or deficient? An informal evaluation is possible only if the assessor has enough prior experience with formal calculations to "see" nutrient amounts in reported food intakes without calculations. Even then, such an informal analysis is best followed by a spot check for key nutrients by actual calculation.

Limitations of Food Intake Analysis Diet histories can be most informative, but the skillful assessor also keeps their limitations in mind. For example, reported portion sizes may not be correct. The person who reports eating "a serving" of greens may not distinguish between ¼ cup and 2 cups; only individuals who have practice measuring food quantities can accurately report serving sizes. Children tend to remember the serving sizes of foods they like as being larger than serving sizes of foods they dislike.

An estimate of nutrient intakes from a food and nutrition history, combined with other sources of information, allows the assessor to confirm or eliminate the possibility of suspected nutrition problems. The assessor must constantly remember that nutrient intakes in adequate amounts do not guarantee adequate nutrient status for an individual. Likewise, insufficient intakes do not always indicate deficiencies, but instead alert the assessor to possible problems. Each person digests, absorbs, metabolizes, and excretes nutrients in a unique way; individual needs vary. Intakes of nutrients identified by diet histories are only pieces of a puzzle that must be put together with other indicators of nutrition status in order to extract meaning.

Anthropometric Measurements

Anthropometrics are physical measurements that reflect body composition and development (see Table E-3). They serve three main purposes: first, to evaluate the progress of growth in pregnant women, infants, children, and adolescents; second, to detect undernutrition and overnutrition in all age groups; and third, to measure changes in body composition over time.

Health-care professionals compare anthropometric measurements taken on an individual with population standards specific for gender and age or with previous measures of the individual. Measurements taken periodically and compared with previous measurements reveal changes in an individual's status.

Mastering the techniques for taking anthropometric measurements requires proper instruction and practice to ensure reliability. Once the correct techniques are learned, taking measurements is easy and requires minimal equipment.

anthropometrics (AN-throw-poe-MET-ricks): relating to measurement of the physical characteristics of the body, such as height and weight.

- **anthropos** = human
- **metric** = measuring

> **FIGURE E-3 Length Measurement of an Infant**

An infant is measured lying down on a measuring board with a fixed headboard and a movable footboard. Note that two people are needed to measure the infant's length.

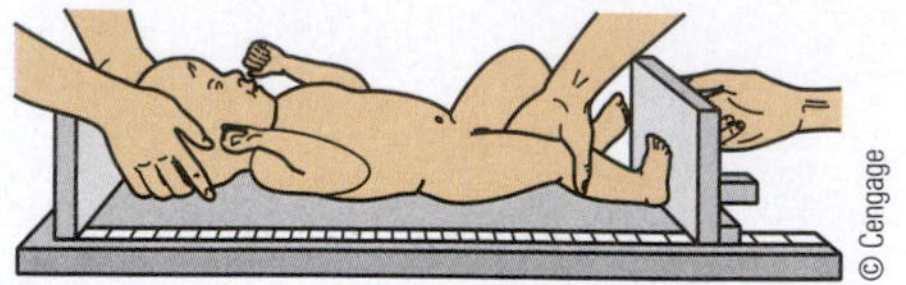

TABLE E-3 Anthropometric Measurements Used in Nutrition Assessments

Type of Measurement	What It Reflects
Abdominal girth measurement	Abdominal fluid retention and abdominal organ size
Height-weight	Overnutrition and undernutrition; growth in children
Head circumference	Brain growth and development in infants and children under age 2
Skinfold	Subcutaneous and total body fat
Waist circumference	Body fat distribution

Height and weight are well-recognized anthropometrics; other anthropometrics include skinfold measurements and various measures of lean tissue. Other measures are useful in specific situations. For example, a head circumference measurement may help assess brain development in an infant, and an abdominal girth measurement supplies information about abdominal fluid retention in individuals with liver disease.

Measures of Growth and Development

Height and weight are among the most common and useful anthropometric measurements. Length measurements for infants and children up to age 3 and height measurements for children over 3 are particularly valuable in assessing growth and therefore nutrition status. For adults, height measurements alone are not critical, but help estimate healthy weight and to interpret other assessment data. Once adult height has been reached, changes in body weight provide useful information in assessing overnutrition and undernutrition.

Height For infants and children younger than 3, health-care professionals may use special equipment to measure length. The assessor lays the barefoot infant on a measuring board that has a fixed headboard and movable footboard attached at right angles to the surface (see Figure E-3). Often two people are needed to obtain an accurate measurement: one to gently hold the infant's head against the headboard, and the other to straighten the infant's legs and move the footboard to the bottom of the infant's feet.

The procedure for measuring a child who can stand erect and cooperate is the same as for an adult. The best way to measure standing height is with the person's back against a flat wall to which a nonstretchable measuring tape or stick has been fixed (see Figure E-4). The person stands erect, without shoes, with heels together. The person's line of sight should be horizontal, with the heels, buttocks, shoulders, and head touching the wall. The assessor places a ruler or other inflexible object on top of the head at a right angle to the wall; carefully checks the height measurement; and records it immediately in either inches or centimeters so that the correct measurement will not be forgotten.

The measuring rod of a scale is commonly used, but is less accurate because it bends easily. The assessor follows the same general procedure, asking the person to face away from the scale and to take extra care to stand erect.

Unfortunately, many health-care professionals merely ask patients how tall they are rather than measuring their height. Self-reported height is often inaccurate and should be used only as a last resort when measurement is impractical (in the case of an uncooperative patient, an emergency admission, or the like).

Weight Valid weight measurements require scales that have been carefully maintained, calibrated, and checked for accuracy at regular intervals. Beam balance and electronic scales are the most accurate. To measure infants' weight, assessors use special scales that allow infants to lie or sit (see Figure E-5). Weighing infants naked, without diapers, is standard procedure. Children who can stand are weighed in the same way as adults (see Figure E-6). To make repeated measures

> **FIGURE E-4 Height Measurement of an Older Child or Adult**

Height is measured most accurately when the person stands against a flat wall to which a measuring tape has been affixed.

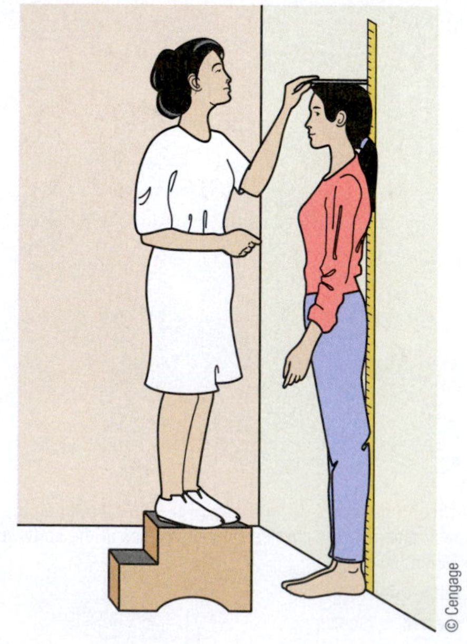

useful, standardized conditions are necessary. Each weighing should take place at the same time of day (preferably before breakfast), in the same amount of clothing (without shoes), after the person has voided, and on the same scale. Special scales and hospital beds with built-in scales are available for weighing people who are bedridden. Bathroom scales are inaccurate and inappropriate in a professional setting. As with all measurements, the assessor records the observed weight immediately in either pounds or kilograms.

Head Circumference Assessors may also measure head circumference to confirm that infant growth is proceeding normally or to help detect malnutrition and evaluate the extent of its impact on brain size. To measure head circumference, the assessor places a nonstretchable tape so that it encircles the largest part of the infant's or child's head: just above the eyebrow ridges, just above the point where the ears attach, and around the occipital prominence at the back of the head. To ensure accurate recording, the assessor immediately notes the measure in either inches or centimeters.

Analysis of Measures in Infants and Children Growth retardation is a sign of poor nutrition status. Obesity is also a sign that dietary intervention may be needed.

Health professionals generally evaluate physical development by monitoring the growth rate of a child and comparing this rate with standard charts. Standard charts compare weight to age, height to age, and weight to height; ideally, height and weight are in roughly the same percentile. Although individual growth patterns may vary, a child's growth curve will generally stay at about the same percentile throughout childhood. In children whose growth has been retarded, nutrition rehabilitation will ideally induce height and weight to increase to higher percentiles. In overweight children, the goal is for weight to remain stable as height increases, until weight becomes appropriate for height.

To evaluate growth in infants, an assessor uses charts such as those in Figures E-7 through E-9 (pp. E-8 through E-10). The assessor follows these steps to plot a weight measurement on a percentile graph:

- Select the appropriate chart based on age and gender.
- Locate the child's age along the horizontal axis on the bottom of the chart.
- Locate the child's weight in pounds or kilograms along the vertical axis.
- Mark the chart where the age and weight lines intersect, and read off the percentile.

To assess length, height, or head circumference, the assessor follows the same procedure, using the appropriate chart. (When length is measured, use the chart for birth to 36 months; when height is measured, use the chart for 2 to 20 years.) Head circumference percentile should be similar to the child's height and weight percentiles. With height, weight, and head circumference measures plotted on growth percentile charts, a skilled clinician can begin to interpret the data.

Percentile charts divide the measures of a population into 100 equal divisions. Thus half of the population falls above the 50th percentile, and half falls below. The use of percentile measures allows for comparisons among people of the same age and gender. For example, a 6-month-old female infant whose weight is at the 75 percentile weighs more than 75 percent of the female infants her age.

Head circumference is generally measured in children under 2 years of age. Because the brain grows rapidly before birth and during early infancy, extreme and chronic malnutrition during these times can impair brain development, curtailing the number of brain cells and the size of head circumference. Nonnutritional factors, such as certain disorders and genetic variation, can also influence head circumference.

Analysis of Measures in Adults For adults, health-care professionals typically compare weights with weight-for-height standards. One such standard is the body mass index (BMI), described in Chapter 8, which is useful for estimating the risk

> FIGURE E-5 Weight Measurement of an Infant

Infants sit or lie down on scales that are designed to hold them while they are being weighed.

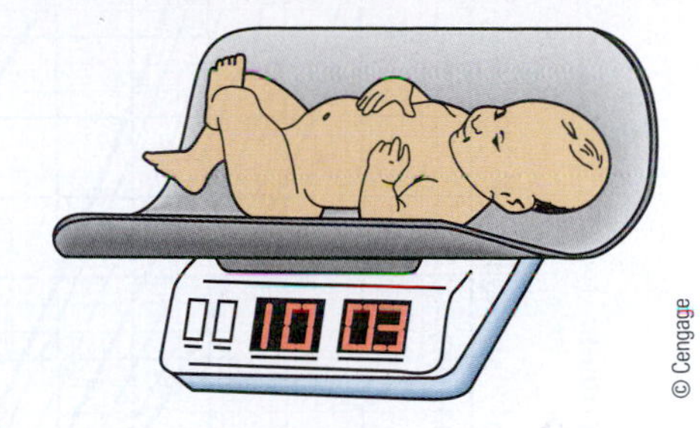
© Cengage

> FIGURE E-6 Weight Measurement of an Older Child or Adult

Whenever possible, children and adults are measured on beam balance or electronic scales to ensure accuracy.

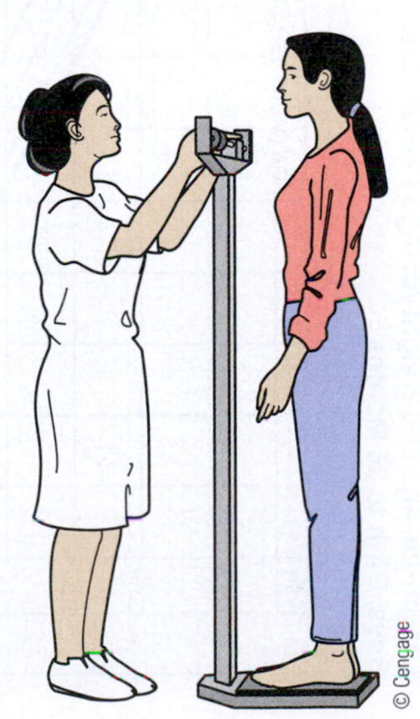
© Cengage

APPENDIX E

> **FIGURE E-7** Length-for-Age and Weight-for-Age Percentiles

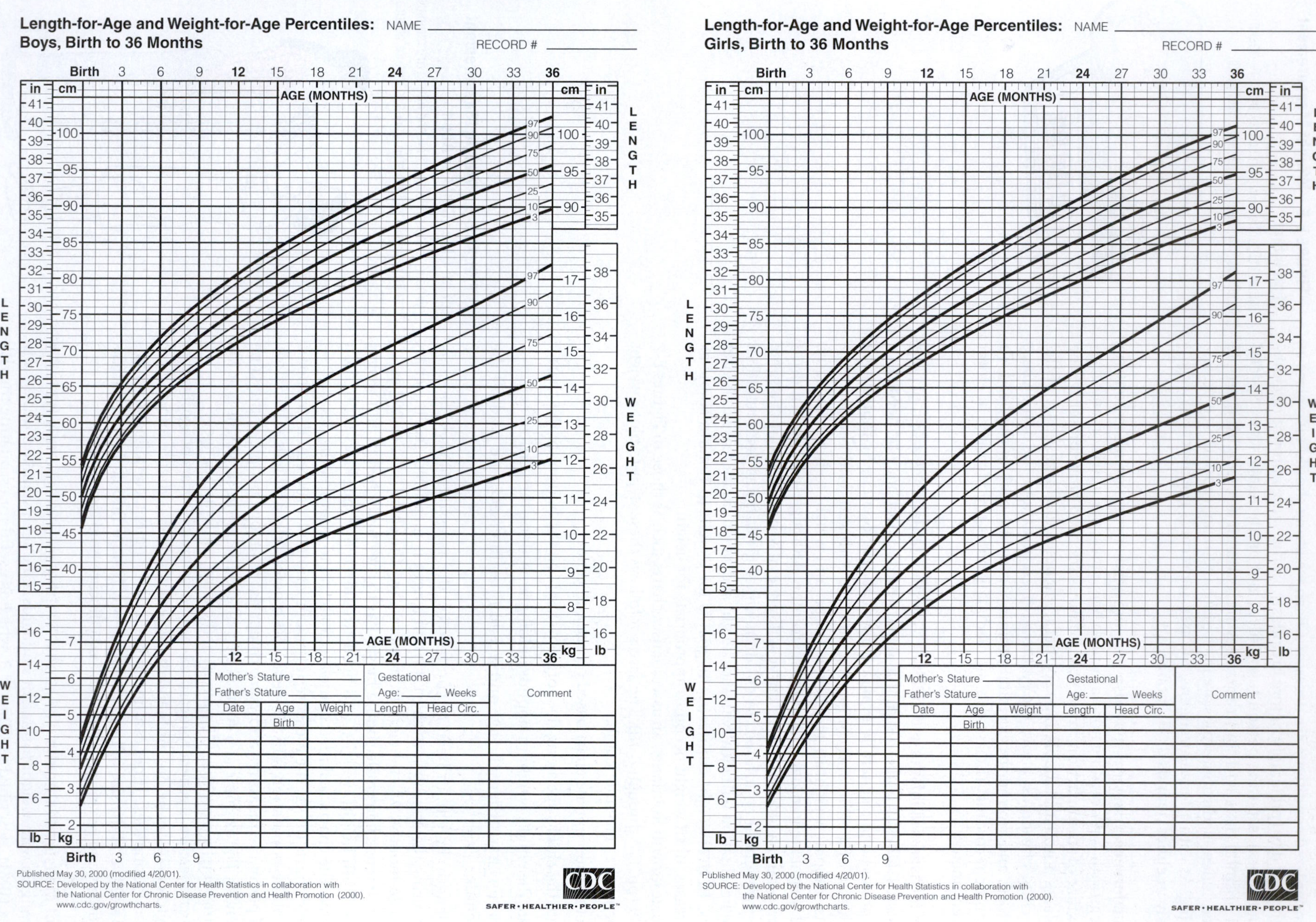
Length-for-Age and Weight-for-Age Percentiles: NAME
Boys, Birth to 36 Months
RECORD #
AGE (MONTHS)
Birth 3 6 9 12 15 18 21 24 27 30 33 36
LENGTH
WEIGHT
in
cm
kg
lb
97 90 75 50 25 10 3
Mother's Stature
Father's Stature
Gestational Age: Weeks
Date
Age
Weight
Length
Head Circ.
Comment
Birth
Published May 30, 2000 (modified 4/20/01).
SOURCE: Developed by the National Center for Health Statistics in collaboration with the National Center for Chronic Disease Prevention and Health Promotion (2000).
www.cdc.gov/growthcharts.
CDC
SAFER • HEALTHIER • PEOPLE™
Length-for-Age and Weight-for-Age Percentiles: NAME
Girls, Birth to 36 Months
RECORD #
AGE (MONTHS)
Birth 3 6 9 12 15 18 21 24 27 30 33 36
LENGTH
WEIGHT
97 90 75 50 25 10 3
Mother's Stature
Father's Stature
Gestational Age: Weeks
Date
Age
Weight
Length
Head Circ.
Comment
Birth
Published May 30, 2000 (modified 4/20/01).
SOURCE: Developed by the National Center for Health Statistics in collaboration with the National Center for Chronic Disease Prevention and Health Promotion (2000).
www.cdc.gov/growthcharts.
CDC
SAFER • HEALTHIER • PEOPLE™

> **FIGURE E-8** Head Circumference-for-Age and Weight-for-Length Percentiles

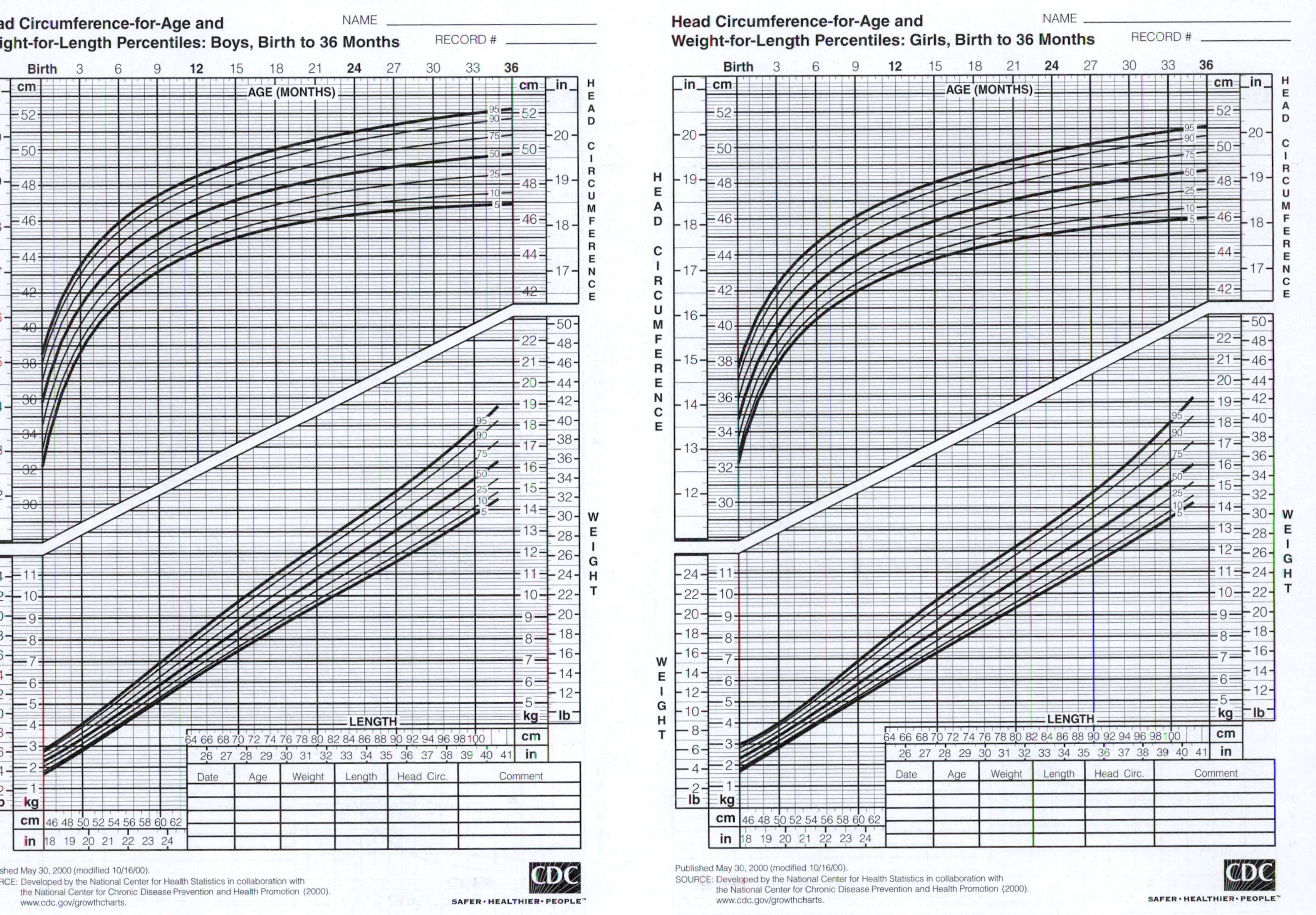

Head Circumference-for-Age and Weight-for-Length Percentiles: Boys, Birth to 36 Months
NAME
RECORD #
AGE (MONTHS)
Birth 3 6 9 12 15 18 21 24 27 30 33 36
HEAD CIRCUMFERENCE
WEIGHT
LENGTH
Date
Age
Weight
Length
Head Circ.
Comment
Published May 30, 2000 (modified 10/16/00).
SOURCE: Developed by the National Center for Health Statistics in collaboration with the National Center for Chronic Disease Prevention and Health Promotion (2000).
www.cdc.gov/growthcharts.
CDC
SAFER • HEALTHIER • PEOPLE™
Head Circumference-for-Age and Weight-for-Length Percentiles: Girls, Birth to 36 Months
NAME
RECORD #
AGE (MONTHS)
Birth 3 6 9 12 15 18 21 24 27 30 33 36
HEAD CIRCUMFERENCE
WEIGHT
LENGTH
Date
Age
Weight
Length
Head Circ.
Comment
Published May 30, 2000 (modified 10/16/00).
SOURCE: Developed by the National Center for Health Statistics in collaboration with the National Center for Chronic Disease Prevention and Health Promotion (2000).
www.cdc.gov/growthcharts.
CDC
SAFER • HEALTHIER • PEOPLE™

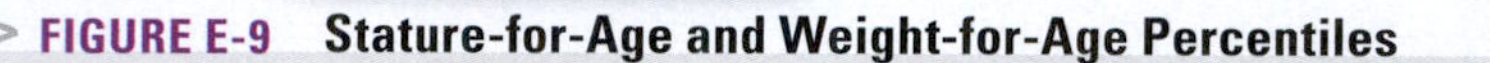
APPENDIX E

> **FIGURE E-9** Stature-for-Age and Weight-for-Age Percentiles

Stature-for-Age and Weight-for-Age Percentiles: Boys, 2 to 20 Years

NAME ______________

RECORD # ______________

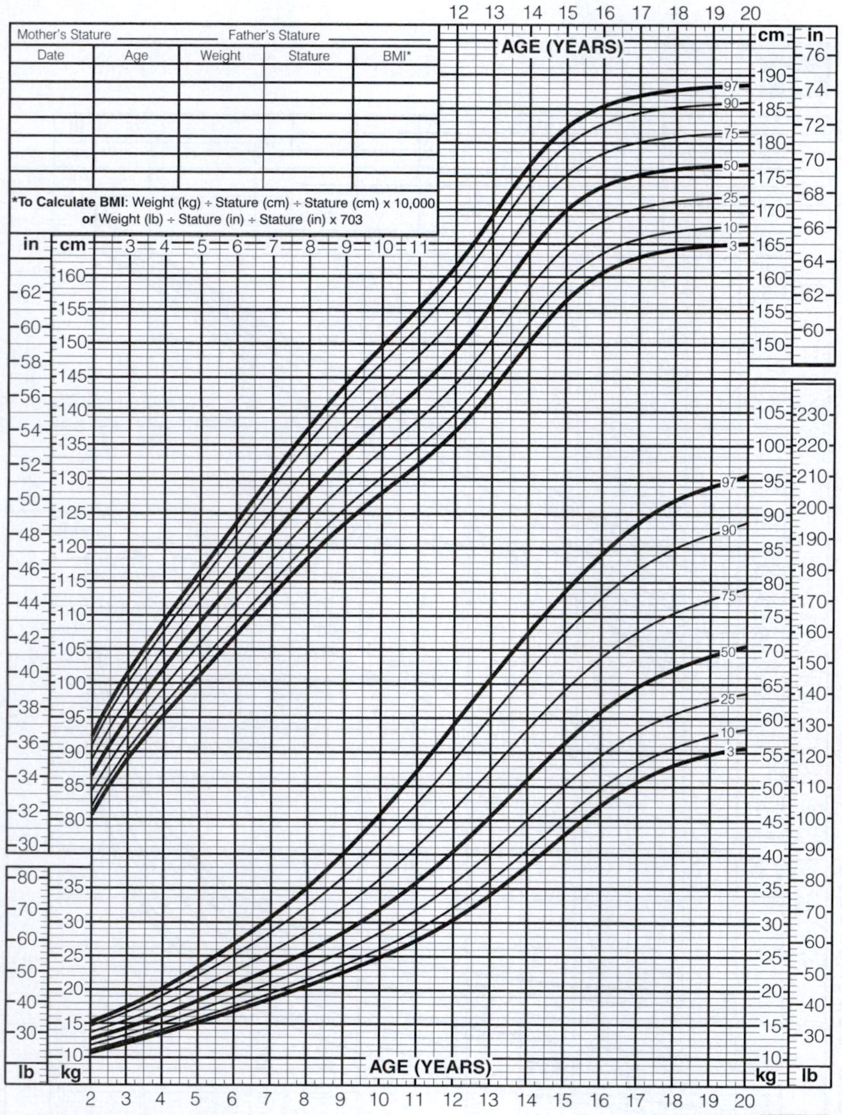

Mother's Stature ______ Father's Stature ______

Date	Age	Weight	Stature	BMI*

*To Calculate BMI: Weight (kg) ÷ Stature (cm) ÷ Stature (cm) x 10,000 or Weight (lb) ÷ Stature (in) ÷ Stature (in) x 703

Published May 30, 2000 (modified 11/21/00).
SOURCE: Developed by the National Center for Health Statistics in collaboration with the National Center for Chronic Disease Prevention and Health Promotion (2000). www.cdc.gov/growthcharts.

CDC SAFER • HEALTHIER • PEOPLE™

Stature-for-Age and Weight-for-Age Percentiles: Girls, 2 to 20 Years

NAME ______________

RECORD # ______________

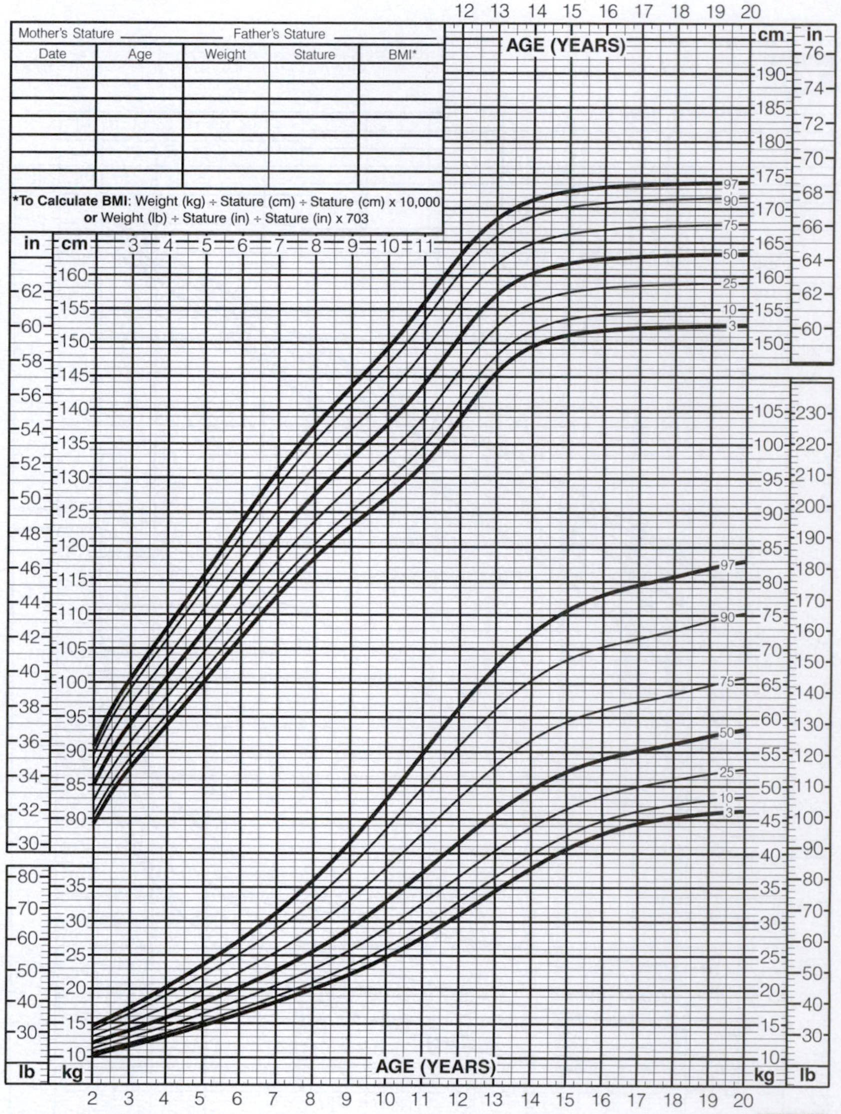

Mother's Stature ______ Father's Stature ______

Date	Age	Weight	Stature	BMI*

*To Calculate BMI: Weight (kg) ÷ Stature (cm) ÷ Stature (cm) x 10,000 or Weight (lb) ÷ Stature (in) ÷ Stature (in) x 703

Published May 30, 2000 (modified 11/21/00).
SOURCE: Developed by the National Center for Health Statistics in collaboration with the National Center for Chronic Disease Prevention and Health Promotion (2000). www.cdc.gov/growthcharts.

CDC SAFER • HEALTHIER • PEOPLE™

to health associated with overnutrition. The insert shows BMI for various heights and weights.

Measures of Body Fat and Lean Tissue

Significant weight changes in both children and adults can reflect overnutrition and undernutrition. To estimate the degree to which fat stores or lean tissues have changed, several anthropometric measurements are useful (review Table E-3, p. E-6).

Skinfold Measures Skinfold measures provide a good estimate of total body fat and a fair assessment of the fat's location. Approximately half the fat in the body lies directly beneath the skin, and the thickness of this subcutaneous fat reflects total body fat. In some parts of the body, such as the back and the back of the arm over the triceps muscle, this fat is loosely attached; a person can pull it up between the thumb and forefinger to obtain a measure of skinfold thickness. (Other common sites for skinfold measures include the biceps, subscapular area below the shoulder blade, suprailiac area above the hip bone, abdomen, and upper thigh.) To measure skinfold, a skilled assessor follows a standard procedure using reliable calipers (illustrated in Figure E-10) and then compares the measurement with standards.

If a person gains body fat, the skinfold increases proportionately; if the person loses fat, it decreases. Measurements taken from central-body sites (around the abdomen) better reflect changes in fatness than those taken from upper sites (arm and back). Because subcutaneous fat may be thicker in one area than in another, skinfold measurements are often taken at several (usually three) different places

> **FIGURE E-10 How to Measure the Triceps Skinfold**

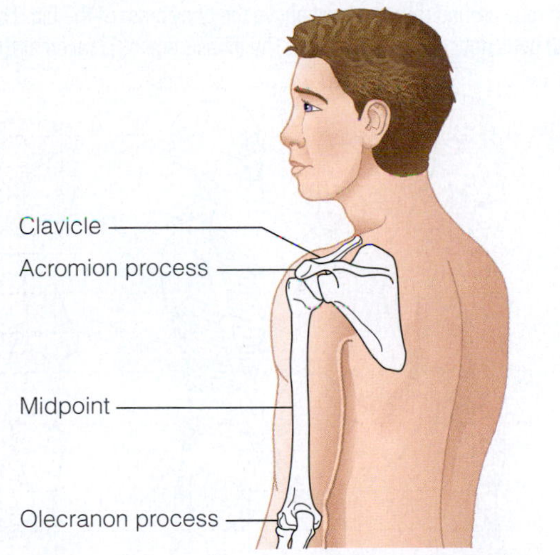
Clavicle
Acromion process
Midpoint
Olecranon process

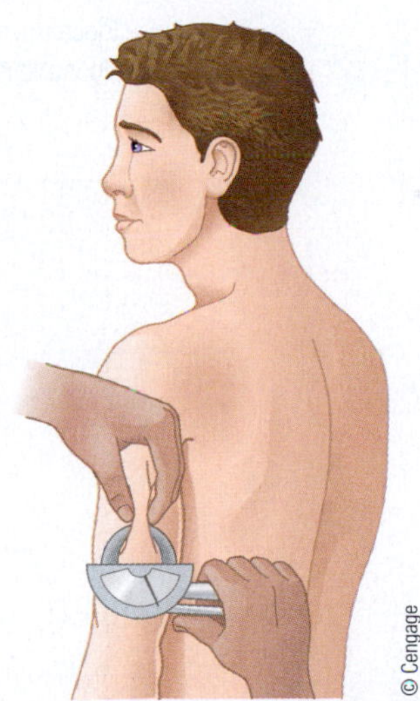
© Cengage

A. Find the midpoint of the arm:
1. Ask the subject to bend his or her arm at the elbow and lay the hand across the stomach. (If he or she is right-handed, measure the left arm, and vice versa.)
2. Feel the shoulder to locate the acromion process. It helps slide your fingers along the clavicle to find the acromion process. The olecranon process is the tip of the elbow.
3. Place a measuring tape from the acromion process to the tip of the elbow. Divide this measurement by 2, and mark the midpoint of the arm with a pen.

B. Measure the skinfold:
1. Ask the subject to let his or her arm hang loosely to the side.
2. Grasp a fold of skin and subcutaneous fat between the thumb and forefinger slightly above the midpoint mark. Gently pull the skin away from the underlying muscle. (This step takes a lot of practice. To be sure you don't have muscle as well as fat, ask the subject to contract and relax the muscle. You should be able to feel if you are pinching muscle.)
3. Place the calipers over the skinfold at the midpoint mark, and read the measurement to the nearest 1.0 millimeter in two to three seconds. (If using plastic calipers, align pressure lines, and read the measurement to the nearest 1.0 millimeter in two to three seconds.)
4. Repeat steps 2 and 3 twice more. Add the three readings, and then divide by 3 to find the average.

on the body (including upper-, central-, and lower-body sites); the sum of these measures is then compared with standards. Multiple measures are not always practical in clinical settings, however, and most often, the triceps skinfold measurement alone is used because it is easily accessible.

Waist Circumference Chapter 8 described how fat distribution correlates with health risks and mentioned that the waist circumference is a valuable indicator of abdominal fat. To measure waist circumference, the assessor places a non-stretchable tape around the person's body, crossing just above the upper hip bones and making sure that the tape remains on a level horizontal plane on all sides (see Figure E-11). The tape is tightened slightly, but without compressing the skin.

Waist-to-Hip Ratio Alternatively, some clinicians measure both the waist and the hips. Like the waist circumference, the waist-to-hip ratio also assesses abdominal obesity, but provides no more information than using the waist circumference alone. To calculate the waist-to-hip ratio, divide the waistline measurement by the hip measurement. For example, a woman with a 28-inch waist and 38-inch hips would have a ratio of 28 ÷ 38 = 0.74. In general, women with a waist-to-hip ratio of 0.80 or greater and men with a waist-to-hip ratio of 0.90 or greater have an increased risk of heart disease and diabetes.

Hydrodensitometry To estimate body density using hydrodensitometry, the person is weighed twice—first on land and then again when submerged under water. Underwater weighing usually generates a good estimate of body fat and is useful in research, although the technique has drawbacks: it requires bulky, expensive, and

> FIGURE E-11 How to Measure Waist Circumference

Place the measuring tape around the waist just above the bony crest of the hip. The tape runs parallel to the floor and is snug (but does not compress the skin). The measurement is taken at the end of normal expiration.

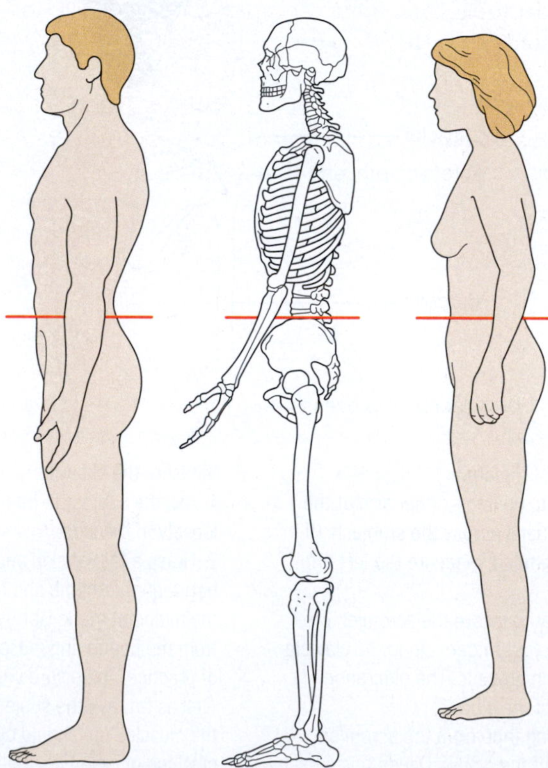

SOURCE: National Institutes of Health Obesity Education Initiative, *Clinical Guidelines on the Identification, Evaluation, and Treatment of Overweight and Obesity in Adults* (Washington, D.C.: U.S. Department of Health and Human Services, 1998), p. 59.

TABLE E-4 Methods of Estimating Body Fat and Its Distribution

Method	Cost	Ease of Use	Accuracy	Measures Fat Distribution
Height and weight	Low	Easy	High	No
Skinfolds	Low	Easy	Low	Yes
Circumferences	Low	Easy	Moderate	Yes
Ultrasound	Moderate	Moderate	Moderate	Yes
Hydrodensitometry	Low	Moderate	High	No
Heavy water tritiated	Moderate	Moderate	High	No
Deuterium oxide, or heavy oxygen	High	Moderate	High	No
Potassium isotope (^{40}K)	Very high	Difficult	High	No
Total body electrical conductivity (TOBEC)	High	Moderate	High	No
Bioelectric impedance (BIA)	Moderate	Easy	High	No
Dual-energy X-ray absorptiometry (DEXA)	High	Easy	High	No
Computed tomography (CT)	Very high	Difficult	High	Yes
Magnetic resonance imaging (MRI)	Very high	Difficult	High	Yes

SOURCE: Adapted from G. A. Bray, a handout presented at the North American Association for the Study of Obesity and Emory University School of Medicine Conference on Obesity. Update: Pathophysiology, Clinical Consequences, and Therapeutic Options, Atlanta, Georgia, August 31–September 2, 1992.

nonportable equipment. Furthermore, submerging some people (especially those who are very young, very old, ill, or fearful) under water is not always practical.

Bioelectric Impedance To measure body fat using the bioelectric impedance method, a very-low-intensity electrical current is briefly sent through the body by way of electrodes placed on the wrist and ankle. Fat impedes the flow of electricity; thus the magnitude of the current is influenced by the body's fat content. Recent food intake and hydration status can influence results. As with other anthropometric techniques, bioelectrical impedance requires standardized procedures and calibrated instruments to provide reliable results.

Chapter 8 (see Figure 8-10, p. 246) illustrated several anthropometric measures of body fat and lean tissue. Clinicians use other methods to estimate body fat and its distribution as well. Each has its advantages and disadvantages as Table E-4 summarizes.

Physical Examinations

An assessor can use a physical examination to search for signs of nutrient deficiency or toxicity. Like the other assessment methods, such an examination requires knowledge and skill. Many physical signs are nonspecific; they can reflect any of several nutrient deficiencies as well as conditions not related to nutrition (see Table E-5, p. E-14). For example, cracked lips may be caused by sunburn, windburn, dehydration, or any of several B vitamin deficiencies, to name just a few possible causes. For this reason, physical findings are most valuable in revealing problems for other assessment techniques to confirm or for confirming other assessment measures.

With this limitation understood, physical symptoms can be most informative about nutrition health. Many tissues and organs can reflect signs of malnutrition. The signs appear most rapidly in parts of the body where cell replacement occurs at a high rate, such as in the hair, skin, and digestive tract (including the mouth and tongue). The summary tables in Chapters 10 through 13 listed additional physical signs of vitamin and mineral malnutrition.

TABLE E-5 Physical Findings Used in Nutrition Assessments

Body System	Signs of Good Health	Signs of Malnutrition	Other Possible Causes
Hair	Shiny, firmly attached to the scalp	Dull, brittle, dry, loose; falls out (severe acute malnutrition); corkscrew hair (vitamin C)	Excessive hair bleaching; hair loss from aging, chemotherapy, or radiation therapy
Eyes	Bright, clear, pink, moist membranes; adjust easily to light	Pale membranes (iron); spots, dryness, night blindness (vitamin A); redness at corners of eyes (B vitamins)	Anemia unrelated to nutrition; eye disorders; allergies; aging
Mouth	No sores, swelling, or bleeding; red tongue; normal sense of taste; no caries; ability to chew and swallow; smooth lips	Bleeding gums (vitamin C); smooth or magenta tongue (B vitamins); poor taste sensation (zinc); dry, cracked, or sores in the corners of the lips (B vitamins)	Sunburn, windburn, excessive salivation from ill-fitting dentures or various disorders, medications, periodontal diseases, poor dental hygiene
Skin	Smooth, firm, good color	Poor wound healing (severe acute malnutrition, vitamin C, zinc); dry, rough, lack of fat under skin (essential fatty acids, vitamin A, B vitamins); bruising or bleeding under skin (vitamin C and vitamin K); pale (iron)	Poor skin hygiene, diabetes mellitus, aging, medications
Nails	Firm, pink, smooth	Spoon-shaped, brittle, pale (iron); rigid (protein malnutrition)	
Other	———	Dementia, peripheral neuropathy (B vitamins); enlarged thyroid gland (iodine); bowed legs (vitamin D)	Disorders of aging (dementia); diabetes (peripheral neuropathy)

Biochemical Analyses

All of the approaches to nutrition assessment discussed so far are external approaches. Biochemical analyses or laboratory tests help determine what is happening to the body internally. Common tests are based on analysis of blood and urine samples, which contain nutrients, enzymes, and metabolites that reflect nutrition status. Other tests, such as blood glucose, help pinpoint disease-related problems with nutrition implications. Tests that define fluid and electrolyte balance, acid-base balance, and organ function also have nutrition implications. Table E-6 lists biochemical tests most useful for assessing vitamin and mineral status.

The interpretation of biochemical data requires skill. Long metabolic sequences lead to the production of the end-products and metabolites seen in blood and urine. No single test can reveal nutrition status because many factors influence test results. The low blood concentration of a nutrient may reflect a primary deficiency of that nutrient, but it may also be secondary to the deficiency of one or several other nutrients or to a disease. Taken together with other assessment data, however, laboratory test results help create a picture that becomes clear with careful interpretation. They are especially useful in helping to detect subclinical malnutrition by uncovering early signs of malnutrition before the clinical signs of a classic deficiency disease appear.

Laboratory tests used to assess vitamin and mineral status are particularly useful when combined with diet histories and physical findings. Vitamin and mineral levels present in the blood and urine sometimes reflect recent rather than long-term intakes. This makes detecting subclinical deficiencies difficult. Furthermore, many nutrients interact; therefore, the amounts of other nutrients in the body can affect a lab value for a particular nutrient. It is also important to remember that nonnutrient conditions such as diseases influence biochemical measures.

It is beyond the scope of this text to describe all lab tests and their relations to nutrition status. Instead, the emphasis is on lab tests used to detect protein malnutrition and nutritional anemias.

Protein Malnutrition

No single biochemical analysis can adequately evaluate protein malnutrition. This discussion focuses on the measures commonly used today—transthyretin, retinol-binding protein, serum transferrin, and IGF-1 (insulin-like growth factor 1). Table E-6 provides standards for these indicators. Although serum albumin is easily and routinely measured, it lacks the sensitivity to assess protein malnutrition because of its long turnover rate.*

TABLE E-6 Normal Values for Serum Proteins

Test	Normal Values
Albumin (g/dL)	3.4–4.8
Transferrin (mg/dL)	200–360
Transthyretin (mg/dL)	20–40
Retinol-binding protein (mg/dL)	3–7
IGF-1 (μg/L)	300

NOTE: Levels less than normal suggest compromised protein status.

Transthyretin and Retinol-Binding Protein

Transthyretin and retinol-binding protein occur as a complex in the plasma.** They have a rapid turnover and thus respond quickly to dietary protein inadequacy and therapy.*** Conditions other than malnutrition that lower transthyretin include metabolic stress, hemodialysis, and hypothyroidism; those that raise transthyretin include kidney disease and corticosteroid use. Conditions other than protein malnutrition that lower retinol-binding protein include vitamin A deficiency, metabolic stress, hyperthyroidism, liver disease, and cystic fibrosis; kidney disease raises retinol-binding protein levels.

Serum Transferrin

Serum transferrin transports iron; consequently, its concentrations reflect both protein and iron status. Using transferrin as an indicator of protein status is complicated when an iron deficiency is present. Transferrin rises as iron deficiency grows worse and falls as iron status improves. Markedly reduced transferrin levels indicate severe protein malnutrition; in mild-to-moderate protein malnutrition, transferrin levels may vary, limiting their usefulness. Conditions other than protein malnutrition that lower transferrin include liver disease, kidney disease, and metabolic stress; those that raise transferrin include pregnancy, iron deficiency, hepatitis, blood loss, and oral contraceptive use. Although transferrin breaks down in the body more quickly than albumin, it is still relatively slow to respond to changes in protein intake and is not a sensitive indicator of the response to therapy.†

IGF-1 (Insulin-like Growth Factor 1)

IGF-1 (insulin-like growth factor 1) declines in protein malnutrition. IGF-1 has a relatively short **half-life** and responds specifically to dietary protein rather than energy.†† For these reasons, it is a sensitive indicator of protein status and response to therapy. Conditions that decrease IGF-1 include anorexia nervosa, inflammatory bowel disease, celiac disease, HIV infection, and fasting.

Nutritional Anemias

Anemia, which can result from a wide variety of nutrition- and nonnutrition-related disorders, is characterized by a significant reduction in the blood's oxygen-carrying capacity. Iron, folate, and vitamin B_{12} deficiencies—caused by inadequate intake, poor absorption, or abnormal metabolism of these nutrients—are the most common nutrition-related anemias. The remainder of this appendix describes laboratory tests that are commonly used in diagnosing and evaluating anemias. Some nonnutrition-related causes of anemia include massive blood loss, infections, hereditary blood disorders such as sickle-cell anemia, and chronic liver or kidney disease.

Assessment of Iron-Deficiency Anemia

Iron deficiency, a common mineral deficiency, develops in stages. First, iron stores diminish, then transport iron decreases, and finally hemoglobin production falls. Chapter 13 described the progression of iron deficiency in detail, as well as the roles of some of the proteins involved in iron metabolism. This section describes the various tests used to assess iron status; Table E-7 (p. E-16) provides normal values. Although other tests are more specific in detecting the early stages of iron deficiency anemia, hemoglobin and

*The half-life of albumin is 14 to 20 days, an indication of a slow degradation rate.
**Transthyretin is also known as *prealbumin* or *thyroxine-binding prealbumin*.
***The half-lives of transthyretin and retinol-binding protein are 2 to 3 days and 12 hours, respectively.
†The half-life of transferrin is 8 to 10 days.
††The half-life of IGF-1 is 12 to 15 hours.

half-life: in blood tests, the length of time that a substance remains in the body. The half-life of albumin, for example, is 14 to 20 days, meaning that half of the albumin circulating in the plasma is degraded in this time period.

TABLE E-7 Normal Values for Iron

Test	Normal Values	
	Female	Male
Hemoglobin (g/dL)	12–16	13.5–17.5
Hematocrit (%)	35–45	39–49
Serum ferritin (ng/mL)	10–120	20–250
Total iron-binding capacity (μg/dL)	250–450	250–450
Serum iron (μg/dL)	50–170	65–175
Mean corpuscualr volume (fL)	80–100	80–100
Transferrin (mg/dL)	200–360	200–360
Transferrin saturation (%)	15–50	20–50
Erythrocyte protoporphyrin (μg/dL RBC)	<70	<70

hematocrit are the most often used because they are relatively inexpensive and easily measured.

Hemoglobin Iron forms an integral part of the hemoglobin molecule that transports oxygen to the cells. In iron deficiency, the body cannot synthesize enough hemoglobin. Table E-7 provides normal hemoglobin values; low hemoglobin values signal depleted iron stores. Hemoglobin's usefulness in evaluating iron status is limited, however, because hemoglobin concentrations drop fairly late in the development of iron deficiency, and other nutrient deficiencies and medical conditions can also alter hemoglobin concentrations.

Hematocrit Hematocrit is commonly used to diagnose iron-deficiency anemia, even though it is an inconclusive measure of iron status. The hematocrit is the percentage of red blood cells in the total blood volume. Table E-7 includes normal values for hematocrit. Low values indicate microcytic (abnormally small-celled), hypochromic (abnormally lacking in color) red blood cells.

Low hemoglobin and hematocrit values alert the assessor to the possibility of iron deficiency. However, many nutrients and other conditions can affect hemoglobin and hematocrit. The following tests of iron status help pinpoint true iron deficiency.

Serum Ferritin In the first stage of iron deficiency, iron stores diminish. Because iron is stored in the protein ferritin, measures of serum ferritin provide an estimate of iron stores. Serum ferritin is not a reliable indicator of iron deficiency, however, because its concentrations are increased by infection, inflammation, alcohol consumption, and liver disease.

The second stage of iron deficiency is characterized by a decrease in transport iron. This is revealed by a decrease in serum iron and an increase in the iron-binding capacity of the protein transferrin. These changes are reflected by the transferrin saturation, which is calculated from the ratio of the other two values as described in the following paragraphs.

Serum Iron Lab technicians can measure serum iron directly. Elevated values indicate iron overload; reduced values indicate iron deficiency. Table E-7 shows the normal values for serum iron.

Total Iron-Binding Capacity (TIBC) Iron travels through the blood bound to the protein transferrin. During iron deficiency, the liver produces more transferrin in an effort to increase iron transport capacity, and therefore iron depletion is characterized by a increase in the total iron-binding capacity (TIBC). Table E-7 includes the normal values for TIBC.

Transferrin Saturation The percentage of transferrin that is saturated with iron is an indirect measure that is derived from the serum iron and total iron-binding capacity measures as follows:

$$\% \text{ Transferrin} = \frac{\text{serum iron}}{\text{total iron-binding capacity}} \times 100$$

Table E-7 shows normal values for transferrin saturation. During iron deficiency, transferrin saturation decreases. The transferrin saturation value is a useful indicator of iron status because it includes information about both the iron and transferrin content of the blood.

The third stage of iron deficiency occurs when the supply of transport iron diminishes to the point that it limits hemoglobin production. It is characterized by increases in erythrocyte protoporphyrin, a decrease in mean corpuscular volume, and decreased hemoglobin and hematocrit (as mentioned earlier).

Erythrocyte Protoporphyrin The iron-containing portion of the hemoglobin molecule is heme, which is formed from iron and protoporphyrin. Protoporphyrin accumulates in the blood when iron supplies are inadequate for the formation of heme. Protoporphyrin may also increase when hemoglobin synthesis is impaired for other reasons, such as lead poisoning or inflammation. Lab technicians can measure erythrocyte protoporphyrin directly in a blood sample. The normal values of erythrocyte protoporphyrin are shown in Table E-7.

Mean Corpuscular Volume (MCV) The hematocrit value divided by the red blood cell count provides a measure of the average size of a red blood cell, referred to as the mean corpuscular volume (MCV). Such a measure helps classify the type of nutrient anemia. In iron deficiency, the red blood cells are smaller than average (microcytic).

Assessment of Folate and Vitamin B_{12} Anemias

Folate deficiency and vitamin B_{12} deficiency present a similar clinical picture—an anemia characterized by abnormally large, misshapen, and mature red blood cells (megaloblastic cells). Distinguishing between folate and vitamin B_{12} deficiency is essential because their treatments differ. Giving folate to a person with vitamin B_{12} deficiency improves many of the lab test results indicative of vitamin B_{12} deficiency, but this is a dangerous treatment because vitamin B_{12} deficiency causes nerve damage that folate cannot correct. Thus inappropriate folate administration masks vitamin B_{12}–deficiency anemia, and nerve damage worsens. For this reason, it is critical to determine whether the anemia results from a folate deficiency or from a vitamin B_{12} deficiency. The following biochemical assessment measures help make this distinction.

Mean Corpuscular Volume (MCV) As mentioned previously, the MCV is a measure of red blood cell size. In folate and vitamin B_{12} deficiencies, the red blood cells are larger than average (macrocytic). Macrocytic cells are not necessarily indicative of nutrient deficiency, however, as they may also result from a high alcohol intake, liver disease, and various medications.

Serum Folate and Vitamin B_{12} Levels Analyses of serum folate and vitamin B_{12} levels are usually among the first tests conducted to determine the cause of macrocytic red blood cells. Low serum levels of either nutrient is consistent with a deficiency, whereas adequate levels can help rule out deficiency. Folate levels are not a specific measure of folate status, however; they increase with folate consumption and decrease with alcohol consumption, pregnancy, or use of anticonvulsant medications. Folate

APPENDIX E

TABLE E-8 Normal Values for Folate and Vitamin B_{12}

Test	Normal Values
Serum folate (ng/mL)[a]	2.6–12.2
Serum homocysteine (µmol/L)	5–14
Erythrocyte folate (ng/mL)[a]	103–411
Serum vitamin B_{12} (pg/mL)	>200
Serum methylmalonic acid (nmol/L)	70–270

NOTE: A nanogram (ng) is one-billionth of a gram; a picogram (pg) is one-trillionth of a gram.
[a]To convert folate values (ng/mL) to international standard units (nmol/L), multiply by 2.266.

depletion is characterized by a fall in the folate concentrations of red blood cells (ery-throcytes). As erythrocyte folate levels diminish, folate-deficiency anemia develops. Because low erythrocyte folate concentrations also occur with vitamin B_{12} deficiency, serum vitamin B_{12} concentrations must also be measured. Table E-8 shows standards for folate and vitamin B_{12} assessment.

Methylmalonic Acid and Homocysteine Levels To determine whether a nutrient is deficient, measures are taken of substances that accumulate when the functions of the nutrient are impaired. For example, the amino acid homocysteine usually increases in both folate and vitamin B_{12} deficiencies because both nutrients are needed for its metabolism. Methylmalonic acid is a breakdown product of several amino acids and requires vitamin B_{12} for its metabolism; consequently, its concentrations are elevated in vitamin B_{12} deficiency, but not in folate deficiency. Thus, this measure is useful in distinguishing between folate and vitamin B_{12} deficiency.

Schilling Test Vitamin B_{12} deficiency usually arises from malabsorption, not from poor intake. To determine whether malabsorption is the cause, a small oral dose of radioactive vitamin B_{12} is given, and urinary excretion is measured. This test is rarely performed, but it measures vitamin B_{12} absorption and is called a Schilling test.

Antibodies to Intrinsic Factor Serum antibodies for intrinsic factor can help confirm a diagnosis of pernicious anemia, an autoimmune disease characterized by destruction of the cells that produce intrinsic factor, the protein required for vitamin B_{12} absorption. These antibodies may be present in various other medical conditions as well.

Cautions about Nutrition Assessment

The tests outlined in this appendix yield information that becomes meaningful only when conducted and interpreted by a skilled clinician. Potential sources of error may be introduced at any step, from the collection of samples and data to their reporting and analyses. Equipment must be regularly calibrated to ensure accuracy of measurements. In addition, the assessor must keep in mind that each assessment measure contributes only one bit of information that may be useful in confirming or eliminating the possibility of suspected nutrition problems. Furthermore, the assessor must constantly remember that a sufficient intake of a nutrient does not guarantee adequate nutrient status for an individual. Conversely, the apparent inadequate intake of a nutrient does not, by itself, establish that a deficiency exists.

Appendix F Estimated Energy Needs

Chapter 8 described how to calculate estimated energy requirements (EER) by using an equation that accounts for gender, age, weight, height, and physical activity level. This appendix presents tables that provide a shortcut to estimating daily energy requirements, as developed by the *Dietary Guidelines for Americans*, and based on the EER equations of the Dietary Reference Intakes (DRI).

Table F-1 describes three activity levels: sedentary, moderately active, and active. Table F-2 presents estimated daily energy needs by age, gender, and these three levels of physical activity. Keep in mind that these values are estimates that have been rounded to the nearest 200 kcalories; an individual's energy needs may be higher or lower than these average estimates. EER equations for this table use reference heights and weights. For children and adolescents, reference heights and weights vary. For adults, the reference man is 5 feet 10 inches tall and weighs 154 pounds and the reference woman is 5 feet 4 inches tall and weighs 126 pounds. Estimates for women do not include women who are pregnant or breastfeeding.

TABLE F-1 Sedentary, Moderately Active, and Active People

Sedentary	A lifestyle that includes only the light physical activity associated with typical day-to-day life.
Moderately active	A lifestyle that includes physical activity equivalent to walking about 1.5 to 3 miles per day at 3 to 4 miles per hour in addition to the light physical activity associated with typical day-to-day life.
Active	A lifestyle that includes physical activity equivalent to walking more than 3 miles per day at 3 to 4 miles per hour in addition to the light physical activity associated with typical day-to-day life.

TABLE F-2 Estimated Daily kCalorie Needs by Age, Gender, and Physical Activity Level

	Gender/Activity Level					
Age (years)	Male/Sedentary	Male/Moderately Active	Male/Active	Female/Sedentary	Female/Moderately Active	Female/Active
2	1000	1000	1000	1000	1000	1000
3	1200	1400	1400	1000	1200	1400
4	1200	1400	1600	1200	1400	1400
5	1200	1400	1600	1200	1400	1600
6	1400	1600	1800	1200	1400	1600
7	1400	1600	1800	1200	1600	1800
8	1400	1600	2000	1400	1600	1800
9	1600	1800	2000	1400	1600	1800
10	1600	1800	2200	1400	1800	2000

(Continued)

TABLE F-2 Estimated Daily kCalorie Needs by Age, Gender, and Physical Activity Level *(continued)*

Age (years)	Gender/Activity Level					
	Male/Sedentary	Male/Moderately Active	Male/Active	Female/Sedentary	Female/Moderately Active	Female/Active
11	1800	2000	2200	1600	1800	2000
12	1800	2200	2400	1600	2000	2200
13	2000	2200	2600	1600	2000	2200
14	2000	2400	2800	1800	2000	2400
15	2200	2600	3000	1800	2000	2400
16–18	2400	2800	3200	1800	2000	2400
19–20	2600	2800	3000	2000	2200	2400
21–25	2400	2800	3000	2000	2200	2400
26–30	2400	2600	3000	1800	2000	2400
31–35	2400	2600	3000	1800	2000	2200
36–40	2400	2600	2800	1800	2000	2200
41–45	2200	2600	2800	1800	2000	2200
46–50	2200	2400	2800	1800	2000	2200
51–55	2200	2400	2800	1600	1800	2200
56–60	2200	2400	2600	1600	1800	2200
61–65	2000	2400	2600	1600	1800	2000
66–75	2000	2200	2600	1600	1800	2000
76+	2000	2200	2400	1600	1800	2000

SOURCE: U.S. Department of Agriculture and U.S. Department of Health and Human Services, *Dietary Guidelines for Americans 2010*, www.dietaryguidelines.gov.

Appendix G Choose Your Foods: Food Lists for Diabetes and Weight Management

CONTENTS

Chapter 2 introduced a meal-planning system based on food lists, and this appendix provides details from the 2014 publications *Choose Your Foods: Food Lists for Diabetes* and *Choose Your Foods: Food Lists for Weight Management*. These lists can help people with diabetes manage their blood glucose levels by controlling the amount and kinds of carbohydrates they consume. These lists can also help in planning diets for weight management by controlling kcalorie intake. In fact because these lists are based on principles of good nutrition, they can be helpful in planning meals for everyone.

The Food Lists

The food lists sort foods by their proportions of carbohydrate, fat, and protein (Table G-1). Some of the food lists are organized into several groups of foods. For example, the carbohydrate list includes:

- Starch
- Fruits

TABLE G-1 The Food Lists

Food Lists	Typical Item/Portion Size	Carbohydrate (g)	Protein (g)	Fat (g)	Energy[a] (kcal)
Carbohydrates					
Starch[b]	1 slice bread	15	3	1	80
Fruits	1 small apple	15	—	—	60
Milk and milk substitutes					
Fat-free, low-fat (1%)	1 c fat-free milk	12	8	0–3	100
Reduced-fat (2%)	1 c reduced-fat milk	12	8	5	120
Whole	1 c whole milk	12	8	8	160
Nonstarchy vegetables	½ c cooked carrots	5	2	—	25
Sweets, desserts, and other carbohydrates	5 vanilla wafers	15	Varies	Varies	Varies
Proteins					
Lean	1 oz chicken (no skin)	—	7	2	45
Medium-fat	1 oz ground beef	—	7	5	75
High-fat	1 oz pork sausage	—	7	8	100
Plant-based	½ c tofu	Varies	7	Varies	Varies
Fats	1 tsp olive oil	—	—	5	45
Alcohol	12 fl oz beer	Varies	—	—	100

[a]The energy value for each food list represents an approximate average for the group and does not reflect the precise number of grams of carbohydrate, protein, and fat. For example, a slice of bread contains 15 grams of carbohydrate (60 kcalories), 3 grams of protein (12 kcalories), and 1 gram of fat (9 calories)—rounded to 80 kcalories for ease in calculating. A ½ cup of nonstarchy vegetables contains 5 grams of carbohydrate (20 kcalories) and 2 grams of protein (8 kcalories), which has been rounded down to 25 kcalories.
[b]The Starch list includes cereals, grains and pasta, breads, crackers and snacks, starchy vegetables (such as corn, peas, and potatoes), and legumes (beans, peas, and lentils).

- Milk and Milk Substitutes (fat-free/low-fat, reduced-fat, and whole)
- Nonstarchy Vegetables
- Sweets, Desserts, and Other Carbohydrates

A serving of any food on a list can be traded for a serving of any other food on the same list without significantly affecting the intake of energy nutrients or total kcalories. The food lists use the term *choice* to describe the specific quantity of each food within a group of similar foods. Note that some foods may count as choices from more than one group. For example, ½ cup black beans counts as 1 starch plus 1 lean protein choice.

Serving Sizes

The serving sizes have been carefully adjusted and defined so that a serving of any food on a given list provides roughly the same amount of carbohydrate, fat, and protein—and therefore total energy. For example, a person may select 17 small grapes or ½ large grapefruit as one fruit choice and either would provide roughly 15 grams of carbohydrate and 60 kcalories. A whole grapefruit, however, would count as two fruit choices.

To apply the system successfully, users must become familiar with the specified serving sizes. A convenient way to remember the serving sizes and energy values is to keep in mind a typical item from each list (review Table G-1).

The Foods on the Lists

Foods do not always appear on the food lists where you might first expect to find them. They are grouped according to their energy–nutrient contents rather than by their source (such as milks), their outward appearance, or their vitamin and mineral contents. For example, cheeses are found among the meats on the Protein lists (not Milk and Milk Substitutes) because, like meats, cheeses contribute energy from protein and fat but provide negligible carbohydrate. For similar reasons, starchy vegetables such as corn, green peas, and potatoes are found on the Starch list with breads and cereals, not with the Nonstarchy Vegetables. Diet planners learn to view mixtures of foods, such as casseroles and soups, as combinations of foods from different food lists.

Managing Energy, Carbohydrate, Fat, and Sodium

The food lists help people manage their intakes of energy nutrients and total kcalories by paying close attention to serving sizes. People wanting to lose weight can easily monitor their energy intake. Similarly, people needing to control blood glucose levels can easily monitor their carbohydrate intake.

The food lists also alert consumers to foods that are unexpectedly high in fat. For example, the Starch list specifies which grain products contain extra fat (such as biscuits, taco shells, and bread stuffing) by marking them with a symbol to indicate high-extra fat (the symbols are explained in the table keys). In addition, foods on the milk and protein lists are separated into categories based on their fat contents (review Table G-1). The Protein list also includes plant-based proteins, which tend to be rich in fiber. Notice that many of these foods (pp. G-11 and G-12) bear the symbol for "good source of fiber."

People wanting to control the sodium in their diets can begin by eliminating any foods bearing the "high in sodium" symbol. In most cases, the symbol identifies foods that, in one serving, provide 480 milligrams or more of sodium. Foods on the Combination Foods or Fast Foods lists that bear the symbol provide more than 600 milligrams of sodium.

Planning a Healthy Diet

To obtain a daily variety of foods that provide healthful amounts of carbohydrate, protein, and fat, as well as vitamins, minerals, and fiber, the meal pattern for adults and teenagers should include at least:

- Three servings of nonstarchy vegetables
- Three servings of fruits
- Six servings of grains (at least three of whole grains), beans, and starchy vegetables
- Two servings of low-fat or fat-free milk or milk substitutes
- No more than 6 ounces of lower-fat protein foods
- No more than 5 to 8 servings of fat, mainly as nuts, seeds, and liquid fats (rather than solid fats)
- *Small* amounts sugar

The actual amounts are determined by age, gender, activity levels, and other factors that influence energy needs. Take time to explore the food lists in Tables G-2 through G-12. Doing so will provide valuable insights about the amounts of energy nutrients and kcalories that various foods provide.

TABLE G-2 Starch

The Starch list includes breads, cereals, grains (including pasta and rice), starchy vegetables, crackers and snacks, and legumes (beans, peas, and lentils).

1 starch choice = 15 grams carbohydrate, 3 grams protein, 1 gram fat, and 80 kcalories.

NOTE: In general, one starch choice is ½ cup of cooked cereal, grain, or starchy vegetable; ⅓ cup of cooked rice or pasta; 1 ounce of bread product, such as 1 slice of bread; ¾ to 1 ounce of most snack foods.

Food	Serving Size
Bread	
Bagel	¼ large (1 oz)
! Biscuit	1 (2½ in. across)
Breads, loaf-type	
white, whole-grain, French, Italian, pumpernickel, rye, sourdough, unfrosted raisin or cinnamon	1 slice (1 oz)
✓ reduced-kcalorie, light	2 slices (1½ oz)
Breads, flat-type (flatbreads)	
chapatti	1 oz
ciabatta	1 oz
naan	3¼-in. square (1 oz)
pita (6 in. across)	½
roti	1 oz
✓ sandwich flat buns, whole-wheat	1 (1½ oz)
! taco shell	2 (each 5 in. across)
tortilla, corn	1 small (6 in. across)
tortilla, flour (white or whole-wheat)	1 small (6 in. across) or ⅓ large (10 in. across)
Cornbread	1¾-in. cube (1½ oz)
English muffin	½
Hot dog bun or hamburger bun	½ (¾ oz)
Pancake	1 (4 in. across, ¼ in. thick)
Roll, plain	1 small (1 oz)
! Stuffing, bread	⅓ cup
Waffle	1 (4-in. square or 4 in. diameter)
Cereals	
✓ Bran cereal (twigs, buds, or flakes)	½ cup
Cooked cereals (oats, oatmeal)	½ cup
Granola cereal	¼ cup
Grits, cooked	½ cup
Muesli	¼ cup
Puffed cereal	1½ cups
Shredded wheat, plain	½ cup
Sugar-coated cereal	½ cup
Unsweetened, ready-to-eat cereal	¾ cup
Grains[a]	
Barley	⅓ cup
Bran, dry	
✓ oat	¼ cup
✓ wheat	½ cup
✓ Bulgur	½ cup
Couscous	⅓ cup
Kasha	½ cup
Millet	⅓ cup
Pasta, white or whole-wheat	⅓ cup
Polenta	⅓ cup
Quinoa, all colors	⅓ cup
Rice, all colors and types	⅓ cup
Tabbouleh (tabouli), prepared	½ cup

(Continued)

TABLE G-2 Starch *(continued)*

Food	Serving Size
Grains *continued*	
Wheat germ, dry	3 Tbsp
Wild rice	½ cup
Starchy Vegetables[b]	
Breadfruit	¼ cup
Cassava or dasheen	⅓ cup
Corn	½ cup
on cob	4- to 4½-in. piece (½ large)
✓ Hominy	¾ cup
✓ Mixed vegetables with corn or peas	1 cup
Marinara, pasta, or spaghetti sauce	½ cup
✓ Parsnips	½ cup
✓ Peas, green	½ cup
Plantain	⅓ cup
Potato	
baked with skin	¼ large (3 oz)
boiled, all kinds	½ cup or ½ medium (3 oz)
! mashed, with milk and fat	½ cup
french-fried (oven-baked)[c]	1 cup (2 oz)
✓ Pumpkin puree, canned, no sugar added	¾ cup
✓ Squash, winter (acorn, butternut)	1 cup
✓ Succotash	½ cup
Yam or sweet potato, plain	½ cup (3½ oz)
Crackers and Snacks	
Crackers	
animal	8
✓ crispbread	2–5 pieces (¾ oz)
graham, 2½-in. square	3
nut and rice	10
Crackers and Snacks—*continued*	
oyster	20
! round, butter-type	6
saltine-type	6
! sandwich-style, cheese or peanut butter filling	3
whole-wheat, baked	5 regular 1½-in. squares or 10 thins (¾ oz)
Granola or snack bar	1 (¾ oz)
Matzoh, all shapes and sizes	¾ oz
Melba toast	4 (2 in. by 4 in.)
Popcorn	
✓ no fat added	3 cups
!! with butter added	3 cups
Pretzels	¾ oz
Rice cakes	2 (4 in. across)
Snack chips	
baked (potato, pita)	~8 (¾ oz)
!! regular (tortilla, potato)	~13 (1 oz)
Beans, Peas, and Lentils[d]	
The choices on this list count as 1 starch + 1 lean protein.	
✓ Baked beans, canned	⅓ cup
✓ Beans (black, garbanzo, kidney, lima, navy, pinto, white), cooked or canned, drained and rinsed	½ cup
✓ Lentils (any color), cooked	½ cup
✓ Peas (black-eyed and split), cooked or canned, drained and rinsed	½ cup
S ✓ Refried beans, canned	½ cup

[a]Serving sizes are for cooked grains, unless otherwise noted.
[b]Serving sizes are for cooked vegetables.
[c]Restaurant-style french fries are on the Fast Foods list.
[d]Also found on the Protein list.

KEY

✓ = Good source of fiber: >3 g/serving

! = Extra fat: +5 grams fat

!! = Extra fat: +10 grams fat

S = High in sodium: ≥480 mg/serving

TABLE G-3 Fruits

Fruit[a]

The Fruits list includes fresh, frozen, canned, and dried fruits and fruit juices.

1 fruit choice = 15 grams carbohydrate, 0 grams protein, 0 grams fat, and 60 kcalories.

NOTE: In general, one fruit choice is ½ cup of canned or frozen fruit or unsweetened fruit juice; 1 small fresh fruit (¾ to 1 cup); 2 tablespoons of dried fruit.

Food	Serving Size
Apple, unpeeled	1 small (4 oz)
Apples, dried	4 rings
Applesauce, unsweetened	½ cup
Apricots	
canned	½ cup
dried	8 halves
fresh	4 (5½ oz total)
Banana	1 extra small, ~4 in. long (4 oz)
✓ Blackberries	1 cup
Blueberries	¾ cup
Cantaloupe	1 cup diced
Cherries	
sweet, canned	½ cup
sweet, fresh	12 (3½ oz)
Dates	3 small (deglet noor) or 1 large (medjool)
Dried fruits (blueberries, cherries, cranberries, mixed fruit, raisins)	2 Tbsp
Figs	
dried	3 small
✓ fresh	1½ large or 2 medium (3½ oz total)
Fruit cocktail	½ cup
Grapefruit	
fresh	½ large (5½ oz)
sections, canned	¾ cup
Grapes	17 small (3 oz total)
✓ Guava	2 small (2½ oz total)
Honeydew melon	1 cup diced
Kiwi	½ cup sliced
Loquat	¾ cup cubed
Mandarin oranges, canned	¾ cup
Mango	½ small (5½ oz) or ½ cup
Nectarine	1 medium (5½ oz)
✓ Orange	1 medium (6½ oz)
Papaya	½ (8 oz) or 1 cup cubed
Peaches	
canned	½ cup
fresh	1 medium (6 oz)
Pears	
canned	½ cup
✓ fresh	½ large (4 oz)
Pineapple	
canned	½ cup
fresh	¾ cup
Plantain, extra ripe (black), raw	¼ (2¼ oz)
Plums	
canned	½ cup
dried (prunes)	3
fresh	2 small (5 oz total)
Pomegranate seeds (arils)	½ cup
✓ Raspberries	1 cup
✓ Strawberries	1¼ cup whole
Tangerine	1 large (6 oz)
Watermelon	1¼ cups diced
Fruit Juice	
Apple juice/cider	½ cup
Fruit juice blends, 100% juice	⅓ cup
Grape juice	⅓ cup
Grapefruit juice	½ cup
Orange juice	½ cup
Pineapple juice	½ cup
Pomegranate juice	½ cup
Prune juice	⅓ cup

[a]The weights listed include skin, core, seeds, and rind.

KEY

✓ = Good source of fiber: >3 g/serving

APPENDIX G

TABLE G-4 Milk and Milk Substitutes

The Milk and Milk Substitutes list groups milks and yogurts based on the amount of fat they contain. Cheeses are on the Protein list because they are rich in protein and have very little carbohydrate; butter, cream, coffee creamers, and unsweetened nut milks are on the Fats list; and ice cream and frozen yogurt are on the Sweets, Desserts, and Other Carbohydrates list.

1 fat-free (skim) or low-fat (1%) milk choice = 12 grams carbohydrate, 8 grams protein, 0–3 grams fat, and 100 kcalories.

1 reduced-fat milk choice = 12 grams carbohydrate, 8 grams protein, 5 grams fat, and 120 kcalories.

1 whole-milk choice = 12 grams carbohydrate, 8 grams protein, 8 grams fat, and 160 kcalories.

1 carbohydrate choice = 15 grams carbohydrate and about 70 kcalories.

1 fat choice = 5 grams fat and 45 kcalories.

NOTE: In general, one milk choice is 1 cup (8 fluid ounces or ½ pint) milk or yogurt.

Food	Serving Size	Choices per Serving
Milk and Yogurts		
Fat-free (skim) or low-fat (1%)		
milk, buttermilk, acidophilus milk, lactose-free milk	1 cup	1 fat-free milk
evaporated milk	½ cup	1 fat-free milk
yogurt, plain or Greek; may be sweetened with artificial sweetener	⅔ cup (6 oz)	1 fat-free milk
chocolate milk	1 cup	1 fat-free milk + 1 carbohydrate
Reduced-fat (2%)		
milk, acidophilus milk, kefir, lactose-free milk	1 cup	1 reduced-fat milk
yogurt, plain	⅔ cup (6 oz)	1 reduced-fat milk
Whole		
milk, buttermilk, goat's milk	1 cup	1 whole milk
evaporated milk	½ cup	1 whole milk
yogurt, plain	1 cup (8 oz)	1 whole milk
chocolate milk	1 cup	1 whole milk + 1 carbohydrate
Other Milk Foods and Milk Substitutes[a]		
Eggnog		
fat-free	⅓ cup	1 carbohydrate
low-fat	⅓ cup	1 carbohydrate + ½ fat
whole milk	⅓ cup	1 carbohydrate + 1 fat
Rice drink		
plain, fat-free	1 cup	1 carbohydrate
flavored, low-fat	1 cup	2 carbohydrates
Soy milk		
light or low-fat, plain	1 cup	½ carbohydrate + ½ fat
regular, plain	1 cup	½ carbohydrate + 1 fat
Yogurt with fruit, low-fat	⅔ cup (6 oz)	1 fat-free milk + 1 carbohydrate

[a]Unsweetened nut milks (such as almond and coconut milks) are on the Fats list.

TABLE G-5 Nonstarchy Vegetables

The Nonstarchy Vegetables list includes vegetables that contain small amounts of carbohydrates and few kcalories; starchy vegetables that contain higher amounts of carbohydrate and kcalories are found on the Starch list. Salad greens (like arugula, chicory, endive, escarole, lettuce, radicchio, romaine, and watercress) are on the Free Foods list.

1 nonstarchy vegetable choice = 5 grams carbohydrate, 2 grams protein, 0 grams fat, and 25 kcalories.

NOTE: In general, one nonstarchy vegetable choice is ½ cup of cooked vegetables or vegetable juice or 1 cup of raw vegetables. Count 3 cups of raw vegetables or 1½ cups of cooked nonstarchy vegetables as one carbohydrate choice.

- Amaranth leaves (Chinese spinach)
- Artichoke
- Artichoke hearts (no oil)
- Asparagus
- Baby corn
- Bamboo shoots
- Bean sprouts (alfalfa, mung, soybean)
- Beans (green, wax, Italian, yard-long)
- Beets
- Broccoli
- Broccoli slaw, packaged, no dressing
- ✓ Brussels sprouts
- Cabbage (green, red, bok choy, Chinese)
- ✓ Carrots
- Cauliflower
- Celery
- Chayote
- Coleslaw, packaged, no dressing
- Cucumber
- Daikon
- Eggplant
- Fennel
- Gourds (bitter, bottle, luffa, bitter melon)
- Green onions or scallions
- Greens (collard, dandelion, mustard, purslane, turnip)
- Hearts of palm
- ✓ Jicama
- Kale
- Kohlrabi
- Leeks
- Mixed vegetables (without starchy vegetables, legumes, or pasta)
- Mushrooms, all kinds, fresh
- Okra
- Onions
- Pea pods
- Peppers (all varieties)
- Radishes
- Rutabaga
- 🧂 Sauerkraut, drained and rinsed
- Spinach
- Squash, summer varieties (yellow, pattypan, crookneck, zucchini)
- Sugar snap peas
- Swiss chard
- Tomato
- Tomatoes, canned
- 🧂 Tomato sauce (unsweetened)
- Tomato/vegetable juice
- Turnips
- Water chestnuts

KEY

✓ = Good source of fiber: >3 g/serving

🧂 = High in sodium: ≥480 mg/serving

APPENDIX G

TABLE G-6 Sweets, Desserts, and Other Carbohydrates

The Sweets, Desserts, and Other Carbohydrates list contains foods with added sugars, added fats, or both.
1 carbohydrate choice = 15 grams carbohydrate and about 70 kcalories.
1 fat choice = 5 grams fat and 45 kcalories.

Food	Serving Size	Choices per Serving
Beverages, Soda, and Sports Drinks		
Cranberry juice cocktail	½ cup	1 carbohydrate
Food drink or lemonade	1 cup (8 oz)	2 carbohydrates
Hot chocolate, regular	1 envelope (2 Tbsp or ¾ oz) added to 8 oz water	1 carbohydrate
Soft drink (soda), regular	1 can (12 oz)	2½ carbohydrates
Sports drink (fluid replacement type)	1 cup (8 oz)	1 carbohydrate
Brownies, Cake, Cookies, Gelatin, Pie, and Pudding		
Biscotti	1 oz	1 carbohydrate + 1 fat
Brownie, small, unfrosted	1¼-in. square, ⅞-in. high (~1 oz)	1 carbohydrate + 1 fat
Cake		
angel food, unfrosted	1/12 of cake (~2 oz)	2 carbohydrates
frosted	2-in. square (~2 oz)	2 carbohydrates + 1 fat
unfrosted	2-in. square (~1 oz)	1 carbohydrate + 1 fat
Cookies		
100-kcalorie pack	1 oz	1 carbohydrate + ½ fat
chocolate chip cookies	2, 2¼ in. across	1 carbohydrate + 2 fats
gingersnaps	3 small, 1½ in. across	1 carbohydrate
large cookie	1, 6 in. across (~3 oz)	4 carbohydrates + 3 fats
sandwich cookies with crème filling	2 small (~2/3 oz)	1 carbohydrate + 1 fat
sugar-free cookies	1 large or 3 small (¾ to 1 oz)	1 carbohydrate + 1–2 fats
vanilla wafer	5	1 carbohydrate + 1 fat
Cupcake, frosted	1 small (~1¾ oz)	2 carbohydrates + 1–1½ fats
Flan	½ cup	2½ carbohydrates + 1 fat
Fruit cobbler	½ cup (3½ oz)	3 carbohydrates + 1 fat
Gelatin, regular	½ cup	1 carbohydrate
Pie		
commercially prepared fruit, 2 crusts	⅙ of 8-in. pie	3 carbohydrates + 2 fats
pumpkin or custard	⅛ of 8-in. pie	1½ carbohydrates + 1½ fats
Pudding		
regular (made with reduced-fat milk)	½ cup	2 carbohydrates
sugar-free or sugar- and fat-free (made with fat-free milk)	½ cup	1 carbohydrate

TABLE G-6 **Sweets, Desserts, and Other Carbohydrates** (*continued*)

Food	Serving Size	Choices per Serving
Candy, Spreads, Sweets, Sweeteners, Syrups, and Toppings		
Blended sweeteners (mixtures of artificial sweeteners and sugar)	1½ Tbsp	1 carbohydrate
Candy		
chocolate, dark or milk type	1 oz	1 carbohydrate + 2 fats
chocolate "kisses"	5 pieces	1 carbohydrate + 1 fat
hard	3 pieces	1 carbohydrate
Coffee creamer, nondairy type		
powdered, flavored	4 tsp	½ carbohydrate + ½ fat
liquid, flavored	2 Tbsp	1 carbohydrate
Fruit snacks, chewy (pureed fruit concentrate)	1 roll (¾ oz)	1 carbohydrate
Fruit spreads, 100% fruit	1½ Tbsp	1 carbohydrate
Honey	1 Tbsp	1 carbohydrate
Jam or jelly, regular	1 Tbsp	1 carbohydrate
Sugar	1 Tbsp	1 carbohydrate
Syrup		
chocolate	2 Tbsp	2 carbohydrates
light (pancake-type)	2 Tbsp	1 carbohydrate
regular (pancake-type)	1 Tbsp	1 carbohydrate
Condiments and Sauces		
Barbecue sauce	3 Tbsp	1 carbohydrate
Cranberry sauce, jellied	¼ cup	1½ carbohydrates
Curry sauce	1 oz	1 carbohydrate + 1 fat
Gravy, canned or bottled	½ cup	½ carbohydrate + ½ fat
Hoisin sauce	1 Tbsp	½ carbohydrate
Marinade	1 Tbsp	½ carbohydrate
Plum sauce	1 Tbsp	½ carbohydrate
Salad dressing, fat-free, cream-based	3 Tbsp	1 carbohydrate
Sweet-and-sour sauce	3 Tbsp	1 carbohydrate
Doughnuts, Muffins, Pastries, and Sweet Breads		
Banana nut bread	1-in. slice (2 oz)	2 carbohydrates + 1 fat
Doughnut		
cake, plain	1 medium (1½ oz)	1½ carbohydrates + 2 fats
hole	2 (1 oz)	1 carbohydrate + 1 fat
yeast-type, glazed	1, 3¾ in. across (2 oz)	2 carbohydrates + 2 fats
Muffin		
regular	1 (4 oz)	4 carbohydrates + 2½ fats
low-fat	1 (4 oz)	4 carbohydrates + ½ fat
Scone	1 (4 oz)	4 carbohydrates + 3 fats
Sweet roll or Danish	1 (2½ oz)	2½ carbohydrates + 2 fats

(*Continued*)

TABLE G-6 Sweets, Desserts, and Other Carbohydrates *(continued)*

Food	Serving Size	Choices per Serving
Frozen Bars, Frozen Desserts, Frozen Yogurt, and Ice Cream		
Frozen pops	1	½ carbohydrate
Fruit juice bars, frozen, 100% juice	1 (3 oz)	1 carbohydrate
Ice cream		
fat-free	½ cup	1½ carbohydrates
light	½ cup	1 carbohydrate + 1 fat
no-sugar-added	½ cup	1 carbohydrate + 1 fat
regular	½ cup	1 carbohydrate + 2 fats
Sherbet, sorbet	½ cup	2 carbohydrates
Yogurt, frozen		
fat-free	⅓ cup	1 carbohydrate
regular	½ cup	1 carbohydrate + 0–1 fat
Greek, lower-fat or fat-free	½ cup	1½ carbohydrates

KEY

S = High in sodium: ≥480 mg/serving

TABLE G-7 Protein

The Protein list groups foods based on the amount of fat they contain.

NOTE: In general, one protein choice is 1 ounce meat, fish, poultry, or hard cheese; serving sizes for meat, fish, and poultry are based on cooked weight after bone and fat have been removed.

Food	Serving Size
Lean Protein	
1 lean protein choice = 0 grams carbohydrate, 7 grams protein, 2 grams fat, and 45 kcalories.	
Beef: ground (90% or higher lean/10% or lower fat); select or choice grades trimmed of fat such as roast (chuck, round, rump, sirloin), steak (cubed, flank, porterhouse, T-bone), tenderloin	1 oz
S Beef jerky	½ oz
Cheeses with ≤3 g fat/oz	1 oz
Curd-style cheeses: cottage-type (all kinds); ricotta (fat-free or light)	¼ cup (2 oz)
Egg substitutes, plain	¼ cup
Egg whites	2
Fish	
fresh or frozen, such as catfish, cod, flounder, haddock, halibut, orange roughy, tilapia, trout	1 oz
salmon, fresh or canned	1 oz
sardines, canned	2 small
tuna, fresh or canned in water or oil and drained	1 oz
S smoked: herring or salmon (lox)	1 oz

Food	Serving Size
Lean Protein—*continued*	
Game: buffalo, ostrich, rabbit, venison	1 oz
S Hot dog[a] with ≤3 g fat/oz	1 (1¾ oz)
Lamb: chop, leg, or roast	1 oz
Organ meats: heart, kidney, liver[b]	1 oz
Oysters, fresh or frozen	6 medium
Pork, lean	
S Canadian bacon	1 oz
S ham	1 oz
rib or loin chop/roast, tenderloin	1 oz
Poultry, without skin: chicken; Cornish hen; domestic duck or goose (well drained of fat); turkey; lean ground turkey or chicken	1 oz
S Processed sandwich meats with ≤3 g fat/oz: chipped beef, thin-sliced deli meats, turkey ham, turkey pastrami	1 oz
S Sausage with ≤3 g fat/oz	1 oz
Shellfish: clams, crab, imitation shellfish, lobster, scallops, shrimp	1 oz
Veal: cutlet (no breading), loin chop, roast	1 oz

TABLE G-7 Protein (*continued*)

Food	Serving Size
Medium-Fat Protein	
1 medium-fat protein choice = 0 grams carbohydrate, 7 grams protein, 5 grams fat, and 75 kcalories.	
Beef trimmed of visible fat: ground beef (85% or lower lean/15% or higher fat), corned beef, meatloaf, prime cuts of beef (rib roast), short ribs, tongue	1 oz
Cheeses with 4–7 g fat/oz: feta, mozzarella, pasteurized processed cheese spread, reduced-fat cheeses	1 oz
Cheese, ricotta (regular or part-skim)	¼ cup (2 oz)
Egg	1
Fish: any fried	1 oz
Lamb: ground, rib roast	1 oz
Pork: cutlet, ground, shoulder roast	1 oz
Poultry with skin: chicken, dove, pheasant, turkey, wild duck, or goose; fried chicken	1 oz
S Sausage with 4–7 g fat/oz	1 oz
High-Fat Protein	
1 high-fat protein choice = 0 grams carbohydrate, 7 grams protein, 8 grams fat, and 100 kcalories. These foods are high in saturated fat, cholesterol, and kcalories and may raise blood cholesterol levels if eaten on a regular basis. Try to eat 3 or fewer choices from this group per week.	

Food	Serving Size
High-Fat Protein—continued	
Bacon, pork	2 slices (1 oz each before cooking)
S Bacon, turkey	3 slices (½ oz each before cooking)
Cheese, regular: American, blue-veined, brie, cheddar, hard goat, Monterey jack, Parmesan, queso, and Swiss	1 oz
! Hot dog: beef, pork, or combination	1 (10 per 1 lb-sized package)
Hot dog: turkey or chicken	1 (10 per 1 lb-sized package)
Pork: sausage, spareribs	1 oz
S Processed sandwich meats with ≥8 g fat/oz: bologna, hard salami, pastrami	1 oz
S Sausage with ≥8 g fat/oz: bratwurst, chorizo, Italian, knockwurst, Polish, smoked, summer	1 oz

[a]May contain carbohydrate.

[b]May be high in cholesterol.

KEY

! = Extra fat: +5 grams fat

S = High in sodium: ≥480 mg/serving (based on the sodium content of a typical 3-oz serving of meat, unless 1 oz or 2 oz is the normal serving size)

Beans, peas, and lentils are also on the Starch list; nut butters in small amounts are on the Fats list. Because carbohydrate content varies among plant-based proteins, read food labels.

1 plant-based protein choice = variable grams carbohydrate, 7 grams protein, variable grams fat, and variable kcalories.

Food	Serving Size	Choices per Serving
Plant-Based Protein		
"Bacon" strips, soy-based	2 (½ oz)	1 lean protein
✓ Baked beans, canned	⅓ cup	1 starch + 1 lean protein
✓ Beans (black, garbanzo, kidney, lima, navy, pinto, white), cooked or canned, drained and rinsed	½ cup	1 starch + 1 lean protein
"Beef" or "sausage" crumbles, meatless	1 oz	1 lean protein
"Chicken" nuggets, soy-based	2 (1½ oz)	½ carbohydrate + 1 medium-fat protein
✓ Edamame, shelled	½ cup	½ carbohydrate + 1 lean protein
Falafel (spiced chickpea and wheat patties)	3 patties (~2 in. across)	1 carbohydrate + 1 high-fat protein
Hot dog, meatless, soy-based	1 (1½ oz)	1 lean protein
✓ Hummus	⅓ cup	1 carbohydrate + 1 medium-fat protein
✓ Lentils, any color, cooked or canned, drained and rinsed	½ cup	1 starch + 1 lean protein

(*Continued*)

TABLE G-7 Protein (*continued*)

Food	Serving Size	Choices per Serving
Meatless burger, soy-based	3 oz	½ carbohydrate + 2 lean proteins
✓ Meatless burger, vegetable- and starch-based	1 patty (~2½ oz)	½ carbohydrate + 1 lean protein
Meatless deli slices	1 oz	1 lean protein
Mycoprotein ("chicken" tenders or crumbles), meatless	2 oz	½ carbohydrate + 1 lean protein
Nut spreads: almond butter, cashew butter, peanut butter, soy nut butter	1 Tbsp	1 high-fat protein
✓ Peas (black-eyed and split peas), cooked or canned, drained and rinsed	½ cup	1 starch + 1 lean protein
✓ 🧂 Refried beans, canned	½ cup	1 starch + 1 lean protein
"Sausage" breakfast-type patties, meatless	1 (1½ oz)	1 medium-fat protein
Soy nuts, unsalted	¾ oz	½ carbohydrate + 1 medium-fat protein
Tempeh, plain, unflavored	¼ cup (1½ oz)	1 medium-fat protein
Tofu	½ cup (4 oz)	1 medium-fat protein
Tofu, light	½ cup (4 oz)	1 lean protein

KEY

✓ = Good source of fiber: >3 g/serving   🧂 = High in sodium: ≥480 mg/serving

TABLE G-8 Fats

Fats and oils have mixtures of unsaturated (polyunsaturated and monounsaturated) and saturated fats. Foods on the Fats list are grouped together based on the major type of fat they contain.

1 fat choice = 0 grams carbohydrate, 0 grams protein, 5 grams fat, and 45 kcalories.

NOTE: In general, one fat choice is 1 teaspoon of oil or solid fat or 1 tablespoon of salad dressing.

When used in large amounts, bacon and nut butters are counted as high-fat protein choices (see Protein list). Fat-free salad dressings are on the Sweets, Desserts, and Other Carbohydrates list. Fat-free products such as margarines, salad dressings, mayonnaise, sour cream, and cream cheese are on the Free Foods list.

Food	Serving Size
Unsaturated Fats—Monounsaturated Fats	
Almond milk (unsweetened)	1 cup
Avocado, medium	2 Tbsp (1 oz)
Nut butters (*trans* fat-free): almond butter, cashew butter, peanut butter (smooth or crunchy)	1½ tsp
Nuts	
almonds	6 nuts
Brazil	2 nuts
cashews	6 nuts
filberts (hazelnuts)	5 nuts
macadamia	3 nuts
mixed (50% peanuts)	6 nuts
peanuts	10 nuts

Food	Serving Size
Unsaturated Fats—Monounsaturated Fats—*continued*	
pecans	4 halves
pistachios	16 nuts
Oil: canola, olive, peanut	1 tsp
Olives	
black (ripe)	8
green, stuffed	10 large
Spread, plant stanol ester-type	
light	1 Tbsp
regular	2 tsp
Unsaturated Fats—Polyunsaturated Fats	
Margarine	
lower-fat spread (30–50% vegetable oil, *trans* fat-free)	1 Tbsp

TABLE G-8 Fats *(continued)*

Food	Serving Size
Unsaturated Fats—Polyunsaturated Fats *continued*	
stick, tub, or squeeze (*trans* fat-free)	1 tsp
Mayonnaise	
reduced-fat	1 Tbsp
regular	1 tsp
Mayonnaise-style salad dressing	
reduced-fat	1 Tbsp
regular	2 tsp
Nuts	
pignolia (pine nuts)	1 Tbsp
walnuts, English	4 halves
Oil: corn, cottonseed, flaxseed, grapeseed, safflower, soybean, sunflower	1 tsp
Salad dressing	
reduced-fat[a]	2 Tbsp
regular	1 Tbsp
Seeds	
flaxseed, ground	1½ Tbsp
pumpkin, sesame, sunflower	1 Tbsp
Tahini or sesame paste	2 tsp
Saturated Fats	
Bacon, cooked, regular or turkey	1 slice
Butter	
reduced-fat	1 Tbsp
stick	1 tsp
Saturated Fats *continued*	
whipped	2 tsp
Butter blends made with oil	
reduced-fat or light	1 Tbsp
regular	1½ tsp
Chitterlings, boiled	2 Tbsp (½ oz)
Coconut, sweetened, shredded	2 Tbsp
Coconut milk, canned, thick	
light	⅓ cup
regular	1½ Tbsp
Coconut milk beverage (thin), unsweetened	1 cup
Cream	
half-and-half	2 Tbsp
heavy	1 Tbsp
light	1½ Tbsp
whipped	2 Tbsp
Cream cheese	
reduced-fat	1½ Tbsp (¾ oz)
regular	1 Tbsp (½ oz)
Lard	1 tsp
Oil: coconut, palm, palm kernel	1 tsp
Salt pork	¼ oz
Shortening, solid	1 tsp
Sour cream	
reduced-fat or light	3 Tbsp
regular	2 Tbsp

[a]May contain carbohydrate.

TABLE G-9 Free Foods

Most foods on the Free Foods list should be limited to 3 servings per day and eaten throughout the day. Eating all 3 servings at one time could raise blood glucose levels. Food and drink choices listed without a serving size can be eaten whenever you like.

1 free food choice = ≤5 grams carbohydrate and ≤20 kcalories.

Food	Serving Size
Low-Carbohydrate Foods	
Candy, hard (regular or sugar-free)	1 piece
Fruits: cranberries or rhubarb, sweetened with sugar substitute	½ cup
Gelatin dessert, sugar-free, any flavor	
Low-Carbohydrate Foods *continued*	
Gum, sugar-free	
Jam or jelly, light or no-sugar-added	2 tsp
Salad greens (such as arugula, chicory, endive, escarole, leaf or iceberg lettuce, purslane, romaine, radicchio, spinach, watercress)	

(Continued)

TABLE G-9 Free Foods (*continued*)

Food	Serving Size
Low-Carbohydrate Foods *continued*	
Sugar substitutes (artificial sweeteners)	
Syrup, sugar-free	2 Tbsp
Vegetables: any **raw** nonstarchy vegetables (such as broccoli, cabbage, carrots, cucumber, tomato)	½ cup
Vegetables: any **cooked** nonstarchy vegetables (such as carrots, cauliflower, green beans)	¼ cup
Reduced-Fat or Fat-Free Foods	
Cream cheese, fat-free	1 Tbsp (½ oz)
Coffee creamers, nondairy	
liquid, flavored	1½ tsp
liquid, sugar-free, flavored	4 tsp
powdered, flavored	1 tsp
powdered, sugar-free, flavored	2 tsp
Margarine spread	
fat-free	1 Tbsp
reduced-fat	1 tsp
Mayonnaise	
fat-free	1 Tbsp
reduced-fat	1 tsp
Mayonnaise-style salad dressing	
fat-free	1 Tbsp
reduced-fat	2 tsp
Salad dressing	
fat-free	1 Tbsp
fat-free, Italian	2 Tbsp
Sour cream, fat-free or reduced-fat	1 Tbsp
Whipped topping	
light or fat-free	2 Tbsp
regular	1 Tbsp
Condiments	
Barbecue sauce	2 tsp
Catsup (ketchup)	1 Tbsp
Chili sauce, sweet, tomato-type	2 tsp
Horseradish	
Hot pepper sauce	
Lemon juice	
Miso	1½ tsp
Condiments *continued*	
Mustard	
honey	1 Tbsp
brown, Dijon, horseradish-flavored, wasabi-flavored, or yellow	
Parmesan cheese, grated	1 Tbsp
Pickle relish (dill or sweet)	1 Tbsp
Pickles	
[S] dill	1½ medium
sweet, bread and butter	2 slices
sweet, gherkin	¾ oz
Pimento	
Salsa	¼ cup
[S] Soy sauce, light or regular	1 Tbsp
Sweet-and-sour sauce	2 tsp
Taco sauce	1 Tbsp
Vinegar	
Worcestershire sauce	
Yogurt, any type	2 Tbsp
Drinks/Mixes	
[S] Bouillon, broth, consommé	
Bouillon or broth, low-sodium	
Carbonated or mineral water	
Club soda	
Cocoa powder, unsweetened	1 Tbsp
Coffee, unsweetened or with sugar substitute	
Diet soft drinks, sugar-free	
Drink mixes (powder or liquid drops), sugar-free	
Tea, unsweetened or with sugar substitute	
Tonic water, sugar-free	
Water	
Water, flavored, sugar-free	
Seasonings	
Flavoring extracts (for example, vanilla, almond, or peppermint)	
Garlic, fresh or powder	
Herbs, fresh or dried	
Kelp	
Nonstick cooking spray	
Spices	
Wine, used in cooking	

Key

[S] = High in sodium: ≥480 mg/serving

TABLE G-10 Combination Foods

Many foods are eaten in various combinations, such as casseroles. Because "combination" foods do not fit into any one choice list, this list of choices provides some typical combination foods.

1 carbohydrate choice = 15 grams carbohydrate and about 70 kcalories.

Food	Serving Size	Choices per Serving
Entrees		
🧂 Casserole-type entrees (tuna noodle, lasagna, spaghetti with meatballs, chili with beans, macaroni and cheese)	1 cup (8 oz)	2 carbohydrates + 2 medium-fat proteins
🧂 Stews (beef/other meats and vegetables)	1 cup (8 oz)	1 carbohydrate + 1 medium-fat protein + 0–3 fats
Frozen Meals/Entrees		
🧂✓ Burrito (beef and bean)	1 (5 oz)	3 carbohydrates + 1 lean protein + 2 fats
Dinner-type healthy meal (includes dessert and is usually <400 kcal)	~9–12 oz	2–3 carbohydrates + 1–2 lean proteins + 1 fat
"Healthy"-type entree (usually <300 kcal)	~7–10 oz	2 carbohydrates + 2 lean proteins
Pizza		
🧂 cheese/vegetarian, thin crust	¼ of a 12-in. pizza (4½–5 oz)	2 carbohydrates + 2 medium-fat proteins
🧂 meat topping, thin crust	¼ of a 12-in. pizza (5 oz)	2 carbohydrates + 2 medium-fat proteins + 1½ fats
🧂 cheese/vegetarian or meat topping, rising crust	⅙ of a 12-in. pizza (4 oz)	2½ carbohydrates + 2 medium-fat proteins
🧂 Pocket sandwich	1 sandwich (4½ oz)	3 carbohydrates + 1 lean protein + 1–2 fats
🧂 Pot pie	1 (7 oz)	3 carbohydrates + 1 medium-fat protein + 3 fats
Salads (Deli-Style)		
Coleslaw	½ cup	1 carbohydrate + 1½ fats
Macaroni/pasta salad	½ cup	2 carbohydrates + 3 fats
🧂 Potato salad	½ cup	1½–2 carbohydrates + 1–2 fats
Tuna salad or chicken salad	½ cup (3½ oz)	½ carbohydrate + 2 lean proteins + 1 fat
Soups		
🧂✓ Bean, lentil, or split pea soup	1 cup (8 oz)	1½ carbohydrates + 1 lean protein
🧂 Chowder (made with milk)	1 cup (8 oz)	1 carbohydrate + 1 lean protein + 1½ fats
🧂 Cream soup (made with water)	1 cup (8 oz)	1 carbohydrate + 1 fat
🧂 Miso soup	1 cup (8 oz)	½ carbohydrate + 1 lean protein
🧂 Ramen noodle soup	1 cup (8 oz)	2 carbohydrates + 2 fats
Rice soup/porridge (congee)	1 cup (8 oz)	1 carbohydrate
🧂 Tomato soup (made with water), borscht	1 cup (8 oz)	1 carbohydrate
🧂 Vegetable beef, chicken noodle, or other broth-type soup (including "healthy"-type soups, such as those lower in sodium and/or fat)	1 cup (8 oz)	1 carbohydrate + 1 lean protein

Key

✓ = Good source of fiber: >3 g/serving

🧂 = High in sodium: ≥600 mg/serving for main dishes/meals and ≥480 mg/serving for side dishes

APPENDIX G

TABLE G-11 Fast Foods

The choices in the Fast Foods list are not specific fast-food meals or items, but are estimates based on popular foods. Ask the restaurant or check its website for nutrition information about your favorite fast foods.

1 carbohydrate choice = 15 grams carbohydrate and about 70 kcalories.

Food	Serving Size	Choices per Serving
Main Dishes/Entrees		
Chicken		
breast, breaded and fried[a]	1 (~7 oz)	1 carbohydrate + 6 medium-fat proteins
breast, meat only[b]	1	4 lean proteins
drumstick, breaded and fried[a]	1 (~2½ oz)	½ carbohydrate + 2 medium-fat proteins
drumstick, meat only[b]	1	1 lean protein + ½ fat
nuggets or tenders	6 (~3½ oz)	1 carbohydrate + 2 medium-fat proteins + 1 fat
thigh, breaded and fried[a]	1 (~5 oz)	1 carbohydrate + 3 medium-fat proteins + 2 fats
thigh, meat only[b]	1	2 lean proteins + ½ fat
wing, breaded and fried[a]	1 wing (~2 oz)	½ carbohydrate + 2 medium-fat proteins
wing, meat only[b]	1 wing	1 lean protein
Main dish salad (grilled chicken–type, no dressing or croutons)	1 salad (~11½ oz)	1 carbohydrate + 4 lean proteins
Pizza		
cheese, pepperoni, or sausage, regular or thick crust	⅛ of a 14-in. pizza (~4 oz)	2½ carbohydrates + 1 high-fat protein + 1 fat
cheese, pepperoni, or sausage, thin crust	⅛ of a 14-in. pizza (~2¾ oz)	1½ carbohydrates + 1 high-fat protein + 1 fat
cheese, meat, and vegetable, regular crust	⅛ of a 14-in. pizza (~5 oz)	2½ carbohydrates + 2 high-fat proteins
Asian		
Beef/chicken/shrimp with vegetables in sauce	1 cup (~6 oz)	1 carbohydrate + 2 lean proteins + 1 fat
Egg roll, meat	1 egg roll (~3 oz)	1½ carbohydrates + 1 lean protein + 1½ fats
Fried rice, meatless	1 cup	2½ carbohydrates + 2 fats
Fortune cookie	1	½ carbohydrate
Hot-and-sour soup	1 cup	½ carbohydrate + ½ fat
Meat with sweet sauce	1 cup (~6 oz)	3½ carbohydrates + 3 medium-fat proteins + 3 fats
Noodles and vegetables in sauce (chow mein, lo mein)	1 cup	2 carbohydrates + 2 fats
Mexican		
Burrito with beans and cheese	1 small (~6 oz)	3½ carbohydrates + 1 medium-fat protein + 1 fat
Nachos with cheese	1 small order (~8)	2½ carbohydrates + 1 high-fat protein + 2 fats
Quesadilla, cheese only	1 small order (~5 oz)	2½ carbohydrates + 3 high-fat proteins
Taco, crisp, with meat and cheese	1 small (~3 oz)	1 carbohydrate + 1 medium-fat protein + ½ fat
✓Taco salad with chicken and tortilla bowl	1 salad (1 lb including bowl)	3½ carbohydrates + 4 medium-fat proteins + 3 fats
Tostada with beans and cheese	1 small (~5 oz)	2 carbohydrates + 1 high-fat protein
Sandwiches		
Breakfast sandwiches		
breakfast burrito with sausage, egg, cheese	1 (~4 oz)	1½ carbohydrates + 2 high-fat proteins
egg, cheese, meat on an English muffin	1	2 carbohydrates + 3 medium-fat proteins + ½ fat
egg, cheese, meat on a biscuit	1	2 carbohydrates + 3 medium-fat proteins + 2 fats

TABLE G-11 Fast Foods (*continued*)

Food	Serving Size	Choices per Serving
Sandwiches ***continued***		
[S] sausage biscuit sandwich	1	2 carbohydrates + 1 high-fat protein + 4 fats
Chicken sandwiches		
[S] grilled with bun, lettuce, tomatoes, spread	1 (~7½ oz)	3 carbohydrates + 4 lean proteins
[S] crispy with bun, lettuce, tomatoes, spread	1 (~6 oz)	3 carbohydrates + 2 lean proteins + 3½ fats
Fish sandwich with tartar sauce and cheese	1 (5 oz)	2½ carbohydrates + 2 medium-fat proteins + 1½ fats
Hamburger		
regular with bun and condiments (catsup, mustard, onion, pickle)	1 (~3½ oz)	2 carbohydrates + 1 medium-fat protein + 1 fat
[S] 4 oz meat with cheese, bun, and condiments (catsup, mustard, onion, pickle)	1 (~8½ oz)	3 carbohydrates + 4 medium-fat proteins + 2½ fats
Hot dog with bun, plain	1 (~3½ oz)	1½ carbohydrates + 1 high-fat protein + 2 fats
Submarine sandwich (no cheese or sauce)		
[S] <6 g fat	1 6-in. sub	3 carbohydrates + 2 lean proteins
[S] regular	1 6-in. sub	3 carbohydrates + 2 lean proteins + 1 fat
[S] Wrap, grilled chicken, vegetables, cheese, and spread	1 small (~4–5 oz)	2 carbohydrates + 2 lean proteins + 1½ fats
Sides/Appetizers		
[S] ! French fries	1 small order (~3½ oz)	2½ carbohydrates + 2 fats
	1 medium order (~5 oz)	3½ carbohydrates + 3 fats
	1 large order (~6 oz)	4½ carbohydrates + 4 fats
[S] Hash browns	1 cup/medium order (~5 oz)	3 carbohydrates + 6 fats
[S] Onion rings	1 serving (8–9 rings, ~4 oz)	3½ carbohydrates + 4 fats
Salad, side (no dressing, croutons, or cheese)	1 small	1 nonstarchy vegetable
Beverages and Desserts		
Coffee, latte (fat-free milk)	1 small (~12 oz)	1 fat-free milk
Coffee, mocha (fat-free milk, no whipped cream)	1 small (~12 oz)	1 fat-free milk + 1 carbohydrate
Milkshake, any flavor	1 small (~12 oz)	5½ carbohydrates + 3 fats
	1 medium (~16 oz)	7 carbohydrates + 4 fats
	1 large (~22 oz)	10 carbohydrates + 5 fats
Soft-serve ice cream cone	1 small	2 carbohydrates + ½ fat

[a]Definition and weight refer to food **with** bone, skin, and breading.
[b]Definition refers to food **without** bone, skin, and breading.

Key

✓ = Good source of fiber: >3 g/serving

! = Extra fat: +5 grams fat

[S] = High in sodium: ≥600 mg/serving for main dishes/meals and ≥480 mg/serving for side dishes

TABLE G-12 Alcohol

NOTE: For those who choose to drink alcohol, guidelines suggest limiting alcohol intake to 1 drink or less per day for women, and 2 drinks or less per day for men. To reduce the risk of low blood glucose (hypoglycemia), especially when taking insulin or a diabetes pill that increases insulin, alcohol should always be consumed with food. While alcohol, by itself, does not directly affect blood glucose, be aware of the carbohydrate (for example, in mixed drinks, beer, and wine) that may raise blood glucose.

1 alcohol equivalent = variable grams carbohydrate, 0 grams protein, 0 grams fat, and 100 kcalories.

Alcoholic Beverage[a]	Serving Size	Choices per Serving
Beer		
light (<4.5% abv)	12 fl oz	1 alcohol equivalent + ½ carbohydrate
regular (~5% abv)	12 fl oz	1 alcohol equivalent + 1 carbohydrate
dark (>5.7% abv)	12 fl oz	1 alcohol equivalent + 1–1½ carbohydrate
Distilled spirits (80 or 86 proof): vodka, rum, gin, whiskey, tequila	1½ fl oz	1 alcohol equivalent
Liqueur, coffee (53 proof)	1 fl oz	½ alcohol equivalent + 1 carbohydrate
Sake	1 fl oz	½ alcohol equivalent
Wine		
champagne/sparkling	5 fl oz	1 alcohol equivalent
dessert (sherry)	3½ fl oz	1 alcohol equivalent + 1 carbohydrate
dry, red or white (10% abv)	5 fl oz	1 alcohol equivalent

[a]The abbreviation "%abv" refers to the percentage of alcohol by volume.

SOURCE: The Food Lists are the basis of a meal planning system designed by a committee of the American Diabetes Association and the Academy of Nutrition and Dietetics. While originally designed for people with diabetes and others who must follow special diets, the Food Lists are based on principles of good nutrition that apply to everyone.

Appendix H Aids to Calculation

Many mathematical problems have been worked out in the "How To" features of the text. This appendix offers additional help and examples.

Conversions

A conversion factor is a fraction that converts a measurement expressed in one unit to another unit—for example, from pounds to kilograms or from feet to meters. To create a conversion factor, an equality (such as 1 kilogram = 2.2 pounds) is expressed as a fraction:

$$\frac{1\text{ kg}}{2.2\text{ lb}} \text{ and } \frac{2.2\text{ lb}}{1\text{ kg}}$$

To convert the units of a measurement, use the fraction with the desired unit in the numerator.

Example 1 Convert a weight of 130 pounds to kilograms. Multiply 130 pounds by the conversion factor that includes both pounds and kilograms, with the desired unit (kilograms) in the numerator:

$$130\text{ lb} \times \frac{1\text{ kg}}{2.2\text{ lb}} = \frac{130\text{ kg}}{2.2} = 59\text{ kg}$$

Alternatively, to convert a measurement from one unit of measure to another, multiply the given measurement by the appropriate equivalent found on the next page of weights and measures.

Example 2 Convert 64 fluid ounces to liters. Locate the equivalent measure from the volume section on the next page (1 ounce = 0.03 liter) and multiply the number of ounces by 0.03:

$$64\text{ oz} \times 0.03\text{ oz/L} = 1.9\text{ L}$$

Percentages

A percentage is a fraction whose denominator is 100. For example:

$$50\% = \frac{50}{100}$$

Like other fractions, percentages are used to express a portion of a quantity. Fractions whose denominators are numbers other than 100 can be converted to percentages by first dividing the numerator by the denominator and then multiplying the result by 100.

Example 3 Express 5/8 as a percent.

$$\frac{5}{8} = 5 \div 8 = 0.625$$

$$0.625 \times 100 = 62.5\%$$

The following examples show how to calculate specific percentages.

Example 4 Suppose your energy intake for the day is 2000 kcalories (kcal) and your recommended energy intake is 2400 kcalories. What percent of the recommended energy intake did you consume?

Divide your intake by the recommended intake.
2000 kcal (intake) ÷ 2400 kcal (recommended) = 0.83
Multiply by 100 to express the decimal as a percent.
0.83 × 100 = 83%

Example 5 Suppose a man's intake of vitamin C is 120 milligrams and his RDA is 90 milligrams. What percent of the RDA for vitamin C did he consume?

Divide the intake by the recommended intake.
120 mg (intake) ÷ 90 mg (RDA) = 1.33
Multiply by 100 to express the decimal as a percent.
1.33 × 100 = 133%

Example 6 Dietary recommendations suggest that carbohydrates provide 45 to 65 percent of the day's energy intake. If your energy intake is 2000 kcalories, how much carbohydrate should you eat?

Because this question has a range of acceptable answers, work the problem twice. First, use 45 percent to find the least amount you should eat.

Divide 45 by 100 to convert to a decimal.
45 ÷ 100 = 0.45
Multiply kcalories by 0.45.
2000 kcal × 0.45 = 900 kcal
Divide kcalories by 4 to convert carbohydrate kcal to grams.
900 kcal ÷ 4 kcal/g = 225 g

Now repeat the process using 65 percent to find the maximum number of grams of carbohydrates you should eat.

Divide 65 by 100 to convert it to a decimal.
65 ÷ 100 = 0.65
Multiply kcalories by 0.65.
2000 kcal × 0.65 = 1300 kcal
Divide kcalories by 4 to convert carbohydrate kcal to grams.
1300 kcal ÷ 4 kcal/g = 325 g

If you plan for between 45 percent and 65 percent of your 2000-kcalorie intake to be from carbohydrates, you should eat between 225 grams and 325 grams of carbohydrates.

Weights and Measures

Length

1 centimeter (cm) = 0.39 inches (in.)
1 foot (ft) = 30 centimeters (cm)
1 inch (in.) = 2.54 centimeters (cm)
1 meter (m) = 39.37 inches (in.)

Weight

1 gram (g) = 0.001 kilograms (kg)
= 1000 milligrams (mg)
= 0.035 ounces (oz)
1 kilogram (kg) = 1000 grams (g)
= 2.2 pounds (lb)
1 microgram (µg) = 0.001 milligrams (mg)
1 milligram (mg) = 0.001 grams (g)
= 1000 micrograms (µg)
1 ounce (oz) = 28 grams (g)
= 0.03 kilograms (kg)
= 1/16 or 0.0625 pound (lb)
1 pound (lb) = 454 grams (g)
= 0.45 kilograms (kg)
= 16 ounces (oz)

Volume

1 cup = 16 tablespoons (tbs or T)
= 0.25 liters (L)
= 236 milliliters (mL, commonly rounded to 250 mL)
= 8 ounces (oz)
1 liter (L) = 33.8 fluid ounces (fl oz)
= 0.26 gallons (gal)
= 2.1 pints (pt)
= 1.06 quarts (qt)
= 1000 milliliters (mL)
1 milliliter (mL) = 0.001 liters (L)
= 0.03 fluid ounces (fl oz)
= 1/5 teaspoon (tsp)
1 ounce (oz) = 0.03 liters (L)
= 30 milliliters (mL)
= 2 tablespoons (tbs)
1 pint (pt) = 2 cups (c)
= 0.47 liters (L)
= 16 ounces (oz)
= 0.5 quarts (qt)
1 quart (qt) = 4 cups (c)
= 0.95 liters (L)
= 32 ounces (oz)
= 1/4 or 0.25 gallon (gal)
= 2 pints (pt)
1 tablespoon (tbs or T) = 3 teaspoons (tsp)
= 15 milliliters (mL)
1 teaspoon (tsp) = 5 milliliters (mL)
1 gallon (gal) = 16 cups (c)
= 3.8 liters (L)
= 128 ounces (oz)
= 8 pints (pt)
= 4 quarts (qt)
1 cup (c) = 8 ounces (oz)
= 16 tablespoons (tbs)
= 250 milliliters (mL)

Energy

1 megajoule (MJ) = 240 kcalories (kcal)
1 kilojoule (kJ) = 0.24 kcalories (kcal)
1 kcalorie (kcal) = 4.2 kilojoule (kJ)
1 g alcohol = 7 kcal = 29 kJ
1 g carbohydrate = 4 kcal = 17 kJ
1 g fat = 9 kcal = 37 kJ
1 g protein = 4 kcal = 17 kJ

Temperature

To change from Fahrenheit (°F) to Celsius (°C), subtract 32 from the Fahrenheit measure and then multiply that result by 0.56.

To change from Celsius (°C) to Fahrenheit (°F), multiply the Celsius measure by 1.8 and add 32 to that result.

A comparison of some useful temperatures is given below.

	Celsius	Fahrenheit
Boiling point	100°C	212°F
Body temperature	37°C	98.6°F
Freezing point	0°C	32°F

Appendix I WHO Nutrition Recommendations

Healthy diets help protect against malnutrition and chronic diseases. Diets may vary depending on an person's needs, cultural traditions, socioeconomic factors, available foods, and dietary preferences, but the basics remain essentially the same. The World Health Organization (WHO) summarized these nutrition recommendations for adults:

- Energy intake: in balance with energy expenditure; sufficient to support growth, physical activity, and a healthy body weight (BMI between 18.5 and 24.9); and limited enough to avoid unhealthy weight gain (greater than 11 pounds) during adult life
- Total fat: <30 percent of total energy
- Saturated fatty acids: <10 percent of total energy
- Polyunsaturated fatty acids: 6 to 10 percent of total energy
- Omega-6 polyunsaturated fatty acids: 5 to 8 percent of total energy
- Omega-3 polyunsaturated fatty acids: 1 to 2 percent of total energy
- *Trans*-fatty acids: <1 percent of total energy
- Total carbohydrate: 55 to 75 percent of total energy
- Sugars: <10 percent of total energy, preferably <5 percent of total energy
- Protein: 10 to 15 percent of total energy
- Cholesterol: <300 mg per day
- Salt (sodium): <5 g salt per day (<2 g sodium per day), appropriately iodized
- Potassium: ≥3510 mg per day
- Fruits and vegetables: ≥400 g per day (about 1 pound); potatoes, sweet potatoes, cassava, and other starchy root vegetables do not count toward this goal
- Total dietary fiber: >25 g per day from foods
- Physical activity: one hour of moderate-intensity activity, such as walking, on most days of the week

Appendix J Healthy People 2020

Chapter 1 introduced the Healthy People 2020 initiative. Table J-1 presents nutrition-related objectives.

TABLE J-1 Nutrition-Related Objectives

Access to Health Services

- Increase the proportion of persons who receive appropriate evidence-based clinical preventive services.

Adolescent Health

- Increase the proportion of schools with a school breakfast program.

Arthritis, Osteoporosis, and Chronic Back Conditions

- Reduce hip fractures among older adults.
- Reduce the proportion of adults with osteoporosis.

Cancer

- Reduce the cancer death rate.
- Increase the mental and physical health-related quality of life of cancer survivors.

Diabetes

- Reduce the annual number of new cases of diagnosed diabetes in the population.
- Reduce the death rate among the population with diabetes.
- Reduce the diabetes death rate.
- Improve glycemic control among the population with diagnosed diabetes.
- Improve lipid control among persons with diagnosed diabetes.
- Increase the proportion of the population with diagnosed diabetes whose blood pressure is under control.
- Increase the proportion of persons with diagnosed diabetes who receive formal diabetes education.
- Increase prevention behaviors in persons at high risk for diabetes with prediabetes.

Early and Middle Childhood

- Increase the proportion of elementary, middle, and senior high schools that require school health education.

Educational and Community-Based Programs

- Increase the proportion of preschool Early Head Start and Head Start programs that provide health education to prevent health problems in the following areas: unintentional injury; violence; tobacco use and addiction; alcohol and drug use, unhealthy dietary patterns; and inadequate physical activity, dental health, and safety.
- Increase the proportion of elementary, middle, and senior high schools that provide comprehensive school health education to prevent health problems in the following areas: unintentional injury; violence; suicide; tobacco use and addiction; alcohol or other drug use; unintended pregnancy, human immunodeficiency virus/acquired immune deficiency syndrome (HIV/AIDS), and sexually transmitted diseases (STD) infection; unhealthy dietary patterns; and inadequate physical activity.
- Increase the proportion of college and university students who receive information from their institution on each of the priority health risk behavior areas (all priority areas; unintentional injury; violence; suicide; tobacco use and addiction; alcohol and other drug use; unintended pregnancy, HIV/AIDS, and STD infection; unhealthy dietary patterns; and inadequate physical activity).
- Increase the proportion of worksites that offer an employee health promotion program to their employees.
- Increase the number of community-based organizations (including local health departments, tribal health services, nongovernmental organizations, and state agencies) providing population-based primary prevention services.

Environmental Health

- Reduce blood lead levels in children.
- Reduce the number of US homes that are found to have lead-based paint or related hazards.

TABLE J-1 Nutrition-Related Objectives *(continued)*

Food Safety

- Reduce infections caused by key pathogens transmitted commonly through food.
- Reduce the number of outbreak-associated infections due to Shiga toxin-producing *Escherichia coli* O157:H7, or *Campylobacter, Listeria*, or *Salmonella* species associated with food commodity groups.
- Reduce severe allergic reactions to food among adults with a food allergy diagnosis.
- Increase the proportion of consumers who follow key food safety practices.
- Improve food safety practices associated with foodborne illness in foodservice and retail establishments.

Heart Disease and Stroke

- Increase overall cardiovascular health in the US population.
- Reduce coronary heart disease deaths.
- Reduce stroke deaths.
- Reduce the proportion of persons in the population with hypertension.
- Reduce the proportion of adults with high total blood cholesterol levels.
- Reduce the mean total blood cholesterol levels among adults.
- Increase the proportion of adults with prehypertension who meet the recommended guidelines.
- Increase the proportion of adults with hypertension who meet the recommended guidelines.
- Increase the proportion of adults with elevated LDL cholesterol who have been advised by a health-care provider regarding cholesterol-lowering management including lifestyle changes and, if indicated, medication.
- Increase the proportion of adults with elevated LDL-cholesterol who adhere to the prescribed LDL cholesterol–lowering management lifestyle changes and, if indicated, medication.

Maternal, Infant, and Child Health

- Reduce low birth weight (LBW) and very low birth weight (VLBW).
- Reduce preterm births.
- Increase the proportion of pregnant women who receive early and adequate prenatal care.
- Increase the proportion of mothers who achieve a recommended weight gain during their pregnancies.
- Increase the proportion of women of childbearing potential with intake of at least 400 micrograms of folic acid from fortified foods or dietary supplements.
- Reduce the proportion of women of childbearing potential who have low red blood cell folate concentrations.
- Increase the proportion of women delivering a live birth who received preconception care services and practiced key recommended preconception health behaviors.
- Increase the proportion of infants who are breastfed.
- Increase the proportion of employers that have worksite lactation support programs.
- Reduce the proportion of breastfed newborns who receive formula supplementation within the first 2 days of life.
- Reduce the occurrence of fetal alcohol syndrome (FAS).
- Reduce occurrence of neural tube defects.

Mental Health and Mental Disorders

- Reduce the proportion of adolescents who engage in disordered eating behaviors in an attempt to control their weight.

Nutrition and Weight Status

- Increase the proportion of adults who are at a healthy weight.
- Reduce the proportion of adults who are obese.
- Reduce iron deficiency among young children and females of childbearing age.
- Reduce iron deficiency among pregnant females.
- Reduce the proportion of children and adolescents who are overweight or obese.
- Increase the contribution of fruits to the diets of the population aged 2 years and older.
- Increase the variety and contribution of vegetables to the diets of the population aged 2 years and older.
- Increase the contribution of whole grains to the diets of the population aged 2 years and older.
- Reduce consumption of saturated fat in the population aged 2 years and older.
- Reduce consumption of sodium in the population aged 2 years and older.
- Increase consumption of calcium in the population aged 2 years and older.
- Increase the proportion of worksites that offer nutrition or weight management classes or counseling.
- Increase the proportion of physician office visits that include counseling or education related to nutrition or weight.
- Eliminate very low food security among children in US households.
- Prevent inappropriate weight gain in youth and adults.
- Increase the proportion of primary care physicians who regularly measure the body mass index (BMI) of their patients.

(Continued)

TABLE J-1 Nutrition-Related Objectives *(continued)*

- Reduce consumption of kcalories from solid fats and added sugars in the population aged 2 years and older.
- Increase the number of states that have state-level policies that incentivize food retail outlets to provide foods that are encouraged by the *Dietary Guidelines*.
- Increase the number of states with nutrition standards for foods and beverages provided to preschool-aged children in child care.
- Increase the percentage of schools that offer nutritious foods and beverages outside of school meals.

Older Adults

- Increase the proportion of the health-care workforce (including dietitians) with geriatric certification.

Oral Health

- Increase the proportion of the US population served by community water systems with optimally fluoridated water.

Physical Activity

- Reduce the proportion of adults who engage in no leisure-time physical activity.
- Increase the proportion of adolescents and adults who meet current federal physical activity guidelines for aerobic physical activity and for muscle-strengthening activity.
- Increase the proportion of the nation's public and private schools that require daily physical education for all students.
- Increase the proportion of adolescents who participate in daily school physical education.
- Increase regularly scheduled elementary school recess in the United States.
- Increase the proportion of children and adolescents who do not exceed recommended limits for screen time.

SOURCE: Adapted from Healthy people 2020: www.healthypeople.gov.

Glossary

Many medical terms have their origins in Latin or Greek. By learning a few common derivations, you can glean the meaning of words you have never heard of before. For example, once you know that "hyper" means above normal, "glyc"" means glucose, and "emia" means blood, you can easily determine that "hyperglycemia" means high blood glucose. The derivations below will help you learn many terms presented in this glossary.

General

a- or **an-** = not, without
ana- = (build) up
ant- or **anti-** = against
ante- or **pre-** = before
bi- or **di-** = two, twice
bio- or **biotic** = life
bovine = of cattle
calor = heat
cata- or **kata-** = (break) down
chele = claw
chroma = color
co- = with, together
dys- or **mal-** = bad, difficult, painful
endo- = inner, within, inside
epi- = upon (over)
erythro- = red
exo- = outside of, without
extra- = outside of, beyond, in addition
gen or **genesis** = producing, arising, making
homeo- = like, similar, the same, constant unchanging state
hyper- = over, above, excessive
hypo- = below, under, beneath, too little
in- = not
inter- = between, in the midst of
intra- = within
lac- or **lacto-** = milk
-lysis = breaking, breakdown
macro- = large, great
malacia = softening
metallo- = metal
micro- = small
mono- = one, single
neo- = new, recent
oligo- = few, small
-osis or **-asis** = condition
para- = near
peri- = around, about
phag- or **phago-** = eat
-philia, -phil, or **-philic** = love
-phobia = fear
phyto- = plant
poly- = many, much
pro- = for, in front of
re- = back, again
semi- = half
-stat or **-stasis-** = stationary, staying
sub- = beneath
tri- = three
xero- = dry

Body

angi- or **vaso-** = vessel
arterio- = artery
cardi-, cardiac, cardio-, or **cardial** = heart
cerebro = brain
cyst = closed sac
-cyte or **-cytic** = cell
encephalic = brain
entero- or **enteric** = intestine
fibro- = fibrous tissue
gastro- = stomach
globin = globular protein
hema-, hemo-, or **-emia** = blood
hepatic = liver
myo- = muscle
nephr- or **renal** = kidney
neuro- = nerve
osteo- = bone
pulmo- = lung
sarco- = flesh
soma = body
ure- or **-uria** = urine
vascular = blood vessels
vena = vein

Chemistry

-al = aldehyde
amino- or **amine** = containing nitrogen
-ase = enzyme
-ate = salt
carbo- = carbon (C)
glyc-, glyco-, glue-, or **gluco-** = sweet (glucose)
glyceride = of glycerol
hydro- or **hydrate** = water
lipo- = lipid
-ol = alcohol
-ose = carbohydrate
peptide = referring to amino acids
saccha- or **sucro-** = sugar

Disease

athero- = porridge, fatty plaque
carcin- = cancer
-itis = infection, inflammation
-osis or **-asis** = condition
thrombo = clot

24-hour dietary recall: a record of foods eaten by a person for one 24-hour period.

A

A1C: a test that measures the percentage of hemoglobin that has glucose attached, which helps diagnose diabetes and evaluate long-term glycemic control.

absorption: the uptake of nutrients by the cells of the small intestine for transport into either the blood or the lymph.

Academy of Nutrition and Dietetics: the professional organization of dietitians in the United States; formerly the American Dietetic Association.

Acceptable Daily Intake (ADI): the estimated amount of a sweetener that individuals can safely consume each day over the course of a lifetime without adverse effect.

Acceptable Macronutrient Distribution Ranges (AMDR): ranges of intakes for the energy nutrients that provide adequate energy and nutrients and reduce the risk of chronic diseases.

accredited: approved; in the case of medical centers or universities, certified by an agency recognized by the US Department of Education.

acetaldehyde (ass-et-AL-duh-hide): an intermediate in alcohol metabolism.

acetyl CoA (ASS-eh-teel or ah-SEET-il, coh-AY): a 2-carbon compound (acetate or acetic acid) to which a molecule of CoA is attached.

acid controllers: medications used to prevent or relieve indigestion by suppressing production of acid in the stomach; also called *H2 blockers.*

acid–base balance: the equilibrium in the body between acid and base concentrations.

acidosis (assi-DOE-sis): higher-than-normal acidity in the blood and body fluids.

acids: compounds that release hydrogen ions (H^+) in a solution.

acne: a chronic inflammation of the skin's follicles and oil-producing glands, which leads to an accumulation of oils inside the ducts that surround hairs; usually associated with the maturation of young adults.

acupuncture (AK-you-PUNK-cher): a technique that involves piercing the skin with long thin needles at specific anatomical points to relieve pain or illness. Acupuncture sometimes uses heat, pressure, friction, suction, or electromagnetic energy to stimulate the points.

acute malnutrition: malnutrition caused by recent severe food restriction; characterized in children by underweight for height *(wasting).*

adaptive thermogenesis: adjustments in energy expenditure related to changes in environment such as extreme cold and to physiological events such as overfeeding, trauma, and changes in hormone status.

added sugars: sugars and other kcaloric sweeteners that are added to foods during processing, preparation, or at the table. Added sugars do not include the naturally occurring sugars found in fruits and milk products.

additives: substances not normally consumed as foods but added to food either intentionally or by accident.

adenosine triphosphate: see *ATP.*

adequacy (dietary): providing all the essential nutrients, fiber, and energy in amounts sufficient to maintain health.

Adequate Intake (AI): the average daily amount of a nutrient that appears sufficient to maintain a specified criterion; a value used as a guide for nutrient intake when an RDA cannot be determined.

ADH: see *antidiuretic hormone.*

ADI: see *Acceptable Daily Intake.*

adipokines (ADD-ih-poe-kines): proteins synthesized and secreted by adipose cells.

adiponectin: a protein produced by adipose cells that inhibits inflammation and protects against insulin resistance, type 2 diabetes, and cardiovascular disease.

adipose (ADD-ih-poce) **tissue:** the body's fat tissue; consists of masses of triglyceride-storing cells.

adolescence: the period from the beginning of puberty until maturity.

adrenal glands: glands adjacent to, and just above, each kidney.

adverse reactions: unusual responses to food (including intolerances and allergies).

aerobic (air-ROE-bic): requiring oxygen.

aerobic physical activity: activity in which the body's large muscles move in a rhythmic manner for a sustained period of time. Aerobic activity, also called *endurance activity,* improves cardiorespiratory fitness. Brisk walking, running, swimming, and bicycling are examples.

AI: see *Adequate Intake.*

alcohol: a class of organic compounds containing hydroxyl (OH) groups.

alcohol abuse: a pattern of drinking that includes failure to fulfill work, school, or home responsibilities; drinking in situations that are physically dangerous (as in driving while intoxicated); recurring alcohol-related legal problems (as in aggravated assault charges); or continued drinking despite ongoing social problems that are caused by or worsened by alcohol.

alcohol dehydrogenase (dee-high-DROJ-eh-nayz): an enzyme active in the stomach and the liver that converts ethanol to acetaldehyde.

alcoholism: a pattern of drinking that includes a strong craving for alcohol, a loss of control and an inability to stop drinking once begun, withdrawal symptoms (nausea, sweating, shakiness, and anxiety) after heavy drinking, and the need for increasing amounts of alcohol to feel "high."

alcohol-related birth defects (ARBD): malformations in the skeletal and organ systems (heart, kidneys, eyes, ears) associated with prenatal alcohol exposure.

alcohol-related neurodevelopmental disorder (ARND): abnormalities in the central nervous system and cognitive development associated with prenatal alcohol exposure.

aldosterone (al-DOS-ter-own): a hormone secreted by the adrenal glands that regulates blood pressure by increasing the reabsorption of sodium by the kidneys. Aldosterone also regulates chloride and potassium concentrations.

alkalosis (alka-LOE-sis): higher-than-normal alkalinity (base) in the blood and body fluids.

alpha-lactalbumin (lact-AL-byoo-min): a major protein in human breast milk, as opposed to *casein* (CAY-seen), a major protein in cow's milk.

alpha-tocopherol: the active vitamin E compound.

Alzheimer's (AHLZ-high-merz) **disease:** a degenerative disease of the brain involving memory loss and major structural changes in neuron networks; also known as *senile dementia of the Alzheimer's type (SDAT), primary degenerative dementia of senile onset,* or *chronic brain syndrome.*

AMDR: see *Acceptable Macronutrient Distribution Ranges.*

amenorrhea (ay-MEN-oh-REE-ah): the absence of or cessation of menstruation. *Primary amenorrhea* is menarche delayed beyond 16 years of age. *Secondary amenorrhea* is the absence of three to six consecutive menstrual cycles.

amino (a-MEEN-oh) **acids:** building blocks of proteins. Each contains an amino group, an acid group, a hydrogen atom, and a distinctive side group, all attached to a central carbon atom.

amino acid pool: the supply of amino acids derived from either food proteins or body proteins that collect in the cells and circulating blood and stand ready to be incorporated in proteins and other compounds or used for energy.

amino acid score: a measure of protein quality assessed by comparing a protein's amino acid pattern with that of a reference protein; also called the *chemical score.*

ammonia: a compound with the chemical formula NH_3, produced during the deamination of amino acids.

amniotic (am-nee-OTT-ic) **sac:** the "bag of waters" in the uterus, in which the fetus floats.

amylase (AM-ih-lace): an enzyme that hydrolyzes amylose (a form of starch). Amylase is a *carbohydrase,* an enzyme that breaks down carbohydrates.

anabolic steroids: drugs related to the male sex hormone, testosterone, that stimulate the development of lean body mass.

anabolism (an-AB-o-lism): reactions in which small molecules are put together to build larger ones. Anabolic reactions require energy.

anaerobic (AN-air-ROE-bic): not requiring oxygen.

anaphylactic (ana-fill-LAC-tic) **shock:** a life-threatening, whole-body allergic reaction to an offending substance.

androstenedione: hormones made in the adrenal glands that serve as precursors to the male sex hormone, testosterone; falsely promoted as burning fat, building muscle, and slowing aging.

anecdote: a personal account of an experience or event; not reliable scientific information.

anemia (ah-NEE-me-ah): literally, "too little blood"; any condition in which there is reduced delivery of oxygen to the tissues. Anemia is not a disease itself but can be a symptom of many different disease conditions, including some nutrient deficiencies.

anencephaly (AN-en-SEF-a-lee): an uncommon and always fatal type of neural tube defect, characterized by the absence of a brain.

aneurysm (AN-you-rizm): an abnormal enlargement or bulging of a blood vessel (usually an artery) caused by damage to or weakness in the blood vessel wall.

angina (an-JYE-nah or AN-ji-nah): a painful feeling of tightness or pressure in and around the heart, often radiating to the back, neck, and arms; caused by a lack of oxygen to an area of heart muscle.

angiotensin I (AN-gee-oh-TEN-sin): an inactive precursor that is converted by an enzyme to yield active angiotensin II.

angiotensin II: a hormone involved in blood pressure regulation.

angiotensinogen: a precursor protein that is hydrolyzed to angiotensin I by renin.

anions (AN-eye-uns): negatively charged ions.

anorexia (an-oh-RECK-see-ah) **nervosa:** an eating disorder characterized by a refusal to maintain a minimally normal body weight and a distortion in perception of body shape and weight.

antacids: medications used to relieve indigestion by neutralizing acid in the stomach.

antagonist: a competing factor that counteracts the action of another factor. When a drug displaces a vitamin from its site of action, the drug renders the vitamin ineffective and thus acts as a vitamin antagonist.

anthropometric (AN-throw-poe-MET-rick): relating to measurement of the physical characteristics of the body, such as height and weight.

antibodies: large proteins of the blood and body fluids, produced by the immune system in response to the invasion of the body by foreign molecules (usually proteins called *antigens*). Antibodies combine with and inactivate the foreign invaders, thus protecting the body.

antidiuretic hormone (ADH): a water-conserving hormone produced by the pituitary gland in response to dehydration (or a high sodium concentration in the blood) that stimulates the kidneys to reabsorb more water and therefore to excrete less. In addition to its antidiuretic effect, ADH elevates blood pressure and so is also called *vasopressin* (VAS-oh-PRES-in).

antigens: substances that elicit the formation of antibodies or an inflammation reaction from the immune system. Examples of antigens include viruses, bacteria, and toxins.

antioxidants: in the body, substances that significantly decrease the adverse effects of free radicals on normal physiological functions.

antioxidants: as a food additive, preservatives that delay or prevent rancidity of fats in foods and other damage to food caused by oxygen.

antipromoters: factors that oppose the development of cancer.

antiscorbutic (AN-tee-skor-BUE-tik) **factor:** the original name for vitamin C.

anus (AY-nus): the terminal outlet of the GI tract.

aorta (ay-OR-tuh): the large, primary artery that conducts blood from the heart to the body's smaller arteries.

appendix: a narrow blind sac extending from the beginning of the colon that contains bacteria and lymph cells.

appetite: the integrated response to the sight, smell, thought, or taste of food that initiates or delays eating.

aquaculture: the practice of fish farming.

arachidonic (a-RACK-ih-DON-ic) **acid:** an omega-6 polyunsaturated fatty acid with 20 carbons and four double bonds; present in small amounts in meat and other animal products and synthesized in the body from linoleic acid.

ARBD: see *alcohol-related birth defects.*

ariboflavinosis (ay-RYE-boh-FLAY-vin-oh-sis): riboflavin deficiency.

ARND: see *alcohol-related neurodevelopmental disorder.*

aroma therapy: a technique that uses oil extracts from plants and flowers (usually applied by massage or baths) to enhance physical, psychological, and spiritual health.

arteries: vessels that carry blood from the heart to the tissues.

artesian water: water drawn from a well that taps a confined aquifer in which the water is under pressure.

arthritis: inflammation of a joint, usually accompanied by pain, swelling, and structural changes.

artificial fats: zero-energy fat replacers that are chemically synthesized to mimic the sensory and cooking qualities of naturally occurring fats but are totally or partially resistant to digestion.

artificial sweeteners: sugar substitutes that provide negligible, if any, energy; sometimes called *nonnutritive sweeteners.*

ascorbic acid: one of the two active forms of vitamin C. Many people refer to vitamin C by this name.

-ase (ACE): a suffix denoting an enzyme. The root of the word often identifies the compounds the enzyme works on. Examples include: *carbohydrase* (KAR-boe-HIGH-drase), an enzyme that hydrolyzes carbohydrates; *lipase* (LYE-pase), an enzyme that hydrolyzes lipids (fats); and *protease* (PRO-tee-ase), an enzyme that hydrolyzes proteins.

atherogenic: able to initiate or promote atherosclerosis.

atherosclerosis (ATH-er-oh-scler-OH-sis): a type of artery disease characterized by plaques (accumulations of lipid-containing material) on the inner walls of the arteries.

atoms: the smallest components of an element that have all of the properties of the element.

ATP or **adenosine** (ah-DEN-oh-seen) **triphosphate** (try-FOS-fate): a common high-energy compound composed of a purine (adenine), a sugar (ribose), and three phosphate groups. ATP = A-P~P~P, with each ~ denoting a "high-energy" bond.

atrophic (a-TRO-fik) **gastritis** (gas-TRY-tis): chronic inflammation of the stomach accompanied by a diminished size and functioning of the mucous membranes and glands. This condition is also characterized by inadequate hydrochloric acid and intrinsic factor—two substances needed for vitamin B_{12} absorption.

atrophy (AT-ro-fee): becoming smaller; with regard to muscles, a decrease in size (and strength) because of disuse, undernutrition, or wasting diseases.

autoimmune disorder: a condition in which the body develops antibodies to its own proteins and then proceeds to destroy cells containing these proteins. In type 1 diabetes, the body develops antibodies to its insulin and destroys the pancreatic cells that produce the insulin, creating an insulin deficiency.

autonomic nervous system: the division of the nervous system that controls the body's automatic responses. Its two branches are the *sympathetic* branch, which helps the body respond to stressors from the outside environment, and the *parasympathetic* branch, which regulates normal body activities between stressful times.

avidin (AV-eh-din): the protein in egg whites that binds biotin.

ayurveda (AH-your-VAY-dah): a traditional Hindu system of improving health by using herbs, diet, meditation, massage, and yoga to stimulate the body, mind, and spirit to prevent and treat disease.

B

bacteriophages (bak-TIR-ee-oh-fayjz): viruses that infect bacteria.

balance (dietary): providing foods in proportion to one another and in proportion to the body's needs.

bariatric: pertaining to the field of medicine that specializes in treating obesity.

basal metabolic rate (BMR): the rate of energy use for metabolism under specified conditions: after a 12-hour fast and restful sleep, without any physical activity or emotional excitement, and in a comfortable setting. It is usually expressed as kcalories per kilogram of body weight per hour.

basal metabolism: the energy needed to maintain life when a body is at complete digestive, physical, and emotional rest.

bases: compounds that accept hydrogen ions in a solution.

B-cells: lymphocytes that produce antibodies. *B* stands for *bone marrow,* where the B-cells develop and mature.

beer: an alcoholic beverage traditionally brewed by fermenting malted barley and adding hops for flavor.

behavior modification: the changing of behavior by the manipulation of antecedents (cues or environmental factors that trigger behavior), the behavior itself, and consequences (the penalties or rewards attached to the behavior).

belching: the release of air or gas from the stomach through the mouth.

benign (bee-NINE): noncancerous.

beriberi: the thiamin-deficiency disease characterized by muscle weakness, edema, or both.

beta-carotene (BAY-tah KARE-oh-teen): one of the carotenoids; an orange pigment and vitamin A precursor found in plants.

beta cells: cells in the pancreas that secrete insulin in response to elevated blood glucose concentration.

beta-alanine: a nonessential amino acid that is the rate-limiting precursor for the synthesis of the dipeptide carnosine. Carnosine acts primarily as a buffer in skeletal muscle. Beta-alanine supplements raise carnosine concentrations, which enhance the muscles' buffering capacity.

beta-hydroxymethylbutyrate (HMB): a metabolite of the amino acid leucine promoted to increase muscle mass and strength.

BGH: see *bovine growth hormone.*

BHA and BHT: preservatives commonly used to slow the development of off-flavors, odors, and color changes caused by oxidation; BHA is butylated hydroxyanisole and BHT is butylated hydroxytoluene.

bicarbonate: an alkaline compound with the formula HCO_3 that is secreted from the pancreas as part of the pancreatic juice. Bicarbonate is also produced in all cell fluids from the dissociation of carbonic acid to help maintain the body's acid-base balance.

bile: an emulsifier that prepares fats and oils for digestion; an exocrine secretion made by the liver, stored in the gallbladder, and released into the small intestine when needed.

binders: chemical compounds in foods that combine with nutrients (especially minerals) to form complexes the body cannot absorb. Examples include *phytates* (FYE-tates) and *oxalates* (OCK-sa-lates).

binge drinking: pattern of drinking that raises blood alcohol concentration to 0.08 percent or higher; usually corresponds to four or more drinks for women and five or more drinks for men on a single occasion, generally within a couple of hours.

binge-eating disorder: an eating disorder characterized by recurring episodes of eating a significant amount of food in a short period of time with marked feelings of lack of control.

bioaccumulation: the accumulation of contaminants in the flesh of animals high on the food chain.

bioavailability: the rate at and the extent to which a nutrient is absorbed and used.

bioelectromagnetic medical applications: the use of electrical energy, magnetic energy, or both to stimulate bone repair, wound healing, and tissue regeneration.

biofeedback: the use of special devices to convey information about heart rate, blood pressure, skin temperature, muscle relaxation, and other body functions to enable a person to learn how to consciously control these medically important activities.

biofield therapeutics: a manual healing method that directs a healing force from an outside source (commonly God or another supernatural being) through the practitioner and into the client's body; commonly known as "laying on of hands."

biological value (BV): a measure of protein quality assessed by measuring the amount of protein nitrogen that is retained from a given amount of protein nitrogen absorbed.

biotechnology: the science of manipulating biological systems or organisms to create or modify their products.

biotin (BY-oh-tin): a B vitamin that functions as a coenzyme in metabolism.

blastocyst (BLASS-toe-sist): the developmental stage of the zygote when it is about 5 days old and ready for implantation.

blind experiment: an experiment in which the subjects do not know whether they are members of the experimental group or the control group.

bloating: uncomfortable abdominal fullness or distention.

blood lipid profile: results of blood tests that reveal a person's total cholesterol, triglycerides, and various lipoproteins.

BMI: see *body mass index.*

BMR: see *basal metabolic rate.*

body composition: the proportions of muscle, bone, fat, and other tissue that make up a person's total body weight.

body mass index (BMI): a measure of a person's weight relative to height; determined by dividing the weight (in kilograms) by the square of the height (in meters).

bolus (BOH-lus): a portion; with respect to food, the amount swallowed at one time.

bomb calorimeter (KAL-oh-RIM-eh-ter): an instrument that measures the heat energy released when foods are burned, thus providing an estimate of the potential energy (kcalories) of the foods.

bone density: a measure of bone strength. When minerals fill the bone matrix (making it dense), they give it strength.

bone meal: crushed or ground bone preparations intended to supply calcium to the diet. Calcium from bone is not well absorbed and is often contaminated with toxic minerals such as arsenic, mercury, lead, and cadmium.

bottled water: drinking water sold in bottles.

botulism (BOT-chew-lism): an often fatal foodborne illness caused by the ingestion of foods containing a toxin produced by bacteria that grow without oxygen.

bovine growth hormone (BGH): a hormone produced naturally in the pituitary gland of a cow that promotes growth and milk production; now produced for agricultural use by bacteria.

bovine spongiform encephalopathy (BOH-vine SPON-jih-form in- SEF-eh-LOP-eh-thee) or **BSE:** an often fatal illness of cattle and wild game that affects the nervous system and is transmitted to people by eating infected meats; commonly called *mad cow disease.*

bran: the protective coating around the kernel of grain, rich in nutrients and fiber.

branched-chain amino acids: the essential amino acids leucine, isoleucine, and valine, which are present in large amounts in skeletal muscle tissue.

breast milk bank: a service that collects, screens, processes, and distributes donated human milk.

breast pump: a device (manual, battery-powered, or electric) that extracts milk from the breast of a lactating woman.

brite adipocytes: white fat cells with brown fat cell characteristics; also called *beige adipocytes.*

brown adipose tissue: masses of specialized fat cells packed with pigmented mitochondria that produce heat instead of ATP.

brown sugar: refined white sugar crystals to which manufacturers have added molasses syrup with natural flavor and color; 91 to 96 percent pure sucrose.

BSE: see *bovine spongiform encephalopathy.*

buffers: compounds that keep a solution's pH constant when acids or bases are added.

bulimia (byoo-LEEM-ee-ah) **nervosa:** an eating disorder characterized by repeated episodes of binge eating usually followed by self-induced vomiting, misuse of laxatives or diuretics, fasting, or excessive exercise.

BV: see *biological value.*

C

caffeine: a natural stimulant found in many common foods and beverages, including coffee, tea, and chocolate; may enhance endurance by stimulating fatty acid release. High doses cause headaches, trembling, rapid heart rate, and other undesirable side effects.

calbindin: a calcium-binding transport protein that requires vitamin D for its synthesis.

calcidiol: vitamin D found in the blood that is made from the hydroxylation of calciol in the liver; also called *25-hydroxyvitamin D.*

calciferol (kal-SIF-er-ol): vitamin D.

calciol: vitamin D from animal-derived foods in the diet or made in the skin from 7-dehydrocholesterol, a precursor of cholesterol, with the help of sunlight; also called *vitamin* D_3.

calcitonin (KAL-seh-TOE-nin): a hormone secreted by the thyroid gland that regulates blood calcium by lowering it when levels rise too high.

calcitriol: vitamin D that is made from the hydroxylation of calcidiol in the kidneys; the biologically active hormone; also called *1,25-dihydroxyvitamin D* or *active vitamin D.*

calcium: the most abundant mineral in the body; found primarily in the body's bones and teeth.

calcium-binding protein: a protein in the intestinal cells, made with the help of vitamin D, that facilitates calcium absorption.

calcium rigor: hardness or stiffness of the muscles caused by high blood calcium concentrations.

calcium tetany (TET-ah-nee): intermittent spasm of the extremities due to nervous and muscular excitability caused by low blood calcium concentrations.

calmodulin (cal-MOD-you-lin): a calcium-binding protein that regulates such cell activities as muscle contractions.

calories or **kcalories:** a measure of *heat* energy. Energy provided by foods and beverages is measured in *kilocalories* (1000 calories equal 1 kilocalorie), abbreviated *kcalories* or *kcal.* One kcalorie is the amount of heat necessary to raise the temperature of 1 kilogram (kg) of water 1°C. The scientific use of the term *kcalorie* is the same as the popular use of the term *calorie.*

CAM: see *complementary and alternative medicine.*

cancers: malignant growths or tumors that result from abnormal and uncontrolled cell division.

capillaries (CAP-ill-aries): small vessels that branch from an artery. Capillaries connect arteries to veins. Exchange of oxygen, nutrients, and waste materials takes place across capillary walls.

carbohydrase (KAR-boe-HIGH-drase): an enzyme that hydrolyzes carbohydrates.

carbohydrates: compounds composed of carbon, oxygen, and hydrogen arranged as monosaccharides or multiples of monosaccharides. Most, but not all, carbohydrates have a ratio of one carbon molecule to one water molecule: $(CH_2O)_n$.

carbonated water: water that contains carbon dioxide gas, either naturally occurring or added, that causes bubbles to form in it; also called *bubbling* or *sparkling water.* The FDA defines seltzer, soda, and tonic waters as soft drinks; they are not regulated as water.

carbonic acid: a compound with the formula H_2CO_3 that results from the combination of carbon dioxide (CO_2) and water (H_2O); of particular importance in maintaining the body's acid-base balance.

carcinogenesis (CAR-sin-oh-JEN-eh-sis): the process of cancer development.

carcinogen (CAR-sin-oh-jen or car-SIN-oh-jen): a substance that can cause cancer; the adjective is *carcinogenic.*

cardiac output: the volume of blood discharged by the heart each minute; determined by multiplying the stroke volume by the heart rate. The stroke volume is the amount of oxygenated blood the heart ejects toward the tissues at each beat. Cardiac output (volume/minute) = stroke volume (volume/beat) × heart rate (beats/minute).

cardiorespiratory conditioning: improvements in heart and lung function and increased blood volume, brought about by aerobic training.

cardiorespiratory endurance: the ability to perform large-muscle, dynamic exercise of moderate to high intensity for prolonged periods.

cardiovascular disease (CVD): diseases of the heart and blood vessels throughout the body. Atherosclerosis is the main cause of CVD. When the arteries that carry blood to the heart muscle become blocked, the heart suffers damage known as *coronary heart disease (CHD).*

carnitine (CAR-neh-teen): a nonessential, nonprotein amino acid made in the body from lysine that helps transport fatty acids across the mitochondrial membrane. As a supplement, carnitine supposedly "burns" fat and spares glycogen during endurance events, but in reality it does neither.

carotenoids (kah-ROT-eh-noyds): pigments commonly found in plants and animals, some of which have vitamin A activity. The carotenoid with the greatest vitamin A activity is beta-carotene.

carrying capacity: the number of people, other living organisms, or crops that a region can support without environmental degradation.

cartilage therapy: the use of cleaned and powdered connective tissue, such as collagen, to improve health.

catabolism (ca-TAB-o-lism): reactions in which large molecules are broken down to smaller ones. Catabolic reactions release energy.

catalyst (CAT-uh-list): a compound that facilitates chemical reactions without itself being changed in the process.

cataracts (KAT-ah-rakts): clouding of the eye lenses that impairs vision and can lead to blindness.

cathartic (ka-THAR-tik): a strong laxative.

cations (CAT-eye-uns): positively charged ions.

CDC (Centers for Disease Control and Prevention): a branch of the Department of Health and Human Services that is responsible for, among other things, monitoring foodborne diseases.

celiac (SEE-lee-ak) **disease:** an intestinal disorder in which the inability to absorb gluten results in an immune response that damages intestinal cells; also called *celiac sprue, nontropical sprue,* or *gluten-sensitive enteropathy.*

cell: the basic structural unit of all living things.

cell differentiation (DIF-er-EN-she-AY-shun): the process by which immature cells develop specific functions different from those of the original that are characteristic of their mature cell type.

cell membrane: the thin layer of tissue that surrounds the cell and encloses its contents, made primarily of lipid and protein.

Centers for Disease Control and Prevention: see *CDC.*

central nervous system: the central part of the nervous system; the brain and spinal cord.

central obesity: excess fat around the trunk of the body; also called *abdominal fat* or *upper-body fat.*

cerebral thrombosis: a clot that blocks blood flow through an artery that feeds the brain.

certified lactation consultants: health-care providers who specialize in helping new mothers establish a healthy breastfeeding relationship with their newborn. These consultants are often registered nurses with specialized training in breast and infant anatomy and physiology.

certified nutritionist or **certified nutritional consultant** or **certified nutrition therapist:** a person who has been granted a document declaring his or her authority as a nutrition professional.

cesarean (si-ZAIR-ee-un) **delivery:** a surgically assisted birth involving removal of the fetus by an incision into the uterus, usually by way of the abdominal wall.

chaff: the outer inedible part of a grain; also called the *husk.*

CHD risk equivalents: disorders that raise the risk of heart attacks, strokes, and other complications associated with cardiovascular disease to the same degree as existing CHD. These disorders include symptomatic carotid artery disease, peripheral arterial disease, abdominal aortic aneurysm, and diabetes mellitus.

cheilosis (kye-LOH-sis or kee-LOH-sis): a condition of reddened lips with cracks at the corners of the mouth.

chelate (KEY-late): a substance that can grasp the positive ions of a mineral.

chelation (kee-LAY-shun) **therapy:** the use of ethylene diamine tetraacetic acid (EDTA) to bind with metallic ions, thus healing the body by removing toxic metals.

chiropractic (KYE-roh-PRAK-tik) **manipulation:** a manual healing method of adjusting the spine to restore health.

chloride (KLO-ride): the major anion in the extracellular fluids of the body. Chloride is the ionic form of chlorine, Cl^-.

chlorophyll (KLO-row-fil): the green pigment of plants, which absorbs light and transfers the energy to other molecules, thereby initiating photosynthesis.

cholecalciferol (KO-lee-kal-SIF-er-ol): vitamin D from animal-derived foods in the diet or made in the skin from 7-dehydrocholesterol, a precursor of cholesterol, with the help of sunlight; also called *vitamin* D_3.

cholecystokinin (COAL-ee-SIS-toe-KINE-in) or **CCK:** a hormone produced by cells of the intestinal wall. Target organ: the gallbladder. Response: release of bile and slowing of GI motility.

cholesterol (koh-LESS-ter-ol): one of the sterols containing a four-ring carbon structure with a carbon side chain.

cholesterol-free: less than 2 milligrams of cholesterol per serving and 2 grams or less of saturated fat and *trans* fat combined per serving.

choline (KOH-leen): a nitrogen-containing compound found in foods and made in the body from the amino acid methionine. Choline is part of the phospholipid lecithin and the neurotransmitter acetylcholine.

chromium: an essential trace mineral that enhances the activity of insulin.

chromosomes: structures within the nucleus of a cell made of DNA and associated proteins. Human beings have 46 chromosomes in 23 pairs. Each chromosome has many genes.

chronic diseases: diseases characterized by slow progression and long duration. Examples include heart disease, diabetes, and some cancers.

chronic malnutrition: malnutrition caused by long-term food deprivation; characterized in children by short height for age (*stunting*).

chronological age: a person's age in years from his or her date of birth.

chylomicrons (kye-lo-MY-cronz): lipoproteins that transport lipids from the intestinal cells to the rest of the body.

chyme (KIME): the semiliquid mass of partly digested food expelled by the stomach into the duodenum.

cirrhosis (seer-OH-sis): advanced liver disease in which liver cells turn orange, die, and harden, permanently losing their function; often associated with alcoholism.

cis: on the near side of; refers to a chemical configuration in which the hydrogen atoms are located on the same side of a double bond.

citric acid cycle: see *TCA cycle.*

clinically severe obesity: a BMI of 40 or greater or a BMI of 35 or greater with additional medical problems. A less preferred term used to describe the same condition is *morbid obesity.*

clone: an organism created without sexual reproduction and genetically identical to one ancestor.

CoA (coh-AY): coenzyme A; the coenzyme derived from the B vitamin pantothenic acid and central to energy metabolism.

coenzymes: complex organic molecules that work with enzymes to facilitate the enzymes' activity. Many coenzymes have B vitamins as part of their structures.

cofactor: a small, inorganic or organic substance that facilitates the action of an enzyme.

colitis (ko-LYE-tis): inflammation of the colon.

collagen (KOL-ah-jen): the structural protein from which connective tissues such as scars, tendons, ligaments, and the foundations of bones and teeth are made.

colonic irrigation: the popular, but potentially harmful practice of "washing" the large intestine with a powerful enema machine; also called *colonic hydrotherapy.*

colostrum (ko-LAHS-trum): a milklike secretion from the breast, present during the first few days after delivery before milk appears; rich in protective factors.

complementary and alternative medicine (CAM): diverse medical and health-care systems, practices, and products that are not currently considered part of conventional medicine; also called *adjunctive, unconventional,* or *unorthodox therapies.*

complementary foods: nutrient- and energy-containing solid or semisolid foods (or liquids) fed to infants in addition to breast milk or infant formula.

complementary proteins: two or more dietary proteins whose amino acid assortments complement each other in such a way that the essential amino acids limited in one are supplied by the other.

complex carbohydrates: polysaccharides (starches and fibers).

compound: a substance composed of two or more different atoms—for example, water (H_2O).

conception: the union of the male sperm and the female ovum; fertilization.

condensation: a chemical reaction in which water is released as two molecules combine to form one larger product.

conditionally essential amino acid: an amino acid that is normally nonessential, but must be supplied by the diet in special circumstances when the need for it exceeds the body's ability to make it.

conditionally essential nutrient: a nutrient that is normally nonessential, but must be supplied by the diet in special circumstances when the need for it exceeds the body's ability to make it.

confectioners' sugar: finely powdered sucrose, 99.9 percent pure.

congregate meals: nutrition programs that provide food for the elderly in conveniently located settings such as community centers.

conjugated linoleic acids: several fatty acids that have the same chemical formula as linoleic acid (18 carbons, two double bonds) but with different configurations (the double bonds occur on adjacent carbons).

constipation: the condition of having infrequent or difficult bowel movements.

contaminants: substances that make a food impure and unsuitable for ingestion.

contamination iron: iron found in foods as the result of contamination by inorganic iron salts from iron cookware, iron-containing soils, and the like.

control group: a group of individuals similar in all possible respects to the experimental group except for the treatment. Ideally, the control group receives a placebo while the experimental group receives a real treatment.

convenient dietary supplements: liquid meal replacers, energy drinks, energy bars, and energy gels that athletes and active people use to replenish energy and nutrients when time is limited.

conventional medicine: diagnosis and treatment of diseases as practiced by medical doctors (MD), doctors of osteopathy (DO), and allied health professionals such as physical therapists and registered nurses; also called *allopathy; Western, mainstream, orthodox,* or *regular medicine;* and *biomedicine.*

cool-down: 5 to 10 minutes of light activity, such as walking or stretching, following a vigorous workout to gradually return the body's core to near-normal temperature.

copper: an essential trace mineral that is part of many enzymes.

Cori cycle: the pathway in which glucose is metabolized to lactate (by anaerobic glycolysis) in the muscle, lactate is converted back to glucose in the liver, and then glucose is returned to the muscle; named after the scientist who elucidated this pathway.

corn sweeteners: corn syrup and sugars derived from corn.

corn syrup: a syrup made from cornstarch that has been treated with acid, high temperatures, and enzymes to produce glucose, maltose, and dextrins. It may be dried and used as *corn syrup solids.* See also, *high-fructose corn syrup (HFCS).*

cornea (KOR-nee-uh): the transparent membrane covering the outside of the eye.

coronary arteries: blood vessels that supply blood to the heart.

coronary heart disease (CHD): the damage that occurs when the blood vessels carrying blood to the heart (the *coronary arteries)* become narrow and occluded.

coronary thrombosis: a clot that blocks blood flow through an artery that feeds the heart muscle.

correlation (CORE-ee-LAY-shun): the simultaneous increase, decrease, or change in two variables. If A increases as B increases, or if A decreases as B decreases, the correlation is *positive.* (This does not mean that A causes B or vice versa.) If A increases as B decreases, or if A decreases as B increases, the correlation is *negative.* (This does not mean that A prevents B or vice versa.) Some third factor may account for both A and B.

cortical bone: the very dense bone tissue that forms the outer shell surrounding trabecular bone and comprises the shaft of a long bone.

coupled reactions: pairs of chemical reactions in which some of the energy released from the breakdown of one compound is used to create a bond in the formation of another compound.

covalent bonds: strong chemical bonds formed between atoms by sharing electrons.

covert (KOH-vert): hidden, as if under covers.

CP: see *creatine phosphate.*

C-reactive protein (CRP): a protein released during the acute phase of infection or inflammation that enhances immunity by promoting phagocytosis and activating platelets. Its presence may be used to assess a person's risk of an impending heart attack or stroke.

creatine (KREE-ah-tin): a nitrogen-containing compound that combines with phosphate to form the high-energy compound creatine phosphate (or phosphocreatine) in muscles.

creatine phosphate (CP): a high-energy compound in muscle cells that acts as a reservoir of energy that can maintain a steady supply of ATP. CP provides the energy for short bursts of activity; also called *phosphocreatine.*

cretinism (CREE-tin-ism): a congenital disease characterized by limited mental and physical development and commonly caused by maternal iodine deficiency during pregnancy.

critical periods: finite periods during development in which certain events occur that will have irreversible effects on later developmental stages; usually a period of rapid cell division.

critical thinking: the mental activity of rationally and skillfully analyzing, synthesizing, and evaluating information to reach an informed conclusion based on evidence.

cross-contamination: the contamination of food by bacteria that occurs when the food comes into contact with surfaces previously touched by raw meat, poultry, or seafood.

CRP: see *C-reactive protein.*

cruciferous vegetables: vegetables of the cabbage family, including cauliflower, broccoli, and brussels sprouts.

crypts (KRIPTS): tubular glands that lie between the intestinal villi and secrete intestinal juices into the small intestine.

cultural competence: having an awareness and acceptance of cultures and the ability to interact effectively with people of diverse cultures.

CVD: see *cardiovascular disease.*

cytokines (SIGH-toe-kines): special proteins that direct immune and inflammatory responses.

cytoplasm (SIGH-toh-plazm): the cell contents, except for the nucleus.

cytosol: the fluid of cytoplasm that contains water, ions, nutrients, and enzymes.

D

Daily Values (DV): reference values developed by the FDA specifically for use on food labels.

deamination (dee-AM-ih-NAY-shun): removal of the amino (NH_2) group from a compound such as an amino acid.

defecate (DEF-uh-cate): to move the bowels and eliminate waste.

deficient: inadequate; a nutrient amount that fails to meet the body's needs and eventually results in deficiency symptoms.

dehydration: the condition in which body water output exceeds water input. Symptoms include thirst, dry skin and mucous membranes, rapid heartbeat, low blood pressure, and weakness.

Delaney Clause: a 1958 amendment to the Food, Drug, and Cosmetic Act of 1938, named after Congressman James Delaney of New York that states that no substance that is known to cause cancer in animals or human beings at any dose level shall be added to foods.

***de minimis* rule:** a guideline that defines risk as a cancer rate of less than one cancer per million people exposed to a contaminant over a 70-year lifetime.

denaturation (dee-NAY-chur-AY-shun): the change in a protein's shape and consequent loss of its function brought about by heat, agitation, acid, base, alcohol, heavy metals, or other agents.

dental caries: decay of teeth.

dental plaque: a gummy mass of bacteria that grows on teeth and can lead to dental caries and gum disease.

deoxyribonucleic acid: see *DNA*.

dextrose: the name food manufacturers use for the sugar that is chemically the same as glucose; *anhydrous dextrose* is similar, differing primarily in the temperature of crystallization.

DFE: see *dietary folate equivalents*.

DHA: see *docosahexaenoic acid*.

DHEA (dehydroepiandrosterone) and **androstenedione:** hormones made in the adrenal glands that serve as precursors to the male sex hormone, testosterone; falsely promoted as burning fat, building muscle, and slowing aging.

DHF (dihydrofolate): a coenzyme form of folate.

DIAAS (digestible indispensable amino acid score): a measure of protein quality similar to PDCAAS, except it determines protein digestibility at the end of the small intestine, which more accurately reflects the extent of amino acid absorption.

diabetes (DYE-uh-BEE-teez): metabolic disorder characterized by elevated blood glucose resulting from insufficient insulin, ineffective insulin, or both; the complete medical term is *diabetes mellitus* (meh-LIE-tus). When blood glucose levels are higher than normal but below the diagnosis of diabetes, the condition is called *prediabetes*.

diarrhea: the frequent passage of watery bowel movements.

diet: the foods and beverages a person eats and drinks.

diet history: a record of eating behaviors and the foods a person eats.

dietary fibers: in plant foods, the *nonstarch polysaccharides* that are not digested by human digestive enzymes, although some are digested by GI tract bacteria.

dietary folate equivalents (DFE): the amount of folate available to the body from naturally occurring sources, fortified foods, and supplements, accounting for differences in the bioavailability from each source. DFE = µg food folate + (1.7 × µg synthetic folate).

dietary nitrate: an inorganic compound composed of nitrogen and oxygen found in water and foods such as spinach, beets, celery, radishes, and lettuce. Dietary nitrate supplementation may reduce the oxygen cost of exercise, thereby improving exercise performance and tolerance.

Dietary Reference Intakes (DRI): a set of nutrient intake values for healthy people in the United States and Canada. These values are used for planning and assessing diets and include: Estimated Average Requirements (EAR), Recommended Dietary Allowances (RDA), Adequate Intakes (AI), and Tolerable Upper Intake Levels (UL).

dietary supplement: any pill, capsule, tablet, liquid, or powder that contains vitamins, minerals, herbs, or amino acids intended to increase dietary intake of these substances.

dietetic technician: a person who has completed a minimum of an associate's degree from an accredited university or college and an approved dietetic technician program that includes a supervised practice experience. See also, *dietetic technician, registered (DTR)*.

dietetic technician, registered (DTR): a dietetic technician who has passed a national examination and maintains registration through continuing professional education.

dietitian: a person trained in nutrition, food science, and diet planning. See also, *registered dietitian nutritionist*.

digestible indispensable amino acid score: see *DIAAS*.

digestion: the process by which food is broken down into absorbable units.

digestive enzymes: proteins found in digestive juices that act on food substances, causing them to break down into simpler compounds.

digestive system: all the organs and glands associated with the ingestion and digestion of food.

dipeptide (dye-PEP-tide): two amino acids bonded together.

diploma mills: entities without valid accreditation that provide worthless degrees.

direct calorimetry: a means of estimating energy expenditure by measuring the amount of heat released.

disaccharides (dye-SACK-uh-rides): pairs of monosaccharides linked together.

discretionary kcalories: the kcalories remaining in a person's energy allowance after consuming enough nutrient-dense foods to meet all nutrient needs for a day.

disordered eating: eating behaviors that are neither normal nor healthy, including restrained eating, fasting, binge eating, and purging.

dispensable amino acids: see *nonessential amino acids*.

dissociates (dis-SO-see-aites): physically separates.

distilled water: water that has been vaporized and recondensed, leaving it free of dissolved minerals.

diverticula (dye-ver-TIC-you-la): sacs or pouches that develop in the weakened areas of the intestinal wall (like bulges in an inner tube where the tire wall is weak).

diverticulitis (DYE-ver-tic-you-LYE-tis): infected or inflamed diverticula.

diverticulosis (DYE-ver-tic-you-LOH-sis): the condition of having diverticula.

DNA (deoxyribonucleic acid): the double helix molecules of which genes are made.

docosahexaenoic (DOE-cossa-HEXA-ee-NO-ick) **acid (DHA):** an omega-3 polyunsaturated fatty acid with 22 carbons and six double bonds; present in fatty fish and synthesized in limited amounts in the body from linolenic acid.

dolomite: a compound of minerals (calcium magnesium carbonate) found in limestone and marble. Dolomite is powdered and is sold as a calcium-magnesium supplement. However, it may be contaminated with toxic minerals, is not well absorbed, and interferes with absorption of other essential minerals.

double-blind experiment: an experiment in which neither the subjects nor the researchers know which subjects are members of the experimental group and which are serving as control subjects, until after the experiment is over.

Down syndrome: a genetic abnormality that causes mental impairment, short stature, and flattened facial features.

DRI: see *Dietary Reference Intakes.*

drink: a dose of any alcoholic beverage that delivers ½ ounce of pure ethanol: 5 ounces of wine, 10 ounces of wine cooler, 12 ounces of beer, or 1½ ounces of liquor (80 proof whiskey, scotch, rum, or vodka).

drug: a substance that can modify one or more of the body's functions.

drug history: a record of all the drugs, over-the-counter and prescribed, that a person takes routinely.

DTR: see *dietetic technician, registered.*

duodenum (doo-oh-DEEN-um or doo-ODD-num): the top portion of the small intestine (about "12 fingers' breadth" long in ancient terminology).

DV: see *Daily Values.*

dysphagia (dis-FAY-jah): difficulty swallowing.

E

EAR: see *Estimated Average Requirement.*

eating disorders: disturbances in eating behavior that jeopardize a person's physical or psychological health.

eating patterns: customary quantities, proportions, and frequencies of consuming various foods and beverages over time.

eclampsia (eh-KLAMP-see-ah): a condition characterized by extremely high blood pressure, elevated protein in the urine, seizures, and possibly coma.

ectopic fat: excess fat in locations other than adipose tissue.

edema (eh-DEEM-uh): the swelling of body tissue caused by excessive amounts of fluid in the interstitial spaces; seen in protein deficiency (among other conditions).

EER: see *Estimated Energy Requirement.*

eicosanoids (eye-COSS-uh-noyds): derivatives of 20-carbon fatty acids; biologically active compounds that help regulate blood pressure, blood clotting, and other body functions. They include *prostaglandins* (PROS-tah-GLAND-ins), *thromboxanes* (throm-BOX-ains), and *leukotrienes* (LOO-ko-TRY-eens).

eicosapentaenoic (EYE-cossa-PENTA-ee-NO-ick) **acid (EPA):** an omega-3 polyunsaturated fatty acid with 20 carbons and five double bonds; present in fatty fish and synthesized in limited amounts in the body from linolenic acid.

electrolyte solutions: solutions that can conduct electricity.

electrolytes: salts that dissolve in water and dissociate into charged particles called ions.

electron transport chain: the final pathway in energy metabolism that transports electrons from hydrogen to oxygen and captures the energy released in the bonds of ATP; also called the *respiratory chain.*

element: a substance composed of atoms that are alike—for example, iron (Fe).

embolism (EM-boh-lizm): the obstruction of a blood vessel by an *embolus* (EM-boh-luss), or traveling clot, causing sudden tissue death.

embryo (EM-bree-oh): the developing infant from 2 to 8 weeks after conception.

emetic (em-ETT-ic): an agent that causes vomiting.

empty-kcalorie foods: a popular term used to denote foods that contribute energy but lack protein, vitamins, and minerals.

emulsifier (ee-MUL-sih-fire): a substance with both water-soluble and fat-soluble portions that promotes the mixing of oils and fats in a watery solution.

endogenous (en-DODGE-eh-nus): from within the body.

endoplasmic reticulum (en-doh-PLAZ-mic reh-TIC-you-lum): a complex network of intracellular membranes. The *rough endoplasmic reticulum* is dotted with ribosomes, where protein synthesis takes place. The *smooth endoplasmic reticulum* bears no ribosomes.

endoscopic procedures: practices that require a physician to insert a medical device into the body (in this case, the gastrointestinal tract) to examine or treat a disorder.

endosperm: the inner edible part of a kernel of grain, rich in starch and proteins.

enema: solution inserted into the rectum and colon to stimulate a bowel movement and empty the lower large intestine.

energy: the capacity to do work. The energy in food is chemical energy. The body can convert this chemical energy to mechanical, electrical, or heat energy.

energy balance: the energy (kcalories) consumed from foods and beverages compared with the energy expended through metabolic processes and physical activities.

energy density: a measure of the energy a food provides relative to the weight of the food (kcalories per gram).

energy-yielding nutrients: the nutrients that break down to yield energy the body can use (carbohydrate, fat, and protein).

enhanced water: water that is fortified with ingredients such as vitamins, minerals, protein, oxygen, or herbs. Enhanced water is marketed as *vitamin water, sports water, oxygenated water,* and *protein water.*

enriched: the addition to a food of specific nutrients to replace losses that occur during processing so that the food will meet a specified standard.

enteropancreatic (EN-ter-oh-PAN-kree-AT-ik) **circulation:** the circulatory route from the pancreas to the intestine and back to the pancreas.

Environmental Protection Agency: see *EPA.*

enzymes: proteins that facilitate chemical reactions without being changed in the process; protein catalysts.

EPA: see *eicosapentaenoic acid.*

EPA (Environmental Protection Agency): a federal agency that is responsible for, among other things, regulating pesticides and establishing water quality standards.

epigenetics: the study of heritable changes in gene function that occur without a change in the DNA sequence.

epiglottis (epp-ih-GLOTT-iss): cartilage in the throat that guards the entrance to the trachea and prevents fluid or food from entering it when a person swallows.

epinephrine (EP-ih-NEFF-rin): a hormone of the adrenal gland that modulates the stress response; formerly called *adrenaline.* When administered by injection, epinephrine counteracts anaphylactic shock by opening the airways and maintaining heartbeat and blood pressure.

epithelial (ep-i-THEE-lee-ul) **cells:** cells on the surface of the skin and mucous membranes.

epithelial tissue: the layer of the body that serves as a selective barrier between the body's interior and the environment. Examples are the cornea of the eyes, the skin, the respiratory lining of the lungs, and the lining of the digestive tract.

ergocalciferol (ER-go-kal-SIF-er-ol): vitamin D derived from plant foods in the diet; also called *vitamin* D_2.

ergogenic (ER-go-JEN-ick) **aids:** substances or techniques used in an attempt to enhance physical performance.

erythrocyte (eh-RITH-ro-cite) **hemolysis** (he-MOLL-uh-sis): the breaking open of red blood cells (erythrocytes); a symptom of vitamin E–deficiency disease in human beings.

erythrocyte protoporphyrin (PRO-toe-PORE-fe-rin): a precursor to hemoglobin.

esophageal (ee-SOFF-ah-GEE-al) **sphincter:** the circular muscle at the upper or lower end of the esophagus. The *lower esophageal sphincter* is also called the *cardiac sphincter* because of its proximity to the heart.

esophagus (ee-SOFF-ah-gus): the food pipe; the conduit from the mouth to the stomach.

essential amino acids: amino acids that the body requires but cannot make, and so must be obtained from the diet; also called *indispensable amino acids.*

essential fatty acids: fatty acids that the body requires but cannot make, and so must be obtained from the diet; both linoleic acid and linolenic acid are essential fatty acids.

essential nutrients: nutrients a person must obtain from food because the body cannot make them for itself in sufficient quantity to meet physiological needs; also called *indispensable nutrients.* About 40 nutrients are currently known to be essential for human beings.

Estimated Average Requirement (EAR): the average daily amount of a nutrient that will maintain a specific biochemical or physiological function in half the healthy people of a given age and gender group.

Estimated Energy Requirement (EER): the average dietary energy intake that maintains energy balance and good health in a person of a given age, gender, weight, height, and level of physical activity.

ethanol: a particular type of alcohol found in beer, wine, and liquor; also called *ethyl alcohol.*

ethnic foods: foods associated with particular cultural groups.

excessive drinking: heavy drinking, binge drinking, or both.

exchange lists: see *food lists.*

exercise: planned, structured, and repetitive body movements that promote or maintain physical fitness.

exogenous (eks-ODGE-eh-nus): from outside the body.

experimental group: a group of individuals similar in all possible respects to the control group except for the treatment. The experimental group receives the real treatment.

extra lean: less than 5 grams of fat, 2 grams of saturated fat and *trans* fat combined, and 95 milligrams of cholesterol per serving and per 100 grams of meat, poultry, and seafood.

extracellular fluid: fluid outside the cells. Extracellular fluid includes two main components—the interstitial fluid between cells and the intravascular fluid inside blood vessels. Extracellular fluid accounts for approximately one-third of the body's water.

F

FAD (flavin adenine dinucleotide): a coenzyme form of riboflavin.

fad diets: popular eating plans that promise quick weight loss. Most fad diets severely limit certain foods or overemphasize others (for example, never eat potatoes or pasta, or eat cabbage soup daily).

faith healing: healing by invoking divine intervention without the use of medical, surgical, or other traditional therapy.

false negative: a test result indicating that a condition is not present (negative) when in fact it is present (therefore false).

false positive: a test result indicating that a condition is present (positive) when in fact it is not present (therefore false).

famine: widespread and extreme scarcity of food in an area that causes starvation and death in a large portion of the population.

FAO (Food and Agriculture Organization): an international agency (part of the United Nations) that has adopted standards to regulate pesticide use, among other responsibilities.

FAS: see *fetal alcohol syndrome.*

FASD: see *fetal alcohol spectrum disorder.*

fasting plasma glucose: a test that measures plasma glucose after a person has fasted (no food or kcaloric beverages) for at least 8 hours.

fat replacers: ingredients that replace some or all of the functions of fat and may or may not provide energy.

fat-free: less than 0.5 gram of fat per serving (and no added fat or oil); synonyms include *zero-fat, no fat,* and *nonfat.*

fats: lipids that are solid at room temperature (77°F or 25°C).

fatty acid oxidation: the metabolic breakdown of fatty acids to acetyl CoA; also called *beta oxidation.*

fatty acids: organic compounds composed of a carbon chain with hydrogens attached and an acid group (COOH) at one end and a methyl group (CH_3) at the other end.

fatty liver: an early stage of liver deterioration seen in several diseases, including obesity and alcoholic liver disease. Fatty liver is characterized by an accumulation of fat in the liver cells.

fatty streaks: accumulations of cholesterol and other lipids along the walls of the arteries.

FDA (Food and Drug Administration): an agency within the Department of Health and Human Services that is responsible for ensuring the safety and wholesomeness of all dietary supplements and foods processed and sold in interstate commerce except meat, poultry, and eggs (which are under the jurisdiction of the USDA); inspecting food plants and imported foods; and setting standards for food composition and product labeling.

female athlete triad: a potentially fatal combination of three medical problems—disordered eating, amenorrhea, and osteoporosis.

fermentable fibers: fibers that can be digested by bacteria in the GI tract.

ferritin (FAIR-ih-tin): the iron storage protein.

fertility: the capacity of a woman to produce a normal ovum periodically and of a man to produce normal sperm; the ability to reproduce.

fetal alcohol spectrum disorder (FASD): an umbrella term used to describe a range of physical, behavioral, and cognitive abnormalities resulting from prenatal alcohol exposure.

fetal alcohol syndrome (FAS): a clinical diagnosis based on specific physical, behavioral, and cognitive abnormalities resulting from prenatal alcohol exposure, including facial malformations, stunted growth, and central nervous disorders.

fetal programming: the influence of substances during fetal growth on the development of diseases in later life.

fetus (FEET-us): the developing infant from 8 weeks after conception until term.

fibrosis (fye-BROH-sis): an intermediate stage of liver deterioration seen in several diseases, including viral hepatitis and alcoholic liver disease. In fibrosis, the liver cells lose their function and assume the characteristics of connective tissue cells (fibers).

filtered water: water treated by filtration, usually through *activated carbon filters* that reduce the lead in tap water, or by *reverse osmosis* units that force pressurized water across a membrane, removing lead, arsenic, and some microorganisms from tap water.

fitness: the characteristics that enable the body to perform physical activity; more broadly, the ability to meet routine physical demands with enough reserve energy to rise to a physical challenge; or the body's ability to withstand stress of all kinds.

flatulence: passage of excessive amounts of intestinal gas.

flavonoids (FLAY-von-oyds): yellow pigments in foods; phytochemicals that may exert physiological effects on the body.

flaxseeds: the small brown seeds of the flax plant; valued in nutrition as a source of fiber, lignans, and omega-3 fatty acids.

flexibility: the capacity of the joints to move through a full range of motion; the ability to bend and recover without injury.

fluid balance: maintenance of the proper types and amounts of fluid in each compartment of the body fluids.

fluorapatite (floor-APP-uh-tite): the stabilized form of tooth crystal, in which fluoride has replaced the hydroxyl groups of hydroxyapatite.

fluoride: an essential trace mineral that makes teeth stronger and more resistant to decay.

fluorosis (floor-OH-sis): discoloration and pitting of tooth enamel caused by excess fluoride during tooth development.

FMN (flavin mononucleotide): a coenzyme form of riboflavin.

FODMAP: a collective term used to describe fermentable oligosaccharides, disaccharides, monosaccharides, and polyols that are commonly found in such foods as wheat, onions, some fruits and vegetables, sorbitol, and some dairy.

folate (FOLE-ate): a B vitamin; also known as folic acid, folacin, or pteroylglutamic (tare-o-EEL-glue-TAM-ick) acid (PGA). The coenzyme forms are *DHF (dihydrofolate)* and *THF (tetrahydrofolate).*

food allergy: an adverse reaction to food that involves an immune response; also called *food-hypersensitivity reaction.*

Food and Agriculture Organization: see *FAO.*

Food and Drug Administration: see *FDA.*

food and nutrition history: a record of eating behaviors and the foods a person eats.

food aversions: strong desires to avoid particular foods.

food banks: facilities that collect and distribute food donations to authorized organizations feeding the hungry.

food chain: the sequence in which living things depend on other living things for food.

food cravings: strong desires to eat particular foods.

food deserts: neighborhoods and communities characterized by limited access to nutritious and affordable foods.

food frequency questionnaire: a checklist of foods routinely consumed. Some questionnaires ask only about the types of food eaten and yield qualitative information; others include questions about portions as well and yield semiquantitative data.

food group plans: diet-planning tools that sort foods into groups based on nutrient content and then specify that people should eat certain amounts of foods from each group.

food insecurity: limited or uncertain access to foods of sufficient quality or quantity to sustain a healthy and active life.

food insufficiency: an inadequate amount of food due to a lack of resources.

food intolerances: adverse reactions to foods that do not involve the immune system.

food lists: diet-planning tools that organize foods by their proportions of carbohydrate, fat, and protein; formerly known as *exchange lists.* Foods on any single list can be used interchangeably.

food poverty: hunger resulting from inadequate access to available food for various reasons, including inadequate resources, political obstacles, social disruptions, poor weather conditions, and lack of transportation.

food record: a detailed log of all foods eaten during a specified time period, usually several days; also called a *food diary.* A food record may also include associated information such as when, where, and with whom each food is eaten as well as details about physical activity, medications, and disease symptoms.

food recovery: collecting wholesome food for distribution to low-income people who are hungry.

food security: access to enough food to sustain a healthy and active life.

foodborne illness: an illness transmitted to human beings through food and water, caused by either an infectious agent (foodborne infection) or a poisonous substance (food intoxication); commonly known as *food poisoning.*

foods: products derived from plants or animals that can be taken into the body to yield energy and nutrients for the maintenance of life and the growth and repair of tissues.

fortified: the addition to a food of nutrients that were either not originally present or present in insignificant amounts. Fortification can be used to correct or prevent a widespread nutrient deficiency or to balance the total nutrient profile of a food.

fossil fuels: coal, oil, and natural gas.

fraudulent: the promotion, for financial gain, of devices, treatments, services, plans, or products (including diets and supplements) that alter or claim to alter a human condition without proof of safety or effectiveness.

free: "nutritionally trivial" and unlikely to have a physiological consequence; synonyms include *without, no,* and *zero.* A food that does not contain a nutrient naturally may make such a claim, but only as it applies to all similar foods (for example, "applesauce, a fat-free food").

free radical: an unstable molecule with one or more unpaired electrons.

fructose (FRUK-tose or FROOK-tose): a monosaccharide; sometimes known as *fruit sugar* or *levulose.* Fructose is found abundantly in fruits, honey, and saps.

fuel: compounds that cells can use for energy. The major fuels include glucose, fatty acids, and amino acids; other fuels include ketone bodies, lactate, glycerol, and alcohol.

full term: births occurring at 39 through 40 weeks of gestation.

functional foods: foods that have a potentially beneficial effect on health when consumed as part of a varied diet on a regular basis at effective levels.

G

g: grams; a unit of weight equivalent to about 0.03 ounces.

galactose (ga-LAK-tose): a monosaccharide; part of the disaccharide lactose.

gallbladder: the organ that stores and concentrates bile. When it receives the signal that fat is present in the duodenum, the gallbladder contracts and squirts bile through the bile duct into the duodenum.

gastric glands: exocrine glands in the stomach wall that secrete gastric juice into the stomach.

gastric aspiration: a technique that uses a tube to empty the contents of the stomach after every meal.

gastric juice: the digestive secretion of the gastric glands of the stomach.

gastrin: a hormone secreted by cells in the stomach wall. Target organ: the glands of the stomach. Response: secretion of gastric acid.

gastroesophageal reflux: the backflow of stomach acid into the esophagus, causing damage to the cells of the esophagus and the sensation of heartburn; commonly known as *heartburn* or *acid indigestion.*

gastrointestinal (GI) tract: the digestive tract. The principal organs are the stomach and intestines.

gatekeepers: with respect to nutrition, key people who control other people's access to foods and thereby exert profound impacts on their nutrition. Examples are the spouse who buys and cooks the food, the parent who feeds the children, and the caregiver in a day-care center.

gene expression: the process by which a cell converts the genetic code into RNA and protein.

gene pool: all the genetic information of a population at a given time.

generally recognized as safe (GRAS): food additives that have long been in use and are believed to be safe. First established by the FDA in 1958, the GRAS list is subject to revision as new facts become known.

genes: sections of chromosomes that contain the instructions needed to make one or more proteins.

genetic engineering: the intentional manipulation of the genetic material of living cells in order to produce some desirable trait not present in the original. Foods produced via this technology are called *genetically modified (GM)* or *genetically engineered (GE) foods.*

genetics: the study of genes and inheritance.

genome (GEE-nome): the complete set of genetic material (DNA) in an organism or a cell. The study of genomes is called *genomics.*

genomics: the study of all the genes in an organism and their interactions with environmental factors.

genotoxicant: a substance that mutates or damages genetic material.

geophagia: see *pica.*

germ: the seed that grows into a mature plant, especially rich in vitamins and minerals.

gestation (jes-TAY-shun): the period from conception to birth. For human beings, the average length of a healthy gestation is 40 weeks. Pregnancy is often divided into 3-month period, called *trimesters.*

gestational diabetes: glucose intolerance with onset or first recognition during pregnancy.

gestational hypertension: high blood pressure that develops in the second half of pregnancy and resolves after childbirth, usually without affecting the outcome of the pregnancy.

ghrelin (GRELL-in): a protein produced by the stomach cells that stimulates appetite and decreases energy expenditure.

GI microbiota: the collection of microbes found in the GI tract; sometimes called the *microflora* or *gut flora.* The collection of genes and genomes of the microbiota is called the *microbiome.*

GI motility (moh-TIL-ih-tee): the spontaneous movement of the GI tract that aids in the digestion and transit of the contents within it.

glands: cells or groups of cells that secrete materials for special uses in the body. Glands may be *exocrine* (EKS-oh-crin) *glands,* secreting their materials "out" (into the digestive tract or onto the surface of the skin), or *endocrine* (EN-doe-crin) *glands,* secreting their materials "in" (into the blood).

glossitis (gloss-EYE-tis): an inflammation of the tongue.

glucagon (GLOO-ka-gon): a hormone secreted by special cells in the pancreas in response to low blood glucose concentration. Glucagon elicits release of glucose from liver glycogen stores.

glucogenic amino acids: amino acids that can make glucose via either pyruvate or TCA cycle intermediates.

gluconeogenesis (gloo-ko-nee-oh-JEN-ih-sis): the making of glucose from a noncarbohydrate source such as amino acids or glycerol.

glucose (GLOO-kose): a monosaccharide; sometimes known as *blood sugar* in the body or *dextrose* in foods.

glucose polymers: compounds that supply glucose, not as single molecules, but linked in chains somewhat like starch. The objective is to attract less water from the body into the digestive tract (osmotic attraction depends on the number, not the size, of particles).

glucose tolerance factors (GTF): small organic compounds that enhance insulin's actions.

gluten (GLOO-tuhn): proteins in grains that give dough its elastic texture; in people with celiac disease, gluten damages the small intestine.

gluten-free: a food that contains less than 20 parts per million of gluten from any source; synonyms include *no gluten, free of gluten,* or *without gluten.*

glycemic (gly-SEEM-ic) **index:** a method of classifying foods according to their potential for raising blood glucose.

glycemic response: the extent to which a food raises the blood glucose concentration and elicits an insulin response.

glycerol (GLISS-er-ol): an alcohol composed of a three-carbon chain, which can serve as the backbone for a triglyceride.

glycobiology: the study of sugars and their derivatives.

glycogen (GLY-ko-jen): an animal polysaccharide composed of glucose; a storage form of glucose manufactured and stored in the liver and muscles. Glycogen is not a significant food source of carbohydrate and is not counted as a dietary carbohydrate in foods.

glycolipids: sugars attached to lipids in a cell's membrane.

glycolysis (gly-COLL-ih-sis): the metabolic breakdown of glucose to pyruvate. Glycolysis does not require oxygen (anaerobic).

glycoproteins: sugars attached to a protein.

goblet cells: cells of the GI tract (and lungs) that secrete mucus.

goiter (GOY-ter): an enlargement of the thyroid gland due to an iodine deficiency, malfunction of the gland, or overconsumption of a goitrogen. Goiter caused by iodine deficiency is sometimes called *simple goiter.*

goitrogens (GOY-troh-jenz): substances that enlarge the thyroid gland and cause *toxic goiter.* Goitrogens occur naturally in such foods as cabbage, kale, brussels sprouts, cauliflower, broccoli, and kohlrabi.

Golgi (GOAL-gee) **apparatus:** a set of membranes within the cell where secretory materials are packaged for export.

good source of: the product provides between 10 and 19 percent of the Daily Value for a given nutrient per serving.

gout (GOWT): a common form of arthritis characterized by deposits of uric acid crystals in the joints.

GRAS: see *generally recognized as safe.*

growth hormone: see *bovine growth hormone* or *human growth hormone.*

GTF: see *glucose tolerance factors.*

H

HACCP: see *Hazard Analysis Critical Control Points.*

half-life: in blood tests, the length of time that a substance remains in the body. The half-life of albumin, for example, is 14 to 20 days, meaning that half of the albumin circulating in the plasma is degraded in this time period.

hard water: water with a high calcium and magnesium content.

hazard: a source of danger; used to refer to circumstances in which harm is possible under normal conditions of use.

Hazard Analysis Critical Control Points (HACCP): a systematic plan to identify and correct potential microbial hazards in the manufacturing, distribution, and commercial use of food products; commonly referred to as "HASS-ip."

HDL (high-density lipoproteins): lipoproteins that help remove cholesterol from the blood by transporting it to the liver for reuse or disposal.

health claims: statements that characterize the relationship between a nutrient or other substance in a food and a disease or health-related condition.

health history: an account of a client's current and past health status and disease risks.

healthy: on food labels, a food that is low in fat, saturated fat, cholesterol, and sodium and that contains at least 10 percent of the Daily Values for vitamin D, potassium, iron, calcium, protein, or fiber.

Healthy Eating Index: a measure that assesses how well a diet meets the recommendations of the *Dietary Guidelines for Americans.*

Healthy People: a national public health initiative under the jurisdiction of the US Department of Health and Human Services (DHHS) that identifies the most significant preventable threats to health and focuses efforts to eliminate them.

heart attack: sudden tissue death caused by blockages of vessels that feed the heart muscle; also called *myocardial* (my-oh-KAR-dee-al) *infarction* (in-FARK-shun) or *cardiac arrest.*

heartburn: a burning sensation in the chest area caused by backflow of stomach acid into the esophagus; medically known as *gastroesophageal reflux.*

heat stroke: a dangerous accumulation of body heat with accompanying loss of body fluid.

heavy drinking: more than three drinks on any day for women and more than four drinks on any day for men.

heavy metals: mineral ions such as mercury and lead, so called because of their relatively high atomic weight. Many heavy metals are poisonous.

Heimlich (HIME-lick) **maneuver** (abdominal thrusts): a technique for dislodging an object from the trachea of a choking person; named for the physician who developed it.

hematocrit (hee-MAT-oh-krit): the percentage of total blood volume that consists of red blood cells.

heme (HEEM) **iron:** the iron in foods that is bound to the hemoglobin and myoglobin proteins; found only in meat, fish, and poultry.

hemochromatosis (HE-moh-KRO-ma-toe-sis): a genetically determined failure to prevent absorption of unneeded dietary iron that is characterized by iron overload and tissue damage.

hemoglobin (HE-moh-GLO-bin): the globular protein of the red blood cells that transports oxygen from the lungs to tissues throughout the body; hemoglobin accounts for 80 percent of the body's iron.

hemolytic (HE-moh-LIT-ick) **anemia:** the condition of having too few red blood cells as a result of erythrocyte hemolysis.

hemophilia (HE-moh-FEEL-ee-ah): a hereditary disease in which the blood is unable to clot because it lacks the ability to synthesize certain clotting factors.

hemorrhagic (hem-oh-RAJ-ik) **disease:** a disease characterized by excessive bleeding.

hemorrhoids (HEM-oh-royds): painful swelling of the veins surrounding the rectum.

hemosiderin (heem-oh-SID-er-in): an iron-storage protein primarily made in times of iron overload.

hepatic portal vein: the vein that collects blood from the GI tract and conducts it to the liver.

hepatic vein: the vein that collects blood from the liver and returns it to the heart.

hepcidin: a hormone produced by the liver that regulates iron balance.

herbal (ERB-al) **medicine:** the use of plants to treat disease or improve health; also known as *botanical medicine* or *phytotherapy.*

HFCS: see *high-fructose corn syrup.*

hGH: see *human growth hormone.*

high: on food labels, 20 percent or more of the Daily Value for a given nutrient per serving; synonyms include *rich in* or *excellent source of.*

high-density lipoproteins: see *HDL.*

high fiber: 5 grams or more of fiber per serving. A high-fiber claim made on a food that contains more than 3 grams of fat per serving and per 100 grams of food must also declare total fat.

high food security: no indications of food-access problems or limitations.

high potency: 100% or more of the Daily Value for the nutrient in a single supplement and for at least two-thirds of the nutrients in a multinutrient supplement.

high-fructose corn syrup (HFCS): a syrup made from cornstarch that has been treated with an enzyme that converts some of the glucose to the sweeter fructose; made especially for use in processed foods and beverages, where it is the predominant sweetener. With a chemical structure similar to sucrose, HFCS has a fructose content of 42 or 55 percent, with glucose making up the remainder.

high-quality proteins: dietary proteins containing all the essential amino acids in relatively the same amounts that human beings require. They may also contain nonessential amino acids.

high-risk pregnancy: a pregnancy characterized by indicators that make it likely the birth will be surrounded by problems such as premature delivery, difficult birth, restricted growth, birth defects, and early infant death.

histamine (HISS-tah-mean or HISS-tah-men): a substance produced by cells of the immune system as part of a local immune reaction to an antigen.

HMB: see *beta-hydroxybetamethylbutyrate.*

homeopathy (hoh-me-OP-ah-thee): a practice based on the theory that "like cures like," that is, that substances that cause symptoms in healthy people can cure those symptoms when given in very dilute amounts.

homeostasis (HOME-ee-oh-STAY-sis): the maintenance of constant internal conditions (such as blood chemistry, temperature, and blood pressure) by the body's control systems. A homeostatic system is constantly reacting to external forces to maintain limits set by the body's needs.

honey: sugar (mostly sucrose) formed from nectar gathered by bees. Composition and flavor vary, but honey always contains a mixture of sucrose, fructose, and glucose.

hormones: chemical messengers. Hormones are secreted by a variety of glands in response to altered conditions in the body. Each hormone travels to one or more specific target tissues or organs, where it elicits a specific response to maintain homeostasis. The study of hormones and their actions is called *endocrinology.*

hormone-sensitive lipase: an enzyme inside adipose cells that responds to the body's need for fuel by hydrolyzing triglycerides so that their parts (glycerol and fatty acids) enter the general circulation and thus become available to other cells for fuel. The signals to which this enzyme responds include epinephrine and glucagon, which oppose insulin.

hourly sweat rate: the amount of weight lost plus fluid consumed during exercise per hour. One pound equals roughly 2 cups (500 milliliters) of fluid.

human genome (GEE-nome): the complete set of genetic material (DNA) in a human being.

human growth hormone (hGH): a hormone produced by the brain's pituitary gland that regulates normal growth and development; also called *somatotropin.*

hunger: the painful sensation caused by a lack of food that initiates food-seeking behavior; a consequence of food insecurity that, because of prolonged, involuntary lack of food, results in discomfort, illness, weakness, or pain that goes beyond the usual uneasy sensation.

husk: the outer inedible part of a grain; also called the *chaff.*

hydrochloric acid: an acid composed of hydrogen and chloride atoms (HCl) that is normally produced by the gastric glands.

hydrogenation (HIGH-dro-jen-AY-shun or high-DROJ-eh-NAY-shun): a chemical process by which hydrogens are added to monounsaturated or polyunsaturated fatty acids to reduce the number of double bonds, making the fats more saturated (solid) and more resistant to oxidation (protecting against rancidity). Hydrogenation produces *trans*-fatty acids.

hydrolysis (high-DROL-ih-sis): a chemical reaction in which one molecule is split into two molecules, with hydrogen (H) added to one and a hydroxyl group (OH) added to the other (from water, H_2O). The noun is *hydrolysis;* the verb is *hydrolyze.*

hydrophilic (high-dro-FIL-ick): a term referring to water-loving, or water-soluble, substances.

hydrophobic (high-dro-FOE-bick): a term referring to water-fearing, or non-water-soluble, substances; also known as *lipophilic* (fat loving).

hydrotherapy: the use of water (in whirlpools, as douches, or packed as ice, for example) to promote relaxation and healing.

hydroxyapatite (high-drox-ee-APP-ah-tite): crystals made of calcium and phosphorus.

hyperactivity: inattentive and impulsive behavior that is more frequent and severe than is typical of others a similar age; professionally called *attention-deficit/hyperactivity disorder (ADHD).*

hypercalcemia: high blood calcium that may develop from a variety of disorders, including vitamin D toxicity. It does *not* develop from a high calcium intake.

hyperglycemia: elevated blood glucose concentrations.

hyperplastic obesity: obesity due to an increase in the *number* of fat cells.

hypertension: consistently higher-than-normal blood pressure. Hypertension that develops without an identifiable cause is known as *essential* or *primary hypertension;* hypertension that is caused by a specific disorder such as kidney disease is known as *secondary hypertension.*

hyperthermia: an above-normal body temperature.

hypertrophic obesity: obesity due to an increase in the *size* of fat cells.

hypertrophy (high-PER-tro-fee): growing larger; with regard to muscles, an increase in size (and strength) in response to use.

hypnotherapy: a technique that uses hypnosis and the power of suggestion to improve health behaviors, relieve pain, and heal.

hypoglycemia (HIGH-po-gly-SEE-me-ah): an abnormally low blood glucose concentration.

hyponatremia (HIGH-poe-na-TREE-mee-ah): a decreased concentration of sodium in the blood.

hypothalamus (high-po-THAL-ah-mus): a brain center that controls activities such as maintenance of water balance, regulation of body temperature, and control of appetite.

hypothermia: a below-normal body temperature.

hypothesis (hi-POTH-eh-sis): an unproven statement that tentatively explains the relationships between two or more variables.

hypothyroidism: underactivity of the thyroid gland that may be caused by iodine deficiency or any number of other causes.

I

ileocecal (ill-ee-oh-SEEK-ul) **valve:** the sphincter separating the small and large intestines.

ileum (ILL-ee-um): the last segment of the small intestine.

imagery: a technique that guides clients to achieve a desired physical, emotional, or spiritual state by visualizing themselves in that state.

immune response: the body's reaction to foreign antigens, which neutralizes or eliminates them, thus preventing damage.

immune system: the body's natural defense against foreign materials that have penetrated the skin or mucous membranes.

immunity: the body's ability to defend itself against diseases.

immunoglobulins (IM-you-noh-GLOB-you-linz): proteins capable of acting as antibodies.

implantation (IM-plan-TAY-shun): the embedding of the blastocyst in the inner lining of the uterus.

indigestion: incomplete or uncomfortable digestion, usually accompanied by pain, nausea, vomiting, heartburn, intestinal gas, or belching.

indirect calorimetry: a means of estimating energy expenditure by measuring the amount of oxygen consumed.

indirect or **incidental additives:** substances that can get into food as a result of contact during growing, processing, packaging, storing, cooking, or some other stage before the foods are consumed; sometimes called *accidental additives.*

indispensable amino acids: see *essential amino acids.*

indispensable nutrients: see *essential nutrients.*

infectious diseases: diseases caused by bacteria, viruses, parasites, or other microorganisms that can be transmitted from one person to another through air, water, or food; by contact; or through vector organisms such as mosquitoes.

inflammation: an immunological response to cellular injury characterized by an increase in white blood cells.

initiators: factors that cause mutations that give rise to cancer, such as radiation and carcinogens.

inorganic: not containing carbon or pertaining to living organisms. The two classes of nutrients that are inorganic are minerals and water.

inositol (in-OSS-ih-tall): a nonessential nutrient that can be made in the body from glucose. Inositol is a part of cell membrane structures.

insoluble fibers: nonstarch polysaccharides that do not dissolve in water. Examples include the tough, fibrous structures found in the strings of celery and the skins of corn kernels.

insulin (IN-suh-lin): a hormone secreted by special cells in the pancreas in response to (among other things) elevated blood glucose concentration. Insulin controls the transport of glucose from the bloodstream into the muscle and fat cells.

insulin resistance: the condition in which a normal amount of insulin produces a subnormal effect in muscle, adipose, and liver cells, resulting in an elevated fasting glucose; a metabolic consequence of obesity that precedes type 2 diabetes.

integrative medicine: care that combines conventional and complementary therapies for which there is some high-quality scientific evidence of safety and effectiveness. Integrative medicine emphasizes the importance of the relationship between the practitioner and the patient and focuses on wellness, healing, and the whole person.

intentional food additives: additives intentionally added to foods, such as nutrients, colors, and preservatives.

international units: see *IU.*

interstitial (IN-ter-STISH-al) **fluid:** fluid between the cells (intercellular), usually high in sodium and chloride. Interstitial fluid is a large component of extracellular fluid.

intestinal ischemia (is-KEY-me-ah): a diminished blood flow to the intestines that is characterized by abdominal pain, forceful bowel movements, and blood in the stool.

intra-abdominal fat: see *visceral fat.*

intracellular fluid: fluid inside the cells, usually high in potassium and phosphate. Intracellular fluid accounts for approximately two-thirds of the body's water.

intragastric balloon: a saline-filled silicone device placed in the stomach to limit food intake.

intravascular fluid: fluid within blood vessels.

intrinsic factor: a glycoprotein (a protein with short polysaccharide chains attached) secreted by the stomach cells that binds with vitamin B_{12} in the small intestine to aid in the absorption of vitamin B_{12}.

invert sugar: a mixture of glucose and fructose formed by the hydrolysis of sucrose in a chemical process; sold only in liquid form and sweeter than sucrose. Invert sugar is used as a food additive to help preserve freshness and prevent shrinkage.

iodide: the ion form of iodine.

iodine: an essential trace mineral that is needed for the synthesis of thyroid hormones; the anion (I^-) form of iodine is *iodide.*

ions (EYE-uns): atoms or molecules that have gained or lost electrons and therefore have electrical charges. Examples include the positively charged sodium ion (Na^+) and the negatively charged chloride ion (Cl^-).

iridology: the study of changes in the iris of the eye and their relationships to disease.

iron: an essential trace mineral that is needed for the transport of oxygen and the metabolism of energy nutrients.

iron deficiency: the state of having depleted iron stores.

iron-deficiency anemia: severe depletion of iron stores that results in low hemoglobin and small, pale red blood cells. Iron-deficiency anemia is a *microcytic* (my-cro-SIT-ic) *hypochromic* (high-po-KROME-ic) *anemia.*

iron overload: toxicity from excess iron.

irradiation: sterilizing a food by exposure to energy waves, similar to ultraviolet light and microwaves; sometimes called *ionizing radiation.*

irritable bowel syndrome: an intestinal disorder of unknown cause. Symptoms include abdominal discomfort and cramping, diarrhea, constipation, or alternating diarrhea and constipation.

IU: international units; an old measure of vitamin activity determined by biological methods (as opposed to new measures that are determined by direct chemical analyses). Many fortified foods and supplements use IU on their labels.

J

jejunum (je-JOON-um): the first two-fifths of the small intestine beyond the duodenum.

joule: a measure of *work* energy; the amount of energy expended when 1 kilogram is moved 1 meter by a force of 1 newton.

K

kcal: abbreviation of kcalories; a unit by which energy is measured.

kcalorie: a measure of *heat* energy. One kcalorie is the amount of heat necessary to raise the temperature of 1 kilogram (kg) of water 1°C. The scientific use of the term *kcalorie* is the same as the popular use of the term *calorie.*

kcalorie (energy) control: management of food energy intake.

kcalorie-free: fewer than 5 kcalories per serving.

keratin (KARE-uh-tin): a water-insoluble protein; the normal protein of hair and nails.

keratinization: accumulation of keratin in a tissue; a sign of vitamin A deficiency.

keratomalacia (KARE-ah-toe-ma-LAY-shuh): softening of the cornea that leads to irreversible blindness; a sign of severe vitamin A deficiency.

Keshan (KESH-an or ka-SHAWN) **disease:** the heart disease associated with selenium deficiency; named for one of the provinces of China where it was first studied. Keshan disease is characterized by heart enlargement and insufficiency; fibrous tissue replaces the muscle tissue that normally composes the middle layer of the walls of the heart.

keto (KEY-toe) **acid:** an organic acid that contains a carbonyl group (C=O).

ketogenic amino acids: amino acids that are degraded to acetyl CoA.

ketone (KEE-tone) **bodies:** acidic compounds produced by the liver during the breakdown of fat when carbohydrate is not available.

ketosis (kee-TOE-sis): an undesirably high concentration of ketone bodies in the blood and urine.

Krebs cycle: see *TCA cycle.*

kwashiorkor (kwash-ee-OR-core or kwash-ee-or-CORE): severe malnutrition characterized by failure to grow and develop, edema, changes in the pigmentation of hair and skin, fatty liver, anemia, and apathy.

L

lactase: an enzyme that hydrolyzes lactose.

lactase deficiency: a lack of the enzyme required to digest the disaccharide lactose into its component monosaccharides (glucose and galactose).

lactate: a 3-carbon compound produced from pyruvate during anaerobic metabolism.

lactation: production and secretion of breast milk for the purpose of nourishing an infant.

lacteals (LACK-tee-als): the lymphatic vessels of the intestine that take up nutrients and pass them to the lymph circulation.

lacto-ovo-vegetarian diet: an eating pattern that includes milk, milk products, and eggs, but excludes meat, poultry, and seafood from the diet.

lactose (LAK-tose): a disaccharide composed of glucose and galactose; commonly known as *milk sugar.*

lactose intolerance: a condition that results from the inability to digest the milk sugar lactose; characterized by bloating, gas, abdominal discomfort, and diarrhea. Lactose intolerance differs from milk allergy, which is caused by an immune reaction to the protein in milk.

lactovegetarian diet: an eating pattern that includes milk and milk products, but excludes meat, poultry, seafood, and eggs from the diet.

large intestine or **colon** (COAL-un): the lower portion of intestine that completes the digestive process. Its segments are the *ascending colon,* the *transverse colon,* the *descending colon,* and the *sigmoid colon.*

larynx (LAIR-inks): the entryway to the trachea that contains the vocal cords; also called the *voice box.*

laxatives: substances that loosen the bowels and thereby prevent or treat constipation.

LBW: see *low birthweight.*

LDL (low-density lipoproteins): lipoproteins that derive from VLDL and transport lipids (primarily cholesterol) in the blood.

lean: less than 10 grams of fat, 4.5 grams of saturated fat and *trans* fat combined, and 95 milligrams of cholesterol per serving and per 100 grams of meat, poultry, and seafood. For mixed dishes such as burritos and sandwiches, less than 8 grams of fat, 3.5 grams of saturated fat, and 80 milligrams of cholesterol per reference amount customarily consumed.

lean body mass: the body minus its fat.

lecithin (LESS-uh-thin): one of the phospholipids. Both nature and the food industry use lecithin as an emulsifier to combine water-soluble and fat-soluble ingredients that do not ordinarily mix, such as water and oil.

legumes (lay-GYOOMS or LEG-yooms): plants of the bean and pea family, with seeds that are rich in protein compared with other plant-derived foods.

leptin: a protein produced by fat cells under direction of the *ob* gene that decreases appetite and increases energy expenditure.

leptin resistance: a condition in which leptin levels are increased and leptin sensitivity is decreased.

less: on food labels, at least 25 percent less of a given nutrient or kcalories than the comparison food; synonyms include *fewer* and *reduced*.

less cholesterol: 25 percent or less cholesterol than the comparison food (reflecting a reduction of at least 20 milligrams per serving), and 2 grams or less of saturated fat and *trans* fat combined per serving.

less fat: 25 percent or less fat than the comparison food.

less saturated fat: 25 percent or less saturated fat and *trans* fat combined than the comparison food.

let-down reflex: the reflex that forces milk to the front of the breast when the infant begins to nurse.

levulose: an older name for fructose.

license to practice: permission under state or federal law, granted on meeting specified criteria, to use a certain title (such as dietitian) and offer certain services. *Licensed dietitians* may use the initials *LD* after their names.

life expectancy: the average number of years lived by people in a given society.

life span: the maximum number of years of life attainable by a member of a species.

light or **lite:** one-third fewer kcalories than the comparison food; 50 percent or less of the fat or sodium than the comparison food; any use of the term other than as defined must specify what it is referring to (for example, "light in color" or "light in texture").

lignans: phytochemicals present in flaxseed that are converted to phytosterols by intestinal bacteria and are under study as possible anticancer agents.

limiting amino acid: the essential amino acid found in the shortest supply relative to the amounts needed for protein synthesis in the body. Four amino acids are most likely to be limiting: lysine, methionine, threonine, and tryptophan.

lingual: pertaining to the tongue.

linoleic (lin-oh-LAY-ick) **acid:** an essential fatty acid with 18 carbons and two double bonds.

linolenic (lin-oh-LEN-ick) **acid:** an essential fatty acid with 18 carbons and three double bonds.

lipases (LYE-pasez): enzymes that hydrolyze lipids (fats). *Lingual lipase* is a fat-digesting enzyme secreted from the salivary gland at the base of the tongue; *gastric lipase* is a fat-digesting enzyme secreted from the cells of the stomach.

lipids: a family of compounds that includes triglycerides, phospholipids, and sterols. Lipids are characterized by their insolubility in water. (Lipids also include the fat-soluble vitamins.)

lipoprotein-associated phospholipase A(2) or **Lp-PLA(2):** a lipoprotein-bound enzyme that generates potent proinflammatory and proatherogenic products such as oxidized free fatty acids and lysophosphatidylcholine. Lp-PLA(2) is a specific marker of plaque inflammation.

lipoprotein lipase (LPL): an enzyme that hydrolyzes triglycerides passing by in the bloodstream and directs their parts into the cells, where they can be metabolized for energy or reassembled for storage.

lipoproteins (LIP-oh-PRO-teenz): clusters of lipids associated with proteins that serve as transport vehicles for lipids in the lymph and blood.

liquor or **distilled spirits:** an alcoholic beverage traditionally made by fermenting and distilling a carbohydrate source such as molasses, potatoes, rye, beets, barley, or corn.

listeriosis (lis-TEAR-ee-OH-sis): an infection caused by eating food contaminated with the bacterium *Listeria monocytogenes*, which can be killed by pasteurization and cooking but can survive at refrigerated temperatures; certain ready-to-eat foods, such as hot dogs and deli meats, may become contaminated after cooking or processing, but before packaging.

liver: the organ that manufactures bile, among many other functions.

longevity: long duration of life.

low: on food labels, an amount that would allow frequent consumption of a food without exceeding the Daily Value for the nutrient. A food that is naturally low in a nutrient may make such a claim, but only as it applies to all similar foods (for example, "fresh cauliflower, a low-sodium food"); synonyms include *little, few,* and *low source of.*

low birthweight (LBW): a birthweight of 5½ pounds (2500 grams) or less; indicates probable poor health in the newborn and poor nutrition status in the mother during pregnancy, before pregnancy, or both. Optimal birthweight for a full-term baby is 6½ to 8 pounds.

low cholesterol: 20 milligrams or less of cholesterol per serving and 2 grams or less of saturated fat and *trans* fat combined per serving.

low-density lipoproteins: see *LDL.*

low fat: 3 grams or less of fat per serving.

low food security: reduced quality of life with little or no indication of reduced food intake; formerly known as *food insecurity without hunger.*

low kcalorie: 40 kcalories or less per serving.

low saturated fat: 1 gram or less of saturated fat and less than 0.5 gram of *trans* fat per serving.

low sodium: 140 milligrams or less per serving.

low-risk pregnancy: a pregnancy characterized by factors that make it likely the birth will be normal and the infant healthy.

LPL: see *lipoprotein lipase.*

lumen (LOO-men): the space within a vessel such as the intestine.

lutein (LOO-teen): a plant pigment of yellow hue; a phytochemical believed to play roles in eye functioning and health.

lycopene (LYE-koh-peen): a pigment responsible for the red color of tomatoes and other red-hued vegetables; a phytochemical that may act as an antioxidant in the body.

lymph (LIMF): a clear fluid that contains infection-fighting white blood cells. Lymph from the GI tract transports fat and fat-soluble vitamins to the bloodstream via lymphatic vessels.

lymphatic (lim-FAT-ic) **system:** network of tissues and organs that transport fluids toward the heart. The GI part of the lymphatic system carries the products of fat digestion into the bloodstream.

lymphocytes (LIM-foh-sites): white blood cells that participate in acquired immunity; B-cells and T-cells.

lysosomes (LYE-so-zomes): cellular organelles; membrane-enclosed sacs of degradative enzymes.

M

macrobiotic diet: a philosophical eating pattern based on mostly plant foods such as whole grains, legumes, and vegetables, with small amounts of fish, fruits, nuts, and seeds.

macrocytic: abnormally large cells.

macronutrients: carbohydrate, fat, and protein; the nutrients the body requires in relatively large amounts (many grams daily).

macrophages (MAK-roe-fay-jez): large phagocytic cells that serve as scavengers of the blood, clearing it of old or abnormal cells, cellular debris, and antigens.

macrosomia (mak-roh-SO-me-ah): abnormally large body size. In the case of infants, a birthweight at the 90th percentile or higher for gestational age (roughly 9 lb—or 4000 g—or more); macrosomia results from prepregnancy obesity, excessive weight gain during pregnancy, or uncontrolled gestational diabetes.

macular (MACK-you-lar) **degeneration:** deterioration of the macular area of the eye that can lead to loss of central vision and eventual blindness. The *macula* is a small, oval, yellowish region in the center of the retina that provides the sharp, straight-ahead vision so critical to reading and driving.

magnesium: a cation within the body's cells, active in many enzyme systems.

major minerals: essential mineral nutrients the human body requires in relatively large amounts (greater than 100 milligrams per day); sometimes called *macrominerals.*

malignant (ma-LIG-nant): describes a cancerous cell or tumor, which can injure healthy tissue and spread cancer to other regions of the body.

malnutrition: any condition caused by excess or deficient food energy or nutrient intake or by an imbalance of nutrients.

malt syrup: a sweetener made from sprouted barley and containing mostly maltose.

maltase: an enzyme that hydrolyzes maltose.

maltose (MAWL-tose): a disaccharide composed of two glucose units; sometimes known as *malt sugar.*

mammary glands: glands of the female breast that secrete milk.

manganese: an essential trace mineral that acts as a cofactor for many enzymes.

maple sugar: a sugar (mostly sucrose) purified from the concentrated sap of the sugar maple tree.

marasmus (ma-RAZ-mus): severe malnutrition characterized by poor growth, dramatic weight loss, loss of body fat and muscle, and apathy.

margarine: a butter substitute made primarily of hydrogenated vegetable oils and sometimes blended with animal fats, emulsifiers, water, milk, salt, vitamins, artificial color, and other ingredients.

margin of safety: when speaking of food additives, a zone between the concentration normally used and that at which a hazard exists. For common table salt, for example, the margin of safety is 1/5 (five times the amount normally used would be hazardous).

marginal food security: one or two indications of food-access problems but with little or no change in food intake.

massage therapy: a healing method in which the therapist manually kneads muscles to reduce tension, increase blood circulation, improve joint mobility, and promote healing of injuries.

matrix (MAY-tricks): the basic substance that gives form to a developing structure; in the body, the formative cells from which teeth and bones grow.

Meals on Wheels: a nutrition program that delivers food for the elderly to their homes.

meat replacements: products formulated to look and taste like meat, fish, or poultry; usually made of textured vegetable protein.

medical history: an account of a patient's current and past health status and disease risks.

medication and supplement history: a record of all the drugs, over-the-counter and prescribed, as well as dietary and herbal supplements that a person takes routinely.

meditation: a self-directed technique of relaxing the body and calming the mind.

megaloblastic: abnormally large immature red blood cells.

menadione (men-uh-DYE-own): the synthetic form of vitamin K.

menaquinone (men-ah-KWYN-own): the bacteria-produced form of vitamin K; also called *vitamin* K_2.

Menkes disease: a genetic disorder of copper transport that creates a copper deficiency and results in mental impairment, poor muscle tone, seizures, brittle kinky hair, and failure to thrive.

MEOS or **microsomal** (my-krow-SO-mal) **ethanol oxidizing system:** a system of enzymes in the liver that oxidize not only alcohol but also several classes of drugs.

meta-analysis: an objective and statistical summary of evidence gathered from multiple selected studies to develop a *quantitative* review; often derived from a systematic review.

metabolic syndrome: a combination of risk factors—insulin resistance, high blood pressure, abnormal blood lipids, and abdominal obesity—that greatly increase a person's risk of developing coronary heart disease.

metabolic water: water generated during metabolism.

metabolism: the sum total of all the chemical reactions that go on in living cells. *Energy metabolism* includes all the reactions by which the body obtains and expends the energy from food.

metalloenzymes (meh-TAL-oh-EN-zimes): enzymes that contain one or more minerals as part of their structures.

metallothionein (meh-TAL-oh-THIGH-oh-neen): a sulfur-rich protein that avidly binds with and transports metals such as zinc.

metastasize (me-TAS-tah-size): the spread of cancer from one part of the body to another.

methylation: the addition of a methyl group (CH_3).

MFP factor: a peptide released during the digestion of meat, fish, and poultry that enhances nonheme iron absorption.

mg: milligrams; one-thousandth of a gram.

mg NE: milligrams of niacin equivalents; a measure of niacin activity.

micelles (MY-cells): tiny spherical complexes of emulsified fat that arise during digestion; most contain bile salts and the products of lipid digestion, including fatty acids, monoglycerides, and cholesterol.

microangiopathies: disorders of the small blood vessels.

microarray technology: research tools that analyze the expression of thousands of genes simultaneously and search for particular gene changes associated with a disease. DNA microarrays are also called *DNA chips.*

microbes (MY-krobes): microscopically small organisms including bacteria, viruses, fungi, and protozoa; also called *microorganisms.*

microcytic (my-cro-SIT-ic) **hypochromic** (high-po-KROME-ic) **anemia:** small, pale red blood cells that develop in iron-deficiency anemia.

microgram (μg): one millionth of a gram.

microgram DFE (μg DFE): micrograms dietary folate equivalents; a measure of folate activity.

microgram RAE (μg RAE): micrograms retinol activity equivalents; a measure of vitamin A activity.

micronutrients: vitamins and minerals; the nutrients the body requires in relatively small amounts (milligrams or micrograms daily).

microvilli (MY-cro-VILL-ee or MY-cro-VILL-eye): tiny, hairlike projections on each cell of every villus that can trap nutrient particles and transport them into the cells; singular *microvillus.*

milk anemia: iron-deficiency anemia that develops when an excessive milk intake displaces iron-rich foods from the diet.

milliequivalents per liter (mEq/L): the concentration of electrolytes in a volume of solution. Milliequivalents reveal characteristics about the solution that are not evident when the concentration is expressed in terms of weight.

mineral oil: a purified liquid derived from petroleum and used to treat constipation.

mineral water: water from a spring or well that naturally contains at least 250 parts per million (ppm) of minerals. Minerals give water a distinctive flavor. Many mineral waters are high in sodium.

mineralization: the process in which calcium, phosphorus, and other minerals crystallize on the collagen matrix of a growing bone, hardening the bone.

minerals: inorganic elements. Some minerals are essential nutrients required in small amounts by the body for health.

misinformation: false or misleading information.

mitochondria (my-toh-KON-dree-uh): the cellular organelles responsible for producing ATP aerobically; made of membranes with enzymes mounted on them. (The singular is *mitochondrion*.)

mmol: millimoles; one thousandth of a mole, the molecular weight of a substance. To convert mmol to mg, multiply by the atomic weight of the substance.

moderate-intensity physical activity: physical activity that requires some increase in breathing and/or heart rate and expends 3.5 to 7 kcalories per minute. Walking at a speed of 3 to 4.5 miles per hour (about 15 to 20 minutes to walk 1 mile) is an example.

moderation (alcohol): up to one drink per day for women and up to two drinks per day for men.

moderation (dietary): providing enough but not too much of a substance.

molasses: the thick brown syrup produced during sugar refining. Molasses retains residual sugar and other by-products and a few minerals; blackstrap molasses contains significant amounts of calcium and iron.

molecule: two or more atoms of the same or different elements joined by chemical bonds. Examples are molecules of the element oxygen, composed of two oxygen atoms (O_2), and molecules of the compound water, composed of two hydrogen atoms and one oxygen atom (H_2O).

molybdenum (mo-LIB-duh-num): an essential trace mineral that acts as a cofactor for many enzymes.

monoglycerides: molecules of glycerol with one fatty acid attached. A molecule of glycerol with two fatty acids attached is a *diglyceride*.

monosaccharides (mon-oh-SACK-uh-rides): carbohydrates of the general formula $C_nH_{2n}O_n$ that typically form a single ring. The monosaccharides important in nutrition are *hexoses*, sugars with six atoms of carbon and the formula $C_6H_{12}O_6$.

monosodium glutamate (MSG): a sodium salt of the amino acid glutamic acid commonly used as a flavor enhancer. The FDA classifies MSG as a "generally recognized as safe" ingredient.

monounsaturated fatty acid: a fatty acid that lacks two hydrogen atoms and has one double bond between carbons; abbreviated *MUFA*. Examples include palmitoleic acid and oleic acid. A *monounsaturated fat* is composed of triglycerides in which most of the fatty acids are monounsaturated.

more: on food labels, at least 10 percent more of the Daily Value for a given nutrient than the comparison food; synonyms include *added* and *extra*.

motility (moh-TIL-ih-tee): see *GI motility*.

mouth: the oral cavity containing the tongue and teeth.

MSG: see *monosodium glutamate*.

MSG symptom complex: an acute, temporary intolerance reaction that may occur after the ingestion of the additive MSG (monosodium glutamate). Symptoms include burning sensations, chest and facial flushing and pain, and throbbing headaches.

mucous (MYOO-kus) **membranes:** the membranes, composed of mucus-secreting cells, that line the surfaces of body tissues.

mucus (MYOO-kus): a slippery substance secreted by cells of the GI lining (and other body linings) that protects the cells from exposure to digestive juices (and other destructive agents). The lining of the GI tract with its coat of mucus is a *mucous membrane*. (The noun is *mucus*; the adjective is *mucous*.)

muscle dysmorphia (dis-MORE-fee-ah): a psychiatric disorder characterized by a preoccupation with building body mass.

muscle endurance: the ability of a muscle to contract repeatedly without becoming exhausted.

muscle power: the product of force generation (strength) and movement velocity (speed); the speed at which a given amount of exertion is completed.

muscle strength: the ability of muscles to work against resistance.

mutations: permanent changes in the DNA that can be inherited.

myoglobin: the oxygen-holding protein of the muscle cells.

myokines: signaling proteins secreted by skeletal muscles.

N

NAD (nicotinamide adenine dinucleotide): the main coenzyme form of the vitamin niacin. Its reduced form is NADH.

NADP (the phosphate form of NAD): a coenzyme form of niacin.

nanoceuticals: substances with extremely small particles that have been manufactured by nanotechnology.

nanotechnology: a manufacturing technology that manipulates atoms to change the structure of matter.

narcotic (nar-KOT-ic): a drug that dulls the senses, induces sleep, and becomes addictive with prolonged use.

natural water: water obtained from a spring or well that is certified to be safe and sanitary. The mineral content may not be changed, but the water may be treated in other ways such as with ozone or by filtration.

naturopathic (nay-chur-oh-PATH-ick) **medicine:** a system that taps the natural healing forces within the body by integrating several practices, including traditional medicine, herbal medicine, clinical nutrition, homeopathy, acupuncture, East Asian medicine, hydrotherapy, and manipulative therapy.

NE: see *niacin equivalents*.

NEAT: see *nonexercise activity thermogenesis*.

nectar: a sugary fluid secreted by plants to encourage pollination by insects.

neotame (NEE-oh-tame): an artificial sweetener composed of two amino acids (phenylalanine and aspartic acid); approved for use in the United States.

net protein utilization (NPU): a measure of protein quality assessed by measuring the amount of protein nitrogen that is retained from a given amount of protein nitrogen eaten.

neural tube: the embryonic tissue that forms the brain and spinal cord.

neural tube defects: malformations of the brain, spinal cord, or both during embryonic development that often result in lifelong disability or death. The two main types of neural tube defects are *spina bifida* (literally "split spine") and *anencephaly* ("no brain").

neurofibrillary tangles: snarls of the threadlike strands that extend from the nerve cells, commonly found in the brains of people with Alzheimer's dementia.

neurons: nerve cells; the structural and functional units of the nervous system. Neurons initiate and conduct nerve impulse transmissions.

neuropeptide Y: a chemical produced in the brain that stimulates appetite, diminishes energy expenditure, and increases fat storage.

neurotransmitters: chemicals that are released at the end of a nerve cell when a nerve impulse arrives there. They diffuse across the gap to the next cell and alter the membrane of that second cell to either inhibit or excite it.

neutrophils (NEW-tro-fills): the most common type of white blood cell. Neutrophils destroy antigens by phagocytosis.

niacin (NIGH-a-sin): a B vitamin. The coenzyme forms are *NAD (nicotinamide adenine dinucleotide)* and *NADP (the phosphate form of NAD)*. Niacin can be eaten preformed or made in the body from its precursor, tryptophan, an essential amino acid.

niacin equivalents (NE): the amount of niacin present in food, including the niacin that can theoretically be made from its precursor, tryptophan, present in the food. 1 NE = 1 mg niacin or 60 mg tryptophan.

niacin flush: a temporary burning, tingling, and itching sensation that occurs when a person takes a large dose of nicotinic acid; often accompanied by a headache and reddened face, arms, and chest.

night blindness: slow recovery of vision after flashes of bright light at night or an inability to see in dim light; an early symptom of vitamin A deficiency.

nitrites (NYE-trites): salts added to food to prevent botulism. One example is sodium nitrite, which is used to preserve meats.

nitrogen balance: the amount of nitrogen consumed (N in) as compared with the amount of nitrogen excreted (N out) in a given period of time.

nitrosamines (nye-TROHS-uh-meens): derivatives of nitrites that may be formed in the stomach when nitrites combine with amines. Nitrosamines are carcinogenic in animals.

nonceliac gluten sensitivity: a poorly defined cluster of digestive symptoms that seem to improve with the elimination of gluten from the diet.

nonessential amino acids: amino acids that the body can make; also called *dispensable amino acids.*

nonexercise activity thermogenesis (NEAT): energy expended in everyday spontaneous activities.

nonheme iron: the iron in foods that is not bound to proteins; found in both plant-derived and animal-derived foods.

nonnutritive sweeteners: sweeteners that yield no energy (or insignificant energy in the case of aspartame).

NPU: see *net protein utilization.*

nucleotide bases: the nitrogen-containing building blocks of DNA and RNA—cytosine (C), thymine (T), uracil (U), guanine (G), and adenine (A). In DNA, the base pairs are A–T and C–G; in RNA, the base pairs are A–U and C–G.

nucleotides: the subunits of DNA and RNA molecules, composed of a phosphate group, a 5-carbon sugar (deoxyribose for DNA and ribose for RNA), and a nitrogen-containing base.

nucleus: a major membrane-enclosed body within cells, which contains the cell's genetic material (DNA), embedded in chromosomes.

nursing bottle tooth decay: extensive tooth decay due to prolonged tooth contact with formula, milk, fruit juice, or other carbohydrate-rich liquid offered to an infant in a bottle.

nutrient claims: statements that characterize the quantity of a nutrient in a food.

nutrient density: a measure of the nutrients a food provides relative to the energy it provides. The more nutrients and the fewer kcalories, the higher the nutrient density.

nutrient profiling: ranking foods based on their nutrient composition.

nutrients: chemical substances obtained from food and used in the body to provide energy, structural materials, and regulating agents to support growth, maintenance, and repair of the body's tissues. Nutrients may also reduce the risks of some diseases.

nutrigenetics: the science of how genes affect the activities of nutrients.

nutrigenomics: the science of how nutrients affect the activities of genes.

nutrition: the science of the nutrients in foods and of their actions within the body. A broader definition includes the study of human behaviors related to food and eating.

nutrition assessment: a comprehensive analysis of a person's nutrition status that uses health, socioeconomic, drug, and diet histories; anthropometric measurements; physical examinations; and laboratory tests.

nutrition screening: a brief assessment of health-related variables to identify people who are malnourished or are at risk for malnutrition.

nutritional genomics: the science of how nutrients affect the activities of genes (*nutrigenomics*) and how genes affect the activities of nutrients (*nutrigenetics*).

nutritive sweeteners: sweeteners that yield energy, including both sugars and sugar alcohols.

O

obese: too much body fat with adverse health effects; BMI 30 or more.

obesogenic (oh-BES-oh-JEN-ick) **environment:** all the factors surrounding a person that promote weight gain, such as increased food intake, especially of unhealthy choices, and decreased physical activity.

obligatory (ah-BLIG-ah-TORE-ee) **water excretion:** the minimum amount of water the body has to excrete each day to dispose of its wastes—about 500 milliliters (about 2 cups or 1 pint).

oils: lipids that are liquid at room temperature (77°F or 25°C).

olestra: a synthetic fat made from sucrose and fatty acids that provides 0 kcalories per gram; also known as *sucrose polyester.*

oligopeptide (OL-ee-go-PEP-tide): string of four to nine amino acids.

omega: the last letter of the Greek alphabet (ω), used by chemists to refer to the position of the closest double bond to the methyl (CH_3) end of a fatty acid.

omega-3 fatty acid: a polyunsaturated fatty acid in which the closest double bond to the methyl (CH_3) end of the carbon chain is three carbons away.

omega-6 fatty acid: a polyunsaturated fatty acid in which the closest double bond to the methyl (CH_3) end of the carbon chain is six carbons away.

omnivorous: an eating pattern that includes foods derived from both animals and plants.

opsin (OP-sin): the protein portion of visual pigment molecules.

oral rehydration therapy (ORT): the administration of a simple solution of sugar, salt, and water, taken by mouth, to treat dehydration caused by diarrhea.

organelles: subcellular structures such as ribosomes, mitochondria, and lysosomes.

organic: in agriculture, crops grown and processed according to USDA regulations defining the use of fertilizers, herbicides, insecticides, fungicides, preservatives, and other chemical ingredients.

organic: in chemistry, substances or molecules containing carbon-carbon bonds or carbon-hydrogen bonds that are characteristic of living organisms. The four classes of nutrients that are organic are carbohydrates, lipids (fats), proteins, and vitamins.

organic: on food labels, that at least 95 percent of the product's ingredients have been grown and processed according to USDA regulations defining the use of fertilizers, herbicides, insecticides, fungicides, preservatives, and other chemical ingredients.

organic halogens: an organic compound containing one or more atoms of a halogen—fluorine, chlorine, iodine, or bromine.

ORT: see *oral rehydration therapy.*

orthomolecular medicine: the use of large doses of vitamins to treat chronic disease.

orthorexia nervosa: an obsession with good nutrition to improve health that is characterized by restrictive diets, ritualized patterns of eating, and rigid avoidance of foods believed to be unhealthy.

osmosis: the movement of water across a membrane *toward* the side where the solutes are more concentrated.

osmotic pressure: the amount of pressure needed to prevent the movement of water across a membrane.

osteoarthritis: a painful, degenerative disease of the joints that occurs when the cartilage in a joint deteriorates; joint structure is damaged, with loss of function; also called *degenerative arthritis.*

osteoblasts: cells that build bone during growth.

osteocalcin (os-teo-KAL-sen): a calcium-binding protein in bones, essential for normal mineralization.

osteoclasts: cells that destroy bone during growth.

osteomalacia (OS-tee-oh-ma-LAY-shuh): a bone disease characterized by softening of the bones. Symptoms include bending of the spine and bowing of the legs. The disease occurs most often in adult women.

osteopenia (OS-tee-oh-PEE-nee-ah): a bone condition in which bone loss is significant, but not as severe as in osteoporosis.

osteoporosis (OS-tee-oh-pore-OH-sis): a disease in which the bones become porous and fragile due to a loss of minerals; also called *adult bone loss.*

outbreaks: two or more cases of a similar illness resulting from the ingestion of a common food.

overload: an extra physical demand placed on the body; an increase in the frequency, duration, or intensity of an activity. A principle of training that states for a body system to improve, it must be worked at frequencies, durations, or intensities that increase by increments.

overnutrition: excess energy or nutrients.

overt (oh-VERT): out in the open and easy to observe.

overweight: body weight greater than the weight range that is considered healthy; BMI 25 to 29.9.

ovum (OH-vum): the female reproductive cell, capable of developing into a new organism upon fertilization; commonly referred to as an egg.

oxaloacetate (OKS-ah-low-AS-eh-tate): a carbohydrate intermediate of the TCA cycle.

oxidants (OKS-ih-dants): compounds (such as oxygen itself) that oxidize other compounds. Compounds that prevent oxidation are called *antioxidants,* whereas those that promote it are called *prooxidants.*

oxidation (OKS-ee-DAY-shun): the process of a substance combining with oxygen; oxidation reactions involve the loss of electrons.

oxidative stress: a condition in which the production of oxidants and free radicals exceeds the body's ability to handle them and prevent damage.

oxytocin (OCK-see-TOH-sin): a hormone that stimulates the mammary glands to eject milk during lactation and the uterus to contract during childbirth.

oyster shell: a product made from the powdered shells of oysters that is sold as a calcium supplement, but it is not well absorbed by the digestive system.

ozone therapy: the use of ozone gas to enhance the body's immune system.

P

pancreas: a gland that secretes digestive enzymes and juices into the duodenum. (The pancreas also secretes hormones into the blood that help maintain glucose homeostasis.)

pancreatic (pank-ree-AT-ic) **juice:** the exocrine secretion of the pancreas that contains enzymes for the digestion of carbohydrate, fat, and protein as well as bicarbonate, a neutralizing agent. The juice flows from the pancreas into the small intestine through the pancreatic duct. (The pancreas also has an endocrine function, the secretion of insulin and other hormones.)

pantothenic (PAN-toe-THEN-ick) **acid:** a B vitamin. The principal active form is part of coenzyme A, called "CoA" throughout Chapter 7.

parasympathetic nervous system: the part of the autonomic nervous system that dominates during nonstressful conditions and includes such effects as normal heart rate, pupil dilation, and peristalsis.

parathyroid hormone: a hormone from the parathyroid glands that regulates blood calcium by raising it when levels fall too low; also known as *parathormone* (PAIR-ah-THOR-moan).

pasteurization: heat processing of food that inactivates some, but not all, microorganisms in the food; not a sterilization process. Bacteria that cause spoilage are still present.

pathogens (PATH-oh-jenz): microorganisms capable of producing disease.

PBB (polybrominated biphenyl) and **PCB (polychlorinated biphenyl):** toxic organic halogens used in pesticides, paints, and flame retardants.

PC (phosphocreatine): see *creatine phosphate (CP).*

PDCAAS (protein digestibility-corrected amino acid score): a measure of protein quality assessed by comparing the amino acid score of a food protein with the amino acid requirements of preschool-aged children and then correcting for the true digestibility of the protein.

peak bone mass: the highest attainable bone density for an individual, developed during the first three decades of life.

peer review: a process in which a panel of scientists rigorously evaluates a research study to ensure that the scientific method was followed.

pellagra (pell-AY-gra): the niacin-deficiency disease, characterized by diarrhea, dermatitis, dementia, and eventually death.

pepsin: a gastric enzyme that hydrolyzes protein. Pepsin is secreted in an inactive form, *pepsinogen,* which is activated by hydrochloric acid in the stomach.

pepsinogen: an inactive compound that is activated by hydrochloric acid in the stomach to form pepsin.

peptic ulcer: a lesion in the mucous membrane of either the stomach (a *gastric ulcer)* or the duodenum (a *duodenal ulcer).*

peptidase: a digestive enzyme that hydrolyzes peptide bonds. *Tripeptidases* cleave tripeptides; *dipeptidases* cleave dipeptides.

peptide bond: a bond that connects the acid end of one amino acid with the amino end of another, forming a link in a protein chain.

PER: see *protein efficiency ratio.*

percent Daily Value (%DV): the percentage of a Daily Value recommendation found in a specified serving of food for key nutrients based on a 2000-kcalorie diet.

percent fat-free: may be used only if the product meets the definition of *low fat* or *fat-free* and must reflect the amount of fat in 100 grams (for example, a food that contains 2.5 grams of fat per 50 grams can claim to be "95 percent fat-free").

perinatal: referring to the time between the twenty-eighth week of gestation and 1 month after birth.

peripheral (puh-RIFF-er-ul) **nervous system:** the peripheral (outermost) part of the nervous system; the vast complex of wiring that extends from the central nervous system to the body's outermost areas. It contains both *somatic* and *autonomic* components.

peripheral resistance: the resistance to pumped blood in the small arterial branches (arterioles) that carry blood to the tissues.

peristalsis (per-ih-STALL-sis): wavelike muscular contractions of the GI tract that push its contents along.

pernicious (per-NISH-us) **anemia:** a macrocytic anemia that reflects a vitamin B_{12} deficiency caused by lack of intrinsic factor and characterized by abnormally large and immature red blood cells. Other symptoms include muscle weakness and irreversible neurological damage.

persistence: stubborn or enduring continuance; with respect to food contaminants, the quality of persisting, rather than breaking down, in the bodies of animals and human beings.

personal and social history: a record of a person's economic and social background, including such factors as education, income, and ethnic identity.

pesticides: chemicals used to control insects on plants, vegetables, fruits, and animals. Used broadly, the term includes herbicides (to kill weeds), insecticides (to kill insects), and fungicides (to kill fungi).

pH: the unit of measure expressing a substance's acidity or alkalinity. The lower the pH, the higher the H^+ ion concentration and the stronger the acid. A pH above 7 is alkaline or base (a solution in which OH^- ions predominate).

phagocytes (FAG-oh-sites): white blood cells (neutrophils and macrophages) that have the ability to ingest and destroy foreign substances.

phagocytosis (FAG-oh-sigh-TOH-sis): the process by which phagocytes engulf and destroy foreign materials.

pharmacological effect: the body's response to a large dose of a nutrient (levels commonly available only from supplements) that overwhelms some body system and acts like a drug.

pharynx (FAIR-inks): the passageway leading from the nose and mouth to the larynx and esophagus, respectively.

phenylketonuria (FEN-il-KEY-toe-NEW-ree-ah) or **PKU:** an inherited disorder characterized by failure to metabolize the amino acid phenylalanine to tyrosine.

phlebotomy: the withdrawal of blood from the body.

phosphocreatine (PC): see *creatine phosphate (CP).*

phospholipid (FOS-foe-LIP-id): a compound similar to a triglyceride but having a phosphate group (a phosphorus-containing salt) and choline (or another nitrogen-containing compound) in place of one of the fatty acids.

phosphorus: a major mineral found mostly in the body's bones and teeth.

photosynthesis: the process in which green plants use the sun's energy to make carbohydrates from carbon dioxide and water.

phylloquinone (FILL-oh-KWYN-own): the plant form of vitamin K; also called *vitamin* K_1.

physical activity: bodily movement produced by muscle contractions that substantially increase energy expenditure.

physiological age: a person's age as estimated from her or his body's health and probable life expectancy.

physiological effect: the body's response to a normal dose of a nutrient (levels commonly found in foods) that provides a normal blood concentration.

physiological fuel value: the number of kcalories that the body derives from a food, in contrast to the number of kcalories determined by calorimetry.

phytic (FYE-tick) **acid:** a nonnutrient component of plant seeds; also called *phytate* (FYE-tate). Phytic acid occurs in the husks of grains, legumes, and seeds and is capable of binding minerals such as zinc, iron, calcium, magnesium, and copper in insoluble complexes in the intestine, which the body excretes unused.

phytochemicals (FIE-toe-KEM-ih-cals): nonnutrient compounds found in plants. Some phytochemicals have biological activity in the body.

phytoestrogens: phytochemicals structurally similar to human estrogen that weakly mimic or modulate estrogen's action in the body. Phytoestrogens include the isoflavones *genistein, daidzein,* and *glycitein.*

pica (PIE-ka): a craving for and consumption of nonfood substances. Pica is known as *geophagia* (gee-oh-FAY-gee-uh) when referring to eating clay, baby powder, chalk, ash, ceramics, paper, paint chips, or charcoal; *pagophagia* (pag-oh-FAY-gee-uh) when referring to eating large quantities of ice; and *amylophagia* (AM-ee-low-FAY-gee-ah) when referring to eating uncooked starch (flour, laundry starch, or raw rice).

pigment: a molecule capable of absorbing certain wavelengths of light so that it reflects only those that we perceive as a certain color.

placebo (pla-SEE-bo): an inert, harmless medication given to provide comfort and hope; a sham treatment used in controlled research studies.

placebo effect: a change that occurs in response to expectations about the effectiveness of a treatment that actually has no pharmaceutical effects.

placenta (plah-SEN-tuh): the organ that develops inside the uterus early in pregnancy, through which the fetus receives nutrients and oxygen and returns carbon dioxide and other waste products to be excreted.

plant-based diets: an eating pattern that derives most of its protein from plant products (although some animal products may be included).

plant sterols: phytochemicals that have structural similarities to cholesterol and lower blood cholesterol by interfering with cholesterol absorption. Plant sterols include *sterol esters* and *stanol esters.*

plaque (PLACK): an accumulation of fatty deposits, smooth muscle cells, and fibrous connective tissue that develops in the artery walls in atherosclerosis. Plaque associated with atherosclerosis is known as *atheromatous* (ATH-er-OH-ma-tus) *plaque.*

platelets: tiny, disc-shaped bodies in the blood, important in blood clot formation.

PLP (pyridoxal phosphate): the primary active coenzyme form of vitamin B_6.

point of unsaturation: the double bond of a fatty acid, where hydrogen atoms can easily be added to the structure.

polar: characteristic of a neutral molecule, such as water, that has opposite charges spatially separated within the molecule.

polypeptide: many (10 or more) amino acids bonded together.

polysaccharides: compounds composed of many monosaccharides linked together. An intermediate string of 3 to 10 monosaccharides is an *oligosaccharide.*

polyunsaturated fatty acid: a fatty acid that lacks four or more hydrogen atoms and has two or more double bonds between carbons; abbreviated *PUFA.* Examples include linoleic acid (two double bonds) and linolenic acid (three double bonds). A *polyunsaturated fat* is composed of triglycerides in which most of the fatty acids are polyunsaturated.

portion sizes: the quantity of a food served or eaten at one meal or snack; *not* a standard amount.

postpartum amenorrhea (ay-MEN-oh-REE-ah): the normal temporary absence of menstrual periods immediately following childbirth.

postpartum depression: moderate to severe depression in a woman after she has given birth.

potable (POT-ah-bul): suitable for drinking.

potassium: the principal cation within the body's cells; critical to the maintenance of fluid balance, nerve impulse transmissions, and muscle contractions.

powdered bone: see *bone meal.*

prebiotics: food components (such as fibers) that are not digested by the human body but are used as food by the GI bacteria to promote their growth and activity.

precursors: substances that precede others; with regard to vitamins, compounds that can be converted into active vitamins; also known as *provitamins.*

prediabetes: condition in which blood glucose levels are higher than normal, but below the diagnosis of diabetes; formerly called *impaired glucose tolerance.* Prediabetes is considered a major risk factor for future diabetes and cardiovascular diseases.

preeclampsia (PRE-ee-KLAMP-see-ah)**:** a condition characterized by high blood pressure and some protein in the urine.

preformed vitamin A: dietary vitamin A in its active form.

prehypertension: blood pressure slightly higher than normal, but below the diagnosis of hypertension.

prenatal alcohol exposure: subjecting a fetus to a pattern of excessive alcohol intake characterized by substantial regular use or heavy episodic drinking.

preservatives: antimicrobial agents, antioxidants, and other additives that retard spoilage or maintain desired qualities, such as softness in baked goods.

pressure ulcers: damage to the skin and underlying tissues as a result of compression and poor circulation; commonly seen in people who are bedridden or chair-bound.

preterm (premature): births occurring before 37 weeks of gestation; births occurring at 37 to 38 weeks of gestation are designated *early term.*

primary deficiency: a nutrient deficiency caused by inadequate dietary intake of a nutrient.

probiotics: living microorganisms found in foods and dietary supplements that, when consumed in sufficient quantities, are beneficial to health.

processed foods: foods that have been intentionally changed by the addition of substances, or a method of cooking, preserving, milling, or such.

processed meat: meat that has been preserved or flavored by additives, curing, fermenting, salting, or smoking. Examples include bacon, ham, hot dogs, jerky, sausages, and some deli meats (such as corned beef); canned meats; and meat-based preparations and sauces.

proenzyme: the inactive form of an enzyme; also called a *zymogen.*

prolactin (pro-LAK-tin)**:** a hormone secreted from the anterior pituitary gland that acts on the mammary glands to promote the production of milk. The release of prolactin is mediated by *prolactin-inhibiting hormone (PIH).*

promoters: factors that favor the development of cancers once they have begun.

proof: a way of stating the percentage of alcohol in distilled liquor. Liquor that is 100 proof is 50 percent alcohol; 90 proof is 45 percent, and so forth.

prooxidants: substances that significantly induce oxidative stress.

proteases (PRO-tee-aces)**:** enzymes that hydrolyze proteins.

protein digestibility: a measure of the amount of amino acids absorbed from a given protein intake.

protein digestibility-corrected amino acid score: see *PDCAAS.*

protein efficiency ratio (PER): a measure of protein quality assessed by determining how well a given protein supports weight gain in growing rats; used to establish the protein quality for infant formulas and baby foods.

protein turnover: the degradation and synthesis of protein.

protein-sparing action: the action of carbohydrate (and fat) in providing energy that allows protein to be used for other purposes.

proteins: compounds composed of carbon, hydrogen, oxygen, and nitrogen atoms, arranged into amino acids linked in a chain. Some amino acids also contain sulfur atoms.

proteome: all proteins produced by an organism. The study of the expression, structure, and function of proteins is called *proteomics.*

puberty: the period in life in which a person becomes physically capable of reproduction.

public health dietitians: dietitians who specialize in providing nutrition services through organized community efforts.

public water: water from a municipal or county water system that has been treated and disinfected.

purified water: water that has been treated by distillation or other physical or chemical processes that remove dissolved solids. Because purified water contains no minerals or contaminants, it is useful for medical and research purposes.

purines: compounds of nitrogen-containing bases such as adenine, guanine, and caffeine. Purines that originate from the body are *endogenous* and those that derive from foods are *exogenous.*

pyloric (pie-LORE-ic) **sphincter:** the circular muscle that separates the stomach from the small intestine and regulates the flow of partially digested food into the small intestine; also called *pylorus* or *pyloric valve.*

pyruvate (PIE-roo-vate)**:** a 3-carbon compound that plays a key role in energy metabolism.

Q

qi gong (chee GUNG)**:** a Chinese system that combines movement, meditation, and breathing techniques to enhance the flow of *qi* (vital energy) in the body.

quality of life: a person's perceived physical and mental well-being.

R

rachitic (ra-KIT-ik) **rosary:** the poorly formed rib attachments that may develop in a vitamin D deficiency; literally, "the rosary of rickets."

RAE: see *retinol activity equivalents.*

randomization (RAN-dom-ih-ZAY-shun)**:** a process of choosing the members of the experimental and control groups without bias.

raw sugar: the first crop of crystals harvested during sugar processing. Raw sugar cannot be sold in the United States because it contains too much filth (dirt, insect fragments, and the like). Sugar sold as "raw sugar" domestically has actually gone through more than half of the refining steps.

RBP: see *retinol-binding protein.*

RDA: see *Recommended Dietary Allowance.*

RDN: see *registered dietitian nutritionist.*

Recommended Dietary Allowance (RDA): the average daily amount of a nutrient considered adequate to meet the known nutrient needs of practically all healthy people; a goal for dietary intake by individuals.

rectum: the muscular terminal part of the large intestine, extending from the sigmoid colon to the anus.

red meat: meat from the muscles of mammals. Examples include beef, goat, horse, lamb, mutton, pork, and veal.

RED-S: see *relative energy deficiency in sport.*

reduced kcalorie: at least 25 percent fewer kcalories per serving than the comparison food.

reference protein: a standard against which to measure the quality of other proteins.

refined: the process by which the coarse parts of a food are removed. When wheat is refined into flour, the bran, germ, and husk are removed, leaving only the endosperm.

refined flour: finely ground endosperm that is usually enriched with nutrients and bleached for whiteness; sometimes called *white flour.*

reflux: a backward flow.

registered dietitian nutritionist (RDN): a person who has completed a minimum of a bachelor's degree from an accredited university or college, has completed approved course work and a supervised practice program, has passed a national examination, and maintains registration through continuing professional education; also called *registered dietitian (RD).*

registration: listing; with respect to health professionals, listing with a professional organization that requires specific course work, experience, and passing of an examination.

relative energy deficiency in sport (RED-S): a syndrome of impaired physiological functions caused by relative energy deficiency (too little energy intake for the energy expended).

remodeling: the dismantling and re-formation of a structure.

renin (REN-in): an enzyme from the kidneys that hydrolyzes the protein angiotensinogen to angiotensin I, which results in the kidneys reabsorbing sodium.

replication (REP-lih-KAY-shun): repeating an experiment and getting the same results.

requirement: the lowest continuing intake of a nutrient that will maintain a specified criterion of adequacy.

residues: whatever remains. In the case of pesticides, those amounts that remain on or in foods when people buy and use them.

resistance training: the use of free weights or weight machines to provide resistance for developing muscle strength, power, and endurance; also called *weight training.* A person's own body weight may also be used to provide resistance such as when a person does push-ups, pull-ups, or abdominal crunches.

resistant starches: starches that escape digestion and absorption in the small intestine of healthy people.

resistin (ree-ZIS-tin): a protein produced by adipose cells that promotes inflammation and causes insulin resistance.

respiratory chain: see *electron transport chain.*

resting metabolic rate (RMR): similar to the basal metabolic rate (BMR), a measure of the energy use of a person at rest in a comfortable setting, but with less stringent criteria for recent food intake and physical activity. Consequently, the RMR is easier to determine, but slightly higher than the BMR.

retina (RET-in-uh): the innermost membrane of the eye, composed of several layers, including one that contains the rods and cones.

retinal (RET-ih-nal): the aldehyde form of vitamin A.

retinoic (RET-ih-NO-ick) **acid:** the acid form of vitamin A.

retinoids (RET-ih-noyds): chemically related compounds with biological activity similar to that of retinol; metabolites of retinol.

retinol (RET-ih-nol): the alcohol form of vitamin A.

retinol activity equivalents (RAE): a measure of vitamin A activity; the amount of retinol that the body will derive from a food containing preformed retinol or its precursor, beta-carotene.

retinol-binding protein (RBP): the specific protein responsible for transporting retinol.

rheumatoid (ROO-ma-toyd) **arthritis:** a disease of the immune system involving painful inflammation of the joints and related structures.

rhodopsin (ro-DOP-sin): a light-sensitive pigment of the retina that contains the retinal form of vitamin A and the protein opsin.

riboflavin (RYE-boh-flay-vin): a B vitamin. The coenzyme forms are *FMN (flavin mononucleotide)* and *FAD (flavin adenine dinucleotide).*

ribonucleic acid: see *RNA.*

ribosomes (RYE-boh-zomes): protein-making organelles in cells that are composed of RNA and protein.

rickets: the vitamin D–deficiency disease in children characterized by inadequate mineralization of bone (manifested in bowed legs or knock-knees, outward-bowed chest, and "beads" on ribs). A rare type of rickets, not caused by vitamin D deficiency, is known as *vitamin D–refractory rickets.*

risk: a measure of the probability and severity of harm.

risk factor: a condition or behavior associated with an elevated frequency of a disease but not proved to be causal. Leading risk factors for chronic diseases include obesity, cigarette smoking, high blood pressure, high blood cholesterol, physical inactivity, and a diet high in added fats and low in vegetables, fruits, and whole grains.

RMR: see *resting metabolic rate.*

RNA (ribonucleic acid): a compound similar to DNA, but RNA is a single strand with a ribose sugar instead of a deoxyribose sugar and uracil instead of thymine as one of its bases.

S

safety: the condition of being free from harm or danger.

saliva: the secretion of the salivary glands. Its principal enzyme begins carbohydrate digestion.

salivary glands: exocrine glands that secrete saliva into the mouth.

salt: a compound composed of a positive ion other than H^+ and a negative ion other than OH^-. An example is sodium chloride (Na^+Cl^-).

sarcopenia (SAR-koh-PEE-nee-ah): loss of skeletal muscle mass, strength, and quality.

satiating: having the power to suppress hunger and inhibit eating.

satiation (say-she-AY-shun): the feeling of satisfaction and fullness that occurs during a meal and halts eating. Satiation determines how much food is consumed during a meal.

satiety (sah-TIE-eh-tee): the feeling of fullness and satisfaction that occurs after a meal and inhibits eating until the next meal. Satiety determines how much time passes between meals.

saturated fat-free: less than 0.5 gram of saturated fat and 0.5 gram of *trans* fat per serving.

saturated fatty acid: a fatty acid carrying the maximum possible number of hydrogen atoms—for example, stearic acid. A *saturated fat* is composed of triglycerides in which most of the fatty acids are saturated.

scurvy: the vitamin C–deficiency disease.

secondary deficiency: a nutrient deficiency caused by something other than an inadequate intake, such as a disease condition or drug interaction that reduces absorption, accelerates use, hastens excretion, or destroys the nutrient.

secretin (see-CREET-in): a hormone produced by cells in the duodenum wall. Target organ: the pancreas. Response: secretion of bicarbonate-rich pancreatic juice.

sedentary: physically inactive (literally, "sitting down a lot").

segmentation (SEG-men-TAY-shun): a periodic squeezing or partitioning of the intestine at intervals along its length by its circular muscles.

selenium (se-LEEN-ee-um): an essential trace mineral that is part of an antioxidant enzyme.

senile dementia: the loss of brain function beyond the normal loss of physical adeptness and memory that occurs with aging.

senile plaques: clumps of the protein fragment beta-amyloid on the nerve cells, commonly found in the brains of people with Alzheimer's dementia.

serotonin (SER-oh-TONE-in): a neurotransmitter important in sleep regulation, appetite control, and sensory perception, among other roles. Serotonin is synthesized in the body from the amino acid tryptophan with the help of vitamin B_6.

serving sizes: the standardized quantity of a food; such information allows comparisons when reading food labels and consistency when following the *Dietary Guidelines.*

set point: the point at which controls are set (for example, on a thermostat). The set-point theory that relates to body weight proposes that the body tends to maintain a certain weight by means of its own internal controls.

sickle-cell anemia: a hereditary form of anemia characterized by abnormal sickle- or crescent-shaped red blood cells. Sickled cells interfere with oxygen transport and blood flow. Symptoms are precipitated by dehydration and insufficient oxygen (as may occur at high altitudes) and include hemolytic anemia (red blood cells burst), fever, and severe pain in the joints and abdomen.

simple carbohydrates: monosaccharides and disaccharides (the sugars).

small for gestational age (SGA): term describing an infant whose birthweight is low compared with the number of weeks in utero, often reflecting growth failure.

small intestine: a 10-foot length of small-diameter intestine that is the major site of digestion of food and absorption of nutrients. Its segments are the *duodenum, jejunum,* and *ileum.*

sodium: the principal cation in the extracellular fluids of the body; critical to the maintenance of fluid balance, nerve impulse transmissions, and muscle contractions.

sodium bicarbonate (baking soda): a white crystalline powder that is used to buffer acid that accumulates in the muscles and blood during high-intensity exercise.

sodium-free and **salt-free:** less than 5 milligrams of sodium per serving.

soft water: water with a high sodium or potassium content.

solanine (SOH-lah-neen): a poisonous narcotic-like substance present in potato skins and sprouts.

solid fats: fats that are not usually liquid at room temperature; commonly found in most foods derived from animals and vegetable oils that have been hydrogenated. Solid fats typically contain more saturated and *trans* fats than most oils.

soluble fibers: nonstarch polysaccharides that dissolve in water to form a gel. An example is pectin from fruit, which is used to thicken jellies.

solutes (SOLL-yutes): the substances that are dissolved in a solution. The number of molecules in a given volume of fluid is the *solute concentration.*

somatic (so-MAT-ick) **nervous system:** the division of the nervous system that controls the voluntary muscles, as distinguished from the autonomic nervous system, which controls involuntary functions.

sperm: the male reproductive cell, capable of fertilizing an ovum.

sphincter (SFINK-ter): a circular muscle surrounding, and able to close, a body opening. Sphincters are found at specific points along the GI tract and regulate the flow of food particles.

spina (SPY-nah) **bifida** (BIFF-ih-dah): one of the most common types of neural tube defects, characterized by the incomplete closure of the spinal cord and its bony encasement.

sports anemia: a transient condition of low hemoglobin in the blood, associated with the early stages of sports training or other strenuous activity.

spring water: water originating from an underground spring or well. It may be bubbly (carbonated), or "flat" or "still," meaning not carbonated. Brand names such as "Spring Pure" do not necessarily mean that the water comes from a spring.

starches: plant polysaccharides composed of many glucose molecules.

sterile: free of microorganisms, such as bacteria.

sterols (STARE-ols or STEER-ols): compounds containing a four-ring carbon structure with any of a variety of side chains attached.

stomach: a muscular, elastic, saclike portion of the digestive tract that grinds and churns swallowed food, mixing it with acid and enzymes to form chyme.

stool: waste matter discharged from the colon; also called *feces* (FEE-seez).

stool softeners: substances that increase the amount of water the stool absorbs in the GI tract, making the stool softer and easier to pass.

stress: any threat to a person's well-being; a demand placed on the body to adapt.

stress fractures: bone damage or breaks caused by stress on bone surfaces during exercise.

stress response: the body's response to stress, mediated by both nerves and hormones.

stressors: environmental elements, physical or psychological, that cause stress.

stroke: an event in which the blood flow to a part of the brain is cut off; also called *cerebrovascular accident (CVA).*

structure-function claims: statements that characterize the relationship between a nutrient or other substance in a food and its role in the body.

subclavian (sub-KLAY-vee-an) **vein:** the vein that provides passageway from the lymphatic system to the vascular system.

subclinical deficiency: a deficiency in the early stages, before the outward signs have appeared.

subcutaneous fat: fat stored directly under the skin.

subjects: the people or animals participating in a research project.

successful weight-loss maintenance: achieving a weight loss of at least 5 to 10 percent of initial body weight and maintaining the loss for at least 1 year.

sucrase: an enzyme that hydrolyzes sucrose.

sucrose (SUE-krose): a disaccharide composed of glucose and fructose; commonly known as *table sugar, beet sugar,* or *cane sugar.* Sucrose also occurs in many fruits and some vegetables and grains.

sudden infant death syndrome (SIDS): the unexpected and unexplained death of an apparently well infant; the most common cause of death of infants between the second week and the end of the first year of life; also called *crib death.*

sugar alcohols: sugarlike compounds that can be derived from fruits or commercially produced from dextrose; also called *polyols.* Examples include *erythritol, isomalt, lactitol, maltitol, mannitol, sorbitol,* and *xylitol.*

sugar-free: less than 0.5 gram of sugar per serving.

sugars: simple carbohydrates composed of monosaccharides, disaccharides, or both.

sulfate: a salt produced from the oxidation of sulfur.

sulfites: salts containing sulfur that are added to foods to prevent spoilage.

sulfur: a mineral present in the body as part of some proteins.

sushi: vinegar-flavored rice and seafood, typically wrapped in seaweed and stuffed with colorful vegetables. Some sushi is stuffed with raw fish; other varieties contain cooked seafood.

sustainable: able to continue indefinitely; using resources at such a rate that the earth can keep on replacing them and producing pollutants at a rate with which the environment and human cleanup efforts can keep pace, so that no net accumulation of pollution occurs.

sustainable agriculture: ability to produce food indefinitely, with little or no harm to the environment.

sustainable diets: patterns of eating that promote health and provide food security for the present population while sustaining environmental resources for future generations.

sympathetic nervous system: the part of the autonomic nervous system that dominates during stressful conditions and includes such effects as increased heart rate, dilated pupils, slowed peristalsis, and secretion of epinephrine and norepinephrine.

synergistic (SIN-er-JIS-tick): multiple factors operating together in such a way that their combined effects are greater than the sum of their individual effects.

systematic review: a critical and integrative summary of evidence gathered from multiple selected studies to answer a specific question and develop a *qualitative* review.

T

tagatose (TAG-ah-tose): poorly absorbed monosaccharide similar in structure to fructose; naturally occurring or derived from lactose.

TCA cycle or **tricarboxylic** (try-car-box-ILL-ick) **acid cycle:** a series of metabolic reactions that break down molecules of acetyl CoA to carbon dioxide and hydrogen atoms; also called the *citric acid cycle* or the *Krebs cycle* after the biochemist who elucidated its reactions.

T-cells: lymphocytes that attack antigens. *T* stands for the *thymus gland,* where the T-cells mature.

TEF: see *thermic effect of food.*

tempeh (TEM-pay): a fermented soybean food, rich in protein and fiber.

teratogen (ter-AT-oh-jen): a substance that causes abnormal fetal development and birth defects.

teratogenic (ter-AT-oh-jen-ik): causing abnormal fetal development and birth defects.

theory: a tentative explanation that integrates many diverse findings to further the understanding of a defined topic.

thermic effect of food (TEF): an estimation of the energy required to process food (digest, absorb, transport, metabolize, and store ingested nutrients); also called the *specific dynamic effect (SDE)* of food or the *specific dynamic activity (SDA)* of food. The sum of the TEF and any increase in the metabolic rate due to overeating is known as *diet-induced thermogenesis (DIT).*

thermogenesis: the generation of heat; used in physiology and nutrition studies as an index of how much energy the body is expending.

THF (tetrahydrofolate): a coenzyme form of folate.

thiamin (THIGH-ah-min): a B vitamin. The coenzyme form is *TPP (thiamin pyrophosphate).*

thirst: a conscious desire to drink.

thoracic (thor-ASS-ic) **duct:** the main lymphatic vessel that collects lymph and drains into the left subclavian vein.

thrombosis (throm-BOH-sis): the formation of a *thrombus* (THROM-bus), or a blood clot, that may obstruct a blood vessel, causing gradual tissue death.

thyroid-stimulating hormone (TSH): a hormone secreted by the pituitary that stimulates the thyroid gland to secrete its hormones—thyroxine and triiodothyronine; also called *thyrotropin.* The release of TSH is mediated by *TSH-releasing hormone (TRH).*

thyrotropin: see *thyroid-stimulating hormone (TSH).*

tocopherols (tuh-KOFF-uh-rawls): members of the vitamin E family having the chemical structure of a complex ring structure with a long saturated side chain.

tocotrienols (TOE-koh-try-EE-nawls): members of the vitamin E family having the chemical structure of a complex ring structure with a long unsaturated side chain.

tofu (TOE-foo): a curd made from soybeans, rich in protein and often fortified with calcium; used in many Asian and vegetarian dishes in place of meat.

Tolerable Upper Intake Level (UL): the maximum daily amount of a nutrient that appears safe for most healthy people and beyond which there is an increased risk of adverse health effects.

tolerance level: the maximum amount of residue permitted in a food when a pesticide is used according to the label directions.

toxicity: the ability of a substance to harm living organisms. All substances are toxic if high enough concentrations are used.

TPP (thiamin pyrophosphate): the coenzyme form of thiamin.

trabecular (tra-BECK-you-lar) **bone:** the lacy inner structure of calcium crystals that supports the bone's structure and provides a calcium storage bank.

trace minerals: essential mineral nutrients the human body requires in relatively small amounts (less than 100 milligrams per day); sometimes called *microminerals.*

trachea (TRAKE-ee-uh): the air passageway from the larynx to the lungs; also called the *windpipe.*

***trans*:** on the other side of; refers to a chemical configuration in which the hydrogen atoms are located on opposite sides of a double bond.

transamination (TRANS-am-ih-NAY-shun): the transfer of an amino group from one amino acid to a keto acid, producing a new nonessential amino acid and a new keto acid.

transcription: the process of messenger RNA being made from a template of DNA.

transcription factors: proteins that bind to specific sites in DNA and alter gene expression.

***trans* fat-free:** less than 0.5 gram of *trans* fat and less than 0.5 gram of saturated fat per serving.

***trans*-fatty acids:** fatty acids with hydrogens on opposite sides of the double bond.

transferrin (trans-FAIR-in): the iron transport protein.

transient ischemic (is-KEY-mik) **attack (TIA):** a temporary reduction in blood flow to the brain, which causes temporary symptoms that vary depending on the part of the brain affected. Common symptoms include light-headedness, visual disturbances, paralysis, staggering, numbness, and inability to swallow.

translation: the process of messenger RNA directing the sequence of amino acids and synthesis of proteins.

trehalose: a disaccharide found in organisms such as fungi and yeast that is about half as sweet as sucrose and is sometimes used as a sweetener in processed foods.

travelers' diarrhea: nausea, vomiting, and diarrhea caused by consuming food or water contaminated by any of several organisms, most commonly, *E. coli, Shigella, Campylobacter jejuni,* and *Salmonella.*

triglycerides (try-GLISS-er-rides): the chief form of fat in the diet and the major storage form of fat in the body; composed of a molecule of glycerol with three fatty acids attached; also called *triacylglycerols* (try-ay-seel-GLISS-er-ols).

tripeptide: three amino acids bonded together.

TSH: see *thyroid-stimulating hormone.*

tumor: an abnormal tissue mass with no physiological function; also called a *neoplasm* (NEE-oh-plazm).

turbinado (ter-bih-NOD-oh) **sugar:** sugar produced using the same refining process as white sugar, but without the bleaching and anticaking treatment. Traces of molasses give turbinado its sandy color.

type 1 diabetes: the less common type of diabetes in which the pancreas produces little to no insulin. Type 1 diabetes usually results from autoimmune destruction of pancreatic beta cells.

type 2 diabetes: the more common type of diabetes in which the cells fail to respond to insulin. Type 2 diabetes usually accompanies obesity and results from insulin resistance coupled with insufficient insulin secretion.

U

UL: see *Tolerable Upper Intake Level.*

ulcer: a lesion of the skin or mucous membranes characterized by inflammation and damaged tissues. See also *peptic ulcer.*

ultrahigh temperature (UHT) treatment: sterilizing a food by brief exposure to temperatures above those normally used.

ultra-processed foods: foods that have been made from substances that are typically used in food preparation, but not consumed as foods by themselves (such as oils, fats, flours, refined starches, and sugars) that undergo further processing by adding a little, if any, minimally processed foods, salt and other preservatives, and additives such as flavors and colors.

umbilical (um-BILL-ih-cul) **cord:** the ropelike structure through which the fetus's veins and arteries reach the placenta; the route of nourishment and oxygen to the fetus and the route of waste disposal from the fetus. The scar in the middle of the abdomen that marks the former attachment of the umbilical cord is the *umbilicus* (um-BILL-ih- cus), commonly known as the "belly button."

uncoupled reactions: chemical reactions in which energy is released as heat.

undernutrition: deficient energy or nutrients.

underweight: body weight lower than the weight range that is considered healthy; BMI less than 18.5.

unsaturated fatty acid: a fatty acid that lacks hydrogen atoms and has at least one double bond between carbons (includes monounsaturated and polyunsaturated fatty acids). An *unsaturated fat* is composed of triglycerides in which most of the fatty acids are unsaturated.

urea (you-REE-uh): the principal nitrogen-excretion product of protein metabolism. Two ammonia fragments are combined with carbon dioxide to form urea.

USDA (US Department of Agriculture): the federal agency responsible for enforcing standards for the wholesomeness and quality of meat, poultry, and eggs produced in the United States; conducting nutrition research; and educating the public about nutrition.

uterus (YOU-ter-us): the muscular organ within which the infant develops before birth.

V

validity (va-LID-ih-tee): having the quality of being founded on fact or evidence.

variables: factors that change. A variable may depend on another variable (for example, a child's height depends on his age), or it may be independent (for example, a child's height does not depend on the color of her eyes). Sometimes both variables correlate with a third variable (a child's height and eye color both depend on genetics).

variety (dietary): eating a wide selection of foods within and among the major food groups.

vasoconstrictor (VAS-oh-kon-STRIK-tor): a substance that constricts or narrows the blood vessels.

vasopressin (VAS-oh-PRES-in): see *antidiuretic hormone.*

vegan (VEE-gan) **diet:** an eating pattern that excludes all animal-derived foods (including meat, poultry, fish, eggs, and dairy products) from the diet; also called *pure vegetarian, strict vegetarian,* or *total vegetarian.*

vegetarian diet: a general term used to describe an eating pattern that excludes meat, poultry, fish, or other animal-derived foods from the diet.

veins (VANES): vessels that carry blood to the heart.

very-low-density lipoproteins: see *VLDL.*

very low food security: multiple indications of disrupted eating patterns and reduced food intake; formerly known as *food insecurity with hunger.*

very low sodium: 35 milligrams or less per serving.

vigorous-intensity physical activity: physical activity that requires a large increase in breathing and/or heart rate and expends more than 7 kcalories per minute. Walking at a very brisk pace (>4.5 miles per hour) or running at a pace of at least 5 miles per hour are examples.

villi (VILL-ee or VILL-eye): fingerlike projections from the folds of the small intestine; singular *villus.*

visceral fat: fat stored within the abdominal cavity in association with the internal abdominal organs; also called *intra-abdominal fat.*

viscous fibers: fibers that have gel-forming properties.

vitamin A: all naturally occurring compounds with the biological activity of *retinol,* the alcohol form of vitamin A.

vitamin A activity: a term referring to both the active forms of vitamin A and the precursor forms in foods without distinguishing between them.

vitamin B_6: a family of compounds—pyridoxal, pyridoxine, and pyridoxamine. The primary active coenzyme form is *PLP (pyridoxal phosphate).*

vitamin B_{12}: a B vitamin characterized by the presence of cobalt. The active forms of coenzyme B_{12} are *methylcobalamin* and *deoxyadenosylcobalamin.*

vitamin D_2: vitamin D derived from plant foods in the diet; also called *ergocalciferol* (ER-go-kal-SIF-er-ol).

vitamin D_3: vitamin D derived from animal foods in the diet or made in the skin from 7-dehydrocholesterol, a precursor of cholesterol, with the help of sunlight; also called *cholecalciferol* (KO-lee-kal-SIF-er-ol) or *calciol.* After hydroxylation in the liver, calciol becomes *calcidiol* and after hydroxylation in the kidneys, calcidiol becomes *calcitriol.*

vitamins: organic, essential nutrients required in small amounts by the body for health. Vitamins regulate body processes that support growth and maintain life.

VLDL (very-low-density lipoproteins): lipoproteins made by the liver that transport lipids (primarily triglycerides) from the liver to other tissues.

VO_{2max}: the maximum rate of oxygen consumption by an individual at sea level.

vomiting: expulsion of the contents of the stomach up through the esophagus to the mouth.

vulnerable plaque: plaque that is susceptible to rupture because it has only a thin fibrous barrier between its lipid-rich core and the artery lining.

W

waist circumference: an anthropometric measurement used to assess a person's abdominal fat.

warm-up: 5 to 10 minutes of light activity, such as easy jogging or cycling, prior to a workout to prepare the body for more vigorous activity.

water balance: the balance between water intake and output (losses).

water intoxication: the rare condition in which body water contents are too high in all body fluid compartments.

water stress: intense demands on water resources by human activities such as municipal water supplies, industries, power plants, and agriculture.

wean: to gradually replace breast milk with infant formula or other foods appropriate to an infant's diet.

weight cycling: repeated loss and regain of body weight; sometimes called *yo-yo dieting* when weight cycling results from sporadic restrictive dieting.

weight management: maintaining body weight in a healthy range by preventing gradual weight gains over time and losing weight if overweight, and by preventing weight losses and gaining weight if underweight.

well water: water drawn from ground water by tapping into an aquifer.

Wernicke-Korsakoff (VER-nee-key KORE-sah-kof) **syndrome:** a neurological disorder typically associated with chronic alcoholism and caused by a deficiency of the B vitamin thiamin; also called *alcohol-related dementia.*

wheat flour: any flour made from the endosperm of the wheat kernel.

whey protein: a by-product of cheese production; falsely promoted as increasing muscle mass. Whey is the watery part of milk that separates from the curds.

white sugar: granulated sucrose or "table sugar," produced by dissolving, concentrating, and recrystallizing raw sugar.

WHO (World Health Organization): an international agency concerned with promoting health and eradicating disease.

whole foods: fresh foods such as vegetables, grains, legumes, meats, and milk that are unprocessed or minimally processed.

whole grain: a grain that maintains the same relative proportions of starchy endosperm, germ, and bran as the original (all but the husk); not refined.

whole-wheat flour: any flour made from the entire wheat kernel.

Wilson's disease: a genetic disorder of copper metabolism that creates a copper toxicity and results in neurologic symptoms such as tremors, impaired speech, inappropriate behaviors, and personality changes.

wine: an alcoholic beverage traditionally made by fermenting a sugar source such as grape juice.

without appreciable risk: practical certainty that injury will not result even after a lifetime of exposure.

World Health Organization: see *WHO.*

X

xanthophylls (ZAN-tho-fills): pigments found in plants responsible for the color changes seen in autumn leaves.

xerophthalmia (zer-off-THAL-mee-uh): progressive blindness caused by inadequate mucus production due to severe vitamin A deficiency.

xerosis (zee-ROW-sis): abnormal drying of the skin and mucous membranes; a sign of vitamin A deficiency.

Y

yogurt: milk product that results from the fermentation of lactic acid in milk by *Lactobacillus bulgaricus* and *Streptococcus thermophilus.*

Z

zinc: an essential trace mineral that is part of many enzymes and a constituent of insulin.

zygote (ZY-goat): the initial product of the union of ovum and sperm; a fertilized ovum.

zymogen (ZYE-mo-jen): the inactive precursor of an enzyme; sometimes called a *proenzyme.*

Index

- Page numbers in bold indicate definition of term.
- Page numbers followed by the letter "f" indicate figures or photographs.
- Page numbers followed by the letter "n" indicate footnotes.
- Page numbers followed by the letter "t" indicate tables.

A

B

C

D

E

J

K

L

M

O

P

Q

R

T

W

X

Y

Z

Daily Values (DV) for Food Labels

The Daily Values (DV) are standards developed by the Food and Drug Administration (FDA) for use on food labels. The values are based on 2000 kcalories a day for adults and children aged 4 years and older. Chapter 2 provides more details.

Nutrient	Current	Proposed
Vitamins		
Biotin	300 µg	30 µg
Choline	550 mg	550 mg
Folate	400 µg	400 µg DFE
Niacin	20 mg	16 mg NE
Pantothenic acid	10 mg	5 mg
Riboflavin	1.7 mg	1.3 mg
Thiamin	1.5 mg	1.2 mg
Vitamin A	1500 µg (5000 IU)	900 µg RAE
Vitamin B_6	2 mg	1.7 mg
Vitamin B_{12}	6 µg	2.4 µg
Vitamin C	60 mg	90 mg
Vitamin D	10 µg (400 IU)	20 µg
Vitamin E (α-tocopherol)	20 mg (30 IU)	15 mg
Vitamin K	80 µg	120 µg
Minerals		
Calcium	1000 mg	1300 mg
Chloride	3400 mg	2300 mg
Chromium	120 µg	35 µg
Copper	2 mg	0.9 mg
Iodine	150 µg	150 µg
Iron	18 mg	18 mg
Magnesium	400 mg	420 mg
Manganese	2 mg	2.3 mg
Molybdenum	75 µg	45 µg
Phosphorus	1000 mg	1250 mg
Potassium	3500 mg	4700 mg
Selenium	70 µg	55 µg
Sodium	2400 mg	2300 mg
Zinc	15 mg	11 mg

NOTE: The proposed Daily Values for updated food labels have been approved and scheduled to be on the market by July 2018, but this deadline may be delayed.

SOURCE: Food and Drug Administration, *Food Labeling: Revision of the Nutrition and Supplement Facts Labels*, https://s3.amazonaws.com/public-inspection.federalregister.gov/2016-11867.pdf (pp. 903–904).

Food Component	Amount	Calculation Factors
Fat	78 g	35% of kcalories
Saturated fat	20 g	10% of kcalories
Cholesterol	300 mg	–
Carbohydrate (total)	275 g	55% of kcalories
Fiber	28 g	14 g per 1000 kcalories
Added sugars	50 g	–
Protein	50 g	10% of kcalories

SOURCE: Food and Drug Administration, *Food Labeling: Revision of the Nutrition and Supplement Facts Labels*, https://s3.amazonaws.com/public-inspection.federalregister.gov/2016-11867.pdf (pp. 905–906).

GLOSSARY
NUTRIENT MEASURES

kcal: kcalories; a unit by which energy is measured (Chapter 1 provides more details).

g: grams; a unit of weight equivalent to about 0.03 ounces.

mg: milligrams; one-thousandth of a gram.

µg: micrograms; one-millionth of a gram.

IU: international units; an old measure of vitamin activity determined by biological methods (as opposed to new measures that are determined by direct chemical analyses). Many fortified foods and supplements use IU on their labels. For those still using IU, the following factors can be used for conversions.

- For vitamin A, 1 IU = 0.3 µg retinol
- For vitamin D, 1 IU = 0.05 µg cholecalciferol
- For vitamin E, 1 IU = 0.67 mg α-tocopherol

mg NE: milligrams niacin equivalents; a measure of niacin activity (Chapter 10 provides more details).

- 1 NE = 1 mg niacin
= 60 mg tryptophan (an amino acid)

µg DFE: micrograms dietary folate equivalents; a measure of folate activity (Chapter 10 provides more details).

- 1 µg DFE = 1 µg food folate
= 0.6 µg folic acid from fortified food or as a supplement taken with food

µg RAE: micrograms retinol activity equivalents; a measure of vitamin A activity (Chapter 11 provides more details).

- 1 µg RAE = 1 µg retinol
= 12 µg β-carotene
= 24 µg other vitamin A carotenoids

mmol: millimoles; one-thousanth of a mole, the molecular weight of a substance. To convert mmol to mg, multiply by the atomic weight of the substance.

- For sodium, mmol × 23 = mg Na
- For chloride, mmol × 35.5 = mg Cl
- For sodium chloride, mmol × 58.5 = mg NaCl